0102517

THE LIBRARY
KENT & SUSSEX HOSPITAL
TUNBRIDGE WELLS
KENT TN4 8AT

FOR
REFERENCE ONLY

Hospital Infections

16.03.93

Κεκτηκα τουτο

Hospital Infections

Third Edition

Edited by

John V. Bennett, M.D.
Professor, Emory University School of Public
Health; Director for Scientific Affairs, Task
Force for Child Survival and Development,
Carter Center, Atlanta

Philip S. Brachman, M.D.
Professor, Emory University School of Public
Health, Atlanta

Foreword by
Jay P. Sanford, M.D.
Dean Emeritus, Uniformed Services University of
the Health Sciences, F. Edward Hébert School of
Medicine, Bethesda, Maryland

Little, Brown and Company
Boston/Toronto/London

Copyright © 1992 by John V. Bennett and Philip S. Brachman

Third Edition

Previous editions copyright © 1979 by Little, Brown and Company (Inc.); 1986 by John V. Bennett and Philip S. Brachman

All rights reserved. No part of this book may be reproduced in any form or by any electronic or mechanical means, including information storage and retrieval systems, without permission in writing from the publisher, except by a reviewer who may quote brief passages in a review.

Library of Congress Cataloging-in-Publication Data
Hospital infections / edited by John V. Bennett, Philip S. Brachman.
  —3rd ed.
     p. cm.
  Includes bibliographical references and index.
    ISBN 0-316-08992-3 :
    1. Nosocomial infections.   2. Nosocomial infections—Prevention.
  I. Bennett, John V.   II. Brachman, Philip.
    [DNLM: 1. Cross Infection—etiology.
  2. Cross Infection—prevention & control.
  WX 167 H8294]
  RA969.H64   1992
  616.9—dc20
  DNLM/DLC
  for Library of Congress
                                91-45980
                                  CIP

Printed in the United States of America
MV-NY

930147

UR 9207066

LIBRARY
KENT & SUSSEX HOSPITAL
MOUNT EPHRAIM
TUNBRIDGE WELLS
TN4 8AT

WX
395

Contents

I. Basic Considerations of Hospital Infections

II. Endemic and Epidemic Hospital Infections

Foreword

Almost 150 years ago in 1847 Ignac F. Semmelweis, then a young assistant to Johann Klein, Professor of Obstetrics at the University of Vienna, through a series of astute clinical observations identified medical practices within hospitals as a major source and mode of spread of infection and demonstrated with modification of such practices that control could be accomplished. His observations remain sufficiently cogent today that a summary may be of interest.

At Vienna General Hospital, there were two obstetrical divisions, exactly the same in every way, each delivering about 3,500 babies per year. There was only one difference between them: In division I, all deliveries were done by obstetricians and medical students, while in division II, all were by midwives and midwifery students. In division I, an average of 600 to 800 mothers died each year from childbed fever; in division II, the average number of deaths was 60. Furthermore, while childbed fever was epidemic within division I, it did not exist elsewhere in Vienna. Mothers delivered at home and mothers self-delivered had essentially no mortality. While pondering these observations, Semmelweis's mentor, Professor Jacob Kolletschka, teacher of forensic pathology, sustained a self-inflicted wound during an autopsy and died quickly of sepsis. Because the pathologic findings on the autopsy of Professor Kolletschka were the same as those observed in patients dying of childbed fever and because sepsis in Professor Kolletschka arose from the inoculation of cadaver particles, Semmelweis concluded that puerperal fever must originate from cadaver particles. The transmitting source was to be found on the hands of the students and attending physicians. In 1847 every medical student and every medical faculty member dissected several cadavers each day while the midwives and their students did not. He concluded that "childbed fever is transmissible, but not a contagious disease." He then instituted the simple measure of washing the hands in a chlorine solution until the skin was slippery and the cadaver smell was gone. In 1846 division I, the physicians' division, had a mortality of 11.4 percent, while mortality in the midwives' division was 2.7 percent. In 1848, the first full year of this hand-washing prophylaxis, division I had a puerperal fever death rate of 1.2 percent and division II 1.3 percent. Unfortunately, Semmelweis's observations were not presented until 1850 and were not published except in abstract form until 1858. About this time he appears to have developed Alzheimer's disease, and he died in an asylum at the age of 47. His approach—sound clinical, epidemiologic and laboratory observations, well-reasoned conclusions, and rational effective intervention— is the cornerstone and forms the template for the control of infection in hospitals today.

In reviewing his observations and reading his biography, anyone who has labored in the field of infection control cannot help but be struck by observations of Niccolo Machiavelli in his 1513 treatise, *The Prince:* "It must be remembered that there is nothing more difficult to plan, more doubtful of success, nor more dangerous to manage than the creation of a new system. For the initiator has the enmity of all who would profit by the preservation of the old institutions and merely lukewarm defenders in those who would gain by the new ones."

While the rate of accrual of knowledge with its application to infection control was not rapid over the ensuing 100 years, before penicillin, major strides were made and the basic foundation was laid. From 1867 to 1875 Sir Joseph Lister recorded the use of carbolic acid topically in the prevention of wound infection. It is of interest to note the genesis of his approach: "In the course of the year 1864 I was much struck with an account of the remarkable effects produced by carbolic acid upon the sewage of the town of Carlisle, the admixture of a very small proportion not only preventing all odour from the lands irri-gated with refuse material, but as it was stated, destroying the entozoa which usually infest cattle fed upon such pastures." In 1875 he demonstrated antiseptic surgery: "We shall first purify the skin with a strong (1 to 20) watery solution of carbolic acid" and "in the next place, we shall have an antiseptic atmosphere provided by means of a spray-producer . . ." which "forms a 1 to 40 spray" of the carbolic acid. While this latter approach to surgical asepsis has been relegated to history, the importance of potential airborne infection within the operating suite is still recognized and has formed the basis of a number of trials involving phenols, ultraviolet irradiation, and the utilization of laminar airflow techniques under specific circumstances including in operating suites and high-level isolation facilities.

While today it is difficult to conceive of performing surgical procedures without gloves, they were introduced relatively recently by Dr. Halsted: "In the winter of 1889 and 1890—I cannot recall the month—the nurse in charge of my operating room complained that the solutions of mercuric chloride produced a dermatitis of her arms and hands. As she was an unusually efficient woman, I gave the matter my consideration and one day in New York requested the Goodyear Rubber Company to make as an experiment two pair of thin rubber gloves with gauntlets. On trial these proved to be satisfactory so that additional gloves were ordered. . . . At first the operator wore them only when exploratory incisions into joints were made. . . . After a time the assistants would remark that they seemed to be less expert with the bare hands than with gloved hands. Thus the operating in gloves was an evolution rather than an inspiration or happy thought, and it is remarkable that during the four or five years as operator I wore them only occasionally. How could we have been so blind as not to have perceived the necessity for wearing them invariably at the operating table." Reread the last sentence in the context of implementation of universal precautions 100 years later. The advent of the surgical mask is more difficult to date. Photographs from the Harvey

Cushing memoirs during World War I show no one in masks, yet by World War II their use was universal.

By the centennial of Semmelweis's observations, surgical asepsis was well defined. Larger metropolitan areas had communicable disease hospitals and sanatoriums for the care of patients with tuberculosis. Infection control in the community hospital was seldom an issue. Concern about nosocomial infection further atrophied following the introduction of penicillin into clinical practice by Abraham, Chain, and associates in 1941. With the further introduction of streptomycin, chloramphenicol, tetracyclines, and erythromycin by 1950, infectious diseases were considered by many, at least in the developed countries, as entities primarily of historical interest. While it was recognized that the hospital represented a locus for the spread of smallpox, nosocomial infections and their prevention reached a nadir. Nosocomial infections returned to the forefront in the late 1950s with the alarming increase in serious staphylococcal infections in the United States and throughout the world. At that time organizations such as the Centers for Disease Control and state health departments became involved in epidemiology, training in control measures, and initiation of much needed research related to hospital infections. Hospitals individually and then under the impetus of the Joint Commission on Accreditation of Hospitals (JCAH) established infection control committees, and infection control personnel became integral members of the hospital. In the face of such efforts, why do we need a third edition of *Hospital Infections*? Have we not identified the problems, learned the solutions, and have only to implement control measures? Clearly no!

Since the second edition, we are faced with an ever increasing number of emerging pathogens, many of which are of major importance as nosocomial pathogens. I have classified such pathogens into four categories based on the mechanisms underlying their recognition or occurrence.

First are infections that were recognized as a result of advances in knowledge. They are not truly new and are not related to antimicrobial resistance or host susceptibility. The etiologic agents span from viruses through bacteria. Examples include parvovirus B-19, now recognized to be the etiologic agent of erythema infectiosum (fifth disease) but now also incriminated in crises of aplastic anemia, hydrops fetalis, and a rubella-like syndrome in adults. Hospital personnel caring for children with sickle cell disease with aplastic crises have become infected. Bacterial etiologies include *Helicobacter pylori*, which has been associated with antral gastritis and may have an important role in the recurrence of duodenal ulcer. The initial occurrence of epidemic gastritis with transient achlorhydria was nosocomial, associated with inadequately sterilized gastroscopes. Legionellosis, now associated with at least 30 species of *Legionellaceae*, is recognized as an important nosocomial pathogen that often contaminates hospital as well as other water systems.

Second are the microorganisms that are not new but have increased or reemerged in clinical importance because of native antimicrobial resistance or acquired antimicrobial resistance. Examples include *Enterobacter* sp. and *Acinetobacter* sp. as major intensive care unit–associated pathogens. Antibiotic-associated colitis due to the production of *Clostridium difficile* toxin is an increasingly important nosocomial problem both in hospitals and nursing homes. Methicillin resistance, more accurately termed beta-lactam resistance, has become the staphylococcal plague of the 1990s in many hospitals. Strains of *Enterococcus faecium*, which have both high-level gentamicin (aminoglycoside) resistance and vancomycin resistance, are being increasingly recognized in Europe and North America. Their spread has been primarily nosocomial. The physician managing the patient with a gentamicin-vancomycin resistant *E. faecium* has returned to the prepenicillin era.

Third are the microorganisms that have emerged because of their ubiquitous nature and ability to invade the immunocompromised host. These include cytomegalovirus, *Staphylococcus epidermidis*, *Pneumocystis carinii*, and *Cryptosporidium* sp., to mention but a few.

Fourth are the agents that appear to be recent in origin, at least in human disease in most of the world, such as HTLV I and HIV I. If no other pathogens had emerged, HIV infection, disease, and its end-stage, AIDS, would suffice as a stimulus to know and practice all one can in infection control.

The third edition of *Hospital Infections* has brought together within its two covers the world's expertise in the multiplicity of disciplines involved in the prevention of nosocomial infections. The information is contemporary and practical. The volume is both encyclopedic in coverage yet handbook in ease of use. Hospital infections and their personal, social, political, legal, and economic impact are with us both as they were in the days of Semmelweis and now, even with the advent of a legion of extremely effective antimicrobial agents.

Jay P. Sanford, M.D.

Preface

Nosocomial infections continue to be a significant public health problem throughout the world, and the threat of their occurrence significantly influences patient care practices in health care facilities sensitive to these problems. During recent years, many advances have been made in our knowledge of nosocomial infections, and health care workers have become skillful in the effective use of available resources for control and prevention. Investigations continue to redefine ongoing problems and describe emerging problems. Laboratory investigations reveal new information related to pathogenicity, diagnostic criteria, and treatment and identify organisms newly associated with the hospitalized patient.

In spite of scientific advances in our knowledge of the prevention and control of nosocomial infections, increasing emphasis on education and training in infection control practices, and the development and publication of guidelines for work practices in health care facilities, nosocomial infections continue to occur, largely because dynamic competing factors increase patient susceptibility and exposure to pathogens. For example, the advancing age of patients and the presence of many chronic diseases can adversely affect a patient's resistance to developing infection. New and improved diagnostic techniques and therapeutic procedures may simultaneously challenge a patient's disease defense mechanisms. Of increasing concern is the HIV/AIDS problem, which affects patients, hospital staff, and others who have contact with health care institutions. The emergence of nosocomial infections caused by multi-drug–resistant tuberculosis organisms is of importance to immunocompromised hosts, including those infected with HIV, other patients, and hospital personnel.

Other areas of concern remain. Infection control staff are not always successful in influencing a change in the behavior of hospital care personnel. We must continue to emphasize the adoption of recommended procedures that will control and prevent infections and the elimination of those that are not effective or are counterproductive.

These areas are discussed in appropriate chapters in this third edition of *Hospital Infections*. All chapters have been revised and references updated, and all reflect new concepts and information. New chapters discuss new areas of emphasis and interest including the role of the hospital epidemiologist, the use of computerized systems in hospital epidemiology, cost effectiveness as related to control and prevention of nosocomial infections, and HIV infection.

Part I reviews the overall problem of nosocomial infections, general principles of control and prevention, and specific areas of concern. Part II focuses on specific nosocomial infection problems related to organ systems and procedures. Epidemiologic principles are stressed throughout the book. Chapters are authored by individuals who have indepth, personal knowledge of the topics they have reviewed.

We are greatly indebted to the contributing authors for their willingness to distill and summarize volumes of data and information into authoritative, succinct, and timely chapters for this third edition. We also appreciate the efforts of authors who contributed only to the first two editions; their contributions have invariably assisted in strengthening the third edition. We also acknowledge the unending direction and support of our publisher, Little, Brown and Company.

J. V. B.
P. S. B.

Contributing Authors

Robert C. Aber, M.D.
Associate Professor, Department of Medicine, Pennsylvania State University College of Medicine; Vice Chairman, Department of Medicine, The Milton S. Hershey Medical Center, Hershey, Pennsylvania

Miriam J. Alter, Ph.D.
Chief, Epidemiology Section, Hepatitis Branch, National Center for Infectious Diseases, Centers for Disease Control, U.S. Public Health Service, Atlanta

Nancy H. Bean, Ph.D.
Chief, Surveillance and Epidemic Investigations Section, Biostatistics and Information Management Branch, National Center for Infectious Diseases, Centers for Disease Control, U.S. Public Health Service, Atlanta

David M. Bell, M.D.
Chief, HIV Infections Branch, Hospital Infections Program, National Center for Infectious Diseases, Centers for Disease Control, U.S. Public Health Service, Atlanta

John V. Bennett, M.D.
Professor, Emory University School of Public Health; Director for Scientific Affairs, Task Force for Child Survival and Development, Carter Center, Atlanta

Lee A. Bland, M.A., M.P.H.
Chief, Dialysis and Medical Devices Section, Hospital Infections Program, National Center for Infectious Diseases, Centers for Disease Control, U.S. Public Health Service, Atlanta

Philip S. Brachman, M.D.
Professor, Emory University School of Public Health, Atlanta

Claire V. Broome, M.D.
Associate Director for Science, Centers for Disease Control, U.S. Public Health Service, Atlanta

John F. Burke, M.D.
  Helen Andrus Benedict Professor of Surgery, Harvard Medical School; Chief of Trauma Services Emeritus, Massachusetts General Hospital, Boston

John P. Burke, M.D.
  Professor of Medicine, University of Utah School of Medicine; Chief, Clinical Epidemiology Department, LDS Hospital, Salt Lake City

David H. Culver, Ph.D.
  Chief, Statistics and Information Systems Branch, Hospital Infections Program, National Center for Infectious Diseases, Centers for Disease Control, U.S. Public Health Service, Atlanta

James W. Curran, M.D., M.P.H.
  Associate Director, HIV/AIDS, Office of the Director, Centers for Disease Control, U.S. Public Health Service, Atlanta

Michael D. Decker, M.D., M.P.H.
  Assistant Professor of Preventive Medicine and Infectious Diseases, Vanderbilt University School of Medicine; Hospital Epidemiologist, St. Thomas Hospital, Nashville, Tennessee

Richard E. Dixon, M.D.
  Associate Professor of Medicine, Hahnemann University School of Medicine, Philadelphia; Medical Director, Helene Fuld Medical Center, Trenton, New Jersey

Herbert L. DuPont, M.D.
  Mary W. Kelsey Professor and Director, Center for Infectious Diseases, The University of Texas Medical School at Houston School of Public Health; Attending Physician, Department of Internal Medicine, Hermann Hospital, Houston

N. Joel Ehrenkranz, M.D.
  Director, Florida Consortium for Infection Control, South Miami, Florida

Theodore C. Eickhoff, M.D.
  Professor of Medicine, University of Colorado School of Medicine; Director of Internal Medicine, AMI Presbyterian-St. Luke's Medical Center, Denver

Martin S. Favero, Ph.D.
  Associate Director for Laboratory Science, Hospital Infections Program, National Center for Infectious Diseases, Centers for Disease Control, U.S. Public Health Service, Atlanta

Jonathan Freeman, M.D.
  Assistant Professor of Epidemiology, Harvard School of Public Health; Assistant Professor of Medicine, Harvard Medical School, Boston

Richard A. Garibaldi, M.D.
  Professor and Vice-Chairman, Department of Medicine, University of Connecticut School of Medicine; Hospital Epidemiologist, The University of Connecticut Health Center, Farmington, Connecticut

Julia S. Garner, R.N., M.N.
  Nurse Consultant, Hospital Infections Program, National Center for Infectious Diseases, Centers for Disease Control, U.S. Public Health Service, Atlanta

Robert P. Gaynes, M.D.
  Chief, Nosocomial Infections Surveillance Activity, Hospital Infections Program, National Center for Infectious Diseases, Centers for Disease Control, U.S. Public Health Service, Atlanta

Donald A. Goldmann, M.D.
  Associate Professor of Pediatrics, Harvard Medical School; Hospital Epidemiologist and Director of Bacteriology Laboratory, Children's Hospital, Boston

Robert W. Haley, M.D.
  Associate Professor, Epidemiology Division, Department of Internal Medicine, University of Texas Health Science Center at Dallas, Southwestern Medical School; Hospital Epidemiologist, Parkland Memorial Hospital, Dallas

Loreen A. Herwaldt, M.D.
  Assistant Professor, University of Iowa College of Medicine; Associate Hospital Epidemiologist, University of Iowa Hospitals and Clinics, Iowa City, Iowa

Patricia L. Hibberd, M.D., Ph.D.
  Assistant Professor of Medicine, Harvard Medical School; Clinical Director, Program in Transplant Infectious Diseases, Massachusetts General Hospital, Boston

Walter J. Hierholzer, Jr., M.D.
  Professor of Medicine and Epidemiology, Department of Internal Medicine, Yale University School of Medicine; Director, Hospital Epidemiology Program, Department of Hospital Epidemiology and Infection Control, Yale-New Haven Hospital, New Haven, Connecticut

James M. Hughes, M.D.
Clinical Assistant Professor, Division of Infectious Diseases, Emory University School of Medicine; Director, National Center for Infectious Diseases, Centers for Disease Control, U.S. Public Health Service, Atlanta

Cynthia A. Hunstiger, R.N., B.S.
Senior Consultant for Materials Management, Lerch Bates Hospital Group, Inc., Littleton, Colorado

Marguerite M. Jackson, R.N., M.S., C.I.C., F.A.A.N.
Assistant Clinical Professor, Department of Community and Family Medicine, University of California, San Diego, School of Medicine; Administrative Director, Medical Center Epidemiology Unit, UCSD Medical Center, San Diego

William R. Jarvis, M.D.
Chief, Investigation and Prevention Branch, Hospital Infections Program, National Center for Infectious Diseases, Centers for Disease Control, U.S. Public Health Service, Atlanta

Andrew M. Kaunitz, M.D.
Associate Professor, Department of Obstetrics and Gynecology, University of Florida College of Medicine, Jacksonville, Florida

Karen Rose Koppel Kaunitz, J.D.
Vice President for Legal Affairs, Methodist Medical Center, Jacksonville, Florida

F. Marc LaForce, M.D.
Professor of Medicine, University of Rochester School of Medicine and Dentistry; Physician-in-Chief, Genesee Hospital, Rochester, New York

William J. Ledger, M.D.
Given Foundation Professor of Obstetrics and Gynecology, Cornell University Medical College; Obstetrician and Gynecologist-in-Chief, The New York Hospital-Cornell Medical Center, New York

Patricia Lynch, R.N., M.B.A, C.I.C.
Clinical Instructor, School of Community Medicine and Public Health, University of Washington; Director, Epidemiology, Harborview Medical Center, Seattle

Dennis G. Maki, M.D.
Ovid O. Meyer Professor of Medicine, and Head, Section of Infectious Diseases, University of Wisconsin at Madison Medical School; Attending Physician, Center for Trauma and Life Support, and Hospital Epidemiologist, University of Wisconsin Hospital and Clinics, Madison, Wisconsin

Stanley M. Martin, M.S.
Chief, Biostatistics and Information Management Branch, Division of Bacterial and Mycotic Diseases, National Center for Infectious Diseases, Centers for Disease Control, U.S. Public Health Service, Atlanta

William J. Martone, M.D.
Director, Hospital Infections Program, National Center for Infectious Diseases, Centers for Disease Control, U.S. Public Health Service, Atlanta

R. Michael Massanari, M.D., M.S.
Adjunct Professor, University of Michigan School of Public Health, Ann Arbor; Medical Director of Hospital Epidemiology, Henry Ford Hospital, Detroit

John F. McGowan, Jr., M.D.
Professor of Pathology and Medicine, Emory University School of Medicine; Director of Clinical Microbiology, Grady Memorial Hospital, Atlanta

Jonathan L. Meakins, M.D., D.Sc.
Professor and Chairman, Department of Surgery, McGill University; Chief of Surgery, Royal Victoria Hospital, Montreal

John D. Nelson, M.D.
Professor of Pediatrics, University of Texas Health Science Center at Dallas, Southwestern Medical School, Senior Attending Physician, Children's Medical Center and Parkland Memorial Hospital, Dallas

Ronald Lee Nichols, M.D., M.S.
William Henderson Professor of Surgery and Professor of Microbiology, Tulane University School of Medicine; Attending Surgeon, Tulane University Medical Center, New Orleans

Brenda A. Nurse, M.D.
Assistant Professor of Medicine, University of Connecticut School of Medicine, Farmington; Chief, Department of Infectious Diseases and Epidemiology, The New Britain Memorial Hospital for Rehabilitation and Chronic Care, New Britain, Connecticut

Jan Evans Patterson, M.D.
Assistant Professor of Medicine (Infectious Diseases) and Laboratory Medicine, Yale University School of Medicine; Associate Hospital Epidemiologist, Yale-New Haven Hospital, New Haven; Hospital Epidemiologist, West Haven Veterans Affairs Medical Center, West Haven, Connecticut

William Petty, M.D.
Professor and Chairman, Department of Orthopedics, University of Florida College of Medicine; Chairman, Department of Orthopedics, Shands Hospital, Gainesville, Florida

Didier Pittet, M.D.
Associate Professor, University of Geneva Medical School; Attending Physician, Department of Internal Medicine, University of Geneva Hospitals, Geneva

Brian D. Plikaytis, M.S.
Chief, Biostatistics Section, Biostatistics and Information Management Branch, Division of Bacterial and Mycotic Diseases, National Center for Infectious Diseases, Centers for Disease Control, U.S. Public Health Service, Atlanta

Jacquelyn A. Polder, B.S.N., M.P.H.
Chief, Guidelines Section, HIV Branch, Hospital Infections Program, National Center for Infectious Diseases, Centers for Disease Control, U.S. Public Health Service, Atlanta

Gina Pugliese, R.N., M.S.
Director, Infection Control and Environmental Safety, American Hospital Association, Chicago

Arthur L. Reingold, M.D.
Professor of Epidemiology, University of California School of Public Health, Berkeley, California

L. Barth Reller, M.D.
Professor of Pathology and Medicine, Duke University School of Medicine; Attending Physician and Director of Clinical Microbiology, Duke University Medical Center, Durham, North Carolina

Frank S. Rhame, M.D.
Associate Professor, Division of Infectious Diseases, University of Minnesota Medical School—Minneapolis, and Division of Epidemiology, University of Minnesota School of Public Health; Hospital Epidemiologist and Director, HIV Clinic, University of Minnesota Hospital and Clinic, Minneapolis

Bruce S. Ribner, M.D., M.P.H.
Associate Professor of Medicine, Medical University of South Carolina College of Medicine; Center Epidemiologist, Ralph H. Johnson Veterans Affairs Medical Center, Charleston, South Carolina

Robert H. Rubin, M.D.
Associate Professor of Medicine, Harvard Medical School; Chief, Program in Transplant Infectious Diseases, and Director, Clinical Investigation Program, Massachusetts General Hospital, Boston

Dennis R. Schaberg, M.D.
Professor of Medicine, University of Michigan Medical School; Staff Physician, Veterans Administration Medical Center, Ann Arbor, Michigan

William Schaffner, M.D.
Professor and Chairman, Department of Preventive Medicine, and Professor of Medicine (Infectious Diseases), Vanderbilt University School of Medicine; Hospital Epidemiologist, Vanderbilt University Hospital, Nashville, Tennessee

Walter E. Stamm, M.D.
Professor of Medicine, University of Washington School of Medicine; Head, Division of Infectious Diseases, Harborview Medical Center, Seattle, Washington

Ofelia C. Tablan, M.D.
Medical Epidemiologist, Hospital Infections Program, National Center for Infectious Diseases, Centers for Disease Control, U.S. Public Health Service, Atlanta

Ronald G. Tompkins, M.D., Sc.D.
Associate Professor of Surgery, Harvard Medical School; Chief, Trauma and Burn Services, Massachusetts General Hospital, Boston

William M. Valenti, M.D.
Clinical Associate Professor of Medicine, University of Rochester School of Medicine and Dentistry; Medical Director, Community Health Network, Rochester, New York

Margarita E. Villarino, M.D., M.P.H.

Medical Epidemiologist, National Center for Infectious Diseases, Centers for Disease Control, U.S. Public Health Service, Atlanta

Duc J. Vugia, M.D.

Medical Epidemiologist, Division of Bacterial and Infectious Diseases, National Center for Infectious Diseases, Centers for Disease Control, U.S. Public Health Service, Atlanta

Robert A. Weinstein, M.D.

Professor of Medicine, University of Illinois College of Medicine; Attending Physician and Director of Infection Control, Humana-Michael Reese Hospital, Chicago

Walter W. Williams, M.D., M.P.H.

Chief, Child and Adult Immunization Section, Division of Immunization, National Center for Prevention Services, Centers for Disease Control, U.S. Public Health Service, Atlanta

Michael L. Wilson, M.D.

Assistant Professor of Pathology, Duke University School of Medicine; Associate Director, Clinical Microbiology Laboratory, Duke University Medical Center, Durham, North Carolina

Basic Considerations of Hospital Infections

I

Notice

The indications and dosages of all drugs in this book have been recommended in the medical literature and conform to the practices of the general medical community. The medications described do not necessarily have specific approval by the Food and Drug Administration for use in the diseases and dosages for which they are recommended. The package insert for each drug should be consulted for use and dosage as approved by the FDA. Because standards for usage change, it is advisable to keep abreast of revised recommendations, particularly those concerning new drugs.

Epidemiology of Nosocomial Infections

Philip S. Brachman

Basic Considerations

This chapter is a review of the basic principles of epidemiology as they relate to nosocomial infections. An understanding of nosocomial infections is necessary for the development and implementation of effective and efficient control and prevention measures. One uses epidemiologic methods to define the factors related to the occurrence of disease, including the relations among the agent, its reservoir and source, the route of transmission, the host, and the environment. Once these relations have been defined for a specific disease, the most appropriate means of control and prevention should be discernible. Without defining each of these relations, control and prevention efforts are, at best, a gamble. Defining the epidemiologic relations introduces science into control and prevention and leads to more effective and economical use of all resources.

Definitions
Epidemiology
The term *epidemiology* is derived from the Greek *epi* (on or upon), *demos* (people or population), and *logos* (word or reason). Literally, it means "the study of things that happen to people"; historically, it has involved the study of epidemics. Epidemiology is the dynamic study of the determinants, occurrence, and distribution of health and disease in a population, which, for nosocomial infections, is the hospital population. Epidemiology defines the relation of disease to the population at risk and involves the determination, analysis, and interpretation of rates. There are many different rates used by epidemiologists; the most common is the attack rate, which is the number of cases of the disease divided by the population at risk. Calculation of other

rates helps define the outbreak—for example, calculation of rates among a selected comparison group to compare with the group in which cases occurred (see Chap. 6, 7).

The principles of epidemiology are also being applied to broaden knowledge of hospital-based occurrences other than infectious disease. Not only are noninfectious disease problems being studied using epidemiologic principles, but the broad area of patient care is being strengthened by the application of epidemiology to the many activities encompassed in quality assurance (see Chap. 2).

Infection

Infection entails the replication of organisms in the tissues of a host; the related development of overt clinical manifestations is known as *disease;* however, if the infection provokes an immune response only, without overt clinical disease, it is a subclinical or inapparent infection. *Colonization* implies the presence of a microorganism in or on a host, with growth and multiplication of the microorganism but without any overt clinical expression or detected immune reaction at the time it is isolated. *Subclinical* or *inapparent infection* refers to a relation between the host and microorganism in which the microorganism is present; there is no overt expression of the presence of the microorganism, but there is interaction between the host and microorganism that results in a detectable immune response, such as a serologic reaction. Therefore, special serologic tests may be needed to differentiate colonization from subclinical infection. In the absence of such information, it is customary to employ the term *colonization. A carrier* (or colonized person) is an individual colonized with a specific microorganism and from whom the organism can be recovered (i.e., cultured) but who shows no overt expression of the presence of the microorganism at the time it is isolated; a carrier may have a history of previous disease due to that organism, such as typhoid. The carrier state may be *transient* (or short-term), *intermittent* (or occasional), or *chronic* (long-term, persistent, or permanent). We have found, for example, in culture studies of hospital staff for nasal carriage of *Staphylococ-*

cus aureus, that approximately 15 to 20 percent are noncarriers, 60 to 70 percent are intermittent carriers, and 10 to 15 percent are persistent carriers. Epidemiologically, the important consideration is whether the carrier is the source of the infection for another individual; any carrier who is disseminating or shedding the organism may subsequently infect another person. Also, the carrier may develop disease with the source of the organism being himself or herself (endogenous source).

Dissemination

Dissemination, or shedding of microorganisms, refers to the movement of organisms from a person carrying them into the immediate environment. To show this, one cultures samples of air or surfaces and swabs objects onto which microorganisms from the carrier may have been deposited. Shedding studies may be conducted in specially constructed chambers designed to quantitate dissemination. While shedding studies have occasionally been useful to document unusual dissemination, they have not generally been useful in identifying carriers whose dissemination has resulted in infection in other persons. In the hospital setting, dissemination is most effectively identified by means of surveillance, in which the occurrence of infection among contacts is noted. When infection is shown to result from dissemination of organisms from a person, that person is referred to as a *dangerous disseminator.*

The demonstration by culturing techniques that an individual is carrying a certain organism defines a potential problem, whereas epidemiologic demonstration by surveillance and investigative techniques defines the real problem. In some hospitals, routine culture surveys of all or selected asymptomatic staff may be conducted in an attempt to identify carriers of certain organisms, but such surveys lack practical relevance unless the results are related to specific cases or an outbreak of disease. This practice only identifies those who are culture-positive and does not in itself reliably separate colonized persons into disseminators as distinct from nondisseminators.

Usually only a fraction of colonized persons are disseminating; thus the nondisseminators are not associated with the actual spread of infection. If disease transmission has occurred and a human source of infection is suspected, culture surveys in conjunction with epidemiologic investigation to identify the potential source are realistic, and additional laboratory studies to confirm the presence of a dangerous disseminator may then be undertaken. Thus culture surveys and microbiologic studies of dissemination in the absence of disease problems are usually inappropriate and wasteful of resources.

In some instances, dissemination from a carrier has been reported to be influenced by the occurrence of an unrelated disease such as a second infection. One report, for example, suggested that infants carrying staphylococci in their nares disseminate staphylococci only after the onset of a viral respiratory infection. Such infants are called *cloud babies* (see Chap. 6). In another instance, a physician disseminated staphylococci from his skin because of a reactivation of chronic dermatitis. Desquamation of his skin led to the transmission of staphylococci to patients with whom he had contact. Dissemination has been reported of tetracycline-resistant *S. aureus* from individuals carrying this organism who were treated with tetracycline. Dissemination may be constant or sporadic. If sporadic, it may result from the intermittent occurrence of some precipitating event, such as a second infection, or it may be due to other, unknown factors. The risk of dissemination is generally greater from individuals with disease caused by that organism than from individuals with subclinical infection or who are colonized with the organism.

Contamination refers to microorganisms that are transiently present on body surface (such as hands) without tissue invasion or physiologic reaction. Contamination also refers to the presence of microorganisms on or in an inanimate object.

Nosocomial Infections

Nosocomial infections are infections that develop within a hospital or are produced by microorganisms acquired during hospitalization. Nosocomial infections may involve not only patients but also anyone else who has contact with a hospital, including members of staff, volunteers, visitors, workers, salespersons, and delivery personnel. The majority of nosocomial infections become clinically apparent while the patients are still hospitalized; however, the onset of disease can occur after a patient has been discharged. As many as 25 percent of postoperative wound infections, for example, become symptomatic after the patient has been discharged (see Chap. 33). In these cases, the patient became colonized or infected while in the hospital, but the incubation period was longer than the patient's hospital stay. This sequence is also seen in some infections of newborns and in most breast abscesses of new mothers. Hepatitis B is an example of a nosocomial disease with a long incubation period; its clinical onset usually occurs long after the patient is discharged from the hospital.

Infections incubating at the time of the patient's admission to the hospital are not nosocomial; they are community-acquired, unless of course they result from a previous hospitalization. However, community-acquired infections can serve as a ready source of infection for other patients or personnel and thus must be considered in the total scope of hospital-related infections.

The term *preventable infection* implies that some event related to the infection could have been altered and that such alteration would have prevented the infection from occurring. A medical attendant who does not wash his or her hands between contacts with the urinary collection equipment of 2 patients, for example, may transmit gram-negative organisms from the first patient to the second, which may result in a urinary tract infection. Hand-washing might have prevented this infection from occurring. The identification of such an event in retrospect, however, is likely to be impossible; at best, the situation is difficult to distinguish from circumstances in which both patients developed infections from their own autogenous flora (e.g., from *Escherichia coli*). It is often impossible to identify the precise mode of acquisition of individual nosocomial infections. More than one mode may contribute to the development of the same infection, and not all modes may be preventable.

A *nonpreventable infection* is one that will occur despite all possible precautions—for example, infection in an immunosuppressed patient due to his or her own flora. It has been estimated that approximately 30 percent of all reported nosocomial infections are preventable. Given ideal circumstances, many infections caused by flora acquired during hospitalization are avoidable by prevention of nosocomial acquisition or avoidance of predisposing procedures in those who have acquired nosocomial strains. Epidemics, especially common-vehicle epidemics, are potentially preventable; however, epidemics account for only a small number of the nosocomial infections that occur. Prompt investigation and the institution of rational control measures should reduce the number of cases involved in outbreaks. Endemic infections account for the majority of nosocomial infections, and the consistent application of recognized, effective control and prevention measures for endemic infections is probably the single most important factor in reducing the overall level of nosocomial infections.

Source: Endogenous (Autogenous) or Exogenous

Organisms that cause nosocomial infections come from either endogenous (autogenous) or exogenous sources. *Endogenous* infections are caused by the patient's own flora; *exogenous* infections result from transmission of organisms from a source other than the patient. Either endogenous organisms are brought into the hospital by a patient (this represents colonization outside the hospital), or the patient becomes colonized after being admitted to the hospital. In either instance, the organisms colonizing the patient may subsequently cause a nosocomial infection. It may not always be possible to determine whether a particular organism isolated from the patient with an infection caused by that organism is

exogenous or endogenous, and the term *autogenous* should be used in this situation. Autogenous infection indicates that the infection was derived from the flora of the patient, whether or not the infecting organism became part of the patient's flora subsequent to admission. Information about current disease problems in the community or in hospital contacts may be useful in differentiating the two sources. Microbiologic determinations of the characteristics of the organism—such as phage typing, antibiograms, biochemical reactions, or genetic analysis—may help identify strains of nosocomial origin (see Chaps. 9, 12, and 14).

Spectrum of Occurrence of Cases

To determine whether a nosocomial infection problem exists in a particular hospital, one must relate the current frequency of cases to the past history of the disease in that institution. To characterize a disease's frequency as sporadic, endemic, or epidemic, investigators must know something of the past occurrence of that disease in relation to time, place, and person. *Sporadic* means that cases occur occasionally and irregularly, without any specific pattern. *Endemic* means that the disease occurs with ongoing frequency in a specific geographic area in a finite population and over a defined time period. *Hyperendemic* refers to what appears to be a gradual increase in the occurrence of a disease in a defined area beyond the expected number of cases; however, it may not be certain whether the disease will occur at epidemic proportions. An *epidemic* is a definite increase in the incidence of a disease above its expected endemic occurrence. *Outbreak* is used interchangeably with epidemic; however, some people use outbreak to mean an increased rate of occurrence but not at levels as serious as an epidemic (see Chap. 5).

An occasional gas gangrene infection among postoperative patients is an example of a sporadic infection. An endemic nosocomial infection is represented by the regular occurrence of infections—either in a particular site or at different sites—that are due to the same organism, occur at a nearly constant rate, and are generally considered by the hospital staff to be within expected and acceptable limits. Surgical wound infections due to a single organism that follow operations classified as "contaminated surgery," for example, could represent the endemic level of postoperative wound infections.

An epidemic classically begins with a sudden increase in the occurrence of disease among susceptible persons who have had contact with a contaminated source, but the onset of disease occurs at an unusually high frequency relative to that expected. On the other hand, an epidemic may also result from prolonged exposure to the source of the organism, with cases occurring irregularly due to irregular dissemination or distribution of the agent, irregular contact between the agent and a susceptible host, or irregular presence of a susceptible host. Cases of salmonellosis, for example, may result from contact with a contaminated food to which patients and staff are exposed over a long period of time, possibly months before it is identified. Only an occasional case of salmonellosis may result from this exposure but, depending on the past history of salmonellosis in the institution, these cases may represent epidemic salmonellosis.

A characteristic sharp and abrupt increase in the number of cases may fail to occur with diseases having a long and variable incubation period. Many people may be exposed to hepatitis B virus at one particular time, for example, but the appearance of the resulting disease may be spread out over weeks, thereby obscuring the presence of an epidemic (see Chap. 6).

Incidence and Prevalence

Occurrence of infection is quantified by calculating its incidence and prevalence. *Incidence* is the number of new cases in a specific population in a defined time period. To determine the true incidence of a disease, culture or serologic surveys may be necessary. *Prevalence* is the total number of current cases of an infection in a defined population at one point in time (point prevalence) or over a longer period of time (period prevalence). The prevalence rate will include cases of recent onset as well as cases of earlier onset that are still clinically apparent (see Chap. 5).

Epidemiologic Methods

There are generally three techniques used in epidemiologic studies—descriptive, analytic, and experimental—all of which may be used in investigating nosocomial infections. The basic epidemiologic method, descriptive epidemiology, is used in most investigations. Once the initial problem has been defined, however, additional studies using one of the other two methods can be conducted to develop more information about the problem, confirm initial impressions, prove and disprove hypotheses, and evaluate the effectiveness of control measures, prevention measures, or both. Additionally, the principles involved in these methods have application to surveillance; surveillance data are commonly analyzed by the descriptive method, and such analysis may suggest the need for analytic studies to identify certain features of a disease. Furthermore, analysis of surveillance data may lead to the development of experimental studies to deal with a specific disease.

Descriptive Epidemiology

Descriptive epidemiology describes the occurrence of disease in terms of time, place, and person; each case of a disease is first characterized by describing these three attributes (see Chap. 6). When data from the individual cases are combined and analyzed, the parameters of the epidemic or disease problem should be characterized.

Time

There are four time trends to consider: secular, periodic, seasonal, and acute. *Secular* trends are long-term trends in the occurrence of a disease—that is, variations that occur over a period of years. The gradual but steady reduction in the incidence of diphtheria in the United States over the past 50 years, for example, is the secular trend of that disease. The secular trend generally reflects the immunologic, socioeconomic, and nutritional levels of the population from which the secular data have been reported. In diphtheria, the downward trend generally reflects the rising immunity and improved socioeconomic and nutritional levels of the overall population.

Periodic trends are temporal interruptions of the secular trend and usually reflect changes in the overall susceptibility to the disease in the population. The upsurge in influenza A activity every 2 to 3 years, for instance, reflects the periodic trend of this disease and is generally the result of antigenic drift of the influenza A virus.

Seasonal trends are the annual variations in disease incidence that are related in part to seasons. In general, the occurrence of a particular communicable disease increases when the circumstances that influence its transmission are favorable. The seasonal pattern of both community-acquired and nosocomial respiratory disease, for example, involves high incidence in the fall and winter months, when transmission through the air is enhanced because people are together in rooms with closed windows and are breathing unfiltered, recirculating air. Thus they have greater contact with one another and with droplets as well as droplet nuclei. There may also be agent and host factors that influence the seasonal trends. The seasonal trend of foodborne disease involves higher incidence in the summer months when ambient temperatures are elevated and refrigeration may be inadequate. Foods contaminated with what normally are non-disease-producing levels of microorganisms may be allowed to incubate, resulting in the attainment of infectious doses.

The fourth type of time variation is the *acute* or epidemic occurrence of a disease with its characteristic upsurge in incidence. The overall shape of the epidemic curve depends on the interaction of many factors: characteristics of the specific agent; its pathogenicity, concentration, and incubation period; the mode and ease of its transmission; host factors, including the susceptibility and concentration of susceptible individuals; and environmental factors, such as temperature, humidity, movement of air, and general housekeeping.

An epidemic can be portrayed by an *epidemic curve*—that is, a graphic representation of the number of cases of the disease plotted against time (see Chap. 6). The time scale will vary according to the incubation or latency period, ranging from minutes, as in an outbreak of disease following exposure to a toxin or a chemical, to months, as in a nosocomial epidemic of hepatitis B. The time scale (abscissa or horizontal scale) should be selected with three facts in mind: (1) The unit time interval should be equal to or less than the average incubation period so that the true nature of the epidemic curve will be apparent (i.e., all the cases will not be bunched together); (2) the scale should be carried out far enough in time to allow all cases to be plotted; and (3) any cases that occurred before the epidemic should be plotted to give a basis for comparison with the epidemic experience.

If the epidemic curve starts with the *index case* (i.e., the first case in the outbreak), the time between the index case and onset of the next case is the *incubation period* if transmission was from the index case directly to the next case—that is, from person to person. The upslope in the curve is determined by the incubation period, the number and concentration of exposed susceptible persons, and the ease of transmission. The height of the peak of the curve is influenced by the total number of cases and the time interval over which they occur. The downslope of the curve is usually more gradual than the upslope; its gradual change reflects cases with longer incubation periods and the decreasing number of susceptible individuals. Cases resulting from *secondary transmission*—that is, resulting from contact with earlier cases in the epidemic—will also be represented on the downslope of the epidemic curve or, occasionally, by a second upswing, which reflects a second, distinct, and usually smaller wave or cluster of disease following the main outbreak. Consecutive clusters of disease may represent ongoing transmission from new focuses or from one focus that is intermittently or periodically infective or from which organisms are periodically disseminated. When consecutive clusters of cases occur resulting from transmission from one cluster to the next, we refer to each cluster as a *generation*— first generation of cases, second generation of cases, and so on. In a common-vehicle epidemic in which contact with the common vehicle is limited to a defined period, the epidemic curve usually rises rather sharply and then gradually falls off. However, if the common vehicle is present consistently or sporadically over a prolonged period, then the epidemic curve will be prolonged over time. In a contact-spread epidemic (person-to-person), the epidemic curve usually rises gradually, has a flatter peak than the common-vehicle curve, and then falls off.

Place

The second feature of descriptive epidemiology is place. In an investigation, there may be three different places that need to be defined: The first is where the patient is when disease is diagnosed, and the second is where contact occurred between the patient and the agent. If a vehicle of infection is involved, the third place is where the vehicle became infected. To implement the most appropriate control and preventive measures, it is necessary to distinguish between these three geographic areas; certain actions may control additional spread from a specific focus but may not prevent new cases from occurring if the source continues to infect new vehicles. Several examples will help to emphasize the importance of carefully describing place or places involved in disease outbreaks.

In an outbreak of nosocomial salmonellosis, the patients were located on various wards throughout the hospital at the time they developed disease. Individual control measures were directed at each patient on the various wards; however, the place of infection was the radiology department, where barium used for gastrointestinal tract roentgenographic examinations was contaminated with salmonella. Because the barium had been contaminated in the radiology department, preventive measures were directed there.

Another example involves outbreaks of septicemia associated with intravenous fluids. In these instances, it is important to determine whether the fluid became contaminated in the process of manufacture (*intrinsic* contamination) or after the fluid had been bottled (*extrinsic* contamination). Extrinsic contamination can occur during shipment to the hospital, after being brought into the hospital, while being prepared for use, or during actual use.

Person

The third major component of descriptive epidemiology is person. Careful evaluation of host factors related to the individual person includes consideration of age, sex, race, immunization status, competence of immune system, and presence of underlying disease that may influence susceptibility (acute or chronic), therapeutic or diagnostic procedures, medications, and nutritional status (see Chap. 6). In essence, any host factor that can influence the development of disease must be considered and described. Those that increase the patient's chance of developing disease are known as *risk factors.*

Age sometimes influences the occurrence of diseases and also provides a clue regarding the cause of an outbreak. Persons at either end of the age spectrum—the young and the elderly—are generally more susceptible to disease. Such susceptibility may reflect levels of immunity, both active and passive, as well as the levels of less specific personal factors of protection against development of disease. Age can also be an important clue to the source of an outbreak of disease. If, in an apparent common-source outbreak, for example, all ages from infancy to old age are involved, then the source of the outbreak must have been available to patients scattered through at least several wards. On the other hand, if all the patients involved in an epidemic are women of childbearing age, then in attempting to identify the place of the exposure, the investigation can be narrowed to the obstetric or, possibly, the gynecologic ward.

Consideration of therapeutic procedures may be of similar importance. If all patients who developed bacteremia due to the same organism have received intravenous fluid therapy, then a common source of intravenous fluids would be suspected as the cause of the outbreak.

These few examples demonstrate that the description of individual host factors among involved patients may point to important information that may lead to a solution of the epidemic problem.

Analytic Epidemiology

The second method of epidemiologic investigation is *analytic epidemiology*, in which the determinants of disease distribution are evaluated in terms of possible causal relations. Two basic methods are used: case-control and cohort studies. In both instances, relations between cause and effect are analyzed: the *case-control* method starts with the effect and searches for the cause: the *cohort* method starts with the cause and evaluates the effect. The case-control and cohort methods have also been referred to as *retrospective* and *prospective* studies, respectively; both methods, however, can be either retrospective or prospective. These terms indicate the temporal frame of reference for the collection of specific data: in a retrospective study, data are collected after the event has occurred; in a prospective study, the data are collected as the event occurs.

Case-Control Study

The case-control method starts with an allocation of persons between a study group (those already affected with the disease) and a comparison control group or groups (see Chap. 6). Any differences between these groups are then determined. In an outbreak of nosocomial urinary tract infections due to *Proteus rettgeri*, for example, a group of patients with this infection was compared to a group that did not have urinary tract infection due to *P. rettgeri*. It was shown that the infected patients were more likely than the comparison group patients to have had indwelling urinary tract catheters, to have been located in the same area of the hospital, and to have previously received systemic antibiotic therapy. Thus it was concluded that in this epidemic, indwelling urethral catheters,

proximity of patients to one another, and previous systemic antibiotic therapy were directly related to the subsequent development of urinary tract infections due to *P. rettgeri*.

The case-control approach has the advantages of being inexpensive, relatively quick, and easily reproducible. It is used most often in acute disease investigations, since the epidemiologist arrives after a problem is recognized and often after the peak of the epidemic has passed. This approach, however, may introduce bias into the selection of the control group since it may be difficult retrospectively to reconstruct the involved and noninvolved populations. In selecting a comparison control group, bias may be introduced if one is unable to exclude patients who are asymptomatically infected with the causative agent being studied. A lesser problem, but a real one, is ascertaining in retrospect that a patient actually had disease and was not asymptomatically infected or colonized. This latter circumstance presents considerable difficulty in categorizing critically ill patients with manifestations that resemble those of infection but stem from other causes. Fortunately, the search for sources can be pursued by including all culture-positive persons in the case definition, and thus it need not be restricted to those with clinical disease. This approach does, however, jeopardize the search for important host factors related to disease occurrence. Another limitation is the memory of the involved patients for past events, the specification of which may be important to the investigation. Also, the hospital records may lack documentation of events important to the investigation. These limitations derive from the retrospective approach rather than deficiencies in the case-control approach per se. Indeed prospective case-control studies can be implemented, but usually they have little usefulness in outbreak investigations.

Cohort Study

In the cohort method, patients exposed to a cause are compared with a group not exposed to the cause to see what the effect will be. In the above outbreak of *P. rettgeri* urinary tract infections, for example, the importance of the proximity of patients with catheters—an infectious risk—was prospectively analyzed by scattering certain patients with urethral catheters throughout the hospital. Inhibition of the nosocomial spread of infection was demonstrated by this cohort approach.

The advantage of the cohort study is that it provides a direct estimate of the risk carried by a particular factor for disease occurrence, and this is relatively easy to accomplish when the incubation period is short. Although bias may still be a problem, it is less likely to be introduced in this type of study, which usually is conducted prospectively. The cohort study, however, is usually more difficult, more expensive, and more time-consuming than retrospective studies. For diseases with long incubation periods, the difficulties may be insurmountable. An example of a prospective cohort study is one in which a cohort of patients who received blood transfusions over a specific period of time is followed to see which patients develop hepatitis B. A retrospective cohort study would involve studying a cohort of patients who developed hepatitis to see which ones received blood transfusions within the past 6 months.

Another technique of analytic epidemiology is a cross-sectional survey, which allows for collection of data over a specific limited period of time. It makes possible accessing the relation between two or more factors, the presence of which can be confirmed at the time of the survey.

Experimental Epidemiology

The third method of epidemiologic investigation is the *experimental method,* which is a definitive method of proving or disproving a hypothesis. The experimental method assumes that causes are followed by effects and that a deliberate manipulation of the cause is predictably followed by an alteration in the effect that could rarely be explained by chance. The two groups selected for study are similar in all respects except for the presence of the study factor in one group. Either the case-control or the cohort method is used to evaluate the interaction between the cause and the effect.

An example of the experimental method is the evaluation of a new drug as treatment for a disease: A group of patients with the disease is randomly divided into two subgroups that are equal in all respects, except one of the subgroups is treated with the drug and the other subgroup (the control group) is given a placebo. If there is no other variation between the two groups, any difference in the course of the disease may be ascribed to the use of the drug.

The experimental method has less direct use in the investigation of outbreaks of nosocomial disease today than the other two methods. This method, however, does have usefulness in assessing general patient care practices and in evaluating new methods to control and prevent disease as long as the patient is not at any increased health risk. It has less use in therapeutic studies because of the need for informed consent and the need to prevent placing the patient at an unjustified or greater risk in attempting to conduct a specific study.

Chain of Infection
General Aspects
Infection results from the interaction between an infectious agent and a susceptible host. This interaction—called *transmission*—occurs by means of contact between the agent and the host. Three interrelated factors—the agent, transmission, and the host—represent the *chain of infection.*

The links interrelate in and are affected by the environment; this relation is referred to as the *ecology of infection*—that is, the relation of microorganisms to disease as affected by the factors of their environment. In attempting to control nosocomial infections, an attack on the chain of infection at its weakest link is generally the most effective procedure. With definition of the links in the chain for each nosocomial infection, future trends of the disease should be predictable, and it should be possible to develop effective control and prevention techniques. Defining the chain of infection leads to specific action, in contrast to the incorporation of nonspecific actions in an attempt to control a nosocomial infection problem.

Disease causation is multifactorial—that is,

disease results from the interaction of many factors related to the agent, transmission, and host. The development of disease reflects the interaction of these factors as they affect a person. Thus some people exposed to an infectious agent develop disease and others do not. For example, among a group of people exposed to β-hemolytic streptococci, usually only some develop disease; this reflects the variability in the various factors related to the development of disease.

Agent

The first link in the chain of infection is the microbial agent, which may be a bacterium, virus, fungus, or parasite. The majority of nosocomial infection problems are caused by bacteria and viruses; fungi occasionally and parasites rarely cause nosocomial infections.

Pathogenicity

The measure of the ability of microorganisms to induce disease is referred to as *pathogenicity,* and it may be assessed by disease-colonization ratios. One organism with high pathogenicity is *Yersinia pestis;* it almost always causes clinical disease in a host. An organism with low pathogenicity is α-hemolytic streptococcus; it commonly colonizes in humans but only rarely causes clinical disease. The pathogenicity of an organism is additionally described by characterizing the organism's virulence and invasiveness.

Virulence is the measure of the severity of the disease. In epidemiologic studies, virulence is defined more specifically by assessing morbidity and mortality rates and the degree of communicability. The virulence of organisms ranges from slightly to highly virulent. Although some organisms are described as avirulent, it appears that any organism can cause disease under certain circumstances. It may be possible to reduce virulence by a deliberate manipulation of the organism (e.g., by repeated subculturing on a specific medium or by exposure to a certain drug or to radiation). Purposeful attempts to develop avirulent strains have been related to efforts to develop a microbial strain for vaccination purposes, such as the attenuated poliomyelitis virus used for oral vaccination. Under certain

host-factor conditions, however, clinical poliomyelitis can result from oral vaccination with the attenuated strain. Some naturally occurring organisms have been considered avirulent or of low virulence; however, under certain conditions—such as high doses, host immunodeficiency, or both—disease has resulted from contact with these organisms. For years, *Serratia marcescens,* for example, was considered to be an avirulent organism; because of this and because certain strains produce easily recognizable red pigment, these organisms were used for environmental studies in hospitals. However, as hospitalized patients became more susceptible to developing infections—due to advancing age, presence of chronic diseases, and the effects of new diagnostic and therapeutic measures—nosocomial disease due to *S. marcescens* organisms subsequently became recognized and reported. It became apparent that this organism could cause disease in individuals with compromised defense systems. Thus *avirulence* is a relative term; whether an organism is avirulent depends on host factors such as susceptibility, agent factors such as dose, and other characteristics of the agent that influence the occurrence of disease.

Invasiveness describes the ability of microorganisms to invade tissues. Some organisms can penetrate the intact integument, whereas other microorganisms can enter only through a break in the skin or mucous membranes. An example of the former is *Leptospira* and of the latter, *Clostridium tetani. Vibrio cholerae* organisms are noninvasive: Once in the gastrointestinal tract, they do not invade the endothelium; rather, they elaborate a toxin that reacts with the mucosal tissue and causes diarrhea. *Shigella* organisms are highly invasive and cause a symptomatic response by invading the submucosal tissue.

Dose

Another important agent factor is *dose*—that is, the number of organisms available to cause infection. The *infective dose* of an agent is that quantity of the agent necessary to cause infection. The number of organisms necessary to cause infection varies from organism to organism and from host to host, and it will be influenced by the mode of transmission. The relation of dose to the onset of typhoid fever, for example, was shown in volunteer studies by Hornick and colleagues [2], who demonstrated that with an inoculum of 10^3 *Salmonella typhosa,* no clinical disease developed in normal volunteers. However, when the inoculum was increased to 10^7 salmonellae, there was a 50 percent attack rate among the volunteers and, with an inoculum of 10^9 organisms, there was a 95 percent attack rate.

Specificity

Microorganisms may be specific with respect to their range of hosts. St. Louis encephalitis virus, for example, has a broad range of hosts, including many avian species, mammals, and mosquitoes. On the other hand, *Rickettsia prowazekii,* the species that causes typhus, has a very narrow host range, involving body lice and humans. *Brucella abortus* is highly communicable in cattle but not in humans. Some *Salmonella* species, such as *S. typhimurium,* are common to both animals and humans, but others have a narrow range of specificity; for example, *S. dublin* primarily infects bovines, and *S. typhosa* is known to infect only humans.

Other Agent Factors

Other characteristics of the organism, such as the production of enzymes, are directed toward overcoming the defense mechanisms of the host. The streptococci, for example, produce leukocidin, hemolysin, and proteinase, all of which are directed toward overcoming humoral and tissue defense mechanisms of the host. Some agents produce polysaccharide capsules and others, toxins, that may give an advantage to the organism.

Certain antigenic variations within species of microorganisms influence the disease-producing potential of the organism. Of the 83 different pneumococcal serotypes, for instance, 14 cause more than 80 percent of human pneumococcal pneumonia infections. Among streptococci, group A organisms are associated with infections of the pharynx, whereas group B organisms are primarily associated with infections of the genitourinary tract.

The antigenic makeup of an organism may change, allowing a new variant to spread through a population because of the lack of host resistance to the new variant. This is seen with influenza A; every 2 to 3 years, a modified variant becomes prevalent and spreads throughout the country. This phenomenon is known as *antigenic drift.* More significant changes in influenza A may occur irregularly; these changes are known as *major antigenic shifts.*

Resistance-transfer plasmids also influence the occurrence of nosocomial disease (see Chap. 14). The transfer of R plasmids from one enteric organism to another has occurred in hospital outbreaks and may account for a change in the antibiotic sensitivity of a strain. The antibiotic sensitivity of hospital organisms is also influenced by the use of antibiotics in the hospital (see Chap. 12); more resistant strains are selected as a result of the increased use of a particular antibiotic (or antibiotics) against which specific resistance plasmids are commonly carried by prevalent nosocomial strains. If a common R plasmid–mediated resistance pattern of *E. coli* in a hospital is ampicillin, tetracycline, and sulfonamide, for example, then the pressures deriving from the use of any one of these drugs will concurrently select for strains with the other two resistances as well. This change in antibiotic sensitivity may make therapy difficult; it can result in an increasing prevalence of the resistant strain, reduce the infecting or colonizing doses of the organism in those receiving drugs to which these strains are resistant, increase the numbers of organisms disseminated from persons colonized with these strains, and subsequently cause a greater frequency of nosocomial infections due to this more resistant strain.

Other organism factors, some plasmid-mediated, include the ability to adhere to intestinal mucosa, resist gastric acid and disinfectants, and produce bacteriocins active against endogenous flora.

Reservoir and Source

All organisms have a reservoir and a source; these may be the same or different, and it is important to distinguish between these potentially different sites if control or prevention measures are to be directed at this aspect of the chain of infection. The *reservoir* is the place where the organism maintains its presence, metabolizes, and replicates. Viruses generally survive better in human reservoirs; the reservoir of gram-positive bacteria is usually a human, whereas gram-negative bacteria may have either a human or animal reservoir (e.g., *Salmonella*) or an inanimate reservoir (e.g., *Pseudomonas* in water). The reservoir may be highly specific: For poliomyelitis virus, for example, the reservoir is always human. On the other hand, *Pseudomonas* species may be found in either an animate or an inanimate reservoir.

The *source* is the place from which the infectious agent passes to the host, either by direct contact or by indirect contact through a vehicle as the means of transmission. Sources also may be animate or inanimate. The reservoir and source may be the same location, or the source may become contaminated from the reservoir. For example, a reservoir for *Pseudomonas* organisms may be the tap water in a hospital; however, the source from which it is transmitted to the patient may be a humidifier that has been filled directly with the contaminated tap water. In a common-source outbreak of measles, the reservoir and source may be the same person.

The source may be mobile or fixed. A susceptible patient may be brought to a fixed source (e.g., a patient who comes to use a contaminated whirlpool bath), or the source may be mobile and brought to the patient (e.g., contaminated food brought from the kitchen to the patient's bedside).

Period of Infectivity

Infectivity refers to the ability of an organism to spread from a source to a host. An infected human may be infective during the incubation period, the clinical disease state, or convalescence. Additionally, an asymptomatic carrier (or colonized person), who does not show evidence of clinical disease, may be infective. An example of a disease that is primarily infectious during the incubation period is hepatitis A: The infected individual is infec-

tive during the latter half of the incubation period and during the first several days of clinical disease. In measles, the patient is infective during the prodromal stage to approximately 4 days after the onset of the rash. In chickenpox, the individual is infective from approximately 5 days before the skin eruption to not more than 6 days after the appearance of the eruption. A disease in which the individual is infective primarily during the initial clinical disease phase is exemplified by influenza, in which the individual is infective for a period of several days after the onset of symptoms. In cases of tuberculosis and typhoid fever, the individual may be infective for essentially the entire pretreatment clinical phase, with infectivity usually significantly decreasing when there is clinical evidence of successful chemotherapy. Examples of diseases that are infectious into the convalescent period are salmonellosis, shigellosis, and diphtheria. In some diseases, such as typhoid fever and hepatitis B, a chronic carrier state may develop in which the individual may be infective for a long time, possibly years, while showing no symptoms of illness. However, the microorganisms that most commonly cause nosocomial infections—such as *E. coli, Klebsiella, Enterobacter,* and *Pseudomonas*—do not demonstrate the same patterns of infectivity or evoke the protective immune responses that typhoid fever and hepatitis B do.

Asymptomatic or subclinical carriers may also be infective for brief periods and continue to be the source of infection for susceptible individuals for long periods. This is seen, for example, in poliomyelitis and hepatitis A. In poliomyelitis, the ratio is approximately 100 carriers to 1 clinical case, and in hepatitis A, 10:1. In spite of not showing clinical evidence of infection, the person with a subclinical infection may be an active transmitter of infection, and clinical disease may result from such transmission. Dissemination from an asymptomatic carrier may be related to a specific event, such as the occurrence of a second disease process (see previous discussion). However, dissemination may also occur that is unrelated to any definable event. The staphylococcus carrier provides a classic example of the asymptomatic dissemination of infectious organisms; in this case, the site of dissemination may be the anterior nares or, at times, the skin. Similarly, the site of asymptomatic streptococcal carriage may be in the pharynx, perianal area, or vagina.

The source of an infection may be an atypical case of a specific disease whose clinical course has been modified by therapy, vaccine (as in measles), or prophylaxis (such as the use of immune serum globulin in hepatitis A). Also, the source may be an abortive case of disease in which the typical expression of the disease has been modified by treatment with antibiotics.

Animals may also provide a source of infection, although this is of less concern in the hospital setting.

Exit
The portal of exit for organisms from humans is usually single, although it may be multiple. It may not always be the obvious portal of exit; in bubonic plague, for example, in which the skin lesions are the most visible concern, exit by the airborne route from unrecognized secondary pneumonia is also of great importance in transmission. In general, the major portals of exit are the respiratory and gastrointestinal tracts as well as the skin and wounds. Blood may also be the portal of exit, as in hepatitis B or human immunodeficiency virus (HIV) infections.

Transmission
Transmission, the second link in the chain of infection, describes the movement of organisms from the source to the host. Spread may occur through one or more of four different routes: contact, common-vehicle, airborne, or vectorborne. An organism may have a single route of transmission, or it may be transmissible by two or more routes. Tuberculosis, for example, is almost always transmitted by the airborne route; measles is primarily a contact-spread disease but may also be transmitted through the air; salmonellae may be transmitted by contact or by the common-vehicle, airborne, or vectorborne routes. Thus in defining the route of transmission, although one

route may be the obvious one involved in a nosocomial infection problem, another route may also be operative. Knowledge regarding the route of transmission for a specific disease can be very helpful in the investigation of a nosocomial infection problem. Such information can point to the source and may allow control measures to be introduced more rapidly.

Contact Spread
In contact-spread disease, the victim has contact with the source, and that contact is direct, indirect, or by droplets. *Direct contact,* of which person-to-person spread is an example, occurs when there is actual physical contact between the source and the victim, such as in the fecal-oral spread of hepatitis A virus. Infections resulting from organisms within the patient may be referred to as *autogenous infections;* that is, the mode of acquisition is autogenous, even though transmission occurred earlier, namely, at the time the host became colonized with the organism. A postoperative cholecystectomy wound infection due to coliform organisms from the patient's own gallbladder, for instance, would represent an autogenous contact infection.

Indirect-contact transmission is distinguished from direct-contact transmission by the participation of an intermediate object (usually inanimate) that is passively involved in the transmission of the infectious agent from the source to the victim. The intermediate object may become contaminated from an animate or inanimate source. An example is the transfer to susceptible hosts of enteric organisms on an endoscope that initially became contaminated when brought in contact with an infected patient (the index patient).

Droplet spread refers to the brief passage of the infectious agent through the air when the source and the victim are relatively near each other, usually within several feet, such as when there is transmission by talking or sneezing. Droplets are large particles that rapidly settle out on horizontal surfaces; thus they are not transmitted beyond a radius of several feet from the source. Examples of droplet-spread infections include measles and streptococcal pharyngitis.

Common-Vehicle Spread

In *common-vehicle-spread* infection, a contaminated inanimate vehicle serves as the vector for transmission of the agent to multiple persons. The victims become infected after contact with the common vehicle. This transmission may be active if the organisms replicate while in the vehicle, such as salmonellae in food, or passive if the organisms are passively carried by the vehicle, such as hepatitis A in food. Other types of common vehicles include blood and blood products (hepatitis B and HIV), intravenous fluids (gram-negative septicemia), and drugs (salmonellosis), in which units or batches of a product become contaminated from a common source and serve as a common vehicle for multiple infections. Thus multiple vehicles may all become contaminated from a single common source. Even though there are multiple vehicles involved, these infections may be considered to be transmitted by a common vehicle because the epidemiologic principles are the same. It should be noted that *common source* and *common vehicle* are not interchangeable terms. A common source is just that: a source common to multiple vehicles from which the vehicles become infected. A common vehicle, on the other hand, is a vehicle of infection associated with two or more cases of a disease. If only a single infection results, the designation of direct-contact or indirect-contact spread, whichever is appropriate for the circumstances, should be used.

Airborne Spread

Airborne transmission describes organisms that have a true airborne phase in their route of dissemination, which usually involves a distance of more than several feet between the source and the victim. The organisms are contained within droplet nuclei or dust particles or on skin squames; the former are airborne particles that result from the evaporation of droplets, are 5 μm or smaller in size, and may remain suspended in air for prolonged periods of time. Dust particles that have settled on surfaces may become resuspended by physical action and may also remain airborne for a prolonged period. Skin squamae may become airborne and provide a mechanism for the airborne transmission of organisms such as staphylococci. Airborne particles may remain suspended for hours or possibly days, depending on environmental factors. Movement may be within a room, or—again depending on environmental factors, especially air currents—transmission may be over a longer distance. The size and density of the airborne particle will also influence the distance it moves.

Airborne spread by means of droplet nuclei is exemplified in the transmission of tuberculosis and, in some instances, staphylococcal infections. The classic experiments of Riley and co-workers [3] demonstrated the airborne route of infection for tubercle bacilli, in which the source of the organisms was disseminating patients with active, sputum-positive, cavitary disease. Some nosocomial staphylococcal disease has been shown to be transmitted by the airborne route. In one report, several postoperative wound infections were said to have resulted from the airborne spread of staphylococci from a staff member who remained at the periphery of the operating room throughout the surgical procedure; the only route for transmission of the organisms was through the air, there being no opportunity in this case for contact or common-vehicle spread [4].

Organisms may be transmitted in dust, as was seen, for example, in an outbreak of salmonellosis, in which transmission occurred by means of contaminated dust contained in a vacuum cleaner bag; the dust became resuspended each time the vacuum cleaner was used [1].

Skin squames are the superficial cells of skin that become airborne by the rubbing of the skin such as by clothing that moves across the skin under normal conditions. The squames may carry organisms such as staphylococci that can be infectious if deposited on a susceptible host. Several outbreaks of streptococcal wound infections have been reported in which the reservoir and source was a hospital staff person.

The airborne route of transmission is more frequently assumed to be the route of an infection than is the case. Creation of an infectious aerosol is more difficult than is usually recognized.

Vectorborne Spread

Vectorborne-spread nosocomial disease, although unreported in the United States, could occur; it includes external and internal vector transmission. *External vectorborne transmission* refers to the mechanical transfer of microorganisms on the body or appendages of the vector; shigellae and salmonellae are transferred in this way by flies, for example. *Internal vectorborne transmission* includes harborage and biologic transmission. In transmission by harborage, there is no biologic action between the vector and the agent; this is seen with *Y. pestis* organisms in the gastrointestinal tract of the flea. *Biologic* transmission occurs when the agent (e.g., a parasite) goes through biologic changes within the vector, as malaria parasites do within the mosquito.

Host

The third link in the chain of infection is the host or victim. Disease does not always follow the transmission of infectious agents to a host. As previously discussed, various agent factors play a part; similarly, a variety of host factors must also be surmounted before infection occurs and disease develops. Host factors that influence the development of infections are the site of deposition of the agent and the host's defense mechanisms, both specific and nonspecific.

Entrance

Sites of deposition include the skin, mucous membranes, and respiratory, gastrointestinal, and urinary tracts. Organisms such as leptospires can gain entrance through normal skin. Other organisms, such as staphylococci, need a minute breach in the integrity of the skin to gain entrance to the body. There may be mechanical transmission through the normal skin, as with hepatitis B or HIV viruses on a contaminated needle or in contaminated blood. Abnormal skin, such as a preexisting wound, may be the site of deposition of organisms such as *Pseudomonas aeruginosa*. Mucous

membranes may be the site of entrance, as the conjunctiva is for adenovirus type 8.

Another site of deposition is the respiratory tract. The exact area of deposition will depend on the size of the airborne particle and the aerodynamics at the time of transmission. Generally, particles 5 μm or larger in diameter will be deposited in the upper respiratory tract, whereas those less than 5 μm in diameter will be deposited in the lower respiratory tract.

Infectious agents may gain entrance to the body through the intestinal tract by means of ingestion of contaminated foods or liquids, contaminated supplemental feedings, contaminated medications, or through contaminated equipment, such as endoscopes inserted into the intestinal tract. Within the gastrointestinal tract, some organisms cause disease by secreting a toxin that is absorbed through the mucosa (enterotoxigenic *E. coli*), whereas others invade the wall of the intestinal tract (*Shigella*). Some microorganisms involve primarily the upper part of the gastrointestinal tract (*Staphylococcus*), and others, the lower part of the tract (*Shigella*). The urinary tract may become infected from contaminated foreign objects such as catheters or cystoscopes inserted into the uretha, or by the retrograde movement of organisms on the external surface of a catheter inserted into the bladder.

Organisms may gain entrance into the host via the placenta, as occurs in rubella and toxoplasmosis. Transplantation is another method by which microorganisms enter the host; infection may follow renal transplantation if the donated kidney is infected with cytomegalovirus.

An organism may colonize one site and cause no disease, but the same organism at another site may result in clinical disease. *E. coli*, for example, routinely colonizes the gastrointestinal tract and under normal circumstances does not cause disease; however, the same organism in the urinary tract may cause infection. *S. aureus* may colonize the external nares without any evidence of disease but, when the same organism colonizes a fresh surgical wound, a postoperative wound infection may develop.

Nonspecific Defense Mechanisms

A host's defense mechanisms may be non-specific or specific; the quantity and quality of these mechanisms will vary from person to person. Nonspecific defense mechanisms include the skin, mucous membranes, and certain bodily secretions. The skin forms the first barrier against infection; it is a mechanical barrier and contains secretions that have an antibacterial action. Tears, a form of epithelial secretion, have an antibacterial action (due to lysozyme), and they also mechanically remove entrapped organisms. The gastrointestinal tract secretes acid that acts as a barrier against enteric organisms. Other secretions, such as mucus and enzymes, bolster the defense mechanisms. The muscular contractions of the intestinal tract act to move the contents through the tract and thus reduce the available time for organisms to invade the mucosa. Within the nose and upper respiratory tract, the cilia act to remove organisms that impinge on them. The blanket of mucus serves to entrap and remove infectious agents. The lower respiratory tract is protected by secretions and macrophages that ingest microorganisms and carry them to regional lymph nodes.

The local inflammatory response provides another nonspecific host defense mechanism. Other nonspecific protective mechanisms include genetic, hormonal, and nutritional factors, as well as behavioral patterns and personal hygiene. Age, as influenced by these nonspecific factors, is associated with decreased resistance at either end of the spectrum; the very young and the very old frequently are more susceptible to infection. Surgery and the presence of chronic diseases—such as diabetes, blood disorders, certain lymphomas, and collagen diseases—alter host resistance, which again reflects the influence of the nonspecific factors just cited.

Specific Defense Mechanisms

Specific immunity results from either natural or artificially induced events. *Natural immunity* results from having had certain diseases—such as rubella and poliomyelitis (type-specific)—and usually persists for the life of the host. Immunity may also develop after inapparent infection, such as in diphtheria or poliomyelitis. With other diseases, there is a latent stage following clinical illness in which immunity is imperfect; the agent will remain in the latent stage until some triggering mechanism initiates disease. Such latency is shown in infection with herpes simplex virus and cytomegalovirus.

Artificial immunity can be either active or passive. *Active* artificial immunity follows the use of vaccines. There are attenuated vaccines, such as those used against poliomyelitis, yellow fever, and tuberculosis; killed vaccines, used against such diseases as typhoid fever and pertussis; and toxoids, which are used against diphtheria and tetanus.

For some vaccines, booster inoculations are recommended. The duration of artificial immunity is variable, depending on the disease. *Passive* immunity results from the use of immune serum globulin (i.e., serum that contains antibody); this is employed, for example, in prophylaxis against hepatitis A infections. Transplacental antibodies, such as measles antibodies, also provide an example of passive antibody protection. Passive antibody protects the individual from disease, but it neither protects against infection nor prevents subsequent spread of the agent to others. Passive protection is of relatively short duration, usually several months at most.

Host Response

The spectrum of the host's response to a microorganism may range from a subclinical (or inapparent) infection to a clinically apparent illness, the extreme being death. The clinical spectrum of disease varies from mild, to a typical course (although a disease may typically be mild), to severe disease and possible death. The degree of host response is determined by both agent and host factors and includes the dose of the infecting organism, its organ specificity, the pathogenicity of the infecting organism, its virulence and invasiveness, and its portal of entry. Host factors include the quantitative and qualitative level of the specific and nonspecific immunologic factors previously discussed.

The same organism infecting different hosts can result in a clinical spectrum of disease that is the same, similar, or different in various individuals. In an epidemic, for example, many cases of what appears to be the epidemic disease may meet the clinical case definition, whereas other cases that epidemiologically are related to the same outbreak may not meet the same case definition. They may, in fact, be cases of the epidemic disease but with a different clinical spectrum (as can occasionally be demonstrated by serologic tests). They may also be cases of other diseases occurring concurrently with the epidemic.

Environment

The environment significantly influences the multiple factors in the chain of infection. The transmission of the agent from its source to the host occurs in an environment that represents the summation of many individual factors; changes in any of these can have an impact on any link in the chain of infection. Some environmental factors are under strict control, such as the air in an operating room, whereas others are not.

At times, too much emphasis is placed on the role of the environment; for example, it is inappropriate to take environmental cultures routinely throughout a hospital (see Chaps. 9, 15). However, in investigating nosocomial infections, it may be appropriate to obtain environmental cultures as suggested by the circumstances of the specific problem under investigation. In other instances, not enough attention is paid to the environment. There needs to be a healthy respect for the environment, with maintenance that does not deliberately promote the transmission of disease-causing agents to hosts but without excessive control measures that impose unnecessary and ineffective actions on the hospital staff and a consequent loss of efficiency and effectiveness, and a wasting of resources such as personnel time and money. Knowledge of environmental factors and their influence on the chain of infection as well as an awareness of adverse changes in the environment should be sufficient to alert one to the need to investigate these environmental factors to ascertain their role in a nosocomial infection problem.

Some environmental factors can influence all the links in the chain of infection, whereas others are more limited in their range of action. Humidity, for example, can influence a multiplicity of factors; it can affect the persistence of an agent as its source, its transmission through the air, and the effectiveness of a host's mucous membranes in resisting infection. Other environmental factors, however, have a more limited effect on the occurrence of infection; for example, the temperature-pressure relation in a specific autoclave affects sterilization within that autoclave, but it has no direct effect on the host.

Certain environmental factors directly affect the agent. Replication of the agent at its reservoir may depend on certain substances in the environment. The agent's survival is influenced by the temperature, humidity, pH, and radiation at its reservoir or source; its survival is even influenced by such factors during its transmission. There may also be toxic substances in the environment that are lethal for the agent.

The transmission of agents will be affected by environmental factors such as temperature and humidity, as mentioned earlier. Airborne transmission is influenced by air velocity and the direction of its movement. The stability and concentration of an aerosol are directly related to environmental factors. In winter, people tend to be indoors with closed windows and reduced air circulation, and this increases the risk of airborne disease compared with summer, when room air is air-conditioned or diluted with outside air. In outbreaks associated with common-vehicle transmission, the temperature of the environment will influence the level of contamination in the vehicle. The spread of vectorborne disease also reflects favorable conditions in the environment for the survival and movement of the vector.

The host's resistance mechanisms are affected by environmental factors; for example, in an excessively dry atmosphere, mucous membranes become dry and are less able to protect against microbial invasion. Also, the host's behavioral patterns are influenced by temperature.

Only after each link in the chain of infection has been carefully described can the most appropriate methods of control and prevention be determined. There may be similarities among cases of disease in different outbreaks; until all the factors involved in the chain of infection are determined for each outbreak, however, it is not possible to be certain that extrapolation of control and preventive measures from one outbreak will be appropriate to another outbreak.

References

1. Bate, J., and James U. *Salmonella typhimurium* infection dust-borne in a children's ward. *Lancet* 2:713, 1958.
2. Hornick, R.B., Greisman, S.E., and Woodward, T.E. Typhoid fever: Pathogenesis and immunologic control. *N. Engl. J. Med.* 283:686, 1970.
3. Riley, R.L., et al. Aerial dissemination of pulmonary tuberculosis: A two-year study of contagion in a tuberculosis ward. *Am. J. Hyg.* 70: 185, 1959.
4. Waller, C.W., Kuntsin, R.B., and Brubaker, M.M. The incidence of airborne wound infections during operation. *J.A.M.A.* 186:908, 1963.

2

The Hospital Epidemiologist

Jan Evans Patterson
Walter J. Hierholzer, Jr.

Historical Perspective

The roots of hospital epidemiology are deeply entwined with those of infectious disease epidemiology and antisepsis. We must acknowledge the contributions of the early hospital epidemiologists, among them Nightingale, Semmelweis, Lister, and Holmes. The term *hospital epidemiologist* was not coined until the late preantibiotic era when it appeared in relation to control measures used for institutional outbreaks of diarrhea [16]. Following the initial successes of antibiotic therapy, use of the term disappeared as institutional medicine produced such positive advances compared to the historical perspective that control of hospital-associated infectious diseases appeared assured.

Hospital epidemiology, both the term and the practice, reappeared with the emergence of penicillinase-producing staphylococci and the associated nosocomial staphylococcal outbreaks of the late 1950s and early 1960s [11]. Organizations such as the American Public Health Association, the New York City Department of Health [19], and the Communicable Disease Center [35] supported the establishment of a hospital staff position for a person knowledgeable about infectious disease epidemiology and related issues. Eventually, the Hospital Infections Branch of the Centers for Disease Control (CDC), was established to assist in dealing with the problem of *nosocomial infections,* a term popularized by members of that group to describe infections associated with hospital care.

First in Great Britain and later in the United States and Canada, there appeared among nursing co-workers the position of nurse epidemiologist. This individual was identified as the critical clinical action person in a program for surveillance and control of nosocomial infections recommended and evaluated by the CDC [15]. A curriculum was defined and a basic training program was funded and offered by the CDC, thereby helping to establish a cadre of professional practitioners with expertise in this increasingly important area of medical practice. As an extension of these programs, a professional organization, the Association for Practitioners in Infection Control (APIC), was established and has grown to a body of more than 8,000 individuals in the United States. Support by the CDC and acceptance of the program and its workers by the American Hospital Association and the Joint Commission on Accreditation of Hospitals (JCAH) were instrumental in the early growth and success of these initiatives.

Physicians were slower to respond to the call for a hospital epidemiologist, but in 1980 the Society of Hospital Epidemiologists of America (SHEA) was formed and has flourished with the increasing need for physicians with expertise in this field. In parallel fashion, professional organizations have appeared in Canada, Great Britain, and many other countries, involving individuals trained in nosocomial infection prevalence studies sponsored by the World Health Organization and its American focus, the Pan American Health Organization.

The Classic Role of the Hospital Epidemiologist

The usual activities of the early hospital epidemiologist were centered around his or her functions as chairperson of the hospital infection control committee. This multidisciplinary professional group was appointed by each hospital and was charged with monitoring and reviewing the infection control–related problems and programs of the institution. The hospital epidemiologist assisted the infection control practitioner (nurse epidemiologist) in formulating, carrying out, and analyzing these programs, including their classic components of surveillance, prevention, and control. To the usual investigative and reporting features of this activity were

added significant political, educational, training, consultative, administrative, and evaluative functions. With the nurse epidemiologist, the hospital epidemiologist became the authoritative action arm of the committee and the program. This unusual authority was recognized and subsequently required and codified in the Standards of the Joint Commission on Accreditation of Healthcare Organizations (JCAHO) [30] and in the public health codes required for licensure of hospitals by many state health departments.

Although no formal training was identified or available for the hospital epidemiologist, his or her functions required an active interest in and some knowledge of microbiology, the epidemiology of infectious disease, disinfection, sterilization, and antisepsis. As the experience and scientific depth and breadth of the field increased through the decades of the sixties through the eighties, the requirements for expertise in these areas grew, and it became apparent that special knowledge in antibiotic resistance and use, occupational health, immunization, and computer data handling was helpful and that special training in epidemiologic methodology was necessary to ensure programs of continuing success. A review of the development of the classic components of the hospital epidemiologist's present-day activities follows.

Infectious Disease Surveillance, Prevention, and Control

The early focus of hospital epidemiologists was on the surveillance, prevention, and control of infectious diseases in the acute-care hospital, and this remains the major emphasis today. Infection control became prominent during the staphylococcal outbreaks in the 1960s but then saw the emergence of multiply drug-resistant, gram-negative enteric bacilli in the 1970s and 1980s. The Enterobacteriaceae and *Pseudomonas aeruginosa* were the nosocomial pathogens of most concern during this era. Multiply resistant strains not only were responsible for nosocomial outbreaks but could persist as endemic and continuing sources of antibiotic-resistant isolates in many institutions [1] (see Chap. 13). During the last decade, gram-positive cocci emerged again as troublesome pathogens. Methicillin-resistant *Staphylococcus aureus* and *Staphylococcus epidermidis* changed empiric anti-staphylococcal therapy and became endemic in many institutions [5]. New mechanisms of resistance in enterococci evolved [27], and nosocomial transmission of these organisms was documented [52] as they became the third most common nosocomial isolate [CDC].

In response to questions about the efficacy of the methods adopted in hospital epidemiologic practice, several studies attributed a decrease in nosocomial infections to effective infection control programs [4, 10, 47]. These were followed by the CDC's Study on the Efficacy of Nosocomial Infection Control (SENIC) in the late 1970s, which affirmed this association in a controlled, nationwide study [23]. SENIC demonstrated a 32 percent reduction in infection rates associated with specific surveillance and infection control components [23]. Indeed a financial incentive for hospital administrations to adopt effective infection control programs became apparent [21].

As important as the early principles of antisepsis and outbreak control measures were (and still are) in infection control programs, the complexity of medical care has increased greatly over the past two decades, and so has the complexity of risk factors for nosocomial infection. Human reservoirs and mechanisms of transmission were emphasized in early control programs, and environmental sources were deemphasized. Routine environmental sampling was discarded as a wasteful and unproductive practice during this period. More recently, the recognition of nosocomial outbreaks of legionellosis and aspergillosis has heightened the hospital epidemiologist's awareness of the environment, with particular regard to architectural and engineering considerations [25, 45]. During the 1970s and 1980s, investigations in the field of infection control have expanded to include the roles of routine use of more and longer indwelling invasive devices, sicker and more highly immunocompromised patients, the implantation of foreign bodies and materials, and use of a broad spectrum of immunomodulating drugs and antimicrobial agents.

Reporting of the Infectious Diseases

One of the surveillance functions adopted by many hospital infection control programs beginning in the 1970s was that of acting as surrogate for the individual physician in reporting to public health authorities communicable diseases in patients seen at the hospital. Such reporting was in response to studies showing very low rates of reporting of these diseases in hospitalized patients by other methods [36]. Reporting through the infection control programs is claimed to have improved the sensitivity of public health data and, in one state, more than 25 percent of communicable disease reports now originate with hospital infection control programs [L. Wintemeir, Iowa State Department of Health, 1985: personal communication].

Infectious Diseases in Medical Care Workers

The classic hospital infection surveillance, prevention, and control program addressed infections in both patients and, in a limited manner, medical care personnel. The hospital epidemiologist usually served in an advisory capacity to the occupational health services of the hospital. Since one of the reservoirs for infectious diseases transmitted to patients in hospitals was the medical care workers, CDC and other programs recommended surveillance, immunization, and control programs for certain communicable diseases in clinical hospital employees and other individuals with patient contact in institutional care [51]. These programs emphasized a tuberculin testing program, immunization for rubella, measles, and other childhood diseases, and policies for restriction of work by individuals with clinical skin, gastrointestinal, and respiratory diseases with potential for transmission to patients.

Impact of the Acquired Immunodeficiency Syndrome Epidemic

The most challenging effort in nosocomial infectious disease control during the past decade has been demonstrated in issues regarding the acquired immunodeficiency syndrome (AIDS) patient and the transmission of the human immunodeficiency virus (HIV) (see Chap. 39). In epidemic areas, the infection control professional was presented with a large number of highly immunocompromised patients, a concomitant increase in serious communicable diseases (e.g., tuberculosis, syphilis) and, early in the epidemic, a general hysteria among the public and health care workers leading to a tendency to quarantine patients with AIDS unnecessarily because the cause of the disease was unknown and the social stigma was great. Decker and Schaffner [11] describe examples of this phenomenon:

> . . . patients were refused admission; physicians and nurses objected to caring for patients with AIDS; once these patients were admitted, health care personnel refused to enter their rooms; nurses falsified vital signs, so as not to have to touch the patients; after a patient was discharged from the hospital, expensive equipment was discarded in the trash, linen was burned, and rooms were obsessively disinfected. It was not the health care profession's finest hour.

CDC epidemiologists advised control measures based on epidemiologic data suggesting that the as-yet-unknown causative agent was likely to have the same mode of transmission as hepatitis B virus. Following this lead, infection control departments led exhaustive and extensive educational efforts in both their hospitals and communities. This was accomplished, in most instances, without an increase in resources or personnel and within an increasingly restrictive medical payment environment. A cooperative cadre of infection control experts facilitated this nationwide educational effort [11].

Even after the causative agent was identified and a readily available antibody test was developed, it became apparent that HIV infection could not be instantaneously detected and that health care workers could become infected from occupational exposure, albeit uncommonly. This led to the concept of universal precautions [20] (see Chap. 11). For health care workers accustomed to dealing with known risks as previously identified by disease-specific isolation, universal precautions required a change in thinking, which met with some resistance [32]. Thus instruction in universal precautions required a

major educational effort by infection control departments in the 1980s.

Despite little evidence of risk of transmission from health care workers to patients during the first decade of the AIDS pandemic, the policy issues regarding the safety and fitness of the HIV-infected health care worker to continue to practice remain a matter of great public interest and debate. Following a model based on the experience for transmission of hepatitis B virus (HBV) from some surgeons and dentists during certain invasive procedures, the CDC has published recommendations for preventing transmission of HIV and HBV to patients during "exposure-prone" invasive procedures [7]. The definition and enumeration of these exposure-prone procedures remain problematic, as does the appropriateness of serologic screening for HIV in either patient or health care worker populations as a means of prevention of transmission in the health care setting. SHEA, APIC, and the infection control community have played an important role in these discussions [2], and the individual hospital epidemiologist will continue to play a crucial role on the expert committees that will determine policies at each institution concerning the HIV-infected individual, whether patient or worker (see Chap. 3).

Concerns about HIV transmission led to public concern about disposal of medical waste. The Medical Waste Tracking Act of 1988 established a demonstration program for the tracking and handling of medical waste in three states [39]. Infection control departments in these states were involved in establishing regulated waste disposal programs in their institutions, another major educational effort.

The Hospital Epidemiologist Then and Now

In a 1975 survey, Haley [22] asked, "Who is the hospital epidemiologist?" and found that the heads of infection surveillance and control programs in U.S. hospitals were a very heterogeneous group, with diverse training backgrounds and epidemiologic approaches. Pathologists comprised 40 percent of the group and clearly predominated as heads of the programs in the formative years. Other groups represented were surgeons (12 percent) and internists (9 percent); infectious disease specialists accounted for only 9 percent at that time but were more likely to be associated with a larger institution. Only 25 percent or so overall had received specific hospital epidemiologic training. Ninety-two percent of the hospital epidemiologists were physicians, and they spent an average of 78 percent of their hospital practice time in infection control efforts, although only 5 percent overall were salaried specifically for these duties [22].

The SENIC Project indicated that the most essential characteristic for the infection control physician in reducing nosocomial infection rates was specific training in infection control [23]. Indeed the skills needed for a modern approach to infection control—epidemiologic principles, biostatistics, surveillance methods, computer skills—are not generally learned in medical training, even in infectious disease fellowships [22].

Although job descriptions have generally been lacking as the infection control physician's role has evolved, Haley [22] outlines six primary infection control functions of the hospital epidemiologist as follows: (1) Develop specific focused surveillance objectives; (2) design surveillance reports relevant to clinicians; (3) interpret surveillance reports to physicians; (4) investigate outbreaks; (5) guide the infection control committee in making policies; and (6) collaborate with the infection control practitioner. The lack of training in infection control and hospital epidemiology also needs to be addressed. Surveillance, epidemiologic investigation, and computer and communication skills required for modern hospital epidemiology programs should be incorporated into infectious disease fellowships and postgraduate courses. Opportunities have been limited but are improving. SHEA and the CDC now sponsor short courses for such a purpose. A few of the infectious disease fellowship training programs emphasize epidemiology and infection control, but most have little or no formal content in this vital area.

Haley [22] compared his 1975 survey with another survey of U.S. hospitals done in 1983

(Table 2-1). Infectious disease physicians were heads of infection control in 11 percent, up from 9 percent in 1975; however, in 1983 they had assumed this position in approximately 50 percent of teaching hospitals, up from 35 percent in 1975 [22]. Infectious disease physicians held this role in 5 percent of nonteaching hospitals in both surveys. More than half of infectious disease physicians were salaried for such a position in 1985, but few physicians with other training were paid. In both surveys, only approximately 25 percent overall received training in infection control. Thus it appears that infectious disease physicians predominate as the hospital epidemiologist in teaching hospitals but not in nonteaching hospitals. They are increasingly being paid for assuming such a role, although many are not adequately trained [22].

An impediment to infectious disease physicians becoming more active in infection control is the failure to pay them for such work. Teaching hospitals have become increasingly aware of the good investment in quality infection control programs, but many nonteaching

Table 2-1. Trends in infectious disease physicians' role in hospital infection control

Trend	Percent participating	
	1975	1983
U.S. hospitals with infectious disease physician as infection control physician		
Teaching hospitals	35	45
Nonteaching hospitals	5	5
All U.S. hospitals	9	11
Infection control physicians paid for such work		
Infectious disease physicians	25	53
Physicians of other specialties	6	9
All infection control physicians	9	17
Infection control physicians with formal training		
Infectious disease physicians	44	35
Physicians of other specialties	25	23
All infection control physicians	28	25

Source: Adapted from R. W. Haley, The role of infectious disease physicians in hospital infection control. *Bull. N.Y. Acad. Med.* 63:597, 1987.

hospitals have not, and these still account for the majority of hospitals in the United States. The SENIC Project [23], increasing pressure from regulatory agencies, financial pressures, and increasing awareness of the capacity of the hospital epidemiologist to contribute to quality assurance should encourage all hospitals to invest in quality hospital epidemiology [22, 24].

New Challenges for the Hospital Epidemiologist
New Microbiologic Methods
New laboratory methods developed and simplified during the past decade can now determine strain relatedness at the molecular level [33]. The ability to isolate plasmid and chromosomal DNA from bacterial organisms, and whole-cell DNA from bacteria as well as viruses and fungi has greatly enhanced the study of nosocomial infections (see Chaps. 9, 13, 14). These techniques have been used to document newly recognized nosocomial pathogens and define new roles for previously recognized ones [43, 44]. The specificity, rapidity, and reproducibility of such methods have now been applied to many organisms and have made epidemiologic typing a current and indispensable tool. In the 1990s, standard nosocomial outbreak investigations will most often involve some type of molecular analysis [28].

Advancement of Epidemiologic Methodology
The epidemiologic methodology used by hospital epidemiologists has expanded along with the complexity of patient and treatment risks for infection in current medical care. Whereas infection control epidemiology was once largely descriptive and analytic (and these methods continue to remain useful), hospital epidemiologists have routinely begun to apply more sophisticated epidemiologic methodology, including relative risk, risk ratio, regression analysis, and correlation coefficients, to the study of nosocomial infections [17, 18, 26, 41]. The availability of the personal computer has made such analysis

routine and accessible. The computerization of infection control surveillance has expanded epidemiology databases and enhanced the study of nosocomial infections (see Chap. 8).

Expanded Occupational Health
The health care worker is exposed to a variety of hazards beyond infectious agents, including chemical exposures, radiation hazard, allergies, stress, and physical injury. In the earlier preantibiotic decades, exposure of the medical worker to streptococcal infection, tuberculosis, and other serious communicable diseases was an expected event, and resultant disease and even death were not rare. Antibiotic and vaccine use lessened the concern with such dangers, but in the past decade no hazard has been discussed more than the risk of occupationally acquired HIV. When such a risk became apparent, the Occupational Safety and Health Administration (OSHA) focused its attention on hospitals and health care worker safety as never before [12]. This challenges hospital occupational health and risk management services to heighten awareness of compliance with all safety issues among employees, trainees, first responders, and all members of the health care team, a long-neglected aspect of health care.

Inherent in the emphasis on protecting the medical worker has been the need to evaluate such interventions and practices to ensure their efficacy and their effectiveness and to affirm that they do not increase the risk of nosocomial transmission to and between patients or result in increased morbidity from lengthened time of procedure or loss of technical finesse. The data collection, analysis, and management tools needed for monitoring, prevention, and control in this area parallel those required for infection control. Therefore, the hospital epidemiologist can contribute much in the way of experience, skill, and especially leadership for these efforts.

The New Hospital Epidemiologist: Quality Assurance and Other Interests
As hospital epidemiologic methodology has matured, it has been increasingly recognized as an early, tested outcome model for poten-

tial application to other programs in related areas of patient care. In the last decade, the field of hospital epidemiology has expanded to encompass interests and demands from other areas in health care that involve study by similar methods. The linking of hospital reimbursement to quality of care and quality assessment by external reviewers such as the Health Care Financing Administration (HCFA) has been a strong incentive to expand the model and the methods of hospital epidemiology to these other so-called quality assurance (QA) or quality improvement (QI) programs. Infection control provides many valuable QA examples, for nosocomial infections are but one of the controllable risks for poor outcome encountered by the institutionalized patient. Other such events may include injuries that are physical, chemical, ergometric, and psychologic in origin [26, 49].

Many analogies may be drawn between the epidemiologic approach to nosocomial infectious and noninfectious risks. Some common noninfectious causal agents include antineoplastics, anticoagulants, intravascular catheterization, blood product administration, surgical procedures, falls, and nutritional problems [8]. Host factors that may predispose to such noninfectious agents include abnormal cardiac physiology, age, mental status, and immobility. Factors contributing to such risks include the experience and skill of practitioners, adequacy of staffing, and equipment [8]. Surveillance for quality assessment of noninfectious risks requires the establishment of risk and outcome definitions, which may be more difficult to qualify than those already established for infection control [9, 32].

The data collection and management required for infection control, occupational medicine, and QA coincide and intersect such that a common, automated database shared by each would increase efficiency and information for each program. The common factors in data acquisition and management and analysis and control methodology suggest that further efficiencies might be achieved by personnel and program coordination within each institution.

Risk Management

One of the formal programs dealing with poor outcome evaluation and control in patients is the liability-centered and malpractice-related risk management program of most U.S. hospitals (see Chap. 26). Although these efforts have their usual focus in attempts to control financial losses based on the indicator sentinel events of poor patient outcomes, recognition is growing that analysis, prevention, and control of the poor outcomes are the keys to improvement and that the infection control model may again be applicable.

Antibiotic Utilization

Antibiotic utilization provides another good example of a common QA issue, and programs for review are well established in many institutions. JCAHO requires that medical staffs develop a systematic process for evaluating the empiric, therapeutic, and prophylactic use of drugs [29]. The Antimicrobial Agents Committee of the Infectious Diseases Society of America has recommended that each hospital provide financial and administrative support for a group concerned with appropriate use of antibiotics [37]. This team should be headed by an infectious disease physician who is a member of the Infection Control Committee and of the Pharmacy and Therapeutics Committee. It is recommended that this individual coordinate a team composed of members of other services, including the clinical microbiologist, pharmacist, and infection control practitioner [37]. Specific audits of antibiotic use are helpful for QA purposes as well as for assessing the need for antibiotic restriction policies and cost-effectiveness of certain agents.

Pharmacoepidemiology

With advances in epidemiologic methods and computerization, agencies and medical payors are requiring monitoring of all drug use, and the ability to detect adverse drug reactions is increasing. In fact, JCAHO now requires that hospitals have the capacity to document and evaluate adverse drug reactions that occur in their patients [34, 50]. The link between antibiotic utilization issues and adverse drug reactions has involved many hospital epidemiologists in pharmacoepidemiology, which studies the effects of drugs, both beneficial and adverse [6]. Again, the role for common databases and for common analysis and control methods is evident.

Emporiatrics

The editorial board of SHEA's journal, *Infection Control and Hospital Epidemiology*, has recently added a regular feature on *emporiatrics*, the study of diseases in the traveler. The physician involved in infection control is often asked for travel advice and is involved in establishing guidelines for returning travelers with communicable diseases [42]. Since approximately 8 million U.S. citizens travel to developing countries each year [31], and it is estimated that 5 percent of the U.S. population is employed in health-related industries, it is relevant for the hospital epidemiologist to stay apprised of current infectious disease events worldwide.

Future Roles for the Hospital Epidemiologist

Clearly, the potential areas of activities for the broadly interested hospital epidemiologist are wide, encompassing roles from consultant microbiologist to clinical epidemiologist. In a presentation at a national APIC conference, Barbara Soule [48] has suggested that the hospital epidemiologist might pursue either the route of specialist focusing on nosocomial microbiology, infection control, and closely related infectious disease areas in hospitals and other health care venues or, alternatively, the role of generalist, expanding the model of nosocomial surveillance, prevention, and control and its epidemiologic methods to the noninfectious QA medical care outcome programs [48]. In either case, it would appear important to protect the proved, highly successful, and cost-effective core of infection control programs in all acute-care hospitals and, as efficacy is demonstrated, in other health care institutions. In a time of financial constraint in medical care institutions, it would appear unwise to disable or dismantle a proved program by attempting to broaden its function beyond the per-

sonnel and financial resources required to continue its effectiveness or to include it under leadership untrained and inexperienced in the methods necessary to continue its success and to expand it into potentially coordinated programs.

The hospital epidemiologist and infection control team are, of necessity, involved in ongoing educational efforts at their own institutions. Additionally, they often serve as regional consultants and educators for other institutions. Consortiums for infection control have been an efficient solution for quality input for some hospitals not affiliated with a university system [13]. This arrangement can serve several such hospitals efficiently and cost effectively [14].

The developing world is recognizing the importance and impact of infection control. Innovative ways of dealing with the overwhelming problems of lack of financial resources and the spectrum of communicable diseases need to be found [40, 46]. Participation of hospital epidemiologists from developed countries in consortiums with those from developing countries is needed [3].

Over three decades of active, modern growth, the role of the hospital epidemiologist has continued to mature and expand, and it seems certain to do so in the future.

References

1. Alford, R. H., and Hall, A. Epidemiology of infections caused by gentamicin-resistant Enterobacteriaciae and *Pseudomonas aeruginosa* over 15 years at the Nashville Veterans Administration Medical Center. *Rev. Infect. Dis.* 9:1079, 1987.
2. The Association for Practitioners in Infection Control and The Society for Hospital Epidemiology of America. Position paper: The HIV-infected health care worker. *Am. J. Infect. Control* 16:371, 1990.
3. Brachman, P. S. Visions for the future. *Am. J. Infect. Control* 12:204, 1984.
4. Britt, M. R., Schleupner, C. J., and Matsumiya, S. Severity of underlying disease as a predictor of nosocomial infection: Utility in the control of nosocomial infection. *J.A.M.A.* 239:1047, 1978.

5. Brumfitt, W., and Hamilton-Miller, J. Methicillin-resistant *Staphylococcus aureus. N. Engl. J. Med.* 320:1188, 1989.

6. Burke, J. P., Tilson, H. H., and Platt, R. Expanding roles of hospital epidemiology: Pharmacoepidemiology. *Infect. Control Hosp. Epidemiol.* 10:253, 1989.

7. Centers for Disease Control. Recommendations for preventing transmission of human immunodeficiency virus and hepatitis B virus to patients during exposure-prone invasive procedures. *M.M.W.R.* 40:1, 1991.

8. Crede, W., and Hierholzer, W. J., Jr. Linking hospital epidemiology and quality assurance: Seasoned concepts in a new role. *Infect. Control Hosp. Epidemiol.* 9:42, 1988.

9. Crede, W., and Hierholzer, W. J., Jr. Surveillance for quality assessment: I. Surveillance in infection control success reviewed. *Infect. Control Hosp. Epidemiol.* 10:470, 1989.

10. Cruse, P. J. E., and Foord, R. The epidemiology of wound infection: A 10-year prospective study of 62,939 wounds. *Surg. Clin. North Am.* 60:27, 1980.

11. Decker, M.D., and Schaffner, W. Changing trends in infection control and hospital epidemiology. *Infect. Dis. Clin. North Am.* 3:671, 1989.

12. Department of Labor, Joint Advisory Notice: Department of Labor/Department of Health and Human Services. HBV/HIV. *Fed. Reg.* 52:41818, 1987.

13. Ehrenkranz, N. J. The efficacy of a Florida hospital consortium for infection control: 1975–1982. *Infect. Control* 7:321, 1986.

14. Ehrenkranz, N. J. South Florida hospital consortium for infection control: Structure and function. *Am. J. Infect. Control* 15:36, 1987.

15. Eickhoff, T. C., and Brachman, P. S., Bennett, J. V., and Brown, J. F. Surveillance of nosocomial infections in community hospitals. I. Surveillance methods, effectiveness, and initial results. *J. Infect. Dis.* 120:305, 1969.

16. Felson, J., and Wolarsky, W. The hospital epidemiologist. *Hospitals* 14:41, 1940.

17. Freeman, J., and McGowan, J. E., Jr. Methodologic issues in hospital epidemiology: I. Rates, case-finding, and interpretation. *Rev. Infect. Dis.* 3:658, 1981.

18. Freeman, J., and McGowan, J. E., Jr. Methodologic issues in hospital epidemiology: III. Investigating the modifying effects of time and severity of underlying illness on estimates of cost of nosocomial infection. *Rev. Infect. Dis.* 6:285, 1984.

19. Fuerst, J. T., Lightman, H. S., and James, G. Hospital epidemiology. *J.A.M.A.* 194:97, 1965.

20. Gerberding, J. L., and the University of California, San Francisco, Task Force on AIDS.

Recommended infection control policies for patients with human immunodeficiency virus infection. *N. Engl. J. Med.* 315:1562, 1986.

21. Haley, R. W. *Managing Hospital Infection Control for Cost-Effectiveness.* Chicago: American Hospital Association, 1986.

22. Haley, R. W. The role of infectious disease physicians in hospital infection control. *Bull. N.Y. Acad. Med.* 63:597, 1987.

23. Haley, R. W., et al. The efficacy of infection surveillance and control programs in preventing nosocomial infections in U.S. hospitals. *Am. J. Epidemiol.* 121:182, 1985.

24. Health Care Financing Administration: Infection Control. Medicare and Medicaid programs; conditions of participation by hospitals; final regulations, effective September 15, 1986. *Fed. Reg.* June 17, 1986. Pp. 22010–22048.

25. Helms, C. M., et al. Legionnaires' disease associated with a hospital water system: A cluster of 24 nosocomial cases. *Ann. Intern. Med.* 99:172, 1983.

26. Hierholzer, W. J., Jr. The practice of hospital epidemiology. *Yale J. Biol. Med.* 55:225, 1982.

27. Hoffman, S. A., and Moellering, R. C. The enterococcus: "Putting the bug in our ears." *Ann. Intern. Med.* 106:757, 1987.

28. John, J. R., Jr. Molecular analysis of nosocomial epidemics. *Infect. Dis. Clin. North Am.* 3:683, 1989.

29. Joint Commission on Accreditation of Healthcare Organizations. *Accreditation Manual for Hospitals.* Chicago: Joint Commission on Accreditation of Healthcare Organizations, 1986. Pp. 205–208.

30. Joint Commission on Accreditation of Healthcare Organizations. *Accreditation Manual for Hospitals.* Chicago: Joint Commission on Accreditation of Healthcare Organizations, 1989. P. 68.

31. Jong, E. C. Medical Approach to the Traveling Patient. In: *The Travel and Tropical Medicine Manual.* Philadelphia: Saunders, 1987.

32. Kearns, K. P. Universal precautions: Employee resistance and strategies for planned organizational change. Hospital and Health Services Administration 33:521, 1988.

33. Koblet, H. Contributions of molecular biology to diagnosis, pathogenesis and epidemiology of infectious diseases. *Experientia* 43:1185, 1987.

34. Koska, M. T. JCAHO accreditation: Top trouble spots for hospitals. *Hospitals* 63:34, 1989.

35. Langmuir, A. D. Significance of epidemiology in medical schools. *J. Med. Educ.* 39:39, 1964.

36. Marier, R. The reporting of communicable diseases. *Am. J. Epidemiol.* 105:587, 1977.

37. Marr, J. J., Moffet, H. L., and Kunin, C. M. Guidelines for improving the use of anti-

microbial agents in hospitals: A statement by the Infectious Diseases Society of America. *J. Infect. Dis.* 157:869, 1988.

38. McGeer, A., Crede, W., and Hierholzer, W. J., Jr. Surveillance for quality assessment: II. Surveillance for noninfectious processes: Back to basics. *Infect. Control Hosp. Epidemiol.* 11:36, 1990.

39. The Medical Waste Tracking Act of 1988. Public Law 100-582 Codified at 42 U.S.C. Section 6992-6992k.

40. Meers, P. D. Infection control in developing countries. *J. Hosp. Infect.* 11 (Suppl. A):406, 1988.

41. Nagachinta, T., Stephens, M., Reitz, B., and Polk, F. Risk factors for surgical-wound infection following cardiac surgery. *J. Infect. Dis.* 156:967, 1987.

42. Nettleman, M. D. Emporiatrics: The study of diseases in travelers. *Infect. Control Hosp. Epidemiol.* 11:157, 1990.

43. Patterson, J. E., et al. Nosocomial transmission of *Hemophilus influenzae* type b in a geriatric unit confirmed by restriction endonuclease analysis. *J. Infect. Dis.* 157:1002, 1988.

44. Patterson, T. F., et al. A nosocomial outbreak of *Branhamella catarrhalis* confirmed by restriction endonuclease analysis. *J. Infect. Dis.* 157:996, 1988.

45. Rhame, F. S. Nosocomial aspergillosis: How much protection for which patients? *Infect. Control Hosp. Epidemiol.* 10:296, 1989.

46. Schlabach, W. E. Dealing with hospital infections in developing countries. *Trop. Doct.* 18:161, 1988.

47. Shoji, K. T., Axnick, K., and Rytel, M. W. Infections and antibiotic use in a large municipal hospital 1970–1972: A prospective analysis of the effectiveness of a continuous surveillance program. *Health Lab. Sci.* 11:283, 1974.

48. Soule, B. The evaluation of our profession: Lessons from Darwin. *Am. J. Infect. Control* 19:45, 1991.

49. Steel, K., et al. Iatrogenic illness on a general medical service at a university hospital. *N. Engl. J. Med.* 304:638, 1981.

50. Strom, B. L., and Tugwell, P. Pharmacoepidemiology: Current status, prospects, and problems. *Ann. Intern. Med.* 113:179, 1990.

51. Williams, W. W. Centers for Disease Control: Guidelines for infection control in hospital personnel. *Infect. Control* 4:326, 1983.

52. Zervos, M. J., et al. Nosocomial infection by gentamicin-resistant *Streptococcus faecalis. Ann. Intern. Med.* 106:687, 1987.

Personnel Health Services

Jacquelyn A. Polder
Ofelia C. Tablan
Walter W. Williams

Persons who work in hospitals are at risk of exposure to communicable diseases in both the workplace and the community. If they develop disease, they may in turn pose a risk for transmission of that disease to patients, other hospital personnel, members of their households, or other community contacts. Health care workers (HCWs)* or others who have frequent and prolonged direct contact with patients may be at the greatest risk of exposure to infectious agents.

This chapter outlines infection control objectives of a hospital personnel health service and discusses important aspects of selected transmissible diseases. General objectives and control measures are set forth, which may need to be broadened for certain personnel groups, depending on the needs of the institution, local and state regulations, and local disease risks.

Infection Control Objectives of a Personnel Health Service

As part of the general program for infection control, hospitals should establish policies to minimize the risk of transmission of infections between HCWs and patients [44]. The personnel health service should coordinate its activities with the infection control program and other hospital departments to ensure prompt implementation of prevention and control measures [44]. The support of the administration, medical staff, and other hospital personnel is essential for goals to be met.

In collaboration with infection control staff, the personnel health service can contribute to infection control activities by establishing

---

*For purposes of this chapter, personnel who work directly with, or in close proximity to, patients will be referred to as *health care workers*.

policies and procedures such as (1) placement evaluations; (2) health and safety education; (3) immunization programs; (4) monitoring potentially harmful infectious exposures and instituting appropriate preventive measures; (5) coordinating plans for managing outbreaks among personnel; (6) providing care to personnel for work-related illnesses or exposures; (7) providing information regarding infection risks related to employment or special conditions; (8) developing guidelines for restricting work because of infectious disease; and (9) maintaining health records on all HCWs.

Placement Evaluations

Placement evaluations should be done before or at the time HCWs are hired. A placement evaluation can be used to assist in ensuring that persons are able to perform job tasks safely and efficiently and that they are not placed in jobs that would pose unusual risk of infection to themselves, other personnel, patients, or visitors. Determining the existence of, or susceptibility to, certain infectious diseases may be an important part of this evaluation and should include determining an HCW's immunization status and history of previous medical conditions such as chickenpox or immunodeficient conditions that may predispose the HCW to acquiring or transmitting infectious diseases. In addition, the preplacement evaluation can be used to educate HCWs about their role in the prevention of nosocomial infections.

Physical examinations for purposes of job placement may help detect unusual susceptibility to infection, conditions that may increase the likelihood of transmitting disease to patients, and presence of communicable diseases or conditions, and may serve as a baseline in the future when evaluating conditions that may be work-related. There are no data, however, to suggest that routine complete physical examinations are needed for infection control purposes. Neither are there data to suggest that routine laboratory testing (such as complete blood cell counts, serologic tests for syphilis, urinalysis, or chest roentgenograms) or preemployment screening for enteric or

other pathogens are cost-beneficial. In some areas, however, local public health ordinances may still mandate that certain screening procedures be employed. Tuberculosis screening should be part of the HCW's initial evaluation and should be completed prior to the HCW having any direct contact with patients (see under the heading Tuberculosis).

Personnel Health and Safety Education

HCW education should be a central focus of the personnel health program, including initial job orientation and ongoing inservice education. In the initial and ongoing educational program, it is important to stress that patient care personnel can decrease the risk of acquiring or transmitting infection by rigorous adherence to infection control practices when caring for patients and, in particular, careful hand-washing after touching patients or materials that are likely to be contaminated [45]. Ongoing educational activities may include the use of lectures, discussion groups, display materials, newsletters, inservice directly on the unit, or any other innovative technique that will assist in maintaining staff awareness of infection control issues.

A mechanism should be in place for HCWs to obtain advice in a timely manner about infections they may acquire or transmit to patients [44]. In addition, this mechanism should address the policy for immediate evaluation following occupational exposure to infectious agents such as human immunodeficiency virus (HIV), hepatitis B virus (HBV), meningitis, or others.

Immunization Programs

Hospital personnel are at risk for exposure to and transmission of certain vaccine-preventable diseases [211]. Using immunizing agents optimally in hospitals will safeguard the health of both personnel and patients, decrease the risk for transmission of preventable infections to others in the hospital setting, and avoid unnecessary work restrictions. Preventing illness through comprehensive personnel immunization policies is far more cost-effective than case management and outbreak control. Mandatory programs are more effective than voluntary programs in ensuring that susceptible persons are vaccinated, and programs in which the hospital bears the cost have had higher vaccination rates. In addition, hospital-based immunization programs for patients can potentially provide an important mechanism for immunizing susceptible persons in the community.

Comprehensive immunization programs should be an essential part of a personnel health and infection control program [44]. Regarding the selection of vaccines to include in immunization programs, one should consider (1) the likelihood of exposure to the agents included in the vaccine; (2) the nature of employment (i.e., type of patient contact); and (3) the potential consequences of not vaccinating.

The Immunization Practices Advisory Committee (ACIP) of the U.S. Public Health Service develops vaccination guidelines for hospital personnel and the general population in the United States. Persons administering immunizing agents should be familiar with ACIP recommendations and be well-informed about indications, storage, dosage, preparation, and contraindications for each of the vaccines, toxoids, and immune globulins [9, 131]. In addition, individual states and professional organizations may have recommendations or regulations regarding vaccination of HCWs that need to be reviewed. Product information should be available at all times, and a pertinent health history should be obtained from each HCW before an agent is given [47]. The most efficient use of vaccine is to immunize personnel before they enter high-risk situations. Table 3-1 summarizes information on the major indications, regimens, and major contraindications of the vaccines and immunobiologic agents generally recommended for HCWs.

Screening for Susceptibility to Hepatitis B, Measles, or Rubella Prior to Vaccination

The decision to screen potential vaccine recipients for susceptibility to HBV prior to vaccination is primarily an economic one. Receipt of HB vaccine is neither hazardous nor beneficial to HB carriers or HB immune persons; the vaccine will not change the recipient's HBV serologic status [80, 192]. In the United States, the cost-effectiveness of screening prior to vaccination is usually determined by balancing the prevalence of previous infection in any targeted group, the cost of screening, and the cost of immunizing personnel without screening [129, 155]. Prevaccination testing in groups with the highest risk for previous HBV infection (HBV marker prevalence greater than 20 percent) may be cost-beneficial as it will identify previously infected persons and prevent unnecessary expensive vaccination of persons who would not benefit from that vaccination. Cost-effectiveness of screening may be marginal for groups at intermediate risk for HBV infection. In groups with a low expected prevalence of HBV serologic markers, such as health professionals in their training years, prevaccination testing is usually not cost-effective. Hepatitis B vaccine, when given in the deltoid, produces antibody in more than 90 percent of healthy susceptible persons. Testing for immunity after vaccination is advised for persons whose subsequent management depends on knowing their immune status (such as dialysis patients and staff) and should also be considered for persons at occupational risk for needle-stick or other blood exposure necessitating postexposure evaluation and prophylaxis. If performed, postvaccination testing should be done between 1 and 6 months after completing the vaccine series.

Routine serologic screening of HCWs to determine measles immunity is not generally recommended, although it may be cost-effective in some situations [126]. Routinely performing serologic tests to ensure that rubella vaccine is given only to proved susceptibles may be very expensive. The ACIP states that rubella immunization of women not known to be pregnant and men is justifiable without serologic testing [130].

Tracking systems should be established to ensure that identified susceptibles return for vaccination or are readily identified in potential outbreak situations so that appropriate preventive measures can be taken.

Table 3-1. Immunizations recommended for health care personnel

Immunization	Major indications*	Dose schedule	Major precautions and contraindications*
Hepatitis B vaccine	Adults at increased risk of occupational, environmental, social, or family exposure to hepatitis B. Certain travelers to foreign countries	2 doses IM (deltoid) 4 weeks apart; third dose 5 months after second; booster doses not routinely recommended (alternative schedules are under consideration)	Pregnancy is not a contraindication if the woman is otherwise eligible
Influenza vaccine	Adults with high-risk conditions, residents of nursing homes or other chronic-care facilities, medical care personnel, healthy persons ≥ 65 yr	Annual vaccination with current vaccine. Either whole- or split-virus vaccine may be used IM	History of anaphylactic hypersensitivity to egg ingestion
Measles vaccine	Adults born after 1956 without verification of adequate measles vaccination with live vaccine, physician-diagnosed measles, or laboratory evidence of immunity. Susceptible travelers to foreign countries	2 doses SC, separated by at least 1 month	Pregnancy; history of anaphylactic reaction following egg ingestion or receipt of neomycin; severe febrile illness; immunosuppression; recent administration of immune globulin
Mumps vaccine	Adults without verification of physician-diagnosed mumps, laboratory evidence of immunity, or proof of vaccination on or after the first birthday. It is reasonable to consider persons born before 1957 immune, but there is no contraindication to vaccinate older persons. Susceptible travelers to foreign countries	1 dose SC; no booster	Pregnancy; history of anaphylactic reaction following egg ingestion or receipt of neomycin; severe febrile illness; immunosuppression; recent administration of immune globulin
Rubella vaccine	Adults without verification of live vaccine on or after first birthday or laboratory evidence of immunity. Susceptible travelers to foreign countries	1 dose SC; no booster	Pregnancy; history of anaphylactic reaction following receipt of neomycin; severe febrile illness; immunosuppression; recent administration of immune globulin
Tetanus-diphtheria toxoid	All adults who have had an initial series should have a booster every 10 years	Initial series: 2 doses IM 4 weeks apart; third dose 6–12 months after second; booster every 10 years	History of a neurologic or hypersensitivity reaction following a previous dose

*Refer to appropriate Immunization Practices Advisory Committee recommendations for more details [126–131].

Work Restrictions and Management of HCW Illnesses and Exposures

A major function of the personnel health service may be to arrange for prompt diagnosis and management of potentially transmissible illnesses or exposures and provide prophylaxis, when appropriate, to HCWs who have experienced an occupational exposure. Hospitals are advised to have well-defined policies for personnel who have transmissible infections [44, 211].

Such policies should address the responsibility of the HCW in using the health service and reporting illness, exclusion from direct contact with patients, and clearance for return to work after recovery from an infec-

tious disease or condition. For any exclusion policy to be enforceable and effective, all personnel—especially department heads, area supervisors, and head nurses—must know when and where an illness is to be reported. Any policy for work restriction should be designed to encourage personnel to report their illnesses or exposures and, as much as possible, not penalize them with loss of wages, benefits, leave time, or job status [44].

Table 3-2 briefly lists recommendations for prophylaxis of hospital workers after certain exposures. Table 3-3 briefly summarizes recommendations and suggested work restrictions for personnel with selected infectious diseases. More detail on selected infectious

Table 3-2. Recommendations for prophylaxis after exposure to various diseases

Disease	Recommendations
General	When prophylactic treatment with drugs, vaccines, or immune globulins is necessary, personnel should be informed of alternative means of prophylaxis, the risk (if known) of infection if treatment is not accepted, the degree of protection provided by the therapy, and the potential side effects.
Hepatitis A	Personnel who have had direct fecal-oral exposure to excretions from a patient found to have been incubating hepatitis A should be given immune globulin (IG) (0.02 ml/kg) as soon as possible. Giving IG more than 2 weeks after exposure is not effective.
	Routine IG prophylaxis for hospital workers is not indicated. Prophylaxis with IG for all personnel who take care of patients with hepatitis A (other than as suggested above) should not be given. Sound hygienic practices should be emphasized.
Hepatitis B	For prophylaxis against hepatitis B after percutaneous (needle-stick) or mucous membrane exposure to blood that might be infective, the recommendations in Table 3-4 should be followed.
Hepatitis C (parenterally transmitted non-A, non-B [NANB] hepatitis)	Results have been equivocal in studies attempting to assess the value of prophylaxis with IGs against parenterally transmitted NANB hepatitis. For persons with percutaneous exposure to blood from a patient with parenterally transmitted NANB hepatitis, it may be reasonable to administer IG (0.06 ml/kg) as soon as possible after exposure.
Meningococcal disease	Antimicrobial prophylaxis against meningococcal disease should be offered immediately to personnel who have had intensive direct contact with an infected patient without using proper precautions. If prophylaxis is deemed necessary, treatment should not await results of antimicrobial sensitivity testing.
Rabies	Hospital personnel who either have been bitten by a human with rabies or have scratches, abrasions, open wounds, or mucous membranes contaminated with saliva or other potentially infective material from a human or animal with rabies should receive a full course of antirabies treatment.

Table 3-3. Work restrictions for hospital workers exposed to or infected with selected infectious diseases

Disease or problem	Relieve from direct patient contact	Partial work restriction	Duration
Conjunctivitis, infectious	Yes		Until discharge ceases
Cytomegalovirus infections	No		
Diarrhea			
Acute stage (diarrhea with other symptoms)	Yes		Until symptoms resolve and infection with *Salmonella* is ruled out
Convalescent stage *Salmonella* (nontyphoidal)	No	Personnel should not care for high-risk patients	Until stool is free of the infecting organism on 2 consecutive cultures not less than 24 hours apart
Enteroviral infections	No	Personnel should not care for infants and newborns	Until symptoms resolve
Group A streptococcal disease	Yes		Until 24 hours after adequate treatment is started
Hepatitis, viral			
Hepatitis A	Yes		Until 7 days after onset of jaundice
Hepatitis B			
Acute	Possibly	Personnel should use barrier precautions for procedures that involve trauma to tissues or contact with mucous membranes or non-intact skin	Until antigenemia resolves
Chronic antigenemia	Possibly	HCWs who are HBeAg-positive may be restricted in certain situations	Until antigenemia resolves
Hepatitis C (parenterally transmitted NANB)	No	Personnel should use barrier precautions for procedures that involve trauma to tissues or contact with mucous membranes or non-intact skin	Period of infectivity has not been determined
Herpes simplex			
Genital	No		
Hands (herpetic whitlow)	Yes	(Note: It is not known whether gloves prevent transmission)	Until lesions heal
Orofacial	No	Personnel should not care for high-risk patients	Until lesions heal
Human immunodeficiency virus	Possibly	HCWs may be restricted in certain situations	
Measles			
Active	Yes		Until 7 days after the rash appears
Postexposure (susceptible personnel)	Yes		From the fifth through the twenty-first day after exposure or 7 days after the rash appears

Table 3-3. *(continued)*

Disease or problem	*Relieve from direct patient contact*	*Partial work restriction*	*Duration*
Mumps			
Active	Yes		Until 9 days after onset of parotitis
Postexposure (susceptible personnel)	Yes		From the twelfth through the twenty-sixth day after exposure or until 9 days after onset of parotitis
Pertussis			
Active	Yes		From the beginning of the catarrhal stage through the third week after onset of paroxysms or until 7 days after start of effective antimicrobial therapy
Postexposure (asymptomatic personnel)	No		
Postexposure (symptomatic personnel)	Yes		Same as active pertussis
Rubella			
Active	Yes		Until 5 days after the rash appears
Postexposure (susceptible personnel)	Yes		From the seventh through the twenty-first day after exposure
Scabies	Yes		Until treated
Staphylococcus aureus (skin lesions)	Yes		Until lesions have resolved
Upper respiratory infections	No	Personnel with upper respiratory infections should not care for high-risk patients	Until acute symptoms resolve
Varicella (chickenpox)			
Active	Yes		Until all lesions dry and crust
Postexposure (susceptible personnel)	Yes		From the tenth through the twenty-first day after exposure and, if varicella occurs, until all lesions dry and crust
Zoster (shingles)			
Active	No, if lesions localized and covered	Appropriate barrier desirable	Until lesions dry and crust, personnel should not care for high-risk patients (regardless if lesions are covered)
Postexposure (personnel susceptible to chicken pox)	Yes		From the tenth through the twenty-first day after exposure and, if varicella occurs, until all lesions dry and crust

HBeAg = hepatitis B e antigen; NANB = non-A, non-B hepatitis.

diseases or conditions that may be transmitted nosocomially and thus require consideration in placement or work restrictions will follow in the remainder of the chapter.

Epidemiology and Control of Selected Infections Transmitted Among Hospital Personnel and Patients

Cytomegalovirus

HCWs may be exposed to patients with cytomegalovirus (CMV) infection, but the risk of acquiring a primary CMV infection from patients appears to be small. There are two principal reservoirs of CMV in the hospital: (1) infants infected with CMV and (2) immunocompromised patients, such as oncology patients, acquired immunodeficiency syndrome (AIDS) patients, and those undergoing kidney or bone marrow transplant (also see Chap. 38). However, available data have shown no evidence of an increased risk of transmission of CMV to personnel working in dialysis units [200], oncology wards [82], or pediatric areas, when compared with personnel with no patient contact [213]. Primary infection with CMV during pregnancy may damage the fetus; however, pregnant women have not been found to be more susceptible to CMV infection than nonpregnant women.

Nosocomially, CMV is transmitted mainly through infected body fluids that come into contact with the hands and are inoculated into the nose or mouth of a susceptible person. Virus can be shed in the urine, saliva, respiratory secretions, tears, feces, breast milk, semen, and cervical secretions.

Screening Programs for CMV Infection

Screening programs to detect CMV-infected patients are not practical, because the tests are time-consuming and costly and would entail screening all high-risk patients, including newborns. Likewise, the drawbacks of mass screening of personnel include its expense and the possibility that a negative result may generate undue fear of acquiring the infection. In addition, since there are no studies to indicate clearly that personnel may be protected by transfer to areas of less contact with infants and children [3, 213], identifying women without antibodies to institute such measures may not reduce the number of primary infections.

Preventing Transmission of CMV

When hygienic practices are used, the risk of acquiring infection through patient contact is low [3]. Therefore, a practical approach to reducing the risk of infection with CMV is to stress careful hand-washing after *all* patient contacts and to avoid direct contact with materials that are potentially infective [45]. Pregnant personnel should be informed of the potential risk to the fetus of primary CMV infection and should practice appropriate precautions (as outlined previously) to minimize the risk of acquiring primary CMV infection.

Personnel who contract illnesses believed to be due to CMV need not be restricted from work [204]. They can reduce the risk of transmission to patients or other personnel by careful hand-washing and by preventing their body fluids from contacting other persons.

Acute Diarrhea

Various agents may cause diarrhea in patients and hospital personnel (see Chap. 30). *Salmonella*, *Shigella*, and *Campylobacter* species are among the common bacterial enteric pathogens. Infection with these agents may produce mild symptoms but is often accompanied by other symptoms, such as abdominal cramps, fever, or bloody diarrhea. Diarrheal illness accompanied by such symptoms suggests a bacterial cause. Rotavirus and the 27-nanometer (Norwalk and Norwalk-like) agents are among the chief causes of sporadic and epidemic viral gastroenteritis. *Giardia lamblia* and other protozoa are also frequent causes of diarrhea. Any of these agents may be transmitted in hospitals via the hands of personnel who are infected.

If personnel develop an acute diarrheal illness accompanied by fever, cramps, or bloody stools, they are likely to be excreting potentially infective organisms in high titer in their feces. The specific cause of acute diarrhea, however, cannot be determined solely on the basis of clinical symptoms; thus, appropriate laboratory tests are important. Evaluation of personnel is usually limited to an initial culture for bacterial pathogens and stool examination for intestinal protozoa; repeat studies may be indicated if the results of the first tests are negative and the illness persists. Whenever appropriate, specific treatment for documented infection with enteric pathogens should be made available to infected personnel. Persons with acute symptoms of diarrheal illness should not provide direct patient care nor should they handle food or items that may go into the patient's mouth [204].

Carriage of Enteric Pathogens by Personnel

Carriage of enteric pathogens may persist after resolution of the acute illness. Once the person has clinically recovered and is having formed stools, however, there should be little hazard to patients, provided good hygienic practices are observed including meticulous hand-washing after toileting activities and prior to handling food or items that may go into the patient's mouth [123]. Existing data suggest that appropriate antibiotic therapy may eradicate fecal excretion of *Shigella* or *Campylobacter*. If persons take antibiotics, any follow-up cultures are best taken 48 hours after the last dose. Carriage of *Salmonella* by personnel, however, calls for special precautions, especially regarding contact with high-risk patients (i.e., newborns, the elderly, immunocompromised patients, and the severely ill) in whom the clinical sequelae of acute salmonellosis are often severe. Antibiotic therapy may prolong *Salmonella* excretion or lead to emergence of resistant strains and is not generally recommended [123]. Thus personnel with typhoidal or nontyphoidal *Salmonella* enteric infections should be excluded from the direct care of any patients until stool cultures are *Salmonella*-free on two consecutive specimens collected not less than 24 hours apart. However, personnel infected by enteric pathogens other than *Salmonella* can normally safely return to patient care duties after symptoms resolve.

Nevertheless, these persons need to be individually counseled, before they return to work, about the importance of meticulous hand-washing [123]. Generally, good personnel hygiene, particularly hand-washing before and after all patient contacts, will minimize the risk of acquiring or transmitting enteric pathogens.

Herpes Simplex Virus

Herpes simplex virus (HSV) can be transmitted among personnel and patients through direct contact with the vesicle fluid or from secretions containing the virus (e.g., saliva, vaginal secretions, and infected amniotic fluid) (see Chap. 38). Exposed areas of the skin, such as the fingers or hands, are the sites of infection that are of most concern in the health care setting.

Transmission of HSV from Patients to HCWs

HCWs may acquire an HSV infection of the fingers (herpetic whitlow or paronychia) from exposure to contaminated secretions. Such exposure is a distinct hazard for nurses, anesthesiologists, dentists, respiratory care personnel, and other HCWs who have direct contact with oral lesions, saliva, or respiratory secretions. Less frequently, HCWs may be exposed to HSV lesions on the skin, genitals, or mucous membranes of patients. To prevent such exposure, HCWs should (1) avoid direct contact with any lesion; (2) wear gloves or use "no-touch" technique with lesion fluid or patient secretions; and (3) always wash hands thoroughly after patient contact [45].

Transmission of HSV from HCWs to Patient

An HCW with active HSV infections should take extreme care to ensure that there is no possibility that patients could have contact with his or her lesion fluid. If lesions are localized and covered, and the infected HCW uses recommended infection control practices (e.g., good hand-washing), it is unlikely that the HCW poses any risk of transmission of HSV to the patient. The risk posed to patients by HCWs with uncovered orofacial lesions is unknown. However, that risk can be reduced by (1) covering the lesion to prevent hand contact; (2) careful hand-washing before all patient contact; and (3) restricting HCWs with active lesions from caring for high-risk patients.

Personnel with herpetic whitlow should not have direct contact with patients until the lesions have healed. Although some have suggested that HCWs should be allowed to perform direct patient care while wearing gloves, the efficacy of wearing gloves to prevent transmission is unknown and the practice is not currently recommended [8, 44, 98].

Hepatitis

Viral hepatitis has long been recognized as a nosocomial hazard (see Chap. 38). The agents that most commonly cause viral hepatitis are hepatitis A virus (HAV), hepatitis B virus, and hepatitis C virus (HCV). Infection with HCV is considered to be the major cause of parenterally transmitted non-A, non-B (NANB) hepatitis.

Hepatitis A Virus

Nosocomial HAV occurs infrequently and is usually associated with two unique circumstances: First, the source of infection is a patient hospitalized for other reasons whose hepatitis is not known or clinically apparent and, second, the patient is fecally incontinent or has diarrhea. These circumstances may occur in adult or pediatric patients.

HAV is primarily transmitted by ingestion of fecally contaminated food or materials. Transmission of HAV has not been reported to occur through accidental or other needle sticks (although it is theoretically possible) but has been reported to occur rarely through blood transfusion [157, 178, 184]. In addition, HAV infection has been associated with illicit drug use, both during needle-sharing and non-needle-sharing activities [49].

In general, fecal excretion of HAV is greatest during the late incubation period of disease and early in the prodromal phase of illness before the onset of symptoms or jaundice. Although the greatest infectivity is during the 2-week period immediately before the onset of symptoms, fecal shedding of HAV, especially in infants and children, may continue after onset of clinical symptoms [41, 73]. In low-birth-weight neonates, viral shedding has been documented by using the polymerase chain reaction, for as long as 4 months after onset [178]. Because anicteric infection is more common than icteric infection, especially in young children, and because the polymerase chain reaction test is not routinely available (to detect duration of fecal HAV shedding), it is often difficult to assess periods of infectivity. There is no evidence supporting the existence of a chronic HAV carrier state.

Personnel can help protect themselves and others from infection with HAV by always maintaining good personal hygiene, practicing thorough hand-washing at all times, and carefully adhering to published infection control recommendations [45]. Personnel who are suspected of being infected with HAV are advised not to take care of patients until 7 days after the onset of jaundice when viral shedding in most adults is complete [44].

Hepatitis B Virus

HBV infection is the major infectious occupational hazard of HCWs, with an estimated 8,000 HCWs becoming infected annually following occupational exposure to blood and serum-derived body fluids. Transmission occurs by parenteral or mucosal exposure to blood positive for hepatitis B surface antigen (HBsAg) from persons who are carriers or who have acute HBV infection.

The principal modes of HBV transmission in the health care setting are given here in order of decreasing efficiency:

1. *Overt parenteral transmission.* Direct percutaneous inoculation by needle or instrument contaminated with serum or plasma (e.g., accidental needle sticks, transfusion of contaminated blood or blood products, and acupuncture)
2. *Inapparent parenteral transmission*
   a. Percutaneous inoculation with infective serum or plasma without overt needle puncture (e.g., contamination of fresh

cutaneous scratches, abrasions, burns, or other lesions)

b. Contamination of mucosal surfaces with infective serum or plasma (e.g., accidental eye splash or other direct contact with mucous membranes of the eyes or mouth, such as hand to mouth or eye when contaminated with infective blood or serum)

c. Transfer of infective material to skin lesions or mucous membranes via inanimate environmental surfaces or contaminated medical devices

d. Contamination of mucosal surfaces with infective secretions other than serum or plasma (e.g., contact involving saliva or semen)

Within the hospital setting, certain work locations and occupational categories have been identified as showing increased risk for acquiring HBV infection [79, 121, 132, 137, 142, 149, 163, 193]. Generally, the highest risk of HBV infection is associated with locations and occupations in which contact with blood or sharps is frequent. Statistically, hospital personnel who are not directly exposed to blood are at no greater risk of HBV infection than the general population.

To prevent transmission of HBV, hospital personnel must be aware of the modes of transmission and utilize appropriate precautions (i.e., universal precautions) in handling blood and certain body fluids of all patients (see Chap. 11). Since droplets from the patient's mouth reach the face of the dentist during certain procedures, dentists should protect their eyes, nose, and mouth from such exposure by using masks and protective eyewear. They can reduce the likelihood of direct contact with infective material in the patient's mouth by routinely wearing gloves during dental procedures [59, 60, 66, 201].

Recommendations for HCWs with HBV Infection　Since the introduction of serologic testing for HBV infection in the early 1970s, reports have been published of 20 clusters in which more than 300 patients were infected with HBV in association with treatment by an HBV-infected HCW. Of these clusters, nine were linked to dentists or oral surgeons [5, 55, 93, 94, 103, 141, 174, 176, 187], and one cluster each was linked to a general practitioner [100, 101], an inhalation therapist [189], and a cardiopulmonary bypass pump technician [74]. None of these 12 HCWs routinely wore gloves, and several had skin lesions that may have facilitated HBV transmission. The clusters associated with the inhalation therapist and the cardiopulmonary bypass pump technician (and possibly some of the other 10 clusters) could have been prevented if current recommendations on universal precautions, including glove use, were in effect. Of the remaining eight clusters, transmission occurred despite glove use by the HCWs; five clusters were linked to obstetricians or gynecologists [21, 42, 70, 140, 207], and three to cardiovascular surgeons [86, 104, 120]. Recent reports indicate HBV transmission from surgeons to patients in 1989 and 1990 during colorectal and other abdominal surgery [120; Centers for Disease Control (CDC): unpublished data].

Seven HCWs linked to the clusters in the United States were allowed to perform invasive procedures following modification of invasive techniques (e.g., double gloving and restriction of certain high-risk procedures) [5, 42, 93, 103, 140, 176]. For 5 HCWs, no further transmission to patients was observed. For 2 HCWs, an obstetrician-gynecologist and an oral surgeon, HBV infection was transmitted to patients even after modification of techniques [94, 140].

A combination of risk factors for transmission of HBV was identified in the 20 published investigations. First, of the HCWs whose hepatitis B e antigen (HBeAg) status was determined (17 of 20), all were HBeAg-positive. The presence of HBeAg in serum is associated with higher levels of circulating virus and therefore greater infectivity of HBsAg-positive individuals [7]; the risk of HBV transmission to an HCW after a percutaneous exposure to HBeAg-positive blood is approximately 30 percent [184, 185]. Second, most of the procedures implicated in transmission were relatively invasive. Finally, in each reported occurrence of transmission, the potential existed for contamination of surgical wounds or traumatized tissue, either from a major break in standard infection control practices (such as not wearing gloves during invasive procedures) or from unintentional injury to the HCW during the procedures (such as needle sticks incurred while palpating needles blindly during suturing).

Most reported U.S. clusters occurred before heightened awareness of the risks of transmission of bloodborne pathogens in health care settings and emphasis on the use of universal precautions and HBV vaccine among HCWs. The infrequency of recent U.S. reports of HBV transmission from HCWs to patients may in part reflect the adoption of universal precautions (also see Chap. 11) and increased HBV vaccine use. However, the rarity of such reports does not preclude the occurrence of undetected or unreported small clusters or individual instances of transmission. Glove use does not prevent most injuries caused by sharp instruments and does not eliminate the potential for exposure of a patient to an HCW's blood and transmission of HBV [21, 22, 42, 74, 86, 104, 120, 140, 207].

The experience with HBV transmission from HCWs to patients indicates that when HCWs adhere to recommended infection control procedures, the risk of transmitting HBV from an HCW to a patient is small. However, the likelihood of exposure of the patient to an HCW's blood is greater for certain procedures as characterized below.* To minimize the risk of HIV or HBV transmission further, recommendations were published [58].

---

*Characteristics of procedures more likely to expose patients to HCWs' blood include digital palpation of a needle tip in a body cavity or the simultaneous presence of the HCW's fingers and a needle, sharp instrument, or other sharp object in a poorly visualized or highly confined anatomic site. Performance of such procedures presents a recognized risk of percutaneous injury to the HCW and, if such an injury occurs, the HCW's blood is likely to contact the patient's body cavity, subcutaneous tissues, or mucous membranes [58].

Hepatitis B (HB) Vaccine Inactivated hepatitis B (HB) vaccines became available in the United States in 1982. The first vaccine, prepared from plasma of HBV carriers, was 85 to 95 percent effective in inducing detectable antibody (anti-HBs) and protecting against HBV infections in adults and was recommended for all health care personnel with regular exposure to blood in the workplace [50, 63, 129]. In 1987, a vaccine produced by recombinant DNA technology in yeast became available. The recombinant vaccine is comparable to the plasma-derived vaccine in potency, efficacy, and safety, although postvaccination antibody titers average approximately half those achieved with the plasma vaccine. The recombinant vaccine was endorsed as an alternative vaccine for use in all risk groups [129, 214]. Both vaccines have been shown to be remarkably free of side effects. The most common side effect observed (5 to 20 percent of vaccinees) has been soreness at the injection site.

Vaccine-induced antibodies decline gradually over time, and approximately 50 percent of those who initially respond to vaccination will lose detectable antibodies over 9 years. However, studies in adults have demonstrated that, despite declining levels of antibody, protection against clinical (or detectable viremic) HBV infection persists. Booster doses are not currently recommended [129]. The possible need for booster doses after longer intervals will be assessed as additional information becomes available.

Development of HB vaccination programs for HCWs has progressed steadily since the HB vaccine became available. By 1985, sixty-five percent of hospitals had established HB vaccination programs, with most employers paying for the vaccination of high-risk personnel [6]. Despite these programs, actual vaccine coverage among high-risk health care professionals has been modest.

Among target groups, including physicians, nurses, and dental practitioners, reasons for not receiving the vaccine have been (1) concern regarding vaccine safety, including unknown low-frequency side effects or unwarranted fear of acquiring HIV infection; (2) need for more information about the vaccine; (3) vaccine cost; (4) possible effects on present or future pregnancies; and (5) not considering oneself to be at risk [6]. Better education of health care personnel about the safety of HB vaccines [50, 63, 214], disease transmission, complications, and indications for vaccination could improve immunization levels.

Hepatitis B prevention programs in the health care setting should include components for both preexposure and postexposure prophylaxis. All HCWs who may have occupational exposure to blood should receive HB vaccine, preferably during their period of professional training and prior to any possible occupational exposures [78, 129]. The possible need for postexposure prophylaxis should be evaluated following percutaneous, mucous membrane, or skin exposure to blood in the workplace. For detailed information regarding postexposure prophylaxis refer to the recommendations of the ACIP [129]. In general, following occupational percutaneous or permucosal exposure to blood that is known to contain or might contain HBsAg, the decision to provide prophylaxis must take into account several factors: (1) the HB vaccination and HB antibody status of the exposed person; (2) whether the source of blood is known or unknown; and (3) whether the HBsAg status of the source is known or unknown. Table 3-4 summarizes recommendations for HBV prophylaxis following occupational percutaneous, mucous membrane, or nonintact skin exposure to blood.

In 1987, in response to a petition by unions representing health care personnel, the Departments of Labor (Occupational Safety and Health Administration [OSHA]) and Health and Human Services issued a Joint Advisory Notice on protection against exposure to bloodborne pathogens in the workplace and began the process of rulemaking to regulate

Table 3-4. Recommendations for hepatitis B prophylaxis following precutaneous or permucosal exposures to hepatitis B virus

Exposed person	Treatment when source is found to be:		
	HBsAg-positive	*HBsAg-negative*	*Not tested or unknown*
Unvaccinated	HBIG × 1[a] and initiate HB vaccine[b]	Initiate HB vaccine[b]	Initiate HB vaccine[b]
Previously vaccinated Known responder	Test exposed for anti-HBs 1. If adequate,[c] no treatment 2. If inadequate, HB vaccine booster dose	No treatment	No treatment
Known nonresponder	HBIG × 2 or HBIG × 1 plus 1 dose HB vaccine	No treatment	If known high-risk source, may treat as if source were HBsAg-positive
Response unknown	Test exposed for anti-HBs (need rapid results) 1. If inadequate,[c] HBIG × 1 plus HB vaccine booster dose 2. If adequate, no treatment	No treatment	Test exposed for anti-HBs 1. If inadequate,[c] HB vaccine booster dose 2. If adequate, no treatment

HBsAg = hepatitis B surface antigen; HBIG = hepatitis B immune globulin; HB = hepatitis B.
[a] HBIG dose 0.06 ml/kg IM.
[b] HB vaccine dose, usual schedule: three doses at 0, 1, and 6 months. For age-specific doses and alternative schedules of currently available vaccines, see [129].
[c] Adequate anti-HBs is $\geq$ 10 sample ratio units (SRU) by radioimmunoassay or positive by enzyme immunoassay.

such exposures [77]. In May 1989, OSHA published a proposed rule in the *Federal Register:* Occupational Exposure to Bloodborne Pathogens; Proposed Rule and Notice of Hearing [78]. The final rule was published December 6, 1991, and mandates that HB vaccine be made available to all at-risk HCWs [78a]. These regulations are expected to accelerate and broaden the use of HB vaccine in HCWs.

Hepatitis C Virus

Infection with HCV is considered to be the major cause of parenterally transmitted NANB hepatitis. Parenterally transmitted NANB hepatitis accounts for 20 to 40 percent of acute viral hepatitis in the United States and has epidemiologic characteristics similar to those of hepatitis B. Multiple episodes of NANB hepatitis have been observed among the same individuals and may be due to different bloodborne agents. An average of 50 percent of patients who have acute parenterally transmitted NANB hepatitis infection later develop chronic hepatitis. Groups at high risk for acquiring this disease include transfusion recipients, parenteral drug users, and dialysis patients [129]. Occupations that entail frequent contact with blood, personal contact with others who have had hepatitis in the past, and contact with infected persons within households have also been documented in some studies as risk factors for acquiring this infection [129]. The role of person-to-person contact in disease transmission has not been well defined. Therefore, recommendations for management of HCV-infected HCWs are not currently available.

The Food and Drug Administration recently licensed two blood screening tests that detect the presence of antibody to HCV in serum or plasma. The tests are used in U.S. blood donation centers to screen, identify, and discard units of blood positive for anti-HCV.

HIV and AIDS
Background

The risk of HIV transmission to an HCW after percutaneous exposure to HIV-infected blood is considerably lower than the risk of

HBV transmission after percutaneous exposure to HBeAg-positive blood (0.3 percent versus approximately 30 percent) [89, 117, 146]. Thus the risk of transmission of HIV from an HCW to a patient during an invasive procedure is likely to be proportionately lower than the risk of HBV transmission from an HBeAg-positive HCW to a patient during the same procedure. As with HBV, the relative infectivity of HIV probably varies among individuals and over time for a single individual (see Chap. 39). Unlike HBV infection, however, there is currently no readily available laboratory test for increased HIV infectivity.

Investigation of a cluster of HIV infections among patients in the practice of one dentist with AIDS strongly suggested that HIV was transmitted to 5 of the approximately 850 patients evaluated through December 1991 [56, 65]. The investigation indicates that HIV transmission occurred during dental care, although the precise mechanisms of transmission have not been determined. In two studies, 75 and 62 patients, respectively, of a general surgeon and a surgical resident with AIDS were tested [24, 168]; all patients were negative at the time of testing. In a third study, evaluation of 143 patients treated by a dental student with HIV infection indicate that none is seropositive [71]. In another investigation, HIV antibody testing was offered to all patients who had a surgical procedure performed by a general surgeon within 7 years before a diagnosis of AIDS was made in the surgeon [153]; the date of the surgeon's HIV infection is unknown. Of 1,340 patients who were contacted, 616 (46 percent) were tested. One patient, a known intravenous drug user, was HIV-positive and may already have been infected at surgery. Excluding this patient, no transmissions were observed in 615 operations (upper limit of the 95 percent confidence interval = 0.5 percent).

The limited number of participants and the differences in procedures performed in these five investigations limit the ability to generalize from them and to define precisely the risk of HIV transmission to patients. A precise estimate of the risk of HIV transmission from infected HCWs to patients can be determined only after careful evaluation of substantially larger numbers of patients who have had invasive procedures performed on them by HIV-infected HCWs.

Blood Exposures Among HCWs and Patients During Surgical Procedures

Despite adherence to the principles of universal precautions, certain invasive surgical and dental procedures have been implicated in the transmission of HBV from infected HCWs to patients. Reported examples include certain oral, cardiothoracic, colorectal [CDC: unpublished data], and obstetric-gynecologic procedures [21, 22, 42, 74, 86, 94, 104, 120, 140, 207]. In a prospective study the CDC conducted in four hospitals, one or more percutaneous injuries occurred among surgical personnel during 96 (6.9 percent) of 1,382 operative procedures on the general surgery, gynecology, orthopedic, cardiac, and trauma services [199]. Percutaneous exposure of the patient to the HCW's blood may have occurred when the sharp object causing the injury recontacted the patient's open wound in 28 (32 percent) of the 88 observed injuries to surgeons (range among surgical specialties, 8 to 57 percent; range among hospitals, 24 to 42 percent).

Recommendations for Minimizing Transmission of HIV and HBV
Investigations of HIV and HBV transmission from HCWs to patients indicates that when HCWs adhere to recommended infection control procedures, the risk of transmitting HBV from an HCW to a patient is small, and the risk of transmitting HIV is likely to be smaller. To minimize the risk of HIV or HBV transmission from HCWs to patients, the CDC published "Recommendations for Preventing Transmission of Human Immunodeficiency Virus and Hepatitis B Virus to Patients During Exposure-Prone Invasive Procedures [58]. In that document, the CDC described certain invasive procedures (termed *exposure-prone*) during which there is a recognized risk for percutaneous injury to the HCW, and if such an injury were to occur, the HCW's blood would be likely to contact the patient's body cavity, subcutaneous tissues, and/or mucous membranes.

Identification of specific procedures was to be accomplished at a later date, based on input from professional organizations whose members performed invasive procedures. The document stated that HCWs who performed such procedures should know their HIV and HBV status and should be evaluated by an expert review panel. The CDC recommended that HCWs who were HIV or HBV (and also HBeAg) positive should not perform such procedures unless an expert review panel had advised them regarding the circumstances, if any, under which they could continue to perform such procedures. Such circumstances were to include notification of prospective patients of the HCW's infection status before they underwent exposure-prone invasive procedures.

Many professional organizations advised that determination of the potential for exposure of a patient to an HCW's blood must include consideration of the HCW's technique, skill, and medical status, in addition to the types of procedures performed. As of January 1992, the CDC was in the process of considering comments and the possible need for additional recommendations.

HCWs Whose Practices Are Modified Because of HIV or HBV Status

HCWs whose practices are modified or restricted because of their HIV or HBV infection status should, whenever possible, be provided opportunities to continue appropriate patient care activities. Career counseling and job retraining should be encouraged to promote the continued use of the HCW's talents, knowledge, and skills. HCWs whose practices are modified because of HBV infection should have their HBeAg status reevaluated periodically to determine whether there is a change due to resolution of infection or as a result of treatment [166].

Meningococcal Disease

Nosocomial transmission of *Neisseria meningitidis* either to hospital personnel taking care of patients with meningococcemia, meningococcal meningitis, or lower respiratory infections, or to laboratory personnel processing specimens containing *N. meningitidis* is uncommon (see also Chap. 32) [52, 53, 175]. In rare instances, transmission in these settings has occurred through intensive direct contact with respiratory secretions or cultures of *N. meningitidis* [52, 53, 175].

In the clinical setting, the most likely mode of spread from a person with respiratory or systemic infections is by large droplets from the respiratory tract. Thus, meningococcal lower respiratory infections may present a greater risk of transmission than meningococcemia or meningitis alone, especially if the patient has an active, productive cough [53, 175]. Airborne transmission and patient-to-patient spread via hands of personnel have been suggested but not well documented [69, 177]. Risk to personnel from casual contact with an infected patient (e.g., as usually occurs with housekeepers) appears to be negligible. To decrease the risk of infection in the clinical setting, personnel taking care of patients with known or suspected *N. meningitidis* infection should wear a mask when close contact with the patient is anticipated [88].

In the laboratory, workers may be exposed to *N. meningitidis* by inoculation, ingestion, and droplet or aerosol exposure of the mucous membranes. It has been recommended that for their protection, laboratory personnel who handle meningococci should wear gloves and gowns, decontaminate all infectious wastes and, when performing procedures that may aerosolize meningococci, use a class II biologic safety cabinet [52].

Prophylaxis After Unprotected Exposure

Antimicrobial prophylaxis can prevent *N. meningitidis* infections in personnel who have unprotected exposure to the organism. Prophylaxis is indicated for persons who, without using appropriate precautions, have intensive direct contact with patients with known or unrecognized meningococcal infection, or in whom cultures are positive for *N. meningitidis* [209].

When prophylaxis is deemed necessary, it is important to begin treatment immediately, before the results of antimicrobial susceptibility testing are available [2, 209]. The ACIP recommends that personnel with mucosal exposure to meningococci receive rifampicin (600 mg orally twice daily for 2 days) for chemoprophylaxis unless the causative organism has been found to be sulfonamide-sensitive [2]. However, rifampicin should not be given to pregnant personnel [2]. Ceftriaxone, recently found to be effective in eradicating pharyngeal carriage of *N. meningitidis*, may be considered in the management of exposed personnel who are pregnant or cannot take rifampicin for other reasons [182].

Carriage of N. meningitidis *by Personnel*

Carriage of *N. meningitidis* in the nasopharynx of healthy persons has been recognized for many years, but the prevalence is variable [26, 99]. Carriage may be transient, intermittent, or chronic. Surveillance of hospital personnel to determine carriage is useful only during special epidemiologic studies. In non-outbreak situations, asymptomatic carriers among personnel need not be identified, treated, or removed from patient care activities [88].

Staphylococcus aureus

Staphylococcal carriage or infection occurs frequently in humans. In nosocomial transmission, there are two sources: a person with a lesion or an asymptomatic carrier (see Chap. 37). Persons with skin lesions due to *Staphylococcus aureus* are most likely to disseminate these organisms. Direct contact is the major route of transmission. Even minor or entirely inapparent skin infections in personnel may represent a hazard to patients. One way to decrease the possibility of dissemination is to not allow patient care personnel to work until skin infection caused by this organism is resolved.

The anterior nares are among the most commonly colonized sites, but carriage of *S. aureus* may occur at other sites, such as any draining or crusted lesion, the nasopharynx and oropharynx, and the skin of the axilla, fingers, and perineum.

Methicillin-susceptible (but penicillin-resistant) *S. aureus* (MSSA) used to account for most staphylococcal infections. However, in recent years, methicillin-resistant *S. aureus*

(MRSA) has become an important nosocomial pathogen. The epidemiology of MRSA does not appear to differ much from that of MSSA except that outbreaks due to MRSA tend to occur more frequently in intensive care and burn units.

Methicillin-Susceptible S. aureus

Culture surveys of personnel can detect carriers of MSSA but do not indicate whether carriers are likely to disseminate the organism. Thus such data are difficult to interpret. A more reasonable approach is to emphasize effective surveillance that permits prompt recognition of MSSA infections in both personnel and patients. If personnel are linked epidemiologically to an increased or unusual cluster of infections, these persons should be cultured and, if positive, removed from patient contact until carriage is eradicated (see Chap. 37).

Methicillin-Resistant S. aureus

MRSA infection and carriage have progressively increased worldwide in the last two decades (see Chap. 37). Although generally the epidemiology of MRSA is similar to that of MSSA [36, 43, 85], nosocomial MRSA infections tend to affect more debilitated patients such as the elderly, the immunocompromised, and those with severe underlying conditions [36, 37, 43]. Consequently, MRSA is more commonly found in certain areas of the hospital—namely, intensive care, burn, and long-term care units [25, 36, 38, 75, 147, 198]. The most important sources in hospitals are infected or colonized patients [35, 36, 143, 152, 186, 206]. Hospital personnel who are infected or colonized with MRSA can also serve as reservoirs and disseminators of MRSA [25, 72, 171] and have been commonly identified as a link for transmission between MRSA-infected or colonized patients and susceptible patients [25, 36, 84, 165]. The main mode of transmission of MRSA is via HCWs' hands, which may become contaminated by contact with colonized or infected sites of patients or personnel themselves [35, 151, 158]. In burn units or in patients with pneumonia or draining skin lesions, large-droplet transmission of

MRSA may occur more frequently [84]. Although the exact role of the environment needs to be further elucidated, heavy contamination of fomites facilitates contact transmission by hand [180].

Because infected skin lesions are associated with increased numbers of microorganisms, one way to decrease the possibility of MRSA dissemination from personnel is not to allow patient care personnel to work until skin infection caused by MRSA is resolved.

As is true in MSSA carriage, culture surveys of personnel can detect MRSA carriers but do not indicate whether carriers are likely to disseminate their microorganisms [27, 158]. However, if personnel are linked to an increased number or unusual cluster of cases of MRSA disease or colonization, these persons should be cultured and, if positive, removed from patient contact until their carriage of MRSA is eradicated. Unless the objective of the hospital is to treat all personnel who are MRSA carriers, whether or not they disseminate MRSA [27], it is prudent to culture only personnel who are implicated in MRSA transmission based on epidemiologic data. If all personnel are cultured routinely to identify MRSA carriers, it is likely that personnel colonized by MRSA but who are not linked to transmission or who may not be disseminators will be identified, subjected to treatment, or removed from patient care unnecessarily. Because of these serious consequences to HCWs, hospitals should weigh the advantages and consequences of routinely culturing personnel before doing so (see Chap. 37).

Streptococcus Groups A and B

Group A and group B streptococci (*Streptococcus pyogenes* and *S. agalactiae*) are important nosocomial pathogens (see Chap. 37).

Group A Streptococci

Patient-to-Personnel Transmission Pharyngeal and skin infections are the most common group A streptococcal infections. Recently, however, clusters of invasive group A streptococcal infections, including the toxic shock–like syndrome (TSLS), have been recognized [183]. Secondary spread and illness (including TSLS, cellulitis, lymphangitis, and pharyngitis) in hospital personnel have occurred following direct contact by personnel with secretions from infected patients [183]. To prevent patient-to-personnel transmission of group A streptococci, personnel should wash their hands thoroughly after each patient contact, wear gloves when contact with potentially contaminated secretions is anticipated, and wear gowns when soiling with infective material is likely [88].

Personnel-to-Patient Transmission Sporadic outbreaks of surgical wound infections or postpartum infections caused by group A streptococci have been associated with carriers among operating room or delivery room personnel [32, 148, 170, 181, 205]. The main reservoirs of group A streptococci in implicated carriers are the pharynx, the skin, the rectum, and the female genital tract. Direct contact and airborne spread are the major modes of transmission of this organism in these settings [32, 148, 170, 181, 205].

Since surgical wound infections or postpartum infections due to group A streptococci occur infrequently, any isolate from cases should be saved for possible serotyping should an outbreak ensue. The occurrence of 2 or more cases should prompt an epidemiologic investigation and a search for a carrier-disseminator. Isolates obtained from personnel and patients should be serotyped to determine strain relatedness. Ideally, only personnel who are epidemiologically linked to cases should have cultures of skin lesions, pharynx, rectum, and vagina and, if positive, should be removed from patient contact until treatment is completed and follow-up cultures are negative. However, in situations in which epidemiologic studies could not establish any links between cases and personnel, the identification of a carrier-disseminator may be facilitated by culturing all personnel associated with cases and by culturing the operating room environment [148]. Routine screening of personnel for group A streptococcal carriage in the absence of cases of nosocomial infection is not recommended [88].

Because experience is limited regarding the treatment and follow-up of personnel-carriers implicated in outbreaks of surgical wound infections due to group A streptococci, and because carriage of the organism by an HCW may be recurrent over long periods of time [32, 205], treatment and follow-up of these personnel-carriers should be individualized.

Group B Streptococci

Personnel who are carriers of group B streptococci may play a role in its nosocomial transmission. However, the epidemiology of early-onset group B streptococcal infections in neonates suggests that maternal colonization with group B streptococci, followed by the infant's acquisition during passage through the birth canal, accounts for most infections. In late-onset neonatal infections, spread of the organism occurs from colonized to uncolonized infants via hands of personnel or by direct contact from colonized hospital personnel. In both types of infections, careful hand-washing will minimize the risk of spread from colonized infants or personnel to uncolonized infants.

Parvovirus

Human parvovirus B19 is the causative agent of erythema infectiosum (EI) or fifth disease which manifests as a rash illness in children or acute arthropathy in adults [18, 19, 30, 167, 172, 208]. Although most B19 infections are mild and self-limited, certain groups of persons are at risk of developing more serious manifestations or complications of B19 infection. Among them are patients with chronic hemolytic anemia, who may develop a pure red-cell aplasia, also known as *transient aplastic crisis* (TAC) [135, 164]; immunodeficient patients, who may develop chronic anemia [96, 133, 134]; and pregnant women, who may have spontaneous abortions and stillbirths [16, 212].

Transmission of B19 has been demonstrated after close-contact exposure (e.g., to susceptible household contacts of patients with EI or TAC [67, 167] or, rarely, to health care personnel caring for patients with B19-associated sickle cell aplastic crisis [30]. It is hypothesized that B19 may be transmitted via one or more of the following means: direct person-to-person contact, fomites, large-particle droplets, or small-particle droplets [19, 30, 61, 67]. Therefore, the following infection control precautions are recommended to prevent transmission of B19 in the health care setting (see Chap. 11): Hands should be washed after contact with a patient with confirmed or suspected B19 infection or with articles potentially contaminated with the patient's secretions; patients with TAC or chronic B19 infection should be admitted to private rooms; masks should be worn by persons in close contact with infected patients; gloves should be worn by persons likely to touch infective material such as respiratory secretions; and gowns should be worn when soiling is anticipated [45, 61].

Transmission of Parvovirus B19 from Patients to Personnel

Isolation precautions are not indicated for most patients with EI because they are already past their period of infectiousness at the time of clinical illness [17, 61, 167]. However, patients in aplastic crisis due to B19 or patients with chronic B19 infection may transmit the virus to susceptible health care personnel or other patients; therefore, patients with chronic hemolytic anemia who are admitted to the hospital with febrile illness and TAC, or patients known or suspected to be chronically infected with B19 should, on admission and until the condition resolves, be placed on the isolation precautions stated above [30].

Pregnant Personnel

Pregnant personnel are at no greater risk of acquiring B19 infection than are nonpregnant personnel; however, if a pregnant woman acquires B19 infection during the first half of pregnancy, the risk of fetal death (spontaneous abortion and stillbirth) is increased [61]. Because of this increased risk, and until a B19 vaccine becomes available,

personnel who are pregnant or who might be pregnant should know the potential risks to the fetus that are associated with B19 infection and the dangers of working with high-risk patient groups, and should practice appropriate infection control precautions when performing their duties [45, 61].

Scabies

Scabies is a disease caused by infestation with the mite *Sarcoptes scabiei*. It is transmitted in hospitals primarily through skin-to-skin contact with an infested person, even when high levels of personal hygiene are maintained [31, 34, 92, 116]. Transmission to personnel has occurred during direct hands-on contact with infested patients. Transmission is especially likely when personnel are exposed to patients with atypical forms of infestation in which large mite populations are present (Norwegian or crusted scabies) or to patients in whom scabies is not suspected [34, 92, 116, 138, 139, 188]. Transmission via infested bedding, clothes, or other fomites probably occurs infrequently and is directly related to the number of mites infesting the source individual(s) [40, 83, 116, 188, 196].

Treatment is recommended for persons with active infestation and their close contacts. In most cases, a single course of therapy (proper skin application of agents that destroy both eggs and the active forms of the mites) is curative and appears to eliminate the risk of transmission immediately after the first treatment [83, 92, 159, 160, 194, 195]. However, more aggressive treatment may be necessary in some cases of Norwegian scabies [124, 139, 173, 188].

Personnel can decrease their risk of acquiring scabies by using appropriate precautions when taking care of infested patients. Such precautions include adequate hand-washing and gloving and gowning when close contact with an infested patient is anticipated. Infested patients with poor hygiene should be admitted to a private room, and the patients' linen and clothing should be handled by gloved personnel and washed thoroughly (in hot cycle) before reuse [139, 173]. Personnel should also have a high index of suspicion for any rash of unknown diagnosis on an immunocompromised or severely ill patient and should practice infection control precautions until the diagnosis of the rash is confirmed (by skin scrapings) not to be scabies [124]. If personnel are infested with the mite, nosocomial transmission can be prevented by exclusion from work until adequate treatment is completed [44].

Tuberculosis

Mycobacterium tuberculosis (TB) continues to pose a serious problem for HCWs. In the hospital, exposure is most likely to occur when a patient has unsuspected pulmonary or laryngeal TB, has bacilli-laden sputum or respiratory secretions, and is coughing or sneezing into air that remains in general circulation (also see Chap. 29). The best ways to protect others from a patient with TB are to maintain a high index of suspicion for TB, to institute appropriate isolation precautions with all known or suspected TB patients, and to institute appropriate chemotherapy promptly [14, 45, 54]. Recent episodes of nosocomial transmission of multidrug-resistant TB to HIV-infected patients and HCWs further emphasize the importance of complying with current guidelines [46, 54].

The most widely accepted approach to the management of infected HCWs or those with active TB disease follows the recommendations for surveillance and control in the general population issued jointly by the American Thoracic Society, the American Lung Association, and the CDC [11], and those of the CDC *Guidelines for Prevention of TB Transmission in Hospitals* [47], CDC *Guideline for Infection Control in Hospital Personnel* [44], and the *Guidelines for Preventing Transmission of Tuberculosis in Health-Care Settings, with Special Focus on HIV-Related Issues* [46].

Screening Programs

Health care facilities providing care to patients at risk for TB should maintain active surveillance for TB among patients and health care facility personnel and for skin-test conversions among HCWs. When TB is suspected or diagnosed, public health authorities should be notified so that appropriate contact investigation can be performed. Data on the occurrence of TB and skin-test conversions among patients and HCWs should be collected and analyzed to estimate the risk of TB transmission in the facility and to evaluate the effectiveness of infection control and screening practices [46].

At the time of employment, all health care facility personnel, including those with a history of bacille Calmette-Guérin (BCG) vaccination, should receive a Mantoux tuberculin skin test (purified protein derivative of tuberculin [PPD]) unless a previously positive reaction can be documented or completion of adequate preventive therapy or adequate therapy for active disease can be documented. Initial and follow-up tuberculin skin tests should be administered and interpreted according to current guidelines [10, 12, 15, 46].

HCWs with a documented history of a positive tuberculin test, or adequate treatment for disease or preventive therapy for infection, should be exempt from further screening unless they develop symptoms suggestive of TB. Periodic retesting of PPD-negative HCWs should be conducted to identify persons whose skin tests convert to positive [46]. In general, the frequency of repeat testing should be based on the individual's risk of developing new infection. HCWs who may be frequently exposed to patients with tuberculosis or who are involved with potentially high-risk procedures (e.g., bronchoscopy, sputum induction, or aerosol treatments given to patients who may have tuberculosis) should be retested at least every 6 months. HCWs in other areas should be retested annually. Data on skin-test conversions should be periodically reviewed so that the risk of acquiring new infection may be estimated for each area of the facility. On the basis of this analysis, the frequency of retesting may be altered [46].

Persons with tuberculous infection can be identified by a significant reaction to a Mantoux method skin test, usually defined as 10 mm or more of induration following administration of 5 tuberculin units (TU) of PPD standard. The Mantoux technique (intracutaneous injection of 0.1 ml PPD-tuberculin containing 5 TU) is the preferred method for screening persons for TB infection [46] because it is the most accurate test available. A two-step procedure requiring administration of two separate tests at least 1 week apart can be used in persons who may have been infected in the distant past and may not respond to the initial test although infected [62]. The first test "boosts" their sensitivity to the PPD and, when the second test is given, they should react if infected [197].

Recommendations for Management of Infected HCWs

HCWs with positive tuberculin skin tests or with skin-test conversions on repeat testing or after exposure should be clinically evaluated for active TB [13]. Persons with symptoms suggestive of TB should be evaluated regardless of skin-test results. If TB is diagnosed, appropriate therapy should be instituted according to published guidelines [14]. Personnel diagnosed with active TB should be offered counseling and HIV-antibody testing [64].

HCWs who have positive tuberculin skin tests or skin-test conversions but who do not have clinical TB should be evaluated for preventive therapy according to published guidelines [14, 62]. Personnel with positive skin tests should be evaluated for risk of HIV infection. If HIV infection is considered a possibility, counseling and HIV-antibody testing should be strongly encouraged [64].

All persons with a history of TB or positive tuberculin tests are at risk for developing TB in the future. These persons should be reminded periodically that they should promptly report any pulmonary symptoms. If symptoms of TB should develop, the person should be evaluated immediately [46].

Routine chest films are not recommended for asymptomatic, tuberculin-negative HCWs. After the initial chest radiograph is taken,

personnel with positive skin-test reactions do not need repeat chest radiographs unless symptoms develop that may be due to TB [29]. Chest radiographs cannot take the place of tuberculin skin tests, as they will not identify persons who are infected but who do not have radiographic evidence of current or past disease.

HCWs with current pulmonary or laryngeal tuberculosis pose a risk to patients and other personnel while they are infectious; therefore, stringent work restrictions for these persons are necessary. They should be excluded from work until adequate treatment is instituted, cough is resolved, and sputum is free of bacilli on three consecutive smears. HCWs with current TB at sites other than the lung or larynx usually do not need to be excluded from work if concurrent pulmonary TB has been ruled out. Personnel who discontinue treatment before the recommended course of therapy has been completed should not be allowed to work until treatment is resumed and they have negative sputum smears on 3 consecutive days.

HCWs who are otherwise healthy and receiving preventive treatment for tuberculous infection should be allowed to continue usual work activities.

HCWs who cannot take or do not accept or complete a full course of preventive therapy should have their work situations evaluated to determine whether reassignment is indicated. Work restrictions may be necessary for otherwise healthy persons who do not accept or complete preventive therapy. These persons should be counseled about the risk of contracting disease and should be instructed to seek evaluation promptly if symptoms develop that may be due to TB, especially if they have contact with high-risk patients (i.e., patients at high risk for severe consequences if they became infected).

Consultation on TB surveillance, screening, and other methods to reduce TB transmission should be available from state health department TB control programs. Facilities are encouraged to use the services of health departments in planning and implementing their surveillance and screening programs.

Varicella-Zoster Virus

Varicella-zoster virus (VZV), a member of the herpesvirus group, is the etiologic agent of varicella (chickenpox) and herpes zoster (shingles). The virus is highly communicable, leading to high attack rates of exanthematous chickenpox among children and the small proportion of adults who are susceptible. Nosocomial transmission of VZV infection among personnel and patients is well recognized (see Chap. 38). Although varicella is usually a benign disease of childhood, it can cause severe illness in patients with impaired immunity. Appropriate isolation precautions for hospitalized patients with known or suspected chickenpox or shingles can reduce the risk of transmission to HCWs or other persons [45]. Only HCWs who have had varicella or those with serologic evidence of immunity should care for patients with infective varicella or herpes zoster. Individuals who may have or may be incubating VZV infection should not enter a hospital unnecessarily.

Varicella is transmitted primarily by inhalation of small-particle aerosols (droplet nuclei) and also by direct contact with respiratory droplets or vesicle fluid. The virus is less likely to be spread by inanimate objects because it is extremely labile in the environment. The incubation period for varicella in the normal host ranges from 10 to 21 days.

Even though personnel who are susceptible to varicella may be few, it is useful to identify such persons at the time of the placement evaluation. Most persons with a clearly positive history of previous varicella are probably immune. Even with negative or unknown histories, most HCWs are immune, but a few may remain susceptible [179]. When available, serologic screening may be used to define susceptibility more precisely. In institutions where patients with varicella are frequently encountered or where there are many high-risk patients, it may be useful to screen those personnel who have a negative or equivocal history of varicella for the presence of serum antibodies to VZV to document susceptibility

or immunity. This knowledge will help in appropriately assigning personnel who are immune to areas where VZV infection may be present, avoiding work restrictions and disruption of patient services if exposure occurs, and reducing the likelihood of nosocomial transmission [115]. Sensitive screening tests, such as the fluorescent antibody to membrane antigen (FAMA), immune adherence hemagglutination (IAH), enzyme-linked immunosorbent assay (ELISA), or varicella skin tests, currently exist but may not be readily available. The complement fixation test is not considered to be reliable for screening purposes because of the false-negative results often obtained by this method.

Shingles results from reactivation of latent VZV acquired during the primary episode of chickenpox. There is little evidence that shingles can be contracted directly from exposure to persons with varicella or zoster. However, VZV (leading to chickenpox in a susceptible person) can be acquired through direct contact with a person with shingles.

If susceptible HCWs are exposed to persons with varicella or herpes zoster, these personnel should be considered potentially infective during the incubation period and should be excluded from work beginning on the tenth day after exposure and remain away from work for the maximum incubation period of varicella (21 days). Personnel who have varicella should be excluded from work until all lesions have dried and crusted [44, 169, 211].

Currently, the only postexposure prophylaxis against VZV infection is varicella-zoster immune globulin (VZIG). VZIG's major effect is to modify infection and prevent serious complications; it does not necessarily prevent infection. Thus susceptible HCWs who have been exposed and receive VZIG still need to be considered potentially incubating (and infectious) and should be reassigned or furloughed during the incubation period. Because VZIG prolongs the VZV incubation interval, if an HCW receives VZIG this period must be extended to 28 days after exposure.

In addition, because of the possibility of transmission to and development of severe illness in high-risk patients, it is advisable to exclude personnel with herpes zoster from taking care of high-risk patients until all lesions are crusted. HCWs with localized zoster may not pose a risk to susceptible patients if the lesions can be covered and there is no chance for exposure of the patient to the HCW's vesicle fluid [44].

A vaccine to prevent VZV infection is not yet currently available for general use. Clinical trials are being conducted [20, 39, 90].

Respiratory Viral Infections

The impact of nosocomial respiratory viral infections has been increasingly recognized in recent years [97, 105, 203] (see Chap. 38). The three chief mechanisms of transmission of respiratory viruses are (1) small-particle aerosols, which can travel over distances greater than 3 ft from the source and thus are truly airborne; (2) large particles (droplets), which require close (within 3 ft) contact between source and recipient; and (3) self-inoculation of viruses after direct (usually hand) contact with infective materials [97, 102, 105, 106, 107, 109, 110, 119, 203]. Different respiratory viruses may vary in the way they are transmitted. The following discussion will focus on two viruses that have been well studied: *respiratory syncytial virus* (RSV), which typifies respiratory viruses that are mainly transmitted by close contact, and *influenza virus*, which spreads mainly by the airborne route.

RSV Infection

RSV is the most important cause of lower respiratory tract disease in infants and young children [97, 105, 203] (see Chap. 38). The disease usually occurs in outbreaks during winter. Infants with congenital diseases of the heart or lung, prematurity, or immunosuppression are at particular risk of severe or fatal RSV infection [68, 112, 113, 118, 144]. RSV infection in adults is usually mild [114, 145, 154]; however, hospital personnel are not spared from illness and usually play a major role in transmitting the virus during nosocomial outbreaks [97, 106, 111].

RSV enters a susceptible host via the conjunctiva or nasal mucosa [107, 110]. The virus appears to be transmitted mainly by hand inoculation of virus onto one's own eye or nose, after the hand has touched RSV-laden secretions or fomites, or by large-droplet deposition as occurs during close contact with an infected individual who sneezes, coughs, or talks [107, 109].

Transmission from Patients to Personnel Hospital personnel acquire RSV infection mainly by self-inoculation with hands that have been contaminated with the virus from infected patients [107]. Direct large-droplet deposition onto the worker's conjunctiva or nasal mucosa during close contact with infected patients may also play a role but probably occurs less frequently [107]. Therefore, measures that deter self-inoculation of the virus by hand, combined with barrier precautions against large-droplet inoculation of the eye and nose, should adequately prevent RSV transmission from patients to personnel. In theory, meticulous hand-washing by staff after each patient contact and after touching potentially contaminated articles should decrease RSV transmission. However, lapses in routine hand-washing practices are common [1], and hand-to-eye or hand-to-nose contact by oneself occurs frequently [119]. Thus additional use of eye-nose barriers (e.g., eye-nose goggles) was found beneficial in decreasing the incidence of RSV infection in personnel at one institution [87]. In contrast, masks, which cover the nose but leave the conjunctivae accessible to viral inoculation by touch or droplet deposition, have not been found to be effective in preventing nosocomial RSV transmission [108, 156].

Transmission from Personnel to Patients RSV-infected personnel may directly transmit RSV to patients during close contact with the patients. Therefore, ideally, personnel with active RSV infection should not have direct contact with infants.

Hospital personnel also may transfer the virus passively by hand, from contaminated fomites or infected patients to other patients [107, 109]. As in patient-to-personnel transmission, careful hand-washing by staff between patient contacts and after contact with RSV-contaminated fomites should significantly decrease transmission of RSV between patients via hands of personnel. Gowns may further decrease the potential for indirect RSV transmission via hands of personnel by decreasing the likelihood of fomite soiling with infectious secretions that may contaminate the hands [88]. Gloves protect the hands of personnel from viral contamination but should be changed between patient contacts to be effective [88, 136]. (Gloves may also discourage the wearer from touching his or her eyes or nose with the hands, thus preventing personnel self-inoculation of RSV infection.)

Recommendations to Prevent Transmission Between Patients and Personnel

1. Hands should be washed after each patient contact and after touching potentially contaminated articles, whether or not gloves are worn.
2. Gloves should be worn when contact with mucous membranes or potentially contaminated secretions or articles is anticipated. Gloves should be changed between patient contacts and after touching infective material.
3. Gowns should be worn when soiling with respiratory secretions is likely.
4. As much as is practicable, personnel who are known to be infected with RSV or who have symptoms of respiratory tract infection during RSV epidemics should not have direct contact with infants. If such personnel must care for infants, they should meticulously follow the preceding recommendations and wear masks.
5. During RSV epidemics, personnel may wear eye-nose goggles to help prevent their acquisition of the virus and its subsequent transmission to susceptible patients [87].

Other infection control measures (e.g., cohorting patients and staff, limiting visitors, using rapid screening tests for RSV) are recommended to prevent patient-to-patient transmission of RSV (see Chap. 11).

Influenza

Influenza is associated with significant morbidity and mortality in the elderly, patients with chronic underlying disease, and immunocompromised patients [28, 91, 125]. Unlike RSV, influenza is spread mainly by small-particle aerosol (i.e., airborne transmission) [81]. Consequently, nosocomial outbreaks of influenza can be explosive once susceptible persons in an institution are exposed to an infected individual [150, 161]. Prevention of nosocomial outbreaks of influenza necessitates prospective immunization of both susceptible personnel and high-risk patients before the influenza season each year [128]. Ideally, efforts to vaccinate high-risk individuals should be directed not only at hospital inpatients and long-term care facilities, but also at high-risk individuals in the community (who may introduce the virus in the hospital if they are admitted with influenza infection) [23, 128].

Once an outbreak occurs within a hospital or long-term care setting, the most effective control measure (against influenza A) is chemoprophylaxis with amantadine [23, 122, 128, 150, 161, 162]. Other measures have been advocated, but their exact roles in controlling influenza outbreaks have not been fully elucidated. These measures include early identification, isolation, or cohorting of infected patients, preferably in rooms with negative air pressure; cohorting of staff; strict hand-washing; gowning when soiling with respiratory secretions is likely; limiting visitors; and avoiding elective admissions and surgery during an influenza outbreak [33, 97, 161, 202] (see Chap. 11).

References

1. Abert, R.K., and Condie, F. Hand-washing patterns in medical intensive-care units. *N. Engl. J. Med.* 304:1465, 1981.
2. Advisory Committee on Immunization Practices, Centers for Disease Control. Meningococcal vaccines. *M.M.W.R.* 34:255, 1985.
3. Ahlfors, K., Ivarsson, S.-A., Johnsson, T., and Renmarker, K. Risk of cytomegalovirus

infection in nurses and congenital infection in their offspring. *Acta Paediatr. Scand.* 70:819, 1981.

4. Ahlfors, K., Ivarsson, S.-A., Johnsson, T., and Svanberg, L. Primary and secondary maternal cytomegalovirus infections and their relation to congenital infection. *Acta Paediatr. Scand.* 71:109, 1082.

5. Ahtone, J., and Goodman, R.A. Hepatitis B and dental personnel. Transmission to patients and prevention issues. *J. Am. Dent. Assoc.* 106:219, 1983.

6. Alexander, P.G., et al. Hepatitis B vaccination programs for health care personnel in U.S. hospitals. *Public Health Rep.* 105:610, 1990.

7. Alter, H.J., et al. Type B hepatitis: The infectivity of blood positive for e antigen and DNA polymerase after accidental needlestick exposure. *N. Eng. J. Med.* 295:909, 1976.

8. American Academy of Pediatrics Committee on Fetus and Newborn. Perinatal herpes simplex viral infections. *Pediatrics* 66:147, 1980.

9. American College of Physicians Task Force on Adult Immunization and Infectious Diseases Society of America: *Guide for Adult Immunization* (2nd ed.). Philadelphia: American College of Physicians, 1990.

10. American Thoracic Society, Ad Hoc Committee of the Scientific Assembly on Tuberculosis. Screening for pulmonary tuberculosis in institutions. *Am. Rev. Respir. Dis.* 115:901, 1977.

11. American Thoracic Society, American Lung Association, and Centers for Disease Control. Preventive therapy of tuberculous infection. *Am. Rev. Respir. Dis.* 110:371, 1974.

12. American Thoracic Society, Centers for Disease Control. Control of tuberculosis. *Am. Rev. Respir. Dis.* 128:336, 1983.

13. American Thoracic Society, Centers for Disease Control. Diagnostic standards and classification of tuberculosis. *Am. Rev. Respir. Dis.* 142:725, 1990.

14. American Thoracic Society, Centers for Disease Control. Treatment of tuberculosis infection in adults and children. *Am. Rev. Respir. Dis.* 134:355, 1986.

15. American Thoracic Society Executive Committee. The tuberculin skin test. *Am. Rev. Respir. Dis.* 124:356, 1981.

16. Anand, A., et al. Human parvovirus infection in pregnancy and hydrops fetalis. *N. Engl. J. Med.* 316:183, 1987.

17. Anderson, M.J., et al. Experimental parvoviral infection in humans. *J. Infect. Dis.* 152:257, 1985.

18. Anderson. M.J., et al. Human parvovirus, the cause of erythema infectiosum (fifth disease) [lett.] ? *Lancet* 1:1378, 1983.

19. Anderson, M.J. et al. An outbreak of erythema infectiosum associated with human parvovirus infection. *J. Hyg.* (Lond.) 93:85, 1984.

20. Andre, F.E., Heath, R.B., and Malpas, J.S. (Eds.). Active immunization against varicella. *Postgrad. Med. J.* 61(Suppl.): 7, 1985.

21. Anonymous. Acute hepatitis B following gynaecological surgery. *J. Hosp. Infect.* 9:34, 1987.

22. Anonymous. Acute hepatitis B associated with gynaecological surgery. *Lancet* 1:1, 1980.

23. Arden, N.H., et al. The roles of vaccination and amantadine prophylaxis in controlling an outbreak of influenza A (H3N2) in a nursing home. *Arch. Intern. Med.* 148:865, 1988.

24. Armstrong, F., Miner, J., and Wolfe, W. Investigation of a health care worker with symptomatic human immunodeficiency virus infection: an epidemiologic approach. *Milit. Med.* 152:414, 1987.

25. Arnow, P.M., et al. Control of methicillin-resistant *Staphylococcus aureus* in a burn unit: Role of nurse staff. *J. Trauma* 22:954, 1982.

26. Aycock, W.L., and Mueller, J.H. Meningococcus carrier rates and meningitis incidence. *Bacteriol. Rev.* 14:115, 1950.

27. Bacon, A.E., Jorgensen, K.A., Wilson, K.H., and Kauffman, C.A. Emergence of nosocomial methicillin-resistant *Staphylococcus aureus* and therapy of colonized personnel during a hospital-wide outbreak. *Infect. Control* 8:145, 1987.

28. Barker, W.H., and Mullooly, J.P. Impact of epidemic type A influenza in a defined adult population. *Am. J. Epidemiol.* 112:798, population. *Am. J. Epidemiol.* 112:798, 1980.

29. Barrett-Connor, E. The periodic chest roentgenogram for the control of tuberculosis in health care personnel. *Am. Rev. Respir. Dis.* 122:153, 1980.

30. Bell, L.M. et al. Human parvovirus B19 infection among hospital staff members after contact with infected patients. *N. Engl. J. Med.* 321:485, 1989.

31. Belle, E.A., et al. Hospital epidemic of scabies: Diagnosis and control. *Can. J. Public Health* 70:133, 1979.

32. Berkelman, R.L., et al. Streptococcal wound infections caused by a vaginal carrier. *J.A.M.A.* 247:2680, 1982.

33. Berlinberg, C.D., Weingarten, S.R., Bolton, L.B., and Waterman, S.H. Occupational exposure to influenza—introduction of an index case to a hospital. *Infect. Control Hosp. Epidemiol.* 10:70, 1989.

34. Bernstein, B., and Mihan, R. Hospital epidemic of scabies. *J. Pediatr.* 83:1086, 1973.

35. Bitar, C.M., et al. Outbreak due to methicillin-resistant *Staphylococcus aureus:* Epidemiology and eradication of the resistant strain from the hospital. *Infect. Control* 8:13, 1987.

36. Boyce, J.M. Methicillin-resistant *Staphylococcus aureus:* Detection, epidemiology and control measures. *Infect. Dis. Clin. North Am.* 3: 901, 1989.

37. Boyce, J.M., Landry, M., Deetz, T.R., and DuPont, H.L. Epidemiologic studies of an outbreak of nosocomial methicillin-resistant *Staphylococcus aureus* infections. *Infect. Control* 2:110, 1981.

38. Boyce, J.M., White, R.L., Causey, W.A., and Lockwood, W.R. Burn units as a source of methicillin-resistant *Staphylococcus aureus* infections. *J.A.M.A.* 249:2803, 1983.

39. Brunell, P.A. (Ed.). Current status of varicella vaccine. *Pediatrics* 78(Suppl.): 721, 1986.

40. Burkhard, C.G. Scabies: An epidemiologic reassessment. *Ann. Intern. Med.* 98:498, 1983.

41. Carl, M., et al. Excretion of hepatitis A virus in the stools of hospitalized patients. *J. Med. Virol.* 9:125, 1982.

42. Carl, M., Francis, D.P., Blakey, D.L., and Maynard, J.E. Interruption of hepatitis B transmission by modification of a gynecologist's surgical technique. *Lancet* 1:731, 1982.

43. Casewell, M.W., and Hill, R.L.R. The carrier state: Methicillin resistant *Staphylococcus aureus. J. Antimicrob. Chemother.* 18(Suppl. A): 1, 1986.

44. Centers for Disease Control. Williams, W.W. CDC guideline for infection control in hospital personnel. *Infect. Control* 4 (Suppl): 326, 1983.

45. Centers for Disease Control. Garner, J.S., and Simmons, B.P. CDC guideline for isolation precautions in hospitals. *Infect. Control* 4 (Suppl): 245, 1983.

46. Centers for Disease Control. Guidelines for preventing the transmission of tuberculosis in health-care settings, with special focus on HIV-related issues. *M.M.W.R.* 39(RR-17): 1, 1990.

47. Centers for Disease Control. Guidelines for Prevention of TB Transmission in Hospitals. Atlanta: U.S. Department of Health and Human Services (HHS publication no. [CDC] 82-8371), 1982.

48. Centers for Disease Control. Guidelines for the Prevention and Control of Nosocomial Infection: Guideline for Handwashing and Hospital Environmental Control. Atlanta: CDC, 1985.

49. Centers for Disease Control. Hepatitis A among drug abusers. *M.M.W.R.* 37:297, 1988.

50. Centers for Disease Control. Hepatitis B virus vaccine safety: Report of an interagency group. *M.M.W.R.* 31:465, 1982.

51. Centers for Disease Control. *HIV/AIDS Surveillance Report.* Atlanta: CDC, April 1991. Pp. 1–18.

52. Centers for Disease Control. Laboratory-acquired meningococcemia—California and Massachusetts. *M.M.W.R.* 40:46, 1991.

53. Centers for Disease Control. Nosocomial meningococcemia—Wisconsin. *M.M.W.R.* 27: 358, 1978.

54. Centers for Disease Control. Nosocomial transmission of multidrug-resistant tuberculosis among HIV-infected persons—Florida and New York, 1988–1991. *M.M.W.R.* 40: 585, 1991.

55. Centers for Disease Control. Outbreak of hepatitis B associated with an oral surgeon, New Hampshire. *M.M.W.R.* 36:132, 1987.

56. Centers for Disease Control. Possible transmission of human immunodeficiency virus to a patient during an invasive dental procedure. *M.M.W.R.* 39:489, 1990.

57. Centers for Disease Control. Public Health Service Statement on management of occupational exposure to human immunodeficiency virus, including considerations regarding zidovudine postexposure use. *M.M.W.R.* 39(RR-1): 1, 1990.

58. Centers for Disease Control. Recommendations for preventing transmission of human immunodeficiency virus and hepatitis B virus to patients during exposure-prone procedures. *M.M.W.R.* 40(RR-8): 1, 1991.

59. Centers for Disease Control. Recommendations for prevention of HIV transmission in health-care settings. *M.M.W.R.* 36:1, 1987.

60. Centers for Disease Control. Recommended infection-control practices for dentistry. *M.M.W.R.*, 35:237, 1986.

61. Centers for Disease Control. Risks associated with human parvovirus B19 infection. *M.M.W.R.* 38:81, 1989.

62. Centers for Disease Control. Screening for tuberculosis and tuberculous infection in high-risk populations, and the use of preventive therapy for tuberculous infection in the United States: Recommendations of the Advisory Committee for Elimination of Tuberculosis. *M.M.W.R.* 39(RR-8): 1, 1990.

63. Centers for Disease Control. The safety of hepatitis B virus vaccine. *M.M.W.R.* 32:134, 1983.

64. Centers for Disease Control. Tuberculosis and human immunodeficiency virus infection: Recommendations of the Advisory Committee for the Elimination of Tuberculosis (ACET). *M.M.W.R.* 38:236, 1989.

65. Centers for Disease Control. Update: Trans-

mission of HIV infection during an invasive dental procedure, Florida. *M.M.W.R.* 40:21, 1991.

66. Centers for Disease Control. Update: Universal precautions for prevention of transmission of human immunodeficiency virus, hepatitis B virus, and other bloodborne pathogens in health-care settings. *M.M.W.R.* 37: 378, 1988.

67. Chorba, T., et al. The role of parvovirus B19 in aplastic crisis and erythema infectiosum (fifth disease). *J. Infect. Dis.* 154:383, 1986.

68. Church, N.R., Anas, N.G., Hall, C.B., and Brooks, J.G. Respiratory syncytial virus–related apnea in infants. *Am. J. Dis. Child.* 138:247, 1984.

69. Cohen, M.S., et al. Possible nosocomial transmission of group Y *Neisseria meningitidis* among oncology patients. *Ann. Intern. Med.* 91:7, 1979.

70. Collaborative study by the Central Public Health Laboratories. Acute hepatitis B associated with gynaecological surgery. *Lancet* 1:1, 1980.

71. Comer, R.W., et al. Management considerations for an HIV positive dental student. *J. Dent. Educ.* 55:187, 1991.

72. Coovadia, Y.M., Bhana, R.H., Haffejee, I., and Marples, R.R. A laboratory-confirmed outbreak of rifampicin-methicillin resistant *Staphylococcus aureus* (RMRSA) in a newborn nursery. *J. Hosp. Infect.* 14:303, 1989.

73. Coulepis, A.G., Locarnini, S.A., Lehmann, N.I., and Gust, I.D. Detection of hepatitis A virus in the feces of patients with naturally acquired infections. *J. Infect. Dis.* 141:151, 1980.

74. Coutinho, R.A., et al. Hepatitis B from doctors. *Lancet* 1:345, 1982.

75. Dacre, J., Emmerson, A.M., and Jenner, E.A. Gentamicin-methicillin-resistant *Staphylococcus aureus:* Epidemiology and containment of an outbreak. *J. Hosp. Infect.* 7:130, 1986.

76. Davis, L.E., Stewart, J.A., and Garvin, S. Cytomegalovirus infection: A seroepidemiologic comparison of nuns and women from a venereal disease clinic. *Am. J. Epidemiol.* 102: 327, 1975.

77. Department of Labor/Department of Health and Human Services Joint Advisory Notice. Protection against occupational exposure to hepatitis B virus (HBV) and human immunodeficiency virus. *Fed. Reg.* 52:41818, Oct. 30, 1987.

78. Department of Labor, Occupational Safety and Health Administration. Occupational exposure to bloodborne pathogens; proposed rule and notice of hearing. *Fed. Reg.* 54:23042, 1989.

78a. Department of Labor, Occupational Safety and Health Administration. Occupational exposure to bloodborne pathogens; final rule. *Fed. Reg.* 56:64004, 1991.

79. Dienstag, J.L., and Ryan, D.M. Occupational exposure to hepatitis B virus in hospital personnel: Infection or immunization? *Am. J. Epidemiol.* 115:26, 1982.

80. Dienstag, J.L., Stevens, C.E., Bhan, A.K., and Szmuness, W. Hepatitis B vaccine administered to chronic carriers of hepatitis B surface antigen. *Ann. Intern. Med.* 96:575, 1982.

81. Douglas, R.G., Jr. Influenza in Man. In: E.D. Kilbourne (Ed.), *Influenza Viruses and Influenza.* New York: Academic, 1975. P. 395.

82. Duvall, C.P., et al. Recovery of cytomegalovirus from adults with neoplastic disease. *Ann. Intern. Med.* 65:531, 1966.

83. Estes, S.A. Diagnosis and management of scabies. *Med. Clin. North Am.* 66:955, 1982.

84. Farrington, M., Ling, J., and French, G.L. Outbreaks of infection with methicillin-resistant *Staphylococcus aureus* on neonatal and burns units of a new hospital. *Epidemiol. Infect.* 105:215, 1990.

85. Fekety, F.R. The epidemiology and prevention of staphylococcal infections. *Medicine* 43:593, 1964.

86. Flower, A.J., et al. Hepatitis B infection following cardiothoracic surgery (abstr.). In: *Proceedings of the 1990 International Symposium on Viral Hepatitis and Liver Diseases,* Houston, 1990. P. 94.

87. Gala, C.L., et al. The use of eye-nose goggles to control nosocomial respiratory virus infection. *J.A.M.A.* 256:2706, 1986.

88. Garner, J.S., and Simmons, B.P. CDC guideline for isolation precautions in hospitals. *Infect. Control* 4 (Suppl.): 245, 1983.

89. Gerberding, J.L., et al. Risk of transmitting the human immunodeficiency virus, cytomegalovirus, and hepatitis B virus to health care workers exposed to patients with AIDS and AIDS-related conditions. *J. Infect. Dis.* 156(1): 1, 1987.

90. Gershon, A.A., et al. Immunization of healthy adults with live attenuated varicella vaccine. *J. Infect. Dis.* 158:132, 1988.

91. Glezen, W.P. Serious morbidity and mortality associated with influenza epidemics. *Epidemiol. Rev.* 4:25, 1982.

92. Gooch, J.J., et al. Nosocomial outbreak of scabies. *Arch. Dermatol.* 114:897, 1978.

93. Goodman, R.A., Ahtone, J.L., and Finton, R.J. Hepatitis B transmission from dental personnel to patients: Unfinished business. *Ann. Intern. Med.* 96:119, 1982.

94. Goodwin, D., Fannin, S.L., and McCracken, B.B. An oral surgeon–related hepatitis B outbreak. *Calif. Morbid.* 14, 1976.

95. Grady, G.F., et al. Hepatitis B immune globulin for accidental exposures among medical personnel: Final report of a multicenter controlled trial. *J. Infect. Dis.* 138:625, 1978.

96. Graeve, J.L.A., deAlarcon, P.A., and Naides, S.J. Parvovirus B19 infection in patients receiving cancer chemotherapy: The expanding spectrum of disease. *Am. J. Pediatr. Hematol. Oncol.*, 11: 441, 1989.

97. Graman, P.S., and Hall, C.B. Epidemiology and control of nosocomial viral infections. *Infect. Dis. Clin. North Am.* 3:815, 1989.

98. Greaves, W.L., Kaiser, A.B., Alford, R.H., and Schaffner, W. The problem of herpetic whitlow among hospital personnel. *Infect. Control* 1:381, 1980.

99. Greenfield, S., Sheehe, P.R., and Feldman, H.A. Meningococcal carriage in a population of "normal" families. *J. Infect. Dis.* 123:67, 1971.

100. Grob, P., Bischof, B., and Naeff, F. Cluster of hepatitis B transmitted by a physician. *Lancet* 2:1218, 1981.

101. Grob, P., and Moeschlin, P. Risk to contacts of a medical practitioner carrying HBsAg. *N. Engl. J. Med.* 293:197, 1975.

102. Gwaltney, J.M., Jr., Mowkalsky, P.B., and Hendley, J.O. Hand-to-hand transmission of rhinovirus colds. *Ann. Intern. Med.* 88:463, 1978.

103. Hadler, S.C., et al. An outbreak of hepatitis B in a dental practice. *Ann. Intern. Med.* 95:133, 1981.

104. Haeram, J.W., et al. HBsAg transmission from a cardiac surgeon incubating hepatitis B resulting in chronic antigenemia in four patients. *Acta Med. Scand.* 210:389, 1981.

105. Hall, C.B. Nosocomial viral respiratory infections: Perennial weeds on pediatric wards. *Am. J. Med.* 70:670, 1981.

106. Hall, C.B. The nosocomial spread of respiratory syncytial viral infections. *Ann. Rev. Med.* 34:311, 1983.

107. Hall, C.B., and Douglas, R.G. Modes of transmission of respiratory syncytial virus. *J. Pediatr.* 99:100, 1981.

108. Hall, C.B., and Douglas, R.G. Nosocomial respiratory syncytial virus infections: The role of gowns and masks on prevention. *Am. J. Dis. Child.* 135:512, 1981.

109. Hall, C.B., Douglas, R.G., and Geiman, J.M. Possible transmission by fomites of respiratory syncytial virus. *J. Infect. Dis.* 141:98, 1980.

110. Hall, C.B., Douglas, R.G., Schnabel, K.C., and Geiman, J.M. Infectivity of respiratory syncytial virus by various routes of inoculation. *Infect. Immun.* 33:779, 1981.

111. Hall, C.B., Geiman, J.M., and Douglas, R.G. Control of nosocomial respiratory syncytial virus infections. *Pediatrics* 62:728, 1978.

112. Hall, C.B., et al. Neonatal respiratory syncytial virus infection. *N. Engl. J. Med.* 300:393, 1979.

113. Hall, C.B., et al. Respiratory syncytial virus infection in children with compromised immune function. *N. Engl. J. Med.* 315:77, 1986.

114. Hall, W.J., Hall, C.B., and Speers, D.M. Respiratory syncytial virus infection in adults: Clinical, virologic, and serial pulmonary function studies. *Ann. Intern. Med.* 88:203, 1978.

115. Hayden, G.F., Meyers, J.D., and Dixon, R.E. Nosocomial varicella: II. Suggested guidelines for management. *West. J. Med.* 130:300, 1979.

116. Haydon, J.R., and Caplan, R.M. Epidemic scabies. *Arch. Dermatol.* 103:168, 1971.

117. Henderson, D.K. et al. Risk for occupational transmission of human immunodeficiency virus type 1 (HIV-1) associated with clinical exposures: A prospective evaluation. *Ann. Intern. Med.* 113:740, 1990.

118. Henderson, F.W., et al. Respiratory-syncytial-virus infections, reinfections and immunity: A prospective, longitudinal study in young children. *N. Engl. J. Med.* 300:530, 1979.

119. Hendley, J.O., Wenzel, R.P. and Gwaltney, J.M. Transmission of rhinovirus colds by self-inoculation. *N. Engl. J. Med.* 288:1361, 1973.

120. Heptonstall, J. Outbreaks of hepatitis B virus infection associated with infected surgical staff in the United Kingdom. *Communicable Disease Reports* 1:R81, 1991.

121. Hirschowitz, B.A., Dasher, C.A., Whitt, F.J., and Cole, G.W. Hepatitis B antigen and antibody and tests of liver function—a prospective study of 310 hospital laboratory workers. *Am. J. Clin. Pathol.* 73:63, 1980.

122. Hoffman, P.C., and Dixon, R.E. Control of influenza in the hospital. *Ann. Intern. Med.* 87:725, 1977.

123. Hook, E.W. *Salmonella* Species. In: G.A. Mandell, R.G. Douglas, and J.E. Bennett (Eds.), *Principles and Practice of Infectious Disease* (3rd ed.). New York: Wiley 1990. Chap. 199.

124. Hopper, A.H., et al. Epidemic Norwegian scabies in a geriatric unit. *Age Ageing* 19:125, 1990.

125. Horman, J.T., et al. An outbreak of influenza in a nursing home. *Am. J. Public Health* 76:501, 1986.

126. Immunization Practices Advisory Committee. Measles prevention. *M.M.W.R.* 38(No. S-9):1, 1989.

127. Immunization Practices Advisory Commit-

tee. Prevention and control of influenza. *M.M.W.R.* 36:373, 1987.

128. Immunization Practices Advisory Committee. Prevention and control of influenza. *M.M.W.R.* 40:1, 1991.

129. Immunization Practices Advisory Committee. Protection against viral hepatitis. *M.M.W.R.* 39(RR-2): 1, 1990.

130. Immunization Practices Advisory Committee. Rubella prevention. *M.M.W.R.* 39(RR-15): 1, 1990.

131. Immunization Practices Advisory Committee. Update: Adult immunization. *M.M.W.R.* 40(RR-12): 1, 1991.

132. Janzen, J., et al. Epidemiology of hepatitis B surface antigen (HBsAg) and antibody to HBsAg in hospital personnel. *J. Infect. Dis.* 137:261, 1978.

133. Kurtzman, G.J., et al. Persistent B19 parvovirus infection as a cause of severe chronic anaemia in children with acute lymphocytic leukaemia. *Lancet* 2:1159, 1988.

134. Kurtzman, G., et al. Pure red-cell aplasia of 10 years' duration due to persistent parvovirus B19 infection and its cure with immunoglobulin therapy. *N. Engl. J. Med.* 321:519, 1989.

135. LaFrere, J.J., et al. Human parvovirus and aplastic crisis in chronic hemolytic anemias: A study of 24 observations. *Am. J. Hematol.* 23:271, 1986.

136. LeClair, J.M., et al. Prevention of nosocomial respiratory syncytial virus infections through compliance with glove and gown isolation precautions. *N. Engl. J. Med.* 317:329, 1987.

137. Leers, W.D., and Kouroupis, G.M. Prevalence of hepatitis B antibodies in hospital personnel. *Can. Med. Assoc. J.* 113:844, 1975.

138. Lempert, K.D., Baltz, P.S., Welton, W.A., and Whittier, F.C. Pseudouremic pruritus: A scabies epidemic in a dialysis unit. *Am. J. Kidney Dis.* 5:117, 1985.

139. Lerche, N.W., et al. Atypical crusted "Norwegian" scabies: Report of nosocomial transmission in a community hospital and an approach to control. *Cutis* 31:637, 1983.

140. Lettau, L.A., et al. Transmission of hepatitis B with resultant restriction of surgical practice. *J.A.M.A.* 255:934, 1986.

141. Levin, M.L., et al. Hepatitis B transmission by dentists. *J.A.M.A.* 228:1139, 1974.

142. Levy, B.S., et al. Hepatitis B in ward and clinical laboratory employees of a general hospital. *Am. J. Epidemiol.* 106:330, 1977.

143. Locksley, R.M., et al. Multiply antibiotic-resistant *Staphylococcus aureus:* Introduction, transmission, and evolution of nosocomial infection. *Ann. Intern. Med.* 97:317, 1982.

144. MacDonald, N.E., et al. Respiratory syncytial viral infection in infants with congenital heart disease. *N. Engl. J. Med.* 307:397, 1982.

145. Mandal, S.K., Joglekar, V.M., and Khan, A.S. An outbreak of respiratory syncytial virus infection in a continuing-care geriatric ward. *Age Ageing* 14:184, 1985.

146. Marcus, R., and CDC Cooperative Needlestick Study Group. Surveillance of health-care workers exposed to blood from patients infected with the human immunodeficiency virus. *N. Engl. J. Med.* 319:1118, 1988.

147. Marples, R.R., and Cooke, E.M. Workshop on methicillin-resistant *Staphylococcus aureus* held at the headquarters of the Public Health Laboratory Service on 8 January 1985. *J. Hosp. Infect.* 6:342, 1985.

148. Mastro, T.D., et al. An outbreak of surgical-wound infections due to group A streptococcus carried on the scalp. *N. Engl. J. Med.* 323:968, 1990.

149. Maynard, J.E. Viral Hepatitis as an Occupational Hazard in the Health Care Profession. In: G.N. Vyas, S.N. Cohen, and R. Schmid, (Eds.), *Viral Hepatitis: A Contemporary Assessment of Epidemiology, Pathogenesis and Prevention.* Philadelphia: Franklin Institute Press, 1978. Pp. 321–331.

150. McDougal, B.A., et al. Nosocomial influenza A infection. *South. Med. J.* 70:1023, 1977.

151. McNeil, M.M., and Solomon, S.L. The epidemiology of methicillin-resistant *Staphylococcus aureus. The Antimicrobic Newsletter* 2:49, 1985.

152. Meers, P.D., and Leong, K.Y. The impact of methicillin-resistant and aminoglycoside-resistant *Staphylococcus aureus* on the pattern of hospital-acquired infection in an acute hospital. *J. Hosp. Infect.* 16:291, 1990.

153. Mishu, B., et al. A surgeon with AIDS: Lack of evidence of transmission to patients. *J.A.M.A.* 264:467, 1990.

154. Morales, F., et al. A study of respiratory infections in the elderly to assess the role of respiratory virus. *J. Infect.* 7:236, 1983.

155. Mulley, A.G., Silverstein, M.D., and Dienstag, J.L. Indications for use of hepatitis B vaccine, based on cost effectiveness analysis. *N. Engl. J. Med.* 307:644, 1982.

156. Murphy, D., et al. The use of gowns and masks to control respiratory illness in pediatric hospital personnel. *J. Pediatr.* 99:746, 1981.

157. Noble, R.C., et al. Posttransfusion hepatitis A in a neonatal intensive care unit. *J.A.M.A.* 252:2711, 1984.

158. Opal, S.M., et al. Frequent acquisition of multiple strains of methicillin-resistant *Staphylococcus aureus* by health-care workers in an endemic hospital environment. *Infect. Control. Hosp. Epidemiol.* 11:479, 1990.

159. Orkin, M., and Mailbach, H.I. Current views of scabies and pediculosis pubis. *Cutis* 33:85, 1984.

160. Orkin, M., and Mailbach, H.I. Modern aspects of scabies. *Curr. Probl. Dermatol.* 13: 109, 1985.

161. Pachucki, C.T., et al. Influenza A among hospital personnel and patients. *Arch. Intern. Med.* 149:77, 1989.

162. Patriarca, P.A., Arden, N.H., Koplan, J.P., and Goodman, R.A. Prevention and control of type A influenza infections in nursing homes. *Ann. Intern. Med.* 107:732, 1987.

163. Pattison, C.P., et al. Epidemiology of hepatitis B in hospital personnel. *Am. J. Epidemiol.* 101:59, 1975.

164. Pattison, J.R., et al. Parvovirus infections and hypoplastic crisis in sickle-cell anaemia (lett.). *Lancet* 1:664, 1981.

165. Peacock, J.E., Jr., Marsik, F.J., and Wenzel, R.P. Methicillin-resistant *Staphylococcus aureus:* Introduction and spread within a hospital. *Ann. Intern. Med.* 93:526, 1980.

166. Perrillo, R.P. et al. A randomized, controlled trial of interferon alfa-2b alone and after prednisone withdrawal for the treatment of chronic hepatitis B. *N. Engl. J. Med.* 323:295, 1990.

167. Plummer, F.A., et al. An erythema infectiosum—like illness caused by human parvovirus infection. *N. Engl. J. Med.* 313:74, 1985.

168. Porter, J., et al. Management of patients treated by a surgeon with HIV infection. *Lancet* 335:113, 1990.

169. Preblud, S.R. Nosocomial varicella: Worth preventing but how? *Am. J. Public Health* 78:13, 1988.

170. Quinn, R.W., and Hillman, J.W. An epidemic of streptococcal wound infections. *Arch. Environ. Health* 11:28, 1965.

171. Reboli, A.C., John, J.F., Platt, C.G., and Cantey, J.R. Methicillin-resistant *Staphylococcus aureus* outbreak at a veterans' affairs medical center: Importance of carriage of the organism by hospital personnel. *Infect. Control Hosp. Epidemiol.* 11:291, 1990.

172. Reid, D.M., et al. Human parvovirus-associated arthritis: A clinical and laboratory description. *Lancet* 1:422, 1985.

173. Reilly, S., Cullen, D., and Davies, M.G. An outbreak of scabies in a hospital and community. *Br. Med. J.* 291:1031, 1085.

174. Reingold, A.L., et al. Transmission of hepatitis B by an oral surgeon. *J. Infect. Dis.* 145: 262, 1982.

175. Riewerts-Eriksen, N.H., et al. Nosocomial outbreak of group C meningococcal disease. *Br. Med. J.* 289:568, 1989.

176. Rimland, D., Parkin, W.E., Miller, G.B., and Schrack, W.D. Hepatitis B outbreak traced to an oral surgeon. *N. Engl. J. Med.* 296:953, 1977.

177. Rose, H.D., Lenz, I.E., and Sheth, N.K. Meningococcal pneumonia: A source of nosocomial infection. *Arch. Intern. Med.* 141:575, 1981.

178. Rosenblum, L.S., et al. Hepatitis A outbreak in a neonatal intensive care unit: Risk factors for transmission and evidence of prolonged viral excretion among preterm infants. *J. Infect. Dis.* 164:476, 1991.

179. Ross, A.H. Modification of chickenpox in family contacts by administration of gamma globulin. *N. Engl. J. Med.* 267:369, 1962.

180. Rutala, W.A., et al. Environmental study of a methicillin-resistant *Staphylococcus aureus* epidemic in a burn unit. *J. Clin. Microbiol.* 18: 683, 1983.

181. Schaffner, W., Lefkowitz, L.B., Jr., Goodman, J.S., and Koenig, M.G. Hospital outbreak of infections with group A streptococci traced to an asymptomatic anal carrier. *N. Engl. J. Med.* 280:1224, 1969.

182. Schwartz, B. Chemoprophylaxis for bacterial infections: Principles of and applications to meningococcal infection. *Rev. Infect. Dis.* 13 (Suppl.): S170, 1991.

183. Schwartz, B., et al. Clusters of invasive group A streptococcal infections: Clinical settings and prevention (abstr. 1054). In: *Abstracts of the 1991 Interscience Conference on Antimicrobial Agents and Chemotherapy*, Chicago. P. 274.

184. Seeberg, S., et al. Hospital outbreak of hepatitis A secondary to blood exchange in a baby (lett.) *Lancet* 1:1155, 1981.

185. Seeff, L.B., et al., Type B hepatitis after needlestick exposure: Prevention with hepatitis B immunoglobulin. Final report of the Veterans Administration Cooperative Study. *Ann. Intern. Med.* 88:285, 1978.

186. Shanson, D.C., Johnstone, D., and Midgley, J. Control of a hospital outbreak of methicillin-resistant *Staphylococcus aureus* infections: Value of an isolation unit. *J. Hosp. Infect.* 6: 285, 1985.

187. Shaw, F.E., et al. Lethal outbreak of hepatitis B in a dental practice. *J.A.M.A.* 255:3261, 1986.

188. Sirera, G., et al. Hospital outbreak of scabies stemming from two AIDS patients with Norwegian scabies (lett.). *Lancet* 335:8699, 1990.

189. Snydman, D.R., et al. Nosocomial viral hepatitis B: A cluster among staff with subsequent transmission to patients. *Ann. Intern. Med.* 85:573, 1976.

190. Snydman, D.R., Greer, C., Meissner, H.C., and McIntosh, K. Prevention of nosocomial transmission of respiratory syncytial virus in a newborn nursery. *Infect. Control Hosp. Epidemiol.* 9:105, 1988.

191. Stagno, S., et al. Congenital cytomegalovirus infection: Occurrence in an immune population. *N. Engl. J. Med.* 296:1254, 1977.
192. Szmuness, W., et al. Hepatitis B vaccine: Demonstration of efficacy in a controlled clinical trial in a high-risk population in the United States. *N. Engl. J. Med.* 303:833, 1980.
193. Tabor, E., Gerety, R.J., Mott, M., and Wilbur, J. Prevalence of hepatitis B in a high risk setting: A serologic study of patients and staff in a pediatric oncology unit. *Pediatrics* 61:711, 1978.
194. Taplin, D., et al. Eradication of scabies with a single treatment schedule. *J. Am. Acad. Dermatol.* 9:546, 1983.
195. Taplin, D., et al. Permethrin five percent dermal clean: A new treatment for scabies. *J. Am. Acad. Dermatol.* 15:995, 1986.
196. Thomas, M.C., Giedinghagen, D.H., and Hoff, G.L. Brief report: An outbreak of scabies among employees in a hospital-associated commercial laundry. *Infect. Control* 8:427, 1987.
197. Thompson, N.J., Glassroth, J.L., Snider, D.E., and Farer, L.S. The booster phenomenon in serial tuberculin testing. *Am. Rev. Respir. Dis.* 119:587, 1979.
198. Thompson, R.L., Cabezudo, I., and Wenzel, R.P. Epidemiology of nosocomial infections caused by methicillin-resistant *Staphylococcus aureus.* *Ann. Intern. Med.* 97:309, 1982.
199. Tokars, J., et al. Percutaneous injuries during surgical procedures. (abstr.). In: *Proceedings of the Seventh International Conference on AIDS, Florence, Italy, 1991;* 108 (2): 83, 1991.
200. Tolkoff-Rubin, N.E., et al. Cytomegalovirus infection in dialysis patients and personnel. *Ann. Intern. Med.* 89:625, 1978.
201. U.S. Department of Health and Human Services: Public Health Service. Infection Control File, Dec. 1989.
202. Valenti, W.M., et al. Nosocomial viral infections: II. Guidelines for prevention and control of respiratory viruses, herpesviruses and hepatitis viruses. *Infect. Control* 1:165, 1981.
203. Valenti, W.M., et al. Nosocomial viral infections: Epidemiology and significance. *Infect. Control* 1:33, 1980.
204. Valenti, W.M., Hruska, J.F., Menegus, M.A., and Freeburn, M.J. Nosocomial viral infections: III. Guidelines for prevention and control of exanthematous viruses, gastroenteritis viruses, picornaviruses, and uncommonly seen viruses. *Infect. Control* 2:38, 1981.
205. Viglionese, A., Nottebart, V.F., Bodman, H.A., and Platt, R. Recurrent group A streptococcal carriage in a health care worker associated with widely separated nosocomial outbreaks. *Am. J. Med.* 91 (Suppl. 3B): 329S, 1991.
206. Walsh, T.J., et al. Prospective microbiologic surveillance in control of nosocomial methicillin-resistant *Staphylococcus aureus.* *Infect. Control* 8:7, 1987.
207. Welch, J., et al. Hepatitis B infections after gynaecological surgery. *Lancet* 1:205, 1989.
208. White, D.G., et al. Human parvovirus arthropathy. *Lancet* 1:419, 1985.
209. Williams, W.W. CDC guideline for infection control in hospital personnel. *Infect. Control* 4 (Suppl.): 326, 1983.
210. Williams, W.W., et al. Immunization policies and vaccine coverage among adults: The risk for missed opportunities. *Ann. Intern. Med.* 108:616, 1988.
211. Williams, W.W., Preblud, S.R., Reichelderfer, P.S., and Hadler, S.C. Vaccines of importance in the hospital setting. *Infect. Dis. Clin. North Am.* 3:701, 1989.
212. Woernle, C.H., Anderson, L.J., Tatersall, P., and Davison, J.M. Human parvovirus B19 infection during pregnancy. *J. Infect. Dis.* 156:17, 1987.
213. Yeager, A.S. Longitudinal, serological study of cytomegalovirus infections in nurses and in personnel without patient contact. *J. Clin. Microbiol.* 2:448, 1975.
214. Zajac, B.A., et al. Overview of clinical studies with hepatitis B vaccine made by recombinant DNA. *J. Infect.* 13 (Suppl. A): 39, 1986.

The Development of Infection Surveillance and Control Programs

Robert W. Haley

Historical Perspective

Nosocomial infections have been a serious problem ever since sick patients were first congregated in hospitals. The explosiveness of spread of the classic epidemic diseases led to the concept of quarantine, from which evolved modern techniques of isolation. The ubiquitous threat of wound infections following surgery stimulated the strigent aseptic tradition of the operating room, including meticulous aseptic surgical technique, environmental cleanliness, and disinfection and sterilization processes. The observations of Semmelweis and Holmes, later bolstered by the popularization of the germ theory of infectious diseases, established the importance of hand-washing for reducing the spread of infection among patients. The unique observations and management abilities of Florence Nightingale established the modern basis for the design of hospitals and the strategies for patient care that minimize infection risks. And finally, the advent and widespread availability of antimicrobial agents in the 1940s revolutionized the treatment of infectious diseases and promised virtually to eliminate infections as a threat to hospitalized patients. Thus by the postwar period of the late 1940s, most of the concepts and tools for preventing nosocomial infections were in the hands of individual physicians and nurses who were to apply them, but no organized group at the hospital level was considered necessary to oversee the activity of infection control.

In the mid-1950s, hospitals in the United States and abroad were struck by a pandemic of staphylococci that were increasingly resistant to available antibiotics and more virulent than previous strains. In response to this widespread problem, hospitals organized Infection Control Committees to develop new strategies for controlling the epidemic and for coordinating the infection control efforts of the diverse groups and departments of the hospital. In addition, the Centers for Disease Control (CDC), then called the Communicable Disease Center, designated a new investigations unit, one purpose of which was to assist Infection Control Committees in investigating hospital epidemics. This nationwide effort was summarized and discussed at two national conferences on the control of staphylococcal disease in 1958. The proceedings of the conferences indicated the leading approaches to be stringent disinfection and monitoring of the inanimate environment, detection and treatment of staphylococcal carriers among the hospital staff, more vigorous encouragement of aseptic technique, and the reporting of staphylococcal infections to the Infection Control Committee [49, 50].

By the mid-1960s, the pandemic began to subside for reasons that are still unclear. It left in its wake, however, a new awareness of nosocomial infections and committees of hospital personnel interested in controlling the problem. At the same time, hospitals were experiencing another strong current of change—the use of increasingly complex technology bequeathed by the World War II technologic "push" and the burgeoning space race. Thus as staphylococcal epidemics declined, new types of infections were seen involving opportunistic pathogens, such as gram-negative rods, fungi, and parasites, infecting an increasing number of highly compromised and immunosuppressed patients undergoing new medical treatments. These developments were described in 1963 at the National Conference on Institutionally Acquired Infections, the name of the conference well illustrating the awareness that a broader problem was emerging [47]. The proceedings of the conference indicated the development of a much wider range of approaches to control of the problem, including the application of epidemiologic methods, the recommendation of organized systems for surveillance of nosocomial infections, and the importance of personnel education [47].

Through the middle and late 1960s, a few hospitals developed organized infection control programs to conduct surveillance, develop control measures, and monitor the control process for the Infection Control Committee, although most hospitals continued to depend on the individual efforts of doctors and nurses. These programs were focused somewhat and encouraged by an infection control manual published and distributed widely by the American Hospital Association's (AHA's) Committee on Infections Within Hospitals [1]. Meanwhile researchers at the CDC were engaged in pilot studies in several community hospitals to develop and test technology for conducting more effective surveillance of nosocomial infections [12]. After demonstrating the futility of depending on voluntary reporting of infections by doctors or nurses, these pilot studies first relied on a physician infection control officer to identify infections. Later, borrowing from the British the concept of the infection control sister [16], which was being tried in two other U.S. hospitals [45, 51], the CDC researchers thoroughly tested the feasibility of surveillance by trained infection control nurses and found that one full-time-equivalent nurse was needed to perform surveillance and control for approximately every 250 beds [6]. On the basis of these findings, the CDC set up a training course for infection control nurses, and the first classes were held in 1968. These developments were summarized and discussed in the First International Conference on Nosocomial Infections held at the CDC in 1970 [7]. The proceedings focused on a debate between the proponents of surveillance of infections by infection control nurses and their critics, who considered the approach infeasible, unnecessary, or too costly.

Following the First International Conference, the CDC developed a strong recommendation for the surveillance approach, which was also supported and promoted by the AHA [2, 44]. Popularized by scientific papers, presentations at scientific meetings and regional and local conferences, practical manuals, training courses, and individual consultations with hospital staffs by medical and nurse epidemiologists from CDC, the approach was adopted in varying degrees by virtually all U.S. hospitals in the early to middle 1970s. For example, although Infection Control Committees had emerged earlier, in 1970 few hospitals had infection control nurses, practiced active surveillance of infections, or had formal policies prescribing aseptic practices; by 1976, however, the majority of hospitals had adopted these and had begun reducing their levels of wasteful routine environmental culturing [26]. Since there were virtually no government or private regulations or standards of much force during those years, this revolution in infection control was entirely a voluntary movement by hospitals to address an emerging problem. Noteworthy signs of the vitality of the movement were the demand for the CDC training course for infection control nurses, the huge circulation of the various books and manuals on infection control, and the formation of a professional society for infection control nurses (the Association for Practitioners in Infection Control [APIC], established in 1972). During the 1970s, the CDC operated a network of 70 voluntary hospitals, the National Nosocomial Infections Surveillance (NNIS) System, to maintain nationwide surveillance of the problem [5].

In 1974, the CDC began a nationwide study to evaluate the effectiveness of the approach that had been adopted throughout the country. Termed the *Study of the Efficacy of Nosocomial Infection Control* (the SENIC Project), the multiphased study had two objectives: first, to measure the extent to which these new programs, labeled *infection surveillance and control programs* (ISCPs), had been adopted by U.S. hospitals; and second, to determine whether these programs had reduced nosocomial infection rates in the country and, if so, to what extent [25]. The study was stimulated by the prediction that future financial pressures on hospitals would cause them to discontinue costly preventive programs of unproved value. If the programs were truly effective, their efficacy should be documented scientifically to perpetuate their support; if not, a demonstration of the lack of efficacy should help to redirect the efforts of the nation's hospitals

toward more effective approaches. (See summary of the results of the SENIC evaluation, following.)

During the ten years (1974–1983) that the SENIC Project was conducted, the infection control movement in U.S. hospitals was going through a maturation phase. In this period, more than 5,000 infection control nurses received training in the CDC training courses, and diverse organizations began sponsoring their own courses for nurses, physicians, and microbiologists. A professional society for physician epidemiologists, the Society of Hospital Epidemiologists of America (SHEA), was formed in 1980. More efficient methods of detecting infections through surveillance were developed. Extensive environmental culturing programs virtually disappeared. National conferences on infection control, including the Second International Conference on Nosocomial Infections in 1980, disseminated new information and provided a forum for infection control personnel to exchange experiences. Finally, a host of new risk factors that predispose patients to infection and cause epidemics were identified and studied. Despite much continued debate over the cost effectiveness of routine infection surveillance, the hospitals that increased the intensity of their surveillance efforts outnumbered those that reduced or discontinued the activity [24].

The early 1980s saw a consolidation of the experiences of the past decade. Of particular importance was the CDC project to record the increasingly complex set of findings and recommendations into a series of guidelines for hospitals. The physician- and nurse-epidemiologists of the CDC Hospital Infections Program had been providing consultation to hospital personnel on diverse technical issues ranging from questions on disinfection techniques to the management of outbreak investigations. By 1980, they were responding to more than 10,000 inquiries per year. The philosophy behind the effort to write guidelines was to provide to all U.S. hospitals simultaneously the answers to the most important and frequently recurring questions [18]. In the end, the effort produced a valuable checklist of the issues that should be addressed in policies of all hospitals [4]. To make the guidelines most useful, each recommendation was classified according to the strength of its backing by scientific evidence or the consensus of experts. This was to allow hospitals to discriminate between approaches very likely to prevent infections and those with a good rationale but of untested value. The intent of the process was to provide a body of useful information and to avoid the aura of governmental regulatory pressures.

Since their initial release from 1981 through 1983, the CDC guidelines have generated widespread interest and discussion. A 1985 nationwide survey to evaluate the diffusion and adoption of the guidelines found that, although 84 percent of infection control personnel across the country were familiar with them, actual adoption varied widely among the specific recommendations [3]. For example, 78 percent of hospitals reported having adopted the recommendation for changing intravenous tubing every 48 hours, whereas only 23 percent reported having adopted the recommendation for computing procedure-specific clean wound infection rates for each surgeon, with feedback of results to the surgeons. Small hospitals were found to have been significantly less likely both to have heard of the guidelines and to have adopted them. It is probable that the guidelines have achieved even wider adoption with the passage of time since the survey.

The late 1980s promised to be a period of innovation in infection control. With the release of the results of the SENIC Project [23] and the financial incentives for hospitals to support infection control created by the national Prospective Payment System [28, 29, 52], it appeared that hospitals would rapidly adopt the new outcome-oriented approaches to surveillance and feedback of epidemiologic data and make major reductions in nosocomial infection risks [20]. The onslaught of the acquired immunodeficiency syndrome (AIDS) epidemic and the growing influence of case review–oriented quality assurance programs, however, seriously distracted infection control personnel in most hospitals, and progress slowed.

Nonetheless, by the early 1990s, most infection control programs had established systems for dealing with AIDS and the resulting personnel health problems. Additionally, they had established the credibility of their epidemiologic methods with their quality assurance supervisors, and the race to implement new surveillance and control strategies began, with the progressive computerization of surveillance leading the new movement [32].

Strategies for Surveillance and Control

The main lesson derived from the past two decades of research and experience is that preventing nosocomial infections and controlling infection outbreaks in hospitals requires an organized management system staffed by dedicated personnel to influence the behavior of practicing doctors, nurses, and paramedical workers [23]. In this respect, the system is similar to an office or department of quality control on the management staff of an industrial corporation [11]. Many nosocomial infections are analogous to product defects resulting from the human errors of workers on the assembly line. Without careful management to ensure quality and without statistical feedback of the product defect rates, quality tends to decline, whereas a system for managing quality usually improves the products. This is the general rationale behind the need for an organized ISCP.

The basic model for an effective ISCP is portrayed in Figure 4-1 [26]. The nosocomial infections that are preventable, perhaps between 30 and 50 percent, are primarily caused by problems in *patient care practices*, such as the use and care of urinary catheters, intravenous and central venous monitoring catheters, and respiratory therapy equipment, as well as hand-washing practices and surgical skill. As in most work situations, in the absence of a system for managing these practices, they are generally determined by the

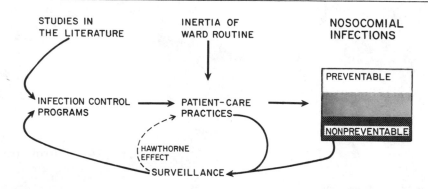

Fig. 4-1. Simplified theoretic model of an infection surveillance and control program. (Reprinted with permission from R. W. Haley, et al., Study on the efficacy of nosocomial infection control (SENIC Project): Summary of study design. *Am. J. Epidemiol.* 111:474, 1980.)

inertia of ward routine—that is, the apprentice system, in which practices are passed on from generation to generation of doctors and other hospital workers. Since old practices become strongly ingrained, changing behavior in the hospital environment meets stiff resistance and, if pursued persistently, generates interpersonal conflict. To change old practices to preventive practices requires an infection control program, consisting of an organized intervention system with specific goals for changing behavior. For this program to be successful it must be guided by sound principles and current information; consequently, the infection control personnel must learn correct preventive practices from studying the published literature, including articles in scientific journals, textbooks, and technical manuals, and they must conduct regular surveillance over the occurrence of nosocomial infections and the patient care practices in their hospital. The information obtained from surveillance not only allows infection control personnel to direct their efforts toward the most serious problems, but also arms them with information with which to obtain the support of hospital workers and provide feedback on the results of preventive changes. Information is power, and the more immediately relevant the information is to the individual hospital's situation, the more powerful it is.

A more detailed model of the infection control process is pictured in Figure 4-2 [26]. There are basically two routes by which the infection control staff can influence patient care practices and reduce infection risks: taking direct action to change behavior without having to rely on the voluntary compliance of hospital personnel (the direct approach) and working with hospital personnel through training or other activities to motivate them to practice correct techniques (the indirect approach). Taking the direct approach—for example, having the purchasing department switch to a new type of phlebotomy needle that reduces the risk of a needle-stick injury to personnel—generally requires a less personnel-intensive effort and is more certain to be effective, but unfortunately only a minority of infection risks are susceptible to this approach.

In contrast, the majority of infection risks require changing behavior, a more difficult and less certain endeavor [38–41]. To change behavior successfully requires a complex management process involving the following steps. First, the preventive practice must be correctly defined; all too frequently medical, nursing, or support service departments use written or informal policies that run counter to proved preventive approaches. Given correct policies, the infection control staff much achieve a unity of purpose among the power brokers of the hospital (e.g., the hospital administrator, nursing service director, chiefs

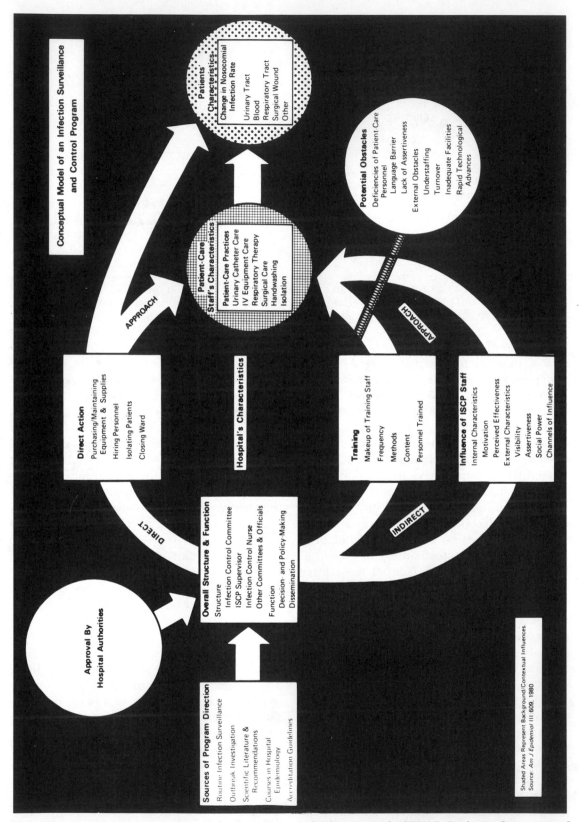

Fig. 4-2. Detailed conceptual model of an infection surveillance and control program (ISCP). Shaded areas represent background-contextual influences. (Reprinted with permission from R. W. Haley et al., Study on the efficacy of nosocomial infection control (SENIC Project): Summary of study design: Appendix A. Conceptual model of an infection surveillance and control program. *Am. J. Epidemiol.* 111:608, 1980.)

of involved medical departments, or directors of support service departments). A dissenting department head will ensure the failure of any attempt to influence patient care in his or her domain. Achieving unity of purpose requires a skillful and diplomatic approach, involving a realistic effort to balance infection control needs against practical constraints. The importance of peer relations must be recognized by having a knowledgeable infection control physician to deal with the medical staff and an influential nurse or other practitioner as the infection control coordinator to work with the nursing and support service staffs.

With unity of purpose established, training efforts must be designed to provide all relevant personnel with the skills and knowledge required to carry out the new preventive practice according to the agreed-on standard. Various motivational techniques can be used to increase compliance; potential obstacles to correct performance, such as understaffing or inadequate hand-washing facilities, must be removed. Once these prerequisite steps are taken, the practice must be monitored to measure compliance, and the results must be reported to department heads and particularly to first-line workers to reward the desired behaviors and focus attention on breakdowns in performance. With unity of purpose among supervisors and department heads *and* quantitative data on performance, correct practice can be maximized. If any of the steps in the process is neglected or fails, the degree of prevention will be reduced. Since halfway programs are often ineffective, a well-organized system to manage the process of infection control is essential to have a substantial effect in the rapidly changing technologic milieu of the modern hospital.

Personnel and Organization
Infection Control Committee

An Infection Control Committee is present in virtually every hospital in the United States and usually functions as the hospital's central decision- and policy-making body [30, 31]. Its decisions are often independent and binding throughout the hospital but may require review and approval by higher authorities such as the hospital administration. Since its purpose is to be the hospital's advocate for prevention of infections, it is usually placed above the various clinical and support service departments. Most committees are composed of representatives from most of the hospital's departments and meet regularly, usually monthly, to deal with current developments and problems. Its multidisciplinary representation is important for at least three reasons. First, since infection problems and control measures often cross departmental lines, effective decision making requires regular participation of members from most departments. Second, to carry out the committee's decisions, it is often most effective to have committee members exert inside influence in their respective departments to ensure agreement and compliance. Third, the multidepartmental representation of the committee bolsters its authority as an advocate for the hospital that transcends the special interests of any single department. When a committee decision is opposed—as, for example, by a strong department head—this overall authority can be very important in ensuring that the final compromise position is in the best interests of patient care in all departments.

The activities of the infection control staff members, such as the infection control practitioner and the hospital epidemiologist or infection control physician (see next section), are generally performed, at least in principle, at the direction of the Infection Control Committee. The job of executive staff of the committee is to provide technical information and surveillance data, to draft policies for the committee's use in the final decision-making process, and to carry out or promote many of the prevention and control measures that are adopted.

Infection Control Physician
Almost all hospitals have a physician acting as the chairperson of the Infection Control Committee [19]. An increasing number of com-

mittees, particularly in the larger hospitals and in those affiliated with medical schools, also have a full- or part-time position for a physician with special training in hospital epidemiology functioning as the hospital epidemiologist. The hospital epidemiologist may be the chairperson of the committee or may occupy a separate position as either a technical advisor or a member of the executive staff of the committee. The former seems preferable in smaller hospitals, whereas the latter creates a separation of the epidemiologic and decision-making roles that could strengthen both activities, particularly in the more complex situations present in larger hospitals.

Most persons occupying the position of hospital epidemiologist are practicing physicians who serve on a part-time basis, often in a 2-year committee assignment [19]. In the mid-1970s, 40 percent were pathologists, 18 percent internists (approximately half of these were infectious disease specialists), 12 percent surgeons, and 20 percent other types of physicians; in 10 percent of U.S. hospitals, the position was held by someone other than a physician, most commonly a microbiologist. By 1983, the tendency was toward increased representation of internists, particularly infectious disease specialists, with a commensurate decrease of nonphysicians and pathologists [unpublished SENIC data]. Infectious disease specialists are increasingly filling the position of epidemiologist in teaching hospitals but not in nonteaching hospitals, and they are more likely to be receiving remuneration for their infection control duties and to have received specific training for the job [21].

The average tenure in this position tends to be 2 to 3 years, and most appointees tend to spend less than 4 hours per week, although pathologists and infectious disease specialists tend to remain much longer and devote more time. An increasing number of hospitals, particularly those that are large and affiliated with medical schools, are creating full-time positions for hospital epidemiologists, some of whom provide the same service for groups of smaller hospitals in the surrounding locale.

The degree of knowledge and interest of these infection control physicians appears to vary widely. In the mid-1970s, only approximately 60 percent of U.S. hospitals had an infection control physician who indicated special interest in the problem, and by 1983 the percentage had not increased [24]. In both periods, only one-third or so of the physicians had taken a training course in infection control. Without a training course, physicians are generally unprepared to manage infection control activities since little, if any, time has been devoted to the subject in the curricula of medical schools, medical residencies, or even infectious disease fellowships. Consequently, the role of the infection control physician appears to be the area of infection control most in need of a focus in the near future.

Following the publication of the results of the SENIC Project in 1985 [20, 23, 24], in which the deficiencies in the number and training of infection control physicians were stressed, there appears to have been an increase in the percentage of U.S. hospitals with a trained physician in this position. A survey of U.S. hospitals in 1988 found that 46 percent had a physician with training in infection control [48]. To increase this further, in 1990 the AHA, SHEA, and CDC began conducting training courses for physicians across the United States. (See Chap. 2.)

Infection Control Practitioner

The infection control practitioner (ICP), or infection control nurse (ICN), occupies the key position in the ISCP. Without a qualified, energetic person in this position, the efforts of the Infection Control Committee will be largely ineffective. This fact has become so apparent that by 1983 virtually 100 percent of U.S. hospitals had established such a position on at least a part-time basis [24], and this has remained true into the late 1980s [48].

These positions have been filled predominantly by nurses. In the mid-1970s, 96 percent were nurses, the rest being mostly trained in microbiology and laboratory technology [13]. This predominance held true through 1983, when 85 percent were nurses and the rest were medical technologists, microbiologists, and from other backgrounds [unpublished data from the 1983 SENIC survey]. The national survey in 1987 by Turner and colleagues [46] found that 75 percent were nurses, but a response rate of only 58 percent leaves the possibility of a large error in the results. The most common job titles for the position are infection control nurse (34 percent of U.S. hospitals in 1983), infection control coordinator (18 percent), nurse epidemiologist (12 percent), and infection control practitioner (5 percent) [unpublished data from the 1983 SENIC survey].

In U.S. hospitals, only approximately one-fourth of the ICPs work on infection control full-time. A much higher percentage (more than 70 percent) work full-time in larger hospitals (more than 300 beds) in contrast to a much lower percentage (14 percent) in smaller hospitals [14]. In 1976 only about one-half of U.S. hospitals met the recommendation for one full-time-equivalent ICP per 250 hospital beds [14]. Since most hospitals tended to have either one half-time or one full-time ICP position, smaller hospitals were more likely to have met this recommendation than large hospitals, even though some larger hospitals have more than one position. By 1983, however, two-thirds of hospitals had established enough ICP positions to meet the recommendation [24]. In small hospitals in which ICPs work less than full-time on infection control, the appointee often has one or more other titles including director or assistant director of nursing service, inservice education coordinator, operating room supervisor, utilization review nurse or, more recently, risk management coordinator [14]. In an increasing number of large medical school–affiliated hospitals, infection control is combined with risk management or utilization review in a single department. Although this situation offers advantages in efficient use of personnel and bringing epidemiologic techniques to the risk management or utilization review activities, it runs the risk of seriously reducing the personnel commitment to infection control if sufficient staff are not

provided to cover all of the added responsibilities. The advent of the AIDS epidemic in the mid-1980s added new responsibilities to the jobs of most ICPs, who were already understaffed. These additional responsibilities varied widely from such duties as monitoring and reducing employee exposures to patients' blood to writing policies for implementing new isolation precautions. In the early 1990s, it appears that the impact of AIDS on the ICP's job has diminished somewhat as the epidemic has become better understood (see Chap. 39).

The ICP position is most often located organizationally in the quality assurance or the nursing service department, although the ICP usually obtains advice and supervision from the infection control physician, if one is present in the hospital [14]. The majority of ICPs hold a nursing position equivalent to nursing supervisor or higher. Choosing more experienced nurses for the job is important to give the ICP a greater insight into the patient care practices that are to be influenced and more experience in the clinical milieu, which facilitates the detection of infections for surveillance and increases rapport with clinical nurses and doctors. In contrast to the levels of training of infection control physicians, almost all ICPs have taken at least one training course in infection control; two-thirds of these were trained in the CDC training course, but an increasing number are taking courses offered by local and national APIC organizations, academic institutions, and private firms [14]. In 1983, as an indication of the increased training opportunities available for ICPs, the CDC, in cooperation with the Association of Schools of Public Health, consulted with a group of infection control training experts and recommended that the CDC reduce or discontinue its direct training efforts and turn these resources toward developing training materials and guidelines for others to use in training [8]. Subsequently, the CDC discontinued training in infection control, and courses were developed by private and professional groups.

ICPs across the country have tended to

spend their time in very similar ways. Regardless of the number of hours per week worked or the size of the hospital, they spend, on the average, approximately half of their time on surveillance of infections, one-fourth on policy development, and the rest about equally divided among training, consulting, and investigating potential outbreaks [14], although time usage of ICPs has not been resurveyed in recent years. Recent task analyses performed by APIC have further specified what the infection control job entails [34, 35, 37, 42].

In the early 1970s, it appeared that there would be a high turnover rate of nurses in the ICP position; however, by the mid-1970s the turnover rate had fallen significantly below that of hospital nurses in general, suggesting that the earlier trend was a temporary feature of the position's formative period [14]. In a 1985 national survey, the rate of turnover of ICPs was found to be 50 percent over 5 years, with a much lower turnover rate (28 percent) in large hospitals (more than 500 beds) than that (54 percent) in small hospitals (fewer than 50 beds) [3].

Efficacy of Surveillance and Control Programs

The question of the efficacy of ISCPs has been posed almost from the beginning of the movement in the 1960s but has been of increasing interest since the First International Conference in 1970. This debate has centered on several issues, including the efficacy and cost-effectiveness of routine infection surveillance over and above vigorous control measures; the need for ICPs; the best ratio of ICPs to hospital beds; the need for interested and trained infection control physicians; and the effectiveness of reporting surgical wound infection rates to surgeons. Although several studies in individual hospitals have demonstrated dramatic reductions of their nosocomial infection rates following the establishment of various combinations of these characteristics, they have not been influential in settling the efficacy questions because of the lack of si-

multaneous control observations, the possibility of selective reporting of positive results in the literature, and other methodologic problems [10, 15, 36, 43, 45].

In the early 1970s, CDC investigators designed the protocol for a large historical prospective study, building in numerous design features to avoid or control for the many potential biases that might be encountered. After clearance through internal scientific peer review at the CDC, presentations at scientific meetings, and formal review in government channels, the project was undertaken by the CDC staff with technical assistance from the Department of Biostatistics of the University of North Carolina School of Public Health, the UCLA Institute for Social Science Research, and the National Center for Health Statistics, with financial support from the CDC, the National Institute of Allergy and Infectious Diseases, the Health Care Financing Administration (HCFA), and the office of the Assistant Secretary for Health, HHS.

After the initial design phase spanning 1974 to 1976, pilot studies were completed to validate the various data collection methods developed specifically for the project [26]. The study was then performed in three phases. First, a questionnaire was mailed to all U.S. hospitals to measure specific surveillance and control characteristics needed to construct indexes of these activities and other measures of the ICP, the infection control physician, and the other components under study. After stratifying all acute-care U.S. hospitals with these two indexes, 338 hospitals were selected randomly from the strata [26]. The sample provided a representative group of hospitals that had established different levels of surveillance and control efforts, including hospitals that had established no programs at all. Second, each of the 338 sample hospitals was visited by trained CDC interviewers to validate the surveillance and control indexes and collect more detailed descriptive information about the programs.

The third phase involved a review by trained CDC medical records analysts of random samples of the medical records of patients admitted in 1970 and in 1975–1976 to the 338 sample hospitals. In each hospital, 500 patients were selected randomly from each of the 2 years, and their records were reviewed to diagnose all nosocomial urinary tract infections, surgical wound infections, pneumonia, and bacteremia from the clinical data found in all parts of the record. These four sites account for more than 80 percent of nosocomial infections. From these data on approximately 339,000 patients, the change of the nosocomial infection rates from 1970 (before any of the hospitals had programs) to 1975–1976 (after the program activities measured in the first two phases had been established) were estimated. In addition, measurements were made of other hospital and patient characteristics, changes in which could have confounded the evaluation. Following the data collection phase (1976–1978), the large computerized database was extensively edited and made ready for analysis (1978–1980),

and the statistical analysis of the influence of the programs on the change in infection rates, controlling for changes in other characteristics, was performed (1980–1983).

The results, published in early 1985 [23], are summarized in Table 4-1. In comparison with hospitals that started no program activities, those that established ISCPs with a full-time-equivalent ICP per 250 occupied beds, an effectual infection control physician with special interest in infection control, and a program for reporting wound infection rates to surgeons reduced their nosocomial infection rates by approximately 32 percent, a result that was highly statistically significant for all four types of infections studied. Separate analyses for cohorts of high- and low-risk patients showed similar results for each type of infection, although programs to prevent infections among low-risk patients had to be somewhat more intensive than those needed

Table 4-1. Percentage of nosocomial infections prevented by the most effective infection surveillance and control programs

Type of infection	Components of most effective programs	Percent prevented
Surgical wound infection (SWI)	An organized hospitalwide program with Intensive surveillance and control Reporting SWI rates to surgeons	20
	plus An effectual physician with special interest and knowledge in infection control	35
Urinary tract infection	An organized hospitalwide program with Intensive surveillance in operation for at least 1 year An ICP per 250 beds	38
Nosocomial bacteremia	An organized hospitalwide program with Intensive control alone	15
	plus Moderately intensive surveillance in operation for at least 1 year An ICP per 250 beds An infection control physician or micro-biologist	35
Postoperative pneumonia in surgical patients	An organized hospitalwide program with Intensive surveillance An ICP per 250 beds	27
Pneumonia in medical patients	An organized hospitalwide program with Intensive surveillance and control	13
All types of nosocomial infections	An organized hospitalwide program with All the components listed above	32

ICP = infection control practitioner.

for high-risk patients. The importance of these results was emphasized by the finding that among hospitals that started no programs, the nosocomial infection rate was increasing at a rate of 18 percent over 5 years, presumably reflecting the increasing infection risks accompanying the continual introduction of invasive and immunocompromising medical technology.

Whereas approximately one-third of nosocomial infections *could* be prevented if all U.S. hospitals had established the programs found to be the most effective, the fact that relatively few hospitals actually had all of the required components meant that in the mid-1970s only 6 percent of nosocomial infections were actually being prevented nationwide [23]. The widespread adoption of the most effective programs might therefore be expected to prevent an additional one-fourth of the infections. A resurvey of a random sample of U.S. hospitals in 1983 found that hospitals had substantially increased the intensity of their surveillance and control activities, but the failure to implement certain specific critical components, such as an adequate staffing ratio for ICPs, training of hospital epidemiologists, or reporting wound infection rates to surgeons, had muted the degree of improvement in prevention to the extent that still only 9 percent of infections were being prevented [24].

Potential Impacts of the SENIC Project

As the first controlled study of the effectiveness of ISCPs, the SENIC Project provided "a powerful justification for the American infection control strategy" [17]. Sufficient time has now passed since the release of the results of the SENIC Project to begin to assess its impact on the practice of infection control in the United States. Evidence to date suggests that the results have favorably influenced at least five areas: (1) preservation of infection control's role; (2) a rekindling of interest in surveillance; (3) a fundamental reorientation of surveillance from process to outcome; (4) an increased emphasis on training for infection control physicians; and (5) the use of multivariate analytic methods in the development of infection risk indexes.

Preservation of Infection Control's Role
When the SENIC results were published in the mid-1980s, the roles of infection control, quality assurance, risk management, utilization review, and other oversight functions of the hospital were undergoing a restructuring under the changing priorities of the Joint Commission on Accreditation of Healthcare Organizations (JCAHO) and the HCFA. In an effort to make these activities more efficient, it was recommended that they be merged, usually under the supervision of the directors of quality assurance. This was unfortunate in many hospitals because most quality assurance programs were strongly oriented toward detecting individual cases of clinical errors and had little involvement with epidemiologic methods. This nationwide change threatened to extinguish the epidemiologic approach from hospitals. The release of the SENIC results, which constituted the first evidence of the efficacy of any of these patient care review functions, gave ICPs ammunition for convincing their quality assurance supervisors and hospital administrators of the need to preserve their epidemiologic orientation. With its survival now guaranteed, the epidemiologic approach appears to be gaining advocates among the other patient care review departments as well.

Rekindling of Interest in Surveillance
In the 1970s, when most hospitals started their organized ISCPs, surveillance of nosocomial infections and calculation of infection rates was a central focus of the programs. In the late 1970s and the early 1980s, however, many hospitals began reducing the intensity of surveillance, some discontinuing it altogether [24]. Since the release of the SENIC findings in early 1985, this trend appears to have been reversed. For example, the practice of feeding back surgeon-specific wound infection rates to individual surgeons—the

surveillance activity found to have had the greatest effect in SENIC [23]—was reportedly performed regularly in 19 percent of U.S. hospitals in 1976 [27], in 13 percent of hospitals in 1983 [24], and in only 6 percent in 1985. But by the end of 1986, Landry and colleagues [33] reported that it had increased to 28 percent of hospitals in Virginia and, in 1987, an independent nationwide survey by the General Accounting Office found a similar prevalence [48]. There may have been further increases since 1987 as a result of policy recommendations for this practice by the Surgical Infection Society [9] and the JCAHO [31], based on the SENIC findings.

Change to Outcome Orientation

Perhaps the most important finding from SENIC, one that was not immediately appreciated, was a strong dissociation of infection control program effectiveness for different types of infections. Programs that were effective in reducing surgical wound infections were usually not the same as those that were effective in reducing urinary tract infections, bacteremias, and pneumonias, and vice versa. Only 0.2 percent of U.S. hospitals had programs that were effective in reducing all four of the main types of infection [23]. This led to the startling and controversial proposal that hospitals should stop doing routine surveillance of all nosocomial infections leading to the overall hospital infection rate and instead develop specific outcome objectives for which separate, targeted surveillance systems ought to be developed [20]. Initially opposed by proponents of routine hospitalwide surveillance, the new concept has been adopted increasingly by U.S. hospitals and was recently incorporated as a recommended model in the 1990 standards for accreditation of hospitals by the JCAHO [31].

Increase in Physician Training

As discussed earlier, the percentage of U.S. hospitals with a physician trained in infection control remained at approximately 25 percent from 1976 to 1983 [24]. Following the release of the SENIC findings, the percent-

age appears to have increased substantially [48], and a new training initiative for physicians has been launched by the AHA, SHEA, and CDC.

Multivariate Risk Indexes

The idea of controlling infection rate comparisons for intrinsic patient infection risk is an old concept, dating back to the late nineteenth century when surgeons confined analysis to "clean" surgical wounds. Before the SENIC Project, analyses were being stratified by wound classification based on the likely level of bacterial contamination of the wound [9]. Using as a model the multivariate analyses of risk factors for wound infection by prior investigators, SENIC investigators applied multivariate analysis to construct a simple, practical risk index combining the traditional wound classification with measures of intrinsic patient susceptibility to infection and predicted wound infection far more powerfully [22]. Whereas the particular multivariate index will undoubtedly be improved in the future, the concept of employing multivariate risk indexes rather than unidimensional risk measures will make nosocomial infection surveillance data far more useful for informing patient care personnel of infection risks in their patients. (See Chap. 8.)

References

1. American Hospital Association. *Infection Control in the Hospital.* Chicago: American Hospital Association, 1968.
2. American Hospital Association. *Infection Control in the Hospital,* rev. ed. Chicago: American Hospital Association, 1970.
3. Celentano, D.D., Morlock, L.L., and Malitz, F.E. Diffusion and adoption of CDC Guidelines for the Prevention and Control of Nosocomial Infections in U.S. hospitals. *Infect. Control* 8(10): 415, 1987.
4. Centers for Disease Control. *Guidelines for the Prevention and Control of Nosocomial Infections.* Springfield, VA: National Technical Information Service, U.S. Department of Commerce, 1982.
5. Centers for Disease Control. *National Nosoco-*

mial Infections Study: Quarterly Reports. Atlanta: Centers for Disease Control, 1970–1983.

6. Centers for Disease Control. *Outline for Surveillance and Control of Nosocomial Infections.* Atlanta: Centers for Disease Control, 1972.

7. Centers for Disease Control. *Proceedings of the First International Conference on Nosocomial Infections, Atlanta, Aug. 5–8, 1970.* Chicago: American Hospital Association, 1970.

8. Centers for Disease Control, Association of Schools of Public Health. *A Report of the Meeting of the CDC/ASPH Working Group on Nosocomial Infection Control Training, April 12–13, 1983.* Atlanta: Centers for Disease Control, 1983.

9. Condon, R.E., Haley, R.W., Lee, J.T., Jr., and Meakins, J.L. Does infection control control infection? *Arch. Surg.* 123:250, 1988.

10. Cruse, P.J.E., and Foord, R. The epidemiology of wound infection: A 10-year prospective study of 62,939 wounds. *Surg. Clin. North Am.* 60:27, 1980.

11. Deming, W.E. The statistical procedure in the SENIC Project. *Am. J. Epidemiol.* 111:470, 1980.

12. Eickhoff, T.C., Brachman, P.S., Bennett, J.V., and Brown, J.F. Surveillance of nosocomial infections in community hospitals: I. Surveillance methods, effectiveness, and initial results. *J. Infect. Dis.* 120:305, 1969.

13. Emori, T.G., et al. Comparison of surveillance and control activities of infection control nurses and infection control laboratorians in United States hospitals, 1976–1977. *Am. J. Infect. Control.* 10:3, 1982.

14. Emori, T.G., Haley, R.W., and Stanley, R.C. The infection control nurse in U.S. hospitals, 1976–1977: Characteristics of the position and its occupant. *Am. J. Epidemiol.* 111:592, 1980.

15. Fuchs, P.C. *Epidemiology of Hospital-Associated Infections.* Chicago: American Society of Clinical Pathologists, 1979. Pp. 74–78.

16. Gardner, A.M.N., Stamp, M., Bowgen, J.A., and Moore, B. The infection control sister. *Lancet* 2:710, 1962.

17. Goldmann, D.A. Nosocomial infection control in the United States of America. *J. Hosp. Infect.* 8:116, 1986.

18. Haley, R.W. CDC guidelines on infection control: Introduction. *Infect. Control* 2:117, 1981.

19. Haley, R.W. The "hospital epidemiologist" in U.S. hospitals, 1976–1977: A description of the head of the infection surveillance and control program. *Infect. Control* 1:21, 1980.

20. Haley, R.W. *Managing Hospital Infection Control for Cost-Effectiveness: A Strategy for Reducing Infectious Complications.* Chicago: American Hospital Publishing, 1986.

21. Haley, R.W. The role of infectious disease physicians in hospital infection control. *Bull. N.Y. Acad. Med.* 63(6): 597, 1987.

22. Haley, R.W., et al. Identifying patients at high risk of surgical wound infection. *Am. J. Epidemiol.* 121(2): 206, 1985.

23. Haley, R.W., et al. The efficacy of infection surveillance and control programs in preventing nosocomial infections in U.S. hospitals. *Am. J. Epidemiol.* 121(2): 182, 1985.

24. Haley, R.W., et al. Hospital infection control: Recent progress and opportunities under prospective payment. *Am. J. Infect. Control* 13 (3): 97, 1985.

25. Haley, R.W., et al. Extra days and prolongation of stay attributable to nosocomial infections: A prospective interhospital comparison. *Am. J. Med.* 70:51, 1981.

26. Haley, R.W., et al. Study on the efficacy of nosocomial infection control (SENIC Project): Summary of study design. *Am. J. Epidemiol.* 111:472, 1980.

27. Haley, R.W., and Shachtman, R.H. The emergence of infection surveillance and control programs in U.S. hospitals: An assessment, 1976. *Am. J. Epidemiol.* 111:574, 1980.

28. Haley, R.W., White, J.W., Culver, D.H., and Hughes, J.M. The financial incentive for hospitals to prevent nosocomial infections under the prospective payment system. *J.A.M.A.* 257(12):1611, 1987.

29. Inglehart, J.K. The new era of prospective payment for hospitals. *N. Engl. J. Med.* 307: 1288, 1982.

30. Joint Commission on Accreditation of Healthcare Organizations. Standards: Infection Control. In: JCAHO, Accreditation Manual for Hospitals. Chicago: Joint Commission on Accreditation of Healthcare Organizations, 1990.

31. Joint Commission on Accreditation of Hospitals. Standards: Infection Control. In: JCAH, *Accreditation Manual for Hospitals.* Chicago: Joint Commission on Accreditation of Hospitals, 1976.

32. LaHaise, S. A comparison of infection control software for use by hospital epidemiologists in meeting the new JCAHO standards. *Infect. Control Hosp. Epidemiol.* 11(4): 185, 1990.

33. Landry, S. Survey of infection control practices in Virginia (abstr.). In *Proceedings of the International Conference of the Association for Practitioners in Infection Control, 1988.* Dallas, TX, May 1–8, 1988.

34. Larson, E., Eisenberg, R., and Soule, B.M. Validating the certification process for infection control practice. *Am. J. Infect. Control* 16: 198, 1988.

35. McArthur, B.J., et al. A national task analysis of infection control practitioners, 1982. Part 1: Methodology and demography. *Am. J. Infect. Control* 12(2): 88, 1984.

36. Moore, W.L., Jr. Nosocomial infections: An overview. *Am. J. Hosp. Pharm.* 351:832, 1974.
37. Pugliese, G., et al. A national task analysis of infection control practitioners, 1982. Part 3: The relationship between hospital size and tasks performed. *Am. J. Infect. Control* 12(4): 221, 1984.
38. Raven, B.H., Freeman, H.E., and Haley, R.W. Social Science Perspectives in Hospital Infection Control. In: A.W. Johnson, O. Grusky, and B.H. Raven (Eds.), *Contemporary Health Services—Social Science Perspectives.* Boston: Auburn House, 1981. Pp. 137–176.
39. Raven, B.H., and Haley, R.W. Social influence in a medical context. *Appl. Soc. Psychol. Annu.,* 1:255, 1980.
40. Raven, B.H., and Haley, R.W. Social influence and compliance of hospital nurses with infection control policies. *Soc. Psychol. Behav. Med.* 17:413, 1980.
41. Seto, W.H., et al. Brief report: The utilization of influencing tactics for the implementation of infection control policies. *Infect. Control Hosp. Epidemiol.* 11:144, 1990.
42. Shannon, R., et al. A national task analysis of infection control practitioners, 1982. Part 2: Tasks, knowledge, and abilities for practice. *Am. J. Infect. Control* 12(3): 187, 1984.
43. Shoji, K.T., Axnick, K., and Rytel, M.W. Infections and antibiotic use in a large municipal hospital 1970–1972: A prospective analysis of the effectiveness of a continuous surveillance program. *Health Lab. Sci.* 11:283, 1974.
44. Stamm, W.E. Elements of an active, effective infection control program. *Hospitals* 50:60, 1976.
45. Streeter, S., Dunn, H., and Lepper, M. Hospital infection—a necessary risk? *Am. J. Nurs.* 67:526, 1967.
46. Turner, J.G., Booth, W.C., Brown, K.C., and Williamson, K.M. National survey of infection control practitioners' educational needs. *Am. J. Infect. Control* 18(2): 86, 1990.
47. University of Michigan School of Public Health, Mayo Foundation, Communicable Disease Center. *Proceedings of the National Conference on Institutionally Acquired Infections, Minneapolis, Sept. 4–6, 1963.* Atlanta: Centers for Disease Control, 1963.
48. U.S. General Accounting Office. *Infection Control: Military Programs Are Comparable to VA and Nonfederal Programs but Can Be Enhanced* (GAO/HRD-90-74). Report to Congressional requestors. Washington, DC: U.S. General Accounting Office, April 1990.
49. U.S. Public Health Service Communicable Diseases Center and the National Academy of Sciences National Research Council. *Proceedings of the National Conference on Hospital-Acquired Staphylococcal Disease, Atlanta, Sept. 15–17, 1958.* Atlanta: Centers for Disease Control, 1958.
50. U.S. Public Health Service Communicable Diseases Center and the National Academy of Sciences National Research Council. *Proceedings of the Conference on Relation of the Environment to Hospital-Acquired Staphylococcal Disease, Atlanta, Dec. 1–2, 1958.* Atlanta: Centers for Disease Control, 1958.
51. Wenzel, K.S. The role of the infection control nurse. *Nurs. Clin. North Am.* 5:89, 1970.
52. Wenzel, R.P. Nosocomial infections, diagnosis-related groups, and the Study on the Efficacy of Nosocomial Infection Control: Economic implications for hospitals under the prospective payment system. *Am. J. Med.* 78(Suppl. 6B): 3, 1985.

5

Surveillance of Nosocomial Infections

Robert W. Haley
Robert P. Gaynes
Robert C. Aber
John V. Bennett

Definition of Surveillance

Surveillance, when applied to disease, may be defined as "the systematic, active, ongoing observation of the occurrence and distribution of disease within a population and of the events or conditions that increase or decrease the risk of such disease occurrence." The term implies that the observational data are regularly analyzed and disseminated to those individuals who need to know them in order to take appropriate actions. Surveillance of disease should be a continuous process that consists of the following elements: (1) defining as concisely and precisely as possible the events to be surveyed; (2) collecting the relevant data in a systematic way; (3) consolidating or tabulating the data into meaningful arrangements; (4) analyzing and interpreting the data; and (5) using the information to bring about change.

In the past, some argued that the concept of surveillance involved only the collection and analysis of data and that the uses of the results were part of a separate control activity. This separation has been widely rejected, however, consequent to cogent criticism of modern infection control programs for collecting large amounts of surveillance data that were never used to change infection risks. Increasingly, the intended uses of surveillance results have become an integral part of the surveillance activity and, in the form of outcome objectives, they have also become the basis for designing surveillance systems.

Historical Perspective

In the decade since the first edition of this book was published, a great deal of discussion and debate has concerned the desirability of continuing routine surveillance, argued by some to be too personnel-intensive in a milieu of constrained hospital budgets. As this discussion continues, an account of how the modern concepts and techniques of surveillance came to be—how we got where we are now—should be considered. Many of these practices were developed to meet emerging problems, and the basic concept has been found effective in reducing infection risks. Knowledge of the historical reasons for these developments may help improve the efficiency and effectiveness of surveillance without discarding well-conceived approaches that remain effective.

The use of surveillance methods to control nosocomial infections dates back at least to the classic work of Dr. Ignaz Semmelweis in Vienna in the 1840s [51]. Although the Semmelweis story is best remembered as the first demonstration of the importance of person-to-person spread of puerperal sepsis and of the effectiveness of washing hands with an antiseptic solution, an equally important achievement was Semmelweis's rigorous approach to the collection, analysis, and use of surveillance data. In contrast, the concurrent work of Dr. Oliver Wendell Holmes on the same subject in the United States was based primarily on the traditional anecdotal case-study approach of clinical medicine.

Semmelweis's investigation constitutes an amazingly contemporary example of the effective use of surveillance in addressing a widespread infection problem. When he assumed the directorship of the obstetric service at the Vienna Lying In Hospital in 1847, the apparent risk of maternal mortality had been at high levels for more than 20 years, so long that the eminent clinicians of the day considered the risks to be no more than the expected endemic occurrence that could not be influenced. Semmelweis first undertook a retrospective investigation of maternal mortality and set up a prospective surveillance system to monitor the problem and the effects of later control measures. The initial results of his retrospective study of annual hospital mortality lists showed clearly that the maternal mortality level, which he measured by simply calculating yearly mortality rates, had indeed increased tenfold following the introduction in the 1820s of the new anatomic school of pathology, which utilized the autopsy as its primary teaching tool. His second discovery, based on the use of ward-specific mortality, was that the risk of death in the ward used for teaching medical students was at least four times higher than that in the ward used for teaching midwifery students. After the septic death of his mentor suggested the presence of a transmissible agent, Semmelweis used the findings from his retrospective surveillance study to implicate the practices of the medical students. After observing their daily routines, he surmised that students might be transferring the infection from their cadavers to the parturient women and that washing hands with a chlorine solution might prevent transmission. Subsequently, his prospective surveillance data documented a dramatic reduction in maternal mortality immediately following the institution of mandatory hand-washing before entering the labor room.

Here the great insights of Semmelweis ended, as often happens to infection control efforts today. Apparently due to his abrasive manner and lack of diplomacy as well as an inability to organize his statistical data into a concise convincing report, Semmelweis failed to win over his clinical colleagues to his discovery. Within 2 years, he was dismissed from the staff of the hospital, and his successor gradually allowed the strict hand-washing measures to decline. In the absence of continuing surveillance, the epidemic promptly resumed and lasted well into the early part of the twentieth century, its severity and means of prevention apparently unappreciated by several more generations of clinicians.

This story well illustrates one of the main impediments to infection control today—namely, that in the absence of careful epidemiologic data and a diplomatic presentation, clinicians, who are oriented almost entirely toward the treatment of their individual patients, often fail to appreciate the severity of the infection transmission problem and sometimes even resist control measures. It also points out the utility of surveillance in identifying problems and developing and applying control measures. From a methodologic viewpoint, Semmelweis's efforts encompassed almost all aspects of the modern surveillance approach: retrospective collection of data to confirm the presence of a problem; analysis of the data to localize the risks in time, place, and person; controlled comparisons of high- and low-risk groups to identify risk factors; formulation and application of control measures; and prospective surveillance to monitor the problem, evaluate the control measures, and detect future recurrences. The main shortcoming of his approach was in not diplomatically educating his powerful colleagues with a careful report of his findings.

As good a model as Semmelweis's work was, the modern era of nosocomial infection surveillance grew as much out of different currents of the midtwentieth century as from the Semmelweis tradition. The importance of surveillance for disease control in general arose as a central concept in the effort to control tropical diseases among troops stationed in the Pacific Theater in World War II. At the end of the war, the core of the epidemiologists of the Malaria Control in War Areas unit were transferred to a civilian facility to apply their surveillance and control strategies to the control of malaria in the southern United States. Located in Atlanta near the endemic areas, the unit was first named the Communicable Diseases Center and later became the Centers for Disease Control (CDC). Since the large number of reports of malaria indicated the disease to be widespread, a surveillance system was immediately set up to define the problem, but as investigators examined each reported case, they found virtually all the reports to be errors in diagnosis. Thus, the mere activity of surveillance "eradicated" the malaria epidemic in the United States.

With this and similar successes fresh in memory, when the pandemic of staphylococcal infections swept the nation's hospitals in the mid-1950s, CDC staff members were quick to apply the concepts of surveillance to the problem [35]. Once asked to assist in

investigating a staphylococcal epidemic in a particular hospital, those early investigators often met strong resistance from clinicians and hospital administrators convinced that no unusual infection problems were present in their hospital. In instances where the CDC staff members were able to continue the investigations, the collection and reporting of surveillance data regularly changed those attitudes to strong concern over the documented problems and eagerness to apply control measures. These initial investigations thus confirmed a nationwide staphylococcal epidemic and led the CDC to sponsor several national conferences to discuss the problem.

As the epidemic subsided in the early 1960s, the CDC's Surveillance Unit continued to develop more effective surveillance methods specifically geared to the hospital situation. By 1970, on the basis of pilot studies, the CDC was recommending that surveillance be practiced routinely in all hospitals. The results were that by the late 1970s almost all U.S. hospitals had adopted the approach, and surveillance culturing of the inanimate environment had been virtually abandoned (see Chaps. 4, 15). In 1976, the Joint Commission on Accreditation of Hospitals (JCAH) incorporated a detailed surveillance system into their standards for accreditation.

By the early 1980s, the pendulum began swinging back in the opposite direction as critics questioned the effectiveness and cost benefit of routine infection surveillance, although more hospitals were still increasing their surveillance efforts than were decreasing them [31]. There is some indication that the inability of some larger hospitals to establish an adequate number of positions for infection control practitioners (at least one full-time-equivalent practitioner per 250 beds) was a major contributor to the disenchantment with routine infection surveillance.

Several factors have influenced contemporary practices favoring a strong surveillance component to infection control programs. First, the continued requirements of the Joint Commission on Accreditation of Healthcare Organizations (JCAHO, formerly JCAH) have legitimized the need for personnel to perform surveillance [37, 38]. Second, the results of the Study on the Efficacy of Nosocomial Infection Control (SENIC) strongly substantiated the essential nature of surveillance along with control measures to reduce infection rates [24, 25, 28]. The strong conclusion was that without an organized, routine, hospitalwide surveillance system, even the most vigorous control policies are unlikely to be successful. To the extent that these results are accepted, the continuing discussions of surveillance can be expected to turn away from questioning the value of surveillance to identifying how to perform surveillance most efficiently without reducing its proved effectiveness. Third, the surveillance practices developed in infection control have begun to influence other aspects of the hospital's patient care review activities. As the concept of targeting surveillance to the reduction of specific endemic problems and monitoring further to ensure an impact [24, 25] were incorporated into the JCAHO's 1990 infection control standards for accreditation [38], the strategy was also applied to hospital quality assurance programs to reduce noninfectious complications [42]. The increasing pressure to continually improve quality is certain to exacerbate the use of surveillance to stimulate change.

The Technique of Surveillance
Reasons for Employing Surveillance
In setting up a new surveillance system or in revamping an old one, it is important to design the surveillance activities to accomplish specific prevention objectives. An all too common, and less desirable, approach has been to examine the surveillance practices of other local hospitals, or those recommended by authoritative experts, and simply begin using them on a routine basis, without defining how they will change infection risks. Unlike intervention or control activities, the mere act of collecting surveillance data does not usually influence infection risks appreciably, although in some serious epidemic situations, a highly visible investigation may change patient care practices and end the problem.

Given the growing financial constraints on hospital budgets and the often limited size of hospital infection control staffs, it has been increasingly necessary to plan surveillance efforts with a different approach. To translate surveillance efforts into infection prevention, it is necessary to identify and state objectives of surveillance before designing and starting surveillance. Many of the uses to which surveillance has been put are summarized as follows.

Establishing Baseline Rates
The most fundamental use of surveillance is the measurement of baseline rates of endemic nosocomial infections. Its prime functions are to provide objective quantitative knowledge of the ongoing infection risks in the hospital and to serve as the basis for the other uses of surveillance. It can also lead directly to the prevention of infections. Finding that endemic infection rates are higher than anticipated often stimulates a search for unsuspected causes that might not otherwise have been made. In the SENIC interview survey in 1976, surveillance was reported to have been used for this purpose in 91 percent of hospitals [15]. This process is aided by analyzing the surveillance data to obtain infection rates that are readily interpretable, such as rates by type of infection, pathogen, or service or hospital area and, in some instances, by individual hospital personnel. Approximately three-fourths of hospitals reported performing these types of analyses of their surveillance data [15].

Identifying Epidemics
The most often discussed use of surveillance is the identification of epidemics. In the SENIC national interview survey, this use was reported by 81 percent of the hospitals [15]. By regularly measuring the infection rates, one can recognize deviations from the baseline rates that sometimes represent epidemics due to a new common source of infection, the introduction of a new virulent pathogen, or increased person-to-person spread from a breakdown in patient care practices.

Justifying the relatively time-consuming activity of routine surveillance and calculation of baseline rates is a complex management issue. On the one hand, when a serious epidemic occurs, particularly when one or more deaths are attributed to it, hospital officials are usually eager to have baseline data with which to confirm quickly the extent of the problem, to pinpoint precisely what changes have occurred in the rates, and to demonstrate that all appropriate measures are being taken. Historically, the usefulness of such data in an epidemic investigation and its perceived value in prevention or earlier recognition of future problems have often been the justification for establishing ongoing surveillance activities. On the other hand, since only a small proportion of nosocomial infections occur in outbreaks or epidemics [34], the justification for routine surveillance must include additional uses that contribute to the control of both endemic and epidemic infections.

Convincing Clinicians

Perhaps the most important use of surveillance—and ironically, the one most often overlooked—is to arm the infection control staff with information that will allow them to convince physicians, nurses, and hospital administrators of the need for preventive actions. Typically, infection control personnel believe that getting hospital personnel to agree when there are serious problems and to adopt the recommended preventive practices is their most difficult task.

Sociologic theory on the means by which people or groups are influenced lists six fundamental bases of social power: (1) providing information that will influence behavior (information power); (2) presenting oneself as an expert whose advice should be followed (expert power); (3) presenting oneself as a legitimate authority with the right to require compliance (legitimacy power); (4) referring to the acceptable conduct of one's peers to obtain his or her compliance (referent power); (5) threatening punishments for failure to conform (coercion power); (6) offering rewards for conformity (reward power). From the SENIC interview survey, it appears that information and expert power were the only

bases of social power used by most infection control nurses, Infection Control Committee chairpersons, and hospital epidemiologists [47]. Staff nurses indicated that their practices would be influenced almost exclusively by these two as well. Conversely, referent, legitimacy, coercion, and reward power were perceived as ineffective and were rarely used by infection control personnel.

How does the infection control staff either obtain sufficiently convincing information or become sufficiently recognized as expert to utilize these two bases of social power fully? A favorite way of achieving both is to become thoroughly familiar with the scientific literature on hospital epidemiology and infection control. Thus, when trying to influence a colleague, one can quote relevant references to establish expertise and to provide convincing information. This approach, however, is only as effective as the information is relevant to the specific situation in question, and since most scientific articles are unable to anticipate the many varied circumstances that affect infection risks in different hospitals, relying entirely on the body of scientific publications is ultimately a losing strategy.

Maintaining current surveillance data allows the infection control staff to present an accurate, quantitative, and timely picture of most infection problems that might arise. Since the epidemiologic analysis of patients in the aggregate is not part of the clinical training of physicians or nurses, having such information elevates the infection control staff to a unique position of expertise and respect. If the data are analyzed correctly and expeditiously and are presented skillfully, clinicians usually come to rely strongly on them for guidance. A particularly effective example is the practice of reporting individual surgeons' wound infection rates to them on a regular basis to allow them to assess their surgical skill in comparison with their peers. In contrast, hospital administrators are accustomed to viewing problems in aggregate statistical terms and often expect proposals, particularly those for money or extra resources, to be formulated in an organized quantitative manner and to be supported by relevant evidence. In short, having routine surveillance data affords the infection control staff both the information and the expert position necessary to influence key hospital staff members in critical situations.

Evaluating Control Measures

Once problems have been recognized through surveillance, potential risk factors have been identified through epidemiologic analysis, and staff members have been influenced to carry out the control measures, continued surveillance is usually necessary to ensure that the problem comes under control and remains so. One of the unfortunate realities of controlling infections is that even the most rational control measures based on the best information and sound judgment sometimes prove to be ineffective. In the absence of continued formal surveillance, it may take a long time to discover that the expected reduction in infections did not occur. Even worse, clinicians recalling the experiences of their own individual patients may disagree over the effects or argue that control is unnecessary or futile. Providing continuing evidence of the progress of the control effort at least places the discussions on a factual basis, with the total picture in view and, at best, points the way to new control strategies that will prove more effective. Even after control measures have been found effective, continuing surveillance can be important. For example, finding a recrudescence of the problem following initial successful control could lead to the identification of a breakdown in the control measures.

Reinforcing Practices

The most important measure in maintaining a sustained reduction in endemic nosocomial infection rates and preventing epidemics due to known risk factors is to perpetuate certain critical patient care practices that reduce infection risks, the so-called preventive patient care practices (e.g., aseptic urinary catheter care, changing intravenous cannulas, coughing and deep breathing in postoperative patients, hand-washing) [6]. Besides the obvious

prerequisites to gaining compliance, such as formulating correct policies, obtaining agreement of key authorities, and training personnel, surveillance can contribute substantially to sustained compliance by providing feedback to the staff on their performance. In the SENIC interview survey, the infection control staff in approximately 80 percent of hospitals claimed they monitored practices and reported surveillance results in inservice education [15].

This feedback can entail either *process evaluations* that report rates of compliance with the policy or *outcome evaluations* that report the changes in infection rates related to the policy. Process evaluations require continuing surveillance of preventive patient care practices, whereas outcome evaluations require surveillance of nosocomial infections. In some circumstances, it may be most appropriate to report these findings directly to the patient care personnel (e.g., wound infection rates to surgeons) and, in others, it might be preferable to report them to the supervisor or chief of service (e.g., a high rate of septicemia in an intensive care unit). For this activity to be most effective, it must be designed to provide relatively immediate positive reinforcement for proper compliance and to identify deficiencies at which corrective action can be directed.

Satisfying Standards

In the 1976 SENIC interview survey, the use of surveillance reported by the largest percentage of hospitals (93 percent) was to satisfy the requirements of the JCAH [15]. In that era, the JCAH directed each Infection Control Committee to develop a practical surveillance system for reporting, evaluating, and keeping records of infections among patients and hospital personnel in order to provide an indication of the endemic level of all nosocomial infections, to identify the sources of infections, and to discover real or potential epidemics [37]. In 1990, the JCAHO standard was altered fundamentally to require hospitals to use surveillance to bring about change in the risk of infection to patients

[38]. With this change the JCAHO has finally legitimized, even required, the use of surveillance for its originally intended purpose— that is, to reduce infection risks.

Defending Against Malpractice Claims

In earlier decades, one of the often voiced criticisms of surveillance was that it created a record that could be used against the hospital in litigation of a malpractice claim related to a nosocomial infection. Based on more extensive experience with malpractice claims and litigation, most legal experts now take just the opposite view, primarily for two reasons. First, in most states the records of internal hospital committees, including the Infection Control Committee, are considered privileged and not discoverable in civil court proceedings. Second, the ability to show that the hospital has a vigorous surveillance system for detecting problems that might occur is believed to be among the most important defenses against unwarranted claims (see Chap. 26). In 1976, fewer than 10 percent of hospital administrators considered surveillance data to be more often a hindrance than a help when faced with a medical malpractice claim or lawsuit [15].

Conducting Research

Apart from their fundamental place in a hospital's infection control effort, surveillance methods have formed the basis for conducting much valuable research in controlling infections in all hospitals. Early studies using surveillance to measure infection risks identified the risk factors on which many of the current infection control policies and recommendations are based. More recently, experiments such as those comparing the safety of different intervals for changing respirator breathing circuits have utilized routine surveillance methods to evaluate alternative practices. The pooling of surveillance data from many hospitals has formed the basis for the CDC's National Nosocomial Infections Surveillance (NNIS) System. The NNIS System allows the detection or confirmation of infection problems with nationwide distribu-

tions. Even though the accuracy of the surveillance data in the NNIS System may vary substantially among its hospitals, consistent definitions and standardized protocols and data collection methods have improved the uniformity of the surveillance data, and this limitation appears to have been of little practical significance in many research efforts [14, 36].

Reducing Nosocomial Infection Rates

While all of the previously mentioned purposes are legitimate reasons for surveillance, the ultimate objective of any surveillance system is to reduce the risks of nosocomial infection. When evaluating the need for particular surveillance activities, one should ask how the activity can be expected to result in the reduction of infection, the *outcome objective*. The activities (e.g., establishing baseline rates, satisfying requirements, etc.) are known as *process objectives* and must not replace the outcome objective in importance. Rather, as part of the design of the surveillance program, activities not directly justified on this basis should probably be discontinued and resources redirected to more clearly outcome objective–oriented activities [24, 25] (see under the heading Priority-Directed Surveillance).

Comparing Hospitals' Nosocomial Infection Rates

Traditionally, surveillance has been recommended solely for gaining understanding of and reducing nosocomial infection rates within individual hospitals. The idea of comparing the infection rates among hospitals, though often suggested by administrators and quality assurance supervisors, has generally been discouraged by infection control physicians and practitioners because the large differences in the mix of intrinsic infection risk of the patients in different hospitals render differences among the rates virtually uninterpretable. Recent studies performed by the CDC, however, have suggested that interhospital comparisons can be useful in reducing infection risks [10, 21, 36] but, for them to be useful, the rate must be specific to a particular site of infection (e.g., urinary tract infection) and must control for variations in the distributions of the major risk factor(s) for that type of infection (e.g., duration of in-dwelling urinary catheterization). Conversely, it must be emphasized that a single number expressing the hospital's overall nosocomial infection rate is not a valid measure of the efficacy of the hospital's infection control programs largely because of the lack of suitable overall risk adjusters for infections of all types [7, 26, 41]. *Therefore, a hospital's overall nosocomial infection rate, as presently derived, should not be used for interhospital comparisons.*

Recently, the JCAHO commissioned an expert task force to formulate and test infection control "indicators" that all accredited U.S. hospitals will ultimately be required to report for the purpose of making useful comparisons among hospitals [26]. The infection control indicators developed initially are carefully formulated and defined nosocomial infection rates that are feasible to collect in most hospitals and reflect the most serious nosocomial infection problems and for which suitable intrinsic risk indexes are available to allow interhospital comparisons to be meaningfully made. It is noteworthy that the task force rejected the overall hospital nosocomial infection rate from the list of indicators because of the infeasibility of doing continuous total-hospital surveillance in many hospitals and the lack of a proved means of controlling for differences in hospitals' mix of patient risk [26].

Hospitals will be expected to analyze the data that they collect for the indicators to make improvements in care and then transmit the infection rate indicators to the JCAHO for analyses comparing hospitals. The distributions of hospitals on the indicator rates, stratified by intrinsic risk indexes, will be reported to hospitals for their use in identifying potential problems in care that could be addressed by further surveillance and control efforts in the hospital. Accreditation decisions will not be made on the basis of the interhospital comparisons but, instead, on the basis of how hospitals responded to the findings of the comparisons.

Methods of Surveillance
Collecting the Data
Defining Events to Be Surveyed   It is of utmost importance, in developing a surveillance system, to define carefully those events to be surveyed and then to apply the accepted definitions systematically in the data-collecting process. In attempting to understand the relationship between urinary tract infection and urinary catheterization, for example, it is necessary first to define or establish criteria to decide what will be called a urinary tract infection and what will be considered urinary catheterization. Once the event to be surveyed has been defined as concisely and precisely as possible and the criteria for determining its presence or absence have been established, then it is imperative that these definitions and criteria be applied systematically and uniformly henceforth. Ideally, all members of the population judged at risk for the occurrence of the event would be systematically and continuously assessed for the presence or absence of the properties specified by the criteria that define the event or the infection being sought. By 1976, written definitions for nosocomial infections were being used in three-fourths of U.S. hospitals [15] and, by 1988, 97 percent of hospitals were using them [52].

The CDC has published guidelines for determining the presence and classification of infection [5, 19]. These guidelines are not rigorous definitions of disease, but rather they serve as practical, operational definitions for most hospitals, regardless of their size or medical sophistication. In constructing the criteria to be used in surveillance, the exact definitions decided on are not as critical as that the Infection Control Committee obtain the concurrence of key hospital staff members. Such widespread advance agreement is necessary to avoid having the results of surveillance later disqualified by disagreements over the definitions.

It is also important that consistent criteria be used in determining the service to which a patient belongs. The service to which the patient was assigned at the time of acquisition of the infection should be used. If this determination is not possible, then the patient should be assigned to the service on which he or she resided at the time of onset of the infection.

Role of the Infection Control Practitioner A number of methods of collecting infection data have been described in the literature. In general, the most satisfactory and practical method at present employs a person (or persons), often called the *infection control practitioner* (ICP), whose job description includes collecting and analyzing surveillance data. Details of the qualifications, functions, and responsibilities of the ICP were given previously (see Chap. 4). The ICP is responsible to the Infection Control Committee and should be under the immediate supervision of the committee chairperson or the hospital epidemiologist, if the hospital has one. The traditional choice of a nurse to fill this position has been primarily based on his or her professional training and ability to interact primarily with other nursing personnel in the data collection process, but experience has shown that persons other than nurses can also function well, particularly in the surveillance process. The original studies of surveillance conducted by the CDC indicated that one full-time-equivalent ICP could conduct surveillance for approximately 250 acute-care hospital beds and have sufficient remaining time for other infection control duties and responsibilities [5]. In recent years, as the average length of a patient's hospital stay has decreased, patient turnover has become more rapid, and patients' severity of illness has increased, the ICP's job has become more demanding. Often with no increase in staffing, ICPs have had to set priorities for the use of their time in ways that will maximize their impact on infection risks; this can be done only by directing efforts at specific outcome objectives [25].

Minimal Data to Collect about Infections The precise information collected in conjunction with each infection may vary according to the institution, service, site of infection, or causative agent. Certain essential identifying data, however, can be recommended: the patient's name, age, sex, hospital identification number, ward or location within the hospital, service, and date of admission; the date of onset of the infection; the site of infection; the organism(s) isolated in culture studies; and the antimicrobial susceptibility pattern of the organisms isolated. Additional information should be collected only if it will be analyzed and used by the hospital. Some institutions may wish to include the primary diagnoses of the infected patients, an assessment of the severity of underlying illness(es), the name(s) of the attending physician(s) or other staff who attended the patient, whether exposure occurred—before the onset of infection—to therapies that may predispose to infection (e.g., surgery; antibiotic, steroid, or immunosuppressive therapy; or instrumentation), what antimicrobial agents were used to treat the infection, and some assessment of mortality related to the infection. Recording the presence or absence of particular exposure factors may be useful for certain types of infections—for example, urinary catheterization for urinary tract infections; respiratory therapy equipment for respiratory infections; and the use of intravenous, subclavian, or arterial catheters for primary bacteremia.

This information may be recorded on a file card or a form by the ICP, and it may subsequently be transferred to a computer for analysis if such is available. It is important to update the infection file—whether it be on cards, forms, or computer disk—as new information becomes available.

Denominators The methods for obtaining the denominators for infection rates have always been the most controversial and have often been the most labor-intensive aspect of generating nosocomial infection rates. In the precomputer era, the usual method was simply to count the number of patients admitted to or discharged from the hospital, or from a particular ward or service, as a crude estimate of the number of patients at risk of infection; later, hospital mainframe computers provided these denominator counts on daily or monthly printouts. Infection rates were generated by dividing the number of infections, obtained from surveillance, by the appropriate denominator to yield the overall hospital infection rate or ward- or service-specific rates. A special use of such "user-supplied denominators" is to count *patient-days* rather than admissions or discharges. Patient-day denominators are derived by summing the number of days that all included patients stayed in the hospital. Since the patient-day denominator includes length of stay, the resulting infection rates are at least partially adjusted for differences among patients' lengths of stay. As with other user-supplied denominators, patient-days for the hospital as a whole and by service can be obtained from most hospitals' medical records department or business office.

In the modern computer era, however, ICPs who have computerized their surveillance data on their own microcomputers often generate the numerators, denominators, and rates all in one step directly from their surveillance database [40]. This is done by entering a computer record for every patient at risk rather than for the infections only. The record contains the risk factors for all patients at risk of infection (e.g., all patients undergoing a surgical operation), and then the information about nosocomial infections is added to the affected patients' records when infections are detected. From this type of complete patient database, the computer simply calculates infection rates for whatever time period and patient population the ICP selects, and the denominators are generated automatically for the calculations. While entering all patients at risk might seem more time-consuming than the traditional method, it is preferable for targeted surveillance projects, such as generating surgeon-specific rates by class or intensive care unit surveillance, because ICPs have far more flexibility in the types of rates that they can generate. With a full database, they can calculate rates by any risk factor, or combination of risk factors, contained in the database. This alternative is made even more attractive by the ability to "download" the denominator records from other hospital computers: For example, the records of all operations can be downloaded daily from the operating room computer. As surveillance becomes increasingly targeted toward specific prevention objectives, user-supplied denominators are expected to be employed less often. (See Chap. 8.)

Sources of Infection Data

The effective ICP must utilize a wide variety of sources of infection information, both from within and outside the hospital, to ensure the most complete enumeration of the infections [1, 15]. The main methods used for detecting cases of infection and the frequency of use of each among U.S. hospitals in the mid-1970s are shown in Figure 5-1. The active techniques of case finding, which are used in almost all hospitals, are strongly preferred to the passive techniques [1]. The active techniques not only allow more complete detection of cases but also provide the opportunity for the ICP to visit the patient care areas regularly, to interact with and provide consultation to the medical and nursing staffs, and to gain firsthand awareness of the infection problems. The passive techniques, particularly the practice of expecting physicians or staff nurses to fill out infection report forms, have been shown to be extremely inaccurate for the routine detection of infections. Hospitals relying on passive techniques typically find extremely low nosocomial infection rates, but these are due to underreporting rather than good practice [1].

The Microbiology Laboratory Of the case-finding methods listed in Figure 5-1, one of the most useful is the periodic (usually daily) review of microbiology laboratory reports. This may be performed each morning prior to making ward rounds, so any new or potential infections can be inspected during ward rounds. Such review requires that the ICP understand the infectious and epidemiologic potential of various microorganisms; such knowledge might be achieved in a laboratory

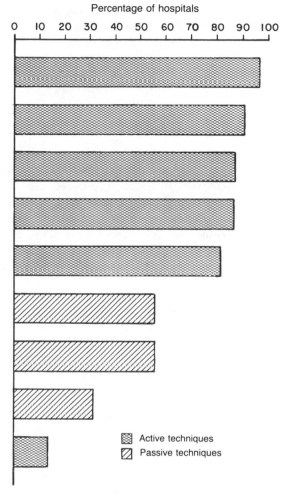

Fig. 5-1. Active and passive case-finding methods used in surveillance. IC = intensive care.

training period at the time of employment and should be reinforced by periodic inservice review sessions. It must be stressed that a review of the microbiology laboratory reports alone is not sufficient for the identification of nosocomial infections, because (1) cultures are not obtained for all infections or may be handled incorrectly; (2) some infectious agents (e.g., viruses) will not be identified in many hospitals' laboratories; and (3) for some types of infections (e.g., surgical wound infections and pneumonia), the identification of a potentially pathogenic organism from a culture specimen does not mean that infection

is present; such infections require clinical detection and verification (see Chap. 9).

Ward Rounds Periodic (preferably daily) ward rounds by the ICP should be included as an integral part of an effective surveillance program. The purposes of such rounds are to identify new infections, to follow up previously identified infections, and to consult with the nursing staff about infection control policies and practices. New infections may be identified outright by physicians or nurses working in the area visited, by review of temperature records, by follow-up of suspicious microbiology laboratory reports, by review of patients having high-risk procedures (such as surgery, urinary tract instrumentation, or indwelling urinary or intravenous catheters), and by review of patients in isolation or receiving antimicrobial therapy. Ward visitation also allows direct inspection and documentation of visible infections, which increases the validity of the data collected.

Postdischarge Follow-up With the progressive reduction in the average length of stay of patients in U.S. hospitals, the percentage of certain nosocomial infections that become manifest after the patient's discharge from the hospital has been increasing. This appears to be true particularly for surgical wound infections, but less so for urniary tract infections, primary bacteremia, and pneumonia, which still occur predominantly before the patient's discharge. In various studies, the percentage of wound infections becoming manifest after discharge has ranged from 20 to 60 percent [8, 43, 48, 53, 56], and at least one study has shown the presence of a strong selection bias in rates based only on in-hospital surveillance [53]. Since the average postoperative length of stay of surgical patients will influence the probability that wound infections will be reconized while the patient is still in the hospital, this variable must be taken into account when analyzing and evaluating a hospital's wound infection rate. Multihospital analyses of wound infection rates in the SENIC Project used length of stay as a covariate in multiple regression analyses [28]; others have suggested using the incidence density (i.e., patient-days in the denominator of the wound infection rates). Increasingly, surgeons are recommending that surgical patients be followed up by postcard or telephone call to the patients or surgeons at 21 to 30 days after the date of the operation to determine whether wound infection occurred [8, 43, 48, 53, 56]. Though this creates additional work for the surveillance staff, the amount of work appears to be commensurate with the gain in completeness and accuracy of the rates.

Other Sources Additional infection information may be obtained through a periodic review of x-ray laboratory reports, records of personnel health clinic visits, and autopsy reports. The exclusive use of alternative methods of infection data collection—such as the review of postdischarge medical records or the use of infection report forms filled out by attending physicians or floor nurses—is less satisfactory from the standpoint of infection control. The former method suffers from its ex post facto nature. Valuable time may be lost between the onset of the infection and its discovery by this method, and such delay may result in excessive morbidity or mortality among patients or hospital personnel. The latter method has been utilized in a number of hospitals, but it suffers from the lack of systematic application of standard definitions and criteria for detecting infection, as well as from great variation from person to person in the completeness of reporting infection.

Consolidating and Tabulating Data
Since it is difficult to recognize potentially important relationships or patterns of infection from the raw data on the file cards, worksheets, or line-listing forms, it is necessary to consolidate the data in ways that make it more understandable. The most effective analyses of surveillance data may take many forms, depending on the objective being addressed by the surveillance. When doing routine, total hospital surveillance, ICPs often simply count and record the number of infections in single-variable frequency tables (e.g., number of infections by service, site, or pathogen) and two-way cross-tabulations (e.g., number of infections by site on each hospital service, by pathogen on each hospital service, and by pathogen for each site), and tally antimicrobial susceptibility patterns for each pathogen by site of infection. In recent years, however, more imaginative analyses are usually done, including three-way rate tables (e.g., pathogen by site by service), four-way rate tables (e.g., susceptibility patterns by pathogen by site by service), and more complex cross-tabulations. Usually these tabulations are per-

formed in subsets of the patients, such as those on a particular service or the patients of a specific surgeon. To do these adequately is increasingly requiring the computerized analysis of patient databases.

Although beginning infection control personnel should first master the standard frequency and cross-tabulation routines mentioned previously, more experienced personnel should begin to try more creative ways of organizing the infection data. The basic purpose of tabulating the infections is to gain a new understanding of when, where, and in whom the infections are occurring. One of the most frequent mistakes made at this stage is to make the initial tabulations hastily and proceed with calculating rates without pausing to examine the data and think about them. It is often very useful just to read over the original listings and the initial simple tabulations to let the mind synthesize the data and suggest additional tabulations, graphs, listings, and so on. For example, finding an increased rate of bacteremias on surgery might call for a tabulation of bacteremias for each surgical subspecialty or for each surgical ward and the surgical intensive care unit, and comparisons with similar rates from previous months or for the same months the previous year. This process of freewheeling exploration of the data has no rigid rules; that is right which works!

Calculating Rates

Definition of Rate   After the intial tabulations of the infections are complete, the infection control staff should have strong suspicions of where infection problems might be occurring. Since these hunches are based solely on examination of infections (numerator data), further analysis involving the calculation of rates is necessary to develop stronger evidence. A practical way of doing this is to write in the denominator data, obtained in the data collection stage, below the appropriate numerator figures in the frequency and cross-tables of infections tabulated earlier. From these numerators (indicating the numbers of infections) and their denominators (indicat-

ing the numbers of patients, or patient-days, at risk for the infections), infection rates can be calculated. Alternatively, currently available computer software can calculate the numerator, denominator, and rate automatically from a database containing all patients at risk and the nosocomial infections that occurred in them.

A *rate* is an expression of the probability of occurrence of some particular event, and it has the form $k(x/y)$, where x, the numerator, equals the number of times an event has occurred during a specific time interval; y, the denominator, equals a population from which those experiencing the event were derived during the same time interval; and k equals a round number (100, 1,000, 10,000, 100,000, and so on) called a *base*. The base that is used depends on the magnitude of x/y, and it is selected to permit the rate to be expressed as a convenient whole number. For example, if 5 infections were found among 100 patients in a given month, the value of x/y would be 0.05 infections per patient per month; to express the rate as a convenient whole number, x/y would be multiplied by the base number 100, giving 5 infections per 100 patients per month. If 50 infections were found among 10,000 patients in a month, the base number 1,000 would be used to express the rate as 5 infections per 1,000 patients per month. It is important to emphasize that in determining a rate, both the time interval and the population must be specified, and these must apply to both the numerator (x) and the denominator (y) of the rate expression.

Types of Rates   Three specific kinds of rates—prevalence, incidence, and attack rate—are fundamental tools of epidemiology and, as such, must be familiar to infection control personnel. *Prevalence* is the number of cases of the disease found to be *active* within a defined population either during a specified period of time (period prevalence) or at a specified point in time (point prevalence); these concepts are discussed in a later section of this chapter. *Incidence* is the number of *new* cases of disease that occur in a defined population during a specified period of time. The incidence rate is obtained by dividing the number of new cases by the number of people in the population at risk during the specified time period. In Figure 5-2, which portrays the infection status of 10 hospitalized patients, the incidence of infection during either time period A or B, for example, would be 3, since 3 new infections began among the 10 patients in each time period. Assuming that period A was 1 month and period B was 3 months, the incidence rates would be 3 infections per 10 patients at risk (30 percent) per month in period A and 10 percent per month in period B (i.e., exactly equivalent to 30 percent per 3 months).

An *attack rate* is a special kind of incidence rate. It is usually expressed as a percentage (i.e., $k = 100$ in the rate expression), and it is used almost exclusively for describing epidemics where particular populations are exposed for limited periods of time (e.g., in common-source outbreaks). Since the duration of the epidemic is reasonably short, the

period of time to which the rate refers is not stated explicitly but is assumed. This is what distinguishes an attack rate from an incidence rate, where the period of time is always stated. If 100 infants in a newborn nursery, for example, were exposed to a contaminated lot of infant formula over a 3-week period, and if 14 of the infants developed a characteristic illness believed to be caused by the contaminated formula, then the attack rate for those infants exposed to the formula would be 14 percent. Notice that the incidence rate would be 14 cases per 100 infants per 3 weeks, preferably expressed as 4.67 cases per 100 infants per week.

Choice of Numerator and Denominator The fact that multiple infections occasionally occur in individual patients somewhat complicates the calculation of rates. Basically two types of incidence rates can be calculated: The *infection ratio* is the number of infections divided by the number of patients at risk during the specified period, and the *infection pro-*

Fig. 5-2. Infection status of 10 hospitalized patients. *Incidence* of infection is 3 during either time period A or B (3 new cases were added during each time period); *prevalence* of infection during

time period A is 40% and during B, 60% (4 cases and 6 cases, respectively, occur in each period of time); and *point prevalence* of infection at time C is 30% (at that point in time, 3 cases exist).

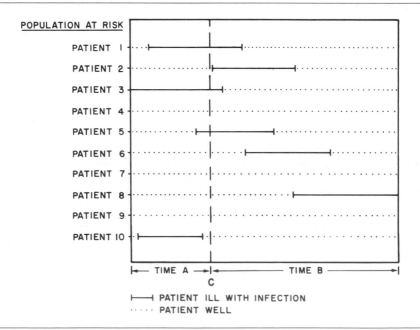

portion is the number of patients with one or more infections divided by the number of patients at risk during the time period. Since approximately 18 percent of patients with nosocomial infections have more than one infection, the infection ratio is usually nearly 1.27 times larger than the infection proportion [30]. In practice, most have found the infection ratio to be far easier to obtain than, and equally as useful as, the infection proportion, and consequently the commonly used term *infection rate* has come to refer specifically to the infection ratio. In either case, however, when presenting the results it is important to specify which method has been used for calculating the rate.

Another approach is to use for the denominator the number of patient-days at risk during the period of surveillance (i.e., the sum of all of the days spent by all patients in the specified area during the time period covered). This rate is referred to as the *incidence density*. To get an idea of how the two types of rates compare, rates based on the number of patient-days (R) are usually smaller than those based on admissions or discharges (r) by a factor approximately equal to the average length of stay of the patients (k); that is,

$$R = k \times r$$

For example, if the infection rate were found to be 5 infections per 100 admissions per month and the patients' average length of stay was 10 days, one would expect to find a rate of approximately 5 infections per 1,000 patient-days. The incidence density is useful primarily in two situations: (1) when the infection rate is a linear function of the length of time a patient is exposed to a risk factor (e.g., indwelling urinary or intravenous catheter) and (2) when the duration of follow-up will influence the measured infection rate (e.g., surgical wound infection rates when no postdischarge surveillance is done). The relative merits of the alternative ways of controlling for differences of stay, including using the incidence density, performing postdischarge follow-up of surgical patients, and

using multivariate analytic methods to control for length of stay, are yet to be clearly defined.

It is especially important that the denominator reflect the appropriate population at risk as precisely as possible. In determining the attack rate of surgical wound infection among patients on the urology service, for example, only those urology patients who actually undergo a surgical procedure that results in a wound capable of being infected would ideally be included in the denominator. Practical difficulties in obtaining such refined denominators, however, often dictate the use of a less precise denominator, such as the total number of admissions or discharges from the urology service during the appropriate period of time.

Device-days (e.g., ventilator-days or central line–days) were collected in hospitals performing surveillance in intensive care units (ICUs) as part of the NNIS System and incorporated in the denominator of rates used for interhospital comparison. The use of device-days may seem like a subtle change, but the choice of denominator was critical for purposes of interhospital comparison. To more fully illustrate this, examine the distribution of several rates for hospital ICUs (Figure 5-3). The top histogram of Figure 5-3 shows the number of central line–associated bloodstream infections per 100 patients, the middle histogram shows the number of central line–days divided by patient-days (i.e., central line utilization), and the bottom histogram shows central line–associated per 1,000 central line–days. Examining the rates for Hospital Unit A on each of the histograms, the rate on the top histogram, which uses the number of patients in the denominator, was nearly five times higher than the median. However, from the middle histogram, Hospital Unit A had the highest central line–utilization rate; that is, more than 80 percent of patient-days were also central line–days. Using central line–days as the denominator of the rate helps to take into account this high utilization of central lines. Hospital Unit A's device-associated, device-day bloodstream infection rate was slightly lower than the median (bottom histo-

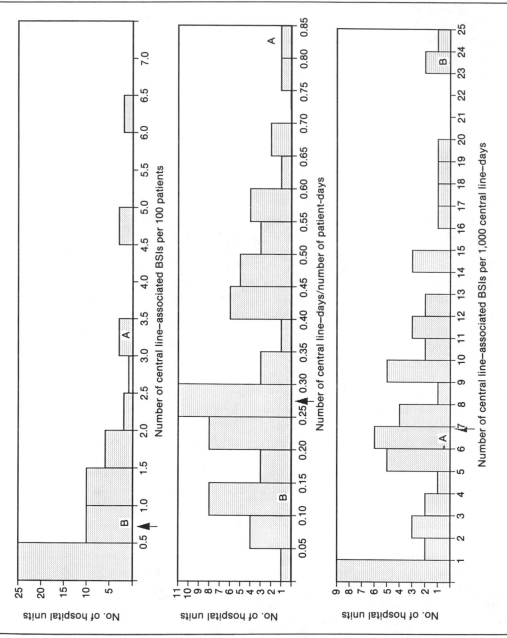

Fig. 5-3. Comparison of the distribution of bloodstream infection (BSI) rates (patient-based and central line–days–based) and central line utilization in combined coronary and medical intensive care units, National Nosocomial Infection Surveillance (NNIS) System, Intensive Care Unit Component, October 1986–December 1990. A and B indicate the specific location of individual hospital unit rates. Arrows indicate median.

gram). Although Hospital Unit A was no longer an outlier, its high central line use may need to be reviewed for appropriateness. On the other hand, for Hospital Unit B, the central line–associated bloodstream infection rate (top histogram) was near the median, and its central line use (middle histogram) was low. When its rate was calculated using central line–days in the denominator, it was quite high, suggesting the need to review central line insertion and maintenance practices.

Analysis

Comparing Patient Groups Analysis implies careful examination of the body of tabulated data in an attempt to determine the nature and relationship of its component parts. This includes comparison of current infection rates to determine whether significant differences exist among different groups of patients. Suppose, for instance, that both the gynecology and general surgery services have had 8 catheter-associated urinary tract infections during a given month; however, during the same month there were 20 patients who had indwelling catheters discharged from the gynecology service and 100 such patients discharged from the general surgery service. Thus, the rates for gynecology and general surgery patients were 40 percent and 8 percent, respectively. Determination of whether the difference observed between these infection rates is significant (i.e., greater than what we would expect by random or chance occurrence alone if indeed no real difference exists) requires the use of a statistical process known as *significance testing* [16].

Several tests of significance—such as the chi-square test and Fisher's Exact test for cross-tables, and Student's *t*-test for comparison of sample means—should be familiar to epidemiologists and ICPs (see chap. 7). Currently available software packages for microcomputers make even the most sophisticated statistical testing procedures very accessible to all infection control departments [23, 40]. In the preceding example, the difference between the observed infection rates (40 percent versus 8 percent) is highly significant at p less than .001 according to the Fisher's Exact test. This means that a difference as large as or larger than that observed (40 percent versus 8 percent) would be expected to occur by chance alone less than 1 time in 1,000. Thus it is very likely that there is a real difference between the infection rates on the two services, and further investigation is indicated to explain why such a difference exists.

Comparing Rates over Time Another type of analysis involves the comparison of current infection rates with those established in the past to determine whether significant changes have occurred over time. Tables of the rates for the present month and each of several preceding months can simply be visually inspected, or the rates can be plotted on graph paper to detect changes of potential importance. Potentially important deviations from baseline rates should then be subjected to tests of statistical significance (see Chap. 7), and further investigation should be undertaken if indicated (see Chap. 6).

An interesting approach to screening large amounts of surveillance data for potential epidemics was developed in the NNIS System [34]. Called *computerized epidemic threshold analysis*, this technique uses the infection experience for the same month over the past several years as a baseline for predicting the rate to be expected in the present month. To allow for random statistical variation in the rates, an upper boundary, or threshold, is set usually at two or three standard deviations above the predicted rate. Any of the current month's rates that significantly exceed their threshold rates are flagged by the program and recorded on a printout as suspicious rate increases to be investigated further. This routine is then repeated automatically for the rates in all of the cells of the various rate tables of interest (e.g., tables of rates by service, ward, site, site by pathogen, etc.). It must be emphasized that establishing thresholds must take place after an experience with an infection rate occurs over a large number of months. Thresholds cannot be arbitrarily established or taken from the experience of others.

One present disadvantage of this method is

the need for sophisticated computer equipment and software to accomplish the large number of comparisons required. Another difficulty is deciding how high to set the threshold. This problem arises from the fact that the sensitivity (the proportion of true outbreaks detected) and the specificity (the proportion of random increases that are falsely called outbreaks) of the method are affected in opposite directions by the level of the threshold. If one raises the threshold, the sensitivity decreases and the specificity increases; this causes fewer true outbreaks to be detected but increases the likelihood that any increase flagged by the program represents a true outbreak. Conversely, decreasing the threshold has the opposite effect of allowing the identification of more true outbreaks but reducing the likelihood that any flagged increase is a true outbreak. Thus, to use the program wisely requires careful judgment so the threshold will be set at just the right level to pick up the most true outbreaks while minimizing the amount of investigation wasted on purely random fluctuations (see Chap. 6).

Clusters Screening for clustering of specific patterns of antimicrobial susceptibility of organisms is another potentially valuable analytic tool for detecting outbreaks, especially when it is applied to particular pathogens on specific wards or in particular geographic areas.

Appropriateness of Medical Care Analysis of surveillance data must not be limited to an analysis of infection rates. For example, if an ICP determines that a hospital's utilization of central lines in ICUs is high compared with that in other hospitals' ICUs (see hospital I in the middle panel of Figure 5-3), a review of appropriateness of device utilization may be needed. Also, after assessing surgical wound infection (SWI) rates, useful information can be obtained by further exploring the distribution of risk factors in each of the risk index categories. For example, while a surgeon with more than the expected number of herniorrhaphies in the higher SWI index categories may be operating on more high-risk patients,

he or she may also be consistently exceeding the seventy-fifth percentile for the duration of surgery for the procedure and thus increasing the patients' risk of SWI. The question must be asked, "Are patients unnecessarily being placed at risk of a nosocomial infection?" Because examination of appropriateness of medical care and device use is a major interest to quality assurance personnel in U.S. hospitals [7, 11, 44, 46], ICPs may find areas for collaboration with their quality assurance colleagues.

Interpretation
Interpretation of the data is considered by many to be the final step in analysis; it is simply an intellectual process by which some meaning is ascribed to the tabulated and analyzed body of information. The interpretation may vary from no significant change in the current infection rates to the detection of a possible outbreak in the hospital. Often, however, more information—particularly that obtained through further investigation directed specifically at problem areas identified by means of the analysis of the surveillance data—will be necessary for final interpretation of the data. Additional uses of other information collected through surveillance, such as the time of onset of infection, are described in Chapters 4 and 6.

Reporting the Data
It is essential that the tabulated data, or at least the analyses and interpretations of the data, get to those people in the hospital who need to know them in order to take appropriate actions. A monthly report containing the tabulated data and the analytic results and their interpretations should routinely be submitted to the Infection Control Committee and maintained on record in the hospital. Of course, weekly or even daily reports may be necessary during epidemics or unusual situations. It is not necessary—in fact, it is often very inefficient—to include a line listing of infections in this report. Also, the analysis of a single month of infection data may yield some tables that contain insufficient data to justify inclusion in the report. These tables

should be retained and a summary table released whenever sufficient monthy data have accumulated.

Calculated rates may be displayed in graphic form to facilitate visual assimilation of the data. Simple, creative, and neatly drawn graphics are particularly effective when presenting important findings to clinicians or administrators to convince them of the existence of a problem and the need for preventive action. The availability of computer software for infection control allows graphic analyses to be performed far more efficiently and accurately than by hand.

Summary reports or graphic representations of the data should also be widely distributed to the professional staff of the hospital. Summary data may be placed on bulletin boards and sent to local or state health departments, to other local hospitals, or elsewhere as judged necessary or desirable by the Infection Control Committee to achieve specific objectives.

In the reporting phase, as well as throughout the surveillance process, measures should be taken to assure the privacy of the information collected on patients and hospital staff members. For example, the ICP should keep all surveillance forms that list patients by name under very tight security, including a locking filing cabinet or other secure storage method. Reports should not mention patients or staff members by name unless there is a good reason and, if it is necessary, the distribution of the reports should be limited. The Infection Control Committee should establish a policy on privacy of information, prescribing the procedures for handling records or reports that identify patients or staff members (e.g., surgeon-specific wound infection rates or laboratory data implicating an employee as a human disseminator of an epidemic organism).

Prevalence
Definition
Prevalence measures the number of all current cases of active disease (new and old) within a specified population at risk during a specific period of time, and the *prevalence rate*

is the prevalence divided by the number of patients at risk during the period. When the period of time used for the calculation is relatively long, usually a month or longer, the measurement is called *period prevalence*. In Figure 5-2, the period prevalence rate of infection during time period A would be 4/10, or 40 percent, and during time period B, 6/10, or 60 percent. When the period of time used for the calculation is relatively short, such as 1 day or less, the measurement is called *point prevalence* (i.e., the frequency of all currently active cases of disease, old and new, at a given instant in time). For example, the point prevalence rate of infection at point C in Figure 5-2 would be 3/10, or 30 percent. It should be apparent that the difference between point and period prevalence is arbitrary; an interval that is considered a point on one time scale may become a period on a different time scale.

The Prevalence Survey
The prevalence survey, as it is applied to nosocomial infections, consists of a systematic study of a defined population for evidence of infection at a given point in time; such a survey derives the point prevalence rate for the population. Typically, after a short period of training to standardize definitions and methods, a team of surveyors visits every patient in the hospital on a single day and detects all active infections from studying the medical record and examining the patient or discussing the case with the clinical staff when necessary. When there are more beds than the survey team can visit in one day, the prevalence study is conducted over several days with care taken to ensure that each bed is visited only once.

If the object is to obtain the prevalence rate of *infections* (the usual procedure), then those infections that have resolved before the day of the visit are not counted, and the point prevalence rate is calculated simply by dividing the number of infections active on the day of the visit by the number of beds visited and multiplying by an appropriate base number (usually 100). If, on the other hand, the object is to obtain the point prevalence rate of *infected patients,* then all patients with currently active or resolved infections contracted during the current hospitalization are counted, and the point prevalence rate is calculated simply by dividing the number of infected patients by the number of beds visited and multiplying by the appropriate base number. To be consistent with the usual way of defining the incidence rate (i.e., the infection ratio), prevalence surveys should be designed to measure the point prevalence rate of infections.

The relative magnitudes of these various measures are complicated but can be deduced from the fundamental relationship between prevalence and incidence [49]:

Prevalence $\propto$ Incidence $\times$ duration

From this general relationship it is apparent that prevalence rates (both point and period prevalence) are always higher than the comparable incidence rates, and the longer the duration of the infections, the greater the difference will become. As explained in the earlier discussion of the two types of incidence rates, the infection ratio is always higher than the infection proportion measured on the same population as long as some patients develop more than one infection. In contrast, the prevalence rate of infections is always lower than the prevalence rate of infected patients, because the duration of an infected patient's remaining in the hospital is almost always longer than the duration of the active infection. Interestingly, point prevalence and period prevalence rates measured on the same population are usually approximately the same although, due to the larger number of patients studied in a period prevalence survey, estimates of period prevalence are usually more precise than those of point prevalence.

In general, the most useful measure to derive from surveillance is the incidence rate, because it provides an estimate of the risk of infection uncluttered by differences in the durations of various infections. The main reason that prevalence rates were used in the past was simply that a point prevalence survey requires much less effort and can be completed much more rapidly than the type of ongoing, daily surveillance needed to obtain incidence rates. There are two main disadvantages of point prevalence surveys: First, due to the complex influence of the duration of infections, the prevalence rate overestimates patients' risk of acquiring infection; and second, except in the largest hospitals, the number of patients included in a point prevalence survey (i.e., the number of beds) is usually too small to obtain precise enough estimates of rates to detect important differences (e.g., a difference between the bacteremia rates on medicine and surgery) with statistical significance. Because of these limitations, prevalence surveys are generally useful primarily when a "quick and dirty" estimate is needed and there is insufficient time or resources to obtain a more useful measure of the incidence [18].

Uses of Prevalence Surveys

Secular Trends   Repeated prevalence surveys in the same institution have been used to document secular trends in the epidemiology of nosocomial infections. Prevalence studies in large hospitals have demonstrated such changes as shifts in the predominant pathogens associated with nosocomial infections and in the patterns of antimicrobial use for hospitalized patients [45]. However, limitations in the numbers of patients studied and variations in the types of prevalence rates determined in the various surveys have complicated the interpretation of these results. In general, incidence rates derived from ongoing surveillance, though more time-consuming, are much better suited for detecting and examining secular trends.

Estimating Surveillance Accuracy   Prevalence surveys have been used to determine the completeness of ascertainment of a hospital's ongoing surveillance system. Typically, a survey team, using the same standard definitions used for routine surveillance by the ICP, visits all patients in the hospital to detect all active infections. By comparing the infections identified by the survey team during the prevalence survey with those detected by the routine surveillance system, and under the assumption that the survey team correctly detected all active infections, an estimate is derived of the percentage of true infections detected by the routine surveillance system. Although this percentage approximates the sensitivity of routine surveillance (i.e., the probability that the routine surveillance system will detect a true infection), the statistic has been referred to as an *efficiency factor* since the difficulty of determining reliably whether infections are active at the time of the prevalence survey introduces some error into the assessment [3]. Because the efficiency factor approximates the sensitivity, it can be used to correct the monthly routine estimates of the incidence rates for the degree of under-ascertainment. Past experience indicates that approximately 60 percent efficiency is usual and that 80 percent or greater is often possible.

One of the weaknesses of this application in past studies has been the failure to estimate the specificity of routine surveillance in addition to its sensitivity (efficiency). Specificity is the probability of correctly classifying a patient as uninfected when he or she in fact develops no infection, and it reflects how often the ICP records an infection when one was not really present. Unfortunately, the specificity of ICPs in estimating incidence rates in routine surveillance has not been thoroughly studied [33, 55]. The process of correcting incidence rates with the efficiency factor assumes that specificity is a perfect 1.0. Corrections for lower levels of specificity would give lower estimates of the incidence rates.

Estimating Incidence from Prevalence Modified prevalence surveys can be used to derive a crude approximation of the incidence rates that would have been obtained from continuous surveillance [54]. Surveys are performed at regular intervals (e.g., weekly) that must be considerably less than the average duration of stay of infected patients. Only infections that began since the preceding survey are tabulated. The denominator of the rates should probably include the number of admissions during the interval plus the census at the start of the period. Obviously, the shorter the interval between prevalence surveys, the more closely the final estimate approximates the true incidence rate. Some loss in completeness, accuracy, and timeliness in detecting infections—as compared to the results of surveillance studies—must be weighed against the potential benefit from a smaller time commitment to case finding.

Alternatively, various formulas have been derived to allow the estimation of incidence rates from data collected in a single prevalence survey [17, 49]. These techniques were of particular interest in the early 1970s when prevalence surveys were being used more commonly. Since incidence rates are currently being obtained by ongoing surveillance in most U.S. hospitals, however, these statistical conversion techniques have not been widely applied.

Other Uses Perhaps the best uses of prevalence studies are to make valuable estimates of antimicrobial usage patterns, to evaluate the adherence to proper isolation practices, to monitor practices related to high-risk procedures such as intravenous and urinary catheters, and so on [45, 50]. In one recent study, the investigators used sequential prevalence surveys to estimate the impact of their infection control program on the risks of nosocomial infection [18]. Prevalence surveys have also been useful for increasing the awareness of nosocomial infection problems in those hospitals without surveillance programs. Indeed, the results of such surveys have often been important in a hospital's decision to institute a more extensive ongoing surveillance system.

Finally, the use of the prevalence survey to establish a single infection prevalence (or incidence) rate for comparison with those of other hospitals is controversial [11]. Since a single overall rate ignores differences in risk in each hospital (i.e., case mix and frequency of exposure to high-risk procedures) and differences in surveillance methodology, it may engender a false sense of complacency or alarm. Certainly, prevalence rates should not be compared with incidence rates. Moreover, no single overall rate should be used to assess the quality of patient care or the effectiveness of intervention measures.

Targeted Surveillance

A recent trend in the development of the concept of surveillance has been to find creative ways of targeting surveillance more directly toward potential infection problems. The purpose of these efforts is to obtain the greatest preventive impact from the effort invested in surveillance. As such, these ideas indicate a greater awareness of the need to direct surveillance efforts toward specific preventive objectives. Although these new approaches were generally motivated by the need to reduce the amount of personnel time devoted to surveillance in hospitals with inadequately staffed programs, the ideas, if proved as effective as routine continuous hospitalwide surveillance, might greatly increase the efficiency of surveillance in all hospitals.

Unit-Directed Surveillance

In some large hospitals faced with insufficient numbers of ICPs to maintain comprehensive surveillance over all of the hospital's beds, one approach has been to direct the available personnel time to the surveillance of infections in areas with the highest infection risks, such as ICUs, oncology units, or the like [12, 55]. For example, in one hospital, the infection rate in the ICU was three times higher than in general medical-surgical patients [12]. By monitoring the ICU, hospitals may follow patients who have devices that are associated with high infection risks. Device-related infection rates (e.g., ventilator-associated pneumonias per 1,000 ventilator-days) may be calculated. This will control for exposure to primary risk factors. These device-related infection rates have proved more useful for interhospital comparison than overall infection rates [21, 36]. ICUs tend to house the patients who are most susceptible to infection: that is, the patients most likely to have

suppressed immunologic systems, to be undergoing invasive diagnostic and therapeutic procedures, and to be receiving intensive nursing and medical care with the attendant risk of person-to-person spread of infection. Focusing scarce resources on a few relatively small units has the advantages of greatly simplifying the surveillance effort and of preventing infections in the patients with the highest risks and the greatest likelihood of suffering severe and life-threatening infections.

Another unit that is worth considering for unit-directed surveillance is the high-risk nursery (HRN). Neonates in the HRN are highly susceptible to nosocomial infection. Host and environmental factors that are unique to patients in this unit contribute to the high infection risk (e.g., low birth weight). Bloodstream infections are among the most common nosocomial infections in all birth-weight groups, this frequency differing dramatically from that in adult patients with nosocomial infections. The specific issues for infection in the ICU and the HRN had led to the development of surveillance components in the NNIS System [13].

Rotating Surveillance

Another approach is to rotate the surveillance efforts around the hospital in an effort to identify and eliminate infection risks in discrete departments or areas in a sequential manner. Typically, in a large hospital with an insufficient number of ICPs, the infection control staff divide the hospital into convenient geographic areas to be surveyed for a month each in sequential fashion. Through the month, the ICP performs careful continuous surveillance of all nosocomial infections occurring among the patients or personnel of the area and of all patient care practices related to infection risks. At the end of the month, the surveillance data are tabulated, analyzed, and discussed by the Infection Control Committee. From the discussion, a final report is written to present the findings, point out the problems, and make recommendations for corrective actions. The report is then given to the appropriate medical, nursing, and other department heads of the area surveyed. After an appropriate time for study, the infection control staff meets with the department heads to achieve a consensus agreement on the corrective actions to take. These are then written officially into procedure manuals, presented to and discussed with the patient care personnel involved, and carried out under the supervision of the regular medical and nursing management staff. Usually within a year or so, this area is resurveyed in a similar fashion according to a rotating schedule, and the degree of adherence to and effectiveness of the recommendations are assessed while simultaneously searching for new problems to correct.

This approach avoids the main disadvantage of the unit-directed approach by sequentially covering all areas, but it sacrifices the ability to detect problems that emerge in the large areas not under surveillance at a given time. Its main attraction lies in the fact that at least once annually every area of the hospital is subjected to a detailed infection control evaluation directed specifically at the objective of eliminating or reducing identified infection risks. When coupled with a commitment to investigating outbreaks or other problems that come to attention in areas not under scrutiny at the time and other regular control measures, this method appears to offer some advantages over the strictly unit-directed approach if resources are limited.

Priority-Directed Surveillance

A third alternative, referred to as surveillance by objectives, attempts to assign the levels of surveillance effort to various infection problems on the basis of priority levels that the problems are assigned [24, 25]. Instead of basing effort on geographic areas, as the previous two alternatives do, the priority-directed approach focuses on the types of infections to be prevented and assigns levels of effort commensurate to the relative seriousness of the problems.

The first prerequisite of this approach is to establish the relative seriousness of the different types of infections to form the basis of the priority rankings. Several possible parameters for setting these priorities are compared in Table 5-1, based on further analysis of data collected in three hospitals in the SENIC pilot studies [32]. In the past, the main parameter used for assessing this has been simply the relative frequency of the different types of infections, since these figures have been familiar for many years. If this measure were used, urinary tract infections would be given the highest priority, followed by SWIs and pneumonia, with primary bacteremia receiving a lower priority just ahead of a large number of relatively rare infections such as hepatitis and tuberculosis.

An alternative parameter that appears to be a better measure of the relative seriousness

Table 5-1. Comparison of the relative frequency of the major types of nosocomial infections and alternative measures of their relative importance

Type of infection	Percent of all nosocomial infections	Total extra days[a] (%)	Total extra charges[a] (%)	Percent preventable[b]
Surgical wound infection	24	889 (57)	$102,286 (42)	35
Pneumonia	10	370 (24)	95,229 (39)	22
Urinary tract infection	42	175 (11)	32,081 (13)	33
Bacteremia	5	59 (4)	7,478 (3)	35
Other	19	69 (4)	8,680 (3)	32
Total (all sites)	100	1,562 (100)	$245,754 (100)	32

[a] Data are drawn from SENIC pilot studies: R. W. Haley et al., Extra days and prolongation of stay attributable to nosocomial infections: A prospective interhospital comparison. *Am. J. Med.* 70:51, 1981. Note that charges are in 1975 dollars.
[b] Data are drawn from SENIC analysis of efficacy: R. W. Haley et al., The efficacy of infection surveillance and control programs in preventing nosocomial infections in U.S. hospitals. *Am. J. Epidemiol.* 121:282, 1984.

of the various types of infections is the total extra hospital costs attributable to each of the infections [24, 25]. This measure reflects both the relative frequency of the infections and the relative degree of morbidity expressed by the costs of the extra days and extra ancillary services necessary to treat the infections. By this criterion, SWIs would constitute the most serious problems, followed by pneumonia, with urinary tract infection and bacteremia in remote third and fourth place (see Table 5-1). Basing time commitments on these priorities, one would concentrate approximately half of available surveillance time on SWIs, one-third on pneumonia, and relatively small amounts of carefully planned time on urinary tract infections and bacteremia, and only occasional effort on the less common infections. These relative levels of effort might be used to the best advantage by the following plan, which uses the surveillance methods likely to produce the greatest amounts of prevention within the times available.

Surgical Wound Infections
With half of the time available for SWIs, all patients undergoing operations would be enrolled into a surveillance registry at the time of the operation, and information on several key risk factors would be recorded at that time. The risk factors that are most likely to be useful in the analysis are the wound classification, type and duration of the operation, and a measure of the severity of the patient's underlying disease, such as the number of underlying diagnoses or the physical status classification of the American Society of Anesthesiologists (ASA) [10, 27, 29, 39]. All of these patients would be visited regularly during hospitalization by the ICP to detect all SWIs. If time permitted, the ICP would also follow up all, or a subset, of the patients for infection occurring after discharge [8, 43, 48, 56].

Each month the tabulation process would involve three steps, ideally accomplished with the aid of a computer (see under the heading The Role of Computers in Surveillance). First, each patient would be assigned to an intrinsic infection risk category, using either the familiar surgical wound classes [2, 9] or a multivariate risk factor scale [10, 29]. Second, the SWI rate would be calculated for each surgeon's patients within *each* category of the infection risk classification—not just for patients with clean wounds or in low-risk categories. Third, two reports would be compiled, one displaying each surgeon's category-specific monthly rates over time (e.g., over 1 or 2 years), and a second comparing the category-specific rates of each surgeon with those of his or her colleagues and for the service overall. Finally, the reports would be discussed at the infection control meeting and given to the chief of the surgical service to distribute among and discuss with the practicing surgeons. With this plan, the half of surveillance time devoted to SWIs would be directed toward the surveillance effort shown to be the most effective in reducing the problem [8, 9, 28].

Pneumonia
With only approximately one-third of the time assigned to the surveillance of pneumonia, a plan more narrowly targeted toward specific prevention objectives must be used. The first consideration is to separate the generically different problems of pneumonia among surgical and medical patients. The vast majority of preventable cases of pneumonia among surgical patients are postoperative pulmonary infections representing progression of the usual atelectasis syndrome most commonly following operations of the upper abdomen. In contrast, most preventable pneumonias among adult medical patients are hypostatic infections related to the failure to turn frequently enough those patients with diminished levels of consciousness. On pediatric and newborn services, the most serious preventable pneumonias follow person-to-person spread of nosocomial infections with viruses such as respiratory syncytial virus (see Chaps. 21, 38).

Since all surgical patients are already being followed closely for wound infections, postoperative pneumonias can be detected with little additional effort. Analysis of these rates within appropriate risk categories can be performed for each nursing unit or for the patients of each surgeon. Reports of these analyses should then be discussed just as the SWI rates are (see preceding section).

For medical patients, a unit-directed approach should be used. The ICP should identify nursing units or ICUs where patients with strokes, drug overdoses, and other patients at high risk of hypostatic pneumonia are congregated. In only these areas, all patients at high risk are followed regularly to detect all cases of pneumonia, and the pneumonia rates among these patients are regularly reported to the head nurse and the charge nurses of the specified nursing units, along with continuing inservice education of the importance of frequently turning these patients to prevent pneumonia.

The ICP should regularly visit units caring for infants or children at high risk of serious pneumonia from respiratory syncytial virus and similar agents to monitor informally the frequency of upper respiratory infections among patients and employees, especially in the fall and winter months. When the frequency of these infections appears to have risen, virologic studies should be done immediately to detect the presence of virulent viruses. When such are found, the staff members should be warned of the imminent danger and instructed in meticulous contact precautions for infected patients and employees [20].

Bacteremia

With little time assigned for the surveillance of bacteremias, the object of the limited surveillance effort must be to detect clusters of nosocomial bacteremia possibly related to correctable errors in patient management, such as failure to change the site of intravenous catheters frequently enough or improper sterilization of arterial pressure–monitoring devices. Since collecting sufficient data to calculate routinely the specific bacteremia infection rates for all of the possible risk factors would be far too time-consuming, the ICP might conduct only "numerator surveillance." This involves merely investigating briefly all cases of bacteremia reported by the microbiology laboratory each day. The object of

this brief daily activity is to recognize common factors that might tie the cases together, such as a single unusual organism, spacial clustering, or a relationship with some diagnostic or therapeutic device. Only when a suspicious cluster or relationship is found would a more detailed investigation involving the calculation of rates be undertaken. Since these problems are likely to occur infrequently, little time will be spent on this problem, but the time spent will be directed so as to maximize the chance of detecting a problem if one occurs.

Urinary Tract Infections

Little time also is assigned to urinary tract infections, so the modest surveillance efforts should be directed toward identifying areas where patient care personnel are not managing urinary catheters or other urinary instrumentations properly. The most efficient way of achieving this would be to perform part-time rotating surveillance on different wards or nursing units to measure catheter-associated urinary tract infection rates (stratified or adjusted by categories of the duration of urinary catheterization) and to assess the indications for inserting and discontinuing catheters and the techniques of aseptically caring for them. By periodically reporting how the urinary tract infection rates of the different units compared, practices could be improved in the units found to have particular problems. Alternatively, the infection control staff could relax other surveillance activities for 1 month each year to devote full time to hospitalwide surveillance of urinary tract infections and catheter care practices. This amount of effort would be commensurate with the magnitude of the problem but would reinforce prevention at least on a yearly basis.

Other Infections

Virtually no time should be routinely spent performing formal surveillance of other infections. Instead, the ICP should depend on other hospital departments to recognize the rare outbreaks of unusual infections. For example, the employee health service should maintain surveillance to recognize problems of tuberculosis transmission to employees; the director of the newborn nursery should be counted on to recognize and notify the ICP of clusters of staphylococcal pyoderma; and someone in the microbiology laboratory should be alert to clusters of unusual pathogens. Again, the level of effort is commensurate with the magnitude of the problems, but the efforts are likely to detect problems if they occur. ICPs must remain alert to such problems regardless of which targeted surveillance approach is employed.

The Role of Computers in Surveillance

Few technologies have offered so much promise in infection control, yet produced so little tangible benefit, as the digital computer. This is ironic since much of the drudgery and time expenditure of surveillance is consumed in keeping lists of patients, counting and recording denominators, and repeating standard infection rate tabulations month after month—jobs that would seem maximally suited for computerization. In most hospitals, however, the past experience was that if you put your data into a computer you could never get it back out.

The reasons for this disappointment are actually rather simple. Computers were designed fundamentally for business and accounting purposes rather than for scientific uses and, until recently, the only computers available to the infection control staff were large mainframe machines owned by and operated solely for the hospital's business office. Given that infection control personnel have been generally inexperienced in the use of computers, it is not surprising that they have been unable to redirect a machine poorly designed for their needs in the first place.

Mainframe Computers

Recently, however, two developments have greatly changed the prospects. First, hospitals have increasingly adopted integrated database management systems for efficiently organizing most information on all hospitalized patients on their mainframe computers. Although administrative efficiency, not infection control, was the objective for these systems, they offer, particularly in large hospitals, a dramatic opportunity to the infection control staff for greatly reducing the work of surveillance. With the demographic, business, pharmacy, laboratory, and other records of all patients residing in one, or a system of, computerized files, only two things are needed to generate surveillance reports directly from the mainframe: first, a mechanism for entering the information on nosocomial infections obtained through surveillance into a file in the database management system; and second, a software package for merging the infection information into the patient database by the patient identification numbers, making the required tabulations and rate calculations, and constructing the various tables and figures for the printed reports.

Although several such systems are commercially available for hospitals' mainframe computers, the initial investment is usually high and operating costs may be prohibitive if the infection control program is charged for computer time and programming. Also, infection data input by infection control staff can itself be time-consuming, although if kept current on a daily basis is often less burdensome (see Chap. 8). To find out whether such a system is available for the computer at a particular hospital, the marketing representative of the company that manufactured the hospital's business computer should be consulted with the assistance of the hospital's data-processing manager.

Microcomputers

The second development is the more recent introduction of the personal microcomputer at prices that have suddenly put potentially powerful computers literally on the desk of the infection control staff. Initially, the usefulness of microcomputers was severely limited by the unavailability of software designed to accomplish the unique tasks required in infection control. More recently, commercial software products have made the microcomputer a very useful tool for the infection surveillance and control activity [4, 22, 40]. In view of the large reductions in hospital length of stay and operating expenses that have been shown by the SENIC Project to be possible [28], hospital administrators are likely to be increasingly willing to invest in microcomputers and software for infection control.

Functions of Microcomputer Software

The best software packages for infection control serve three important functions: learning aid, planning guide, and "workhorse" for entering, analyzing, and reporting surveillance data. To serve as a learning aid, a good software package must be designed by infection control experts who structure the computer functions and the user's manual to teach the approaches that are proved effective. In this way, software products become a powerful vechicle for increasing the sophistication of infection control staff members in all types of hospitals.

To serve as a planning guide, the software package must have the versatility to create special surveillance files and user-defined codes that allow the infection control staff to design new surveillance systems aimed at achieving specific prevention objectives. The user's manual should include sections that assist the infection control staff step by step through the process of planning a new surveillance system and the versatility to support most foreseeable surveillance functions. The infection control staff should be particularly skeptical of packages that are oriented mainly toward microbiologic information or that have objectives which are too broad (e.g., infection control plus risk management, quality assurance, and employee health) unless their usefulness and efficiency for infection control per se are demonstrated. Also, the infection control staff must be prepared to devote sometimes considerable time and effort to becoming familiar with a software package (see Chap. 8).

To serve as a workhorse for surveillance, the software system must be designed to handle the required data quickly while minimizing the time required to enter data, edit the files, and produce reports. To run efficiently, it should be programmed in an efficient language (e.g., assembly language or the C language), and the choice of data items to be collected and processed should be limited to those essential for preventing infections, with only a few nonspecific fields that can be defined by the user for special purposes. For efficiency of entering data, it should have a menu-driven format with appropriate help screens, and the data entry fields should fit on as few screens as possible to reduce time-consuming page turning. All fields, except perhaps a comments field, should have structured codes with internal edit checks to prevent entry of invalid responses. Since open-ended (noncoded) responses cannot be analyzed easily, such data are rarely used and only reduce efficiency of storage and processing. Codes should be user-designed wherever possible. The package should allow the creation of separate files for special surveillance projects such as surgical wound, ICU, or procedure surveillance and, ideally, infections entered into any special file should be automatically added to an infection master file to facilitate overall hospital analysis if needed. Efficient file structures should be provided for entering, storing, and retrieving large denominator files (e.g., a record for each surgical operation) and later adding infection information to those cases in which infections occurred (e.g., wound infection data). Likewise, it should be possible to enter only numerator data (e.g., infections) and supply numerical denominators in the analysis stage. An effective report generator should be able to select records based on a string of search criteria, sort the resulting file, and print line listings of cases, two- and three-way cross-tabulations, and selected rates for virtually all variables in the database. It should also have the ability to display graphics, including epidemic curves, line graphs, and bar charts, on the computer screen as well as in printed form, and the ability to output data files to other computers or statistical packages.

Developing the type of compact and highly efficient software systems needed for routine use in community hospitals is made difficult by the need to limit the amount of information collected to maximize efficiency of computer usage and staff time. To limit the amount of information appropriately, software designers must make very difficult judgment decisions about what is the bare minimum of information essential for effective infection control. They must then be ruthless about excluding extra data fields that might have research or other appeals but have only marginal or no actual infection control impact. Since this requires astute epidemiologic insights into the priorities and functioning of infection control programs rather than statistical or computer-programming judgments, one can expect slower progress and fewer good products to emerge in this class of software packages. This fact will necessitate great care in choosing an infection surveillance software package.

Selecting the Best Software Package

As discussed earlier, the most important decisions that must be made before selecting a software system are the objectives to be achieved by the surveillance activity. In view of the substantial differences among the packages available for testing at the time this chapter went to press, it is apparent that a system selected before one's objective are written and agreed on may not meet the needs when it is put into use. For example, if the objectives of surveillance include research, the best software package might be one of the general-purpose database management packages that allow complete flexibility but require far greater computer skills and more time. On the other hand, if the objectives are limited to routine aspects of preventing and controlling infections, one of the software packages designed specifically for infection control would probably be the best choice. Furthermore, a significant change in the infection control program's objectives may require the acquisition of a new software package. Various methods have been used for comparing computer software packages for use in accomplishing the specified objectives of the infection surveillance and control program [4, 22, 40]. These have highlighted broad differences in speed of computation, time required for the ICP to complete analyses, and accuracy of numerical computations.

Starting a Computerized Surveillance System

Perhaps the greatest impediment to the effective use of microcomputers in infection control is the lack of computer literacy among adults. Not uncommonly, microcomputers and powerful software systems have been purchased and placed in the infection control office only to sit idle amid growing disillusionment with computers. Often this is due to the inability of the staff to master the basic workings of the computer rather than deficiencies in the hardware or software. (See Chapter 8 for additional problems in implementing surveillance by computer.) To avoid this common pitfall, the infection control staff should either take a computer course at a local college or computer store or find a friend or colleague who could act as a personal advisor in beginning computer skills. After mastering the basics, one should schedule at least a month to read the infection control software manual thoroughly, become familiar with its functions, and design the surveillance system, including the types of surveillance studies to perform, the user-defined variables and codes, and the types of reports that will be needed. All of this planning should be based on the objectives to be accomplished and should be approved by the Infection Control Committee before the system is put into operation. If introduced in this carefully planned manner, the microcomputer can indeed become the fundamental tool for infection surveillance in the hospital.

References

1. Abrutyn, E., and Talbot, G.H. Surveillance Strategies: A primer. *Infect. Control* 8(11):459, 1987.
2. Altemeir, W.A., et al. *Manual on the Control of Infection in Surgical Patients.* Philadelphia: Lippincott, 1976. Pp. 29–30.
3. Bennett, J.V., Scheckler, W.E., Maki, D.G., and Brachman, P.S. Current National Patterns:

United States. In: P.S. Brachman and T.C. Eickhoff (Eds.), *Proceedings of the International Conference on Nosocomial Infections.* Chicago: American Hospital Association, 1971.

4. Berg, R. Reviews: Software. *Am. J. Infect. Control* 14:139, 1986.

5. Centers for Disease Control. *Outline for Surveillance and Control of Nosocomial Infections.* Atlanta: Centers for Disease Control, 1972.

6. Centers for Disease Control. *Guidelines for the Prevention and Control of Nosocomial Infections.* Springfield, VA: National Technical Information Service, U.S. Department of Commerce, 1982.

7. Chassin, M.R., et al. Does inappropriate use explain geographic variations in the use of health care services? A study of three procedures. *J.A.M.A.* 258:2533, 1987.

8. Condon, R.E., Haley, R.W., Lee, J.T., and Meakins, J.L. Does infection control control infection? *Arch. Surg.* 123:250, 1988.

9. Cruse, P.J.E., and Foord, R. The epidemiology of wound infection: A 10-year prospective study of 62,939 wounds. *Surg. Clin. North Am.* 60:27, 1980.

10. Culver, D.H., and National Nosocomial Infection Surveillance System. Surgical wound infection rates by wound class, operation, and risk index in U.S. hospitals, 1986–90. *Am. J. Med.* 91(Suppl. 3B):152S, 1991. hospitals, 1986–90. *Am. J. Med.* 1991 (in press).

11. Donabedian, A. Contributions of epidemiology to quality assessment and monitoring. *Infect. Control Hosp. Epidemiol.* 11:117, 1990.

12. Donowitz, L.G., Wenzel, R.P., and Hoyt, J.W. High risk of hospital-acquired infection in the ICU patient. *Crit. Care Med.* 10:355, 1982.

13. Emori, T.G., et al. National Nosocomial Infections Surveillance System (NNIS): Description of surveillance methodology. *Am. J. Infect. Control* 19:19, 1991.

14. Emori, T.G., et al. Nosocomial infections in elderly patients in the United States, 1986–90. *Am. J. Med.* 91(Suppl. 3B):294S, 1991.

15. Emori, T.G., Haley, R.W., and Garner, J.S. Techniques and uses of nosocomial infection surveillance in U.S. hospitals, 1976–77. *Am. J. Med.* 770:933, 1981.

16. Fleiss, J.L. *Statistical Methods for Rates and Proportions.* New York: Wiley, 1973.

17. Freeman, J., and McGowan, J.E., Jr. Day-specific incidence of nosocomial infection estimated from a prevalence survey. *Am. J. Epidemiol.* 114:888, 1981.

18. French, G.L., et al. Repeated prevalence surveys for monitoring effectiveness of hospital infection control. *Lancet* 2:1021, 1989.

19. Garner, J.S., et al. CDC definitions for nosocomial infections. *Am. J. Infect. Control* 16:128, 1988.

20. Garner, J.S., and Simmons, B.P. (Eds.). CDC guideline for isolation precautions in hospitals. *Infect Control* 4:245, 1983.

21. Gaynes, R.P., et al., and National Nosocomial Infections Surveillance System. Comparison of rates of nosocomial infections in neonatal intensive care units in the United States. *Am. J. Med.* 91(Suppl. 3B):192S, 1991.

22. Gaynes, R.P., Friedman, C., Copeland, T.A., and Mauck-Thiele, G. A methodology to evaluate a computer-based system for surveillance of hospital-acquired infections. *Am. J. Infect. Control* 18:40, 1990.

23. Gustafson, T.L. *True Epistat.* (4th ed). Richardson, TX: Epistat Services, 1991.

24. Haley, R.W. Surveillance by objectives: A priority-directed approach to the surveillance of nosocomial infection. *Am. J. Infect. Control* 13:78, 1985.

25. Haley, R.W. *Managing Hospital Nosocomial Control for Cost-Effectiveness.* Chicago: American Hospital Publishing, 1986.

26. Haley, R.W. JCAHO infection control indicators, parts 1 and 2. *Infect Control Hosp. Epidemiol.* 11:545, 1990.

27. Haley, R.W. Nosocomial infections in surgical patients: Developing valid measures of intrinsic patient risk. *Am. J. Med.* 91(Suppl. 3B):145S, 1991.

28. Haley, R.W., et al. The efficacy of infection surveillance and control programs in preventing nosocomial infections in U.S. hospitals. *Am. J. Epidemiol.* 121:282, 1984.

29. Haley, R.W., et al. Identifying patients at high risk of surgical wound infection: A simple multivariate index of patient susceptibility and wound contamination. *Am. J. Epidemiol.* 121:206, 1984.

30. Haley, R.W., et al. Nosocomial infections in U.S. hospitals, 1975–76: Estimated nationwide frequency by selected characteristics of patients. *Am. J. Med.* 70:947, 1981.

31. Haley, R.W., et al. Hospital infection control: Recent progress and opportunities under prospective payment. *Am. J. Infect. Control* 13:97, 1985.

32. Haley, R.W., et al. Extra days and prolongation of stay attributable to nosocomial infections: A prospective interhospital comparison. *Am. J. Med.* 70:51, 1981.

33. Haley, R.W., et al. The accuracy of retrospective chart review in measuring nosocomial infection rates: Results of validation studies in pilot hospitals. *Am. J. Epidemiol.* 111:534, 1980.

34. Haley, R.W., et al. How frequent are outbreaks of nosocomial infection in community hospitals? *Infect. Control Hosp. Epidemiol.* 6:233, 1985.

35. Hughes, J.M. Nosocomial infection surveil-

lance in the United States: Historical perspective. *Infect. Control* 8(11):450, 1987.

36. Jarvis, W.R., Edwards, J.R., and National Nosocomial Infections Surveillance System. Nosocomial infections in adult and pediatric intensive care units in the United States, 1986–90. *Am. J. Med.* 91(Suppl. 3B):185S, 1991.

37. Joint Commission on Accreditation of Healthcare Organizations, Standards: Infection Control. In: *JCAHO, Accreditation Manual for Hospitals.* Chicago: Joint Commission on Accreditation of Healthcare Organizations, 1990.

38. Joint Commission on Accreditation of Hospitals. *Accreditation Manual for Hospitals, 1976.* Chicago: Joint Commission on Accreditation of Hospitals, 1976.

39. Keats, A.S. The ASA classification of physical status—a recapitulation. *J. Anesthesiol.* 49:233, 1978.

40. LaHaise, S. A comparison of infection control software for use by hospital epidemiologists in meeting the new JCAHO standards. *Infect. Control Hosp. Epidemiol.* 11:185, 1990.

41. Larson, E. A comparison of methods for surveillance of nosocomial infections. *Infect. Control* 1:377, 1980.

42. Lynch, P., and Jackson, M.M. Monitoring: Surveillance for nosocomial infections and uses for assessing quality of care. *Am. J. Infect. Control* 13(4):161, 1985.

43. Manian, F.A., and Meyer, L. Comprehensive surveillance of surgical wound infections in outpatient and inpatient surgery. *Infect. Control Hosp. Epidemiol.* 11(10):515, 1990.

44. McGeer, A., Crede, W., and Hierholzer, W.J., Jr. Surveillance for quality assessment: II. Surveillance for noninfectious processes: Back to basics. *Infect. Control Hosp. Epidemiol.* 11:36, 1990.

45. McGowan, J.E., Jr., and Finland, M. Infection and usage of antibiotics at Boston City Hospital: Changes in prevalence during the decade 1974–1973. *J. Infect. Dis.* 129:421, 1974.

46. Myers, S.A., and Gleicher, N. A successful program to lower caesarean section rates. *N. Engl. J. Med.* 319:1511, 1988.

47. Raven, B.H., and Haley, R.W. Social Influence and Compliance of Hospital Nurses with Infection Control Policies. In: J.R. Eiser (Ed.), *Social Psychology and Behavioral Medicine.* New York: Wiley, 1982.

48. Reimer, K., Gleed, C., and Nicolle, L.E. Impact of postdischarge infection in surgical wound infection rates. *Infect. Control* 8(6):237, 1987.

49. Rhame, F.S., and Sudderth, W.D. Incidence and prevalence as used in the analysis of the occurrence of nosocomial infections. *Am. J. Epidemiol.* 113:1, 1981.

50. Scheckler, W.E., Garner, J.S., Kaiser, A.B., and Bennett, J.V. Prevalence of Infections and Antibiotic Usage in Eight Community Hospitals. In: P.S. Brachman and T.C. Eickhoff (Eds.), *Proceedings of the International Conference on Nosocomial Infections.* Chicago: American Hospital Association, 1971.

51. Semmelweis, I.P. *The Etiology, the Concept and the Prophylaxis of Childbed Fever.* Leipzig: C.A. Hartleben, 1861.

52. U.S. General Accounting Office. *Infection Control: Military Programs Are Comparable to VA and Nonfederal Programs but Can Be Enhanced* (GAO/HRD-90-74). Report to Congressional Requestors. Washington, DC: U.S. General Accounting Office, 1990.

53. Weigelt, J.A., Dryer, D., and Haley, R.W. The necessity and efficiency of wound surveillance after discharge. *Arch. Surg.* 152:77, 1992.

54. Wenzel, R.P., et al. Hospital-acquired infections in intensive care unit patients: An overview with emphasis on epidemics. *Infect. Control* 4:371, 1983.

55. Wenzel, R.P. Osterman, C.A., Hunting, K.J., and Gwaltney, J.M., Jr. Hospital-acquired infections: I. Surveillance in a university hospital. *Am. J. Epidemiol.* 103:251, 1976.

56. Zoutman, D., et al. Surgical wound infections occurring in day surgery patients. *Am. J. Infect. Control* 18(4):277, 1990.

Investigation of Endemic and Epidemic Nosocomial Infections

Richard E. Dixon

Although effective infection control programs reduce the incidence of nosocomial infections, these infections continue to be a problem even in hospitals with very effective programs. Some nosocomial infections are unavoidable using techniques now available, but many can be prevented, and a hospital's infection control program should be designed to identify preventable infections, determine why they occur, and reduce the probability of their occurrence.

This chapter provides guidelines that hospital infection control personnel can use to determine when epidemiologic investigations should be initiated and introduces techniques that can be used in those investigations.

Criteria for Initiating Investigations

An epidemiologic investigation may be useful whenever a hospital has a potential nosocomial infection problem, such as when the incidence of infections is excessively high. Because no hospital can, or should, investigate every nosocomial infection that occurs, infection control programs should focus efforts on preventable infections rather than waste time and money evaluating issues that cannot be affected by changes in hospital practices. Frequently, however, neither clinical nor epidemiologic findings indicate whether specific infections are preventable; therefore, the hospital epidemiologist must establish additional criteria to identify the kinds of infections to investigate.

In many instances, definitive criteria do not exist to identify problems that require evaluation, and hospitals are so variable that it is unlikely that absolute criteria can be established. As a result, the decision to investigate a potential problem depends ultimately on the judgment of the hospital epidemiologist, who must decide whether a problem exists but may not have definitive criteria on which to make that decision. The epidemiologist must recognize that it is usually possible to find some reasonable explanation to discount the possibility of a problem. Reasons commonly advanced to argue that a *potential* problem is not a *real* problem and therefore does not need evaluation include the following: The hospital has recently been treating more susceptible patients than in the past, surveillance has been especially vigorous, or infecting strains do not all share the same characteristics. Infection control programs should guard against accepting these explanations too readily. The epidemiologist should generally assume that a potential problem is both real and important until evidence is collected to indicate otherwise, since the goal of the infection control program is to prevent infections, not explain them away.

The following information may be useful to epidemiologists when setting priorities for investigations.

Epidemic Infections

Infections that occur as part of an epidemic are traditionally considered to be among the most preventable of all infections, and any cluster of infections that appears to be epidemic should be evaluated. On occasion, however, it may be difficult to decide, before an assessment has been conducted, whether a cluster of infections actually represents an epidemic. By definition, a classic epidemic is marked by an unusual, statistically significant increase in the incidence of a particular disease; it usually occurs during a brief interval, involves a specific patient population with defined susceptibility factors, and is caused by a single microbial strain.

This classic definition is useful for identifying some problems, but it fails to characterize all nosocomial and community-acquired infection epidemics. For example, the epidemiologist may not know whether an apparent increase in infection incidence indicates the presence of an epidemic or merely reflects an appropriate fluctuation associated with varia-

tions in the host susceptibility characteristics of hospitalized patients. Nor can the epidemiologist rely on the criterion that a single disease and unique microorganism are seen in a typical epidemic, since nosocomial infection epidemics often involve several diseases or multiple pathogens, such as occurs when an especially virulent strain causes infection at multiple sites or when a breakdown in routine patient care practices allows the spread of several different microorganisms. Finally, the epidemiologist should not always expect to see an abrupt rise in the incidence of infections since the rates of infection may have been excessive for prolonged periods without recognition. Thus, although recognized epidemics almost always require an assessment, the epidemiologist will also need to consider investigating other infections that do not fulfill classic epidemic criteria.

Endemic Infections

Sporadic (endemic) infections represent the bulk of preventable nosocomial infections, and their control should be a primary objective of ongoing infection control activities. Comparisons of infection rates in similar hospitals show variations that cannot be explained by differences in epidemic experiences, patient characteristics, kinds of treatment provided, or other hospital characteristics. Some of these differences in infection rates can be explained by the existence of more effective infection control programs in some hospitals than in others. Therefore, the hospital epidemiologist should also consider endemic infections worthy of epidemiologic investigation if the local rates of infection appear to be higher than they should be.

Specific Criteria
Infection Rate Is Greater than Accepted Threshold

Few published criteria define acceptable epidemic or endemic infection rate thresholds in hospitals. One such criterion has been offered by the American Public Health Association, which stated that "The occurrence of two or more concurrent cases of staphylococcal disease related to a nursery or a maternity ward is presumptive evidence of an epidemic and warrants investigation" [1].

Recently, increasing numbers of epidemiologic studies have described infection rates for certain defined patient populations, such as patients undergoing specific surgical procedures or exposed to particular medical devices or treatments. Although such reports often fail to control for degree of host susceptibility or other factors that may influence infection risk, they may provide useful benchmarks against which the epidemiologist may compare local endemic infection rates.

As hospitals increasingly use techniques to evaluate severity of illness and other case mix characteristics of their patients, additional data may become available that will control, at least in part, for variations in the extent of underlying illnesses and thereby allow more meaningful comparisons than have previously been possible.

Recognized Problem in Other Hospitals
Hospitals generally have similar practices and use similar therapeutic approaches, so the recognition of an infection control problem in another hospital should prompt an evaluation of local practices. For example, infection control programs began to recognize epidemics of bacteremia associated with use of arterial pressure–monitoring devices as they became widely used in intensive care units, and within a brief period a variety of problems and infection control measures were reported in the literature. These reports stimulated other hospitals to evaluate their use of these devices, and similar problems were found on occasion.

The infection control staff is not obligated to institute every infection control measure suggested in the literature, however, for some may not be appropriate for widespread application. The epidemiologist may wish to conduct an epidemiologic study to determine whether new procedures are needed, in light of local infection experiences.

Significant Increase in Infection Rate
The need to conduct ongoing, total hospital surveillance for nosocomial infections re-

mains controversial, and many excellent infection control programs have instituted limited or targeted surveillance (see Chap. 5). Nonetheless, systematic and rigorously applied surveillance remains a powerful technique for recognizing subtle but important changes in a hospital's infection experience. Such surveillance may be unnecessary to identify explosive or very large problems leading to clinically serious disease, but more subtle problems, such as gradual increases in infection rates, outbreaks caused by several pathogens, and serious problems occurring in small patient populations (such as surgical wound infections associated with a single surgeon or procedure) may be difficult to identify without systematic data collection.

Sophisticated statistical analysis of epidemiologic data is within reach of all hospitals now that statistics programs have been developed for microcomputers (see Chap. 8) but, even without formal statistical analyses, an infection control program can establish its own thresholds for evaluating potential problems. For example, a 2- to 2.5-fold increase in the infection rate of any site, pathogen, or site-pathogen combination would almost always justify an evaluation. For infections with a high baseline incidence, a smaller rise in infection rate would call for investigation.

Figure 6-1 provides a statistical guideline that might be used to establish general thresholds for concern. The number of infections is plotted against the population at risk. A family of curves for a range of baseline infection rates, ranging from 1 per thousand to 20 per thousand, indicates the upper 95 percent limit of the expected number of infections for each baseline rate. For example, if the expected baseline incidence of an infection is believed to be 5 cases per thousand and if 1,000 patients have been at risk of acquiring that infection, we would expect to observe fewer than 10 cases of infection 95 percent of the time. If a larger number is seen, an investigation might profitably be instituted.

Although Figure 6-1 may be useful as a guideline, it must be used cautiously. It cannot be used arbitrarily as a criterion for deciding when to evaluate a potential problem

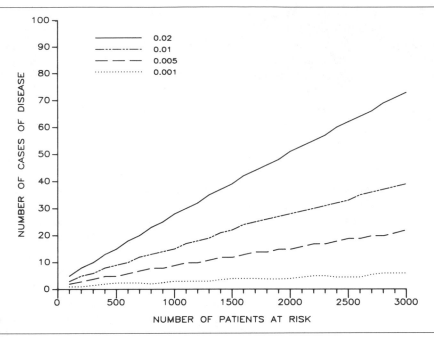

Fig. 6-1. Upper limits of expected number of infections for selected endemic infection rates. For each endemic infection rate (0.001, 0.005, 0.01, 0.02), the upper limit of numbers of infections that would be expected to occur is plotted against the number of patients at risk of infection. In 5% of instances or fewer, a larger number of infections might be expected to occur by chance alone. The formula used to calculate the plots is

$$p_x = \frac{e^{-N\lambda}(N\lambda)^x}{x!}$$

where e = base of natural log, x = number of observed infections, N = number of subjects available, λ = baseline level of occurrence, and p = probability of occurrence. The probabilities (p) were summed until the cumulative probability reached or exceeded .95. (The author gratefully acknowledges the assistance of Stanley M. Martin, M.S., Centers for Disease Control, in constructing this figure.)

since fewer than the threshold number of cases may represent an important problem on occasion and, in approximately 5 percent of instances, a larger number may be due to chance alone.

Selected High-Priority Infections

Certain nosocomial infections are either so uncommon or sufficiently important that their occurrence almost invariably suggests a potential problem without regard to the size of the hospital or the characteristics of the host population. In modern U.S. hospitals, for example, group A streptococcal infections occur rarely, and the occurrence of two or more nosocomial infections with this pathogen within a brief period of time usually suggests an infection control problem.

Multiply drug-resistant microorganisms,

once established in a hospital, complicate patient management and have been notoriously difficult to eradicate (see Chap. 13). Many hospitals consider the isolation of a new antimicrobial-resistant strain to require investigation and control, even if the strain does not produce disease. The identification of multiple isolations of a new nosocomial strain may similarly call for an epidemiologic assessment, even if the strain does not obviously cause patient illness, since this may also be an indication that a new mechanism of transmission or a new reservoir has become established.

Although every hospital epidemiologist would undoubtedly identify different high-priority infections, selected site-pathogen combinations that frequently suggested infection control problems during Centers for Disease Control (CDC) investigations are listed in Table 6-1.

Principles of Epidemiologic Investigations

For an infection to occur, a sufficient number of pathogenic microorganisms (the agent) must be present; an individual (the host) must be susceptible to infection; and a means for the agent to have appropriate contact with the host (mode of transmission) must be present (see Chap. 1). An infection may be prevented by altering any one of these factors. The goal of an epidemiologic investigation is to determine which of these factors may be most easily altered to prevent disease.

When a potential problem is first recognized, many factors may seem important. There may be, for example, many potential reservoirs, numerous possible host susceptibility factors, and various modes of transmission that might be responsible for disease acquisition. Which of these is actually related to the occurrence of disease is unknown, and it is therefore difficult to know how to control the problem. An investigation is designed to

Table 6-1. Site-pathogen combinations suggestive of infection problems

Pathogens	Systemic and blood	Surgical wound	CNS	Respiratory	UTI	Skin	Gastro-enteritis
Bacteria							
Acinetobacter			*				
Citrobacter	*		*				
Clostridium perfringens		*					
Corynebacterium diphtheriae	*			*		*	
Enterobacter	*		*				
Escherichia coli			*				
Klebsiella			*				
Legionella				*			
Listeria monocytogenes	*		*				
Neisseria meningitidis	*		*	*			
Pseudomonas aeruginosa		*	*				
Pseudomonas cepacia	*	*	*	*	*		
Salmonella	*	*	*		*		*
Serratia	*						
Shigella		*					*
Staphylococcus aureus			*				
Staphylococcus epidermidis			*				
Streptococcus, group A	*	*	*			*	
Streptococcus, group B	*		*				
Other microorganisms and diseases							
Aspergillus	*	*		*			
Herpes simplex virus	*	*					
Pneumocystis				*			
Varicella-zoster virus	*					*	

CNS = central nervous system; UTI = urinary tract infection.
Note: The combinations of microorganisms and sites of infection shown with an asterisk are unusual or serious in most U.S. hospitals, without regard to hospital size or type. The occurrence of 2 or more cases of nosocomial disease in a 30-day period generally deserves an evaluation. Isolation of *Corynebacterium diphtheriae* deserves assessment even if not associated with disease.

discover which factors are relevant so that control efforts can be efficiently instituted and concern about irrelevant factors discarded.

In the classic, formal investigation, identification of important factors is accomplished by comparing the characteristics of affected persons (the case population) with those of a similar group of unaffected persons (the control population). The major differences between the case and control populations are assumed to play a role in determining the occurrence of disease.

As discussed in the next section, on occasion effective control measures may be confidently designed without a formal investigation. In these settings, control measures can generally be taken because formal investigations have previously identified the important variables and have demonstrated effective control measures.

Epidemiologic investigations use the same basic study design and analytic principles as are used in other kinds of biomedical research. Several principles must be emphasized, however.

First, an investigation may show association but be unable to prove causation. For example, the risk of nosocomial pneumonia may be demonstrated to be strongly associated with recent thoracic or abdominal surgery. This does not prove that the surgery causes pneumonia; it merely indicates that something about the surgery—or the patients who typically undergo that kind of surgery—increases the risk of pneumonia. In some instances, however, the epidemiologic associations are sufficiently strong to allow a conclusion to be drawn about causation. A very strong association between exposure to a particular intravenous medication and primary bacteremia implies that the medication may be contaminated, especially if no other strong association is demonstrable. If the weight of epidemiologic evidence finds very strong associations and if those associations are biologically plausible as causal factors, the epidemiologist should be able to draw strong conclusions about causes of illness, and these conclusions can reasonably become the basis for institution of control measures.

Second, the epidemiologist should not expect to find that every case patient is exposed to the factor that is implicated as causing disease. Even in epidemics, in which specific factors are often proved responsible for disease, one occasionally identifies case patients who fulfill the criteria for being part of the outbreak but have no demonstrable association with the presumed causal factor. It must be remembered that even in epidemic situations, sporadic, endemic disease continues to occur and that these patients may be difficult to separate from the epidemic cases on clinical or epidemiologic grounds. This is illustrated in the epidemiologic studies showing the relation between cigarette smoking and the development of lung cancer. Not everyone who smokes will acquire cancer, and some persons acquire lung cancer without exposure to cigarette smoking. Nonetheless, the associations between smoking and development of cancer are exceedingly strong and, moreover, the possibility that smoking causes lung cancer is biologically plausible. Therefore, most observers have concluded that a direct, causal link exists, and efforts to encourage less smoking have been widely adopted.

Third, the epidemiologist uses clinical data somewhat differently from the clinician. If a nursing mother has a breast abscess, for example, her physician would prefer microbiologic proof before making the diagnosis of staphylococcal infection. In contrast, if the same patient's records are reviewed by an epidemiologist during the investigation of a nursery staphylococcal outbreak and if the woman's infant had staphylococcal disease, the epidemiologist should assume that she, too, had a staphylococcal infection, whether or not a culture was obtained.

Protocol for Epidemiologic Investigations in the Hospital

Some investigations of nosocomial infection problems are highly complex, requiring that investigators be skilled in epidemiology and statistics, that resources be available for sophisticated analyses of complex data, or that specialized laboratory facilities be readily available. Most epidemiologic investigations of nosocomial infections do not require special resources, however, and every hospital's infection control staff should be able to perform at least the initial phases of most investigations.

Each epidemiologic study is different, and there is no simple, standardized approach to conducting an investigation. Not only is each epidemiologist likely to approach a problem differently, but the relative importance and sequence of steps will necessarily differ according to the nature of the problem. Nonetheless, there are general approaches to epidemiologic investigation that have proved practical and effective when employed by CDC epidemiologists in investigating nosocomial infection problems, and these steps are summarized in this section.

Figure 6-2 illustrates a decision pathway to help determine whether a formal, classic, case-control investigation (a *major* investigation) is required or whether a more limited

Fig. 6-2. Decision pathway to select between a basic and major epidemiologic investigation.

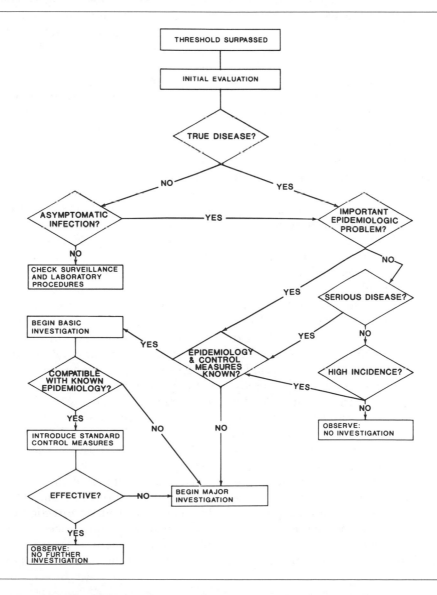

study (a *basic* investigation) will suffice. The basic investigation is adequate to solve most nosocomial infection problems and should be within the capabilities of most infection control programs. The major investigation is required for unique, very serious, or complex problems, and such investigations may require outside assistance in many institutions. The initial steps are similar for both kinds of investigations, however.

Initial Evaluation

As illustrated in Figure 6-2, an initial investigation should be instituted whenever the hospital's established threshold of concern, as described earlier, is surpassed.

Conduct Preliminary Case Review

The epidemiologist first reviews the clinical and epidemiologic characteristics of affected patients. At this stage, the epidemiologist may choose to study a convenient sample of patients; the purpose of the review is to establish the nature and seriousness of the potential problem in general terms, not to characterize it completely. This patient sample may include persons present in the hospital, those identified by routine surveillance, or those whose medical records are conveniently available.

It is important to remember, however, that study subjects who are selected because they are readily available (i.e., a sample of convenience) may not accurately reflect the characteristics of other affected patients and may introduce bias into the investigation that can be misleading. For example, neonatal staphylococcal infection has an incubation period of approximately 7 days. As a result, staphylococcal disease in full-term infants often begins after hospital discharge, and disease with onset during hospitalization occurs more often in hospitalized infants with prolonged stay. Therefore, although a nursery staphylococcal problem may initially seem to be limited to premature infants or those born by cesarean section, thorough case finding may identify a large number of term infants also affected. The epidemiologist who relies solely on a sample of convenience—in this example,

hospitalized infants—may fail to recognize the full scope of a problem. More systematic case finding is generally required at later stages for all but the simplest outbreaks.

Evaluate Clinical Severity

During the initial clinical and epidemiologic review, the epidemiologist should determine whether disease is present. The absence of actual disease does not indicate the absence of an infection control problem, however, and the epidemiologist often needs to continue an investigation even in such circumstances.

Approximately 11 percent of formal nosocomial epidemiologic investigations conducted by CDC investigators between 1956 and 1979 were determined to be pseudo-epidemics, generally caused by surveillance artifacts or laboratory errors [3]. Although pseudoepidemics may not be associated with patient illness, they are nonetheless important to identify since they may affect the quality of patient care. Errors in processing or interpreting laboratory specimens should be identified since they may lead to faulty clinical diagnoses or inappropriate patient treatment. Faulty surveillance should be corrected so that actual infections are not missed and infection control information is reliable.

On occasion, microbial colonization without disease may reflect an important problem, such as when a colonizing strain is resistant to multiple antimicrobial agents and may serve as a source for subsequent transmission. In other instances, an epidemic of colonization may indicate a breakdown in basic infection control techniques that allows the colonizing strain to spread from patient to patient. In a setting such as this, more virulent strains might also be easily spread, so an investigation into the mechanism of transmission may be useful.

The epidemiologist may choose not to investigate a problem that involves few patients, causes inconsequential disease, or does not seem likely to result from a fundamental breakdown of routine infection control practices. In such circumstances, implementation of empiric control measures or continued monitoring of the problem using surveillance may be all that is necessary. Serious disease or infections affecting large numbers of persons will usually call for an active investigation.

If, on the other hand, serious clinical disease occurs, infections occur at high frequency, or a potentially serious infection control problem is identified, either a basic or major investigation is indicated.

If the epidemiologist's initial assessment suggests that the hospital's problem is similar to ones that have previously occurred and that effective infection prevention and control measures are well known, it is reasonable to begin a basic investigation. A major investigation should be begun at this point if the problem seems to be unusual and control measures are not readily apparent.

As is illustrated in Figure 6-2, a basic investigation may be begun during which the epidemiologist may decide that a formal case-control evaluation is required. Additional evaluation during the basic investigation may show that the problem is actually unique or that the control measures that initially seemed reasonable are inappropriate. Later, those standard control measures that have been implemented may not be effective in solving the problem. In each circumstance, a major investigation should be begun.

The Basic Investigation

The basic epidemiologic investigation is a useful and efficient technique for evaluating simple, uncomplicated, and generally nonserious infection problems. It allows the hospital to implement reasonable control measures that have been previously developed, evaluated, and found to be effective. The majority of common problems in hospitals can be managed by this approach.

The basic investigation is especially useful when the clinical and epidemiologic characteristics of case patients are similar to those described elsewhere and when prevention and control measures have been documented to be effective.

In the basic investigation, unlike the major investigation, prevention and control techniques that are likely to be effective are applied empirically. Furthermore, epidemio-

logic techniques are not used to demonstrate differences between case and control patients. As a result, the basic investigation is unlikely to provide scientific evidence about the cause of the problem being investigated and should not be used if the problem requires continuing scientific study or if the investigator wishes to publish the result of the investigation.

Collect Critical Data and Specimens

Early in the investigation, the epidemiologist needs to ensure that critical data, specimens, and observations that may be needed during the subsequent phases of the investigation are preserved. Samples of microbial strains believed to be implicated in the problem (epidemic strains) should be saved by the microbiology laboratory. Hospital practices prevailing during the period should be documented since widespread changes in practices often occur once an investigation is begun, and it may not be possible to reconstruct the procedures later in the investigation. Any commercially supplied medications, devices, or materials that may be associated with the problem should be placed in quarantine and saved for public health authorities such as those of the Food and Drug Administration (FDA); all too frequently, such materials are discarded or returned to the manufacturer during the early phases of investigations, making them unavailable for subsequent independent testing if they are implicated in causing disease. Selected specimens of materials likely to be relevant should be collected for testing, since such materials are often cleaned or discarded early in investigations. Although it is very uneconomical and generally unrewarding to initiate widespread, indiscriminate culturing of specimens from patients, personnel, or the inanimate environment, the epidemiologist must judiciously select for sampling those sources that are highly suspect on the basis of past experiences.

Institute Empiric Control Measures

The epidemiologist should institute control measures based on previous experiences with similar problems and that are appropriate to the problem as defined in the patient case review. It is sometimes impossible to implement any reasonable control measure until an epidemiologic investigation has identified the cause of the problem, and in such instances a major investigation is warranted. In other instances, the problem may have many potential causes, and it is impractical to institute control measures for each; here too a major investigation is useful. For most problems, however, a large body of experience exists to guide the epidemiologist in selecting the appropriate prevention and control measures and to assist in deciding their priorities.

Identify Affected Patients

The epidemiologist initiates a systematic attempt to identify as many affected patients as possible, recognizing, as discussed earlier, that readily available case patients may not represent the actual affected population. Formulation of a *tentative case definition* will help guide the search for potential patients with disease. The case definition is simply the epidemiologist's best description of the probable characteristics of case patients. It often includes descriptions of the host group affected and a definition of the kind of disease that occurs; at this point, it must be based on the findings of the preliminary review. For example, the case definition in a nursery staphylococcal outbreak might simply be: An infant, born in the past 3 months, with (1) skin lesions characteristic of staphylococcal pustulosis or (2) a positive culture for *Staphylococcus aureus* from any site, or (3) both.

At this early phase in the investigation, the case definition should be broad since the full scope of the outbreak cannot be known with certainty. An overly broad case definition may lead to a review of patients who are not part of the problem, but they can be subsequently excluded from analysis. An excessively restrictive case definition tends to exclude patients from being evaluated, and the failure to study such patients may seriously jeopardize the investigation.

Case-finding methods are determined by the problem being investigated but, in the majority of epidemiologic investigations in hospitals, a reasonably complete listing of probable case patients can be readily obtained by reviewing surveillance and microbiology records.

Carefully collected surveillance data are a prime resource, but case finding should not be limited to these data since surveillance typically fails to identify all nosocomial infections even when excellent surveillance methods are employed. Surveillance is especially likely to miss patients with mild or asymptomatic infection or those who have onset of clinical disease after discharge.

Microbiology records should generally be reviewed as a matter of course to identify other potentially affected individuals. The investigator should seek not only to identify patients with infection at the site or with the microorganism that prompted the investigation, but also to review similar strains and potentially related sites of infection to ensure that the problem is not more widespread than was originally thought. On occasion patients who have had negative results on laboratory studies may need to be evaluated, for they too may be part of the outbreak.

In certain outbreaks, specialized case-finding techniques are required. A carefully designed questionnaire or telephone survey of selected physicians or recently discharged patients may be useful if a characteristic clinical syndrome, unlikely to be identified by hospital surveillance or culturing, is being investigated. If onset of disease may occur after hospital discharge, inquiries to other hospitals, community physicians, and local health departments may be particularly helpful. Clinical examination, culture surveys, skin tests, or serologic surveys may also be useful in some instances.

Review Characteristics of Representative Case Patients

The epidemiologist next reviews a sufficient number of case patients to define the clinical and epidemiologic characteristics of the potential problem. In this review, the epidemiologist is particularly interested in identifying common host or exposure features of case patients.

When possible, all potentially affected patients should be reviewed. In very large outbreaks (e.g., involving more than 50 patients), it is appropriate to study a sample of patient cases.

Various techniques are available to select samples of patients for review. Whatever scheme is used, the epidemiologist must take care that the sampling process selects a group for study that is *representative* of the total population. In general, randomized sampling is least likely to introduce bias and therefore should be used unless there are strong arguments for using an alternative technique. Systematic sampling can be used in hospital studies if the investigator can be assured that the systematic sampling interval does not correspond to patterns within the hospital that might bias case selection. Samples of convenience—the selection of patients who are readily available—should generally be avoided.

Basic patient-identifying information should be recorded that will allow subsequent retrieval of clinical records, and selected clinical and epidemiologic data should be abstracted. The data to be abstracted fall into several categories that are considered epidemiologically in terms of time, place, and person (see also Chap. 1).

Time   The time course of an infection problem provides valuable epidemiologic information. An *epidemic curve*—a graph showing the number of cases of disease according to the time of onset—should be plotted. This curve allows ready comparison of an epidemic period with a preepidemic, or baseline, period and, in addition, may allow identification of temporal clusters of cases of disease. The characteristics of the epidemic curve often suggest how disease is spread. An abrupt increase in the number of cases suggests a single exposure to a point source of contamination, as is shown in Figure 6-3A. A more protracted course may be compatible with person-to-person spread (Fig. 6-3B). Mixed modes of transmission may be implied by curves such as that shown in Figure 6-3C and, as in Figure 6-3D, the epidemic curve is occasionally consistent with several distinct modes of spread.

When the epidemic curve is drawn, the time-scale intervals should be shorter than the presumed incubation period of the disease since person-to-person spread may appear to be common-source spread if longer intervals are used (Fig. 6-4).

Similar plots showing dates of exposure to potential sources of disease, rather than dates of clinical onset, may be especially useful when the disease has a long or variable incubation period. Such plots may suggest common exposures that are not apparent in curves showing the dates of disease onset.

Place   Geographic clustering should also be evaluated. Pictorial representation in the form of *spot maps* is useful: Each case of disease is located by its geographic point of onset or acquisition. This simple technique often makes prominent otherwise inapparent clustering and may also suggest the mode of spread. Clustering in a single ward implies a common source or person-to-person spread. Hospital airflow patterns may explain the spatial clustering of disease, as is shown in Figure 6-5 [2]; this spot map shows the distribution of cases of smallpox in a German hospital (see also Chap. 38). The index case (patient 1) had no direct or indirect contact with any of the other cases (secondary and tertiary cases). All secondary and tertiary cases, however, occurred in rooms that received air that flowed from the room of the index case.

A disease scattered at random throughout the hospital is compatible with an autogenous source, widespread distribution of a contaminated common source, or an extensive breakdown in patient care practices.

Not only should the place of primary residence of patients be considered, but their exposures to other hospital areas should also be evaluated. Surgical wound infections, for example, may be specifically associated with a particular operating room.

Time and place descriptions can be combined to reconstruct the dynamic spread of infection through the hospital. Here again, graphic or pictorial representation may be useful. Geographic exposures may be added to a standard epidemic curve, or sequential

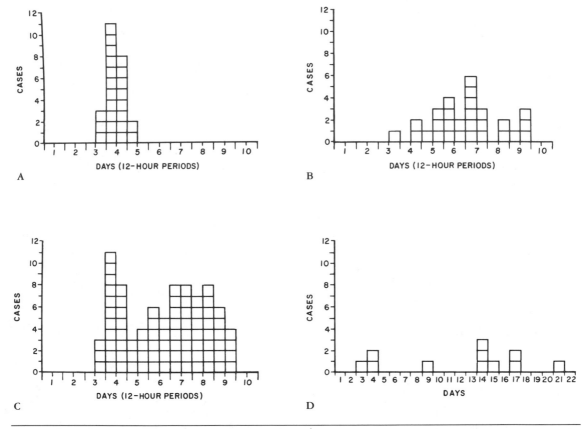

Fig. 6-3. Epidemic curves depicting commonly observed temporal characteristics of outbreaks in hospitals. *A.* A common-source outbreak of disease with an incubation period of 18–36 hours. Disease occurrence reaches its peak rapidly. *B.* Person-to-person transmission of a disease with a similar incubation period. The first case of disease (index case) is followed by increasing numbers of cases as the disease spreads. *C.* Mixed common-source and person-to-person transmission of the same disease. The initial peak represents those patients exposed to the contaminated common source, and the later, broader peak represents secondary spread of the disease. *D.* Intermittent exposure to a common source is represented by an indeterminate pattern. This pattern is also consistent with that of a common-source outbreak of disease with a variable incubation period, that of spread from asymptomatic carriers, or that of spread from infected persons who have prolonged carriage. This pattern may also be seen when many persons have asymptomatic infection and only few have clinically apparent disease.

spot maps may be constructed to trace the spread of disease.

Person A thorough description of the case population is the most important part of this phase of the investigation. The goals of this description are to define the specific underlying host characteristics that predispose to infection and to evaluate all exposures that may alter susceptibility or provide an opportunity for contact with the infecting agent.

Here a deliberate, exhaustive search for common features shared by the cases of infection is crucial. Patient host factors that may influence susceptibility to disease should be recorded, such as age, sex, nutritional status, types of underlying diseases, history of active or passive immunization, and the receipt of antimicrobial or immunosuppressive medications. For some diseases, specific host factors are important. Patients with gastric achlorhydria are especially susceptible

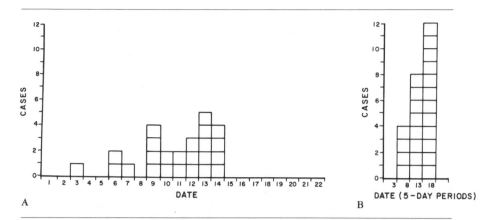

Fig. 6-4. Effects of the time scale on the appearance of the epidemic curve. The epidemic curves represent the same outbreak caused by a pathogen with a 2-day incubation period. *A.* The curve can correctly suggest person-to-person spread if the time scale has intervals slightly shorter than the incubation period. *B.* When long intervals are used, the curve incorrectly suggests a common-source exposure.

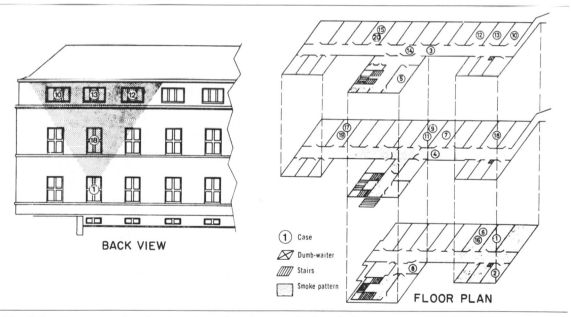

Fig. 6-5. Spot map showing location of patients with nosocomial smallpox and relation to airflow patterns in a hospital in Meschede, Germany. Patient 1 was the index case. Shaded areas show flow of air from the room of patient 1 to other areas of the hospital. (From Centers for Disease Control. Follow-up smallpox—Federal Republic of Germany. *M.M.W.R.* 19:234, 1970. [Adapted from World Health Organization, Smallpox surveillance. *Weekly Epidemiol. Rec.* 45:249, 1970.])

to shigellosis and other enteric diseases, for example.

Exposure factors should also be recorded, both animate and inanimate. Contacts with people should be considered, even when disease is usually considered to be acquired from

autogenous sources. The source for gram-negative microorganisms such as *Escherichia coli,* for example, is usually believed to be autogenous carriage or exogenous acquisition from the inanimate environment. These infections may, however, be transmitted from person-to-person; frequently, such spread occurs by way of patient care personnel.

Therapeutic measures may alter intrinsic host susceptibility or provide the opportunity for contact with the infecting pathogen. Antimicrobial therapy should generally be considered, since it may predispose to colonization or disease if the infecting strain is resistant or it may prevent disease if the strain is susceptible. Specific treatments may provide a portal of entry for the infecting microorganism: Urinary catheterization, for example, provides a direct route by which bacteria may enter the bladder, and intravenous cannulas provide direct access to the vascular system. Knowledge of such exposures may point to the source of the infecting strain.

Methods to Obtain and Process Data
The case review may be aided by careful design of the data collection forms. It should be remembered that the goal of the investigation is to characterize selected aspects of the entire affected population, not every detail about each individual case. Thus simple descriptive characteristics (e.g., age, sex, nature of underlying diseases) and notations as to the presence or absence of selected exposures (e.g., geographic areas, personnel, medications, procedures) are all that are generally required.

A simple line-listing form is usually the most efficient way to record these data (Fig. 6-6). Each patient is listed on the form, and

the appropriate characteristics are checked off or otherwise summarized.

If many patients must be evaluated or numerous host and exposure factors analyzed, data-processing techniques may aid in the analysis of data. Minicomputers or microcomputers and sophisticated data-base management and statistical software programs are widely available in hospitals (see Chap. 8), and infection control personnel may elect to develop skills in their use. Unless extensive data are collected and the investigators are familiar with computerized data-processing techniques (or have readily available support from others who can assist with the design of computer-based analytic programs), however, computerization of the investigation is likely to entail more work and require more time than manual tabulation.

Refine the Case Definition
After the patient case review has been completed, the epidemiologist should be able to define the general nature of the problem. This is usually done by refining the preliminary case definition developed at the beginning of the investigation. The case definition should now describe the essential features of affected patients: Are the illnesses nosocomial or community-acquired; what particular patient populations are affected; what are the clinical sites of infection; what microorganisms are involved; during what period of time does the problem occur?

Fig. 6-6. Portion of a typical line-listing form used to tabulate data during an epidemiologic investigation. The items to be tabulated are determined by the nature of the problem under investigation.

CASE NO.	PATIENT I.D. NO.	DATES Adm	DATES Disch	DATES Death	AGE	SEX	SERVICE	WARD	SITE INFCT	DATE ONSET	1	2	3	4	5	6	7	8	9	10	11	12	IV	URINE CATH
1	42266	4/27	6/1		46	M	Surg	4B	Blood	5/16	X	X		X	X	X		X	X	I	X	X	5/15-5/28	4/27-6/1
2	05819	5/17		5/24	32	F	OB	6A	Blood	5/18	X	X		X	X	X		X	X	I	X	X	5/18-5/19	
3	38776	5/8		5/18	76	M	Med	2B	Blood	5/18	X	X		X	X	X		X	X	X	X	X	5/8-5/18	5/12-5/18

(ANTIMICROBIAL RESISTANCE (X) spans columns 1–12)

As a rule, the full extent of the problem is seldom recognized early in the investigation. Patients initially considered to be cases may now need to be discarded from the study population, and additional patients may need to be added to the study group as the investigation proceeds and the epidemiologist develops a better understanding of the characteristics of the problem.

Although the epidemiologist may reasonably decide to take expedient shortcuts in many phases of the epidemiologic investigation, great care should be taken at this stage to establish an accurate case definition since this definition guides all subsequent phases of the investigation. If this case definition is inaccurate, the conclusions drawn from the investigation are likely to be faulty, and control measures may not be accurately identified.

An overly restrictive case definition will exclude true case patients and make it more difficult to show statistically significant differences between case and control patients. An inappropriately inclusive case definition will dilute true case patients with those who are not a part of the problem and may obscure associations with disease. In general, it is best to be overly inclusive during the early stages of the investigation but as restrictive as possible at this stage. If it is impossible to determine whether some patients should be included as case patients, the epidemiologist may label them as possible or probable cases and conduct analyses with those patients both included and excluded from the analysis group.

Reconsider Whether Major Investigation Is Needed

After collecting epidemiologic and clinical data from case patients, the epidemiologist should decide whether the characteristics of the problem are similar to those described in other institutions and whether reasonable control measures have already been established elsewhere. If the problem is not unique, empiric control measures should be implemented. If, on the other hand, the characteristics of the cases are not consistent with what

is known about similar problems, a major investigation should be initiated.

Institute Appropriate Control Measures

Steps to prevent or control disease are often taken immediately—even before the investigation is begun—especially when the problem is serious. If such control measures have not been introduced, the epidemiologist should consider whether any are likely to be effective on the basis of what has been learned from the patient case review. Numerous control measures are frequently available for use, varying in cost, complexity, and efficacy.

A decision about the kinds of control measures to implement should be based on the urgency of control. Major, disruptive, or costly control measures may not be indicated if the clinical and epidemiologic problems are not serious. If effective control measures have not been established or established measures appear to be inappropriate to the epidemiologic situation, the epidemiologist may elect to initiate a major investigation.

Monitor Effectiveness of Control Measures

The institution of control measures may be followed by an apparent resolution of the problem. It must be recognized that the control measures may have had no actual effect and that a temporary reduction in disease occurrence may be fortuitous. The infection control program must continue to monitor the problem, therefore, to ensure that it does not recur. Although standard surveillance techniques occasionally are adequate to monitor a problem, specific techniques are frequently necessary, including careful follow-up of high-risk patients, ongoing surveillance of patient care techniques, or selective culturing of patients or their environment. Ultimately, control measures should be judged successful only if an acceptable rate of patient infection is maintained.

If control measures reduce the incidence of disease to acceptable levels for an appropriate period of time, no additional investigation is required, but if the control measures are ineffective or the problem recurs while those control measures are in effect, a major epidemiologic investigation should be instituted immediately.

The Major Epidemiologic Investigation

The major investigation—a more rigorous scientific evaluation than the basic investigation, typically involving careful comparisons of case and control populations—should be conducted when a problem is unusual, complex, or of substantial scientific importance, or when the basic investigation has been unsuccessful.

Many of the studies conducted in the early portion of the basic investigation are also done in the major investigation but, as noted in Table 6-2, the strategies diverge after the epidemiologist has reviewed the clinical and epidemiologic characteristics of case patients. Rather than institute empiric control measures, as in the basic investigation, the epidemiologist attempts to identify the causes of the problem through a series of case-control studies and analyses.

Table 6-2.　Steps in initial, basic, and major epidemiologic investigations

Initial investigation
　Conduct preliminary case review
　Evaluate severity of problem
　Select basic or major investigation
Basic investigation
　Collect critical data and specimens
　Institute control measures
　Identify affected patients
　Review case characteristics (time, place, person)
　Refine case definition
　Reconsider major investigation
　Institute control measures
　Monitor effectiveness of control measures
　Reconsider major investigation
Major investigation
　Collect critical data and specimens
　Consider institution of control measures
　Identify affected patients
　Review case characteristics (time, place, person)
　Refine case definition
　Determine if consultation needed
　Formulate tentative hypotheses
　Test hypotheses
　Institute control measures
　Evaluate control measures

If a major investigation is undertaken after a basic investigation has failed to solve a problem, the steps already conducted need not be repeated. However, the investigator should reevaluate the methods used in the basic investigation to be certain that shortcuts were not taken that might impair the validity of the more rigorous evaluation. In particular, the epidemiologist should review the adequacy of previous attempts to (1) develop a case definition, (2) identify all infected patients, and (3) characterize the case patients clinically and epidemiologically.

Refine Case Definition

If a preliminary basic investigation has failed to identify the problem, the preliminary case definition may have been faulty. Commonly, the initial working case definition is too restrictive and has thereby failed to identify major segments of the affected population. When beginning a formal investigation, the initial case definition should be reconsidered and broadened if necessary. The revised case definition will continue to be refined as the investigation progresses, and patients can be removed from the case group if the subsequent investigation indicates they are not part of the problem.

Refine Case-Finding Techniques

During a basic investigation, the epidemiologist often takes expedient shortcuts, such as identifying and reviewing only a sample of affected patients. On beginning a major investigation, aggressive steps should be taken to identify *all* potential cases. It is especially important that a broad case definition be used for case finding so that few cases of infection will be missed. Case finding should extend sufficiently into previous time periods to identify when the first cases of disease occurred, since the most recently occurring cases may have different epidemiologic characteristics from those of cases occurring earlier.

Review Cases of Disease

In all but the largest outbreaks, the epidemiologist conducting a major investigation should attempt to review all identified cases of disease. In very large outbreaks, this may be impractical, but special care must then be taken to ensure that the sample of patients reviewed is representative. Again, random sampling techniques are preferred, and patients should be selected for review from the complete potential case listing. On occasion, stratified random sampling can compensate for small numbers of patients in important risk groups.

It is useful to reevaluate the case records of all affected patients, even if they have been previously evaluated during an earlier, more limited assessment. For those patients, as well as for new patients not previously studied, a thorough tabulation of epidemiologic characteristics (time, place, and person) is necessary. The epidemiologist should not only look for factors that have been documented as important in previous investigations but also be prepared to identify previously unrecognized associations.

If a major investigation is undertaken from the start, the steps listed in Table 6-2 and described for the basic investigation should be completed.

Determine Whether Consultation Is Required

Early in the major investigation, the epidemiologist should consider whether outside assistance is likely to be necessary; the investigation may require a substantial investment of time as well as sophisticated laboratory or statistical support. Many state and local health departments are able to advise hospitals regarding epidemiologic investigations and often can assist in arranging epidemiologic and laboratory support when indicated. Universities with an academic and research interest in nosocomial infections as well as private consulting epidemiologists provide additional sources for assistance. State health departments may request direct assistance from the CDC if needed, and the CDC also provides advice to hospital personnel about strategies that can be used in investigation.

When contamination of a commercially supplied medication or device is suspected, public health authorities should be notified immediately. In particular, the FDA and CDC should be notified; other hospitals may also be affected, and these federal agencies are responsible for evaluation and control of such problems.

Formulate Tentative Hypotheses

After completing the review of the clinical and exposure data available for affected patients, the epidemiologist prepares a profile of cases, which is a summary of host factors and exposures of patient cases developed by tabulating the presence or absence of the time, place, and person characteristics previously described. In this profile, the epidemiologist seeks to identify common features among the bases, the assumption being that at least one of these common features will account for the susceptibility to infection.

The list of common features may be short or long. On rare occasions, one feature is so prominent among cases that only a single explanation for the infection problem need reasonably be considered. More often, a large list is developed, and there are numerous reasonable hypotheses that may be advanced to explain the problem. The following hypothetical example illustrates the process of hypothesis formulation.

An investigation of epidemic *Proteus rettgeri* urinary tract infection (UTI) shows that all patients infected with the epidemic strain were hospitalized on a single ward, and each had indwelling urinary catherization before the onset of infection. The epidemic strain neither had been isolated elsewhere in the hospital nor had caused disease other than UTI.

From the case review, the problem appears uniquely to affect patients on a single ward who have been catheterized. These two associations suggest a number of hypotheses, some of which follow. The geographic clustering may have several explanations: It may result from practices in obtaining culture specimens that are unique to the affected ward; a common source such as a medication or an infected staff member may be present on the ward; or ward patients themselves who are already infected may provide a source for the epidemic strain. The association with urinary catheterization also suggests several hypotheses. The catheter may be related because it leads to a breach in bladder defenses. Alternatively, the catheter or some agent associated with catheter insertion may be contaminated with the epidemic strain. The catheter may be a proxy for the true risk factor, urinary irrigation, which is not routinely recorded in the patient record. Finally, if every patient on the ward is catheterized, catheterization may be unrelated to the risk of disease.

No factor can be excluded as unimportant simply because it is not present in each patient defined as a case. Rarely are all host and exposure factors identified with certainty. Furthermore, sporadic cases of disease—those that are, in fact, unrelated to the problem being investigated—may occur during an outbreak, and these cases may be difficult to distinguish from the outbreak cases.

Test the Hypotheses

A valid hypothesis should explain not only why some patients acquire disease but also why other patients do not. Most of the explanations in the example just provided are reasonable to explain UTI due to *Proteus* organisms, but if information is obtained only about the infected patients, the absence of disease in other patients remains an enigma. The crucial next step of the major investigation allows refinement of the hypotheses so that fortuitous associations can be discarded and causal factors more clearly delineated.

Three basic techniques are commonly used to refine hypotheses: case-control, cohort, and prospective intervention studies.

Case-Control Study Retrospectively conducted case-control evaluation is the most effective technique for investigating most hospital epidemics, and it is also often useful for investigating hyperendemic problems (see Chap. 1). In such a study, a group of un-

infected patients (the *control group*) is compared with infected patients (the *case group*), and differences in susceptibility and exposure factors are examined. If a proper control group is selected, statistically significant differences between groups are likely to identify the cause of the problem. The value of the case-control study is illustrated in the following example which, although simplified, is based on an actual investigation.

Over a 4-month period, 50 patients on a urology service had UTI due to *Pseudomonas cepacia*. A review of the charts of the patient cases showed that 48 (96 percent) had urinary tract irrigation before infection. No other factor was seen as often: Previous cystoscopy was performed in 45 (90 percent), no single physician treated more than 20 percent of infected patients, and only 62 percent could be documented to have had contact with another known case.

From the case data, urinary tract irrigation appeared to be strongly implicated. To test this hypothesis, a control population composed of 84 uninfected urology patients hospitalized in the same period was evaluated. In this control population, it was found that irrigation was indeed common; uninfected control patients had irrigation almost as often as did cases (Table 6-3). Only 24 of the 84 control patients, however, had previous cystoscopy. This suggested that the cystoscopy procedure may have been more important. Even this association, however, did not prove that cystoscopy was responsible for the outbreak. Why did some cystoscopy patients develop infection, whereas others did not?

Uninfected cystoscopy patients were used as a second control group, and comparison of the data pointed up yet another significant as-

Table 6-3. *Pseudomonas cepacia* urinary tract infection outbreak: exposures of cases and controls

Patient category	Cases (%)	Controls (%)
Total patients	50	84
Exposed to urinary irrigation	48 (96)	80 (95)
Exposed to cystoscopy	45 (90)	24 (29)

sociation: There was a marked difference between the groups of physicians who treated the cases and controls (Table 6-4). In this analysis, treatment by one group of urologists (group A) was associated with only 2 cases of infection, but these physicians treated 12 of the uninfected control patients. In contrast, infection occurred in 43 of 55 cystoscopy patients treated by the other group (group B) of urologists. Additional investigation revealed that the group having fewer cases disinfected cystoscopy instruments with glutaraldehyde, whereas the group with the higher attack rate preferred the use of an aqueous quaternary ammonium disinfectant. On culture, the quaternary ammonium disinfectant yielded the epidemic strain of *P. cepacia.*

This hypothetical example, based on an actual outbreak, illustrates that several control groups are often required to identify the susceptibility and exposure factors responsible for an outbreak of disease. It is also apparent that the epidemiologist selects each control group to test one or more specific hypotheses. A basic strategy for selecting control groups in a stepwise manner can now be described.

First, the epidemiologist should identify important host factors that influence susceptibility to infection. How, for example, do case patients differ from other hospitalized patients in terms of age, sex, underlying disease, immune status, and antimicrobial therapy. Often it is not necessary to select a formal control group to evaluate some of these factors. If disease occurs only in neonates, it is not necessary to use a formal control group

of the general hospital population to show that age is an important factor. It may be necessary, however, to compare gestational age, birth weight, or Apgar score of infected and uninfected infants.

Since susceptibility alone is not sufficient to explain infection (appropriate exposure to a pathogen is also required), one must next evaluate exposure factors. As with the case review, time, place, and person characteristics should be studied. In this phase of the investigation, susceptibility factors can be controlled by using patients in the control group with similar susceptibility factors; for example, if patients with disease are significantly older than control patients, subsequent control populations should be selected to contain an age distribution comparable to that found for cases. As another example, if patients with gastroenteritis due to *Salmonella* have a significantly higher occurrence of peptic ulcer disease, subsequent control groups should be selected to include a comparable proportion of patients with ulcer.

If all cases have a single susceptibility factor, all controls should have that factor. More commonly, several susceptibility factors occur in varying proportions and with varying degrees of statistical significance when case populations are compared with controls. To deal with this problem, the control populations should be stratified to ensure comparability. Age is one such susceptibility variable that is amenable to stratification. Table 6-5

Table 6-4. *Pseudomonas cepacia* urinary tract infection outbreak: exposures to two physician groups (A and B), cystoscopy cases versus cystoscopy controls

Patient category	Cystos-copy cases	Cystos-copy controls	Total exposed	Infection rates (%)
Total patients	45	24	69	—
Exposed to group A	2	12	14	14
Exposed to group B	43	12	55	78

Table 6-5. Percentage distribution of patient ages: cases of disease compared with random control population

Age range (years)	Cases (%)	Controls (%)
Birth−9	0	7
10−19	0	4
20−29	0	12
30−39	2	9
40−49	22	18
50−59	26	21
60−69	28	18
70−79	18	8
80 and older	4	3

shows the distribution of ages for hypothetical case and control populations. Although the patients with cases of disease are significantly older than the patients in the control population, young patients also have disease. To control for age adequately, subsequent control populations should be stratified to ensure that they have a similar age distribution to the case group.

If an outbreak occurs during a discrete period, two control populations are possible. First, uninfected patients hospitalized before or after the outbreak may be compared with those with disease to identify significantly different exposures to people, procedures, or other factors. Next, uninfected patients hospitalized during the epidemic period may be studied to test whether these differences are important; that is, if the differences remain, such exposures may be important.

Exposure to various hospital locations can be similarly examined. If hemodialysis patients with hepatitis B had a significantly higher exposure to a single dialysis station than dialysis patients without hepatitis who were treated during the same period, the dialysis station is implicated as potentially important.

Finally, exposures to personnel, other patients, procedures, and medications should be evaluated. Using a control population that is similar to the case group in terms of disease susceptibility and time and place characteristics, the exposure to the infecting pathogen should be found to occur significantly more frequently among cases than controls.

This progressive use of multiple control populations, controlling at each step for previously identified significant factors, may seem tedious and arduous. This description of the process, however, overemphasizes the number of separate steps required. The steps listed separately can often be combined, for it is usually possible to evaluate several time, place, and person exposures at the same time by using the same carefully selected control group. It must be recognized, however, that the process described previously should not be ignored lest the chance of bias, with the resulting risk of deriving a faulty conclusion, be introduced.

On rare occasions, no difference in host susceptibility can be established on comparison of cases and controls. This occurs most frequently when the infecting agent is virulent or when the portal of infection is such that, on exposure, every patient develops disease. Similarly, the case-control evaluation may fail to demonstrate significant differences in exposures between infected and uninfected patients. Most commonly, this occurs when there is widespread or unrecognized infection in the control population, when the disease results from endogenous colonization present at the time of admission, or when case records do not document the truly significant exposure. Each of these possibilities must be evaluated with the prospective techniques described on page 130.

Hospitalization itself can have a profound effect on host susceptibility, and this can complicate the interpretation of case-control studies. As an illustration, patients with lymphoma may have similar susceptibilities to infection at time of admission to the hospital. After treatment is initiated, however, their susceptibilities are altered. If infected and uninfected lymphoma patients are compared for host factors apparent at the time of their admission, no major differences in susceptibility may be apparent. To obtain a clearer definition of susceptibility factors, it may be necessary to compare these factors after a period of hospitalization. In this example, the epidemiologist might calculate the average interval between the time of admission and that of the onset of disease in case patients and then compare the host characteristics of cases and controls at that point.

Methods for Selection of Control Groups　Before selecting the members of a control group, the epidemiologist must decide the number of control patients required and the specific technique for determining which uninfected patients will be selected. (See Chap. 7.)

The number of control patients required to show differences between case and control patients depends on a number of factors, including the relative frequencies with which the factor to be compared occurs in each population and the statistical certainty required by the investigator in showing differences or no differences. Statistical techniques are available for estimating the size of control groups, but it is often unnecessary to calculate the control group size precisely. If the factor to be compared occurs either very frequently or very infrequently in patients with disease, one control patient for each case patient is usually sufficient; on the other hand, if the factor occurs in approximately half of the case patients, several control patients for each case are usually necessary. Almost always, at least one control patient for each case patient should be chosen.

Next, the epidemiologist must select a method by which to choose control patients. Individual control patients may be selected by including all in the pool of appropriate uninfected patients (a universal sample) or by taking a portion of that pool according to a sampling scheme.

When small populations are studied, all available controls may be required. If the potential pool of control patients is large, this universal sampling method is inefficient, since more control patients than are necessary will be evaluated. In such circumstances, matched, random, or stratified random-sampling schemes may be used.

A *matched sample* may be used when there are only a few general factors that must be controlled, such as age or date of hospitalization. With the matching procedure, each case patient is matched with one or more uninfected control patients according to specified matching characteristics. It is relatively easy to find an appropriate match when a single factor needs to be controlled. As the number of factors increases or the matching factors become more specific (e.g., the type and duration of surgical procedure), matching becomes more difficult. Even if successful, large numbers of records of potential control patients must be reviewed and discarded to obtain each successful match.

A *random sample* does not require the tedious selection process used in developing a matched sample. Instead, the epidemiologist relies on the powerful effect of chance to ensure that a representative, nonbiased population is selected. Various randomization schemes are available, but the use of a random number system is probably simplest for the hospital epidemiologist. Widely available computer programs will generate a series of random numbers, or a table of random numbers may be used. To use a random number table for selecting 20 patients from a pool of 200 potential controls, for example, each potential control is given a number between 001 and 200. The first 20 three-digit numbers found in the table that fall within the range 001 to 200 identify the patients to be selected. Other techniques have been used, such as using patient record numbers, selecting control patients admitted just before or after case patients, or selecting every nth patient (e.g., every fifth bacteremia case or every seventh admission). These systematic sampling methods may lead to nonrandom selection, however; for example, patients are neither admitted nor operated on randomly, few elective surgical patients are admitted on Saturdays, and more difficult surgical procedures are usually scheduled early in the day.

The random selection of control patients is most useful when one does not need to control for specific factors within the pool of patients available as controls. If there are no age, sex, or other susceptibility factors identified as important in an outbreak of wound infection following cardiac surgery, for example, one can quickly obtain an appropriate control group by randomly selecting uninfected patients who had cardiac surgery in the appropriate period.

How can a control population be selected if it is necessary to control for numerous factors such as age, sex, and type of operation? As noted, matching on these factors would be very tedious and, furthermore, one might have difficulty finding control patients who match appropriately each case patient with regard to each factor. For this problem, a *stratified random sample* can be used. It is almost as convenient to select as is a true random sample, and it allows almost the same degree of control over important variables as does the matching strategy. To draw a stratified random sample, the potential pool of control patients is divided into groups that correspond to the factors that must be controlled. Then, from each group, a separate random sample is chosen. To illustrate, consider the need to control for the type of operation when 50 percent of case patients had cholecystectomy, 30 percent had herniorrhaphy, and 20 percent had chest surgery. Potential control patients would be divided into groups according to the type of surgery. The epidemiologist would then select, with a separate random pick, half of the controls from the cholecystectomy group, 30 percent from the herniorrhaphy group, and the remainder from the chest surgery group.

Analysis of Case-Control Data   The frequencies of various susceptibility and exposure factors among cases and controls are tabulated. All differences between the two groups are considered potentially important. When possible, statistical techniques should be used to calculate the probabilities that the observed differences could have occurred by chance. Statistically significant differences are highly suggestive, but of course the presence or absence of statistical significance does not prove or disprove causation.

The case-control study may not provide the solution for a problem. Under such circumstances, other epidemiologic techniques—such as a cohort study or a prospective intervention study—may be employed.

Cohort Study   A cohort study may be conducted prospectively or retrospectively (see Chap. 1). For the investigation of nosocomial infections problems, a retrospective cohort study is seldom useful, since case-control techniques are generally more powerful. If, however, a case-control review fails to solve a problem because the data available retrospectively are inadequate or, as noted in the

next section, it is necessary to confirm the results of the case-control study, then a defined high-risk population (the cohort) may be identified and followed prospectively. Necessary clinical and laboratory observations can then be made. After a period of time, differences in susceptibility or host factors among ill and well patients may become apparent that will identify the source of the infection problem.

Rarely is a cohort study conducted independently of a retrospective case-control study. Usually, the case-control study is used to narrow the list of hypotheses and to identify the high-risk populations that are studied prospectively.

Prospective Intervention Study   The prospective trial (an experimental epidemiologic study), like the cohort study, is rarely used primarily in studying nosocomial infection problems (see Chap. 1). It also usually grows out of the findings of a retrospective case-control study. Here, a hypothesis is tested experimentally by intervening with specific measures to correct a presumed infection problem and measuring the impact of that intervention on infection rates. When feasible, such trials should be controlled—that is, the intervention should be applied to one segment of the population at risk but not to a comparable group of control patients. Only by comparing disease risk in the treated group versus the control group can one reliably interpret the results of such a trial.

Illustrations of the ways that uncontrolled trials have been misleading are legion and fall into several broad groups. First, disease occurrence may decline independently of the intervention; without a control group, the drop in infection rate may inappropriately be attributed to a beneficial effect of the intervention. Of course, it is also possible that the treatment regimen may be harmful; again, the use of an untreated control group allows documentation of this effect. It is also possible that an intervention may be beneficial but fail to alter the observed disease risk in the treated population. This might occur if the benefit were offset by some new event that independently increased the disease risk. When a control group is used for comparison, disease risk would also increase more in the untreated population, thereby indicating benefit in the treated group. Of course, there are situations in which a controlled trial is difficult to justify; this occurs, for example, when the disease under study is very serious and when the intervention measures are highly likely to be useful. Even in these circumstances, however, a controlled trial should be strongly considered for the reasons outlined.

Microbiologic Study It is a common mistake, when an infection problem is first investigated, to obtain large numbers of microbiologic cultures. As noted earlier, some carefully selected culture specimens may be obtained from persons or the inanimate environment if they will not be available later because of the institution of control measures. It must be stressed, however, that such surveys should supplement the epidemiologic investigation, not direct it. Furthermore, the cultures should be obtained only from sites that are likely to be epidemiologically relevant. (See Chap. 9.)

Beginning epidemiologists at CDC are cautioned, only partly in jest, that if the epidemiologic and laboratory data disagree, they should disregard the laboratory data. This advice may seem radical, especially to those who consider laboratory data to be "hard" and real and who view statistical and epidemiologic data as "soft" and speculative. The CDC's advice, however, is valuable for several reasons.

First, the isolation of a microorganism by itself rarely explains the occurrence of a disease. The hospital is not a sterile environment, and viable pathogenic microorganisms may be isolated from most hospital locations. For example, large numbers of personnel are often colonized by the epidemic strain during a staphylococcal outbreak. However, these personnel are often, like the affected patients, victims of the outbreak rather than its causes. Similar arguments can be made about isolation of microorganisms from sink drains, floors, air, or whatever. Unless there is an epidemiologic link between the source of the isolate and the occurrence of patient disease, the mere isolation of a microorganism, even of an epidemic strain, may mean little.

Second, the failure to isolate a microorganism from a presumed source or reservoir does not vindicate that site. The culture determinations may be negative because they were improperly collected or processed, because adequate technologic procedures were not available for primary isolation, or because too few specimen samples were obtained. This last possibility is dramatically illustrated by the outbreaks of disease caused by contaminated, commercially supplied intravenous medications. In several of these outbreaks, contamination had occurred in a very small proportion of individual units (approximately 1 in 5,000 to 10,000 units in some outbreaks), and many negative culture specimens were processed before the first positive result was obtained. If the epidemiologic data had not strongly implicated intrinsic contamination of such fluids, extensive culturing could not have been justified and would not have been undertaken. With direction provided by the epidemiologic findings, however, examinations continued until positive results were obtained.

As another example, several outbreaks of group A streptococcal surgical wound infections have been traced to medical personnel who had negative pharyngeal culture specimens for group A streptococci. Because of the epidemiologic association of the disease with these persons, extensive examinations were conducted, and asymptomatic anal carriage of the epidemic strain was documented. The initial failure to isolate a strain does not discredit the epidemiologic findings; instead, it requires that both the epidemiologic and microbiologic techniques be reevaluated.

Institute and Evaluate Control Measures

As soon as the explanation for a nosocomial infection problem is found, control measures should be vigorously applied. These control measures may be used to confirm the validity of that explanation. The effectiveness of such control measures should be evaluated by continued surveillance for disease and, if necessary, by prospective study.

Evaluate Other Hospital Practices

A thorough epidemiologic investigation of a nosocomial infection problem often leads to improved infection control practices not only in the areas where the problem occurred but also throughout the hospital. An outbreak of disease might be considered to be an experiment of nature; that is, the factors that permit epidemic infections to occur are often responsible for endemic infections as well. Investigations of UTIs caused by multiply drug-resistant Enterobacteriaceae, for example, have documented that many of these infections are transmitted by way of personnel from infected, catheterized patients to neighboring patients who are also catheterized. It is highly likely that infections with other microorganisms are also transmitted by this mechanism, but the mode is more difficult to recognize if common pathogens are involved. Thus measures to control the spread of an epidemic strain may also be expected to control the spread of other strains. The epidemiologist should therefore review practices and procedures throughout the hospital when an epidemiologic study is completed and should institute reasonable control or preventive measures throughout the institution. Hospital personnel should be informed about the investigation and its results.

Responsibilities for Dissemination of Information

Hospitals are an integral part of larger communities, and their personnel and patients come from and return to that community. Infection problems in the community influence the hospital, and, conversely, infection problems within the hospital may be spread to the community by patients or personnel. Because of this intimate association between the community and the hospital, the institution's infection control personnel must cooperate with local public health authorities by reporting and assisting in the investigation of problems.

Each hospital is also a part of the larger community of other hospitals. Patients may be transferred from one institution to another and carry their infections with them. Accordingly, frank and frequent exchanges of information between hospitals are important. Although each hospital has its unique practices and policies, a problem in one institution may also be a problem in other hospitals that have the same practices. Thus the results of epidemiologic investigations should be disseminated widely. Finally, hospitals may be affected by outbreaks caused by a contaminated common vehicle that is commercially available to other institutions. When problems with such products are discovered, the hospital epidemiologist has the responsibility to notify promptly not only the manufacturer or distributor of the product but also the appropriate public health authorities. Local and state health authorities, the FDA, and the CDC cooperate closely in monitoring and attempting to control the contamination of such products and, if such a problem is suspected, these agencies should be notified immediately.

Administrative Aspects

An epidemiologic investigation requires vigorous action by hospital personnel. Because of this, each hospital should have an administrative structure that will allow uninhibited investigation of infection problems. The requirements are several.

First, the hospital must have access to someone trained and interested in hospital epidemiology. Often responsibilities for infection control are delegated to an infection control team composed of one or more infection control nurses and a physician hospital epidemiologist (see Chap. 2). This team should be given adequate resources to conduct investigations. Their continuing education should be supported. Sufficient time should be set aside in advance, and adequate financial backing must be available to support investigations. The infection control team should have the administrative authority to conduct efficient and wide-range investigations and should specifically have the authority to evaluate patients, take appropriate culture specimens from patients and personnel, and consult with outside experts. That administrative authority must also provide a mechanism that allows the team to make emergency decisions when an infection problem threatens the health and safety of patients and personnel.

Most important, the infection control effort must have adequate support from other departments in the hospital. The microbiology laboratory must maintain the ability to process the specimens required for an epidemiologic investigation, and laboratory personnel should be able to serve as expert consultants in selecting the appropriate microbiologic and serologic techniques required in these investigations (see Chap. 9). The hospital's engineering and housekeeping departments must be ready to provide consultation regarding environmental control. Nursing services must work with the infection control program in conducting epidemiologic studies as well as in applying control measures. Finally, the infection control program must have the wholehearted support and assistance of the medical staff. If the infection control effort takes place without the interest or support of other personnel in the hospital, little can be accomplished.

References

1. Benenson, A. S. (Ed.). *Control of Communicable Diseases in Man* (15th ed.). New York: American Public Health Association, 1990. P. 408.
2. Centers for Disease Control. Follow-up smallpox—Federal Republic of Germany. *M.M.W.R.* 19:234, 1970. (Adapted from World Health Organization. Smallpox surveillance. *Weekly Epidemiol. Rec.* 45:249, 1970.)
3. Stamm, W. E., Weinstein, R. A., and Dixon, R. E. Comparison of Endemic and Epidemic Nosocomial Infections. In: R. E. Dixon (Ed.), *Nosocomial Infections*. New York: Yorke Medical Books, 1975. Pp. 9–13.

Statistical Considerations for Analysis of Nosocomial Infection Data

Stanley M. Martin
Brian D. Plikaytis
Nancy H. Bean

Data that have been collected in a study of nosocomial infections must be reduced from observations on every included patient to summary statistics describing particular groups of patients. While culture results or other information about 1 or 2 patients can be important in understanding the cause of infection, information from more patients is needed to determine which of several potentially important factors contributed to the infection. A transition from clinical diagnosis of illness in a single patient to understanding illness in populations of patients must underlie the study of nosocomial infections; the physician's diagnosis of illness in single patients must change to the statistical "diagnosis" of illness in the population of patients.

This chapter describes some basic statistical considerations for understanding nosocomial infection data from the collection phase through the interpretation. Several study design considerations are presented as reminders of necessary precursors of a good study. Among these, control group selection by either an independent or matched procedure influences which statistical test should be used in the analysis. Emphasis is placed on data collection procedures because of the need for careful definition of data to be collected and as much standardization of the collection process as possible. Finally, a scheme for choosing appropriate significance tests is presented.

Data Collection

In many epidemiologic studies, the inability of investigators to reach conclusions can be attributed to the collection of data with little or no previous planning of the objectives of the study, the failure to collect data relevant to the objectives, the lack of a defined population for study, failure to identify the best locations in the hospital in which to find the data, the absence of understanding about who will record the data, and improper selection of the period to be covered. In the investigation of possible outbreaks of a particular infection type, the investigator should also consider whether it is necessary to extend the scope of investigation beyond the inpatient population of the hospital to the outpatient department, beyond the primary hospital of interest to other hospitals of a similar type or in the same location, or beyond hospitals to the community.

Studies of nosocomial infections previously have involved the collection of data from personal interviews, patient examinations, patient chart reviews, laboratory records, personnel health clinic records, or autopsy data. These sources of data, singly or in combination with one another, continue to provide reliable information for many hospitals. However, the proliferation of computing equipment in the management of patient-related data in hospitals offers a source of more easily obtainable data for investigating nosocomial infections. The investigator of nosocomial infections should learn about the administrative processes within the hospital that can generate useful "machine-readable" patient records. For example, admissions office personnel may enter demographic data and admitting diagnoses on all patients via a computer terminal or keypunched record. Other hospital locations such as the pharmacy and various laboratories may generate additional records that arrive in the central computer area for the same patients. Medical procedures, operations, diagnoses, and costs may be entered into the computer system from still other sources, possibly for billing purposes; discharge diagnoses and other information may be added as well (see Chap. 5).

These records can provide a valuable resource in hospitals having well-planned computer systems and local area networks. They can be available with relatively little work beyond determining from administrative personnel, the accounting office, laboratories,

and pharmacy what data are part of the hospital computer system, and from the computer center how to gain access to the needed data. Preliminary inquiries of this kind can offer the potential for larger and better-controlled studies because of less cost and time in the data collection phase.

Control Groups

Little information about the association of any factor that may predispose a patient to infection can be gained by studying only a group of patients who have been exposed to the factor. Similarly, studying cases only is descriptive but may not lead to assessment of risks associated with a factor. For example, an attempt to study the association of excisional surgical wound infections caused by *Staphylococcus aureus* with operations by a particular surgeon will be of limited benefit unless a suitable comparison group is also studied. The surgeon performing the operation may be only one of several factors that can potentially influence the risk of incisional infections. Therefore, a suitable control group should include patients receiving the same operation from another surgeon or patients receiving the operation from any of the entire surgical staff performing operations in the hospital other than the suspect surgeon. The control group should include patients expected to be like the infected group with respect to all known possible risk factors except for the surgeon performing the operation. Differences in infection rates between the control group and the group receiving the operation from the suspect surgeon could then be associated with this surgeon.

Studies of this kind can be successfully controlled within a hospital because both exposed and nonexposed patients are present. However, the study of association of infection with the use of a particular, possibly contaminated, product or apparatus may require a multihospital study or an intervention study within a single hospital. It would be impossible to study the association of pneumonia with cleaning techniques of respiratory therapy equipment within a single hospital if the hospital's policy dictates one particular cleaning technique for all such apparatus. This is because no control group would be available unless, for purposes of the study, the policy could be changed for at least a portion of the equipment. Intervention in the hospital policy regarding the cleaning of respiratory therapy equipment would allow the investigator to design a study to compare pneumonia rates between a group of patients using respiratory therapy equipment cleaned in the usual way and a group of patients using the same type of equipment during the same period but cleaned by a different technique. Of course intervention studies of this kind must be preceded by careful attention to ethical concerns for the welfare of the patient.

Even though patients can be stratified into groups according to exposure or nonexposure to the factor under consideration, comparability of the patients included in each group must be ensured. The underlying risks of patients for acquiring the infection under study can differ drastically even without considering exposure to a single factor. For example, patients with a particular diagnosis may be immunosuppressed and more susceptible to infection. Other factors such as catheterization, exposure to respiratory therapy equipment, prophylactic or therapeutic antibiotics, and intravenous fluids can predispose patients to a greater risk of infection. A well-designed study will attempt to balance the patients in the control and study groups with respect to such known factors that can alter the patients' risk to infection. This may require that control patients be matched to the study patients on these factors. The objective, whether control patients are selected by an independent selection process or matched to the study patients, is to remove the effect of underlying factors that might mask or exaggerate the effect of a particular factor under study (see Chap. 6).

Multihospital studies require more than a single study hospital and a single control hospital. Generally, it is not reasonable to expect many of the same potentially important, but not necessarily obvious, factors to exist in any

two hospitals. Studies involving more than one hospital must include adequate numbers of hospitals in both the study group and the control group. Factors such as number of beds, hospital policies, ratio of staff to patients, patient characteristics, numbers of discharges, and hospital type must be considered in selecting suitable study and control groups of hospitals. The scope of this chapter is limited to studies within a single hospital to avoid lengthy discussions of the sampling problems and other statistical problems accompanying multihospital studies.

Summary Statistics

When confronted with pages of written observations on infected and noninfected patients, little can be learned about the association between infection and a factor under study until an appropriate summary statistic is found to describe a "typical" value of the factor for the whole group. For example, the proportion of patients who became infected shortly after urinary catheterization can be compared with the proportion of a similar group of patients who were not catheterized and became infected. The proportion summarizes the infection experience in each of the two groups, catheterized and noncatheterized patients. It relates the number of infected patients to the total number at risk of becoming infected in the two groups. The at-risk population usually includes all patients exposed to a factor or combination of factors. It can include all patients admitted or discharged (e.g., exposed to the hospital or a particular service) during a particular period, only patients with a particular diagnosis, or only patients who received a particular procedure or drug.

The actual number of patients at risk may be the best available denominator; however, some investigators can measure the at-risk portion of the summary statistic in terms of the duration of each patient's exposure to risk. This can be the number of days hospitalized, number of hours with inserted catheter, or other time of exposure. If the numerator represents the number of patients with a particular infection, the investigator should subtract from the at-risk period in the denominator the total time patients were exposed after they were infected since, for purposes of the study, exposure while a patient is infected contributes no additional risk: However, this additional exposure should be included in the denominator if the numerator represents the number of episodes for infections for each patient.

The numerator of the summary statistic also can be formed in different ways. A single patient may experience more than one infection episode due to the same organism. In this case, one must decide whether these patients have had a recurrence of infection from the initial organism or a reinfection with the same organism. If multiple infections occur, the summary statistic can be a count of the total number of infections relative to the total number of patients for whom the numerator was counted. This statistic would be the average number of infections per patient. Decisions about the association of a particular factor with infection can usually be made using the number of infected patients for the numerator and the number of patients at risk (or patient-time exposure) for the denominator.

Study Design

Proportions or other summary statistics are obtained to decide whether hospitalized patients exposed to the factor under consideration are at higher risk of infection than patients who are not exposed to the factor. A significance test is used to determine the probability that a difference as large as the observed difference between the two proportions could have occurred by chance. A small probability of chance occurrence of a difference as large as the observed difference leads the observer to conclude that patients exposed to the factor are likely to be at higher risk of infection. The question then becomes: How small should the probability be so that a conclusion associating infection with the fac-

tor is correct? In fact there are two probabilities of primary concern in significance testing [16]; these are stated below as questions for the investigator of nosocomial infections.

Type 1. Given that there actually is *no difference* between the proportion of patients infected among those exposed to the factor and the proportion of patients infected among those not exposed to the factor, what is the probability that the particular samples of patients observed in this study would indicate a *difference by chance?*

Type 2. Given that there actually is a *difference* between the proportion of patients infected among those exposed to the factor and the proportion of patients infected among those not exposed to the factor, what is the probability that the particular samples of patients observed in this study would indicate *no difference* by chance?

These two probabilities of error form the basis for decisions from significance tests and are determined by the investigator in the planning stage of the study. A summary of the major steps leading to significance testing for the difference between proportions is presented below. All these should be considered in planning studies of nosocomial infections.

State Hypothesis to Be Tested and Alternative Hypothesis

As an example, the hypothesis (H) that there is no difference between the proportions versus the hypothesis that there is a difference between the proportions (the alternative hypothesis [AH]) can be written as

$$H_0: P_E = P_{NE}$$

$$AH: P_E \neq P_{NE}$$

where P_E and P_{NE} are the proportions infected in the exposed and nonexposed groups, respectively. H_0, the "null" hypothesis, states that the proportion infected in the exposed group is the same as the proportion infected in the nonexposed group. The alternative hypothesis states that the proportion infected in the exposed group is not the same as the proportion infected in the nonexposed group. Because the alternative hypothesis does not state the direction of the difference (and would be favored whether P_E were significantly greater than or significantly less than P_{NE}), significance tests used to test these hypotheses must consider differences in both directions. These are called two-tailed tests and are generally useful when the investigator does not know before the data are collected whether to expect exposure to the factor to increase or diminish the patients' risk of infection. When the investigator has reason to believe that exposure to the factor would increase (or decrease) the patients' risk of infection, a one-tailed test should be used. The hypotheses may be stated as

$$H_0: P_E \leq P_{NE}$$
$$AH: P_E > P_{NE}$$

In this case, the null hypothesis states that P_E is less than or equal to P_{NE}, whereas the alternative hypothesis states that P_E is greater than P_{NE}. This is a directional difference because the investigator expects exposure to increase the patient's risk of infection, if a difference exists at all. Considering the purpose of studies of infection outbreaks within the hospital, one must conclude that one-tailed tests of significance are generally appropriate.

State Desired Probability Levels for Type 1 and Type 2 Errors

These probabilities are not based on statistical computations but on the investigator's willingness to chance an error of either kind. Stating the type 2 error indirectly states another probability that is also important in determining how likely the study is to succeed. This probability, defined by

$$p = (1 - \text{type 2 error})$$

is called the power of the test and p is the probability that, if a difference actually exists (i.e., the alternative hypothesis is true), the significance test will reject the null hypothesis in favor of the alternative hypothesis. The power of the test is used in initial planning of the study to ensure an adequate study size to achieve the objectives.

Determine Study Design to Achieve Desired Objective

A primary consideration in study design is that of deciding whether the study and control groups should be selected independently or whether patients selected for the control group should be matched on certain variables to patients in the study group: That is, for each study patient, one or more control patients could be selected to match the study patient on factors determined ahead of time. Many studies of nosocomial infections have required that patients be matched for validity on factors such as age, sex, underlying diagnoses, and predisposing therapeutic factors. In outbreak investigations, it may not be possible to know the specific factors that should be studied; therefore, the study population may consist of all patients who were infected and the control population may include patients who were like the infected patients but were not infected. The proportion exposed to particular factors would then be determined from samples of each of these two populations. Whether patients are matched or unmatched, most studies of nosocomial infection outbreaks involve comparisons of these proportions. The single direction hypotheses would be written as

$$H_0: P_I \leq P_{NI}$$
$$AH: P_I > P_{NI}$$

where P_I and P_{NI} are the proportions exposed to the factor under study in the infected and noninfected groups of patients, respectively.

Study design must include consideration of study size. This should be based on the requirements to test certain hypotheses or estimate certain parameters and to achieve predetermined error probability levels. Sometimes the size of the study is limited by the time or resources available. In this case, it should be understood that a low power or large type 2 error may be associated with the study because inadequate sample sizes are involved, and a decision must be made about the value of doing the study under these circumstances. Approaches to determining sample size requirements for testing the difference between two proportions often involve approximation formulas that can be programmed relatively easily [20].

Plan Data Collection Procedures and Train Data Collectors

A main consideration in planning the study is the choice of personnel to collect the data. Deciding whether a patient is infected requires a level of medical knowledge that may be beyond that of a secretary or clerical person. Regardless of who the data collectors are, they must be given standard procedures for deciding about each data item such as the case definition. Some verification of the data collection process should be planned to avoid problems such as drifting away from established procedures, misunderstanding procedures, inability to follow procedures, and random errors. Too often inadequate attention is given to quality of data collection because data checking and editing require extra effort for the investigator. Often it is tempting to assume good data quality when the data are collected as computer records. Without close scrutiny, computer summary tables and statistics based on incorrect data entries can appear as if they were valid because the formatting of computer output is often independent of the data quality. When this happens, the study can become a victim of poor or misleading data instead of contributing valuable information for control of nosocomial infections. Decisions about data handling must be planned in advance to avoid delays. If computer records are involved, coordination with a programmer or other computer personnel is necessary before the study begins.

Collect Data and Begin Data Processing

One early consideration in study design is the data collection instrument. Designing the form with the intention to use present computer technology requires knowledge of computer input mechanisms and coding schemes that can be employed. A common tendency is to ask for too much data on a form, but a well-planned study will pare down the questionnaire to include the important questions only. Simplicity for understanding, recording data, and tabulating is the key to a successful data collection document. Data processing may involve no more than hand tabulation, but it can involve detailed computer programs for sophisticated analyses. Realizing beforehand that substantial time of nursing staff or other personnel may be required in both the collection and processing phases, and planning for this, can avoid overburdening these people at what may be an inopportune time.

Perform Analysis and Report Results

A common error of an investigator heading a study is to spend unlimited effort collecting data but to allow only a very short time for the analysis. However, analyses must take into account all the design considerations, hypotheses to be tested, and level of measurement of the data. Enough analysis time should be allocated to understand thoroughly what the data say. Simply summarizing findings with p values is usually an indication that the data have not been thoroughly analyzed. Studies planned to meet some types of objectives can begin with examination of the stated hypotheses, followed by determination of other features of the data that support the conclusions. However, the analysis of data from nosocomial infection outbreaks can require a different approach. Usually there is not a single hypothesis to be tested, and the study objective for infection outbreak data is to determine which factors increase the patients' risk of infection. One approach is to test several factors, looking for an association of any factor with infection. When this procedure is used and the seemingly important factors tested, attention must be given to the effect of multiple significance testing on the overall type 1 error. One way to compensate for several significance tests is to set the type 1 error probability for each test low enough to yield a specified type 1 error over all tests. For example, if it is desired to perform k tests with an overall type 1 error of α, then the type 1 error for each test could be set approximately to

$$A = \frac{\alpha}{k}$$

where A is the approximate significance level for each test [15].

Significance Testing

Before presenting directions for choosing a significance test for a particular study, it is necessary to mention briefly two statistical terms. Significance tests can be separated into two categories—*parametric* and *nonparametric*. Use of parametric statistics requires assumptions about the parent population from which the study samples were drawn. For example, observations of urine output volume on a sample of infected patients could be assumed to have come from a population of urine output volumes that were normally distributed around a mean, μ, and variance, σ^2. Because the assumption is made that these values are normally distributed, the significance testing procedure involves a parametric test. On the other hand, if one is not willing to make assumptions about the parameters of the parent distribution, one may choose a nonparametric test.

The parametric test is usually preferred as long as it is reasonable to make the assumptions for it, because there is an associated gain in power. Although the loss of power accompanying the use of a nonparametric test can be substantial, some of the nonparametric tests actually offer power comparable to parametric tests. When both parametric and nonparametric tests are presented in this chapter, the power of the nonparametric test is reasonably close to that of the corresponding parametric test; the tests mentioned here are commonly used in the analysis of nosocomial infection data.

The decision of which of the many statistical tests to use requires, in addition to thought about the hypotheses and study design, consideration of the level of measurement of the observations. For the sake of simplicity, the discussion in this chapter of level of measurement will be limited to two classifications, *attributes* and *measurements*. Usually, data collected on nosocomial infections involve answers to questions such as:

Was the patient infected or not infected?
Was the patient exposed or not exposed?
Was the change in a measurement positive or negative?

Attribute responses—yes or no, plus or minus, zero or one—simply give the direction of differences, whereas measurement data—height, weight, blood sugar level—give the direction and magnitude of the differences. The scheme shown in Figure 7-1 for selecting an appropriate test takes into account the issues just mentioned and should help the investigator choose a significance test by making three simple choices [12]. This scheme uses a partial list of tests and is not intended to limit broader choices that are available [19].

Two sets of data will be used to illustrate the test procedures listed in Figure 7-1. First, assuming that the samples were selected independently, the tests listed for independent samples will be illustrated. Next the tests listed for matched samples will be illustrated, using the assumption that the same samples were selected with control (noninfected) patients matched to study (infected) patients.

Example 1—Attribute data. Suppose 100 patients on the general medicine service acquired *Escherichia coli* urinary tract infections during a 6-month period. A sample of 30 of these patients is randomly selected to determine whether the infection is associated with urinary catheterization. A control group of 30 noninfected patients is selected from among all other patients on the general medicine service during the same 6-month period. The status of patients in

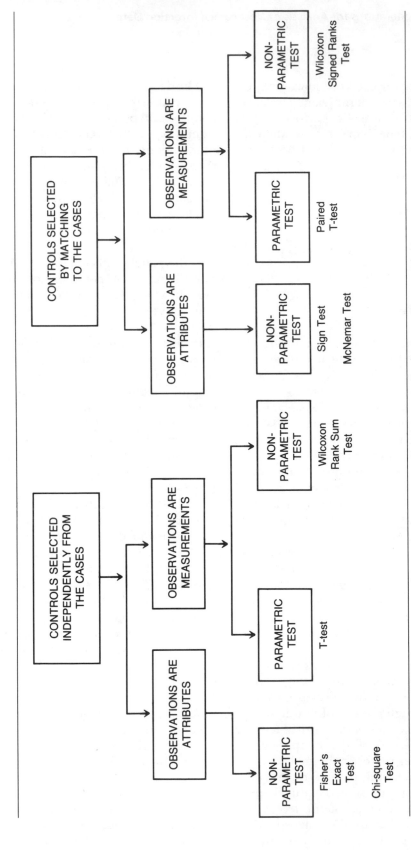

Fig. 7-1. Scheme for selecting an appropriate significance test. (Reprinted with permission from S. M. Martin, Choosing the Correct Statistical Tests. In R. P. Wenzel (Ed.), *Handbook of Hospital-Acquired Infections*. Boca Raton, FL: CRC Press, 1981.)

each group with respect to catheterization is presented in Table 7-1.

Example 2—Measurement data. Suppose times from admission to onset of *E. coli* urinary tract infection for the 30 infected patients and times from admission to discharge of the 30 noninfected patients from example 1 are observed to determine whether infection occurred at about the time the patients who were infected would have been discharged if they had not been infected. The time in hours observed for each patient is given in Table 7-2.

The examples will be used first to illustrate the tests employed when the samples of infected and noninfected persons are independently selected. Since studies of nosocomial infection outbreaks usually involve one-tailed tests, the tests illustrated here, except for the chi-square tests, will be one-tailed.

The observations from example 1 can be summarized into a 2 × 2 table to determine whether there is an association of catheters with infection. A high proportion (22/30) of infected patients and a low proportion (5/30)

of noninfected patients were catheterized (Table 7-3). The purpose of the significance test of these data is to determine whether the proportion catheterized was significantly larger among infected patients (P_I) than among noninfected patients (P_{NI}). The single-direction hypotheses can be stated as

$$H_0: P_I \leq P_{NI}$$
$$AH: P_I > P_{NI}$$

Fisher's Exact Test

Fisher's Exact test [6] computes the probability of occurrence of the observed arrangement of the data in Table 7-3 plus the probability of occurrence of all other arrangements more divergent than the observed data in the direction of the alternative hypothesis, subject to the condition that all marginal totals of the tables remain fixed. The formula for computing the test probability for each derived table can be stated in terms of the cell values given in Table 7-4. The probability of the observed arrangement for each table is computed by

$$p_k = \frac{(a + b)! \, (c + d)! \, (a + c)! \, (b + d)!}{a! \, b! \, c! \, d! \, n!}$$

Table 7-1. Catheterization status of patients on general medicine service (example 1)

	Infected patients						Noninfected patients				
Pt. no.	Cath.	No cath.	Pt. no.	Cath.	No cath.	Pt. no.	Cath.	No cath.	Pt. no.	Cath.	No cath.
1.	X		16.	X		1.		X	16.		X
2.	X		17.	X		2.		X	17.		X
3.	X		18.	X		3.		X	18.		X
4.		X	19.	X		4.	X		19.		X
5.	X		20.	X		5.		X	20.	X	
6.		X	21.	X		6.		X	21.		X
7.		X	22.	X		7.		X	22.		X
8.		X	23.		X	8.		X	23.		X
9.	X		24.	X		9.		X	24.		X
10.	X		25.		X	10.		X	25.	X	
11.	X		26.	X		11.		X	26.		X
12.		X	27.	X		12.	X		27.		X
13.	X		28.	X		13.		X	28.		X
14.		X	29.	X		14.		X	29.		X
15.	X		30.	X		15.	X		30.		X

Pt. no. = patient number; Cath. = catheterization.

Table 7-2. Intervals of exposure to the hospital for infected and noninfected patients (example 2)

Time (in hours) from admission to onset of infection (infected patients)				Time (in hours) from admission to discharge (noninfected patients)			
Pt. no.	*Hrs.*	*Pt. no.*	*Hrs.*	*Pt. no.*	*Hrs.*	*Pt. no.*	*Hrs.*
1.	216	16.	234	1.	253	16.	242
2.	187	17.	205	2.	82	17.	233
3.	88	18.	136	3.	125	18.	133
4.	280	19.	253	4.	138	19.	342
5.	310	20.	165	5.	137	20.	102
6.	239	21.	340	6.	116	21.	93
7.	344	22.	325	7.	232	22.	82
8.	315	23.	178	8.	327	23.	248
9.	280	24.	153	9.	171	24.	113
10.	293	25.	355	10.	338	25.	294
11.	200	26.	338	11.	335	26.	304
12.	229	27.	77	12.	109	27.	211
13.	208	28.	335	13.	126	28.	104
14.	233	29.	261	14.	182	29.	261
15.	190	30.	93	15.	247	30.	269

Pt. no. = patient number.

Table 7-3. Catheterization status of infected and noninfected patients (example 1)

	Infected	Noninfected	Total
Catheter	22	5	27
No catheter	8	25	33
Total	30	30	60

Table 7-4. General table for summarizing the association of a factor with infection

	Infected	Noninfected	Total
Catheter	a	b	$a + b$
No catheter	c	d	$c + d$
Total	$a + c$	$b + d$	n

where $p_k = 0$ is the probability computed for the observed table, $p_k = 1$ is the probability computed for the next most divergent table, and so on, until the probabilities for all such tables are computed. The next most divergent tables can be generated easily by successively adding 1 to the a and d cells while subtracting 1 from the b and c cells, when the data are

arranged as shown in Table 7-4. Note that this procedure leaves the marginal totals unchanged, a requirement for this test. The probability is computed for each successive table and the final probability is determined by summing these.

$$p_0 = \frac{27!\ 33!\ 30!\ 30!}{22!\ 5!\ 8!\ 25!\ 60!} = .0000094776297$$

$$p_1 = \frac{27!\ 33!\ 30!\ 30!}{23!\ 4!\ 7!\ 26!\ 60!} = .0000006339551$$

$$p_2 = \frac{27!\ 33!\ 30!\ 30!}{24!\ 3!\ 6!\ 27!\ 60!} = .0000000273931$$

$$p_3 = \frac{27!\ 33!\ 30!\ 30!}{25!\ 2!\ 5!\ 28!\ 60!} = .0000000007044$$

$$p_4 = \frac{27!\ 33!\ 30!\ 30!}{26!\ 1!\ 4!\ 29!\ 60!} = .0000000000093$$

$$p_5 = \frac{27!\ 33!\ 30!\ 30!}{27!\ 0!\ 3!\ 30!\ 60!} = \frac{.0000000000013}{}$$

$$p_{Tot} = .00001014$$

Because the total probability ($p_{Tot} = .00001014$) is small (less than .05), the conclusion is that there is an increased risk of *E. coli* infection among catheterized patients in this hospital.

It is important to note that the two-tailed probability for testing the hypothesis—

$$H_0: P_I = P_{NI}$$

$$AH: P_I \neq P_{NI}$$

—can be computed by repeating the computations for the opposite direction, determining the appropriate tables for the other tail of the test. This is accomplished by determining the probabilities for tables for which the proportion of catheterized patients is lower in the infected group than in the noninfected group subject to the condition that the marginal totals remain fixed (i.e., the total numbers of infected and noninfected patients is kept constant). Then the second tail of the test is computed by summing the probabilities for all tables in the second direction that have probabilities less than or equal to the probability for the observed table. The probability for the two-tailed test would then be found by summing the probabilities for each of the two tails. When the number of infected patients sampled, n_1, is equal to the number of noninfected patients sampled, n_{NI}, simply doubling the probability for one tail will produce the two-tailed probability [13].

Chi-Square for Independent Samples

Computations for the Fisher's Exact test are tedious without the assistance of a programmable calculator or computer. Chi-square is a suitable approximation when the expected cell frequencies of the 2 × 2 table are sufficiently large. Some authors [20] have recommended that the approximation is inadequate if the total sample size, $n = n_1 + n_{NI}$, is less than 20 or if the total sample size is between 20 and 40 with one or more expected cell frequencies as small as 5. Chi-square is a test of independence of the factor and infection or, equivalently, a test of the hypotheses:

$$H_0: \quad P_I = P_{NI}$$

$$AH: \quad P_I \neq P_{NI}$$

A simple computational formula makes this test easy to compute:

$$X^2 = \frac{(n) \times \left(|ad - bc| - \dfrac{n_1 + n_{NI}}{2}\right)^2}{(a + b)(c + d)(a + c)(b + d)}$$

$$= \frac{(60) \times \left(|22 \times 25 - 8 \times 5| - \dfrac{60}{2}\right)^2}{27 \times 33 \times 30 \times 30}$$

$$= \frac{13,824,000}{801,900}$$

$$= 17.239$$

This value is greater than the tabulated value of the chi-square distribution (readily available in standard statistical tables) corresponding to a significance level (type 1 error) of 0.05 ($\chi^2 = 3.84$). Therefore, the test leads to the conclusion that $P_I \neq P_{NI}$, or that infection is not independent of catheterization.

t-test

Example 2 will be used to illustrate two tests for measurement data. The assumption that time intervals were sampled from a normal distribution of time intervals permits use of the *t*-test. This is a parametric test of the difference between two means from independent samples. The hypotheses can be written as follows:

$$H_0: \mu_I \leq \mu_{NI}$$

$$AH: \mu_I > \mu_{NI}$$

where μ_I and μ_{NI} are the means of time intervals for the infected and noninfected populations, respectively, from which the samples were drawn. The definitions of symbols used in the formula for the *t*-test are given below and are more completely discussed elsewhere [21].

x_{I_i} = one time interval measured for the ith selected infected patient

x_{NI_i} = one time interval measured for the ith selected noninfected patient

n_1 = number of infected patients selected

n_{NI} = number of noninfected patients selected

The mean interval from the sample of infected patients is calculated as

$$\bar{x}_I = \frac{\sum_{i=1}^{n_I} x_{I_i}}{n_I}$$

The mean interval from the sample of noninfected patients is calculated as

$$\bar{x}_{NI} = \frac{\sum_{i=1}^{n_{NI}} x_{NI_i}}{n_{NI}}$$

The variance estimate from the sample of infected patients is calculated as

$$s_I^2 = \frac{\sum_{i=1}^{n_I} (x_{I_i} - \bar{x}_I)^2}{n_I - 1} = \frac{\sum_{i=1}^{n_I} x_{I_i}^2 - \frac{\left(\sum_{i=1}^{n_I} x_{I_i}\right)^2}{n_I}}{n_I - 1}$$

The variance estimate from the sample of noninfected patients is calculated as

$$s_{NI}^2 = \frac{\sum_{i=1}^{n_{NI}} (x_{NI_i} - \bar{x}_{NI})^2}{n_{NI} - 1} = \frac{\sum_{i=1}^{n_{NI}} x_{NI_i}^2 - \frac{\left(\sum_{i=1}^{n_{NI}} x_{NI_i}\right)^2}{n_{NI}}}{n_{NI} - 1}$$

The variance of the difference between sample means is calculated as

$$s_{(\bar{x}_I - \bar{x}_{NI})}^2 = \frac{(n_I - 1)\, s_I^2 + (n_{NI} - 1)\, s_{NI}^2}{(n_I + n_{NI} - 2)}$$
$$\times \left(\frac{1}{n_I} + \frac{1}{n_{NI}} \right)$$

The *t*-statistic is calculated as

$$t = \frac{\bar{x}_I - \bar{x}_{NI}}{s_{(\bar{x}_I - \bar{x}_{NI})}}$$

These values for the data of example 2 (Table 7-2) are given below:

$$\bar{x}_I = \frac{7,060}{30} = 235.33$$

$$\bar{x}_{NI} = \frac{5,949}{30} = 198.30$$

$$s_I^2 = \frac{1,846,916 - \frac{7,060^2}{30}}{30 - 1} = 6,395.2644$$

$$s_{NI}^2 = \frac{1,398,207 - \frac{5,949^2}{30}}{30 - 1} = 7,535.1828$$

$$s_{(\bar{x}_I - \bar{x}_{NI})}^2 = \frac{(29)\,(6,395.2644) + (29)\,(7,535.1828)}{58}$$
$$\times \left(\frac{1}{30} + \frac{1}{30} \right)$$

$$= 464.3482$$

$$t = \frac{235.33 - 198.30}{21.5487} = 1.718$$

A comparison of this computed value of *t* with tabulated values of the *t* distribution ($n_I + n_{NI} - 2$ degrees of freedom) reveals that the probability of a chance occurrence of the observed data is less than .05, the value often used as a criterion for judging significance. Therefore, the null hypothesis is rejected, and the mean time from admission to onset of infection in the infected group is considered significantly greater than the mean time from admission to discharge in the noninfected group.

If, on the other hand, the investigator decides it is unreasonable to assume that the samples were drawn from normally distributed populations, a nonparametric test can be chosen to test the difference between the means. In the following section, the data from example 2 are used without the normality assumption to demonstrate a nonparametric test for comparing two sample means, again assuming that the samples were independently selected.

Wilcoxon Rank Sum Test

This test procedure begins by ranking the individual observations of numbers of hours from 1 to n ($n = n_I + n_{NI}$), with the least number of hours receiving a rank of 1. The ranks are assigned without regard for the sample from which the observations are drawn. When the original values are tied, equal ranks are assigned as the average of the ranks that would have been assigned to the tied observations if they had not been tied. One of several ties in the example occurred between the time intervals for infected patient number 19 and noninfected patient number 1 (Tables 7-2, 7-5). Each of these was assigned a rank of 39.5, the average of the next two ranks that would have been assigned if they had not been tied. The ranking (Table 7-5) begins with the assignment of rank 1 to infected patient number 27 and ends with the assignment of rank 60 to infected patient number 25.

After the ranking is completed, the ranks are separated into two groups corresponding to the original samples (Table 7-5). The sum of ranks for the sample having the fewer number of observations is obtained. Since, in this example, the number of observations is the same for both the infected and noninfected groups, the sum of ranks of either of these can be used.

The sum of ranks for the infected and noninfected groups are 1,070 and 812, respectively. Referring to the tables for the Wilcoxon Rank Sum test [22, 23] for a one-tailed probability at $p = .05$, the upper boundary is 1,027. Since the sum of ranks for this example is greater than 1,027, the investigator would conclude that the average time from admission to onset for infected patients is significantly longer than the time from admission to discharge of noninfected patients.

In the design of a study of nosocomial infections, it is usually necessary to match the controls (noninfected patients) to the infected patients. It is difficult to interpret conclusions about the association of factors with nosocomial infection when controls and study groups are selected independently. If the groups are independent, as in the previous examples, no information is available to allow the investigator to determine whether in-

Table 7-5. Intervals and ranks for infected and noninfected patients (example 2)

Ranks and time (in hours) from admission to onset of infection (infected patients)						Ranks and time (in hours) from admission to discharge (noninfected patients)					
Pt. no.	Hrs.	Rank	Pt. no.	Hrs.	Rank	Pt. no.	Hrs.	Rank	Pt. no.	Hrs.	Rank
1.	216	29	16.	234	34	1.	253	39.5	16.	242	36
2.	187	23	17.	205	26	2.	82	2.5	17.	233	32.5
3.	88	4	18.	136	15	3.	125	12	18.	133	14
4.	280	44.5	19.	253	39.5	4.	138	19	19.	342	58
5.	310	49	20.	165	19	5.	137	16	20.	102	7
6.	239	35	21.	340	57	6.	116	11	21.	93	5.5
7.	344	59	22.	325	51	7.	232	31	22.	82	2.5
8.	315	50	23.	178	21	8.	327	52	23.	248	38
9.	280	44.5	24.	153	18	9.	171	20	24.	113	10
10.	293	46	25.	355	60	10.	338	55.5	25.	294	47
11.	200	25	26.	338	55.5	11.	335	53.5	26.	304	48
12.	229	30	27.	77	1	12.	109	9	27.	211	28
13.	208	27	28.	335	53.5	13.	126	13	28.	104	8
14.	233	32.5	29.	261	41.5	14.	182	22	29.	261	41.5
15.	190	24	30.	93	55.5	15.	247	37	30.	269	43

Pt. no. = patient number.

fected patients really had onset of infection at approximately the same time as noninfected patients were being discharged. If the noninfected patients generally were admitted with more serious underlying illness than the infected patients, their length of stay in the hospital could have been prolonged on the average longer than their length of stay had they been admitted with illnesses comparable to those of the infected patients. The time from admission to onset of infection could have appeared, from the data, to be nearly the same as the interval from admission to discharge of noninfected patients, yet in truth could have exceeded the admission-to-discharge interval. In this case, the investigator could overlook an important feature of the observations under study—that is, that infections were occurring after prolonged stay beyond the usual length of stay for patients with underlying illnesses like those of the infected group. Matching the noninfected patients to the infected patients on such important variables can avoid this problem.

If we discard the assumption that the samples from examples 1 and 2 were independent and assume that patients in the noninfected group were matched to patients in the infected group on the basis of day of admission, underlying diagnosis, age, and sex, then a new group of tests can be introduced (see Fig. 7-1). Although these examples illustrate the situation for one-to-one matching of controls to cases only, testing procedures are available for situations in which a variable number of controls is matched to cases [17].

First, two tests for attribute data from matched samples are illustrated using example 1. The data from example 1 must be summarized and tested differently if the patients are matched [2]; the arrangements of Tables 7-3 and 7-4 are for the unmatched situation. Infected–noninfected pairs rather than individual patients are counted in the 2×2 table for matched studies (Table 7-6).

There were 20 pairs in which the infected patient was catheterized but the matched, noninfected patient was not catheterized. There were only three pairs in which infected patients were not catheterized while their noninfected matches were catheterized. The

Table 7-6. General table for summarizing the association of a factor with infection-matched data

		Infected		
		Catheter	No catheter	Total
Noninfected	Catheter	a	b	a + b
	No catheter	c	d	c + d
	Total	a + c	b + d	n

two cells (Table 7-7) that count the number of pairs having both patients catheterized or neither of the patients catheterized (two and five pairs, respectively) contribute no information about whether infected or noninfected patients were catheterized more often. Therefore, these two cells are not used in the significance tests for attributes. Only the cells counting discordant pairs add information about the association of infection and catheterization. The effective sample size for this example, therefore, is 23 pairs.

Sign Test

The sign test takes into account only the direction of differences between members of each pair and has a relatively low power. If there were no difference in the frequency of catheterization among infected and noninfected patients, there would be as many pairs in which the infected patient was catheterized and the matched, noninfected patient not catheterized as there were pairs with the infected patient not catheterized and the matched, noninfected patient catheterized. For this example of 23 untied pairs, it is expected that, if no difference in the frequency of catheterization exists between infected and

Table 7-7. Pairs of patients by catheterization status (example 1)

		Infected		
		Catheter	No catheter	Total
Noninfected	Catheter	2	3	5
	No catheter	20	5	25
	Total	22	8	30

noninfected patients, there should be 11.5 pairs with a catheterized, infected patient and a noncatheterized, noninfected patient, and 11.5 pairs with a noncatheterized, infected patient and a catheterized, noninfected patient. The probability of observing a given number of pairs or fewer having a non-catheterized, infected patient and a catheterized, noninfected patient is given by the sum of binomial probabilities:

$$p_{\text{Tot}} = \sum_{x=0}^{c} \frac{n!}{x!\,(n-x)!} (.5)^x (1 - .5)^{n-x}$$

where n is the number of untied pairs [16], and c is the smaller of the two cells (b and c) in Table 7-6. The formula sums the probabilities of obtaining 0, 1, . . ., c noncatheterized, infected patients paired with a catheterized, noninfected patient, when half the total untied pairs, 11.5, are expected to be in this cell. The probabilities for example 1 are:

$$p_x = \frac{23!}{x!\,(23 - x)!} (.5)^x (1 - .5)^{23-x}$$

$$p_0 = \frac{23!}{0!\,(23 - 0)!} (.5)^x (1 - .5)^{23-0}$$

$$= 1.19209290 \times 10^{-7}$$

$$p_1 = \frac{23!}{1!\,(23 - 1)!} (.5)^x (1 - .5)^{23-1}$$

$$= 2.74181366 \times 10^{-6}$$

$$p_2 = \frac{23!}{2!\,(23 - 2)!} (.5)^x (1 - .5)^{23-2}$$

$$= 3.01599503 \times 10^{-5}$$

$$p_3 = \frac{23!}{3!\,(23 - 3)!} (.5)^x (1 - .5)^{23-3}$$

$$= 2.11119652 \times 10^{-4}$$

$$p_{\text{Tot}} = 2.44140625 \times 10^{-4}$$

This low probability leads to a rejection of the null hypothesis:

$$H_0: P_I \le P_{NI}$$

in favor of the alternative hypothesis:

$$AH: P_I > P_{NI}$$

The conclusion is that catheterized patients were at higher risk of infection.

McNemar Test

The McNemar test [14] is a chi-square test that uses pairs of patients rather than individuals; therefore, it differs from the ordinary chi-square test presented earlier. As in the sign test, the McNemar test uses only those pairs with untied observations for the infected and noninfected patients. The formula presented below and the previous formula for chi-square for independent observations both include a correction for continuity. Many elementary statistics textbooks present discussions of appropriate use of the continuity correction [20, 21].

$$\chi^2 = \frac{(|b - c| - 1)^2}{b + c}$$

$$= \frac{(|3 - 20| - 1)^2}{23}$$

$$= \frac{(|-17| - 1)^2}{23}$$

$$= \frac{16^2}{23}$$

$$= 11.13$$

Again, this is a two-tailed test for an association between infection and catheterization in either direction (i.e., more risk associated with catheterization or less risk associated with catheterization). Although computed from matched samples, the value of chi-square from the McNemar test should be compared to the same tabulated values of the chi-square distribution that were used for the chi-square test computed from independent samples. The inference about the populations from which the samples from example 1 were drawn, if they were matched, would be that catheterization is associated with infection, since the probability associated with a chi-square of 11.13 is only .00085.

Next, tests for measurement data from matched samples are presented, using example 2 and assuming that the noninfected patients were selected by matching to the infected patients. These tests use the differences between observations for members of the pairs instead of the two observations separately. The hypotheses to be tested are

$$H_0 : \mu_I \leq \mu_{NI}$$

$$AH : \mu_I > \mu_{NI}$$

The hypothesis that the mean of the intervals from admission to onset of infection for infected patients is less than or equal to the mean of the intervals from admission to discharge for noninfected patients is tested against the alternative hypothesis that the mean interval from admission to onset of infection for the infected patients exceeds the mean interval from admission to discharge of noninfected patients. The investigator wishes to decide whether the risk of infection is increased because hospital stay is longer than it would have been if the patients had not acquired infections, or whether the length of stay for infected patients is increased because of infection. If the mean time from admission to onset of infection is approximately the same as the mean time from admission to discharge of noninfected patients, the investigator could conclude that prolonged stay in the hospital is not the underlying cause of infection. Additional study such as examining the distribution of intervals from onset of infection to discharge would then be necessary to understand to what extent infections actually increased the length of stay. The assumption that the sample observations were selected from a population of normally distributed time intervals must be made for the parametric test presented next.

Paired t-test

The paired t-test uses the statistical theorem that the distribution of differences between two normally distributed, random variables (the sample time intervals) is also normal. Once these differences (Table 7-8) between the time intervals of the two members of each pair are determined, the t-test can be used to

decide whether the mean difference is greater than zero. The formula for this t-test is

$$t = \frac{\bar{d}}{s_{\bar{d}}}$$

where $\bar{d} = \dfrac{\sum\limits_{i=1}^{n} d_i}{n} = \dfrac{1,111}{30} = 37.0333$

d_i being the difference between time intervals for the members of the ith pair,

and $s^2 = \dfrac{\sum\limits_{i=1}^{n}(d_i - \bar{d})^2}{n(n-1)} = \dfrac{\sum\limits_{i=1}^{n} d_i^2 - \dfrac{\left(\sum\limits_{i=1}^{n} d_i\right)^2}{n}}{n(n-1)}$

$$= \dfrac{397,253 - \dfrac{(1,111)^2}{30}}{30\,(30-1)}$$

$$= 409.3206$$

$\bar{d}$ and s^2 being the mean and standard error of the mean of differences in the time intervals, and where n is the number of pairs. Then

$$t = \frac{37.0333}{20.2317} = 1.83$$

is greater than 1.699, the tabulated value of t with $n - 1 = 29$ degrees of freedom corresponding to a one-tailed probability of .05. The null hypothesis that the interval from admission to onset of infection is less than or equal to the interval from admission to discharge of noninfected patients is rejected in favor of the alternative hypothesis, that $\mu_I > \mu_{NI}$. These data would support the hypothesis that infections occurred after a prolonged stay in the hospital rather than that prolonged stay resulted from infection.

Wilcoxon Signed Ranks Test

If the assumption of normality is not acceptable, the hypothesis can be tested from matched data using a nonparametric test. The Wilcoxon Signed Ranks test [23] is easy to apply in this case. The results of each step

Table 7-8. Summary of differences for the paired t-test (example 2)

Pair no.	Infected patient	Noninfected patient	Difference	Pair no.	Infected patient	Noninfected patient	Difference
1.	216	253	−37	16.	234	242	−8
2.	187	82	105	17.	205	233	−28
3.	88	125	−37	18.	136	133	3
4.	280	138	142	19.	253	342	−89
5.	310	137	173	20.	165	102	63
6.	239	116	123	21.	340	93	247
7.	344	232	112	22.	325	82	243
8.	315	327	−12	23.	178	248	−70
9.	280	171	109	24.	153	113	40
10.	293	338	−45	25.	355	294	61
11.	200	335	−135	26.	338	304	34
12.	229	109	120	27.	77	211	−134
13.	208	126	82	28.	335	104	231
14.	233	182	51	29.	261	261	0
15.	190	247	−57	30.	93	269	−176

in the test procedure are given in Table 7-9. First the differences are determined (column 4) for all pairs without considering the sign of the difference. Then these unsigned differences are ranked from lowest to highest (column 5), with the smallest difference receiving rank 1 (pair number 18). Differences of 0 (e.g., pair number 29) are omitted from the test procedure. Tied differences are assigned the average value of the ranks that would have been assigned if the differences had not been tied (e.g., pair number 1 and pair number 3). Finally, the signs of differences are assigned to the ranks (column 6) and the sums of absolute values of positive and negative ranks are obtained separately. The value of the smaller of the two sums is compared to the critical value [22] for a one-tailed test at the .05 level. This value, 140, is exceeded by the sum of negative ranks in this example, supporting the hypothesis that the mean interval from admission to onset was greater than the mean interval from admission to discharge of the noninfected patients.

Relative Risk and Odds Ratios

Another approach to analyzing hospital-acquired infection data uses estimates of rela-tive risk and odds ratios. These two quantities measure the association between the infection status and exposure histories of two groups of individuals. Referring to Table 7-4, the in-fection rate or risk of infection in the exposed (catheterized) group is

$$I_E = \frac{a}{(a + b)}$$

and this rate in the unexposed (noncathe-terized) group is

$$I_{NE} = \frac{c}{(c + d)}$$

The relative risk measures the strength of the exposure effect and is defined as

$$R = \frac{\text{Risk of disease, exposed group}}{\text{Risk of disease, unexposed group}} = \frac{I_E}{I_{NE}}$$

$$= \frac{\dfrac{a}{(a + b)}}{\dfrac{c}{(c + d)}}$$

Prospective Cohort Versus Case-Control Studies

If the data in Table 7-1 had been collected by identifying two groups of patients—one

Table 7-9. Summary of the ranking procedure for Wilcoxon Signed Ranks test (example 2)

Pair no.	Infected patient	Noninfected patient	Difference (unsigned)	Rank (unsigned)	Rank (signed)*
1.	216	253	37	6.5	−6.5
2.	187	82	105	17	17
3.	88	125	37	6.5	−6.5
4.	280	138	142	24	24
5.	310	137	173	25	25
6.	239	116	123	21	21
7.	344	232	112	19	19
8.	315	327	12	3	−3
9.	280	171	109	18	18
10.	293	338	45	9	−9
11.	200	335	135	23	−23
12.	229	109	120	20	20
13.	208	126	82	15	15
14.	233	182	51	10	10
15.	190	247	57	11	−11
16.	234	242	8	2	−2
17.	205	233	28	4	−4
18.	136	133	3	1	1
19.	253	342	89	16	−16
20.	165	102	63	13	13
21.	340	93	247	29	29
22.	325	82	243	28	28
23.	178	248	70	14	−14
24.	153	113	40	8	8
25.	355	294	61	12	12
26.	338	304	34	5	5
27.	77	211	134	22	−22
28.	335	104	231	27	27
29.	261	261	0	Omit	Omit
30.	93	269	176	26	−26

*Sum of positive ranks = 292; sum of negative ranks = 143.

group of catheterized patients and the other group not catheterized—these two groups could have been observed prospectively to determine which ones would develop a urinary tract infection. Using the data summarized in Table 7-3, the risk of acquiring a urinary tract infection would be $^{22}/_{27} = 0.8148$ for catheterized patients and $^8/_{33} = 0.2424$ for noncatheterized patients. The ratio of these two risks, or the relative risk of acquiring a urinary tract infection for those patients who were catheterized, is $^{0.8148}/_{0.2424} = 3.36$. Thus,

in this example, catheterized patients were 3.36 times more likely to have developed a urinary tract infection than those who were not catheterized.

Relative risks greater than 1 imply an association of the exposure factors with infection. If there is no increased risk of acquiring an infection associated with a particular exposure, then

$$\frac{a}{(a + b)} = \frac{c}{(c + d)}$$

and the relative risk is 1.0. If there is a decreased risk in acquiring an infection for a particular exposure, then

$$\frac{a}{(a + b)} < \frac{c}{(c + d)}$$

and the relative risk is between 0.0 and 1.0. This implies a potentially protective effect of the exposure because the exposed group has proportionally fewer infected individuals than the unexposed group. In general, relative risk can be interpreted according to the following summary:

Relative risk	Possible interpretations
<1	Exposure protects against infection.
1	There is no association between exposure and infection.
>1	Exposure is associated with infection.

The second measure for describing the relationship between infection status and exposure is the odds ratio. If an infection occurs with probability p, the odds of that infection occurring is defined as

$$\frac{p}{(1 - p)}$$

For example, if a particular infection occurs with 3 : 1 odds, this means it occurs with a .75 probability and that the odds are

$$\frac{.75}{(1.0 - .75)} = \frac{.75}{.25} = \frac{3}{1}$$

This is expressed as 3 : 1 odds.

Referring to Table 7-4, the odds of acquiring an infection for the exposed group of patients are expressed as

$$\frac{\dfrac{a}{(a + b)}}{\dfrac{b}{(a + b)}} = \frac{a}{b}$$

The odds of acquiring an infection for patients in the unexposed group are

$$\frac{\dfrac{c}{(c + d)}}{\dfrac{d}{(c + d)}} = \frac{c}{d}$$

The ratio of the odds of acquiring an infection for the exposed group to the odds for the unexposed group is the infection-odds ratio:

$$\frac{\dfrac{a}{b}}{\dfrac{c}{d}} = \frac{ad}{bc}$$

Using Table 7-3, the odds ratio for acquiring an infection for catheterized patients is

$$\frac{(22 \times 25)}{(8 \times 5)} = 13.75$$

Therefore, the odds of acquiring an infection are 13.75 times greater for the catheterized patients than for the noncatheterized patients.

If the infection in question is rare, then $a + b$ can be estimated by b, and $c + d$ can be estimated by d. This provides a simple estimate of the relative risk using the odds ratio:

$$\hat{R} = \frac{\dfrac{a}{(a + b)}}{\dfrac{c}{(c + d)}} \simeq \frac{\dfrac{a}{b}}{\dfrac{c}{d}} = \frac{ad}{bc}$$

The numbers in Table 7-3 indicate that a urinary tract infection is common in the two groups of patients. For this reason, the odds ratio is not a good approximation of the relative risk for these data.

In a *prospective cohort study*, cohorts are defined as the two exposure groups, patients are assigned to each group according to their catheterization status, and the patients' infection outcomes are recorded. Relative risks can then be calculated. Typically, these studies are difficult to perform for both economic and logistic reasons. If the incidence of the particular infection is low, the groups must be large to ensure the inclusion of infected patients in the study. These large groups of patients must be followed for extended periods to acquire reliable estimates for risk of disease. Often the number of required patients can exceed the population at hand in the hospital. Also, in the hospital setting, ethical and practical considerations often make it impossible to assign individuals randomly to two different treatment or exposure groups.

One mechanism to circumvent these problems is to use the concepts outlined previously and identify all individuals with a particular infection, and then select a suitable group of noninfected patients for a comparison group. Each patient in these two groups is then classified as exposed or unexposed to the factor in question. This design is known as a *retrospective case-control study,* in that infected (case) and noninfected (control) patients are identified and their exposure histories are tabulated retrospectively.

In this situation, the numbers of infected and noninfected patients may be determined by the resources available to do the study and may not reflect the actual frequencies in the hospital population. For this reason, it is not possible to calculate the risk of disease in the two exposure categories. In fact, in this context,

$$\frac{a}{(a + b)} \text{ and } \frac{c}{(c + d)}$$

are meaningless, and relative risk cannot be calculated.

Odds ratios, however, can be determined by calculating the odds of exposure among the infected group as

$$\frac{\dfrac{a}{(a + c)}}{\dfrac{c}{(a + c)}} = \frac{a}{c}$$

and the odds of exposure among the noninfected group as

$$\frac{\dfrac{b}{(b + d)}}{\dfrac{d}{(b + d)}} = \frac{b}{d}$$

This leads to the summary exposure-odds ratio, which expresses the exposure in the infected group relative to the exposure in the noninfected group, as

$$\frac{\dfrac{a}{c}}{\dfrac{b}{d}} = \frac{ad}{bc}$$

Summarizing these results, the odds ratio is the same for both the prospective cohort study and the retrospective case-control study. For rare diseases, it closely approximates the relative risk, which can be calculated only in the prospective cohort study. In the case-control study, the relative risk can only be approximated using the odds ratio (see Chap. 1).

Testing the Significance of Odds Ratios

A variety of methods are available [3, 8] to determine whether the infection-odds ratio is statistically greater than unity. The Fisher's Exact test described earlier can be used to make this determination. The hypotheses can be stated as

$$H_0: \text{odds} \leq 1$$

$$AH: \text{odds} > 1$$

From the earlier analysis of these data, chi-square was 17.239, indicating that the proportion of infected patients who were catheterized was not equal to the proportion of noninfected, catheterized patients. Likewise, the hypothesis that the odds ratio is less than or equal to unity would be rejected by Fisher's Exact test in favor of the alternative hypothesis that the odds ratio is greater than unity. The resulting conclusion would be that the odds of infected patients being catheterized are greater than the odds of noninfected patients being catheterized.

In addition to investigating exposure factors or underlying predisposing factors that increase the risk of infection, infection control personnel may wish to examine the possibility that a factor decreased the risk of acquiring the infection. Since these "protective" factors have odds ratios of less than 1, the hypotheses to be tested are

$$H_0: \text{odds} \geq 1$$

$$AH: \text{odds} < 1$$

Fisher's Exact test, discussed earlier, is appropriate to evaluate these hypotheses.

Confounding Factors

Although the odds ratio is easy to compute, it can give misleading results if other factors are present that are related to both the risk of infection and the exposure. These other associated factors are called *confounding factors*. For example, patients may be catheterized for the same reasons that they are treated with antibiotics, and their treatment with antibiotics can affect their infection status. To evaluate confounding, the investigator could stratify the patients into two groups—those receiving antibiotic treatment and those not receiving antibiotic treatment—and then compute the odds ratios for each stratum separately. If the odds ratios obtained in the two strata are different from the odds ratio obtained in the nonstratified analysis (both antibiotic treatment groups combined), the investigator would conclude that antibiotic treatment status modified the relationship between catheterization and infection. The statistical procedures to evaluate the effects of stratification on odds ratio estimates are described by Mantel and Haenszel [11].

Confidence Intervals for Odds Ratios

The odds ratio calculated from a sample of patients from the hospital provides a single number that is an estimate of the true odds ratio, the ratio that would be observed if all patients in the hospital population were used in the calculations. Since only a sample of patients was used, the odds ratio is a point estimate of the true odds for that setting. In addition to the point estimate, the investigator can calculate an interval of values that will include, with a particular level of confidence (often 99 percent or 95 percent), the true odds ratio. This interval is known as a *confidence interval* for the odds ratio and can be interpreted in the following way: If the investigator could take many samples—100, for example—from this population and compute the confidence interval (e.g., 95 percent confidence interval) from each sample, then 95 of the intervals would be expected to include the true odds ratio. Loosely stated, the investigator would be 95 percent confident that the true odds ratio would be included in the interval calculated from the sample.

One method of estimating the confidence interval is based on the $\ln(\text{odds})$ [24]. In large samples, the $\ln(\text{odds})$ has a normal distribution and the variance of the $\ln(\text{odds})$ is defined as

$$\text{var}[\ln(\text{odds})] = \left[\frac{1}{a} + \frac{1}{b} + \frac{1}{c} + \frac{1}{d}\right]$$

This procedure provides a reasonable estimate of the variance when all cell frequencies are relatively large; when cell sizes are small, other procedures are more appropriate [3, 5]. The upper and lower confidence limits of an approximate $1 - \alpha$ confidence interval for $\ln(\text{odds})$ are

$$\text{Lower} = \text{Odds} \times \exp\left\{-Z_\alpha \sqrt{\text{var}[\ln(\text{odds})]}\right\}$$

$$\text{Upper} = \text{Odds} \times \exp\left\{+Z_\alpha \sqrt{\text{var}[\ln(\text{odds})]}\right\}$$

where α is the type 1 error described earlier and Z_α is the point corresponding with the standard normal distribution that is exceeded with $\alpha/2$ probability. These values may be readily found in statistical tables that present the cumulative normal frequency distribution. In most applications, α is set at .01 corresponding to $Z_\alpha = 2.58$, or .05 corresponding to $Z_\alpha =$

1.96, and would provide a 99 percent or 95 percent confidence interval, respectively.

The odds ratio for the data in Table 7-1 was 13.75, and the variance of the odds was determined by

$$\text{var } [ln(\text{odds})] = \frac{1}{22} + \frac{1}{5} + \frac{1}{8} + \frac{1}{25} = 0.4105$$

The lower and upper limits of the 95 percent confidence interval are

$$\text{Lower limit} = 13.75 \times \exp\left[-1.96\sqrt{.4105}\right]$$
$$= 3.92$$

$$\text{Upper limit} = 13.75 \times \exp\left[1.96\sqrt{.4105}\right]$$
$$= 48.27$$

The investigator would be 95 percent confident that the population odds ratio estimated from the sample is included in the interval 3.92 to 48.27. Other methods for calculating these confidence intervals are available [3, 5].

Other Considerations in Retrospective Studies

Several things must be considered before extrapolating the results of a retrospective study to the entire hospital population or to patients from a group of hospitals. One major concern is the degree to which the infected and noninfected patients in the study represent infected and noninfected patients in the target population with respect to the exposure factors being evaluated. Commonly, in a case-control study, all infected patients are included and a suitable sample of noninfected patients is then selected as controls. Since the infected patients are not randomly chosen and the noninfected patients are often chosen to match certain characteristics of the selected infected patients, the degree to which these groups in the study represent the population in the hospital will determine the appropriateness of inferences about that hospital population. If a study were conducted in a hospital serving a limited portion of the population (e.g., a Veterans Administration hospital or a municipal hospital serving a crowded urban area), any inferences made from the study subjects might not be applicable to other hospital populations (e.g., those patients treated at university-affiliated hospitals) [9].

Another concern about using odds ratios or relative risk estimates in a retrospective study is ascertainment bias when recording exposure histories for infected and noninfected patients. In a prospective cohort study, where the exposures are predetermined, if the infection control nurse, hospital epidemiologist, or other investigator is not aware of the exposure status of a study subject, the determination of infection status can more likely be made in an unbiased fashion. However, in a retrospective case-control study, if the infection status is known to the data collector, determination of risk factors can be more prone to bias. Also, infected patients may more easily recall exposure histories than will noninfected patients; hospital charts may be incomplete or unavailable; and the time required to review charts or other documents may add stress to overworked staff and result in a less thorough review. Investigators should take care to avoid these sources of bias.

Another important consideration in ensuring a successful retrospective study is that data related to the infected group should be obtained in the same manner as data for the noninfected group. If exposure histories are collected through questionnaires, the interviewers should not question the infected patients more vigorously than the noninfected patients. Indeed, to the extent possible, data collectors should be kept unaware of the infection status of the patient to guarantee impartiality in this regard. Interviewers and chart reviewers should each collect data on infected and noninfected patients so that the same techniques and interpretations are used for both groups.

Finally, the data source should be the same for both groups. If hospital records are used for data collection on the infected patients, then hospital records should also be used for the noninfected patients. If relatives or other surrogate respondents answer questions for the infected patients, they should provide the same information for the noninfected patients [9].

Interpretation of Statistically Significant Differences

The practical implications of a statistical result on hospital policies must involve the judgment of the investigator in conjunction with hospital staff. Strictly setting policies contingent on the result of a statistical test or the size of the odds ratio is not a prudent strategy, since many factors discussed earlier can affect statistical results (e.g., sample size, confounding factors, study design, and measurement error).

For example, if the odds ratio from a particular study is determined to be not significant when the size of the odds ratio is large enough to indicate a possible association between exposure and infection, several questions should be addressed. First, what was the power of the study; was the sample size large enough to detect a statistically significant result if a real association was present? If not, the investigator may wish to perform an additional study with a larger sample size. If an increase in sample size is not possible but another study with the same sample size could be performed, then results from both studies would help in deciding about an association. If results from the second study were similar to those of the first study, there would be more reason to believe the earlier study results. If the second study results did not support the findings from the first study, the results of the two studies would be difficult to interpret, and the first study's results would be questionable.

Second, what was the level of significance in the study: Were the significance tests probabilities close to .05, hinting at an association, or were they remarkably greater, indicating that no association existed? The investigator may not wish to use the .05 level of significance as the only determining factor because other events may have influenced the study's outcome.

Third, what was the width of the confidence interval? If the odds ratio confidence interval was narrow, the investigator could be more confident about the value of the true odds ratio. Otherwise, the true value would be difficult to ascertain.

Discussion

Several principles of study design have been presented to remind those responsible for studying nosocomial infections of ways to improve their studies and potentially gain access to computer records for selecting study and control patients. Some simple testing procedures and a scheme for deciding when each is appropriate have been presented. The investigator must be careful to avoid oversimplification of the problems associated with data on nosocomial infections. The use of a simple significance test without understanding the underlying assumptions, without considering the study design, and without giving attention to possible confounding variables can lead to meaningless interpretation of the data. The significance tests presented in this chapter are in no way intended as a complete list of available tests. They were chosen as commonly used examples that are available in each of the situations presented. The objective has been to show the readers, presumably hospital personnel, how the approach to analyzing nosocomial infection data is affected by assumptions, study design, and level of measurement of data. There is no intention to limit analyses to a single factor in any study. Although the scope of this chapter is limited to the single factor (univariate) case, help for analyses of multiple factors (multivariate) can be found in the references cited.

The selection scheme (see Fig. 7-1) is intended to assist with correct application of common test procedures, but even the correct choice of test for a single variable (univariate test) may not produce an accurate conclusion about the association of the factor and infection. There are two reasons for this. First, conclusions from hypothesis testing are based on error probabilities that the investigator sets before the data are collected. Second, the investigator must understand the complete data set, possibly including interrelations among several factors. For the data of example 1, inquiring into the possible increased risk of infection caused by catheterization would include examination of underlying illnesses and other factors that might be considered confounding factors. A factor that may itself be associated with exposure to the factor under study and with the risk to infection should be considered as a potential confounding factor. One might ask whether the catheterized patients were infected as a result of catheterization or whether their infections occurred as a result of serious underlying illness that not only predisposed the patients to infection but also required that the patients be catheterized. Questions like these can sometimes be answered on the basis of a scan of cross-tabulations of the data. Some of these possible confounding variables can be handled in the study design by matching [4]. However, multivariate statistical tools are also available to help in understanding the effects of several variables at the same time.

One of these methods is the Mantel-Haenszel procedure [11], which tests the hypothesis of association of a single variable with infection while keeping a second variable fixed. This allows the second variable to be tested in the presence of the first variable.

Another method for examining more than one variable and even joint effects of variables involves regression techniques. Multiple linear logistic regression techniques have been applied to a variety of situations, including matched study designs [1, 7, 18]. These procedures permit the investigator to develop models including potentially important variables and interaction terms for determining possible joint effects of variables. This is a particularly helpful development for the study of nosocomial infection outbreaks when the causative factors are unknown, because one can explore the data for associations of several potential factors with infection. However, the computations are beyond those that can be done practically with a small calculator. Computer programs that require access to a large computer have been published for this procedure [10], and versions of these programs are presently being developed for personal computers.

The study of nosocomial infections can be simplified, as previously suggested, by taking advantage of data that may be routinely collected in machine-readable form. Rarely do such data contain judgments of infected or noninfected status of patients; therefore, many data items such as culture results, pharmaceuticals, or other indicators must be used to signal that a particular record may be for an infected patient. Usually the infection control practitioner, the hospital epidemiologist, or the Infection Control Committee must solicit the hospital computer center to make provision for entry of the infection status and data about the infection. Of course, this requires active infection surveillance or comprehensive record review by the infection control practitioner. The return in simplified selection of study and control groups from computer files and the potential for computer-assisted analysis can, in many instances, easily offset the cost of additional data collection efforts to obtain machine-readable records.

References

1. Breslow, N.E., and Day, N.E. *Statistical Methods in Cancer Research, vol. 1. The Analysis of Case-Control Studies* (International Agency for Research on Cancer, Scientific Publications, No. 32). Lyon, France: International Agency for Research on Cancer, 1980. Pp. 192–279.
2. Cochran, W.G. The comparison of percentages in matched samples. *Biometrika* 37:256, 1971.
3. Cornfield, J. A Statistical Problem Arising from Retrospective Studies. In: J. Neyman (Ed.), *Proceedings of the Third Berkeley Symposium, vol. IV*. Berkeley: University of California Press, 1956. Pp. 135–148.
4. Cornfield, J., and Haenszel, W. Some aspects of retrospective studies. *J. Chronic Dis.* 11:523, 1960.
5. Fisher, R.A. Confidence limits for a cross-product ratio. *Aust. J. Stat.* 4:41, 1962.
6. Fisher, R.A. *Statistical Methods for Research Workers.* Darien, CT: Hafner, 1970. Pp. 96–97.
7. Gail, M.H., Lubin, J.H., and Rubenstein, L.V.

Likelihood calculations for matched case-control studies and survival studies with tied death times. *Biometrika* 68:703, 1981.

8. Gart, J.J. The comparison of proportions: A review of significance tests, confidence intervals and adjustments for stratification. *Rev. Int. Stat. Inst.* 39:148, 1971.

9. Kahn, H.A., and Sempos, C.T. *Statistical Methods in Epidemiology.* New York: Oxford University Press, 1989.

10. Lubin, J.H. A computer program for the analysis of matched case-control studies. *Comput. Biomed. Res.* 14:138, 1981.

11. Mantel, N., and Haenszel, W. Statistical aspects of the analysis of data from retrospective studies of disease. *J. Natl. Cancer Inst.* 22:719, 1959.

12. Martin, S.M. Choosing the Correct Statistical Tests. In R.P. Wenzel (Ed.), *Handbook of Hospital-Acquired Infections.* Boca Raton, FL: CRC Press, 1981.

13. Maxwell, A.E. *Analysing Qualitative Data.* London: Methuen, 1971. P. 23.

14. McNemar, Q. *Psychological Statistics.* New York: Wiley, 1955.

15. Miller, R.B., Jr. *Simultaneous Statistical Inferences* (2nd ed.). New York: Springer-Verlag, 1981. P. 67.

16. Ostle, B. *Statistics in Research.* Ames, IA: Iowa State University Press, 1954.

17. Pike, M.C., and Morrow, R.H. Statistical analysis of patient-control studies in epidemiology, factor under investigation an all-or-none variable. *Br. J. Prev. Soc. Med.* 24:42, 1970.

18. Schlesselman, J.J. *Case-Control Studies.* New York: Oxford University Press, 1982. Pp. 227–280.

19. Siegel, S. *Nonparametric Statistics for the Behavioral Sciences.* New York: McGraw-Hill, 1956.

20. Snedecor, G.W., and Cochran, W.G. *Statistical Methods.* Ames, IA: Iowa State University Press, 1968.

21. Steel, G.D., and Torrie, J.H. *Principles and Procedures of Statistics.* New York: McGraw-Hill, 1960.

22. Wilcoxon, F., Kattie, S.K., and Wilcox, R.A. *Critical Values and Probability Levels for the Wilcoxon Rank Sum Test and the Wilcoxon Signed Rank Test.* Pearl River, NY: American Cyanamid Co. and Florida State University, 1963.

23. Wilcoxon, F., and Wilcox, R.A. *Some Rapid Approximate Statistical Procedures.* Pearl River, NY: American Cyanamid Co. 1964.

24. Woolf, B. On estimating the relation between blood group and disease. *Ann. Hum. Genet.* 19:251, 1955.

8

The Use of Computerized Systems in Hospital Epidemiology

Jonathan Freeman

When properly designed, computerized systems can be tireless slaves that do error-free fetching, sorting, ordering, and calculating. On the other hand, poorly planned computerized systems can be voracious consumers of resources that never justify their cost [2]. The informed epidemiologist-consumer must be able to determine in what settings computerized systems will be helpful and when computerization will result in a net loss of time, money, and efficiency [2, 6]. The computerized system, and not the computer itself, is the functional unit. In most situations, the cost of the software and the personnel resources required to computerize some function far exceed the cost of the computer hardware. Merely buying computer hardware without effective planning for the continuing financial support for personnel and software is worse than useless.

Recent History

The recession in the computer industry in the mid-1980s was a direct result of the fact that actual usefulness of computers had been misrepresented, because the effort required to computerize any task had been minimized and underestimated. Computerized systems had been oversold for activities these systems *could* perform and also for tasks they *could not* accomplish in a realistic manner at that time. The computer hardware was not faulty, but software programs either had never been written or had not been developed to the point where they were functional at a practical level for nonexperts. Furthermore, rarely was a potential user sophisticated enough to be able to estimate accurately the human resources that would be required to create and maintain a computerized system. Wishful thinking replaced objective testing and balanced judgments when the time came to consider the purchase of computer hardware and software. Hospital epidemiology is arriving at the altar of computerization a decade after the business community performed its initial experiments, and we must heed the expensive lessons of the past if we are not to repeat them.

It is the purpose of this chapter to describe which functions in hospital epidemiology might reasonably be accomplished with a computerized system, what advantages might accrue, and the additional resources that will be required. Many erstwhile computer users will be surprised to find that computerization of a task will generally involve an *increase* in cost, so the potential gain in usefulness of information that can be manipulated by an electronic slave must be compared with the substantially added cost of creating and maintaining the system in which the electronic slave can function effectively. In most settings, hospital epidemiology units will find that the paper- or card-based data systems they are currently using are relatively inexpensive. The cost of computerizing an already functioning paper-based system must be weighed against any potential gains.

Epidemiology units will find computers to be very useful for word processing and for accessing literature databases such as Medline, because these expensive databases were created and are maintained by other agencies. Beyond those two functions, the potential usefulness of computers must be weighed objectively for each individual job and setting. For example, with substantial additional investment of resources, it is possible to create an electronic surveillance database from the paper-based system for one's own hospital. In addition, for those few epidemiology units that regularly publish the results of serious epidemiologic research, acquiring one of the statistical packages and teaching someone to apply it might be useful. In each instance, the real needs and abilities of the potential users must be assessed. Working systems in use at other similar institutions or hospitals should

be tried and evaluated prior to making any purchase.

Research in Computerized Systems for Hospital Epidemiologic Use

Several groups of investigators have pioneered in the investigation of the application of computerized systems to hospital epidemiology [8, 12, 24, 25]. These research systems have been developed over decades at a cost of tens of millions of dollars and apply only to the institutions in which they were developed. Each of these systems is based on the incorporation of electronic databases created and maintained by other departments of the hospital, such as microbiology, clinical pathology, pharmacy, radiology, and administration. Data from these different departments within each hospital are kept in different ways, and the development of functional systems to download, recode, combine, and analyze data from these diverse sources in a timely manner is what has made these systems so expensive.

The resources required to create or acquire such systems are far beyond the capability of most hospital epidemiology units. Rather, we can simply look to these systems as the initial steps in the development of generally applicable systems in the distant future. Accurately differentiating between these costly research systems and what is currently practical for the daily work of an individual hospital epidemiology unit will prevent epidemiologists from making the major errors in judgment that characterized the introduction of computers into the business world.

The Nature of Past Disappointment Engendered by the Computer Industry
Personification of the Computer

There are many reasons why computers, especially personal computers, failed to live up to the expectations of eager consumers. A common error made by naive potential computer users was personification of computers. Somehow people attributed active human thought patterns to computers when these machines first became readily available. A mistaken belief existed that a computer would somehow just reach out and take over large portions of an individual's work. Computers are completely passive, however, and do not imitate human thought patterns. They do exactly what they are programmed to do, including performing all the errors written into a program, at great speed with outstanding accuracy. Unfortunately for naive users, the titles of articles about computers tend to support this erroneous view of the computer as an active entity (e.g., "Computer surveillance of . . .").

Ultimately, a computer can do an extraordinary number of mindless tasks that are regarded by humans as drudgery, but there is a steep price. First, simply learning to use a computerized system takes much longer than inexperienced purchasers might anticipate. Second, computerizing an epidemiologic database, for example, requires substantial additional resources for data entry, editing, and correction. In fact, the cost of the human resources necessary for creating a usable database will far exceed the initial expense of the necessary hardware and software. The fact that computerization, in most situations, will substantially increase costs is an unpleasant surprise for many potential buyers.

Misleading Advice from Enthusiastic Sources

Many current magazines, published for virtually every type of computer, provide helpful advice on choosing computers, peripherals, and software. The potential consumer must remember the enthusiasm and biases of those who work in the computer industry. Advice from well-intentioned and knowledgeable hobbyists has been, and will continue to be, seriously misleading to the episodic or occasional computer user. Whereas a computer hobbyist might describe a piece of software as easy to use and the manual as well organized, an occasional user might find this same program to be very complicated and the manual opaque and inaccessible. A computer hobbyist who reads manuals and experiments with software as a form of recreation probably would not consider attending a course to learn to use an operating system or a new piece of software. In contrast, occasional users are hesitant to tackle a fat reference manual on a complex program and would gladly attend a short course that concentrates on the core elements of using an operating system or program. Furthermore, once learned, a complex operating system or program not used daily is easily forgotten and, a year later, might have to be relearned.

The Difficulty of Learning to Use Common Software

Essential software such as some operating systems and elaborate word-processing, database, and spreadsheet programs took much longer to learn to use than advertisements and computer hobbyists acknowledged. One of the best-kept secrets among the manufacturers of these complex and expensive word-processing, database, and spreadsheet programs manufactured for business use is that no more than 10 to 15 percent of the software packages that they sell are ever used. In fact, the difficulty of learning to use these programs spawned a whole new industry of schools for teaching the use of common programs, especially programs used on IBM-compatible personal computers. Casual inspection of the shelves of colleagues in the hospital epidemiology field reveals numbers of unused and even unopened packages of costly software, indicating that epidemiology users are no different from business users in their lack of ability to judge beforehand what uses computers will actually serve in their profession.

Computerized systems can be extremely helpful, for they can augment the writing and editing process, manipulate large databases, and perform complex calculations with seemingly magical speed and accuracy. However, this magic comes at a much higher price than inexperienced purchasers might imagine.

Pitfalls of Computerization
Potential Computer Users: Hobbyists Versus Occasional Users

The computer user is the most important element determining the success or failure of any attempt to computerize a task. This same computer user is also the most variable aspect of any computerized system. Before making decisions regarding the computerization of any task in hospital epidemiology, it is essential to consider the interests and capabilities of the identified computer operators. There are many levels of sophistication among potential computer users, from computer hobbyists and "hackers" at one extreme to occasional and even reluctant users at the other. Computer hobbyists spend days and weeks playing with hardware and software as a form of entertainment, whereas most potential computer users in the business and medical worlds see computer use as a form of work, not recreation.

There are several choices open to a hospital epidemiology unit that wishes to implement a computerized system. Personnel involved in hospital epidemiology usually have arrived at their calling through their interest and expertise in medical areas and thus are generally only occasional users of computers. Rarely, one may have access to a gifted computer hobbyist or hacker who is willing to undertake the large job of system design and personnel education. Unfortunately, hobbyists may overestimate both their ability and the amount of time they are willing to devote to such an enterprise. In the absence of free services, substantial resources will have to be invested in training casual or occasional computer users if they are to become facile operators of the complex programs that are standard in the business arena of the personal computer industry. The other alternative is to seek out computerized systems that are specifically designed for simplicity.

The Added Costs of Computerizing Almost Any Function

If the computer user views learning to use software programs as recreation, to be performed in spare time outside of working hours, then there is little additional time cost associated with this phase of instituting a computerized system. On the other hand, when the days or weeks required to become facile with a complex piece of new software are taken from other activities normally performed during the working day, then the salary costs of learning about a new program may reach many thousands of dollars, far exceeding the purchase price of the computer hardware and software.

Furthermore, even after one has learned to use new software, there are usually costs associated with continued use of a program. The clearest example is the database that would arise from normal surveillance activities in a hospital. The data are originally recorded on paper forms or cards and are immediately useful as a paper or card system. If the decision is made to enter these data into an electronic database, then there will be the additional ongoing expense of data entry, data editing, and data correction. Although surveillance data may be more useful in an electronic format, for many hospitals the cost of computerizing surveillance data will far exceed any possible benefit.

Estimating Total Costs of Computerization Beforehand

Wishful thinking has allowed many an epidemiologist to become enslaved, at least for a time, by a computer. To avoid making repeated costly errors with respect to computerized systems, it is necessary to understand what human, software, and hardware resources are required to set up and maintain a computerized system [6]. By far the most important resources for any computerized system are the human resources required. This is the area in which inexperienced but hopeful computer users make the most errors. Next most important is the availability of suitable software, and least important is the hardware, or the computer itself.

How does one obtain a realistic estimate of the resources required to create and maintain computerized systems? This process requires estimating the resources required to perform an activity with a paper or card system and then formulating a realistic estimate of the additional costs of utilizing a computerized system to accomplish the same result. The added cost of computerizing a function includes the cost of acquiring the software and the hardware, the cost of installing the system, the cost of learning to use the software, the cost of entering, editing, and correcting data, the costs of repeating these procedures as more data are added periodically, and the cost of maintaining the system.

Let us look at a common example, the desire to computerize a hospital surveillance database. Most hospital epidemiology units currently conduct some sort of formal surveillance for nosocomial infections. The data are recorded as line lists on paper forms or on individual cards, and monthly or weekly tallies may be made of infections by site, service, procedure, and various patient characteristics. Those involved in the monthly shuffling, sorting, and counting of paper forms or cards may envision an easier solution that includes use of a computer to replace paper shuffling with electronic accounting. This certainly is possible, but computerization of a database involves a number of extra steps, and a practical decision would depend on where the extra resources could be found.

In most hospitals, the budget for hospital epidemiology is fixed, so the extra resources required to computerize the surveillance database would have to be taken from some other activities within an epidemiology unit. Specifically, it would be necessary to allocate time every week to enter all of the data from the paper forms into the computerized database, to edit the data that have been entered, and to correct keypunching errors. The time saved in sorting and summarizing data in a computerized system at the end of each month may be overshadowed by the even greater amount of time required to enter the data into the electronic database.

If additional clerical resources are made available for data entry, then computerizing a database may be a real advantage. On the other hand, when resources are fixed, and a trained epidemiologist would have to be removed from some clinical activities on wards

in order to keypunch data, then computerization of a surveillance database may result in a net loss of clinical functionality for a hospital epidemiology unit. These judgments need to be made individually for every hospital.

Appropriate Applications of a Computerized System
Tasks for Which Computers Are Always Useful

As was mentioned earlier, there are two sorts of tasks for which computers are almost universally useful, and these are word processing and searching a database (such as Medline, a literature database) that somebody else created and maintains [5]. These two tasks are computerized functions that any hospital epidemiology unit, no matter how small, will probably need. They require minimal investment in hardware and software and, if there is a medical library nearby, literature searches may be free. Minimal effective hardware and software requirements for these two essential functions are discussed later.

Additional Tasks for Which Computers May Sometimes Be Useful

There are three additional specialized tasks for which computers also can be useful: (1) creating, maintaining, and updating simple statistical reports from an individual hospital database; (2) performing complex or repeated epidemiologic or statistical calculations; and (3) desktop publishing, or producing a newspaper or newsletter at regular intervals. Computerization of these last three functions will only be cost-effective for hospital epidemiology units under relatively unusual circumstances. The nature, selection, and training of potential computer operators has been described earlier, and the characteristics of computers and their interaction with humans are described next.

Characteristics of Computers

Although a detailed description of the technical aspects of computers is beyond the scope of this chapter, a brief description of their general characteristics will help explain common vocabulary. A few basic definitions are common to all computer systems.

Definitions

The core of any computer is the actual *computing chip* or *processor,* which performs all data processing and calculations. Each computing chip functions at a specified clock speed, measured in megahertz (MHz), and can perform one operation with each tick of its clock. Data to be used by the computing chip come in elements called *bits.* Eight bits form one *byte,* which corresponds roughly to one character or one digit. The computing chip handles data in chunks of specific size, 4 bits (½ byte), 8 bits (1 byte), 16 bits (2 bytes), 32 bits (4 bytes), or 64 bits (8 bytes) at once. Computing chips or processors thus have two defining characteristics, a clock speed and a size in bits.

Information is stored in two general types of memory: primary memory and secondary memory. The *primary memory* is the memory in which the computing or processing chip does its active computing or figuring. This primary memory consists of memory chips called *random access memory* (RAM), which is instantly available to the processor. *Secondary memory* is made up of magnetic media such as hard disks, floppy disks, or tape. The contents of secondary memory must be read into primary memory before they can be used by the processor. Memory capacity is measured in kilobytes (kB) or megabytes (MB). Therefore, any particular piece of information can be picked out of the RAM primary memory by the computing chip immediately when needed, but data are available from secondary magnetic media after a delay determined by the mechanics of the device. Information can be read from a hard disk relatively rapidly and from a floppy disk approximately one-tenth as fast. Tape is a very inexpensive storage medium, but retrieval of information from tape is very slow.

Data are moved around inside the computer between the computing chip and RAM via a roadway called a *bus.* The size of the bus, which corresponds to the width of the road-

way, usually matches the size of the computing chip, so a computer with a 16-bit processor usually has a 16-bit bus. With one tick of its clock, a 16-bit computer can move 2 bytes of information from RAM to the processor. Other parts that complete a computer system include an *input device,* such as a keyboard, and *output devices,* such as a monitor and printer. A *modem* is used to transmit information over telephone lines between two distant computers. These are discussed later under specific applications.

Evolution of Computers

A brief description of the evolution of computers will help explain the current array of choices. Traditional distinctions among types of computers are becoming less meaningful as the performance of personal computers has increased and prices have dropped. Generally useful categories of computers are mainframe computers, workstations, personal computers, and programmable calculators.

Mainframe Computers

Mainframe computers have the largest and fastest processors and have relatively unlimited chip and hard-disk memory capacity. Mainframes have operating systems that allow multiple users to share the same large and fast machines. Although mainframes are least limited in their range of capabilities, they remain the most expensive to buy, require skilled professional operators to maintain, and have the most complex programs and operating systems. As a result, most medical investigators still are forced to employ professional programmers as intermediaries to make effective use of mainframe computers, and thus they remain one step removed from direct use of the computer system.

Other disadvantages to mainframes are that individual users must wait while control of the single shared mainframe passes among multiple users. Access is determined by the priority system for the computer and, during busy periods, long jobs submitted by low-priority users may wait for undefined periods before being executed. Access to a shared mainframe may be instantaneous late at night or early in the morning, but many users want access during the standard workday and find unpredictable delays difficult to manage.

Beginning mainframe users were particularly annoyed when their terminal screens repeatedly froze and unfroze as control of the machine passed among many simultaneous users. Keystrokes made while the screen was frozen were stored electronically and executed all at once when control returned to an individual terminal. It was a common experience for an impatient amateur to want to backspace over a letter or two, hold down the backspace key in frustration while the terminal screen was frozen, and then watch helplessly as lines or pages of work disappeared when the terminal became active again and all the stored backspaces were executed at once. These unpleasant aspects of communal mainframe computer use led to the development of the personal computer.

Personal Computers

Though the first personal computers lacked the ability to perform many of the tasks of the mainframe, they were dedicated to the individual user. An operator never had to wait while a screen froze, because control of a personal computer never passed to another user. This was particularly important for word processing, which became essentially instantaneous on a personal computer. In the last decade, simple personal computers have become common and the software for word processing so well developed that the way we write in the medical world has changed dramatically. Individual medical practitioners and researchers have learned to write and edit drafts, and former secretaries now function more effectively in administrative capacities because typewriting is no longer their most time-consuming occupation.

Historically, Apple developed the first practical personal computer, and the machines in the Apple II line are the simple but highly functional descendants of this first personal computer. The Visicalc spreadsheet was invented for the original Apple, and business users eagerly sought these machines because

large interdependent sets of numbers in accounting sheets could be recalculated in seconds instead of hours. After a few years, the giant IBM Corporation decided that the personal computer was not a fad and designed the IBM PC, which quickly became the standard of the business world. IBM has since extended this line to include the AT and a series of smaller, more powerful computers called System/Two.

The high profits reaped by IBM lured a number of competitors into the field, who built so-called IBM clones or IBM compatibles. Many competitors built machines that duplicated the functions of the original IBM computers but were less costly. Another competitor, Compaq, developed personal computers that cost as much as the IBM line but were portable or offered more features or were more powerful. Still other companies developed very small "laptop" personal computers that were powered by batteries and could be carried and used almost anywhere. IBM is now only one of many manufacturers in this marketplace, and the consumer has an extremely wide choice in price and function among IBM compatibles.

The original Apple and IBM computers were controlled by conventional text commands typed on the keyboard, and the pointer or cursor was moved around the monitor screen with the arrow keys. Apple then developed the graphic user interface (GUI) for its Macintosh line of personal computers. Instead of addressing the computer in words, the Macintosh allowed an operator to use pictures or symbols, and the cursor could be moved around the screen freehand through the use of a drawing device called a *mouse*. It soon was clear that there were many potential users of personal computers who were frightened by the conventional command line text interface, and these individuals were drawn to the picture and symbol interface of the Macintosh line.

Programmers in the IBM-compatible world have been busy developing similar graphic interfaces for their lines of machines, but these new graphic interfaces for IBM compatibles are still very cumbersome and require that they be installed on substantially more expensive machines in order for them to function reasonably. Apple, IBM, and their competitors now have lines of very powerful personal computers with similar capabilities. The two original computer companies have been joined by a multitude of others that have made this one of the most fertile areas for creativity and the inventive spirit.

Workstations

The workstation is intermediate between a mainframe computer and a personal computer and shares some attributes of both. A workstation is actually a small mainframe designed for a single user or a small number of users. Although workstations retain most of the capabilities and complexities of mainframes, little or no waiting is involved in their use. The most powerful of the personal computers are now beginning to approach the capabilities of workstations in their speed and capabilities. Complex computing projects in epidemiology, such as complex statistical analyses of large sets of categorical data, may exceed the limits of commonly available personal computers and are conveniently performed on workstations.

Programmable Calculators

Before the personal computer reached a practical stage of development, the programmable calculator had already revolutionized data analysis in small and moderately sized epidemiologic projects [37]. The original programmable calculators had relatively slow computer chips that processed information 4 bits at once but, since they could be programmed, they were real computers and are still widely used by those who deal with numbers.

History of Data Management
Functional Speed and Accuracy of Computers

It is important to appreciate the relative speeds with which sorting and calculating have been done during this century. Before the advent of electronic computing devices, some epidemiologists and statisticians kept large data sets in giant tables on the backs of rolls of wallpaper. These were unrolled in living rooms and down corridors in academic buildings, and researchers crawled around on their hands and knees counting exposures, attributes, and events for study subjects. Accuracy depended on how long the investigator was willing to spend on his or her knees recounting and checking numbers in these vast tables.

Various card systems were also developed as more efficient paper-based systems of data storage and manipulation. Decks of common index cards are frequently used to store data, and multiple sorts can be accomplished more quickly than with the wallpaper-based systems just mentioned. This is especially true if the index cards are marked in color along the edges. A more sophisticated card system is available as McBee cards, which have holes punched along the edges. Once stacked in trays, McBee cards can be sorted quickly and accurately with a long rod resembling a knitting needle.

When the first mainframe computers were developed, they also incorporated a card system for the storage and sorting of data. The ubiquitous computer punch card, or Hollerith card, was actually developed in the previous century to program patterns for weaving on mechanical looms, and its almost universal adoption as the media for computers was inevitable. The early mainframes allowed neater card storage of data on attributes and events, which could then be sorted and counted with complete accuracy by mechanical card sorters. However, the early mainframes were not easily accessed, even by professionals.

After the data were sorted by a computerized mechanical card sorter, complex statistical and epidemiologic computations could be carried out. Because of the expense, the threatened devastation of forests, and the very slow speeds at which cards could be sorted mechanically, the punch card and the mechanical card sorter are now a part of computing history, and data entry is carried out on magnetic media. Currently, sorting is done electronically, and final calculations are easily accomplished with programmable calculators [37] or statistical packages [11, 39, 41, 42].

Even the slowest computer is incredibly fast and accurate compared with a human performing the same tasks. The problems with speed and accuracy inherent in a system that depended on the investigator crawling around on the back of a roll of wallpaper are evident. Data storage and sorting on cards, either by hand or by mechanical card sorters, is quicker. For large, complex data sets, the gains realized in moving from rolls of wallpaper to a mainframe computer were extreme. However, in the medical world, data sorting on mainframes generally continues to require professional programmers as intermediaries, an aspect that has not changed appreciably since the early days of the mainframe.

Because of the intermediary, the turnaround time from formulation of the request until delivery of the results of a successful mainframe sort might be days to weeks. However, one can do other work in the interim, and if the program is correctly written, the accuracy of the sorting procedure is assured. Analyses of these sorted data can then be carried out expeditiously with a programmable calculator or personal computer.

Shortly after the programmable calculator came into wide use, the original Visicalc spreadsheet was developed for the simplest Apple computer. The early spreadsheets could deal with only relatively small data sets but, after data were entered into the spreadsheet, this combination could perform in a minute or two computations that would have taken an experienced user with a calculator a whole day to complete. This represents a five-hundred-fold jump in speed, and an increase of this magnitude has never been approached since. The fastest and most expensive 32-bit personal computers now available are only twenty to forty times as fast as the original 8-bit machines available a decade earlier.

An additional benefit that accrued from the use of an electronic spreadsheet was that once the data were entered and checked for accuracy, no further errors in data entry or calculation could occur. Since data had to be reentered for many repeat calculations with early calculators, use of a spreadsheet also represented an enormous decrease in errors in data entry. Shortly after the invention of the spreadsheet, electronic databases were developed for personal computers that, given enough time, could faultlessly sort data sets of almost any size but had limited abilities to perform calculations. There is now a series of programs for storing and manipulating surveillance data in hospital epidemiology that is based on electronic databases.

The functional speed and efficiency of a computerized system is determined by a myriad of variables. In practice, speed differences on the order of four- or fivefold are noticeable to operators, but smaller differences are difficult to detect. Many claims about computer speed involve differences so minor that they would not be apparent to the average user. Most advertisements and technical discussions of computers focus on the clock speed of the processor, which is also frequently misleading. The top speed of a computer chip is discussed in the same manner as the top speed of an automobile and has about as much relevance in daily use. Automobiles almost never reach top speed and, similarly, computers rarely are limited by chip speed.

The efficiency with which a computer can accomplish a particular task is dependent on a multitude of other factors, primarily the presence of a hard disk and disk speed. After that, the amount of RAM, the scratchpad on which the computer works, is important, as is the size of the bus. Perceived speed also depends on how well different parts of a computer keep up with one another. The speed of operation of some programs is limited by the way in which they use the monitor screen, so functional speed is determined by how rapidly the monitor screen can be renewed. Chip speed is one of the least important practical determinants of computer speed as it is perceived by the user.

Functional Computer Speed Primarily Dependent on Mechanical Functions

Computerized systems involve an integrated mixture of components, many electronic but some mechanical. Electronic processing generally takes place at high speed on a computer, whereas the mechanical tasks progress much more slowly. Most computer programs make extensive use of secondary data storage by reading from a hard disk and writing to a hard disk. Functions performed slowly on mechanical components can be accomplished at an accelerated level by switching to faster mechanical components. This will bring notable increases in the functional speed of a computer, and moving this same function to the electronic level will enhance performance further still. We will look at the use of floppy disks, hard disks, and electronic RAM disks as secondary memory.

Floppy disks are inexpensive and convenient storage devices for large amounts of text, data, or programs. Hundreds of pages of text may be stored on a single floppy, and the equivalent of a long paper or 40 pages of text can be written to or read off a floppy disk in a period of a few seconds to a minute or two. In mechanical terms, this seems very fast; however, it is glacially slow compared with the electronic capabilities of even the simplest computer.

A hard disk spins ten times as fast as a floppy disk, and information is transferred on and off a hard disk ten or twenty times as rapidly. Nevertheless, the mechanical hard disk is still most likely to be the rate-limiting component of a computer system. To circumvent the speed limits imposed by mechanical disk drives, electronic storage on extra RAM may be used to replace mechanical disks. This can be accomplished in a personal computer by organizing extra RAM to function as an artificial disk drive called a *virtual disk*. Data can flow to and from an electronic disk at the top speed available from that electronic device. Switching secondary memory storage from floppy disk drives to a hard disk involves an order of magnitude increase in speed, and switching from a mechanical hard disk to an electronic RAM disk will increase speed by approximately another order of magnitude. Only at the electronic level of operation of a RAM disk will the speed of the computer be limited by chip speed and bus size.

Computer Speed for Various Types of Programs

For word processing, the most common task for personal computers, chip speed plays almost no role in how well and easily writing, editing, and printing can be accomplished. Likewise, the speed in using a literature database is not determined by the chip in the personal computer, because the database is being searched by a time-sharing mainframe computer at the other end of a telephone line. Functional speed in using a literature database is most often limited by the nature of the modem used to connect with the central mainframe and the quality of the telephone line over which the transmissions take place.

A database program that might be used to manipulate hospital surveillance information and make simple statistical calculations stores data on a hard disk, and the efficiency of such a database program depends primarily on the speed of data exchange between the processor and the hard disk in the computer. This is usually limited by the mechanical speed with which the hard disk can access stored information but may also be influenced by the design of the database program itself and the size of the bus.

Spreadsheets do generally calculate at chip speed, and even the slowest computer can produce recalculation results with stunning speed and accuracy compared with the time required to perform the same operations on a programmable calculator. Large spreadsheets are recalculated in a minute or two on even the slowest machine. Investigators in hospital epidemiology generally do not make giant spreadsheets, and even a major difference in speed of recalculation is not likely to save very many minutes in a year.

Academic research for publication in the hospital epidemiology field may involve the use of one of the large statistical packages [11, 39, 41, 42], and this is the only setting in which chip speed and machine architecture will have a major influence on the practical functionality of a computerized system. Statistical calculations generally are the most difficult type of operation for a computer, because many significant figures have to be carried along in classic analysis of variance, and long iterative processes are involved in performing analyses such as logistic regression. These academic enterprises are the only situations in which an expensive and fast personal computer is likely to make a real difference. However, one should never consider the purchase of a machine such as this until the data are already in hand and the immediate need for statistical computation is clear. As will be discussed later, computer technology is evolving fast and prices continue to fall. Since data collection for most research projects in epidemiology takes a year or more to complete, major gains in computing power may be realized simply by postponing purchase of an expensive machine until the end of a research project rather than acquiring a computer at the outset.

Reliability of Computerized Systems
From the point of view of the reliability of a computerized system, it is convenient to divide system components into two groups, electrical and mechanical. In general, if the electronic components of a computerized system—the circuit boards and chips—function perfectly in the beginning, they will continue to function that way for a long time. However, the power supply may have a shorter lifetime, especially if it was relatively small to start, and if the user has added a number of extra boards to the computer that have relatively high energy requirements. Also, computer hackers who repeatedly plug and unplug chips and boards from their machines may eventually mechanically disrupt some electrical connections on the circuit boards.

Because the electronic components of computerized systems are so trouble-free, beginning users tend to forget that there are also essential mechanical components in a computerized system, such as disk drives and printers. All mechanical devices need regular service, just like an automobile and, like an automobile, will break down on occasion. Because hard disks work so well and are so fast, beginners tend to depend on them completely and store everything on the hard disk. Modern hard disks are very reliable, and most run for years without trouble, but hard disk drives are also mechanical components. Computer sages repeat that there are only two kinds of hard disk drives: Those that have already failed, and those that are about to fail.

Every computer user must be prepared to lose the entire contents of the hard disk periodically. If the hard disk contained months or years of work, and there are no other copies, then a hard disk crash is a major catastrophe. In monetary terms, a hard disk may contain data that are worth tens or even hundreds of thousands of dollars. The obvious safeguard is to make multiple copies of all important files on floppy disks or cassette tape and to update them regularly. There are a number of programs for the speedy backup of hard disks and special tape drives that will accomplish the backup of tens of megabytes in a few minutes. Although backup takes time, it is obviously cost-effective to back up a hard drive at least weekly.

General Considerations in Choosing a Computer System
There is no such thing as the best computer, there is only the simplest and least expensive computerized system to be used by a specific operator that will perform the tasks essential for the defined needs. The most important single determinant of success with a computerized system is the inclination and training of the identified computer operator. Proponents of the two major standards for personal computers, IBM and Apple, tout their favorite systems with religious fervor. Historically, less expensive IBM compatibles generally have provided more computing power for the hardware dollar but require more in the way of human resources to learn. Apple systems are more expensive to purchase but are substantially easier for nonexperts to use.

Apple has brought out a new line of less expensive Macintosh computers to compete more directly with the large array of low-cost IBM compatibles.

The reason most of the complex programs sold for personal computers were never used is that competent operators did not exist at the proposed site of use and the purchaser never had the resources to become facile with the program. Since the functionality of any personal computer system is determined by the facility of the operator, even substantial differences in hardware and software costs ultimately become trivial in comparison with the expense of training and maintaining the operator. If extensive resources are not available within a hospital epidemiology unit for sustaining a computer operator, it is essential to seek out a simple system, one that can be operated by a range of nonexpert employees. Otherwise, a complex and expensive computerized system may become useless when the trained operator is lost.

Business users usually can hire professional full-time computer operators and, in this setting, the cost of training such an individual can be amortized over years. In contrast, hospital epidemiology units are composed of full-time health care workers and rarely can dedicate a whole salary to computer operation. The computerized system that is most accessible to multiple amateur and occasional users in a hospital epidemiology unit may be far different from the optimal system selected for business use.

Using Existing Computer Facilities

Most, if not all, computer systems needed by hospital epidemiology units may already be available within the hospital at no cost. A number of tasks are more efficiently carried out on preexisting computer systems. Many hospitals use mainframe computers for accounting and billing and are willing to allow use of these for hospital epidemiology. The availability of these mainframes and programs varies markedly. Most hospital and medical school libraries already have access to literature databases through personal computers and modems. For use in hospital epidemi-

ology, it is far more efficient and less expensive to conduct occasional literature searches through utilization of these standard facilities.

Minimizing Cost

There are three considerations for minimizing expenses associated with computer hardware acquisition; borrowing time on underused systems, looking for free personal computers, and postponing computer purchase until the last possible moment. There tend to be many unused and underused personal computers of various ages sitting in offices and laboratories around hospitals, and borrowing time on an already functioning computer is the best way to learn about the use of simple word processing or a spreadsheet program.

The original Macintosh systems and the Apple II systems popular in schools are the simplest personal computers to use and represent excellent initial systems for those who are uncertain what role computers may play in their professional lives. Epidemiologists should constantly be on the lookout to salvage free personal computers from offices and laboratories within a hospital. This is especially true for Apple II computers, because they were incorporated as part of many pieces of laboratory equipment commonly used in hospitals. Many of these machines become available from laboratories as equipment is replaced. Although they are no longer fashionable, with the addition of some RAM or a hard disk they are excellent word processors and work fine with modems used to address literature databases. Both of these tasks make minimal demands on any computer: That is, the personal computer needed for 90 to 100 percent of the functions of most hospital epidemiology units may well be found free or for little additional cost.

Technical advances are being made at a remarkable pace in the personal computer industry, and the amount of computing power available per dollar has continued to double approximately every 2 years: That is, in 2 years the same functionality will be available for approximately half of the cost today, or twice the power can be purchased for the same price in 2 years. Never buy a machine or a piece of software for its potential or for some purpose it might serve in the undefined future. The history of the computer industry is characterized by wishful thinking. Most proposed programs never are written or never reach their potential level of usefulness. It makes sense to delay the purchase of a computerized system until the last possible moment when the actual needs are most clearly defined. Then, buy exactly the hardware and software available at the moment that fulfill the needs of the immediate task at hand.

Interfaces: First Barrier to Personal Computer Use

The computer interface is simply the way an operator communicates with a computer. In the world of IBM compatibles, the interface with the computer is text typed in on the command line via the keyboard. In the Macintosh line, Apple went to a graphic interface, in which basic operations are represented by picture symbols termed *icons*. The popularity of this graphic interface indicates how many potential computer users were put off by the classic command line interface. The world of IBM compatibles is now racing to catch up in the area of graphics, but graphic-based systems for IBM compatibles involve substantially more complexity and expense.

Operating Systems: Second Barrier to Personal Computer Use

The operating system and utilities are the primary programs that tell the computer how to control all of its components and how to perform basic housekeeping and accounting chores, such as allocating disk space and moving files around. These seem so central to computer use that beginners are surprised that a separate program is needed to accomplish these essential functions. The nature of the operating systems available for the various computer systems is emblematic of the relative ease of use of the system in general.

PC DOS and MS DOS are the functionally equivalent primary operating systems for IBM and IBM-compatible personal computers, respectively. There are many sequential versions of these programs extant, and version 3.3 or greater is needed to use all of the common types of disk drives. These operating system programs are difficult for beginners to master and contain many traps for the unwary. It is still relatively easy for an amateur inadvertently to destroy files or even whole disks with a nonspecific use of a FORMAT, COPY, or DELETE command. These operating systems deliver insufficient warning when catastrophic changes are about to take place, and these unfortunate tendencies have given rise to a whole industry devoted to the development of programs to protect the user from the DOS operating system for IBM compatibles.

By far the easiest way to learn to use the DOS operating system is to take a course for beginners. Otherwise, days of study will be required to become familiar with the complexities of these operating systems. The same warning concerning how to learn a program holds true for most of the complex word-processing, spreadsheet, or database programs for the IBM compatibles that are popular in the business world. Many of these programs have tried to minimize the difficulties with the DOS operating system by incorporating simplified DOS functions within the other programs. As a result, some beginners have found it easier to move files around on a hard disk with a word-processing program than with the DOS operating system. Although IBM compatibles represent a good value of computer power for cost of hardware, one must set aside substantial additional resources in the form of time and money to support educating users to employ such a system safely.

Apple systems have much simpler and more intuitive operating systems that are accessible to most users without taking a course. The high-end Apple Macintosh systems are the functional equivalents of the expensive IBM compatibles, and word-processing, spreadsheet and database programs with similar capabilities are available for both. Apple systems are ahead when it comes to the interface, the operating system, and programs that use graphics, such as desktop publishing. In contrast, the statistical packages moved from mainframes to personal computers have been adapted to the IBM systems first and for some years were available only on IBM-compatible computers. However, these statistical packages are currently becoming available for the powerful machines at the high end of the Macintosh line as well.

If no free equipment is available and some purchases must be made, then one should try an installed version of any system being considered for purchase to determine what level of sophistication is required from the operator. Remember that personnel costs and not hardware or software will ultimately represent the major expense involved in the implementation of any computerized system.

Practical Computerized Systems in Hospital Epidemiology
First Programs for Hospital Epidemiology

There are many personal computers available, and almost any of them will serve most needs among hospital epidemiology units. The best beginning computer is the computer one already owns or can use for nothing. Make sure there is no other choice before spending any money on hardware. In the following sections, hardware needs, according to application, are reviewed with each function.

Simple but very effective programs for word processing, spreadsheets, databases, and telecommunications are available for every computer system in combinations called *integrated packages*. The names of many of these integrated programs end in the suffix *-works*. These integrated programs generally are inexpensive simplified versions of more complex programs and offer the beginner an opportunity to try using a word processor, a communications program, a spreadsheet, and a database with a common set of commands. Almost everyone will find a simple word processor to be cost-efficient but, if personnel in a hospital epidemiology unit never use the simple spreadsheet or database programs in an integrated package, then there will be no need to consider the purchase of

more expensive and complex versions of the same programs.

Word Processing

Somewhere in excess of 90 percent of all computer use by hospital epidemiology units is for word processing. Memos and letters are written daily, and minutes of meetings and manuals have to be revised repeatedly. All of this is facilitated by the use of a simple word-processing program. At the most, scientific documents require underlining, subscripting, and superscripting, and the simplest current word-processing programs included in integrated packages provide these functions. Furthermore, word processing makes minimal demands on the computing chip, so computer speed considerations are almost irrelevant for word processing.

As long as they have sufficient memory to hold a reasonably sized program either in RAM or on a hard disk, the simplest of personal computers can serve as highly functional and efficient word processors. An expensive personal computer that is forty times faster than an elementary personal computer at performing complex statistical calculations will not be notably better for word processing. Furthermore, the added complexity of alleged state-of-the-art programs that beginners tend to purchase along with expensive high-end machines actually interferes with the accessibility and general utility of a computerized system. It is possible for almost anybody to master a simple word-processing program, and hospital epidemiology personnel should not hesitate to acquire simple hardware and software for word processing.

Searching a Literature Database

Because a literature database is searched by the computer at the other end of the telephone line, the power and speed of the personal computer used to address the distant computer is irrelevant. The quality and speed of the modem used for transmission of messages between computers over telephone lines determine the functional speed of the system. Modem speeds are rated in *baud*, which are approximately bits per second. Remember that 8 bits form 1 byte, or 1 character. Cheap modems are available to transmit at the lowest speeds—300 baud—and reasonably priced modems have the ability to transmit and receive at all common speeds—300 baud, 1,200 baud, and 2,400 baud. Higher-speed modems are available at higher prices for special purposes.

Electronic noise on telephone lines is the factor that most often limits the speed at which communication can take place between computers. Modems have built-in electronic circuitry to filter out unwanted noise, and the higher-speed modems have better filter systems. Almost any modem will work at 300 baud, but this is only about the speed at which one types, and it takes an annoyingly long time to collect a screen full of text at 300 baud. Furthermore, the total cost of telecommunication between computers includes the cost of the modem and software plus the cost of using the telephone line. If telephone charges are considered as well, a 300-baud modem is not an economically wise choice. A 2,400-baud modem may work at 2,400 baud for good telephone connections, but it will work better than a 1,200-baud modem at 1,200 baud because of its improved filter system. Unlike most areas in computing reviewed in this chapter, the purchase of the more expensive item in this case, a 2,400-baud modem, will rapidly prove cost-effective in any situation where a modem is used even a moderate amount and results in extra measurable monthly telephone charges.

Communication between computers also requires a telecommunications program to connect the modem with the computer. Many modems are packaged with usable software, and most of the integrated packages include a telecommunications program as well, so there is little need to buy a separate program for searching a literature database.

Creating and Managing a Database

An electronic database is simply a program for recording and sorting data. Simple databases such as the ones included with integrated packages can be used effectively to store and sort data from a study or outbreak investigation. Data sets with dozens of vari-

ables for every subject can be sorted rapidly according to one or several variables at once with complete accuracy. This is the electronic equivalent of instant shuffling and reshuffling of paper data forms. Using a simple electronic database system for a limited study will acquaint the beginning user with the potential costs and benefits of such a computerized system.

Since surveillance is an integral function of the hospital epidemiology unit, it is also natural to consider the creation of a surveillance database for storing and accessing surveillance information. Several companies market database systems that are designed and customized for hospital epidemiology. These are expensive to acquire initially, and substantial time must be invested in order to learn how to use an electronic database. Furthermore, these require additional investment of time daily or weekly to enter all of the surveillance data. Once the program has been mastered and the data are entered, it is relatively easy to generate reports and summaries of the data. The potential usefulness of such a system for keeping records of an entire hospital depends on the balance between the time and money costs of entering the data into the electronic database versus the savings that might be realized when the data have to be sorted and summarized. It is substantially more difficult to master and maintain a database than a word processor, and thoughtful reflection is necessary before investing in an expensive database.

The New Hospital Accreditation Program Scoring Guidelines

In 1975, the Joint Commission on the Accreditation of Healthcare Organizations (JCAHO) issued the first-generation standard for hospital epidemiology. The major thrust of the original standard was the creation of Infection Control Committees and clear organizational lines of authority and responsibility for infection control activities within each hospital. Also included in the first-generation standard was a stipulation that separate infection control manuals be written for different clinical services and different geographic areas in each hospital. The quality and timely updating of these infection control manuals became a major focus of attention for JCAHO surveyors. There was also a nonspecific requirement for surveillance of antibiotic use and nosocomial infections. In the original standard, the data to be collected were not specified, and no use for these data was defined.

As was pointed out by critics from Europe, the line lists of nosocomial infections automatically produced for a decade or more in this country were generally not used for any productive purpose [33]. The collection of surveillance data that are never used for any purpose represents a waste of resources. The intermediate level of detail included in these line lists, and in most routine surveillance systems, is an unhappy compromise between the low level of information required to determine whether anything unusual is happening among subgroups of hospitalized patients and the very high level of detail required to interrupt, analyze, or resolve an epidemic.

Fifteen years later, a second-generation standard has been issued, and the new *Accreditation Manual for Hospitals* issued by the JCAHO includes a specific set of scoring guidelines on which the compliance of a hospital will be judged [1]. To obtain the highest score, an individual hospital must provide evidence of an ongoing and effective surveillance system based on validated clinical data that produces rates of nosocomial infection for different subgroups of patients and links these rates with a hospitalwide quality assurance program [1]. The explicit scoring system that will be used by surveyors from the JCAHO has highlighted the need to reevaluate the manner in which hospital epidemiology units collect, sort, analyze, and store surveillance data. Of central importance will be the practical operational functionality of the database.

Attributes Defining the Functionality of a Database System

A user of any database system must be able to enter, store, retrieve, and sort those data accurately in order to allow analyses of the data and the timely generation of reports. All of this must take place with minimal expenditure of resources. After data have been collected, all database systems require some form of data entry, data editing, and error correction prior to data sorting. A number of hospitals have been maintaining paper or card-based systems for decades that have been used to analyze nosocomial infection data on various subgroups such as those suggested in the new standard issued by the JCAHO [1]. The manner in which each of these steps is accomplished for paper, card, and electronic database systems and mixtures of such systems is outlined here.

Paper-Based Systems The original paper databases consisted of sheets of lined paper listing individuals in rows down the side with attributes defined as column headings along the top. This produced the traditional line lists of nosocomial infections. The infection control officers could take the duplicate microbiology laboratory slips and line lists onto the wards every day as they reviewed Kardexes, temperature sheets, and medical records, interviewed nurses and physicians, and examined patients. Daily updating of line lists was accomplished in this manner, and line lists are still in common use because they are the simplest to create, maintain, and store. Different types of line lists are easily made for various types of patients.

Potential disadvantage of line lists are that complex analyses may require reentry of data onto another medium because paper forms may not stand up well to repeated handling, and counting and page turning is done by hand and is subject to human error. Furthermore, if substantial additional patient data are taken from other offices in the hospital, these additional data must then be copied by hand onto the line lists. The benefits of line lists are that data entry is immediate and the organization self-evident, so that virtually no training time or user sophistication is required. Paper and pencils are very inexpensive, and updated line lists are immediately useful for simple report generation.

Card-Based Systems Decks of common index cards are relatively efficient when used for analyzing moderately sized to large data sets.

The data for one subject is recorded on each card, and then colored marks can be made in specified locations along the edges of each card to indicate the presence of various exposures, attributes, or events. These color-coded cards can then be sorted and counted quickly by hand and will stand up to repeated hand sortings.

The next level of sophistication involves McBee cards that have holes punched along the edges. When the cards are stacked in a tray, the holes line up and a long rod can be used to sort cards by passing it through any specified hole location. Thus sorting of McBee cards is much faster and more accurate than sorting color-coded index cards, and large data sets are conveniently handled using this system.

One disadvantage of a card-based system is similar to the problem with the paper-based system described previously—namely, data from other offices in the hospital must still be transferred onto cards by hand. However, cards retain the inherent organizational simplicity of line lists and have some additional advantages. A card system is particularly efficient when the card is also the primary data collection form and cards rather than line lists are carried onto the wards. No additional steps of data transfer are required, and analyses can be carried out directly on the primary data collection form. Cards hold up well to multiple sortings and can be regrouped and resorted repeatedly. Cards are likewise very inexpensive, and sorting and counting cards is faster and more accurate than shuffling papers and counting ticks on line lists. As with the paper-based systems, data on cards remain immediately available for the timely production of reports.

Combining Numerators from Cards with Denominators from the Hospital Administrative Database An efficient system for small- to moderately large-sized hospitals can be created simply by combining nosocomial infection surveillance data from cards with data taken from the administrative or discharge abstract electronic database already maintained by the hospital. If a card is used to record the data related to each patient who acquires a nosocomial infection, then these specific infection numerator data can be used in conjunction with other denominator data generally available from the electronic database maintained by the administrative offices of a hospital.

For example, denominator data for all surgical procedures of a specific type or all procedures performed by an individual surgeon or all patients with a specific diagnosis in a year are often readily available from an administrative electronic database. Detailed information on the nosocomial infections experienced by these subgroups of patients can be taken from surveillance data recorded on cards to provide procedure- or surgeon- or diagnosis-specific incidences of nosocomial infection.

A mixed system such as this is relatively inexpensive because it combines numerator data on nosocomial infections from the hospital epidemiology unit with denominator data from an electronic database maintained by someone else, in this instance the hospital administration. Experience with such mixed systems suggests that they are practical if the number of discharges who acquire a nosocomial infection during hospitalization is not more than 500 to 1,000 per year. That is, a mixed system is reasonable so long as the number of cards that need to be sorted in the process of creating procedure- or surgeon- or site-specific nosocomial infection reports is not greater than 500 to 1,000. If approximately 5 percent of discharges experience a nosocomial infection, then hospitals with as many as 10,000 to 20,000 discharges annually could consider using a mixed system.

Dedicated Infection Control Electronic Databases Now that nosocomial infection rates for subgroups of patients must be produced, computer enthusiasts have incorrectly suggested that dedicated computerized database systems have become essential in hospital epidemiology [28]. In fact, the actual usefulness of electronic database systems has become the focus of a major controversy. Nosocomial infection rates according to site, service, physician, geographic location, and risk factors have been produced for decades using the paper- and card-based systems already described, and the issuance of the new infection control standards has not altered the basic balance between the added personnel, hardware, and software expense of creating and maintaining an electronic database and the increased functionality of the data available from such a system.

Dedicated computerized database systems for record keeping and sorting of hospital epidemiologic surveillance data have been tested and reviewed by various groups [3, 19, 28, 34] and have provoked editorials and record numbers of letters to the editor [29]. Whereas data entry and organization are immediate and self-evident for paper- or card-based systems, the same is not true for an electronic database. The real usefulness of these dedicated computerized databases will depend on the long-term availability of extra resources to enter, edit, and correct data from original data collection forms and the resources to train and maintain an operator to manipulate the electronic database. In addition, the computer hardware and software must be purchased, the system assembled, and the programs installed.

One exceptional potential advantage to an electronic database is that computerized data from other offices in the hospital may be captured and downloaded into the system without the necessity of reentry of data by hand. The availability of computerized data from other sources such as administration and billing, laboratories, radiology, and the pharmacy will vary among hospitals, and the ease with which such data can be captured varies among database programs. At the expense of tens of millions of dollars, some research institutions have been able to create systems with interfaces to access virtually all of the information available in tertiary care hospitals as it becomes available and to feed back the information to physicians and epidemiologists in real time, so that it can be utilized immediately in patient care [8, 12, 25].

However, the creation of an electronic database that will be useful in the timely analysis of data and production of reports is far from a trivial undertaking. At the Centers

for Disease Control, the National Nosocomial Infections Surveillance (NNIS) System was created as a standardized electronic database system for recording the data generated from line lists in multiple individual hospitals nationwide. Although this was a very desirable ambition, because of the inherent difficulties of setting up and maintaining an electronic database, by the end of the 1980s the NNIS System had fallen a number of years behind in summarizing data and generating reports. The goal of maintaining an electronic database that will be useful in the timely analysis of data and generation of reports has eluded even experienced central authorities with substantial resources.

Features of an Individual Hospital that Determine the Usefulness of a Dedicated Electronic Database

Each hospital epidemiology unit must judge individually whether it has the additional resources that will be required to create and maintain a large electronic database dedicated to infection control and whether such an investment would result in a reasonable return. Two extreme situations are presented here, and most hospitals will fall somewhere in between.

A hospital that already maintains administrative, billing, laboratory, radiology, and pharmacy data in computerized format and is willing to supply a programmer who will make these data easily downloadable into a hospital epidemiology database is an ideal setting in which to switch to an electronic database. In such a setting, large amounts of information will already be available for each patient, and infection control personnel need only add their own data to what already exists. The extra time required to enter data into this system will be more than compensated by the vast amount of information already available from other sources within the hospital. Currently, this situation exists in only a few research settings [8, 12, 25], but the potential to create another should not be overlooked. An appropriately maintained and updated electronic database is a joy to use when it is time to generate routine reports and can also facilitate investigations of unusual events.

On the other hand, for many small and moderately sized hospitals and for hospitals with no additional resources for programming and data entry, the use of a dedicated infection control electronic database would require removing personnel from clinical responsibilities to enter, edit, and correct data. Furthermore, if data were not easily accessible electronically from other offices in the hospital, then these additional data would have to be entered manually into the electronic database. If clinical personnel would have to be withdrawn from clinical responsibilities and forced to devote a substantial portion of their time to the clerical work involved in data entry, a dedicated electronic database would probably be far less functional than a card-based system.

It would have to be judged individually within each hospital whether the implementation of a dedicated electronic database system would result in a net gain or loss of efficiency. In a hospital epidemiology unit with fixed resources and no practical electronic availability of data from other offices in the hospital, the change to a dedicated electronic database would certainly detract from time spent on the wards.

Safeguards for Implementing an Electronic Database System

If it is decided that a hospital epidemiology unit will switch from a paper or card system to an electronic database for surveillance, there are certain safeguards that are routinely practiced in the professional computing world. It can never be assumed that it will be possible to switch from one system to another in an instant or even over a short interval. For a period, the old paper- or card-based system and the new electronic database must be run side by side, until all involved are convinced that the new system can be used to analyze data accurately and produce the desired reports without unreasonable delays.

Several kinds of backup for an electronic system are also essential. Hard disks on personal computers are simple to use and thus easy to ignore. Hard disks are precision mechanical devices and will fail eventually, so all data on hard disks must be backed up at least weekly onto tapes or diskettes. If a hard disk is not religiously backed up, then a routine hard-disk crash will result in a catastrophic loss of data and subsequent loss of function of the epidemiology unit. Additionally, if data are collected on cards, then the card-based system can be retained as a precaution in case of computer malfunction or lack of availability of the trained database operator.

The Balance of Benefit Versus Harm in Implementing Computerized Systems in Hospital Epidemiology

When a computerized system is thoughtfully planned, purchased, and utilized, then substantial benefit will accrue from this change. An example of a computerized system that is virtually always of major benefit to a hospital epidemiology unit is a simple word processor. This technology has been so well developed over the last decade that it is virtually impossible to fail in setting up a word-processing system, and the gains in efficiency will be substantial.

In contrast, the use of a complex and costly program such as a dedicated database or statistical package will be of net benefit only under specific circumstances. The successful implementation of a computerized system can result in great benefit, but active harm will result from having wasted time and money in purchasing expensive software and hardware that are never used. The major reason that so many naive users have failed to implement complex computerized systems successfully is that they did not include in the planned purchase price of the computerized system the substantial personnel costs of learning to use and maintain intricate programs.

A major recession occurred in the computer industry when business users discovered this very real problem and noted that only a small minority of the costly programs they purchased were ever successfully applied. With this background, it is now possible for hospital epidemiologists to make realistic plans when contemplating the substantial investments in computerized systems.

Computerized Systems in Advanced Epidemiologic Research
Computerized Systems for Different Purposes
The computerized system that is optimal for effective analysis of a complex data set originating from a disease outbreak, or for the analysis of data for research into an endemic problem, is different from the software described earlier. The area in which computers can be most helpful in advanced epidemiologic research is in the removal of distortions from confounding [15, 27, 36].

Confounding
We like to think of epidemiology in simple terms, such as the occurrence of cholera in Snow's London depending on the source of drinking water, or measles in a second-grade classroom. In these stark examples, only two things really mattered: who was susceptible and who was exposed. Most diseases in epidemiology, including hospital epidemiology, are diseases of multiple causation. That is, many factors acting jointly produce the outcome, and the factors that produced the outcome in one subject may not be the factors that produced the same outcome in another. In actuality, we are always dealing with multiple causes or determinants of the same outcome.

For the sake of understanding, we prefer to estimate the magnitude of the effect of one determinant at a time. The bench biologist has control of the environment and can set up experiments to change one variable at a time. To accomplish that same end in observational epidemiology, we must somehow nullify or correct for the effects of multiple other unwanted determinants or exposures that are actually acting jointly with the exposure under study.

Since several factors or determinants acting jointly are almost invariably responsible for a single outcome in hospital epidemiology, confounding can be seen as the distortion of the estimate of the magnitude of the effect of one cause of an outcome when it is mixed with some of the effects of other causes of the same outcome [15, 27, 36]. We know that older age, female gender, and instrumentation of the urinary tract are all determinants or causes of nosocomial urinary tract infections. In a hospital population, patients with nosocomial urinary tract infections tend to be older and are more likely to be female than the patients without urinary tract infections. The urinary tract infections that occurred would have been jointly determined by all three of these exposures. If we want to measure the effect of instrumentation alone, then we must somehow nullify the effect of age and gender. If we fail to adjust for the effect of age and gender, then our estimates of the effect of instrumentation of the urinary tract will be distorted or confounded by the effects of these other unwanted extraneous variables.

Variation in the Severity of Underlying Disease
The most overarching problem in the analysis of data from observational studies in hospital epidemiology is confounding by severity of underlying disease [15]. In many institutions, hospital epidemiology has recently been broadened to include the relatively new area of quality assurance [9, 10, 30], and difficulties with confounding have been best illustrated by the initial efforts of a government agency to judge quality of hospital care through monitoring and reporting hospital death rates and rates of nosocomial infections. Both death and infection have many causes, and to measure the effect of one of these—say, the effect of quality (or lack of quality) of hospital care—in the analysis, one must adjust successfully for the effects of all of the other determinants of death or infection. (See Chap. 2.)

The first attempts of this government agency demonstrate the hazard of failing to consider the confounding effect of different degrees of severity of underlying illness in the comparison of crude hospital death rates. Despite the fact that the need for adjusting for severity of underlying disease was clearly demonstrated when comparing hospital death rates [23], this agency failed to adjust for variations in the severity of underlying illness and so identified a hospice as the hospital with the highest "abnormal" mortality in the country, without consideration of the terminal nature of the illnesses of patients admitted to a hospice [7]. Increasingly sophisticated means for adjusting for severity of illness (case mix) are now being employed by this agency. However, perhaps because of the errors in the initial effort, the intended consumers of these data—the hospital leaders—still generally reject these results [4]. Further research has indicated that after adjustment for severity of illness, using objective comparisons, it remains extremely difficult to detect differences in hospital care that lead to excess mortality [32].

Sicker patients are more likely to acquire nosocomial infections and, similarly, these same sicker patients are more likely to have adverse outcomes of hospitalization. One way to create groups of generally similar risk is through systematic assignment of study subjects into comparable groups, as in randomized intervention trials. Intervention trials are rare in hospital epidemiology. When randomization of exposure can be imposed on a study population, then the randomization process usually will ensure that the two groups being compared are similar and do not differ by other extraneous variables that could cause the outcome under study.

Unfortunately, most studies in hospital epidemiology are observational in nature. In any comparison in an observational study, no matter whether the subjects are neonates [14, 20, 21] or adults [15, 16, 18], separating the effects of severity of illness from the effects of the exposure under study remains the major challenge. Sicker patients have more exposures and more bad outcomes, and the interpretability of almost any study in hospital epidemiology depends on how well adjustment can be made for varying degrees of severity of illness [15].

At the Second International Conference on Nosocomial Infections held in 1980, there was but a single paper on the effects of differential risks of nosocomial infection [17], whereas a large number of such papers were presented at the Third International Conference held a decade later [13]. Despite the clear importance of underlying disease in determining nosocomial infection, the same government agency that failed to adjust for underlying illness when comparing hospital death rates also concluded that nosocomial infection should be used as a generic screen for quality of hospital care. In their view, every nosocomial infection indicated a problem with quality of care, irrespective of the underlying illness of the patient [22]. This reasoning erroneously suggested that a patient with a terminal underlying illness and compromised host defenses who acquired an infection with his or her own flora suffered a nosocomial infection that was somehow preventable. The degree to which the unalterable characteristics of the patient himself or herself determine the inherent susceptibility to infection and probability of death are not yet well defined but clearly are of major importance in modern hospital epidemiology. Stratification is the simplest, most intuitive way to approach this problem, and a simple logical scheme for analyzing complex epidemiologic data sets has been published [15, 27, 36]. In these references, confounding and a related concept, effect modification, are defined, and multiple examples of analysis using these concepts are provided.

Multiway stratification has long been the favorite analytic tool of the epidemiologist, but sophisticated programs for producing adjusted summary estimates of risk ratios and 95 percent confidence intervals have appeared only relatively recently [37], and now there are a number of programs for personal computers that focus on the epidemiologic analysis of categorical data. These are followed and reviewed regularly [42]. In addition, versions of programs suitable for sophisticated analysis of categorical data are now beginning to be included in the standard statistical packages [11, 37, 39, 41, 42].

Introduction to Multivariate Modeling Using Statistical Packages

Complex epidemiologic data sets containing data on many variables have commonly been analyzed by multiway stratification, without fitting multivariate models [15, 37]. Canned statistical programs are available that make the fitting of such models relatively easy for beginners and experts alike [11, 39, 41, 42]. All three common statistical packages have versions for both mainframes and personal computers. The personal computer versions are readily available for the IBM compatibles, although they are still limited in the amount of RAM that can be used because of the DOS operating system. The limitations in RAM usage for the personal computer versions inhibit some of the memory-intensive procedures for analyzing categorical data.

The programming necessary to use these statistical packages is much more complex than the programming required for the other uses of computers described previously in this chapter, so a potential user should definitely experiment with a statistical package before spending any money. The least expensive way to investigate the potential usefulness of one of these statistical packages is to borrow time on a hospital or university mainframe in which one of these packages is already installed. Statistical packages for personal computer use can be purchased but are very expensive. At least one company makes personal computer versions available through local lease of site licenses rather than through purchase [39], which is much less costly.

Many practitioners in the field of hospital epidemiology have chosen to use regression models, either multiple linear regression or multiple logistic regression. The general availability of these programs is a mixed blessing, because substantial expertise in statistics and epidemiology is essential for understanding what the programs do, understanding what assumptions underlie the models, and understanding how to interpret the output. The essential assumptions are often impossible to verify, which renders the interpretation difficult.

What One Should Know Before Attempting to Use Multivariate Models

Many of the ideas in biostatistics and epidemiology are represented in the world of multivariate models, some explicitly but most implicitly. If one is not informed on the workings of a program for fitting a multivariate

model, and if one is not knowledgeable about the structure and meaning of the model itself, then most of the assumptions underlying the model remain unknown to the investigator, and the interpretation of the analysis remains obscure. Subsequently, if the results of a multivariate analysis are reported in the literature, the confusion is spread to the public at large. A partial list of issues is provided next, and some brief explanations follow. This is by no means intended as a primer on multivariate analysis; it simply lists some of the major ideas with which an investigator must be familiar to use these processes. For more specific details, advanced textbooks and the individual manuals must be consulted [11, 31, 38, 39, 41, 42].

In biostatistics, there is a clear separation between the use of data to suggest and generate hypotheses and the use of data to test hypotheses already generated from previous data sets [26, 40]. Although all programs for fitting multivariate models automatically generate test statistics, these are interpretable only in clear hypothesis-testing situations.

Common analytic processes, including stratification and the fitting of linear regression models and logistic regression models, assume either an additive or a multiplicative model for effects. The difference must be clear in the mind of the investigator, and the biologic interpretation of the model altered to conform with the underlying structure. Effect modification, for example, has a different representation in additive and multiplicative models.

The formulation of terms that might be entered into a multivariate model indicate the investigator's belief in the nature of the effect of each variable. For example, a variable entered only as a single term constrains the relationship between that exposure and the outcome to be linear. If a quadratic term in the same variable is constructed, then the relationship may be curvilinear. If product terms are constructed, then interactions or effect modification can be investigated.

Each type of regression model or analysis requires particular assumptions about distributions and variances for interpretation of the model. Linear regression, for example, must have an outcome that is normally distributed in order for probabilities to be interpretable in hypothesis testing. All regression models assume noncolinearity, or that exposure variables are independent predictors of the outcome, and one exposure variable must not be similar to another with simply a different name.

Also, the order in which these terms are entered has meaning for the epidemiologist. In an hypothesis-testing setting, the variable whose association with the outcome is being tested must be held out and entered last. To adjust for confounding, all of the potential confounders must be forced into the model before the exposure variable being tested. The probability that this last variable could be associated with the outcome by chance alone is the appropriate probability to report for a significance test.

Avoiding Problems Caused by Automatic Stepwise Algorithms

Statistical packages usually provide two different ways to construct regression models. Optimally, the investigator should specify the variables to be included in the model and the order in which they are to be entered. The other alternative is to allow canned automatic stepwise algorithms for constructing regression models to employ statistical criteria for including or excluding variables. These statistical criteria are unrelated to epidemiologic interpretation and epidemiologic criteria for causality [26, 27, 36]. Rather, they consider strength of association (probability [p] values), so the automatic algorithms are unable to evaluate potential confounders according to the basic definition of how confounders alter the magnitude of the effect being investigated. These statistical criteria are also blind to biologic causation and cannot distinguish which exposure must precede which other on a causal pathway [26, 27, 36].

Since p values rather than logic specify the order in which terms are entered into a multivariate model by an automatic stepwise algorithm, the algorithm may select a square term containing information on a variable, or

an interaction term, before it chooses the main term for that variable. Since that variable is then only partially in the model, the interpretation is unclear.

It is not generally recognized that if automatic stepwise algorithms are applied in building linear regression models for complex data sets, a forward stepwise procedure will generally produce a different result from a backward stepwise procedure applied to the same data set [31, 38]. In addition, two more different models will result if backward and forward automatic stepwise algorithms for logistic regression are applied to the same data set. This will happen because logistic regression assumes a multiplicative model, whereas linear regression assumes an additive model. Unfortunately, four different models from four different procedures on the same data set will produce four different sets of predictors and four different constructs of "truth." The blind application of an automatic stepwise statistical regression algorithm is never recommended in epidemiology.

Summary of the Epidemiologic Use of Statistical Packages

Many statistical packages contain excellent programs for the analysis of categorical data, especially multiway stratification. These programs are indispensable for the analysis of complex data sets. Additionally, despite this long list of very real problems with the naive application of multivariate models in epidemiology, there are a number of appropriate uses of multivariate analysis.

There are two steps to understanding what is happening in a complex observational data set: (1) elimination of the myriad of variables that have no bearing on the outcome under investigation, and (2) elucidation of the biologic influence of the few variables that actually are causally related to the outcome [14, 17, 18, 26, 27, 35, 36]. Statistical packages on computers are efficient at fitting multivariate models to sort through and discard as unimportant many variables in complex data sets. Although an epidemiologist may be hesitant to render a positive biologic interpretation of the results of a multivariate model, the same model will be very helpful in indicating which variables are of no importance and can be ignored in future analyses of the same data set. In this manner, multivariate models can be used to identify variables that merit further analysis by methods such as stratification, which more easily lend themselves to the causal interpretation of results.

References

1. American Hospital Association. *1990 Accreditation Manual for Hospitals.* Chicago: American Hospital Association, 1990.
2. Barr, R.L., and Gerzoff, R.B. Controlling urges and infections—computer system design for epidemiology. *Infect. Control Hosp. Epidemiol.* 6:317, 1985.
3. Berg, R. Reviews: Software. *Am. J. Infect. Control* 14:139, 1986.
4. Berwick, D.M., and Wald, D.L. Hospital leaders' opinions of the HCFA mortality data. *J.A.M.A.* 264:247, 1990.
5. Birnbaum, D. Computers in hospital epidemiology practice. *Infect. Control Hosp. Epidemiol.* 9:81, 1988.
6. Bowen, W. The puny payoff from office computers. *Fortune* 113:20, 1986.
7. Brinkley, J. U.S. releasing lists of hospitals with abnormal mortality rates. *The New York Times* March 12:1, 1986.
8. Broderick, A., et al. Nosocomial infections: Validation of surveillance and computer modeling to identify patients at risk. *Am. J. Epidemiol.* 131:734, 1990.
8a. Classen, D.C., et al. Surveillance for quality assessment: IV. Surveillance using a hospital information system. *Infect. Control Hosp. Epidemiol.* 12:239, 1991.
9. Crede, W., and Hierholzer, W.J. Surveillance for quality assessment: I. Surveillance in infection control success reviewed. *Infect. Control Hosp. Epidemiol.* 10:470, 1989.
10. Crede, W.B., and Hierholzer, W.J. Surveillance for quality assessment: III. The critical assessment of quality indicators. *Infect. Control Hosp. Epidemiol.* 11:197, 1990.
11. Dixon, W.J., Brown, M.B., Engleman, L., and Jennrich, R.I. *BMDP Statistical Software Manual.* Berkeley, CA: University of California Press, 1990.
12. Evans, R.S., et al. Computer surveillance of hospital-acquired infections and antibiotic use. *J.A.M.A.* 256:1007, 1986.
12a. Foster, D., and Sullivan, K. Software. In: R.H. Bernier and V.M. Mason (Eds.), *Epi-*

source: A Guide to Resources in Epidemiology. Roswell, GA: The Epidemiology Monitor, 1991. Pp.973–1064.
13. Final program and abstracts of the Third International Conference on Nosocomial Infections, July 31–Aug. 3, 1990, Atlanta, GA.
14. Freeman, J., et al. Association of intravenous lipid emulsion and coagulase-negative staphylococcal bacteremia in neonatal intensive care units. *N. Engl. J. Med.* 323:301, 1990.
15. Freeman, J., Goldmann, D.A., and McGowan, J.E., Jr. Methodologic issues in hospital epidemiology: IV. Risk ratios, confounding, effect modification, and the analysis of multiple variables. *Rev. Infect. Dis.* 10:1118, 1988.
16. Freeman, J., and McGowan, J.E., Jr. Risk factors for nosocomial infection. *J. Infect. Dis.* 138:811, 1978.
17. Freeman, J., and McGowan, J.E., Jr. Differential risks of nosocomial infection. *Am. J. Med.* 70:915, 1981.
18. Freeman, J., and McGowan, J.E., Jr. Methodologic issues in hospital epidemiology: III. Investigating the modifying effects of time and severity of underlying illness on estimates of the cost of nosocomial infection. *Rev. Infect. Dis.* 6:285, 1984.
19. Gaynes, R., Friedman, C., Copeland, T.A., and Thiele, G.H. Methodology to evaluate a computer-based system for surveillance of hospital-acquired infections. *Am. J. Infect. Control* 18:40, 1990.
20. Goldmann, D.A., Durbin, W.A., Jr., and Freeman, J. Nosocomial infections in the neonatal intensive care unit. *J. Infect. Dis.* 144:449, 1981.
21. Goldmann, D.A., Freeman, J., and Durbin, W.A., Jr. Nosocomial infection and death in a neonatal intensive care unit. *J. Infect. Dis.* 147:635, 1983.
22. Health Care Financing Administration. Generic quality screens. Peer Review Organization, Third Scope of Work, Attachment 1. September 1989.
23. Hebel, R.J., Kessler, I.I., Mabuchi, K., and McCarter, R.J. Assessment of hospital performance by use of death rates: A recent case history. *J.A.M.A.* 248:3131, 1982.
24. Hierholzer, W.J., Jr. The practice of hospital epidemiology. *Yale J. Biol. Med.* 55:225, 1982.
25. Hierholzer, W.J., Jr., Miller, S.P., Streed, S.A., and Wood, D. On-Line Infection Control System Using PCS/IMS. In: J.T. O'Neill (Ed.), *Proceedings of the Fourth Annual Symposium on Computer Applications in Medical Care, Washington, D.C., Nov. 2–5, 1980.* Washington, DC: Center for Health Sciences Research, 1980. P.540.

26. Hill, A.B. *Principles of Medical Statistics* (9th ed.). New York: Oxford University Press, 1971.

27. Keinbaum, D.G., Kupper, L.L., and Morgenstern, H. *Epidemiologic Research: Principles and Quantitative Methods.* Belmont, CA: Lifetime Learning Publications, 1982.

28. LaHaise, S. A comparison of infection control software for use by hospital epidemiologists in meeting the new JCAHCO standards. *Infect. Control Hosp. Epidemiol.* 11:185, 1990.

29. Letters to the editor. *Infect. Control Hosp. Epidemiol.* 11:400, 1990.

30. McGeer, A., Crede, W., and Hierholzer, W.J. Surveillance for quality assessment: II. Surveillance for noninfectious processes: Back to basics. *Infect. Control Hosp. Epidemiol.* 11:36, 1990.

31. Mosteller, F., and Tukey, J.W. *Data Analysis and Regression: A Second Course in Statistics.* Reading, MA: Addison-Wesley, 1977.

32. Park, R.A., et al. Explaining variations in hospital death rates: Randomness, severity of illness, quality of care. *J.A.M.A.* 264:484, 1990.

33. Proceedings of the International Symposium on Control of Nosocomial Infection, Jerusalem, Israel, April 28–May 2, 1980. *Rev. Infect. Dis.* 3:635, 1981.

34. Reagan, D.R. The choice of microcomputer software for infection control. *Infect. Control Hosp. Epidemiol.* 11:178, 1990.

35. Rinehart, E., et al. Rapid dissemination of β-lactamase-producing, aminoglycoside-resistant *Enterococcus faecalis* among patients and staff on an infant-toddler surgical ward. *N. Engl. J. Med.* 323:1814, 1990.

36. Rothman, K.J. *Modern Epidemiology.* Boston: Little, Brown, 1986.

37. Rothman, K.J., and Boice, J.D., Jr. *Epidemiologic Analysis with a Programmable Calculator.* Washington, DC: Department of Health, Education, and Welfare, 1979.

38. Sall, J. *Technical Report: A-102: SAS Regression Applications.* Cary, NC: SAS Institute, 1981.

39. *SAS/STAT Users Guide* (release 6.03 ed.). Cary, NC: SAS Institute, 1988.

40. Snedecor, G.W., and Cochran, W.G. *Statistical Methods* (7th ed.). Ames, IA: Iowa State University Press, 1980.

41. *SPSS-X Users Guide* (3rd ed.). Chicago, IL: SPSS, 1988.

42. Sullivan, K. Epiware. *Epidemiology Monitor* 8:1, 1987; 9:1, 1988; 12:7, 1991. (*Epiware is a frequent column that updates reviews of software.*)

The Role of the Laboratory in Control of Nosocomial Infection

John E. McGowan, Jr.
Robert A. Weinstein

Nosocomial infections continue to present a major problem in hospitals today. Because of the importance of this subject, each hospital laboratory has the responsibility of supporting activities related to surveillance, control, and prevention of nosocomial infections. Each laboratory can make major contributions toward infection control, as long as the persons responsible for infection control efforts and those in charge of the clinical microbiology laboratory cooperate closely to attack this problem. Often the same persons have both of these responsibilities; nearly half of those who chair Infection Control Committees are laboratory personnel [185].

Laboratory personnel attempt to minimize the occurrence of nosocomial infection in the following seven ways: (1) participation in hospitalwide infection control activities, especially those of the hospital Infection Control Committee; (2) accurate identification of responsible organisms; (3) careful attention to antibiotic susceptibility testing; (4) timely reporting of laboratory data and participation in surveillance of nosocomial infection; (5) provision of additional studies, when necessary, to establish similarity or difference of organisms; (6) provision, on occasion, of microbiologic studies of the hospital environment; and (7) training of infection control personnel.

In the past decade, improvements in laboratory instrumentation and procedures have provided dramatic aid to infection control efforts in several ways. Among these are techniques for more rapid detection and differentiation of organisms and improved systems of reporting for both patient data and trend analysis. Perhaps the most dramatic advances have come in special procedures for examining ("typing") hospital organisms for similarity or difference; here, molecular and other techniques have permitted more definitive examination of a wider range of organisms than was possible before.

Participation in Hospitalwide Infection Control Activities

Relationship of the Laboratory to the Infection Control Committee

A clinically oriented member of the laboratory staff can contribute significantly by serving on the Infection Control Committee. Such participation is essential in contributing to a harmonious relationship among clinical, infection control, and microbiology personnel [149].

In the typical hospital, the majority of members of the Infection Control Committee do not have a background in microbiology. Thus it is of great importance for the representative of the laboratory to provide the microbiologic expertise that is critical to many decisions of the group. This knowledge may be required for the assessment of the significance of culture data, for determining the validity of laboratory techniques used to identify cases of nosocomial infection, and in the design and implementation of investigations and survey projects.

The diagnostic microbiology laboratory is engaged primarily in the evaluation of cultures related to infection. Because these are crucial data for successful infection control, the laboratory activities should be closely coordinated with the Infection Control Committee. For example, the adequacy of the basic techniques for primary isolation, speciation, and antimicrobial susceptibility testing should be discussed by the microbiologists and the Infection Control Committee. Laboratory resources often are stretched by patient care requirements, especially in smaller hospitals [23]. Laboratory support for infection control activities must be given with discretion. For example, use of laboratory resources to assess colonization or to sample personnel and the environment for bacterial or other organisms should never be permitted when the epidemiologic indications are unclear.

Major changes have occurred in reimbursement methods for hospitals in the United States [39]. In view of these changes, there seems to be an added service that the laboratory microbiologist can provide to the Infection Control Committee and other hospital committees concerned with infection control. Under prospective reimbursement, there will continue to be new and intensive attempts to evaluate the validity and usefulness of hospital programs such as infection control [13, 147]. Techniques for assessment are the bread and butter activity of clinical microbiology personnel, who have to make similar cost-benefit judgments for laboratory equipment, instruments, and procedures almost daily [145]. The insights and methods used for such laboratory activities should be helpful to the infection control team and the various committees (infection control, quality assurance, pharmacy and therapeutics, etc.) as they review the benefit of their activities and attempt to improve the productivity of the program [13, 147].

Budgetary Considerations

Costs for laboratory procedures that are not related directly to care of patients (e.g., bacteriologic sampling of personnel and the environment) should be borne by a budget separate from that of the laboratory. To facilitate all the microbiologic activities necessitated by an outbreak, the laboratory (or the hospital epidemiologist, or the Infection Control Committee, depending on the organizational structure of the hospital) should have a contingency fund to enable personnel, materials, and space to be temporarily assigned to epidemic aid support. An investigation of an outbreak should not be financed by charging individual patients for cultures taken during the study.

Accurate Identification of Organisms Involved in Nosocomial Infection

Infection control personnel search constantly for evidence that a common organism has spread from patient to patient or from employee to patient. Thus information permitting the successful tracing of organism movements within the hospital may be of value to the hospital infection control team, whether the positive cultures represent episodes of infection or indicate colonization of the patient [1]. Though some clinical features of illness provide information about etiology, the main sources for this determination usually are the data provided by the clinical laboratory. Thus the ability of the laboratory staff to isolate and identify responsible microorganisms is crucial to infection control [73].

The spectrum of organisms causing nosocomial infection has changed dramatically during the past decade [97, 144]. Among the patterns of special concern are the appearance of fungi and viruses as more frequent agents of nosocomial infection [76, 146]. Fortunately, technologic developments in the laboratory during the past decade have continued to increase the efficiency with which nosocomial organisms can be recognized and recovered [73, 219]. There are three main aspects to this. First, new instruments and devices have become widely available. These permit easier detection of the presence of organisms in blood cultures, organism identification, and testing of susceptibility to antimicrobials [219]. Some of these devices are automated, permitting the laboratory to provide these improved services with the same or fewer personnel [106]. Many of the instruments can be cost-effective for limited numbers of specimens; as a result, smaller laboratories as well as large ones can now include some of these methods in their program. Use of these instruments and devices also has led to a more standard approach throughout the United States to the identification and susceptibility testing of nosocomial pathogens.

Second, nonculture tests have permitted identification of agents of nosocomial infection that would not have been recognized in earlier years [24]. Immunologic and nucleic acid testing methods have added to our ability to recognize viruses and other organisms that are difficult or impossible to grow in culture; some of these are involved in nosocomial infection [24, 48, 53, 206]. Techniques such as polymerase chain reaction promise to make immunologic diagnosis of infection even more sensitive in the future [29, 175].

Third, these newer tests and instruments

not only permit identification of additional agents but also allow more rapid diagnosis of both new and old pathogens. This speedier testing should provide earlier recognition of outbreaks and more efficient handling of organisms in endemic nosocomial and community-acquired infection [111], which should reduce the likelihood for community-acquired organisms to serve as a source for nosocomial infection.

Even with these new technologic developments, certain basic principles of operation remain crucial to producing reliable microbiologic data. Several of these are discussed here.

Collection and Transport of Specimens

Specimen collection, transport, and handling must be of sufficiently high quality to provide valid data. Specimens that are not collected or transported properly may give inaccurate results, even when handled as well as possible once they reach the laboratory. In turn these inaccurate results may lead to improper clinical decisions by physicians, unnecessary labor by laboratory personnel, and unnecessary patient charges. Yet, according to Matsen [138], "in the whole of the clinical microbiology laboratory operation, the weakest link is likely to be specimen collection." The laboratory must monitor specimen handling continually and work closely with the wards and clinics to make sure that the possibility of contaminated specimens is minimized. This is a necessity to ensure that laboratory information presented to the hospital epidemiologist reports organisms actually associated with the patient's site of culture rather than contaminants.

Certain laboratory findings suggest specific handling errors [219]. For example, a frequent failure to isolate organisms from deep wounds or abscesses of patients who are not on antibiotics, or inability to recover pathogens seen on Gram stain in cases of presumed anaerobic infections, suggests inadequate anaerobic transport media, delay or inappropriate refrigeration of specimens in transit, or use of inadequate techniques for isolating anaerobes. The frequent recovery of three or more different organisms in clean-voided midstream urine specimens in patients without chronic indwelling urinary catheters suggests unsatisfactory technique in collecting specimens, a delay in transporting specimens to the laboratory, or a delay in culturing the specimens. The finding of negative cultures from a high percentage of patients with positive smears for bacteria suggests unsatisfactory specimen collection or handling, errors in staining, contaminated reagents, or errors in culture techniques [152].

Specimen collection and handling should be assessed regularly to detect and correct such problems; the frequency with which probable contaminants are isolated from clinical specimens can be a measure of the quality of specimen collection in a specific hospital area. For example, determining frequency of urine specimens with characteristics that suggest specimen contamination permits wards with high rates to be singled out for evaluation and, if necessary, for inservice education programs instituted by laboratory or infection control personnel. In addition, identifying persons who draw blood cultures that frequently contain diphtheroids, coagulase-negative staphylococci, or other probable skin contaminants may permit reinstruction of these personnel in aseptic technique. Periodic review of the relative incidence of false-positive smears for acid-fast bacilli or of specimens with heavy bacterial contamination may highlight problems in sputum collection and processing [222].

Some hospitals use laboratory slips with space to record both the time the specimen was collected and the time the laboratory received it so that transport time can be monitored periodically or continuously and the culturing of old specimens avoided. Evaluation of turnaround time has become an important element of laboratory quality assurance [213].

Initial Evaluation of Specimens

Assessment of specimens at the time they are received in the laboratory is one of the best ways to evaluate their suitability. For example, microscopic review of Gram stain of sputum specimens remains the best way to determine whether these specimens are contaminated [72, 121]; specimens identified as inadequate are not processed further and do not confuse either clinician or epidemiologist. A new specimen should be requested unless the clinician provides notice of special circumstances (e.g., immunosuppression) that might make it worthwhile to proceed with culture [111].

Culture or smear results for other types of specimens may also suggest contamination at the time of collection. For example, urine specimens with more than two different organisms present ordinarily suggest contamination in patients without chronic indwelling urine catheters. Such specimens should be held for 2 to 3 days without further processing. The patient's physician should be notified so that unusual clinical situations requiring further identification of the specimen can be recognized. Scoring systems for use in determining acceptable wound, vaginal, cervical, and other specimens also have been described [13]. Application of such criteria will ensure that the information generated from the specimens that are processed completely will more likely correlate with true infecting organisms and will reduce unnecessary laboratory costs. Repeat specimen collection should be requested for these inadequate specimens, and additional processing of organisms isolated from poor specimens (for example, speciation, susceptibility testing) should be limited. The culture report should alert the clinician about the questionable value of the specimen so that results will be used cautiously, if at all, for guidance in diagnosis and therapy.

For specimens from sputum and wounds, reporting of the morphologic characteristics of bacteria seen on Gram stain may be misleading if no statement is made regarding the presence or absence of white blood cells. Both sites may be extensively contaminated with skin, oropharyngeal, or intestinal bacterial flora. When organisms are found only in the presence of abundant squamous epithelial cells, it is unlikely that they are the causative agents, and reports of such mixed flora without qualification about the accompanying cells may lead the clinician falsely to assume mixed flora as the cause of the infection. Substantial effort will be conserved and superior information ultimately provided if repeat collection is requested for such specimens.

Microscopy at the time of specimen submission can help other aspects of microbiologic diagnosis. For example, examination on Gram stain for morphology can identify organisms that might be epidemiologically important but not reflected by culture. Thus presence of a mixed flora on Gram stain of a sputum specimen, when coupled with an aerobic culture yielding only *Hemophilus influenzae*, may indicate possible mixed aerobic-anaerobic infection rather than pneumonia due to *Hemophilus*. Because infection control implications of these two causes may differ, evaluations of this type by the laboratory can be important. Similarly, nonculture methods for identifying the presence of parvovirus B19 (e.g., demonstration by electron microscopy or gene probe) have helped us learn more about this organism as a cause of nosocomial infection [160].

Anaerobic culture of specimens should be limited to (1) those that show leukocytes on Gram stain, (2) those with no evidence of contaminating squamous cells and organisms suggestive of anaerobic species, or (3) specimens from patients whose unusual circumstances suggest a need for anaerobic culture. This limitation results in reporting of isolates that have a much higher probability of association with infection. The application of sensitive techniques for culturing and identifying anaerobes to specimens containing endogenous flora is costly and productive of misleading information [219]. Large numbers of anaerobic organisms are present in the normal flora of skin, oral cavity, and genital and gastrointestinal tracts. Thus swabs from superficial portions of skin or mucous membrane lesions, specimens of expectorated sputum, and any materials contaminated with feces should be considered inappropriate for anaerobic culture [219]. Submission for anaerobic culture of such specimens or of specimens from sites that are rarely infected by anaerobes (e.g., urine) suggests the need for inservice education of hospital personnel.

Efforts such as those outlined will substantially reduce errors in diagnosis and use of unnecessary antimicrobial therapy. Such an approach will also improve the specificity of infection surveillance data, which otherwise might include isolates of questionable etiologic significance.

Identification of Isolates

Once a specimen has been received in the laboratory, it must be processed in a way that will maximize the likelihood of recovering older agents as well as the many newer agents causing hospital cross-infection.

Often it is difficult to determine the causative agents in nosocomial infection. Recovery of an organism does not ensure that it is the causative agent of the nosocomial infection [111]. Thus etiologic diagnosis cannot be made with certainty in many cases. The majority of cases today for which the cause is known involve gram-positive cocci and gram-negative aerobic bacilli [97]. Most frequent among these gram-negative rods are *Klebsiella, Enterobacter, Pseudomonas, Serratia, Proteus,* and *Escherichia coli* (in approximately that order). In recent years, organisms such as *Acinetobacter, Flavobacterium, Legionella,* and *Pseudomonas* species other than *Pseudomonas aeruginosa* have become increasingly prominent [144].

Anaerobic bacterial organisms (usually found in mixed aerobic-anaerobic infections) have become less frequent in nosocomial infection in the past decade. However, viral agents (e.g., rotavirus) and fungi and parasites such as *Pneumocystis* and *Toxoplasma* have been identified as important causes of nosocomial infection [139]. This expansion of the list of possible microbial pathogens for hospitalized patients has made it more difficult for both microbiologist and clinician to deal effectively with hospital infection. Effective handling of such problems requires the laboratory staff to keep up with the steadily unfolding panorama of organisms important in cross-infection and to implement and maintain culture and other techniques that will bring these to light.

Need for Complete Identification

The degree to which organism identification routinely is carried can be important to nosocomial infection control efforts. Infection control personnel constantly are searching for evidence that a common organism has spread from patient to patient [148]. The ability to detect such an event is enhanced by identification of the organism at least to the level of species. Reporting of "biotyping" information (pattern of response to biochemical testing) on occasion can be of value in differentiating organisms that are frequently encountered, but this identification is not needed on a routine basis [73, 148].

When organisms are to be identified completely, it is important that standard criteria and nomenclature be consistently applied. Otherwise, attack rates for nosocomial infections with various species may identify false problems (e.g., because of previously unreported species or strains) or fail to identify true problems. Furthermore, such surveillance data may not be comparable to data developed in other institutions or in cooperative surveillance programs.

Even more important, incomplete or incorrect identification of organisms may obscure real problems and make retrospective epidemiologic investigation impossible. For example, a report of "*Klebsiella-Enterobacter* group" (formerly "*Klebsiella-Aerobacter* group") fails to distinguish between two organisms (*Klebsiella* and *Enterobacter*) that have different epidemiologic patterns of infection within the hospital [182]. Similarly, identifying an isolate as *Pseudomonas cepacia*, an organism frequently associated with illness or pseudoepidemics caused by contaminated water or other solutions [90], provides more useful epidemiologic information than identifying the organism only as "*Pseudomonas* species," in which the strain is lumped with a group of organisms that may not have as characteristic a hospital reservoir.

Because of these considerations, laboratories should maintain the capability to identify gram-negative aerobic bacilli to the genus level with at least 95 percent accuracy, and such identification should be a routine part of laboratory procedure. The laboratory should also have the capability of identifying these organisms to the species level when special or recurring problems in a given institution

make such information useful for dealing with nosocomial infection problems.

Many hospitals find it advantageous to employ commercial, multiple test media for biochemical testing that provide this degree of characterization. Acceptable methods for microbiologic identification procedures are described in detail elsewhere [11]; additional assistance in identifying unusual isolates beyond the stated expertise of an individual laboratory is available from state and national reference laboratories.

Sometimes it is the pattern of susceptibility to antimicrobials that discriminates epidemiologically significant organisms from other apparently similar hospital organisms. For example, many U.S. hospitals currently encounter nosocomial infections due to *Staphylococcus aureus* strains resistant to methicillin [19]. Such organisms can be the subject of infection control activities only if the laboratory maintains effective and efficient means for their identification [16, 82].

Need for Accuracy and Consistency

Many spurious outbreaks have been traced to inaccurate or inconsistent microbiologic procedures. An "outbreak" of *S. aureus* infection, for example, may be caused by delayed reading of coagulase tests, resulting in misidentification of coagulase-negative organisms as coagulase-positive. Unfortunately, most of the rapid tests available identify organisms that are not common nosocomial pathogens. Thus one challenge for the 1990s is the need to develop rapid testing methods for the organisms closely associated with nosocomial infection (especially staphylococci, enterococci, and gram-negative aerobic bacilli).

To date, performance characteristics (sensitivity, specificity, reproducibility, etc.) of some of the rapid tests for identification of hospital pathogens are not good [107, 125]. These tests provide information of such doubtful value that often the epidemiologist will not act on the data [47, 57]. This means that the rapid tests are used only as an adjunct to other testing. Such tests tend to *increase* care costs rather than decrease them, and their utility is not clear. Improving test methodology will be essential if tests such as these are to assume a strong role in infection control.

The renaming of organisms that results from better knowledge of organism relationships also can cause confusion. For example, the renaming as *Xanthomonas maltophilia* of the emerging nosocomial pathogen formerly called *Pseudomonas maltophilia* gave false alarm to institutions not used to seeing or dealing with what appeared to be a new intruder [136].

Introduction of New Procedures

The laboratory must also consider whether additional laboratory techniques can make testing results more relevant. For example, cultures of intravenous catheter tips may become positive because of contamination at the time of catheter removal or from the intravascular device becoming infected. Several semiquantitative and quantitative methods for culture of intravenous catheters [27, 115, 189] have been shown to be useful in distinguishing between these possibilities (see Chap. 40). Similar claims of usefulness have been made for cultures of other fluids [226], burn wounds (see Chap. 34) and surgical wounds [34] (see Chap. 33). It is not so clear that these special techniques generate useful information.

Quality Control

Just as an effective clinical microbiology laboratory is essential to an effective infection control program, adequate quality control is essential to the practice of good clinical microbiology [8, 13]. Such a quality program begins with a comprehensive procedure manual that establishes standards for performance, including definition of acceptable and unacceptable quality of specimens and specimen containers, permissible delay between collection and receipt of the specimen in the laboratory, and times during which specimens are accepted for processing. The action to be taken by workers when specimens are not in accord with these standards also must be defined. These standards should be communicated to clinicians and nurses as well as to laboratory personnel.

The procedure manual also should cover administrative aspects of laboratory operation related to infection control and employee safety [8, 176]. Minimum standards for identification of isolates should be provided, including a listing of the equipment and reagents to be monitored and the measures to be made to ensure reproducible and accurate performance. The periodic evaluation of skills of all workers, including evening, night, and weekend workers, should be included in the program.

Participating in proficiency testing programs helps the laboratory maintain competence, particularly if proficiency test specimens are submitted to the laboratory in a blind fashion and are handled by routine procedures. If problems develop with such evaluation, the identity of the problem specimens should be made known and the personnel challenged to deal with the specimen in as careful a fashion as possible, to ensure that the laboratory actually has within its capability the correct handling and identification of the organisms.

In addition to such outcome-oriented projects, periodic review of selected laboratory materials, media, and other equipment should be performed. On occasion, erroneous microbiologic results related to the inadvertent use of contaminated or faulty materials may occur. For example, nonviable contaminants were found in specimen tubes in commercial lumbar puncture trays; these resulted in the assumption that an outbreak was occurring of nosocomial meningitis when the contaminants were seen on Gram stains of cerebrospinal fluid [221]. Specimen tubes, skin preparation solutions, slides, transport media, laboratory media, and pipettes all have been implicated as sources of contamination [43]. Such "pseudo-outbreaks" must be considered when laboratory culture or stain results do not correlate with clinical or epidemiologic findings.

Hospital-supported continuing education is essential for quality work in the microbiology laboratory. It is especially important for personnel in smaller hospital laboratories to stay abreast of technologic advances and trends in nosocomial infection occurrence and diagnosis [23]. Fortunately, a number of organizations, including the American Society for Microbiology, the Association for Practitioners in Infection Control, and the American Society of Clinical Pathlogists, provide frequent programs on nosocomial infection topics.

Accurate Characterization of Antimicrobial Susceptibility of Many Nosocomial Pathogens

A standardized method of antimicrobial susceptibility testing subject to quality control evaluation is essential in any clinical microbiology laboratory and is equally critical to infection control studies. Occasionally, the epidemiologist will suspect that a group of nosocomial infections with organisms of the same species have a common origin. To investigate whether strains in this cluster are common or different, the usual practice is to examine results of speciation, biochemical tests, and the pattern of susceptibility to antimicrobial agents [75, 148]. Often these results will answer the question of relationships. Occasionally, additional tests are needed; these are described in a later section of this chapter.

New patterns of antimicrobial resistance have been characteristic of the organisms causing hospital infection in the recent past (see Chaps. 12 through 14). Organisms that consistently had been susceptible to older antimicrobials have developed resistance to these drugs, and some nosocomial organisms have developed resistance to new antimicrobials almost as soon as the drugs have been marketed [146]. Methicillin-resistant *S. aureus* (MRSA) and coagulase-negative strains are involved in hospital infection nationwide [19]. *S. aureus* strains have developed resistance to the newer fluoroquinolone drugs almost as soon as they were marketed, and strains of coagulase-negative staphylococci (*S. hemolyticus*) resistant to vancomycin also have been seen. Enterococci have increased in importance as nosocomial pathogens; some of these strains developed high-level resistance to aminoglycoside antibiotics, others now

produce β-lactamase enzymes that inactivate many of the common antibiotics used for therapy, and yet a few others have become resistant to vancomycin. Enterbacteriaceae, a common source of nosocomial infection, have developed resistance to some of the newer β-lactam antibiotics through small modifications in the structure of the enzymes they already possessed. The sequential appearance and persistence of these resistant organisms suggests spread of the resistant organisms within the hospital. Gram-negative aerobic bacilli of the intestinal tract also have continued to develop plasmid-mediated resistance to aminoglycosides, a mainstay of therapy against nosocomial infection. All these problems of resistance in bacteria are well-known and easily controlled in comparison to our ability to understand and to control resistance in viruses [56].

Several of these current resistance patterns require new or modified laboratory techniques for detection. For example, detection of MRSA requires several modifications of susceptibility testing techniques and is especially a problem for automated systems of detection [82, 179]. The enterococcal strains with high-level resistance to aminoglycosides also require special testing [163]. Detection of resistance to newer cephalosporins, ureidopenicillins, and β-lactamase inhibitor compounds in enterobacteriaceal strains poses special problems as well, although the role of automated testing systems seems more secure [220].

The Kirby-Bauer single-disk diffusion method or an equivalent test system is used in many laboratories for routine testing of antimicrobial susceptibility of bacteria [179]. However, many laboratories are now routinely performing a more quantitative evaluation of sensitivity, using broth-dilution or agar-dilution test methods [179]. In addition, tube dilution or other methods of establishing minimum inhibitory concentration or susceptibility to "gate" concentrations of antibiotic must be used for testing organisms that have not been standardized for testing by a disk method. The latter include a number of anaerobic bacteria, fungi, and yeasts. Other sources may be consulted for detailed discussion of the performance and quality control of these procedures [11, 161–163, 179].

Some microorganisms can be additionally differentiated by indicating the relative degree to which susceptibility or resistance to antimicrobials is present [148]. This can be done by noting the absolute value of zone size in agar-diffusion testing or by providing assessment of minimum inhibitory concentration or minimum bactericidal concentration [179]. Situations in which this more quantitative information would be useful should be delineated jointly by the laboratory and infection control team.

Selection of Strains for Susceptibility Testing

Applications of susceptibility tests to bacteria that are doubtfully related to infection must be avoided, and specific guidelines for the selection of isolates for susceptibility determination should be established by the laboratory. For example, the request for testing of susceptibility should be carefully evaluated when the organisms isolated are endogenous flora present at sites in which they are not normally pathogens. Similarly, the testing of organisms from mixed culture should be avoided in most cases because of the unclear role of the various isolates [219]. Direct testing of urine and spinal fluid is not essential in most cases. Direct testing of susceptibility of isolates from blood culture can be useful as long as the results are confirmed by standardized techniques [179]. Potential pathogens with well-established susceptibility to antimicrobials should not be tested routinely; this group currently includes *Streptococcus pyogenes* and *Streptococcus pneumoniae,* but isolates of the latter from spinal fluid probably should be tested for penicillin susceptibility, in view of the relatively resistant strains being reported in many parts of the United States and other countries [179].

Selection of Drugs for Routine and Special Testing

The selection of drugs for routine testing should be undertaken by the laboratory after consultation with the Infection Control Committee and the Pharmacy and Therapeutics Committee; the chosen agents should reflect both common usage practices of physicians in the hospital and the spectrum of pathogens that are frequently encountered [179]. Occasionally, testing of susceptibility to certain drugs will be performed for epidemiologic purposes; results of such testing may be omitted from routine clinical reporting. Similarly, certain antimicrobials for which the hospital wishes to control usage may be tested but not reported routinely, or tested only after consultation [134, 162].

Different groups of antimicrobials often are used for gram-negative and gram-positive aerobic organisms. Drugs included in each panel should be periodically evaluated and updated. The epidemiologic value of susceptibility patterns may be enhanced by inclusion of certain antibiotics that are not in routine clinical use. Such additional information can also provide valuable taxonomic and quality control information [148], but these benefits must be weighed against the extra time and cost required for testing and recording of the additional studies.

For some of the newer nosocomial pathogens, susceptibility testing methods are not very good. For example, susceptibility testing methods for fungi do not correlate well with clinical outcome [179]. Thus another challenge for the 1990s is the need to develop susceptibility testing methods for some of the newer organisms closely associated with nosocomial infection, especially gram-negative nonfermentive bacilli, fungi, and viruses.

Quality Control

Consistent and accurate identification of organisms over time is necessary for susceptibility data to be useful for clinical and epidemiologic purposes. In addition, errors in performance of susceptibility tests may result in information that is misleading about diagnosis or therapy. To minimize this possibility, detailed quality control procedures must be maintained for all elements of the susceptibility testing process [161, 162, 179]. Special attention must be given to storage of reagents, control of batch-to-batch variation in media, use of control strains for testing, and monitoring of incubation temperatures and atmosphere. When results of these quality control tests exceed acceptable limits, reports on clinical isolates can be withheld until satisfactory control results are obtained. The reproducibility of susceptibility tests can also be assessed by participation in quality control programs of groups such as the College of American Pathologists or the Centers for Disease Control, which periodically distribute unknown specimens for evaluation. Such testing programs focus on clinically and epidemiologically important strains; correct identification assures the laboratory and infection control personnel that the laboratory applies proper techniques and skills.

Timely Reporting of Laboratory Data and Participation in Surveillance of Nosocomial Infection

To deal with individual problems of nosocomial infection in the hospital as they arise, control measures must be taken as quickly as possible and must be based on accurate assessment of the problem and its causes [148]. Without rapid identification and reporting of the organisms involved, control measures cannot be efficiently designed and implemented.

Laboratory records are an important tool for infection control practitioners [149]. Development of computerized laboratory information systems has progressed rapidly during the past decade, and this has led to major improvements in several ways that the laboratory can provide infection control information.

Surveillance
Laboratory records are an important tool for surveillance of infections. More than 80 percent of infections defined by other criteria as nosocomial may be identified by review of positive cultures from the microbiology laboratory [65, 119]. Review of laboratory records is the most common method for surveillance of hospital infection carried out in the United States [185]. Thus data gathered by infection control personnel during laboratory visits form an important base to which additional

surveillance data from clinical rounds must be added. Both sources must be used to obtain an accurate estimate of the true rate of occurrence of nosocomial infection in a given hospital (see Chap. 5).

For both endemic and epidemic nosocomial infection, microbiologic and immunologic reports may be the starting point for additional epidemiologic investigations. These investigations often require information about attributes of the patient, the personnel involved in care, or the diagnostic and therapeutic procedures provided to the patient. Obtaining these nonlaboratory data usually is easier when the patient is still present in the hospital or at least is fresh in the minds of hospital personnel. Prompt reporting of pertinent laboratory results facilitates information retrieval of this type.

Computer programs have been developed to identify clusters of infections with the same organism and susceptibilities that occur at the same time in the same patient care area (ward or service) [185]. Such programs have permitted identification of outbreaks; whether they provide such information in rapid enough fashion to permit use of control measures remains open to question [223].

The laboratory can indicate only which organisms were present in culture. The epidemiologist must supplement this information with clinical data to determine whether organisms found in culture indicate infection or colonization. If colonization is present, the identification of organisms in the culture may be of little help to the clinician. To the epidemiologist, however, both the organisms involved in episodes of exogenous colonization and those of infection are of interest. Either may be evidence of spread of organisms from one site to another, indicating an area in which control measures may halt transmission. Data used for this purpose must be accurate, which emphasizes the role of continuing quality control studies in the laboratory.

Reporting of Results
To facilitate the surveillance of nosocomial infections and of all infections requiring isolation or notification of public health authori-

ties, a copy of positive culture results should be provided to the infection control personnel. Physicians and nurses sometimes are lax about notifying public health authorities of reportable diseases. Isolation of such organisms will be reported to health authorities more efficiently if the responsibility for reporting is delegated to the infection control nurse or some other person designated by the Infection Control Committee (see Chap. 10).

Availability of a computerized laboratory information system can make it possible for the laboratory routinely to produce frequent and tailored reports for the infection control practitioner (see Chap. 5). For example, we generate such a report at the start of each day at Grady Memorial Hospital [149]. The report lists selected positive cultures and immunologic tests from the previous day, sorted by ward in the order in which each practitioner makes daily rounds. The *only* culture results selected and printed on this report are those specified as relevant by the infection control personnel. This maintains a relatively concise report, while ensuring that the infection control officer has access to all information of current interest. The list of results to be selected is changed on a periodic basis to make sure that current needs are addressed (e.g., when the name of an organism has changed or when a new nosocomial pathogen has arisen at the institution).

Prompt reporting by telephone to both clinicians and infection control personnel is essential when presumptive identification is made of isolates of nosocomial significance; this is the only way to ensure proper treatment of the patient and the application of proper control measures [129]. Occasions for reporting include incidents such as the presumptive identification of certain agents in meningitis, isolation of salmonellae or shigellae from stool specimens, positive smears and cultures of tuberculosis bacilli from any patient or employee, and isolation of *S. aureus* from any culture taken of an employee or from lesions of a newborn.

Laboratory studies may provide early warning of the emergence within a hospital of highly infectious microorganisms, multiply drug-resistant organisms, and clusters of unusual infections. In some hospitals, laboratory workers may be the first to detect these and other trends of infection. When findings suggest a possible outbreak, notification requires quicker action than a final report, because useful epidemiologic investigations triggered by the first preliminary data from the laboratory often are profitable. The major elements needed in any early warning are the interest and expertise of the laboratory worker in calling results to the attention of infection control colleagues. This may be done by telephone or page, if urgent; if not, a mention during the daily visit of the infection control staff usually suffices.

Such reporting facilitates the efforts of the infection control personnel. At the same time, early warning must not be requested for so many situations that this becomes an unreasonable burden for the laboratory personnel. The key here is consultation between laboratory and infection control personnel to establish which findings need to be given critical-value status [129].

Laboratory Records

In addition to instituting control measures, infection control workers often need to analyze laboratory data from various periods to try to detect patterns of infection [145]. To assist in this effort, it is helpful if the laboratory can provide an archival summary of organisms on a periodic basis. Data of particular usefulness here might include compiled listings of organisms by culture site, date, patient, and ward; a summary of susceptibility testing results for various species of organisms for given time periods might also be of help. Computer storage and retrieval of all results can aid this process considerably. Some newer laboratory information systems permit downloading of information pertinent to infection control to a personal computer [153, 223]. These data then can be used both by the laboratory and in infection control, if these departments have a compatible personal computer. The specific laboratory data that can aid epidemiologic analyses vary from hospital to hospital. The information to be included and the frequency with which such summaries are made should be determined by the people providing and working with the data in each hospital.

Laboratory records should be retained in such a way that they facilitate such retrospective epidemiologic investigations and quality control activities. The source of each specimen, date of collection, patient identification, hospital number, hospital service, ward, and organisms identified in the final report should be recorded. Records also should be kept of results of antimicrobial sensitivity tests and of any special biochemical or typing reactions.

All cultures should be recorded so that results are readily available by date, type of specimen, and pathogens isolated. Culture data on inpatients and outpatients should be maintained separately. Computer storage and retrieval of all results is optimal [153, 223]. These records also can be maintained in simple, inexpensive, and epidemiologically useful fashion by bound log books, which are kept chronologically for each major type of specimen (e.g., blood, wound, skin, cerebrospinal fluid, urine, stool, sputum). Sole reliance on a filing system of loose laboratory slips is not desirable because specific data are difficult to retrieve and easily lost.

The permanent records of the microbiology laboratory should include dates and other details of any major changes in culturing techniques or laboratory procedures. Dates of changes in the criteria for identification and taxonomic designations applied to isolates should be recorded as well.

Retention Period for Records
No analysis of previous data can be made if the records are not available. To this end, it is incumbent on the laboratory staff to maintain the microbiologic records in some accessible format (e.g., final report sheets, disc or tape storage) for a reasonable period. The length of time such records can be maintained depends on hospital size, work volume of the laboratory, and available storage facilities, as well as on infection control needs. Thus storage time should be determined by laboratory

personnel after consultation with the hospital infection control staff. One author considers 18 months to be a reasonable minimum [73].

Summary Reports for Clinical Use
Development of profiles for susceptibility of frequently tested pathogens to drugs commonly in use can be of considerable assistance in guiding therapy for sepsis of unclear cause and other infections. Testing other organisms (e.g., slow-growing bacteria or organisms requiring special test procedures) may be performed at intervals to develop a profile of their susceptibility. As long as susceptibility patterns can be presumed to remain stable, such testing may be a useful substitute for testing each isolate at the time of recovery.

These summaries of susceptibility patterns should be available to the medical staff on at least an annual basis [134]. In addition to the hospital epidemiologist, any or all of the Infection Control Committee, medical staff committees, and quality assurance committee may also wish to receive susceptibility summaries to guide their review of antibiotic utilization (see Chap. 2) [147, 149]. The use of a laboratory information system to tabulate the data directly or to download the raw data to a personal computer for calculation of results [153] has eased the burden of performing this task by hand. The laboratory information system also can be employed to provide information about proper use of antimicrobial agents; in one study, this had a dramatic effect on the appropriateness of antimicrobial therapy [59].

Tabulations that may be of particular use include frequency of susceptibility to individual drugs by site of infection (which may provide guidance to the clinician for empiric therapy of infection before the causative organism has been identified) and tabulation of frequency of susceptibility to individual antimicrobials by pathogen (which may be used to direct therapy after an organism has been identified but before susceptibility tests have been completed).

A listing of the relative costs of the currently employed antimicrobials may be developed with cooperation of the pharmacy;

inclusion of this information with suscepti-bility summaries may enhance the incentive to reduce costs of antimicrobial usage [134].

Additional Studies to Establish Similarity or Difference of Organisms

On occasion, the epidemiologist will suspect that a group of nosocomial infections with or-ganisms of the same species have a common origin. To investigate whether strains in this cluster [181] are common or different, the usual practice is to examine results of specia-tion, biochemical tests, and pattern of suscep-tibility to antimicrobial agents. However, for organisms commonly encountered in the hos-pital (e.g., *S. aureus* or *Klebsiella*), the general pattern of these results may be similar on the basis of chance alone. Conversely, for other organisms (e.g., *P. aeruginosa*), the variation in these characteristics from strain to strain is so small that the tests provide little informa-tion about similarity or difference of tested strains [1]. Testing of additional antimicro-bials not ordinarily included, or of suscep-tibility to other antibacterial substances (e.g., silver) may differentiate strains in some cases. In situations in which no differences can be shown for the above tests, examination ("typing") of additional organism characteris-tics (markers) can be of great assistance [73, 145, 148].

Although hospital laboratory personnel may not have the facilities to perform special-ized typing procedures, they should know which organisms can be typed and which can-not and where specific procedures can be performed. When epidemiologically impor-tant isolates require special typing, it may be necessary to forward them to public health or private reference laboratories. Potentially pathogenic materials should be packaged for air transport in conformance with federal regulations [44, 211].

Methods for Typing of Isolates

A variety of techniques have been used for typing isolates [62, 73, 145, 170, 201]. Se-lected typing systems of special value in inves-tigating nosocomial infection problems are summarized in Tables 9-1 through 9-3. So many typing systems are being used today for so many organisms that only a few examples can be provided in the tables. Many are be-yond the capabilities of the usual clinical labo-ratory, but a number can be conducted when circumstances dictate.

A number of organisms involved in noso-comial infection have been differentiated suc-cessfully by *antimicrobial susceptibility testing* (see Table 9-1). This technique was discussed earlier in this chapter. Test antimicrobials not usually employed for routine clinical use can be of assistance here [75]. As noted earlier, a quantitative assessment of the relative degree to which susceptibility or resistance to anti-microbials is present may help make this differentiation [148]. In the past, bacterial strains acquired in the hospital often were more likely to be resistant to antimicrobials than were community-acquired strains of the same organism; this is not necessarily the case today [151]. The antibiogram of strains in the same clone can change over time [62]. Susceptibility to various chemicals, especially heavy metals (*resistotyping*) also has proved of value in selected instances.

Biotyping is the use of certain characteristic biochemical reactions to identify subgroups of bacteria. Typing schemes using this method have been devised for a variety of bacterial organisms, both anaerobes and aerobes, and found to be useful in infection control inves-tigations (see Table 9-1). These schemes often are used in conjunction with pattern analy-sis of antimicrobial susceptibility results to attempt discrimination of isolates. Unfortu-nately, the biotype codes generated by many of the commercial identification systems are poorly reproducible [62]. The method is most useful when unusual biotypes characterize the nosocomial pathogen.

Susceptibility to bacteriophages (*phage typ-ing*) is a characteristic used for typing a num-ber of organisms of nosocomial importance (see Table 9-1). The technique is especially handy for grouping strains of *S. aureus*. This procedure usually is available only in refer-ence laboratories, and plasmid transfer of

Table 9-1. Typing systems for selected organisms causing nosocomial infection: susceptibility testing, biotyping, and phage testing

Organism	*Antimicrobials or heavy metals*	*Biotyping*	*Phage susceptibility*
Acinetobacter spp.	[3, 215]*	[18, 215]	[18]
Candida spp.	[100]	[30, 194]	
Clostridium difficile	[225]		[9]
Coagulase-negative staphylococci	[20, 128]	[20, 128, 135]	[128, 177]
Diphtheroids	[159]	[159]	
Enterobacter spp.	[141]	[64]	[64, 69]
Enterococcus spp.		[101]	
Escherichia coli	[126]	[67]	[154]
Hemophilus influenzae	[187, 218]	[187, 218]	
Klebsiella spp.	[113]	[113]	[68]
Listeria spp.			[205]
MRSA	[71, 114]	[37]	[114, 155]
Mycobacteria	[217]	[26]	
Proteus spp.	[5, 45]	[5]	[92]
Providencia stuartii	[94, 202]	[94, 202]	
Pseudomonas aeruginosa	[130, 181]		[80]
Pseudomonas cepacia	[174]	[174]	
Salmonella spp.	[166, 216]	[109, 166]	[109, 216]
Serratia spp.	[116, 142]	[116, 142]	[77]
Shigella spp.	[54]		[108]
Staphylococcus aureus	[17, 177]	[73]	[17, 89, 177]
Staphylococcus epidermidis	[63]	[63]	[10]

MRSA = methicillin-resistant *Staphylococcus aureus*.
*Numbers refer to references citing use of the indicated typing scheme for the indicated organism.

phage characteristics apparently can occur, but the procedure continues to be of value in relating isolates under epidemic conditions [150]. It often has been desirable to determine the bacteriophage types of *S. aureus* isolates obtained just before an outbreak for comparison with the pattern of the epidemic strain. Although routine typing of all strains is not cost-effective, some laboratories store isolates for later typing should it prove desirable. Isolates may be conveniently and inexpensively stored by placing a small amount of growth on a blank paper disk that is placed in a 2-ml glass screw-cap vial containing a few granules of silica gel. If the vial is kept tightly closed, isolates may be held up to 6 months; they can then be easily retrieved by placing the disk in broth.

Serotyping is a major technique used for typing of many gram-negative aerobic bacilli, especially *Klebsiella pneumoniae* isolates (see Table 9-2). Serotyping is probably the single most valuable technique for typing *P. aeruginosa*. The technique can be of great help for other organisms shown in the table as well, in both outbreak situations and research investigations [1]. However, when reagents are not readily available, or when typing procedures are complex, the techniques are available only in referral laboratories. The cost of routine serotyping of isolates in the absence of an outbreak has not been justified by demonstration of benefit to patient diagnosis or therapy. See Chapter 30 for a discussion of the value of serotyping of enteropathogenic strains of *E. coli*.

Many bacteria produce products that can kill or inhibit the growth of other organisms. Production of such bacteriocins by an epidemic strain, or susceptibility of the organism in question to those produced by other bacteria, can be used as a typing tool for a number

Table 9-2. Typing systems for selected organisms causing nosocomial infection: serotyping and bacteriocin testing

Organism	Serotyping	Bacteriocin production or susceptibility
Acinetobacter spp.	[210]*	[6]
Astrovirus	[122]	
Clostridium difficile	[208]	[9]
Enterobacter spp.	[64, 69, 141]	[64, 69]
Escherichia coli	[15, 154]	[91]
Hemophilus influenzae	[218]	
Klebsiella spp.	[165]	[14]
Legionella spp.	[224]	
Listeria spp.	[196]	
Mycobacterium avium	[50, 93]	
Proteus spp.	[5, 169]	[5]
Providencia spp.	[94, 202]	
Pseudomonas aeruginosa	[78, 212]	[80, 184]
Pseudomonas cepacia	[174]	[174]
Rotavirus	[203, 214]	
Salmonella spp.	[109]	
Serratia spp.	[116, 142]	[116]
Shigella spp.	[51]	[156]
Staphylococcus aureus	[35]	
Staphylococcus epidermidis	[35]	
Streptococcus spp.	[83]	

*Numbers refer to references citing use of the indicated typing scheme for the indicated organism.

Table 9-3. Typing systems for selected organisms causing nosocomial infection: plasmid profiles and restriction endonuclease testing

Organism	Plasmid profiles	Restriction endonuclease[a]
Acinetobacter spp.	[2, 70, 215][b]	[3]
Antibiotic plasmids	[190]	[190]
Candida spp.		[186, 197]
Citrobacter spp.	[140, 216]	
Clostridium difficile	[33]	[33, 105]
Coagulase-negative staphylococci	[10, 20, 128]	[10, 20]
Cytomegalovirus		[32, 46]
Enterobacter spp.	[140, 141]	
Enterococcal spp.	[183]	[158, 168]
Escherichia coli	[126, 154, 188]	[126, 216]
Hemophilus influenzae	[140, 187]	[167]
Herpes simplex virus		[87]
Klebsiella spp.	[103, 140]	
Lactobacillus spp.	[204]	
Legionella spp.	[140, 209]	[167, 209]
Listeria spp.	[60]	[60, 164]
MRSA	[71, 124, 227]	[25, 37, 227]
Mycobacterial spp.	[140, 217]	[31]
Providencia spp.	[140, 216]	[167]
Pseudomonas aeruginosa	[103, 130, 140]	[3, 80, 167]
Pseudomonas cepacia	[103]	[174]
Salmonella spp.	[109, 166, 216]	[109, 166]
Serratia spp.	[142]	[142]
Shigella spp.	[127, 140, 173]	
Staphylococcus aureus	[140, 177, 183]	[89]

MRSA = methicillin-resistant *Staphylococcus aureus*.
[a] Digestion of plasmid or genomic material.
[b] Numbers refer to references citing use of the indicated typing scheme for the indicated organism.

of organisms (see Table 9-2). The method requires careful use of controls, and widespread agreement on standards for reagents and interpretation is unusual. Reproducibility of results is a problem; all strains should be tested at the same time [62, 170].

During the past decade, molecular and other newer techniques (see Table 9-3) have permitted more definitive typing of a wider range of organisms than ever before [48, 53, 61, 170, 175, 206]. These methods have helped immeasurably in defining mode of spread, reservoirs, and asymptomatic and unsuspected sources of infection [103]. It is now clear that these techniques can provide an epidemiologic picture different from that of prior methods [87, 197].

A number of other systems for typing have been proposed for organisms important in cross-infection (Table 9-4). Many of the methods shown in this table have been employed

Table 9-4. Additional typing methods for organisms causing nosocomial infection

Typing system	Organism studied	Reference
Enzyme electrophoresis	Various	[53]
	Citrobacter spp.	[123]
	Serratia spp.	[103, 116]
	Pseudomonas aeruginosa	[78]
	Salmonella spp.	[109]
	Staphylococcus aureus	[17, 21]
	MRSA	[21]
	Candida spp.	[120]
	Mycobacteria (rapid grower)	[217]
Whole-cell electrophoresis	*Acinetobacter* spp.	[2]
	Serratia spp.	[85]
	Staphylococcus aureus	[41]
	MRSA	[16, 41]
	Coagulase-negative staphylococci	[207]
Protein electrophoresis	Coagulase-negative staphylococci	[171]
	Hemophilus influenzae	[55]
Ribosomal RNA electrophoresis	Rotavirus	[28, 203]
Ribosomal RNA sequencing	Respiratory syncytial virus	[198]
Chromosomal DNA probes	Respiratory syncytial virus	[199]
	Mycobacteria	[180]
Enzyme content	*Staphylococcus aureus*	[150]
	MRSA	[114, 124]
Marker proteins	*Staphylococcus aureus*	[36]
	Acinetobacter spp.	[18]
	Citrobacter spp.	[112]
	Serratia spp.	[66]
Nucleic acid by polymerase chain reaction	Rotavirus	[74]
Dienes reaction	*Proteus mirabilis*	[45]
Serum opacity	Streptococcal spp.	[104]
Lipopolysaccharide immunotype	*Pseudomonas aeruginosa*	[40]
Colony morphology	Diphtheroids	[159]
	Staphylococcus epidermidis	[10]
Extracellular products	Coagulase-negative staphylococci (slime)	[63, 178]
	MRSA (exported proteins)	[37]
Killer-system analysis	*Candida albicans*	[172]
Cytotoxicity assay	*Clostridium difficile*	[225]
Lectin analysis	Multiple	[193]
Electrophoretic karyotyping	*Candida albicans*	[132]
	Pneumocystis carinii	[96]
Pilin type	*Pseudomonas aeruginosa*	[195]
Cell-surface hydrophobicity	Coagulase-negative staphylococci	[137]
Pyrolysis mass spectrometry	*Streptococcus pyogenes*	[131]
Fatty-acid analysis	*Pseudomonas cepacia*	[157]

MRSA = methicillin-resistant *Staphylococcus aureus.*

in only a small number of reports, and their relative usefulness is not yet determined.

Choosing Typing Systems
While the potential benefit of these new techniques for hospital infection control is great,

some cautions are needed regarding their use [148]. Sometimes the new systems for analysis have impeded rather than aided in outbreak investigations. For example, pseudoepidemics of nosocomial infection may occur in association with use of newer diagnostic techniques

[118]. Incorrect results also may arise from contamination of reagents, a special concern with use of newer techniques such as the polymerase chain reaction, with which sensitivity is so great that the chance of contamination is high [175]. Some typing methods provide data of doubtful value or results that are difficult to interpret for a given epidemiologic situation. To improve these, further information is needed to evaluate their validity as a tool for infection control [148].

Even if the methods are valid, overinterpretation or underinterpretation of the results is a potential problem. Typing never proves that organisms are the same [53]. On the other hand, the use of too many individual markers in several typing methods can cause problems as well. For example, use of 20 different antibiotics in typing a series of specimens in which organisms are defined as different if their pattern of susceptibility varies by more than one drug almost guarantees that organisms that actually are part of the outbreak will be identified as different and thus considered unrelated [148].

Results from some typing methods may be redundant; if so, this needs to be discovered, so that the cheaper method can be used. An important question for current investigation should be not *whether* new tests provide additional discrimination but *how much* discriminating ability they add to tests that are readily available [99]. For example, in a study of infections with coagulase-negative staphylococci, antibiogram, biotyping, phage typing, and plasmid profiling all were performed. The antibiogram, selected as the first stage of the scheme because it was the simplest and cheapest test, proved to be the most discriminatory stage, providing 66 percent of the discriminating ability between strains [128]. A related issue is how often most hospitals really will need these newer techniques. Most of the newer methods are used today for research (detailing routes of transmission or reservoirs of organisms) rather than for acting on outbreaks. Use of these typing methods should be reserved for the unusual situations in which routine, inexpensive methods fail [61]. For most of the newer molecular testing methods, instruments and reagents are not readily available [102]. The expertise to perform and interpret the tests is not widespread. In addition, outbreak organisms rarely are all isolated at once so typing procedures are performed at separate times; the need for control of batch-to-batch variation in media, reagents, phages, and the like is especially crucial with many of these typing procedures. These considerations explain why many newer typing procedures should not be performed in the routine clinical laboratory. In some cases, one may need to go back and type isolates recovered at different time periods together on the same media to remove confounding variables of the testing process [148]. Thus, not every laboratory must be able to perform every, or even most, of these tests. The laboratory director must be aware of the tests that are available, determine which can be performed on site when needed, and identify referral laboratories (friend, state, private, etc.) where other methods are available on request.

Storage of Strains

For supplemental tests to be performed, such as those described in the preceding section, the organisms must be available. Thus a related duty of the clinical laboratory staff is to retain strains that may relate to nosocomial infection for a given period while it is determined whether additional testing is needed. In cooperation with infection control personnel, the laboratory staff should subculture and save epidemiologically important isolates, whether such isolates are from outbreaks or from single cases of unusual or potentially epidemic diseases. A system for reviewing and periodically discarding these isolates also must be established. How long a storage period is required for this purpose will vary from hospital to hospital and should be agreed on between epidemiologist and clinical laboratory supervisor [73, 149]. The technique used to ensure the viability of the organisms (e.g., freezing, lyophilization) should be determined by the laboratory staff after considering the equipment and personnel that are available for this task.

Occasional Microbiologic Studies of Hospital Personnel or Environment

In some situations, nosocomial infection may result from environmental or personnel sources. In evaluating such episodes, the infection control staff may ask the laboratory staff to process specimens from employees, environmental sources, or hospital equipment (e.g., respiratory therapy machines) as part of the investigation [143]. It should be emphasized, however, that such environmental culturing should focus on investigation of documented infections in patients. When such culturing is necessary, its costs should be considered part of the hospitals' infection control program, and charges for the cultures should not be billed to the patients involved in the outbreak [148].

A few procedures of this type should be done routinely (Table 9-5). Others are elective, performed in association with episodes of patient illness or as part of an educational program. A third group is specifically not recommended. Each will be dealt with in turn.

Table 9-5. Microbiologic studies of hospital personnel and the hospital environment

I. Recommended for routine performance
  A. Monitoring of sterilization
    1. Steam sterilizers
    2. Ethylene oxide sterilizers
    3. Dry-heat sterilizers
  B. Sampling of infant formula prepared in the hospital and other specific high-risk hospital-prepared products
  C. Monitoring of dialysis fluid (if required by regulatory agencies)
II. Elective environmental monitoring
  A. Surveys to investigate a specific problem of patient infection
  B. Surveys for educational purposes
III. Procedures not recommended
  A. Routine culture surveys of patients or hospital personnel
  B. Routine culture of commercial products labeled as sterile
  C. Routine testing of antiseptics and disinfectants
  D. Routine culture of blood units
  E. Routine monitoring of disinfection process for respiratory therapy equipment

Routine Environmental Sampling

Surveillance cultures of the hospital environment and personnel once were advocated on a routine basis. During the 1970s, studies found these programs to be of minimal value in infection control; by 1980, most institutions took the approach that routine environmental culturing should be severely limited [143]. During the past decade, limiting cultures of the environment has become even more imperative because of changes in the economics of health care in the United States. Fortunately, further studies of cultures of the neutropenic patient [200], infants in intensive care units [58], and preoperative cultures of surgical patients [177] have supported this selective approach. Close communication between epidemiologist and microbiologist about the need for such cultures continues to be essential to keep from wasting valuable resources [138].

In the absence of an epidemic, sampling should be minimal; microbiology and infection control personnel should be firm in not conducting indiscriminate routine microbiologic sampling and testing (see Chap. 15). However, routine checks on the adequacy of sterilizer function, culture of dialysis infusates and the water used to prepare them, culture of infant formula and some other products prepared in the hospital, and periodic checks on the effectiveness of disinfection of certain equipment that directly contacts tissues other than skin may help prevent infections from these sources.

Monitoring of Sterilization

All steam and ethylene oxide gas sterilizers should be checked at least once each week with a suitable live-spore preparation [191]; if sterilization is performed less often, testing should be done on each day that sterilization is done (see Chap. 16). Ethylene oxide gas sterilizers also should be checked with each load of items that will come into contact with blood or other tissues. In addition, each load in either type of sterilizer should be monitored with a spore test if it contains implantable objects. These implantable objects should not be used until the spore test is reported as negative, usually at 48 hours of incubation.

Guidelines from the Centers for Disease Control additionally recommend that dry-heat sterilizers be monitored at least once each month [191].

All sterilizers should be equipped with time-temperature recorders to provide evidence of adequate exposure for each load. However, evidence that a sterilizing temperature has been held for an adequate time does not prove that sterilization took place; the temperature is measured at the outlet valve and does not reflect whether adequate sterilization occurred within dense volumes of fluid or large, dense, fabric-wrapped packs. The use of chemical monitors (e.g., test tapes or heat-sensitive color indicators) within the autoclave is recommended for the outside of each package sterilized [191]. This provides an indication that a sterilizing temperature may have been reached, although such monitors do not show whether there was an adequate duration of exposure. Thus additional monitoring systems are required, which ordinarily involve the laboratory: Biologic monitoring with spore strips generally has been accepted as the most effective way to determine successful sterilization (see Chap. 16).

Microorganisms chosen for spore strip tests are more resistant to sterilization than are most naturally occurring pathogens. The test organisms are provided in relatively high concentrations to ensure a margin of safety. The spores may be provided either in impregnated filter-paper strips or in solution in glass ampules. For steam sterilization, the thermophile *Bacillus stearothermophilus* is used, and, for ethylene oxide and dry-heat sterilizers, *B. subtilis* (strain *globigii*, variety *niger*) is employed. Both species frequently are incorporated simultaneously in the test strips, and these can be used to test for adequate sterilization with either procedure.

Most spore strip preparations are packaged in envelopes that contain one or two test strips and a control strip. The test strips are packaged in separate envelopes and are removed and sterilized at the time other material is processed. Subsequently, the test strips and control strip are cultured by placing the strips in a tube of tryptic-digest casein-soy (TS) broth that is incubated at 37°C (99°F) for *B. subtilis* and 56°C (133°F) for *B. stearothermophilus*. It is not necessary to culture a positive control strip for each test; if strips are obtained from a single lot, only 10 percent of the positive control strips need be tested.

Spore solutions are prepared in sealed glass ampules for testing the adequacy of sterilization fluids. These ampules should be incubated at 56°C (133°F) in a water bath. If there is no change in the indicator by 7 days, the test is reported as negative. Alternatively, the fluid may be inoculated with a test culture, which may be subcultured after autoclaving.

Other types of spore preparations are commercially available and require different handling. In each case, the manufacturer's directions should be followed closely.

Test strips or spore solutions should always be placed in the center of the specimen to be tested, never on an open shelf in the autoclave. The center of a pack located near the bottom front exhaust valve will be exposed for the least adequate duration and temperature of sterilization and thus provides the best location for a test measurement. Testing of sterilization of fluids is accomplished by placing an ampule containing a spore solution in the largest vessel.

Use of ampules containing spore solutions is not appropriate for checking sterilization of microbiologic culture media, because these media do not require the duration of exposure that is required for sterilization of material known to contain large populations of bacteria. Heating of bacteriologic culture media to a temperature sufficient to ensure sterilization of a test strip or spore ampule will result in damage to the medium through overheating.

The likelihood of cross-contamination can be reduced by minimizing the handling of the strip after sterilization. Test strips can be removed from their envelopes and placed in sterile glass tubes before sterilization. The tube then is sterilized with the screw-cap removed or with other closures permeable to steam in place. After sterilization, the tube is sent to the laboratory, where the nutrient broth is added.

The handling of spore strips in the laboratory requires considerable care to prevent secondary contamination. The transfer should be made in a laminar-flow cabinet if available, using sterile forceps and scissors. The forceps and scissors are common sources of contamination, which may be insufficiently sterilized by flaming or wiping with alcohol. Alcohol may contain viable spores that might not be killed by flaming, and flaming may be insufficient to heat instruments to a temperature that will destroy viable spores. Care should be taken not to cross-contaminate the sterilized spore strips with the control strips.

Condensation on the cover of a 56°C (133°F) water bath may cause contamination of the caps and closures of tubes. A heating block may be used to avoid this, or the bath may be left uncovered; the latter will make it necessary to provide a reservoir to maintain the water level, as the evaporation rate is high at this temperature. Uninoculated culture media should be incubated at 35°C (95°F) or at 56°C (133°F) to ensure that contamination will not yield false-positive reports.

Gram staining and subculturing should be performed to detect secondary contamination of test cultures. If organisms other than gram-positive bacilli are observed, the test should be repeated and reported as "possible laboratory contamination, test being repeated."

Whenever positive results are obtained, the sterilizers should be checked immediately for proper use and function [191]. Careful examination must be made of thermometer and pressure-gauge readings, and recent time and temperature records must be reviewed. If any deficiency is observed or if the repeat sterility test still results in growth, engineering personnel and experts in autoclave maintenance and function should be consulted promptly. Objects other than those used for implants do not need to be recalled at this point unless defects are discovered in the sterilizer or its use; if spore tests remain positive after proper use of the sterilizer is documented, the machine should be removed from service until the defects are corrected (see Chap. 16).

Sampling of Infant Formula and Other Products Prepared in the Hospital

Infant formula prepared in the hospital kitchen should be monitored on a weekly basis [191]. A guideline for interpretation of culture suggests that fewer than 25 organisms per milliliter be present and that no virulent bacteria, such as *Salmonella* or *Shigella*, be present [191]. The guideline is an arbitrary one, however, and should be a matter of local preference.

Other products prepared in hospitals that have been demonstrated to have a potential for causing nosocomial infection also should be monitored. At one hospital, these consisted of hyperalimentation fluid prepared in the hospital and breast milk collected for group use [143]. Whether any products fit into this category and the frequency of monitoring for any identified should be determined by the individual hospital.

Culture of Blood Components

The American Association of Blood Banks [4] does not recommend routine culturing of transfusion components.

Culture of Dialysis Fluid

The water used for preparation of dialysis fluid should be tested by colony count at least once per month, according to requirements of the Centers for Disease Control [191]. Guidelines of the Association for Advancement of Medical Instrumentation [7] specify that the fluid should contain fewer than 200 viable organisms per milliliter, and the dialysate fewer than 2,000 colony-forming units (cfu) per milliliter. Defined methods for such testing vary from one regulatory body to the next; in general, the correlation between the specified levels and occurrence of patient disease is poor [49]. Counts obtained vary markedly with media and conditions of incubation [88] (see Chap. 19).

Periodic Sampling of Disinfected Equipment

Any article that makes direct contact with the vascular system or tissue other than unbroken skin should be sterile. Whenever possible, steam or gas sterilization should be applied. If chemical disinfection or pasteurization rather than sterilization is used on equipment such as cystoscopes and other endoscopes or anesthesia equipment, some authorities recommend (and some require) that periodic microbiologic sampling be done to ensure the absence of pathogens after processing.

The frequency of sampling such disinfected devices depends on the results of intermittent sampling, any evidence that nosocomial infection is associated with their use, and an assessment by the Infection Control Committee of the adequacy of standards for control of contamination of such equipment. There is little agreement on which items of this type should be tested, or how often. If such a monitoring program is begun, it may be possible to cut back on the frequency of culturing after a period of time in which cultures are negative, as long as no changes are made in equipment and techniques used [143]. Samples of reusable equipment should be taken after the product has been disinfected and made ready for use on patients.

On occasion, local or regional regulations will require routine culture of transplant organs (e.g., eye, bone, and porcine heart valves), laminar flow hoods, or pharmacy admixture solutions.

Elective Environmental Monitoring

A wide variety of items and substances can be responsible for cross-infection. Thus environmental surveys may be useful during investigation of specific problems within a hospital and should be instituted in response to, and specifically address, epidemiologic findings [143]. Elective culturing programs may also be instituted in association with educational efforts.

Support for Investigation of Specific Problems

Outbreaks of nosocomial infection must be dealt with as rapidly as possible [148]. This means that the laboratory may face exceptional demands for service at the beginning of, and throughout, an epidemic period [73]. Advance preparation for such situations makes response easier in the time of need. The laboratory personnel should prepare contingency plans for the types of outbreaks that have occurred most frequently in the past in the hospital so that they are ready to deal with these exceptional requests in a smooth fashion.

Investigation of an outbreak of nosocomial infection may require isolation and identification of isolates in specimens not only from patients but also from personnel who might be colonized with the outbreak strain and from environmental objects that might be similarly contaminated [148]. Such activity may require the laboratory staff to process and evaluate large numbers of cultures, and special techniques may be necessary to accomplish such projects. For example, reliable detection of *Salmonella* carriage, rather than infection with this organism, requires enhancement of growth by use of selective media [11]. The laboratory staff and the infection control team can process this work efficiently by making careful assessment of the sites to be cultured and determining which culture media and techniques will be employed.

A detailed description of suitable culture techniques for every possible vehicle of cross-infection is beyond the practical scope of this chapter. The development of selective media and techniques for culture of environmental objects has continued during the past decade as new potential reservoirs and vectors of hospital infection have been recognized [73, 148]. Methods for sampling sites relevant to infections caused by specific pathogens are described in the appropriate chapters of Part II of this text. The infection control worker and laboratorian must be familiar with general aspects of culture procedures discussed in the following sections, but they should not obtain or process such cultures unless surveillance of infections in patients specifically implicates these items as potential sources of nosocomial infection.

Because standard methods for the microbiologic evaluation of such culture procedures do not exist or are of doubtful validity, considerable expense may be incurred in the production of information that is worthless or misleading. Thus requests for such cultures should be approached with caution, and the infection control staff should be clear regarding how the culture results will affect patient care or epidemiologic control measures before undertaking such tasks [143].

Culture of Blood Products After a Transfusion Reaction Bacteria present in blood components can cause a septic transfusion reaction; fortunately, this is a very rare occurrence. Such reactions usually are due to endotoxin produced by organisms that can grow in the cold. If transfusion reaction is suspected by clinical signs, the transfusion should be halted immediately and the unit examined. If further evaluation of the signs, symptoms, and clinical course of the patient then suggests bacterial contamination of the blood product, cultures of the suspect component(s) may be indicated, at refrigerator, room, and body temperatures [4]. It is desirable as well at this time to collect blood culture specimens by venipuncture from the patient.

Cultures of Parenteral Fluids and Intravascular Therapy Equipment The investigation of bacteremia associated with parenteral therapy may require investigation of the needle or catheter, portions of the administration set, the fluid being administered, and portions of the cap or closure provided with the fluid [189] (see Chap. 40). Blood culture specimens should be collected simultaneously from the patient. It is especially important to keep careful track of lot numbers, which should be recorded on the patient's chart as well as on all subsequent laboratory records.

Needles and catheters must be submitted separately from the hubs and other portions of the administration set that may have been exposed to superficial contamination. If portions of the administration set are suspected, these must be received properly capped to exclude spurious contamination. The bottle and administration set should remain connected and be placed in a plastic bag to minimize contamination during delivery to the laboratory.

The standard method for culture of catheters and needles has been the semiquantitative method in which the catheter tip is rolled across a plate containing solid media. Recently, authors have suggested flushing the inside with nutrient broth [115] or a quantitative sonication method for culture of the catheter [189] instead of (or in addition to) a semiquantitative culture. Substitution of hub cultures and cultures of the skin around the insertion point has been suggested to provide as much clinical information without requiring removal of the catheter [27]. Quantitative cultures are time-consuming and are a drain on personnel resources; the need to employ them rather than the more efficient semiquantitative methods has not been demonstrated [226]. Options for culture of the catheter are discussed further in Chapter 40.

Culture methods for intravenous fluids in containers or collected from administration lines are described in Chapter 40 as well. Careful aseptic technique is critical.

Methods for Culturing Hands and Skin Several methods are suitable for culture of hands. The simplest is to take a sterile swab, moisten it with sterile saline or a culture broth appropriate to skin organisms (brain-heart infusion broth [BHIB] is one), and then swab the palmar surface of the hand or hands. A rapid and simple way to obtain these cultures also is provided by pressing the subject's palm gently on a large culture plate containing a suitable agar medium (or a Rodac plate, described below in the section on culture of floors and other surfaces). When a more quantitative estimate of the organisms present is desired, 50 ml of culture broth can be poured into a sterile container or plastic bag. The person to be cultured is asked to rub hands together in the broth for 30 seconds. An estimate of colony-forming units per milliliter can be obtained [98].

In contrast to these simple methods, sampling of hands associated with testing of antiseptics or disinfectants is a more complicated process and requires special techniques [117].

Monitoring of antibiotic-resistant organisms frequently has involved investigation of skin of patients or health care workers as potential sources of resistant organisms. To quantify skin microflora, several methods have been developed [52, 86]. The methods, which are used for toe web cultures as well, involve streaking of cotton swabs for a prescribed period of time in areas delineated by an aluminum foil template. Such methods are useful for investigation of adults but are not suitable for neonates; alternatives are described elsewhere [110].

Methods for Culturing Tubes and Containers
Cultures of external surfaces or internal cavities (e.g., tubes and containers) may be conducted by a swab-rinse technique [145]. BHIB supplemented with 0.5% beef extract is used. The broth should contain 0.07% lecithin and 0.5% polysorbate 80 as neutralizers whenever the cultured objects are likely to contain residual disinfectants. A cotton applicator swab is immersed in this broth in a screw-cap tube, wrung out, and used to swab the surface to be sampled. The swab is returned to the tube after sampling; the portion of the stick handled by the operator should be broken off.

Containers and the lumens of tubular structures may be sampled by a rinse technique, which is a better and more convenient sampling method than the swab method for such equipment. The rinse technique involves introducing a suitable quantity of BHIB into the lumen of tubular structures (40 to 50 ml for respiratory therapy tubing) and manually tilting the object to produce a rinsing action. Up to 50 agitations are desirable. Following this, a sample of the broth is placed in a screw-cap tube. Bottles and containers such as nebulizer reservoirs may be sampled by adding 10 to 15 ml of rinse broth, inserting a sterile stopper if required, and shaking vigorously for approximately 30 seconds. The broth then is decanted or pipetted into a sterile container and sample tubes thoroughly agitated to ensure a homogeneous suspension.

If a colony count is desired, prepare a series of tenfold dilutions in tubes of TS broth using 1 ml of the test sample for the first dilution. From each tube of the dilution series, 0.5 ml are pipetted onto the surface of a TS agar plate, which is supplemented with 5% sheep or rabbit blood. The plate is rocked until the inoculum is thoroughly distributed and then is allowed to dry at 35°C (95°F). The plates are then inverted and incubated for 24 hours, after which colony counts are made if colonies appear to be coalescing or spreading; otherwise, counts are made after 48 hours of incubation.

For specific identification of isolates, the original broth sample should be subcultured at 4 hours and 24 hours after removal of the 1 ml that was used for the dilution count. To perform each subculture, 0.5 ml are pipetted onto the surfaces of culture media suitable for the target organisms. They are rocked to distribute the inoculum and allowed to dry before incubation at 35°C (95°F). At 24 hours, media are inoculated from the original BHIB rinse sample, which has been incubated at 35°C (95°F). If growth seems apparent because the broth already is turbid, a loopful should be subcultured and streaked to provide isolated colonies.

Sampling of Respiratory Therapy Equipment
In situations of high endemic or epidemic levels of occurrence of nosocomial respiratory infections, sampling of respiratory therapy apparatus may be of value [192]. Methods listed earlier for culturing tubes or containers may be employed. A direct-dilution method of sampling has been reported by one group of investigators to be satisfactory for detection of organisms in the range of 10^1 to 10^6 cfu/ml [133].

Methods for Sampling of Air
Air sampling may be performed with either settling plates or more sophisticated equipment [79]. Airborne spread of nosocomial bacterial or viral infection is known to occur [81] but is probably uncommon; air sampling should be required infrequently. Perhaps the most common recent indications for use of this technique have involved *Legionella* [22] and *Aspergillus* [12] infections or monitoring of operating room infections [95].

Particles suspended in hospital air vary greatly in size and in the number of microorganisms they contain. The average diameter of airborne microbial particles in ward air is approximately 13 μm, but 7 percent are less than 4 μm in size and 30 percent are greater than 18 μm. Particles with a mean size of 13 μm settle at a rate of approximately 1 foot per minute. Since the surface of a standard 100-mm Petri dish represents an area of approximately $\frac{1}{15}$ square foot, and assuming that the air in the study area contains particles of average size, an open Petri dish in still air will sample microbial particles from nearly 1 cubic foot of air during 15 minutes of exposure [145]. Brain-heart infusion (BHI) or trypticase-soy agar (TSA) are recommended media for such sampling [145].

Although this is an inexpensive way to evaluate airborne microbial contamination, quantitative results may correlate poorly with those obtained with mechanical, volumetric air samplers because of variation in particle size and unknown influences of air turbulence. Under low-humidity conditions, droplet nuclei of approximately 3 μm can remain suspended indefinitely and can be collected only with high-velocity, volumetric air samplers.

A slit sampler is suitable for many precise air sampling applications [145]. BHI or TSA media should be used in the sampling plates. A staged sampler [79] should be needed only when there is some reason to determine the size distribution of the particles, which should be an extremely infrequent event in most U.S. hospitals. Efficient vacuum sources must be used for both samplers, and the rate of flow of air must be properly calibrated to ensure accurate results.

The total number of airborne microbial particles will not be measured precisely by observing growth after impaction on an agar plate, as an airborne microbial particle may contain more than one viable cell. Air-sampling techniques in which volumetric samples are taken by bubbling air through collection fluid will break up airborne particulate matter and better reflect the total number of organisms than will air samplers that impinge contaminated particles on agar.

Culture of Floors and Other Surfaces Methods for sampling of floors and other surfaces have been described in detail [42, 145]. One method is an adaptation of the swab technique previously described. In this case, a 2 × 2–inch square hole is cut from the center of a sheet of heavy paper, which subsequently is sterilized and wrapped. The culture is collected by placing the paper on the surface to be sampled. The swab is rubbed slowly in close, parallel streaks across the exposed area. This procedure is repeated after moving the swab in a direction perpendicular to the first streaks.

Such surfaces also may be sampled conveniently by use of Rodac plates, which are designed to permit direct contact of agar with flat surfaces. Such plates should be filled with 16.5 ml of TSA containing 0.07% lecithin and 0.5% polysorbate 80 as neutralizers of disinfectant. Both the plates and the surface to be sampled should be dry at the time the sample is collected. Plates are pressed firmly against the surface, avoiding a rotary or sliding motion. Colonies are counted after incubation at 35°C to 37°C (95°F to 99°F) for 48 hours. The use of various types of automatic or semiautomatic colony counters will save time in counting large numbers of plates.

Standards for acceptable levels of contamination of floors and bedside tables as sampled by the Rodac plate technique have been suggested by a committee of the American Public Health Association [38]. There is no evidence, however, that any particular level of contamination is directly correlated with an increased risk of infection, and such standards probably are useful only in assessing the adequacy of housecleaning procedures.

Sampling Methods for Water and Ice Water that meets U.S. Public Health Service standards for drinking water frequently contains up to 1 million or more microorganisms per milliliter, and some of these organisms are potential pathogens. Ice also can contain organisms that can pose a threat of infection, especially in patients with compromised host defenses. However, correlation of levels of microorganisms with occurrence of patient illness has been rare.

Samples of water or melted ice can be obtained by collection in a sterile container. If chlorine is present, it can be inactivated by thiosulfate. The specimen is cultured by passing large quantities through a 0.45-μm (or 0.22-μm) Millipore filter and culturing the filter in broth or directly on agar. More than 4 colonies per 100 ml is considered abnormal by this test [145].

Developing Selective Media for Surveys　To reduce the workload in the laboratory and to expedite the processing of specimens, selective survey media should be used whenever possible for culturing specimens during outbreak investigations. Susceptibility data on known or suspected epidemic strains may be used to identify an appropriate selective medium for use in surveys of the animate and inanimate environment of the hospital. Once the implicated organism is isolated and tested on appropriate media containing one or more antibiotics to which it is resistant, the media can be used to exclude numerous bacteria unrelated to the outbreak. This may accelerate the detection of contaminated equipment or infected patients. Pretesting of the media is essential because of possible synergy or antagonism between the added antimicrobials or between these drugs and the media; such interactions could cause inhibition of growth of the epidemic strain or failure to inhibit growth of nonimplicated organisms.

Other selective media also may be useful. For example, cetrimide medium may be helpful in selectively isolating *P. aeruginosa* from contaminated material or mixed cultures. Similarly, tetrathionate broth is an excellent medium for selective preenrichment of *Salmonella* cultures. Mueller-Hinton agar containing sorbitol, a pH indicator, and antibiotics (vancomycin, colistin, and nystatin) provides selective differentiation of *Serratia* species. Many epidemic strains of *S. aureus* are resistant to mercuric chloride, and the incorporation of small amounts of this compound

in TSA can be helpful in inhibiting nonepidemic strains of *S. aureus, S. epidermidis,* and most gram-negative organisms except *Pseudomonas.* Methicillin-resistant strains of *S. aureus* have become a problem in many U.S. hospitals; agar containing small concentrations of methicillin have been of use in investigating hospital problems due to these strains [19]. The resistance of epidemic microorganisms to other heavy metals, dyes, disinfectants, and other antimicrobial substances also may be used to identify and construct selective media for surveys.

Surveys for Educational Purposes
Sampling techniques that are not directly related to epidemiologic surveys may prove useful in educational programs; visible evidence of contamination of hands, clothing, equipment, and surfaces may serve to teach the need for effective aseptic technique and sanitation.

Sampling that Is Not Recommended
Routine Culture Surveys of Patients and Personnel
Routine culturing of patients or hospital personnel is not recommended (see Chap. 3). Surveys may be useful during investigation of specific problems within a hospital and should be instituted in response to, and specifically address, epidemiologic findings.

Routine Culture of Commercial Products
Although commercial patient care items that are labeled *sterile* (e.g., intravascular catheters and fluids) occasionally have been contaminated with viable organisms that can cause patient disease, routine sampling of these items is not recommended, because the low frequency of contamination makes it difficult (because of the large number of specimens that would have to be taken) and expensive to perform adequate sterility testing.

Routine Testing of Antiseptics and Disinfectants
In-use testing of antiseptics and disinfectants should not be a routine procedure for hospi-

tal microbiology laboratories [191]. If contamination of commercial products sold as sterile is suspected, infection control personnel should be notified and the nearest office of the U.S. Food and Drug Administration contacted immediately [145]. State regulations may require immediate notification of state health authorities as well.

Random Culture of Blood Units

The American Association of Blood Banks [4] does not recommend random culture of blood units to ensure sterility.

Routine Monitoring of Disinfection Process for Respiratory Therapy Equipment

Guidelines from the Centers for Disease Control recommend that "in the absence of an epidemic or high endemic rate of nosocomial pulmonary infections, the disinfection process for respiratory therapy equipment should not be monitored by cultures; that is, routine sampling should not be done" [192]. Disinfection of respiratory therapy and anesthesia equipment is discussed additionally in Chapter 29.

Routine sampling of respiratory therapy equipment while it is being used by a patient is not recommended [192].

Teaching Microbiologic Aspects of Nosocomial Infection to Infection Control Personnel

The persons responsible for infection control usually are not trained in clinical laboratory procedures. Since the key to success in infection control efforts is communication, it is necessary that all involved speak the same language. For this purpose, training of epidemiology personnel in the language of the clinical laboratory microbiologist is important. The training of many infection control personnel in microbiology is inadequate or out-of-date [84]. The goal of such teaching is not necessarily to make the infection control staff accomplished laboratory workers but rather to familiarize them with the procedures and practices of the laboratory, the micro-

organisms involved in nosocomial infection, the validity of test procedures used in identifying these pathogens, and the strengths and weaknesses of the resulting data.

Similarly, it is important for the microbiologist to learn some of the concepts of the epidemiologist, since few laboratory directors or technologists have adequate grounding in epidemiology [84]. Especially important are exposure to techniques used for measuring frequency of infection and the concept of colonization versus infection.

Such joint efforts permit ready communication between the two groups of colleagues. Teaching of this type can be done in a formal fashion but is also effective when included as part of the day-to-day informal contacts between the infection control staff and laboratory personnel.

References

1. Aber, R.C., and Mackel, D.C. Epidemiologic typing of nosocomial microorganisms. *Am. J. Med.* 70:899, 1981.
2. Alexander, M., Rahman, M., Taylor, M., and Noble, W.C. A Study of the value of electrophoretic and other techniques for typing *Acinetobacter calcoaceticus. J. Hosp. Infect.* 12:273, 1988.
3. Allardet-Servent, A., et al. Use of low-frequency-cleavage restriction endonucleases for DNA analysis in epidemiological investigations of nosocomial bacterial infections. *J. Clin. Microbiol.* 27:2057, 1989.
4. American Association of Blood Banks. *Technical Manual* (10th ed.). Arlington, VA: AABB, 1990.
5. Anderson, R.L., and Engley, F.B., Jr. Typing methods for *Proteus rettgeri:* Comparison of biotype, antibiograms, serotype, and bacteriocin production. *J. Clin. Microbiol.* 8:715, 1978.
6. Andrews, H.J. *Acinetobacter* bacteriocin typing. *J. Hosp. Infect.* 7:169, 1986.
7. Association for Advancement of Medical Instrumentation. *Water Requirements for Dialysis.* Arlington, VA: AAMI, 1984. Pp.1–47.
8. August, M.J., Hindler, J.A., Huber, T.W., and Sewell, D.L. (with Weissfeld, A.S., Coord. Ed.). *Cumitech 3A—Quality Control and Quality Assurance Practices in Clinical Microbiology.* Washington, D.C.: American Society for Microbiology, 1990. Pp.1–14.

9. Bacon, A.E., Fekety, R., Schaberg, D.R., and Faix, R.G. Epidemiology of *Clostridium difficile* colonization in newborns: Results using a bacteriophage and bacteriocin typing system. *J. Infect. Dis.* 158:349, 1988.

10. Baddour, L.M., et al. Phenotypic variation of *Staphylococcus epidermidis* in infection of transvenous endocardial pacemaker electrodes. *J. Clin. Microbiol.* 28:676, 1990.

11. Balows, A., et al. (Eds.). *Manual of Clinical Microbiology* (5th ed.). Washington, DC: American Society for Microbiology, 1991.

12. Barnes, R.A., and Rogers, T.R. Control of an outbreak of nosocomial aspergillosis by laminar air-flow isolation. *J. Hosp. Infect.* 14:89, 1989.

13. Bartlett, R.C. *Quality Assurance in Clinical Microbiology*. Skokie, IL: American Society of Clinical Pathologists, 1989. Pp.1–11.

14. Bauernfeind, A., Petermuller, C., and Schneider, R. Bacteriocins as tools in analysis of nosocomial *Klebsiella pneumoniae* infections. *J. Clin. Microbiol.* 14:15, 1981.

15. Bettelheim, K.A., and Thompson, C.J. New method of serotyping *Escherichia coli:* Implementation and verification. *J. Clin. Microbiol.* 25:781, 1987.

16. Bigelow, N., Ng, L.-K., Robson, H.G., and Dillon, J.R. Strategies for molecular characterization of methicillin- and gentamicin-resistant *Staphylococcus aureus* in a Canadian nosocomial outbreak. *J. Med. Microbiol.* 30:51, 1989.

17. Bouvet, A., et al. Epidemiological markers for epidemic strain and carrier isolates in an outbreak of nosocomial oxacillin-resistant *Staphylococcus aureus*. *J. Clin. Microbiol.* 28:1338, 1990.

18. Bouvet, P.J.M., Jeanjean, S., Vieu, J.-F., and Dijkshoorn, L. Species, biotype and bacteriophage type determinations compared with cell envelope protein profiles for typing *Acinetobacter* strains. *J. Clin. Microbiol.* 28:170, 1990.

19. Boyce, J.M. Methicillin-resistant *Staphylococcus aureus:* Detection, epidemiology, and control measures. *Infect. Dis. Clin. North Am.* 3:901, 1989.

20. Boyce, J.M., et al. A common-source outbreak of *Staphylococcus epidermidis* infections among patients undergoing cardiac surgery. *J. Infect. Dis.* 161:493, 1990.

21. Branger, C., Goullet, P., Boutonnier, A., and Fournier, J.M. Correlation between esterase electrophoretic types and capsular polysaccharide types 5 and 8 among methicillin-susceptible and methicillin-resistant strains of *Staphylococcus aureus*. *J. Clin. Microbiol.* 28:150, 1990.

22. Breiman, R.F., et al. Role of air sampling in investigation of an outbreak of Legionnaires' disease associated with exposure to aerosols from an evaporative condenser. *J. Infect. Dis.* 161:1257, 1990.

23. Britt, M.R. Infectious diseases in small hospitals: Prevalence of infections and adequacy of microbiology. *Ann. Intern. Med.* 89:757, 1978.

24. Buck, G.E. Nonculture methods for detection and identification of microorganisms in clinical specimens. *Pediatr. Clin. North Am.* 36:95, 1989.

25. Burnie, J.P., Matthews, R.C., Lee, W., and Murdoch, D. A comparison of immunoblot and DNA restriction patterns in characterising methicillin-resistant isolates of *Staphylococcus aureus*. *J. Med. Microbiol.* 29:255, 1989.

26. Casal Roman, M., and Linares Sicilia, M.J. Preliminary investigation of *Mycobacterium tuberculosis* biovars. *J. Clin. Microbiol.* 20:1015, 1984.

27. Cercenado, E., et al. A conservative procedure for the diagnosis of catheter-related infections. *Arch. Intern. Med.* 150:1417, 1990.

28. Chan, R.C.K., Tam, J.S., Fok, T.F., and French, G.L. RNA-electrophoresis as a typing method for nosocomial rotavirus infection in a special-care baby unit. *J. Hosp. Infect.* 13:367, 1989.

29. Chapman, N.M., Tracy, S., Gauntt, C.J., and Fortmueller, U. Molecular detection and identification of enteroviruses using enzymatic amplification and nucleic acid hybridization. *J. Clin. Microbiol.* 28:843, 1990.

30. Childress, C.M., Holder, I.A., and Neely, A.N. Modifications of a *Candida albicans* biotyping system. *J. Clin. Microbiol.* 27:1392, 1989.

31. Chiodini, R.J. Characterization of *Mycobacterium paratuberculosis* and organisms of the *Mycobacterium avium* complex by restriction polymorphism of the rRNA gene region. *J. Clin. Microbiol.* 28:489, 1990.

32. Chou, S. Reactivation and recombination of multiple cytomegalovirus strains from individual organ donors. *J. Infect. Dis.* 160:11, 1989.

33. Clabots, C.R., Peterson, L.R., and Gerding, D.N. Characterization of a nosocomial *Clostridium difficile* outbreak by using plasmid profile typing and clindamycin susceptibility testing. *J. Infect. Dis.* 158:731, 1988.

34. Claesson, B.E.B., and Holmlund, D.E.W. Dip slide culture of intraoperative peritoneal irrigation fluid for prediction of septic complication in elective surgery. *J. Clin. Microbiol.* 24:922, 1986.

35. Cohen, J.O. Serotyping of Staphylococci. In: J.O. Cohen (Ed.), *The Staphylococci*. New York: Wiley Interscience, 1972.

36. Cohen, M.L., et al. Toxic shock syndrome: Modification and comparison of methods for detecting marker proteins in *Staphylococcus aureus*. *J. Clin. Microbiol.* 18:372, 1983.

37. Coia, J.E., Thomson-Carter, F., Baird, D., and

Platt, D.J. Characterisation of methicillin-resistant *Staphylococcus aureus* by biotyping, immunoblotting, and restriction enzyme fragmentation patterns. *J. Med. Microbiol.* 31:125, 1990.

38. Committee on Microbial Contamination of Surfaces, Laboratory Section, American Public Health Association. A comparative microbiological evaluation of floor-cleaning procedures in hospital patient rooms. *Health Lab. Sci.* 7:3, 1970.

39. Conn, R.B. The golden age of American medicine. *Am. J. Clin. Pathol.* 91:725, 1989.

40. Conroy, J.V., et al. Bacteremia due to *Pseudomonas aeruginosa:* Use of a combined typing system in an eight-year study. *J. Infect. Dis.* 148:603, 1983.

41. Costas, M., Cookson, B.D., Talsania, H.G., and Owen, R.J. Numerical analysis of electrophoretic protein patterns of methicillin-resistant strains of *Staphylococcus aureus. J. Clin. Microbiol.* 27:2574, 1989.

42. Craythorn, J.M., et al. Membrane filter contact technique for bacteriological sampling of moist surfaces. *J. Clin. Microbiol.* 12:250, 1980.

43. Cunha, B. Pseudomeningitis—another nosocomial headache. *Infect. Control Hosp. Epidemiol.* 9:391, 1988.

44. Daggett, P.-M. Safe transport of etiologic agents. *A.S.M. News* 54:650, 1988.

45. Dance, D.A.B., Pearson, A.D., Seal, D.V., and Lowes, J.A. A hospital outbreak caused by a chlorhexidine and antibiotic-resistant *Proteus mirabilis. J. Hosp. Infect.* 10:10,1987.

46. Demmler, G.J., et al. Nosocomial cytomegalovirus infections within two hospitals caring for infants and children. *J. Infect. Dis.* 156:9, 1987.

47. Dennehy, P.H., et al. Lack of impact of rapid identification of rotavirus-infected patients on nosocomial rotavirus infections. *Pediatr. Infect. Dis. J.* 8:290, 1989.

48. DNA technology and rapid diagnosis of infection. Leading-Article. *Lancet* 2:897, 1989.

49. Doern, G.V., et al. Quantitative microbiological monitoring of hemodialysis fluids: Evaluation of methods and demonstration of lack of test relevance in single-pass hemodialysis machines with automatic dialysate proportioning with reverse osmosis-treated tap water. *J. Clin. Microbiol.* 16:1025, 1982.

50. duMoulin, G.C., et al. Concentration of *Mycobacterium avium* by hospital hot water systems. *J.A.M.A.* 260:1599, 1988.

51. Edwards, P.R., and Ewing, W.H. *Identification of Enterobacteriaceae.* Minneapolis: Burgess Publishing, 1972.

52. Ehrenkranz, N.J., Eckert, D.G., Alfonso, B.C., and Moskowitz, L.B. Proteeae groin skin carriage in ambulatory geriatric outpatients. *Infect. Control Hosp. Epidemiol.* 10:150, 1989.

53. Eisenstein, B.I. New molecular techniques for microbial epidemiology and the diagnosis of infectious diseases. *J. Infect. Dis.* 161:595, 1990.

54. Elek, S.D., Davies, J.R., and Miles, R. Resisto-typing of *Shigella sonnei. J. Med. Microbiol.* 6:329, 1973.

55. Elliott, J.A., et al. Separation of *Haemophilus influenzae* type b subtypes by numerical analysis. *J. Clin. Microbiol.* 25:1476, 1987.

56. Erice, A., et al. Progressive disease due to ganciclovir-resistant cytomegalovirus in immunocompromised patients. *N. Engl. J. Med.* 320:289, 1989.

57. Escuro, R.S., et al. Prospective evaluation of a *Candida* antigen detection test for invasive candidiasis in immunocompromised adult patients with cancer. *Am. J. Med.* 87:621, 1989.

58. Evans, M.E., et al. Sensitivity, specificity, and predictive value of body surface cultures in a neonatal intensive care unit. *J.A.M.A.* 259:248, 1988.

59. Evans, R.S., et al. Computer surveillance of hospital-acquired infections and antibiotic use. *J.A.M.A.* 256:1007, 1986.

60. Facinelli, B., Varaldo, P.E., Casolari, C., and Fabio, U. Cross-infection with *Listeria monocytogenes* confirmed by DNA fingerprinting. *Lancet* 2:1247, 1988.

61. Falkiner, F.R. Epidemiological typing: A user's view. *J. Hosp. Infect.* 11:303, 1988.

62. Farmer, J.J., III. Conventional typing methods. *J. Hosp. Infect.* 11 (Suppl. A): 309, 1988.

63. Fidalgo, S., et al. Bacteremia due to *Staphylococcus epidermidis:* Microbiologic, epidemiologic, clinical, and prognostic features. *Rev. Infect. Dis.* 12:520, 1990.

64. Flynn, D.M., et al. Patients' endogenous flora as the source of "nosocomial" enterobacter in cardiac surgery. *J. Infect. Dis.* 156:363, 1987.

65. Freeman, J., and McGowan, J.E., Jr. Methodologic issues in hospital epidemiology. I. Rates, case-finding, and interpretation. *Rev. Infect. Dis.* 3:658, 1981.

66. Gargallo-Viola, D., and Lopez, D. Numerical analysis of electrophoretic periplasmic protein patterns, a possible marker system for epidemiologic studies. *J. Clin. Microbiol.* 28:136, 1990.

67. Gargan, R., Brumfitt, W., and Hamilton-Miller, J.M.T. A concise biotyping system for differentiating strains of *Escherichia coli. J. Clin. Pathol.* 35:1366, 1982.

68. Gaston, M.A., Ayling-Smith, B.A., and Pitt, T.L. New bacteriophage typing scheme for subdivision of the frequent capsular serotypes

of *Klebsiella* spp. *J. Clin. Microbiol.* 25:1228, 1987.

69. Gaston, M.A., Strickland, M.A., Ayling-Smith, B.A., and Pitt, T.L. Epidemiological typing of *Enterobacter aerogenes*. *J. Clin. Microbiol.* 27:564, 1989.

70. Gerner-Smidt, P. Frequency of plasmids in strains of *Acinetobacter calcoaceticus*. *J. Hosp. Infect.* 14:23, 1989.

71. Gillespie, M.T., Lyon, B.R., and Skurray, R.A. Typing of methicillin-resistant *Staphylococcus aureus* by antibiotic resistance phenotypes. *J. Med. Microbiol.* 31:57, 1990.

72. Gleckman, R., et al. Sputum gram stain assessment in community-acquired bacteremic pneumonia. *J. Clin. Microbiol.* 26:846, 1988.

73. Goldmann, D.A. New microbiologic techniques for hospital epidemiology. *Eur. J. Clin. Microbiol.* 6:344, 1987.

74. Gouvea, V., et al. Polymerase chain reaction amplification and typing of rotavirus nucleic acid from stool specimens. *J. Clin. Microbiol.* 28:276, 1990.

75. Graham, D.R., Dixon, R.E., Hughes, J.M., and Thornsberry, C. Disk diffusion antimicrobial susceptibility testing for clinical and epidemiologic purposes. *Am. J. Infect. Control* 13:241, 1985.

76. Graman, P.S., and Hall, C.B. Epidemiology and control of nosocomial viral infections. *Infect. Dis. Clin. North Am.* 3:815, 1989.

77. Gransden, W.R., Webster, M., French, G.L., and Phillips, I. An outbreak of *Serratia marcescens* transmitted by contaminated breast pumps in a special care baby unit. *J. Hosp. Infect.* 7:149, 1986.

78. Griffith, S.J., et al. The epidemiology of *Pseudomonas aeruginosa* in oncology patients in a general hospital. *J. Infect. Dis.* 160:1030, 1989.

79. Groschel, D.H. Air sampling in hospitals. *Ann. N.Y. Acad. Sci.* 353:230, 1980.

80. Grothues, D., Koopmann, U., Von der Hardt, H., and Tummler, B. Genome fingerprinting of *Pseudomonas aeruginosa* indicates colonization of cystic fibrosis siblings with closely related strains. *J. Clin. Microbiol.* 26:1973, 1988.

81. Gundermann, K.D. Spread of microorganisms by air-conditioning systems—especially in hospitals. *Ann. N.Y. Acad. Sci.* 353:209, 1980.

82. Hackbarth, C.J., and Chambers, H.F. Methicillin-resistant staphylococci: Detection methods and treatment of infections. *Antimicrob. Agents Chemother.* 33:995, 1989.

83. Hahn, G., and Nyberg, I. Identification of streptococcal groups, A, B, C, and G by slide coagglutination of antibody-sensitized protein A–containing staphylococci. *J. Clin. Microbiol.* 4:99, 1976.

84. Haley, R.W. The "hospital epidemiologist" in U.S. hospitals, 1976–1977: A description of the head of the infection surveillance and control program. *Infect. Control* 1:21, 1980.

85. Hamadeh, R.M., Mandrell, R.E., and Griffiss, J.M. Immunophysical characterization of human isolates of *Serratia marcescens*. *J. Clin. Microbiol.* 28:20, 1990.

86. Hambraeus, A., Hoborn, J., and Whyte, W. Skin sampling—validation of a pad method and comparison with commonly used methods. *J. Hosp. Infect.* 16:19, 1990.

87. Hamory, B., Jones, M., Greene, W., and Wigdahl, B. Use of DNA restriction endonuclease technology to investigate a possible HSV outbreak in a nursery. *Am. J. Infect. Control* 18:138, 1990.

88. Harding, G.B., et al. Bacterial contamination of hemodialysis center water and dialysate: Are current assays adequate? *Artif. Organs* 13:155, 1989.

89. Hartstein, A.I., et al. Restriction enzyme analysis of plasmid DNA and bacteriophage typing of paired *Staphylococcus aureus* blood culture isolates. *J. Clin. Microbiol.* 27:1874, 1989.

90. Henderson, D.K., Baptiste, R., Parrillo, J., and Gill, V.J. Indolent epidemic of *Pseudomonas cepacia* bacteremia and pseudobacteremia in an intensive care unit traced to a contaminated blood gas analyzer. *Am. J. Med.* 84:75, 1988.

91. Hettiaratchy, I.G.T., Cooke, E.M., and Shooter, R.A. Colicine production as an epidemiologic marker of *Escherichia coli*. *J. Med. Microbiol.* 6:1, 1973.

92. Hickman, F.W., and Farmer, J.J., III. Differentiation of *Proteus mirabilis* by bacteriophage typing and Dienes reaction. *J. Clin. Microbiol.* 3:350, 1976.

93. Hoffner, S.E., et al. Serovars of *Mycobacterium avium* complex isolated from patients in Sweden. *J. Clin. Microbiol.* 28:1105, 1990.

94. Hollick, G.E., et al. Characterization of endemic *Providencia stuartii* isolates from patients with urinary devices. *Eur. J. Clin. Microbiol.* 3:521, 1984.

95. Holton, J., Ridgway, G.L., and Reynoldson, A.J. A microbiologist's view of commissioning operating theatres. *J. Hosp. Infect.* 16:29, 1990.

96. Hong, S.-T., et al. *Pneumocystis carinii* karyotypes. *J. Clin. Microbiol.* 28:1785, 1990.

97. Horan, T., et al. Pathogens causing nosocomial infections: Preliminary data from the National Nosocomial Infections Surveillance System. *Antimicrobic Newsletter* 5:65, 1988.

98. Horn, W.A., Larson, E.L., McGinley, K.J., and Leyden, J.J. Microbial flora on the hands of health care personnel: Differences in composition and antibacterial resistance. *Infect. Control Hosp. Epidemiol.* 9:189, 1988.

99. Hunter, P.R. Reproducibility and indices of discriminatory power of microbial typing methods. *J. Clin. Microbiol.* 28:1903, 1990.

100. Hunter, P.R., and Fraser, C. Use of modified resistogram to type *Candida albicans* isolated from cases of vaginitis and from faeces in the same geographical area. *J. Clin. Pathol.* 40:1159, 1987.

101. Hussain, Z., Kuhn, M., Lannigan, R., and Austin, T.W. Microbiological investigation of an outbreak of bacteraemia due to *Streptococcus faecalis* in an intensive care unit. *J. Hosp. Infect.* 12:263, 1988.

102. Isenberg, H.D. Typing and nosocomial candidiasis. *J. Clin. Microbiol.* 28:1086, 1990.

103. John, J.F., Jr. Molecular analysis of nosocomial epidemics. *Infect. Dis. Clin. North Am.* 3:683, 1989.

104. Johnson, D.R., and Kaplan, E.L. Microtechnique for serum opacity factor characterization of group A streptococci adaptable to the use of human sera. *J. Clin. Microbiol.* 26:2025, 1988.

105. Johnson, S., et al. Nosocomial *Clostridium difficile* colonisation and disease. *Lancet* 336:97, 1990.

106. Jorgenson, J.H. (Ed.), *Automation in Clinical Microbiology.* Boca Raton, FL: CRC Press, 1987.

107. Jungkind, K., Serlen, R., and Forrer, J. Clinical and diagnostic dilemmas related to respiratory syncytial virus laboratory testing. *Am. J. Infect. Control* 18:143, 1990.

108. Kallings, L.O., Lindberg, A.A., and Sjoberg, L. Phage typing of *Shigella sonnei. Arch. Immunol. Ther. Exp. (Warsz.)* 16:280, 1968.

109. Kapperud, G., et al. Comparison of epidemiological marker methods for identification of *Salmonella typhimurium* isolates from an outbreak caused by contaminated chocolate. *J. Clin. Microbiol.* 27:2019, 1989.

110. Keyworth, N., Millar, M.R., and Holland, K.T. Swab-wash method for quantitation of cutaneous microflora. *J. Clin. Microbiol.* 28:941, 1990.

111. Kiehn, T.E., Ellner, P.D., and Budzko, D. Role of the microbiology laboratory in care of the immunosuppressed patient. *Rev. Infect. Dis.* 11 (Suppl. 7): S1706, 1989.

112. Kline, M.W., Mason, E.O., Jr., and Kaplan, S.L. Epidemiologic marker system for *Citrobacter diversus* using outer membrane protein profiles. *J. Clin. Microbiol.* 27:1793, 1989.

113. Kolmos, H.J. Epidemiological characterization of *Klebsiella* isolates from patients in a renal department. *J. Hosp. Infect.* 11:144, 1988.

114. Kozarsky, P.E., Rimland, D., Terry, P.M., and Wachsmuth, K. Plasmid analysis of simultaneous nosocomial outbreaks of methicillin-

resistant *Staphylococcus aureus. Infect. Control* 7:577, 1986.

115. Kristinsson, K.G., Burnett, I.A., and Spencer, R.C. Evaluation of three methods for culturing long intravascular catheters. *J. Hosp. Infect.* 14:183, 1989.

116. Larose, P., et al. Nosocomial *Serratia marcescens* individualized by five typing methods in a regional hospital. *J. Hosp. Infect.* 15:167, 1990.

117. Larson, E., and Rotter, M.L. Handwashing: Are experimental models a substitute for clinical trials? Two viewpoints. *Infect. Control Hosp. Epidemiol.* 11:63, 1990.

118. Laussucq, S., et al. False-positive DNA probe test for *Legionella* species associated with a cluster of respiratory illness. *J. Clin. Microbiol.* 26:1442, 1988.

119. Laxson, L.B., Blaser, M.J., and Parkhurst, S.M. Surveillance for the detection of nosocomial infections and the potential for nosocomial outbreaks: I. Microbiology culture surveillance is an effective method of detecting nosocomial infection. *Am. J. Infect. Control* 12:318, 1984.

120. Lehmann, P.F., Kemker, B.J., Hsiao, C.-B., and Dev, S. Isoenzyme biotypes of *Candida* species. *J. Clin. Microbiol.* 27:2514, 1989.

121. Lentino, J.R., and Lucks, D.A. Nonvalue of sputum culture in the management of lower respiratory tract infections. *J. Clin. Microbiol.* 25:758, 1987.

122. Lewis, D.C., Lightfoot, N.F., Cubitt, W.D., and Wilson, S.A. Outbreaks of astrovirus type 1 and rotavirus gastroenteritis in a geriatric in-patient population. *J. Hosp. Infect.* 14:9, 1989.

123. Li, J., et al. Genotypic heterogeneity of strains of *Citrobacter diversus* expressing a 32-kilodalton outer membrane protein associated with neonatal meningitis. *J. Clin. Microbiol.* 28:1760, 1990.

124. Licitra, C.M., et al. Use of plasmid analysis and determination of aminoglycoside-modifying enzymes to characterize isolates from an outbreak of methicillin-resistant *Staphylococcus aureus. J. Clin. Microbiol.* 27:2535, 1989.

125. Lipson, S.M., et al. Occurrence of nonspecific reactions among stool specimens tested by the Abbot TestPack rotavirus enzyme immunoassay. *J. Clin. Microbiol.* 28:1132, 1990.

126. LiPuma, J.J., et al. DNA polymorphisms among *Escherichia coli* isolated from bacteriuric women. *J. Infect. Dis.* 159:526, 1989.

127. Litwin, C.M., et al. Molecular epidemiology of *Shigella sonnei* in Pima County, Arizona: Evidence for a Mexico-related plasmid. *J. Infect. Dis.* 161:797, 1990.

128. Ludlam, H.A., Noble, W.C., Marples, R.R., and Phillips, I. The evaluation of a typing scheme for coagulase-negative staphylococci suitable for epidemiological studies. *J. Med. Microbiol.* 30:161, 1989.

129. Lundberg, G.D. Critical (panic) value notification: An established laboratory practice policy (parameter). *J.A.M.A.* 263:709, 1990.

130. MacArthur, R.D., Lehman, M.H., Currie-McCumber, C.A, and Shlaes, D.M. The epidemiology of a gentamicin-resistant *Pseudomonas aeruginosa* on an intermediate care unit. *Am. J. Epidemiol.* 128:821, 1988.

131. Magee, J.T., Hindmarch, J.M., Burnett, I.A., and Pease, A. Epidemiological typing of *Streptococcus pyogenes* by pyrolysis mass spectrometry. *J. Med. Microbiol.* 30:273, 1989.

132. Mahrous, M., et al. Electrophoretic karyotyping of typical and atypical *Candida albicans*. *J. Clin. Microbiol.* 28:876, 1990.

133. Malecka-Griggs, B., and Reinhardt, D.J. Direct dilution sampling, quantitation, and microbial assessment of open-system ventilation circuits in intensive care. *J. Clin. Microbiol.* 17:870, 1983.

134. Marr, J.J., Moffitt, H.L., and Kunin, C.M. Guidelines for improving the use of antimicrobial agents in hospitals: A statement by the Infectious Diseases Society of America. *J. Infect. Dis.* 157:869, 1988.

135. Marshall, R.J., Davies, A.J., Kirk, R., and Reeves, D.S. The laboratory interpretation of coagulase-negative staphylococcal bacteremia in neonates. *J. Hosp. Infect.* 13:295, 1988.

136. Marshall, W.F., Keating, M.R., Anhalt, J.P., and Steckelberg, J.M. *Xanthomonas maltophilia:* An emerging nosocomial pathogen. *Mayo Clin. Proc.* 64:1097, 1989.

137. Martin, M.A., Pfaller, M.A., Massanari, R.M., and Wenzel, R.P. Use of cellular hydrophobicity, slime production, and species identification markers for the clinical significance of coagulase-negative staphylococcal isolates. *Am. J. Infect. Control* 17:130, 1989.

138. Matsen, J.M. The role of the infectious disease physician in hospital clinical microbiology. *Bull. N.Y. Acad. Med.* 63:605, 1987.

139. Mayer, K.H., and Opal, S.M. Unusual nosocomial pathogens. *Infect. Dis. Clin. North Am.* 3:883, 1989.

140. Mayer, L.W. Use of plasmid profiles in epidemiologic surveillance of disease outbreaks and in tracing the transmission of antibiotic resistance. *Clin. Microbiol. Rev.* 1:228, 1988.

141. McConkey, S.J., et al. *Enterobacter cloacae* in a haematology/oncology ward—first impressions. *J. Hosp. Infect.* 14:277, 1989.

142. McGeer, A., et al. Use of molecular typing to study the epidemiology of *Serratia marcescens*. *J. Clin. Microbiol.* 28:55, 1990.

143. McGowan, J.E., Jr. Environmental factors in nosocomial infection: A selective focus. *Rev. Infect. Dis.* 3:760, 1981.

144. McGowan, J.E., Jr. Changing etiology of nosocomial bacteremia and fungemia and other hospital-acquired infections. *Rev. Infect. Dis.* 7 (Suppl. 3): S357, 1985.

145. McGowan, J.E., Jr. Role of the Microbiology Laboratory in Prevention and Control of Nosocomial Infection (Chapter 11). In: E.H. Lennette, A. Ballows, W.J. Hausler, Jr., and H.J. Shadomy. (Eds.), *Manual of Clinical Microbiology* (4th ed.). Washington, D.C.: American Society for Microbiology, 1985. P.110.

146. McGowan, J.E., Jr. Gram-positive bacteria: Spread and antimicrobial resistance in university and community hospitals in the USA. *J. Antimicrob. Chemother.* 21 (Suppl. C): 49, 1988.

147. McGowan, J.E., Jr. Infection control—a plan for the 1990's. *Am. J. Infect. Control* 18:29, 1990.

148. McGowan, J.E., Jr. Laboratory Approach to an Outbreak of Nosocomial Infection: Systems and Techniques for Investigation. In: K.R. Cundy, B. Kleger, E. Hinks, and L.A. Miller (Eds.), *Infection Control: Dilemmas and Practical Solutions*. New York: Plenum, 1990. P.21.

149. McGowan, J.E., Jr. Communication with Hospital Staff. In: A. Balows, et al., (Eds.), *Manual of Clinical Microbiology* (5th ed.). Washington, DC: American Society for Microbiology, 1991. Pp.151–158.

150. McGowan, J.E., Jr., et al. Nosocomial infections with gentamicin-resistant *Staphylococcus aureus:* Plasmid analysis as an epidemiologic tool. *J. Infect. Dis.* 140:864, 1979.

151. McGowan, J.E., Jr., Hall, E.C., and Parrott, P.L. Antimicrobial susceptibility in gram-negative bacteremia: Are nosocomial isolates really more resistant? *Antimicrob. Agents Chemother.* 33:1855, 1989.

152. Medcraft, J.W., and New, C.W. False-positive Gram-stained smears of sterile body fluids due to contamination of laboratory deionized water. *J. Hosp. Infect.* 16:75, 1990.

153. Molnar, P.A. Epidemiology system for clinical microbiology. *Clin. Microbiol. Newsletter* 11:172, 1989.

154. Monsur, K.A., Begum, Y.A., Ahmed, Z.U., and Rahman, S. Evidence of multiple infections in cases of diarrhea due to enterotoxigenic *Escherichia coli. J. Infect. Dis.* 159:144, 1989.

155. Morgan, M.G., and Harte-Barry, M.J. Methicillin-resistant *Staphylococcus aureus:* A

ten-year survey in a Dublin hospital. *J. Hosp. Infect.* 14:357, 1989.

156. Morris, G.K., and Wells, J.G. Colicin typing of *Shigella sonnei. Appl. Microbiol.* 27:312, 1974.

157. Mukwaya, G.M., and Welch, D.F. Subgrouping of *Pseudomonas cepacia* by cellular fatty acid composition. *J. Clin. Microbiol.* 27:2640, 1989.

158. Murray, B.E., et al. Comparison of genomic DNAs of different enterococcal isolates using restriction endonucleases with infrequent recognition sites. *J. Clin. Microbiol.* 28:2059, 1990.

159. Murray, J.E., Karchmer, A.W., and Moellering, R.C., Jr. Diphtheroid prosthetic valve endocarditis: A study of clinical features and infecting organisms. *Am. J. Med.* 69:838, 1980.

160. Naides, S.J. Infection control measures for human parvovirus B190 in the hospital setting. *Infect. Control Hosp. Epidemiol.* 10:326, 1989.

161. National Committee for Clinical Laboratory Standards. *Methods for Dilution Antimicrobial Susceptibility Tests for Bacteria that Grow Aerobically (M7–A2)* (2nd ed.). Villanova, PA: NCCLS, 1990.

162. National Committee for Clinical Laboratory Standards. *Performance Standards for Antimicrobial Disk Susceptibility Tests (M2–A4)* (4th ed.). Villanova, PA: NCCLS, 1990.

163. Neumann, M.A., Sahm, D.F., Thornsberry, C., and McGowan, J.E., Jr. *Cumitech 6A—New Developments in Antimicrobial Susceptibility Testing. A Practical Guide.* Washington, DC: American Society for Microbiology, February, 1991.

164. Nocera, D., et al. Characterization by DNA restriction endonuclease analysis of *Listeria monocytogenes* strains related to the Swiss epidemic of Listeriosis. *J. Clin. Microbiol.* 28: 2259, 1990.

165. Onokodi, J.K., and Wauters, G. Capsular typing of *Klebsiella* by coagglutination and latex agglutination. *J. Clin. Microbiol.* 13:609, 1981.

166. Opal, S.M., et al. Investigation of a foodborne outbreak of salmonellosis among hospital employees. *Am. J. Infect. Control* 17:141, 1989.

167. Owen, R.J. Chromosomal DNA fingerprinting—a new method of species and strain identification applicable to microbial pathogens. *J. Med. Microbiol.* 30:89, 1989.

168. Patterson, J.E., et al. Gentamicin resistant plasmids of enterococci from diverse geographic areas are heterogeneous. *J. Infect. Dis.* 158:212, 1988.

169. Penner, J.L., and Hennessy, J.N. O-antigen grouping of *Morganella morganii (Proteus morganii)* by slide agglutination. *J. Clin. Microbiol.* 10:8, 1979.

170. Pfaller, M.A. Typing Methods for Epidemiological Investigation. In: A. Balows, et al. (Eds.), *Manual of Clinical Microbiology* (5th ed.). Washington, DC: American Society for Microbiology, 1991. Pp.171–182.

171. Pierre, J., et al. Identification of coagulase-negative staphylococci by electrophoretic profile of total proteins and analysis of penicillin-binding proteins. *J. Clin. Microbiol.* 28:443, 1990.

172. Polonelli, L., Archibusacci, J., Sestito, M., and Morace, G. Killer system: A simple method for differentiating *Candida albicans* strains. *J. Clin. Microbiol.* 17:774, 1983.

173. Prado, D., Murray, B.E., Cleary, T.G., and Pickering, L.K. Limitations of using the plasmid pattern as an epidemiological tool for clinical isolates of *Shigella sonnei. J. Infect. Dis.* 155:314, 1987.

174. Rabkin, C.S., et al. *Pseudomonas cepacia* typing systems: Collaborative study to assess their potential in epidemiologic investigations. *Rev. Infect. Dis.* 11:600, 1989.

175. Remick, D.G., Kunkel, S.L., Holbrook, E.A., and Hanson, C.A. Theory and applications of the polymerase chain reaction. *Am. J. Clin. Pathol.* 93(Suppl. 1): S49, 1990.

176. Richardson, J.H., and Barkley, W.E. (Eds.). *Biosafety in Microbiological and Biomedical Laboratories.* Washington, DC: U.S. Government Printing Office Publication 1983-646-010/8285, 1983.

177. Ridgway, E.J., Wilson, A.P.R., and Kelsey, M.C. Preoperative screening cultures in the identification of staphylococci causing wound and valvular infection in cardiac surgery. *J. Hosp. Infect.* 15:55, 1990.

178. Rimland, D., and Alexander, W. Absence of factors associated with significant urinary tract infections caused by coagulase-negative staphylococci. *Diagn. Microbiol. Infect. Dis.* 12:123, 1989.

179. Sahm, D.F., Neumann, M.A., Thornsberry, C., and McGowan, J.E., Jr. *Cumitech 25—Current Concepts and Approaches to Antimicrobial Agent Susceptibility Testing.* Washington, DC: American Society for Microbiology, 1988. Pp.1–17.

180. Saito, H., et al. Identification of various serovar strains of *Mycobacterium avium* complex by using DNA probes specific for *Mycobacterium avium* and *Mycobacterium intercellulare. J. Clin. Microbiol.* 28:1694, 1990.

181. Schaberg, D.R., et al. Nosocomial bacteriuria: A prospective study of case clustering and antimicrobial resistance. *Ann. Intern. Med.* 93:420, 1979.

182. Schaberg, D.R., Weinstein, R.A., and Stamm, W.E. Epidemics of nosocomial urinary tract infection caused by multiply resistant gram-negative bacilli: Epidemiology and control. *J. Infect. Dis.* 133:363, 1976.

183. Schaberg, D.R., and Zervos, M.R. Plasmid analysis in the study of epidemiology of nosocomial gram-positive cocci. *Rev. Infect. Dis.* 8:705, 1986.

184. Schable, B., Olson, D.R., and Smith, P.B. Improved, computer-generated system for pyocin typing of *Pseudomonas aeruginosa*. *J. Clin. Microbiol.* 24:1017, 1986.

185. Schifman, R.B. *ASCP Check Sample— Microbiology: Surveillance for Nosocomial Infections: the Laboratory Component.* Check Sample No. MB89-1 (MB182). Skokie, IL: American Society of Clinical Pathologists, 1989. Pp.1–10.

186. Schmid, J., Voss, E., and Soll, D.R. Computer-assisted methods for assessing strain relatedness in *Candida albicans* by fingerprinting with the moderately repetitive sequence Ca3. *J. Clin. Microbiol.* 28:1236, 1990.

187. Scott, G.M., et al. Outbreaks of multiresistant *Haemophilus influenzae* infection. *Lancet* 335:925, 1990.

188. Senerwa, D., et al. Colonization of neonates in a nursery ward with enteropathogenic *Escherichia coli* and correlation to the clinical histories of the children. *J. Clin. Microbiol.* 27:2539, 1989.

189. Sherertz, R.J., et al. Three-year experience with sonicated vascular catheter cultures in a clinical microbiology laboratory. *J. Clin. Microbiol.* 28:76, 1990.

190. Shlaes, D.M., and Currie-McCumber, C.A. Plasmid analysis in molecular epidemiology: A summary and future directions. *Rev. Infect. Dis.* 8:738, 1986.

191. Simmons, B.P. Centers for Disease Control guidelines for hospital environmental control: Microbiologic surveillance of the environment and of personnel in the hospital. *Infect. Control* 2:145, 1981.

192. Simmons, B.P., and Wong, E.S. Guideline for prevention of nosocomial pneumonia. *Infect. Control* 3:327, 1982.

193. Slifkin, M., and Doyle, R.J. Lectins and their application to clinical microbiology. *Clin. Microbiol. Rev.* 3:197, 1990.

194. Soll, D.R., et al. Multiple *Candida* strains in the course of a single systemic infection. *J. Clin. Microbiol.* 26:1448, 1988.

195. Speert, D.P., et al. Use of a pilin gene probe to study molecular epidemiology of *Pseudomonas aeruginosa*. *J. Clin. Microbiol.* 27:2589, 1989.

196. Stamm, A.M., et al. Listeriosis in renal transplant recipients: Report of an outbreak and review of 102 cases. *Rev. Infect. Dis.* 4:665, 1982.

197. Stevens, D.A., Odds, F.C., and Scherer, S. Application of DNA typing methods to *Candida albicans* epidemiology and correlations with phenotype. *Rev. Infect. Dis.* 12:258, 1990.

198. Storch, G.A., Park, C.S., and Dohner, D.E. RNA fingerprinting of respiratory syncytial virus using ribonuclease protection. Application to molecular epidemiology. *J. Clin. Invest.* 83:1894, 1989.

199. Sullender, W.M., Anderson, L.J., Anderson, K., and Wertz, G.W. Differentiation of respiratory syncytial virus subgroups with cDNA probes in a nucleic acid hybridization assay. *J. Clin. Microbiol.* 28:1683, 1990.

200. Surveillance cultures in neutropenia. Leading-Article. *Lancet* 1:1238, 1989.

201. Sutherland, S. Viral typing. *J. Hosp. Infect.* 11 (Suppl. A): 315, 1988.

202. Swiatlo, E., et al. Survey of multiply resistant *Providencia stuartii* in a chronic care unit. *J. Hosp. Infect.* 9:182, 1987.

203. Tam, J.S.L., et al. Distinct populations of rotaviruses circulating among neonates and older infants. *J. Clin. Microbiol.* 28:1033, 1990.

204. Tannock, G.W., Fuller, R., Smith, S.L., and Hall, M.A. Plasmid profiling of members of the family *Enterobacteriaceae*, lactobacilli, and bifidobacteria to study the transmission of bacteria from mother to infant. *J. Clin. Microbiol.* 28:1225, 1990.

205. Taylor, A.G., et al. Hospital cross-infection with *Listeria monocytogenes* confirmed by phage-typing. *Lancet* 2:1106, 1981.

206. Tenover, F.C. Diagnostic deoxyribonucleic acid probes for infectious diseases. *Clin. Microbiol. Rev.* 1:82, 1988.

207. Thomson-Carter, F.M., and Pennington, T.H. Characterization of coagulase-negative staphylococci by sodium dodecyl sulfate— polyacrylamide gel electrophoresis and immunoblot analyses. *J. Clin. Microbiol.* 27:2199, 1989.

208. Toma, S., et al. Serotyping of *Clostridium difficile*. *J. Clin. Microbiol.* 26:426, 1988.

209. Tram, C., et al. Molecular typing of nosocomial isolates of *Legionella pneumophila* serogroup 3. *J. Clin. Microbiol.* 28:242, 1990.

210. Traub, W.H. *Acinetobacter baumannii* serotyping for delineation of outbreaks of nosocomial cross-infection. *J. Clin. Microbiol.* 27:2713, 1989.

211. U.S. Postal Service. Proposed rule on the mailability of etiologic agents. *Fed. Reg.* 54(March 23): 11970, 1989.

212. Vale, T.A., Gaston, M.A., and Pitt, T.L. Subdivision of O serotypes of *Pseudomonas*

aeruginosa with monoclonal antibodies. *J. Clin. Microbiol.* 26:1779, 1988.

213. Valenstein, P. Turnaround time—can we satisfy clinicians' demands for faster service? Should we try? *Am. J. Clin. Pathol.* 92:705, 1989.

214. Vial, P.A., Kotloff, K.L., and Losonsky, G.A. Molecular epidemiology of rotavirus infection in a room for convalescing newborns. *J. Infect. Dis.* 157:668, 1988.

215. Vila, J., Almela, M., and Jimenez de Anta, M.T. Laboratory investigation of hospital outbreak caused by two different multiresistant *Acinetobacter calcoaceticus* subsp. *anitratus* strains. *J. Clin. Microbiol.* 27:1086, 1989.

216. Wachsmuth, K. Molecular epidemiology of bacterial infections: Examples of methodology and of investigations of outbreaks. *Rev. Infect. Dis.* 8:682, 1986.

217. Wallace, R.J., Jr., et al. Diversity and sources of rapidly growing mycobacteria associated with infections following cardiac surgery. *J. Infect. Dis.* 159:708, 1989.

218. Wallace, R.W., Jr., et al. *Haemophilus influenzae* infections in adults: Characterization of strains by serotypes, biotypes, and beta-lactamase production. *J. Infect. Dis.* 144:101, 1981.

219. Washington, J.A., II. Effective use of the microbiology laboratory. *J. Antimicrob. Chemother.* 22(Suppl. A): 101, 1988.

220. Washington, J.A, II, Knapp, C.C., and Sanders, C.C. Accuracy of microdilution and the AutoMicrobic system in detection of beta-lactam resistance in gram-negative bacterial mutants with derepressed beta-lactamase. *Rev. Infect. Dis.* 10:824, 1988.

221. Weinstein, R.A, et al. Factitious meningitis. *J.A.M.A.* 233:878, 1975.

222. Weinstein, R.A., Stamm, W.E., and Anderson, R.L. Early detection of false-positive acid-fast smears. *Lancet* 2:174, 1975.

223. Wenzel, R.P., and Streed, S.A. Surveillance and use of computers in hospital infection control. *J. Hosp. Infect.* 13:217, 1989.

224. Wilkinson, H.W., et al. Reactivity of serum from patients with suspected legionellosis against 29 antigens of *Legionellaceae*, and *Legionella*-like organisms by indirect immunofluorescence assay. *J. Infect. Dis.* 147:23, 1983.

225. Wust, J., Sullivan, N.M., Hardegger, U., and Wilkins, T.D. Investigation of an outbreak of antibiotic-associated colitis by various typing methods. *J. Clin. Microbiol.* 16:1096, 1982.

226. Yagupsky, P., and Nolte, F.S. Quantitative aspects of septicemia. *Clin. Microbiol. Rev.* 3:269, 1990.

227. Zuccarelli, A.J., et al. Diversity and stability of restriction enzyme profiles of plasmid DNA from methicillin-resistant *Staphylococcus aureus. J. Clin. Microbiol.* 28:97, 1990.

10

The Relationship Between the Hospital and the Community

Michael D. Decker
William Schaffner

The hospital has always been, in its essence, an act of community. Hospitals, the structural embodiment of hospitality, originally were established to provide shelter to medieval pilgrims. The hospital's subsequent status as a charitable institution for the housing of the needy, destitute, and infirm in Renaissance times has evolved into its modern role as the institution supported by the community to provide care to the seriously ill. The hospital continues to be a linchpin of the local community—an important social symbol, a focus of community pride, and a major employer, as well as a beneficiary of charitable effort. On a personal level, virtually all persons are born and most will die in a hospital.

This rich 600-year relationship between the hospital and the community has become vastly more complex in the past few decades as a result of changes in the scientific, commercial, and governmental determinants of health care. Hospitals are where the latest laboratory research results are applied to patient care and, as such, they are never very far from the glare of news media attention. Hospitals are big businesses and are regulated as such. They are viewed as important sources of hazardous or offensive—even infectious—waste and are regulated as such. They are viewed as major employers whose employees are at risk of serious occupational illness and are regulated as such. They are viewed as sentinels (and occasionally sources) of infection and are regulated as such.

Although some of these regulatory relationships do not involve infection, an optimum response to any of them will (or ought to) call on the talents of hospital epidemiologists and infection control practitioners. Such persons are the reservoir of expertise within the hospital regarding the collection and evaluation of surveillance data, as well as being those charged with infection control and, often, employee health.

Spread of Infections Between the Hospital and the Community

The hospital is an organic part of the community and, although the characteristic pattern of infections in each differs, infectious events in either may influence the occurrence of infections in the other. This integrated relationship was not appreciated when nosocomial infections first received serious attention.

History of Nosocomial Infection Recognition and Spread

Before World War II and for a short period thereafter, hospital-acquired infections were recognized as an occasional problem, but usually they were believed to be caused by microorganisms that originated in the community. During the decade of the 1950s, hospitals around the world were struck by the well-known nosocomial pandemic of *Staphylococcus aureus* infections. Thus attention shifted to the hospital as a special environment, separate from the community. No matter what was "going around" in the community, staphylococcal infections were prevalent within the hospital. These dire circumstances stimulated intensive laboratory, clinical, and epidemiologic investigation and resulted in the discipline of hospital epidemiology [6].

The nature of nosocomial infections, however, did not remain constant. As the staphylococcal problem receded during the 1960s and other nosocomial infections were recognized, it became clear that infections that occurred within the hospital had consequences for the surrounding populace. The proverbial street was found to run both ways. Microorganisms acquired in the community continued to pose problems of spread within hospitals, but some infections that were acquired in the hospital only appeared after the patient was discharged and now were capable of spreading from former patients to community contacts. As these circumstances became known, hospitals began to fear the adverse

publicity and lawsuits that could result from nosocomial infections, and patients expressed concern about their admission to institutions that no longer were perceived as completely benign (see Chap. 26).

Recent Trends Affecting Nosocomial Infection Spread

Recent trends have exacerbated the potential for transport of infection between the hospital and the community. In particular, the drive to shorten inpatient hospitalizations will mean that nosocomial infections of all types increasingly will become clinically manifest only after discharge. Such infections can be problematic for the community physician, who may not immediately recognize their derivation and that their causative bacteria are likely to be resistant to usual first-line antibiotics. In addition, resistant hospital-acquired organisms have been demonstrated to spread from patients to their community contacts. For example, infants colonized by enteric organisms containing antibiotic-resistance plasmics were followed after their discharge from an intensive care nursery. After 12 months, nearly half of the infants continued to carry these multiresistant organisms, and one-third of their family members also had acquired the same plasmid-positive strains in their fecal flora. No family members of a control group of infants were colonized with such bacilli [3].

Increasingly, discharge from the hospital—particularly for the debilitated patients most likely colonized with nosocomial pathogens—is to a nursing home. It has become evident that nursing homes all too frequently have their own endemic problems of infection with resistant organisms (see Chap. 24). Inevitably, some such patients are readmitted to an acute-care hospital, carrying with them their resistant flora. Although resistant gram-negative bacilli participate in this cycle, it is more often methicillin-resistant *Staphylococcus aureus* (MRSA) (see Chap. 13) [13]. In some communities, this cycle has led to an adversarial situation, with both hospital and nursing home resisting accepting the patients of the other. This is a battle often won by the nursing home, to the detriment of the economic health of the hospital. The diplomatic skill of the infection control staff can be essential to the hospital in managing these situations.

The national trend toward performing increasingly elaborate surgical procedures on an outpatient basis and toward early discharge of inpatients further increases the likelihood that substantial numbers of nosocomial infections will become manifest in the community rather than in the hospital. This carries two important consequences. First, the infection control team is much less likely to become aware of the infection and thus less likely to detect adverse trends and implement corrective actions promptly. Second, those witnessing the clinical manifestations of the infections (e.g., family rather than nursing staff) are less likely to appreciate their implications immediately or to institute appropriate management.

Indications for Improved Surveillance and Control of Nosocomial Infections

Procedures for the surveillance and control of nosocomial infections were developed and tested for hospitalized patients, and they are not directly applicable to patients outside the hospital (see Chap. 4). Because the emphasis on both prompt discharge and ambulatory care will not likely abate, infection control staff now are exploring strategies to allow better detection of nosocomial infections in patients who have left the hospital building [12]. In one of our institutions, every patient undergoing an outpatient surgical procedure is sent home with a simple postage-paid form to return to the epidemiology department in the event of fever, wound redness or discharge, or symptoms of urinary tract infection or pneumonia; the form also urges the patient to contact his or her physician promptly. Such a patient-based surveillance system complements physician-based reporting of postdischarge nosocomial infections; we have found that neither alone is adequate.

The substantial success of the national childhood immunization programs has produced a growing cohort of young adults who were never exposed to the natural illnesses

that now are vaccine-preventable. It is clear, however, that a substantial proportion of young adults remain susceptible to measles, mumps, rubella, or other vaccine-preventable diseases because they neither received the vaccine nor were ever exposed to the natural infection. Not surprisingly, some of these young adult susceptibles find employment within hospitals, and hospital staff have played important roles in the propagation of these infections (see Chap. 3).

An early example occurred at the University of Colorado Medical Center, where two small outbreaks of pertussis that originated among children in the community spread to house officers and nurses, then spread additionally from them to children in the outpatient department and to other adults [11]. Thus the disease originating in the community was transmitted in the hospital and spread back out into the community.

Before rubella immunization of hospital personnel became commonplace, there were several reports of physicians and nurses transmitting this viral infection to patients, some of whom were pregnant [9]. Measles has provided the most dramatic recent example: Major outbreaks in several large cities have involved spread within hospitals, both to staff and susceptible patients [4]. Immunization of susceptible staff remains the mainstay of prevention (see Chap. 3) [7].

Community outbreaks of chickenpox are an almost annual event. Introductions of varicella into the hospital occur rather commonly, and the ease with which chickenpox can spread on pediatric wards makes it an especially vexing problem [10, 16]. Children who are incubating the infection may be admitted for elective surgery, for example, and move freely about the ward, exposing numerous patients and staff. We also have observed hospital personnel who continued to work despite their having chickenpox. Typically this occurred because they had mild illnesses with modest fever and only a few skin lesions. Nosocomial chickenpox presents a serious threat to immunocompromised children, who constitute a growing proportion of the hospitalized pediatric population.

The long-term decline in tuberculosis case rates has had the paradoxical effect of increasing the occupational risk of tuberculosis for hospital staff (see Chap. 3). First, virtually all of the old tuberculosis hospitals have been closed, thereby requiring that general hospitals undertake the care of patients with active tuberculosis. Second, hospital workers are now more apt to be susceptible (tuberculin-negative) and thus at risk of acquiring infection when exposed to tubercle bacilli. Third, the diagnosis of subtle forms of reactivation tuberculosis among the elderly may be delayed, resulting in the close exposure of personnel. Fourth, the acquired immunodeficiency syndrome (AIDS) epidemic has brought into the hospital a new cohort of patients with a remarkable prevalence of contagious tuberculosis. Contemporary technology may amplify the hazard: Air-handling systems can efficiently spread airborne disease, and innovative therapy such as inhaled pentamidine can place nearby workers and patients at risk both for tuberculosis and for toxic exposures [2].

Salmonella infections are notorious for their ability to spread within hospitals. A few years ago, a pediatric ward of a midwestern hospital experienced a prolonged outbreak of salmonellosis that was initiated when a child with *Salmonella* gastroenteritis was admitted. Transmission was accomplished by contact spread, most likely by the hands of medical attendants. It is of special interest that the epidemic extended beyond the hospital to a foundling home and to another hospital when infected patients or their community contacts were admitted to those secondary facilities.

Relationship of the Hospital with External Authorities

As mentioned previously, it is no longer sufficient for the hospital epidemiology staff to limit their responsibility regarding relations with outside authorities to the traditional contacts with the public health authorities. New regulatory initiatives in the areas of solid waste, toxic discharges, occupational health, and review of the quality and utilization of medical care demand the involvement of the epidemiology team. Some of these initiatives relate directly to the classic functions of the infection control unit; others are best managed with strong input from those with epidemiologic expertise. Indeed, these nontraditional regulators are likely to occupy an extraordinary measure of the energies of the infection control team in the next decade. Table 10-1 delineates some of the more important external authorities and the focus of their activities.

The Public Health Authorities

The most well-developed and collaborative of these relationships remain those between the hospital and the public health authorities. The health authorities look to the hospital for the reporting of specified sporadic or epidemic diseases. In turn, the hospital looks to health authorities for assistance in three infection control areas: consultation on the establishment of a useful program, training of personnel to carry out the program, and assistance in the investigation of epidemics.

It has long been recognized that a system of prompt and accurate notification of the occurrence of certain communicable diseases was a requisite to their control. In 1883, the state of Michigan adopted legislation establishing a system of communicable disease reporting, and all other states have since followed suit. These laws have been determined by the courts on numerous occasions not to violate the special nature of the doctor-patient relationship.

These reporting systems are pluralistic: Typically, physicians, hospitals, and laboratory directors (even those within hospitals) each have an independent obligation to notify the public health authorities of any patients known or reasonably suspected to have certain illnesses. It is important for several reasons that hospitals develop a system of disease notification. First, not only do these reporting requirements have the force of law

Table 10-1. A sample of external accrediting, regulating, licensing, or standards-setting entities that affect hospitals

Identity	*Purpose and examples*
Federal agencies	
Bureau of Alcohol, Tobacco and Firearms	License for ethanol in pharmacy
Drug Enforcement Administration	Regulate dispensing of controlled drugs
Environmental Protection Agency	Regulate waste disposal
Food and Drug Administration	Audit institutional review board
Federal Aviation Administration	License heliport
Federal Communications Commission	License radio communications systems
Health Care Financing Administration (Medicare, PROs, etc.)	Regulate quality and utilization for Medicare/Medicaid
Occupational Safety and Health Administration	Regulate workers' exposure to bloodborne hazards, chemicals, radiation
State agencies	
Various entities, usually included within the state health department	Hospital license
	Broad regulation of hospital activities
	Certificates of need for capital expenditures
	Air resources management (incinerators)
	Solid-waste management
	Water resources management (liquid effluents and nearby waterways)
	Trauma center designation and coordination
	Licensure of laboratory and other components
	Radiologic materials licenses and inspection
	Elevator inspection and licensure
	Boiler inspection and licensure
Agriculture department	Pest control inspections
Board of pharmacy	License pharmacy
Insurance commissioner	Self-insurance for workers' compensation
Municipal agencies	
Fire department	Inspect fire pump, local hydrants, codes compliance
Health department	Inspect boilers, incinerators, cafeteria, etc.
Solid-waste management department	Regulate solid-waste disposal
Water and sewer department	Inspect meters and backflow preventers; regulate conduct
Private agencies	
Joint Commission on Accreditation of Healthcare Organizations	Overall accreditation
American Association of Blood Banks	Blood bank standards and accreditation
College of American Pathologists	Laboratory standards and accreditation
National accrediting agencies for in-house training programs	Accredit medical student, house staff, nursing, technologist training programs

but, further, compliance with them is usually reviewed by licensing authorities and is a component of the recently revised standards for infection control of the Joint Commission on Accreditation of Healthcare Organizations (JCAHO). Second, by reporting promptly, hospitals can be of assistance to the public health authorities in the control of communicable disease in their own communities. Third, by educating the staff physicians and employees of this responsibility, the hospital becomes an advocate of good preventive medical practice. Fourth, the hospital's unique role enables it to be a major contributor to the state and national morbidity data collection mechanism, which determines funding priorities for research and control activities. Finally, as medicine's capacity to prevent disease increases, there will be a consequent increasing need for precise information on disease occurrence. The recent histories of Legionnaires' disease, toxic shock syndrome, AIDS, and measles resurgence illustrate these points all too clearly. Table 10-2 provides a representative list of reportable conditions.

We have recently reviewed the procedures for disease reporting in our institutions and have found that the traditional mechanisms were no longer sufficiently comprehensive (see Chap. 4). Reporting based on laboratory isolates or serologic results is vital, yet a system based solely on laboratory reports misses all those diseases for which diagnosis does not depend on the laboratory. Reports from the emergency room are essential for those reportable diseases that often do not require admission (animal bites and foodborne illnesses, for example). Reports generated from routine infection control surveillance are valuable, but in few institutions would the infection control team be assured of reviewing every pertinent chart. Medical records–based surveillance represents the final opportunity to detect the reportable illness; however, not only is it tardy but it often misses a reportable diagnosis that is secondary to the principal problem. We have established a surveillance and reporting system incorporating each of these elements, with all internal reporting directed to the epidemiology department, which has sole responsibility for reporting to the public health authorities. This minimizes duplicate reporting, ensures the earliest possible reports, generates a comprehensive centralized log of reports for review by relevant agencies, and ensures that those charged with infection control are cognizant of the presence in the hospital of patients with these reportable (and, usually, communicable) diseases.

In addition to the foregoing, we participate in several special surveillance programs including an influenza surveillance system organized by the state health department, and the National Nosocomial Infection Surveillance (NNIS) System of the Centers for Disease Control (CDC) (see Chap. 27). Through such programs, we enhance our own skills and further our community's ability to coordinate the prevention of illness.

So much for the hospital's assistance to the

Table 10-2. Reportable diseases in Tennessee

Reportable by name, address, race, sex, and age of the patient
Acquired immunodeficiency syndrome
Botulism
Brucellosis
Campylobacteriosis
Cholera
Congenital rubella syndrome
Diphtheria
Encephalitis
   Arthropodborne
   Other infectious forms
Giardiasis, acute
Gonorrhea
Legionellosis
Leprosy
Leptospirosis
Lyme disease
Malaria
Measles
Meningitis
   Meningococcal
   Other bacterial forms
Plague
Poliomyelitis
Psittacosis
Rabies, human
Reye's syndrome
Rocky Mountain spotted fever
Rubella
Salmonellosis
   Typhoid fever
   Other
Shigellosis
Syphilis
Tetanus
Toxic shock syndrome
Trichinosis
Tuberculosis, all forms
Tularemia
Typhus
Disease outbreaks
Foodborne
Related to industrial substances
Waterborne
Reportable by number of cases
Chickenpox
Influenza
Meningitis, aseptic

public health authorities; what of the authorities' assistance to hospitals? The first level of support is the closest—the local, regional, or state public health departments. Although the interest and ability of these entities to provide meaningful help to hospital infection control programs has increased considerably in recent years, it still varies widely from jurisdiction to jurisdiction. Health departments and hospitals have largely gone their separate ways in our society, the first concerned with public health and the second with diagnostics and therapeutics. Therefore, the infection control affairs of the hospital often are not believed to be a major concern of the health department. Even when such an interest is acknowledged, implementation may be difficult for several reasons. Health departments have traditional responsibilities of impressive diversity and must work within the constraints of tight budgets. Furthermore, the doctors and nurses in the health department may not be comfortable in the highly technologic milieu of the contemporary hospital. Small wonder, then, that local health authorities have been hesitant to open the Pandora's box of nosocomial infection. Hospitals, in turn, value their independence and frequently are wary of close associations with government agencies.

Appropriate laboratory support is essential to the investigation of all but the simplest hospital outbreaks (see Chap. 9). Most health department laboratories are reference laboratories, although they may process clinical specimens in such circumscribed areas as *Salmonella, Shigella,* and gonococcal bacteriology. The techniques required to perform primary isolation of hospital pathogens from diverse clinical specimens, environmental sampling, and antimicrobial susceptibility testing usually are not in the public health laboratory's repertoire. On the other hand, state laboratories usually can assist in identifying unusual organisms and can often provide specialized assays useful in investigating suspected outbreaks. Furthermore, the pathway to the reference laboratories of the CDC generally lies through the state laboratory.

Some state health departments have invested considerable effort in establishing programs for the control of nosocomial infections. Their program content varies, but most have sponsored training courses that emphasize the basic epidemiologic and laboratory aspects of infection control. Some also employ infection control practitioners who are able to provide advice to individual hospitals about their infection control problems.

A recent example has demonstrated that imaginative local health department officials can provide dynamic leadership in circumstances that combine aspects of nosocomial infection control and community public health. Physicians in New York were among the first to recognize patients with the syndrome now known as AIDS. In addition to their many other contributions to the investigation of this new disease entity, health officials in New York offered a unique service: The Department of Health provided a monthly forum in which the many investigators in the city could share their new information about the clinical and laboratory features of AIDS. The forum met with immediate success and became a vital communications link among the investigators and with the health department. As Sencer [15] has aptly stated, "Here, the health department has acted . . . as skeleton, with the muscle coming from the community." This example can serve as a model for the synergistic collaboration that can result when health departments and hospitals join resources for a common purpose.

The CDC, through its Hospital Infections Branch, is an important national resource for infection control programs. It generates guidelines that are widely followed, provides assistance to local hospitals and health departments in developing effective programs, offers training courses for personnel, provides sophisticated surveillance of nosocomial infections, and assists in the investigation and control of such infections.

The Food and Drug Administration (FDA) has regulatory authority over industry and the responsibility for recalling products suspected of being contaminated, as well as intervening in the marketing of those products associated with undue adverse reactions. The surveillance systems of hospital epidemiology programs may detect either type of event.

The Regulators of Waste: EPA and Others

Fortunate is the infection control program that has not yet had to wrestle with the issues of infectious waste—fortunate and rare. The New Jersey beach trash washups in the summer of 1988 ultimately were found to be nearly entirely unrelated to hospital waste, yet they unmasked an extraordinary level of public and legislative anxiety on this issue. All hospitals are subject to both municipal and state regulation of solid-waste disposal; most are subject to special regulations for medical or infectious waste; and some are subject to the regulations of the Environmental Protection Agency (EPA) demonstration project (the Medical Waste Tracking Act of 1988: 40 CFR 22, 259) mandated by Congress following the New Jersey debacle.

It must be acknowledged that in the past many hospitals and physicians' offices have been less than rigorous in their disposal of solid wastes. There likely were numerous reasons for this casual approach, including the fact that medical waste had not been associated with either disease or contamination of groundwater as well as the increased costs of more elaborate waste-handling procedures. Nevertheless, in the AIDS era, communities have demanded that hospitals go to great lengths to protect the environment and the populace from feared contamination. Unfortunately, overly elaborate procedures offer no increased protection against infection, but they are very expensive. Hospital infection control programs have two challenges in this regard: to assist in their institution's compliance with local waste disposal regulations and to involve themselves in their community's planning on these issues. To do so may not prevent much infection, but it surely may prevent much waste [14].

The Regulators of Employee Health: OSHA and Others

The Occupational Safety and Health Administration (OSHA) recently has launched a major effort to ensure the safety of employees in the health care industry, with particular focus on infectious and toxic hazards. Under the authority of both the General Duty clause of the OSHA Act (29 USC 651(5)(a)(1)) as well as the OSHA Bloodborne Hazard Standard (*Fed Reg.* 56: 64003–64174, December 6, 1991) hospitals will undergo regular rigorous inspections. Failure to meet the applicable standards may result in adverse publicity and substantial fines.

An OSHA inspection will consist of at least the following components: an evaluation of the infection control plan, the employee health program, the employee training program, and of the monitoring and management of toxic, radioactive, infectious, sharp, and other wastes; a walkaround inspection of the facility; inspection of employee health charts, immunization records, and injury logs; verification of the availability of personal protective equipment; and private interviews of randomly selected employees to establish that they know the policies, know how to follow them, are able to follow them, and agree that they are followed. Hospitals commonly prepare for periodic JCAHO accreditation visits by conducting their own mock surveys; we recommend similar preparation for an OSHA inspection.

The Regulators of Quality and Utilization: JCAHO, HCFA, and Others

It may seem that the issues of quality assurance and utilization review are of little pertinence in a textbook on infection control. However, it is clear that major changes are occurring in these areas that can have profound implications for infection control practitioners and hospital epidemiologists. Both the Health Care Financing Administration (HCFA) and especially the JCAHO are developing an entirely new approach to accreditation review. Spurred by the revolution in industrial quality control initiated in postwar Japan by W. Edwards Deming [8] and others, which now has been adopted widely in U.S. industry, the JCAHO's *Agenda for Change* will depend heavily on the concepts of statistical process control and continuous quality improvement [1]. These new approaches are strongly dependent on those analytical thought processes and skills that have served infection control and hospital epidemiology so successfully. Therefore, it is likely that many engaged in these traditional activities will seek or be sought to broaden their role in the hospital through participation in these new activities as well (see Chap. 2).

Broader Influence of the Hospital Epidemiologist

As a person in the medical community with a heightened interest in preventive medicine, the hospital epidemiologist is occasionally in a position to influence decisions in areas beyond those already described (see Chap. 2). The abolition of tobacco use within the hospital is one example, which has been accomplished at our own and many other institutions. Not only does this present a consistent health message, but it may promote a decrease in tobacco use throughout the community.

Similarly, a number of hospitals that provide pediatric or obstetric services are establishing programs to promote the use of child passenger safety seats among their clients; indeed, in many instances the hospitals provide the seats. It is well known that motor vehicle crashes are the principal cause of death for children and that safety seats are highly successful in preventing such deaths; these programs are in the finest traditions of preventive medicine [5].

Another area in which the epidemiologist can be of assistance is in the immediate management of community contacts of patients with certain infections. A 26-year-old married father of two children, for example, is admitted with meningococcal meningitis. Who is responsible—the attending internist, the pediatrician, or the local health officer—for providing antibiotic prophylaxis to his wife and children? There is no absolute rule, but the hospital epidemiologist can act as an arbiter, providing assurance that this essential preventive medical service is not overlooked.

Finally, it is paradoxical that hospitals, so-ciety's most visible health care institutions, have lagged in providing preventive medical services for their employees. Although OSHA regulations will compel minimum standards in certain aspects of employee health, hospital epidemiologists have the opportunity to persuade hospitals to provide screening programs for hypertension and other coronary risk factors and cervical and breast cancer, as well as to provide comprehensive immunization programs and even family planning services (see Chap. 3). If these were combined with an educational effort, hospitals, long admired for their sophisticated care of sick patients, could make a more comprehensive contribution to medicine's highest goal, the prevention of disease.

References

1. Berwick, D. M. Continuous improvement as an ideal in health care. *N. Engl. J. Med.* 320: 53, 1989.
2. Centers for Disease Control. Guidelines for preventing the transmission of tuberculosis in health-care settings, with special focus on HIV-related issues. *M.M.W.R.* 39(RR-17), 1990.
3. Damato, J. J., Eitzman, D. V., and Baer, H. Persistence and dissemination in the community of R-factors of nosocomial origin. *J. Infect. Dis.* 129:205, 1974.
4. David, R. M., et al. Transmission of measles in medical settings 1980 through 1984. *J.A.M.A.* 255:1295, 1986.
5. Decker, M. D., et al. Failure of hospitals to promote the use of child restraint devices. *Am. J. Dis. Child.* 142:656, 1988.
6. Decker, M. D., and Schaffner, W. Changing trends in infection control and hospital epidemiology. *Infect. Dis. Clin. North Am.* 3:671, 1989.
7. Decker, M. D., and Schaffner, W. Immunization of hospital personnel and other health care workers. *Infect. Dis. Clin. North Am.* 4:211, 1990.
8. Deming, W. E. *Quality, Productivity, and Competitive Position.* Cambridge, MA: Massachusetts Institute of Technology, Center for Advanced Engineering Study, 1982.
9. Greaves, W. L., et al. Prevention of rubella transmission in medical facilities. *J.A.M.A.* 248:861, 1982.
10. Gustafson, T. L., et al. An outbreak of air-

borne nosocomial varicella. *Pediatrics* 70:550, 1982.

11. Kurt, T. L., Yeager, A. S., Guenette, S., and Dunlop, S. Spread of pertussis by hospital staff. *J.A.M.A.* 221:264, 1972.

12. Manian, F. A., and Meyer, L. Comprehensive surveillance of surgical wound infections in outpatient and inpatient surgery. *Infect. Control Hosp. Epidemiol.* 11:515, 1990.

13. Muder, R. R., et al. Methicillin-resistant staphylococcal colonization and infection in a long-term care facility. *Ann. Intern. Med.* 114:107, 1991.

14. Rutala, W. A. Infectious waste. *Infect. Control* 5:149, 1989.

15. Sencer, D. J. Major urban health departments: The ideal and the real. *Health Affairs* 2:88, 1983.

16. Weber, D. J., Rutala, W. A., and Parham, C. Impact and costs of varicella prevention in a university hospital. *Am. J. Public Health* 78:19, 1988.

Universal Precautions and Isolation Systems

Julia S. Garner

Historical Review

Isolation precautions were used in hospitals in the United States even before recommendations for such precautions were published. So-called fever hospitals were opened in the 1700s, primarily during epidemics such as yellow fever, to prevent infection transmission. These were usually closed after the epidemics disappeared or waned [5].

Published recommendations for isolation of patients with communicable diseases appeared in the United States as early as 1877, when a hospital handbook recommended placing patients with communicable diseases in isolation huts [34]. Although patients with communicable diseases were segregated, problems with cross-infection soon resulted because infected patients were not separated from one another according to their disease, and few, if any, aseptic procedures were practiced. As early as 1889, communicable disease hospitals gradually began to combat the problems of cross-infection by setting aside a floor or ward for housing patients with similar communicable diseases [19] and by putting into practice aseptic procedures recommended in nursing textbooks published from 1890 to 1900 [34].

In 1910, isolation practices in the United States were altered by the introduction of the cubicle system for isolating individual patients [19]. With the cubicle system, patients in multiple-bed wards were managed for the first time as if they were in a room by themselves; in addition, hospital personnel used separate gowns, washed their hands with antiseptic solutions after patient contact, and disinfected objects contaminated by the patient. The nursing procedures used with the cubicle system were designed to prevent transmission of pathogenic organisms to other patients and personnel; these procedures became known as *barrier nursing*.

In the 1950s, the contagious disease hospitals and wards gradually began to close, and patients with communicable diseases were provided care in the general hospital setting. In the mid-1960s, tuberculosis hospitals also began to close, partly because general hospital or outpatient treatment became preferred for patients with tuberculosis. Thus, by the late 1960s, patients needing isolation precautions were housed in wards in the general hospital, either in specially designed, single-patient isolation rooms or in regular single- or multiple-patient rooms.

To assist general hospitals with patient isolation procedures, the Centers for Disease Control (CDC) in 1970 published *Isolation Techniques for Use in Hospitals* and revised it in 1975 [8]. This publication was a detailed manual of isolation procedures that could be applied in small community hospitals with limited resources as well as in large metropolitan university-associated medical centers. The manual suggested that hospitals use isolation categories that were determined almost entirely by the epidemiologic features of the diseases, primarily the routes of disease transmission. Certain isolation techniques, believed to be the minimum necessary to prevent transmission of *all* diseases in the category, were indicated for each isolation category. Because all diseases in a category did not have exactly the same epidemiology and some required fewer precautions than others, more precautions were suggested for some patients than were necessary. This disadvantage of "overisolation" for some patients was offset by the convenience of having a small number of categories, all easily understood by most hospital personnel. By the mid-1970s, 93 percent of U.S. hospitals had adopted this approach for isolation precautions [27].

By 1980, despite these precautions, hospitals were experiencing endemic and epidemic nosocomial infection problems, some caused by multiply drug-resistant microorganisms and some caused by newly recognized syndromes, which required different isolation precautions from those specified for an existing category of isolation. Moreover, precautions needed to be directed more specifically at nosocomial infections in special-care units rather than at the intrahospital spread of classic contagious diseases acquired in the community [37]. Furthermore, new facts about the epidemiology of some patients made it appropriate for the CDC to revise the isolation manual. Toward that end, during 1981–1983, CDC Hospital Infections Program personnel consulted with infectious disease specialists in medicine, pediatrics, and surgery, hospital epidemiologists, and infection control practitioners to get advice on revising the isolation precautions.

In 1983, the *CDC Guideline for Isolation Precautions in Hospitals* [23, 24] (hereafter referred to as the *isolation guideline*) was published to take the place of the 1975 isolation manual. In the isolation guideline, recommendations for isolation precautions were modified substantially to reflect new knowledge. For example, many infections were assigned to new categories and three new categories of isolation were added: contact isolation, tuberculosis (acid fast bacilli [AFB]) isolation, and blood and body fluid precautions. In addition, the old isolation category of protective isolation was deleted because it did not appear to be any more effective than strong emphasis on hand-washing when caring for immunologically compromised patients [35].

The most important change in the 1983 isolation guideline, however, was the increased emphasis on decision making. Unlike the 1975 manual [8], which encouraged few decisions on the part of users, the isolation guideline encouraged decision making at several levels [21, 26]. First, hospital Infection Control Committees were offered a choice between category-specific or patient-specific isolation precautions. Second, the physician or nurse who places a patient on isolation precautions was encouraged to make decisions about the individual precautions to be taken (e.g., whether the patient's age, mental status, or condition indicates that a private room is needed to prevent sharing of contaminated articles). Third, personnel taking care of patients on isolation precautions were encouraged to decide whether they would need to wear masks, gowns, or gloves based on the likelihood of exposure to infective material. Such decisions are necessary to isolate the disease but not the patient and to reduce the costs associated with unnecessary isolation precautions.

Recent Developments

In 1985, largely because of the human immunodeficiency virus (HIV) epidemic, isolation practices in the United States were dramatically altered by the introduction of a new strategy to minimize the risk of transmitting bloodborne pathogens in the workplace. The strategy placed emphasis for the first time on applying blood and body fluid precautions universally to all persons regardless of their infection status [10]. Until this time, most patients placed on isolation precautions were those for whom a diagnosis of an infectious disease had been made or suspected. Applying blood and body fluid precautions to *all* persons is now referred to simply as *universal precautions*. In addition to emphasizing the prevention of needle-stick injuries and the use of traditional barriers such as gloves and gowns, universal precautions expanded the old isolation category of blood and body fluid precautions to include use of masks and eye coverings to prevent mucous membrane exposures during certain procedures and use of ventilation devices where the need for resuscitation is predictable. This approach, particularly prevention of mucous membrane exposures, was reemphasized in subsequent CDC reports that contained recommendations for the prevention of transmission of HIV in health care settings [9, 11, 13].

In 1987, one of these reports updated portions of the 1983 CDC isolation guideline [11]. The report stated that implementation of universal precautions for *all* patients eliminates the need for blood and body fluid precautions, as recommended for use in the CDC isolation guideline, for patients known or suspected to be infected with bloodborne pathogens. However, the report stated that other category- or disease-specific isolation precautions recommended in the CDC guideline should be used as necessary for prevention of nonbloodborne pathogens.

The 1987 report was updated in 1988 to include, in addition to HIV, hepatitis B virus (HBV) and other bloodborne pathogens [14]. The 1988 report emphasized two important points: (1) Blood is the single most important source of HIV, HBV, and other bloodborne pathogens in the occupational setting, and (2) infection control efforts for preventing transmission of bloodborne pathogens in the workplace must focus on preventing exposures to blood as well as on delivery of HBV immunization. The report also clarified that universal precautions, as recommended by the CDC, apply to blood, to body fluids that have been implicated in the transmission of bloodborne infections (semen and vaginal secretions), to body fluids from which the risk of transmission is unknown (amniotic, cerebrospinal, pericardial, peritoneal, pleural, and synovial fluids), and to any body fluid visibly contaminated with blood.

In 1987, an alternative system of isolation and universal precautions, called *body substance isolation,* was proposed by the Harborview Medical Center in Seattle and the University of California at San Diego [33]. Unlike the universal precautions recommended by the CDC, which focus primarily on blood and body fluids that have been implicated in the transmission of bloodborne pathogens, body substance isolation focuses on the isolation of all moist body substances (blood, feces, urine, sputum, saliva, wound drainage, and other body fluids) from all patients. Additional precautions are recommended for diseases that have an airborne component of transmission. Body substance isolation is described in more detail later in this chapter.

In 1989, continuing concerns about transmission of bloodborne pathogens in the workplace prompted the Occupational Safety and

Health Administration (OSHA) to publish proposed regulations regarding exposure to bloodborne pathogens in hospitals and other health care settings [15]. The proposed regulations are based on the CDC concept of universal precautions, and they contain many of the recommendations published by the CDC for preventing the transmission of bloodborne pathogens in the workplace. Although the regulations are not yet enforceable, OSHA has the authority to conduct inspections of hospitals to ensure safe working environments. Until OSHA's final regulations become official, at a minimum CDC recommendations for universal precautions should be implemented in health care settings in the United States.

Universal Precautions

Universal precautions are intended to prevent parenteral, mucous membrane, and nonintact skin exposures to bloodborne pathogens in health care settings. In addition, immunization with HBV vaccine is recommended as an important adjunct to universal precautions for persons who have exposures to blood (see Chap. 3).

Universal precautions include the following components:

1. Gloves should be worn for touching blood and other specified body fluids requiring universal precautions (amniotic fluid, pericardial fluid, peritoneal fluid, pleural fluid, synovial fluid, semen, vaginal secretions, and any body fluid visibly contaminated with blood); for touching mucous membranes and nonintact skin of *all* patients; for handling items or surfaces soiled with blood or body fluids requiring universal precautions; and for performing vascular access or invasive procedures. Gloves should be changed after contact with each patient. Hands should be washed immediately after gloves are removed.
2. Hands and other skin surfaces should be washed immediately and thoroughly if contaminated with blood or other body fluids requiring universal precautions.
3. Special care should be taken to prevent injuries caused by needles, scalpels, and other sharp instruments or devices during procedures and during handling, cleaning, or disposal after procedures. To prevent needle-stick injuries, needles should not be recapped, purposely bent or broken by hand, removed from disposable syringes, or otherwise manipulated by hand. After they are used, disposable syringes and needles, scalpel blades, and other sharp items should be placed in puncture-resistant containers for disposal; the puncture-resistant containers should be located as close as practical to the use area. Large-bore reusable needles should be placed in a puncture-resistant container for transport to the reprocessing area.
4. Masks and protective eyewear or face shields should be worn to prevent exposure of mucous membranes of the mouth, nose, and eyes during procedures that are likely to generate droplets of blood or other body fluids requiring universal precautions.
5. Gowns or aprons should be worn during procedures that are likely to generate splashes or sprays of blood or other body fluids requiring universal precautions.
6. Mouthpieces, resuscitation bags, or other ventilation devices should be available for use in areas in which the need for resuscitation is predictable.
7. Health care workers who have exudative lesions or weeping dermatitis should refrain from all direct patient care and from handling patient care equipment until the condition resolves.
8. Linen and articles soiled with blood or bloody body fluids should be placed and transported in bags that prevent leakage.
9. Category-specific or disease-specific isolation precautions, described later in this chapter, should be used as necessary if infections other than bloodborne infections are diagnosed or suspected.

Definition of Isolation Precautions

The term *isolation precautions* is being used in its broadest sense—that is, to define steps to prevent the spread of an infectious agent from an infected or colonized person to another person. In this context, isolation precautions should be considered a continuum ranging from the most to the least demanding. They include private rooms or roommate selection; protective barriers such as masks, gowns, and gloves; special emphasis on hand-washing; and special handling of contaminated articles. Primarily because of epidemiologic differences among diseases, these precautions may be critical to prevent spread of some diseases but may not be necessary for other diseases. No attempt is made here to define the epidemiology of individual infections because such information is available in many standard references. However, the uses of the most important isolation precautions are discussed.

Hand-Washing

Hand-washing is the single most important means of preventing the spread of infection. Hands should be washed, even if gloves are used, after touching any infective material and after taking care of any infected patient or patient colonized by multiply drug-resistant bacteria. If done properly, hand-washing generally removes organisms acquired from infected patients. Use of antimicrobial-containing products for hand-washing is not necessary when caring for infected patients, but these agents may provide an extra margin of safety.

Patient's Room

Private rooms are useful as an isolation precaution because they separate patients and lessen the chance of infection transmission by any route. Most patients infected with organisms that can be transmitted by air should be placed in private rooms. However, patients infected with organisms spread by direct contact do not need private rooms unless the organisms frequently cause serious disease if transmitted or the infected patient has poor hygienic habits. A patient with poor hygienic habits is defined as a patient who does not wash hands after touching infective material (blood, feces, purulent drainage, or secretions), contaminates the environment, or shares contaminated articles. Such patients may include children, patients who have altered mental status, and those who are likely to bleed profusely and cause environmental contamination. Even when private rooms are indicated, patients infected or colonized by the same organism can share a room if no other secondary infection or condition is present that would preclude such sharing. Sharing a room (cohorting) may be necessary during epidemics when private rooms are not readily available.

Sometimes a private room with special ventilation is indicated as an isolation precaution because the organism is spread by air and frequently causes severe infections. Special ventilation is characterized by (1) negative air pressure in the room in relation to the anteroom or hall, (2) a minimum of six air changes per hour, and (3) special handling of ventilation air from the room, either by discharging the air outdoors where it will be well diluted or subjecting it to high-efficiency filtration before circulating it to other areas. Proper installation, testing, and meticulous maintenance are critical if a high-efficiency filtration system is used [2]. Additional specifications that reduce microbial contamination of air are recommended for hospitals or other inpatient facilities that provide treatment or care for patients known or suspected to have infectious tuberculosis [6].

Even when a private room is not indicated as an isolation precaution, special emphasis is placed on choosing the room and roommate for an infected patient. Generally, infected patients should not share a room with a patient who is likely to become infected or for whom consequences of infection are likely to be serious. Such patients include those who are immunocompromised or who are about to undergo extensive surgery with insertion of prosthetic devices.

Protective Clothing and Equipment for Health Care Personnel

Use of masks is intended to prevent transmission of infectious agents through the air. Masks protect the wearer from inhaling (1) large-particle aerosols (droplets) that are transmitted by close contact and generally travel only short distances (up to approximately 3 feet) and (2) small-particle aerosols (droplet nuclei) that remain suspended in the air and thus may travel longer distances. High-efficiency disposable surgical masks are more effective than cotton-gauze or paper-tissue masks in preventing airborne and droplet spread. Masks generally lose some efficiency when they are wet or after being worn for prolonged periods. When masks are used, they should fit well and cover both the nose and the mouth. Disposable particulate respirators have recently been recommended for use by health care workers who must share air space with a patient who has infectious tuberculosis because standard surgical masks may not fit well enough to provide a tight face seal and to filter out particulates of the droplet nucleus size [6]. Although particulate respirators provide a better facial fit and better filtration capability than standard surgical masks, the efficiency of particulate respirators in protecting susceptible persons from infection with tuberculosis has not been demonstrated.

Gowns are indicated as an isolation precaution when soiling of clothes with infective material is likely, because such soiling can potentially transmit infection to personnel or patients. When gowns are indicated, they should be worn only once and discarded rather than saved for reuse. If large splashes or quantities of infective material are present or anticipated, impervious gowns or aprons should be worn.

Gloves are used for several reasons. First, gloves should reduce the incidence of hand contamination with infective material. Second, gloves reduce the possibility that personnel will become infected with organisms from infected patients; for example, gloves may prevent personnel from developing herpetic

whitlow after touching mucous membranes or oral secretions contaminated by herpes simplex virus. Third, gloves also reduce the likelihood that personnel will transmit microbial flora from their hands to patients, either their own endogenous flora or that transiently acquired from infected patients or the environment. However, gloves are not the only means to prevent transmission of transiently acquired organisms; good hand-washing eliminates these organisms and interrupts transmission without the use of gloves. Nonetheless, gloves are often recommended as an extra isolation precaution, because personnel frequently do not wash hands when they should [1].

Special Handling of Articles and Equipment

Isolation precautions often include special handling of used articles. Some used articles may need to be enclosed in a bag before they are removed from the room or cubicle. Such bagging is intended to prevent inadvertent exposures of personnel to articles contaminated with infective material and to prevent contamination of the environment. Most articles do not need to be bagged unless they are contaminated (or likely to be contaminated) with infective material. One bag is adequate if the bag is sturdy (not easily penetrated) and prevents leaking of infective material and if the article can be placed in the bag without contaminating the outside of the bag; otherwise, two bags (double bagging) should be used.

Disposable or reusable patient care equipment can be used for patients on isolation precautions. Using disposable equipment reduces the possibility that equipment will serve as a vehicle for transmission, but such equipment must be disposed of safely and adequately. Disposable equipment that is contaminated (or likely to be contaminated) with infective material should be bagged, labeled or color-coded, and disposed of according to hospital policy for disposal of infective waste (see Chap. 15). Local regulations may call for incineration or disposal in an authorized sanitary landfill. Ideally, reusable patient care equipment should be returned to a central processing area for decontamination and reprocessing by trained personnel (see Chap. 16). When contaminated with infective material, equipment should be bagged and labeled or color-coded before being removed from the patient's room or cubicle and should remain bagged until it is ready for decontamination and reprocessing.

Although soiled linen may be contaminated with pathogenic microorganisms, the risk of actual disease transmission is negligible. Rather than rigid procedures and specifications, hygienic storage and processing of clean and soiled linen is recommended. Soiled linen from all patients should be handled as little as possible and with minimum agitation to prevent gross microbial contamination of the air and of persons handling the linen. Soiled linen should be put in a laundry bag in the patient's room or cubicle or at the location where it is used and, if wet, should be transported in bags that prevent leakage.

Disposable or reusable dishes can be used for patients on isolation precautions. The combination of water temperature and dishwasher detergents used in hospital dishwashers is sufficient to decontaminate dishes; therefore, no special precautions are generally indicated for dishes.

Other Considerations

The same general cleaning schedules and methods that are used in other hospital rooms can be used for patients on isolation precautions. Cleaning of walls, blinds, and curtains is not indicated unless they are visibly soiled. Disinfectant fogging is not recommended, and airing the room is not necessary.

Other precautions may be necessary with certain infections but are too specific to be discussed in detail in this chapter [6, 7].

CDC Systems for Isolation Precautions

The CDC currently recommends that hospitals use either category-specific or disease-spe-

cific isolation precautions. Category-specific isolation precautions, recommended by the CDC since 1970, group diseases for which similar isolation precautions are indicated. Disease-specific isolation precautions, recommended by the CDC since 1983, consider each infectious disease individually so that only those precautions (private room, masks, gowns, and gloves) indicated to interrupt transmission of that disease are recommended. Although data on the efficacy of the traditional category-specific isolation precautions and the more recently recommended disease-specific isolation precautions are lacking, few cases of disease transmission are reported when these recommendations are followed. The two systems are compared in Table 11-1.

In deciding between the two systems, hospitals should consider the relative advantages and disadvantages of each approach. Most importantly, the category-specific system is a simpler system requiring personnel to learn only a few established routines for applying isolation precautions. However, because many different diseases are grouped into six categories, unnecessary precautions will be applied to some diseases. Alternatively, the disease-specific system ensures that the only isolation precautions applied are those required to interrupt transmission of the specific infection. Because the set of precautions is individualized to each disease, this system requires more initial training and inservice education and a much higher level of attention from patient care personnel. Disease-specific isolation precautions eliminate overisolation, but personnel may be prone to mistakes in applying them. Adapting disease-specific isolation precautions to a hospital computerized information system has resulted in more accurate use of this system [28]. Both isolation systems use a card displayed near the patient to alert personnel and visitors that special precautions are necessary. In the disease-specific system, an individualized card is prepared that lists the precautions indicated for a given patient. In the category-specific system, standard, preprinted, color-coded instruction cards are

Table 11-1. Comparison of category-specific and disease-specific isolation precautions

Feature	*Category-specific precautions*	*Disease-specific precautions*
Isolation precautions	Six categories, each with a different set of precautions	Individualized for each disease
Instruction card for door or cubicle	Separate, preprinted, color-coded card for each category	One all-purpose card to be individualized for each patient
Advantages	Simpler system; less diagnostic information needed to assign precautions Less decision making needed to assign precautions	Minimizes unnecessary precautions; may reduce cost of placing patient on isolation precautions May encourage compliance, especially by physicians
Disadvantages	Unnecessary precautions taken for some diseases May increase cost of isolation	Requires more skill and responsibility to assign precautions Requires more diagnostic information about disease to assign precautions

used that list the recommended precautions for diseases in a given category.

Category-Specific Isolation Precautions

Six isolation categories are currently recommended for category-specific isolation precautions: strict isolation, contact isolation, respiratory isolation, tuberculosis (AFB) isolation, enteric precautions, and drainage/secretion precautions. A previous category, blood and body fluid precautions [23, 24], was superseded by CDC recommendations for universal precautions in 1987 [11]. In general, a category ending with the term *isolation* is used when a private room is indicated; a category ending with the term *precautions* is used when a private room is optional or not indicated. Let us review the purpose of and specifications for each isolation category.

Strict Isolation

Strict isolation is designed to prevent transmission of highly contagious or virulent infections that may be spread by both air and contact. Rarely indicated, this category is used for patients with pharyngeal diphtheria, Lassa fever or other viral hemorrhagic fevers, pneumonic plague, varicella (chickenpox), and zoster that occurs in an immunocompromised host or is disseminated.

Specifications include the following: a private room is indicated and the door should be

kept closed. Patients infected by the same organism may share a room. Ideally, patients on strict isolation should be placed in a private room with special ventilation (negative air pressure in the room in relation to the anteroom or hall, a minimum of six air changes per hour, and special handling of ventilation air from the room). Masks, gowns, and gloves are indicated for all persons entering the room. Hands must be washed after gloves are removed and before taking care of another patient. Articles contaminated with infective material should be discarded or bagged and labeled before being sent for decontamination and reprocessing.

Contact Isolation

Contact isolation is designed to prevent transmission of highly transmissible or epidemiologically important infections (or colonizations) that do not warrant strict isolation. All diseases or conditions included in this category are spread primarily by close or direct contact. Contact isolation is indicated for (1) pediatric patients with acute respiratory infections, pharyngitis, or pneumonia; (2) newborns with gonococcal conjunctivitis, herpes simplex virus infection, or staphylococcal skin infections; (3) any patient with group A streptococcal endometritis, pneumonia, or skin infection; and (4) any patient with cutaneous diphtheria, disseminated herpes simplex virus infection, infection or colonization by epidemiologically significant multiply drug-resistant bacteria, staphylococcal pneumonia or major skin infections, pediculosis, scabies, rabies, rubella, or vaccinia. Regardless of the pathogens involved, contact isolation is indicated for patients with major skin infections that are draining and cannot be covered adequately with dressings. The inclusion of pediatric respiratory syncytial virus (RSV) infections in this category was based on theoretic reasons and on results of studies available at the time the isolation guideline was being prepared for publication. Since then, several studies comparing the efficacy of measures to control nosocomial transmission of RSV have been published [4, 20, 30, 31, 38]. However, controversy still exists about which isolation precautions should be used for RSV.

Specifications include the following: A private room is indicated. Patients infected by the same organism may share a room unless otherwise contraindicated. During outbreaks, infants and young children with the same respiratory clinical syndrome may share a room. Masks are indicated for those who come close to the patient. Gowns are indicated if soiling is likely. Gloves are indicated for touching infective material. Hands must be washed after removal of gloves and before taking care of another patient. Articles contaminated with infective material should be discarded or bagged and labeled before being sent for decontamination and reprocessing.

Respiratory Isolation

Respiratory isolation is designed to prevent transmission of infectious diseases over short distances through the air (droplet transmission). Direct or indirect contact transmission occurs with some infections in this category but is infrequent. Respiratory isolation is indicated for patients with measles; *Hemophilus influenzae* epiglottiditis, meningitis, or pneumonia in children; serious meningococcal disease (pneumonia, meningitis, sepsis); mumps; and pertussis (whooping cough). The previous recommendation of respiratory isolation for acute erythema infectiosum [23, 24] has

been superseded by a recent report that recommends respiratory isolation for human parvovirus B19 (the causative agent for erythema infectiosum) only when patients are in transient aplastic crisis or are immunodeficient due to chronic human parvovirus B19 infections [12].

Specifications include the following: A private room is indicated. Patients infected with the same organism may share a room unless otherwise contraindicated. Masks are indicated for those who come close to the patient. Gowns and gloves are not indicated. Hands must be washed after touching the patient or potentially contaminated articles and before taking care of another patient. Articles contaminated with infective material should be discarded or bagged and labeled before being sent for decontamination and reprocessing.

Tuberculosis Isolation

Tuberculosis isolation is used for patients suspected or known to have infectious tuberculosis, including laryngeal tuberculosis. This category can be referred to as *AFB* to protect the patient's confidentiality.

Specifications have recently been updated because of heightened concern about preventing nosocomial transmission of multiply drug-resistant tuberculosis, in settings in which persons with HIV infection receive care [6]. The new guidelines emphasize reducing microbial contamination of air by dilution and removal of airborne contaminants, air mixing, and directional air flow, and the importance of wearing appropriate masks when health care workers must share air space with a patient who has infectious tuberculosis. Because some surgical masks may not be effective in preventing inhalation of droplet nuclei, personnel should consider using disposable particulate respirators, which provide a better facial fit and better filtration capability. However, the efficacy of particulate respirators in protecting susceptible persons from infection with tuberculosis has not been demonstrated [6].

In hospitals or other inpatient facilities, any patient suspected or known to have infectious tuberculosis should be placed on AFB isolation in a private room. The room should have at least six total air changes per hour, including at least two outside air changes per hour, with sufficient within-room air distribution to dilute or remove tuberculosis bacilli from locations where health care facility personnel or visitors are likely to be exposed. The direction of air flow should be set up, maintained, and monitored so that air flows into the room from the hallway (negative pressure) to minimize possible spread of tuberculosis bacilli into the general health care setting. Air from the room should be exhausted directly to the outside of the building and away from intake vents and people in accordance with federal, state, and local regulations concerning environmental discharges. Isolation-room doors must be kept closed to maintain control over the direction of air flow. Persons who enter a room in which AFB isolation precautions are in place should wear particulate respirators [6]. Gowns are indicated only if needed to prevent gross contamination of clothing. Gloves are not indicated. Hands must be washed after touching the patient or potentially contaminated articles and before taking care of another patient. Articles are rarely involved in transmission of tuberculosis. However, articles should be thoroughly cleaned, disinfected, or discarded. The CDC guidelines for preventing the transmission of tuberculosis in health care settings [6] should be consulted for additional details beyond the scope of this chapter.

Enteric Precautions
Enteric precautions are designed to prevent infections that are transmitted primarily by direct or indirect contact with fecal material. Enteric precautions are indicated for patients with infectious diarrhea or gastroenteritis caused by amebae, cholera and other *Vibrio* species, *Campylobacter, Cryptosporidium, Dientamoeba, Escherichia coli, Giardia, Salmonella, Shigella, Yersinia enterocolitica,* and other bacteria, enteroviral infections (e.g., pleurodynia, viral meningitis, and poliomyelitis); enterocolitis caused by *Clostridium difficile* or

Staphylococcus aureus; necrotizing enterocolitis of newborns; and hepatitis A.

Specifications include the following: A private room is not indicated unless patient hygiene is poor. Masks are not indicated. Gowns are indicated if soiling is likely. Gloves are indicated for touching infective material. Hands must be washed after removing gloves. Articles contaminated with infective material should be discarded or bagged and labeled before being sent for decontamination and reprocessing.

Drainage/Secretion Precautions
Drainage/secretion precautions are designed to prevent infections transmitted by direct or indirect contact with purulent material or with drainage from an infected body site. Infectious diseases in this category include those resulting in production of infective purulent material, drainage, or secretions, unless the disease is included in another isolation category requiring more rigorous precautions.

Specifications include the following: A private room is not indicated. Masks are not indicated. Gowns are indicated if soiling is likely. Gloves are indicated for touching infective material. Hands must be washed after removing gloves and before taking care of another patient. Articles contaminated with infective material should be discarded or bagged and labeled before being sent for decontamination and reprocessing.

Disease-Specific Isolation Precautions
Specific isolation precautions are indicated to prevent the transmission of most of the common infectious agents and diseases that are likely to be found in U.S. hospitals. Because specific precautions are indicated for more than 150 different diseases, syndromes, or conditions, space does not permit them to be listed in this chapter. They are, however, listed in the CDC isolation guideline [23, 24], along with other pertinent comments about disease-specific isolation precautions. Previously mentioned updates [6, 11, 12, 14], however, must be consulted to ensure that recommendations are current.

Alternative Isolation Systems
Body Substance Isolation

Body substance isolation [33], briefly described earlier, has been proposed as an alternative isolation system to those recommended by the CDC. As its name implies, the system focuses on the isolation of potentially infectious moist body substances (blood, feces, urine, sputum, saliva, wound drainage, and other body fluids).

Body substance isolation, initially described in 1987, is composed of two parts. The first and primary part focuses on the isolation of moist body substances through the use of barrier precautions, primarily gloves; this part is used for all patients regardless of their diagnosis. A single universal reminder sign that defines body substances and describes the barrier precautions to be taken is placed in each single patient room or at the bedside in intensive care units. The second part of body substance isolation is a diagnosis-driven component that is used for patients who have some of the diseases that are transmitted exclusively or in part by airborne transmission; a "stop sign alert" is placed on the doors of patients that have these diseases. The sign instructs anyone wishing to enter the room to check with the floor nurse; the floor nurse then determines whether the person wishing to enter the room needs to wear a mask.

Body substance isolation includes the following [33]:

1. Gloves should be worn for anticipated contact with blood, secretions, mucous membranes, nonintact skin, and moist body substances of all patients. Hand-washing is not necessary when gloves are worn unless the hands become visibly soiled. Gloves should be changed before another patient is treated.
2. After other types of patient contact, hands should be washed.
3. Gowns, plastic aprons, masks, or goggles should be worn when secretions, blood, or body fluids are likely to soil or splash on clothing, skin, or the face.
4. Soiled reusable items, linen, and trash should be contained to prevent leaking. Double bagging is not necessary unless the outside of the bag is visibly soiled.
5. Needles (without recapping them) and sharp items should be placed in puncture-resistant, rigid containers.
6. Private rooms are indicated for patients with some diseases transmitted exclusively or in part by the airborne route, such as pulmonary tuberculosis and other diseases listed in the strict isolation category of the *CDC Guideline for Isolation Precautions in Hospitals* [23, 24]. Private rooms are also indicated for patients who soil articles in the environment with body substances.

In addition to the above, personnel should be immune to or immunized against infectious agents transmitted by airborne or droplet routes (measles, mumps, rubella, and varicella) or should not enter rooms of patients with these infections [33]. Other issues related to implementing body substance isolation in a university teaching hospital have been described [32].

Comparison of Body Substance Isolation with CDC-Recommended Systems

Body substance isolation replaces some, but not all, of the isolation categories and disease specific isolation precautions recommended by the CDC. Body substance isolation does not appear to eliminate the need for contact isolation and respiratory isolation or corresponding disease-specific isolation precautions for diseases that are transmitted by droplet contact occurring as a result of coughing or sneezing by an infected person who has clinical disease or is a carrier of the infectious agent. Transmission of infectious agents by droplets is considered close-contact, rather than airborne, transmission since droplets usually travel no more than 3 feet. Moreover, body substance isolation does not eliminate the need for strict isolation and tuberculosis isolation or corresponding disease-specific isolation precautions recommended by the CDC for diseases that are transmitted by the airborne route of transmission. Airborne transmission occurs by dissemination of either droplet nuclei or dust particles in the air containing the infectious agent.

Body substance isolation incorporates many of the features of universal precautions to prevent transmission of bloodborne pathogens in health-care settings. However, there is one important difference in the indications for glove use and hand-washing. Under universal precautions, gloves are worn for anticipated contact with blood and specified body fluids requiring universal precautions, and hands are washed immediately after gloves are removed. Under body substance isolation, gloves are worn for anticipated contact with any moist body substance, but hand-washing after glove removal is not required unless the hands become visibly soiled due to punctures in the gloves [33]. The lack of emphasis on hand-washing when gloves are removed has been cited as one of the theoretic disadvantages of body substance isolation [22, 25]; using gloves as a substitute for hand-washing may provide a false sense of security, result in less hand-washing, and increase the risk of nosocomial transmission of pathogens because hands are easily contaminated in the process of removing gloves [25]. Although use of gloves may be better than no hand-washing, the efficacy of using gloves as a substitute for hand-washing has not been demonstrated.

Current and Future Trends

During the past several years, most hospitals and health care facilities in the United States and Canada have revised their isolation precautions. Many hospitals have added universal precautions to their traditional isolation system and have incorporated subsequent updates recommended by the CDC. Other hospitals have adopted body substance isolation [33]. Some hospitals have taken components of both and developed systems tailored to their unique needs. Consequently, various universal precautions and isolation systems with various names are being used in hospitals and health care facilities in the United States and Canada [3, 36].

In the future, the final OSHA standard to prevent transmission of bloodborne pathogens in occupational settings may dictate that hospitals and health care facilities make additional changes in their policies and procedures for universal precautions and isolation systems. Further changes may be indicated by new scientific knowledge regarding the epidemiology, transmission, and prevention of infectious diseases in hospitals and health care facilities (for example, the recently published *Guidelines for Preventing the Transmission of Tuberculosis in Health-Care Settings, with Special Focus on HIV-Related Issues* [6]). Concern about the costs of universal precautions [17] and the theoretically even more costly body substance isolation will continue to be raised as more studies assessing their direct costs begin to appear in the scientific literature [16]. Finally, only a few reports have appeared in the literature that address the complex issues of the efficacy of universal precautions and body substance isolation [18, 29, 32, 39].

References

1. Albert, R.K., and Condie, F. Hand-washing patterns in medical intensive care units. *N. Engl. J. Med.* 304:1465, 1981.
2. American Society of Heating, Refrigerating, and Air Conditioning Engineers. *1987 ASHRAE Handbook: Heating, Ventilating, and Air-Conditioning Systems and Applications.* Atlanta: American Society of Heating, Refrigerating, and Air Conditioning Engineers, Inc., 1987. 23.1.
3. Birnbaum, D., et al. Adoption of guidelines for universal precautions and body substance isolation in Canadian acute-care hospitals. *Infect. Control Hosp. Epidemiol.* 11:465, 1990.
4. Brawley, R.L. Infection control practices for preventing respiratory syncytial virus infections. *Infect. Control Hosp. Epidemiol.* 9:103, 1988.
5. Bordley, J. *Two Centuries of American Medicine, 1776–1976.* Philadelphia: Saunders, 1976.
6. Centers for Disease Control. Guidelines for preventing the transmission of tuberculosis in health-care settings, with special focus on

HIV-related issues. *M.M.W.R.* 39(RR-17):1, 1990.

7. Centers for Disease Control. Management of patients with suspected viral hemorrhagic fever. *M.M.W.R.* 37(Suppl. 3):1, 1988.

8. Centers for Disease Control. *Isolation Techniques for Use in Hospitals* (2nd ed.). Washington, DC: U.S. Government Printing Office, DHEW, Publ. No. (CDC) 76-8314, 1975.

9. Centers for Disease Control. Recommendations for preventing transmission of infection with human T-lymphotropic virus type III/lymphadenopathy-associated virus during invasive procedures. *M.M.W.R.* 35:221, 1986.

10. Centers for Disease Control. Recommendations for preventing transmission of infection with human T-lymphotropic virus type III/lymphadenopathy-associated virus in the workplace. *M.M.W.R.* 34:681, 1985.

11. Centers for Disease Control. Recommendations for prevention of HIV transmission in health care settings. *M.M.W.R.* 36 (Suppl. 2S):1S, 1987.

12. Centers for Disease Control. Risks associated with human parvovirus B19 infection. *M.M.W.R.* 38:81, 1989.

13. Centers for Disease Control. Update: Human immunodeficiency virus infections in health-care workers exposed to blood of infected patients. *M.M.W.R.* 36:285, 1987.

14. Centers for Disease Control. Update: Universal precautions for prevention of transmission of human immunodeficiency virus, hepatitis B virus, and other bloodborne pathogens in health care settings. *M.M.W.R.* 37:377, 1988.

15. Department of Labor. Occupational Safety and Health Administration. Occupational exposure to bloodborne pathogens; proposed rule and notice of hearings. *Fed. Reg.* 54(102):23042, 1989.

16. Doebbeling, B.N., and Wenzel, R.P. The direct costs of universal precautions in a teaching hospital. *J.A.M.A.* 264:2083, 1990.

17. Eickhoff, T.C. The cost of prevention. *Infect. Dis. News* 4:6, 1991.

18. Fahey, B.J., Koziol, D.E., Banks, S.M., and Henderson, D.K. Frequency of nonparenteral occupational exposures to blood and body fluids before and after universal precautions training. *Am. J. Med.* 90:145, 1991.

19. Gage, N.D., Landon, J.F., and Sider, M.T. *Communicable Disease.* Philadelphia: Davis, 1959.

20. Gala, C.L., et al. The use of eye-nose goggles to control nosocomial respiratory syncytial virus infection. *J.A.M.A.* 256:2706, 1986.

21. Garner, J.S. Comments on CDC guideline for isolation precautions in hospitals 1984. *Am. J. Infect. Control* 12:163, 1984.

22. Garner, J.S., and Hughes, J.M. Options for isolation precautions. *Am. Intern. Med.* 107:248, 1987.

23. Garner, J.S., and Simmons, B.P. CDC guideline for isolation precautions in hospitals. *Am. J. Infect. Control* 12:103, 1984.

24. Garner, J.S., and Simmons, B.P., CDC guideline for isolation precautions in hospitals. *Infect. Control* 4:245, 1983.

25. Goldman, D., Platt, R., and Hopkins, C. Control of Hospital-Acquired Infections. In: S.L. Gorbach, J.G. Bartlett, and N.R. Blacklow (Eds.), *Infectious Diseases in Medicine and Surgery.* Philadelphia: Saunders, 1992 (in press).

26. Haley, R.W., Garner, J.S., and Simmons, B.P. A new approach to the isolation of patients with infectious diseases: Alternative systems. *J. Hosp. Infect.* 6:128, 1985.

27. Haley, R.W., and Shachtman, R.H. The emergence of infection surveillance and control programs in U.S. hospitals: An assessment, 1976. *Am. J. Epidemiol.* 111:574, 1980.

28. Jacobson, J.T., et al. Adapting disease-specific isolation guidelines to a hospital information system. *Infect. Control* 7:411, 1986.

29. Klein, R.S. Universal precautions for preventing occupational exposures to human immunodeficiency virus type 1. *Am. J. Med.* 90:141, 1991.

30. Krasinski, K., et al. Screening for respiratory syncytial virus and assignment to a cohort at admission to reduce nosocomial transmission. *J. Pediatr.* 116:894, 1990.

31. LeClair, J.M., et al. Prevention of nosocomial respiratory syncytial virus infections through compliance with gown and glove isolation precautions. *N. Engl. J. Med.* 317:329, 1987.

32. Lynch, P., et al. Implementing and evaluating a system of generic infection precautions: Body substance isolation. *Am. J. Infect. Control* 18:1, 1990.

33. Lynch, P., Jackson, M.M., Cummings, M.J., and Stamm, W.E. Rethinking the role of isolation precautions in the prevention of nosocomial infections. *Am. Intern. Med.* 107:243, 1987.

34. Lynch, T. *Communicable Disease Nursing.* St. Louis: Mosby, 1949.

35. Nauseef, W.M., and Maki, D.G. A study of the value of simple protective isolation in patients with granulocytopenia. *N. Engl. J. Med.* 304:448, 1981.

36. Pugliese, G., Lynch, P., and Jackson, M.M. *Universal Precautions: Policies, Procedures, and Resources.* Chicago: American Hospital Association, 1991.

37. Schaffner, W. Infection control: Old myths and new realities. *Infect. Control* 1:330, 1980.

38. Snydman, D.R., Greer, C., Meissner, H.C., and McIntosh, K. Prevention of nosocomial transmission of respiratory syncytial virus infection in a newborn nursery. *Infect. Control Hosp. Epidemiol.* 9 : 105, 1988.

39. Wong, E.S., et al. Are universal precautions effective in reducing the number of occupational exposures among health care workers? *J.A.M.A.* 265 : 1123, 1991.

Antibiotics and Nosocomial Infections

Theodore C. Eickhoff

The era of chemotherapy for infectious disease is now almost 50 years old. Those 50 years have been marked by the continuous development and introduction of new and potent antimicrobial agents and by the relentless development and spread of significant antibiotic resistances among pathogenic bacteria. Today the contemporary clinician has available a broad array of potent antibiotic agents of proved efficacy against susceptible pathogens and sometimes of significant toxicity.

During these 50 years, significant changes have occurred in the character of nosocomial infections. The available data strongly suggest that in the 1940s and 1950s nosocomial infection was generally synonymous with gram-positive coccal infection, most notably with β-hemolytic streptococci and staphylococci. In the 1950s, staphylococci—particularly those resistant to the antimicrobial drugs in common use, such as penicillin G, tetracycline, erythromycin, chloramphenicol, and streptomycin—emerged to cause epidemic infection in hospitals. For reasons that are poorly understood, staphylococci subsided somewhat in importance as the major cause of nosocomial infection in the early 1960s, to be replaced by enteric gram-negative bacilli, enterococci, and fungi [11]. This pattern has continued for the last two decades, with some variations.

It is tempting to relate the changing character of nosocomial infections, as briefly sketched, to the sequential introduction of new antimicrobial agents and to impute a cause-and-effect relation. No one can seriously doubt that antimicrobial drugs have had a profound effect in shaping the character of nosocomial infections, but such an explanation is greatly oversimplified and fails to take into account the enormous changes in the technology of medicine and patterns of health care delivery that have also taken place in the past 50 years.

This chapter will explore more fully the way in which antimicrobial drugs are used in hospitals and consider the epidemiologic effects of such drug use on both the host and the microorganism. The biochemical mechanisms of antimicrobial drug resistance and the spread of such resistances among bacteria are fully discussed in Chapters 13 and 14. In addition, several excellent reviews have recently been published [22, 41].

Antibiotic Use in Hospitals

Data on the overall patterns of antibiotic use within hospitals have appeared in the literature frequently in the last several decades. The general thrust of such data indicates that from 25 to 35 percent of hospitalized patients receive systemic antibiotics at any given time [6, 28]. Furthermore, sequentially obtained data suggest that there is a trend toward increasing, rather than decreasing, antibiotic use with hospitals.

A series of four prevalence surveys carried out at the Boston City Hospital during January or February of the years 1964, 1967, 1970, and 1973 provides interesting comparative data [37]. In 1964, 26 percent of patients in that hospital were receiving at least one systemic antibacterial agent; in 1967, the figure was 27 percent; in 1970, it was 34 percent and, in 1973, 36 percent. In the 1973 survey, 76 percent of patients receiving antibiotics were considered to have an active infection at the time.

Scheckler and Bennett [49] reported on antibiotic use in seven community hospitals scattered throughout the United States; they employed a survey technique comparable to that used in the Boston City Hospital surveys. Twenty-four such prevalence studies carried out between November 1967 and June 1969 indicated that more than 30 percent of patients were receiving one or more systemic antibiotics but that only 38 percent of patients

receiving antibiotics surveyed in 1969 had recorded evidence of infection.

Kunin and co-workers [29] reported a study of antibiotic use carried out in 1969 at the University of Virginia Hospital. During a 3-month period, all antibiotic therapy given to patients on the medical and surgical services was reviewed by the infectious disease resident and staff, and the use of antibiotics in any given patient was judged by the group to be appropriate or inappropriate. During the survey period, 27 percent of patients admitted to the medical service and 29 percent of patients admitted to the surgical service were given antibiotics. Among patients on the surgical service, 48 percent of the antibiotic therapy given was for prophylaxis, whereas on the medical service, only 6 percent of antibiotic therapy was for prophylaxis.

Inappropriate therapy included instances in which a different drug was believed to be preferable, the dose was considered inappropriate, or the administration of any antimicrobial therapy or prophylaxis was considered unjustified. In the reviewers' judgment, 52 percent of all antimicrobial therapy was inappropriate. On the medical service, 42 percent of all antimicrobial drug use was judged inappropriate, whereas 62 percent of all antibiotic therapy on the surgical service was considered inappropriate.

A survey carried out in 1979, which was part of a series of prevalence surveys of infections and antibiotic use at the Latter Day Saints Hospital in Salt Lake City, revealed that the use of systemic antimicrobial agents had increased to 37 percent of all hospitalized surveyed patients, compared to 23 percent of patients found in a comparable survey conducted in 1971 [56]. These investigators found that the increase in antibiotic use could be attributed mainly to increased use of cephalosporin antibiotics for surgical prophylaxis. Their definition of *appropriate use* was somewhat less stringent than that of Kunin [29] and, overall, 31 percent of antibiotic use was judged to be inappropriate.

Such massive use of antibacterial drugs in hospitals, whether appropriate or inappropriate, has profound effects on both the hosts who receive these drugs and the bacteria exposed to them. In addition to the ecologic consequences of this massive use of antibiotics, to be discussed in subsequent sections, Kunin [28] has clearly identified the economic consequences and pointed out the enormous pressures brought to bear by the pharmaceutical industry in the direction of increased antibiotic use. In 1983, the total world market for antibiotics was $9.0 billion (U.S.). It was estimated that this would increase to $18.0 billion in 1990 and to $40.5 billion by the year 2000. The United States and Canada, with approximately 6 percent of the world population, account for nearly 20 percent of worldwide pharmaceutical sales [31].

Drug Resistance of Bacteria in Hospitals

Current problems of resistance of bacteria to antimicrobial drugs become more understandable if one recalls some of the history of the development of antibacterial drug resistance. In Paul Ehrlich's laboratory, trypanosomes became resistant to the drug *p*-rosaniline after repeated exposures [40]. Similarly, it was shown that pneumococci could develop resistance to hydrocupreine derivatives following repeated exposure [12]. In the mid-1940s, shortly after the introduction of penicillin G, it was recognized that certain strains of staphylococci elaborated a potent β-lactamase, an enzymatic inactivator of penicillin, and that penicillin G had no therapeutic activity in patients with infections caused by such staphylococci. This recognition surely came as a major disappointment but not as a total surprise. In the 50 years that have elapsed since that time, it has become abundantly clear that the major nosocomial pathogens either are naturally resistant to clinically useful antimicrobial drugs or possess the ability to acquire resistance. The best-known examples are the staphylococci and aerobic gram-negative bacilli, which together regularly account for the majority of nosoco-

mial infections. Every major class of bacterial pathogens has thus far demonstrated an ability to develop resistance to one or more commonly used antimicrobial agents [10].

Selective pressures favoring drug-resistant bacteria conferred by antibiotic therapy may indeed be principally focused in the institutional setting, but they extend widely into the community as well. The increasing prevalence of ampicillin-resistant *Hemophilus influenzae,* the increasing frequency of β-lactamase-producing gonococci, the widespread dissemination of methicillin-resistant staphylococci, and the emergence of penicillin-insensitive pneumococci are recent examples. Maxwell Finland [10] wrote in 1978, "Little by little, we are experiencing the erosion of the strongest bulwarks against serious bacterial infection."

Virulence of Antibiotic-Resistant Bacteria

The occurrence of nosocomial infection due to multiply drug-resistant organisms is governed by a number of factors including antibiotic selection pressure, the nature of the resistance determinant, whether the plasmid is conjugative or nonconjugative or is a transposon, and possible linkage with other antibiotic resistances and genetic determinants governing adhesion and pathogenicity [9]. Evidence is conflicting regarding the altered virulence—whether enhanced or diminished—of drug-resistant bacteria compared to that of drug-susceptible organisms. There may prove to be no single answer to such a question, the answer rather being dependent on the particular bacterial species involved, the specific genetic determinants present, and what these genetic determinants contribute to the metabolic activities of the cell and the specific antigens located on the bacterial cell surface.

Although it is generally true that serious infection, such as bacteremic infection, caused by drug-resistant bacteria results in higher mortality than would be true of comparably serious infections caused by drug-susceptible bacteria, it is not at all clear whether the increased mortality is a reflection of increased virulence, diminished effectiveness of antibiotic therapy, or both. Jessen and colleagues [23], for example, who studied the occurrence of methicillin-resistant staphylococci and staphyloccal bacteremia in Denmark, showed that the combined effects of lysogenicity, transduction, and selection not only influenced the phage type and antibiotic resistance of staphylococci, but also involved properties more directly connected with pathogenicity, such as lipase production, which is believed to facilitate the development of abscesses and to affect adversely the prognosis in bacteremia. The authors could not determine, however, whether the poorer prognosis was due to the shortcomings of antibiotic therapy or to correlated bacterial properties that enhanced virulence.

Holmberg and his associates [18] at the Centers for Disease Control recently reviewed the health and economic impacts of antimicrobial resistance. Working from a database of 175 reports of investigations of outbreaks, both community and nosocomial, of selected pathogens, they compared mortality, likelihood of hospitalization, and duration of hospital stay in patients in outbreaks of antibiotic-resistant pathogens to patients involved in outbreaks of antibiotic-susceptible pathogens. Included in the database were outbreaks of salmonellosis, shigellosis, staphylococcal infection, *Serratia* infections, and other gram-negative bacillary infections. As expected, there were many possible con-

founding variables in such a retrospective analysis but, nonetheless, mortality, likelihood of hospitalization, and hospital stay were at least two-fold higher in patients infected with drug-resistant pathogens as compared to patients infected with drug-susceptible pathogens. This was true for both community outbreaks and hospital outbreaks.

Thus, at the clinical level, the consequences of antimicrobial drug resistance are profound and measurable, even though there may not be in vitro evidence of enhanced virulence. The adverse consequences of antimicrobial drug resistance were due both to ineffective antibiotic therapy and to the higher risk of drug-resistant infection in patients who had been on previous antibiotic therapy as a result of other underlying conditions.

Parallels in Antibiotic Use and Antibiotic Resistance

Evidence from a number of studies suggests that the proportion of bacteria resistant to a given antibiotic may increase as use of the drug increases or, conversely, may decrease if there is decreased use or cessation of use of the drug. Examples of such studies are shown in Tables 12-1 and 12-2.

Lepper and co-workers [30] found that after 5 months of intensive use of erythromycin for the treatment of all susceptible infections, three-fourths of the strains were highly resistant to that drug. When all erythromycin

Table 12-1. Studies demonstrating a temporal relationship between increased use of antimicrobial agents and increased prevalence of resistant hospital organisms

Year	Setting for use of antimicrobials	Organisms	Antimicrobials
1953	General	*Staphylococcus aureus*	Erythromycin
		S. aureus	Penicillin
		S. aureus	Chlortetracycline
1956	Burn ward	*S. aureus*	Chloramphenicol
		S. aureus	Chlortetracycline
1967	Surgical prophylaxis	*S. aureus*	Neomycin cream
1971	Burn ward	*Pseudomonas aeruginosa*	Gentamicin
1978	Surgical prophylaxis	*P. aeruginosa*	Gentamicin
		Serratia species	Gentamicin
1979	Postoperative	*Serratia* species	Gentamicin

Source: Adapted from J.E. McGowan, Jr., Antimicrobial resistance in hospital organisms and its relation to antibiotic use. *Rev. Infect. Dis.* 5 : 1033, 1983.

Table 12-2. Studies demonstrating a temporal relationship between decreased use of antimicrobial agents and decreased prevalence of organisms

Year	Setting for use of antimicrobials	Organisms	Antimicrobials
1953	General	*Staphylococcus* species	Chloramphenicol
1954	General	*S. aureus*	Erythromycin
1956	Burn ward	*S. aureus*	Chlortetracycline
		S. aureus	Chloramphenicol
1960	General	*S. aureus*	Penicillin
1960		*S. aureus*	Tetracycline
1966	Pediatric ward	*S. aureus*	Erythromycin
1967	Surgical prophylaxis	*S. aureus*	Neomycin cream
1970	General	*Escherichia coli* species	Streptomycin
		Klebsiella, Enterobacter species	Streptomycin
1970	Neurosurgical unit	*Klebsiella* species	All
1970	General	*S. aureus*	Erythromycin
		S. aureus	Novobiocin
1971	Burn wound	*Pseudomonas aeruginosa*	Gentamicin
1972	Burn ward	Enterobacteriaceae	Carbenicillin
		P. aeruginosa	Carbenicillin
1973	Nursery	Enterobacteria	Kanamycin
1974	Urology ward	Gram-negative bacilli	Five agents
1975	Nursery	*E. coli*	Kanamycin
1978	Surgical prophylaxis	*P. aeruginosa*	Gentamicin
		Serratia species	Gentamicin

Source: Adapted from J.E. McGowan, Jr., Antimicrobial resistance in hospital organisms and its relation to antibiotic use. *Rev. Infect. Dis.* 5:1033, 1983.

therapy was discontinued and penicillin and tetracycline therapy resumed, the proportion of erythromycin-resistant strains decreased, whereas the proportion of penicillin-resistant strains, which had declined while erythromycin was used exclusively, rose again rapidly. Similar results were found for tetracycline, to which resistance had increased sharply while it was used for susceptible infections and subsequently declined as its use decreased. Gibson and Thompson [15] described a similar phenomenon with staphylococci from burn wounds that had become highly resistant to tetracycline while that drug was used. When chloramphenicol was substituted for tetracycline, the proportion of chloramphenicol-resistant staphylococci rose sharply during the succeeding 6 months, whereas the proportion of tetracycline-resistant staphylococci fell. When chloramphenicol therapy was discontinued, the proportion of chloramphenicol-resistant strains dropped sharply. Bauer and colleagues [4] reported an entirely comparable experience and demonstrated a cor-

relation between the extent of resistance and use of antibiotics. In an extensive study of staphylococci and staphylococcal infection in Great Britain, Barber and her colleagues [1] documented not only a decline in the incidence of staphylococcal infection per patient when a number of anti-cross-infection measures and a controlled antibiotic policy were put into effect, but also a sharp reversal of penicillin and tetracycline resistance of isolates toward increased susceptibility.

Prevailing drug resistance of gram-negative bacilli is also susceptible to alteration by restriction or cessation of use of a given drug. When kanamycin was replaced by gentamicin in an effort to control an outbreak of nosocomial infections caused by kanamycin-resistant enteric organisms, kanamycin-resistant organisms were virtually eliminated from the nursery within a month, which suggested that the selective pressure provided by the extensive use of kanamycin was a major factor in causing and propagating the outbreak. As gentamicin was increasingly used, a significant increase in gentamicin resistance of the infants' intestinal flora occurred [13].

Sogaard and colleagues [53], in studying antibiotic-resistant gram-negative bacilli in a urologic ward in Denmark, found a progressive decrease in the incidence of antibiotic resistance among enteric bacteria over a 9-year period that was coincident with a decreasing use of antibiotics in response to a restrictive antibiotic use policy. In addition, the number of more resistant organisms, such as *Pseudomonas aeruginosa, Proteus, Providencia, Klebsiella, and Enterobacter,* declined during the period of study. Bulger and co-workers [7], in surveying resistance among strains of *Escherichia coli* and *Klebsiella-Enterobacter* over a 10-year period, observed a decline in the frequency of resistance to antibiotics; they attributed their findings in part to conservative and selective use of antibiotics and in part to the development of an overall hospital infection control program.

Working in the Birmingham Accident Hospital Burn Unit, Lowbury and associates [33] studied the emergence of strains of *P. aeruginosa* and Enterobacteriaceae that carried a resistance (R) factor conferring resistance to tetracycline, kanamycin, carbenicillin, ampicillin, and cephaloridine. These strains emerged under the selective pressure of carbenicillin therapy, which was widely used on the burn unit. After discontinuation of all use of carbenicillin and restriction of the use of tetracycline, kanamycin, ampicillin, and cephaloridine, strains of *P. aeruginosa* and Enterobacteriaceae carrying this linked multiply drug-resistant pattern disappeared. Price and Sleigh [44] reported an unusually dramatic experience in attempting to control an epidemic *Klebsiella* infection by a neurosurgical unit; the epidemic was not curtailed by radical measures for the prevention of cross-infection, and the epidemic strain disappeared only when the use of all antibiotics, both prophylactic and therapeutic, was discontinued in the unit. Based on data such as those reviewed previously, many individuals believe that a policy of restricting the use of the newest and most broadly active antibiotics would minimize the development of resistance to

those drugs and hence prolong their useful life span.

In an excellent review, McGowan [36] has summarized seven types of evidence linking antimicrobial use in the hospital with antimicrobial resistance in hospital bacteria:

1. Antimicrobial resistance is more prevalent among bacteria causing infection in the nosocomial setting than among bacteria causing community-acquired infection. Although exceptions exist, they have been relatively few, and most of the data support the generalization.
2. In outbreak situations in the nosocomial setting, patients infected with resistant outbreak strains are more likely to have received previous antibiotic therapy than are patients colonized or infected with susceptible strains of the same species. This has been particularly illustrated in recent outbreaks of methicillin-resistant *Staphylococcus aureus.*
3. Changes in antimicrobial use may lead to parallel changes in the prevalence of resistance to that antibiotic.
4. Areas of most intense antibiotic use within the hospital generally also have had the highest prevalence of antibiotic-resistant bacteria. These are also generally the areas of the hospital in which the most highly susceptible patients are encountered and include intensive care units, burn units, oncology units, and other special-care units.
5. Increased duration of exposure to antibiotics in the hospital generally increases the likelihood of colonization of infection with resistant organisms. This factor may, however, also simply act as a marker for more highly susceptible hosts.
6. The higher the dose of antibiotic given, the greater the likelihood of superinfection or colonization with resistant organisms. Evidence in support of this contention is not well controlled and is most convincing in the case of respiratory tract infection.
7. Finally, the notion of a cause-effect relation seems to fit the existing data, in biologic terms. That is, antibiotic therapy

produces marked effects on the host's endogenous flora and exerts selective pressure in favor of resistant organisms. As emphasized by McGowan [36], however, antibiotic therapy appears to act primarily by selecting a drug-resistant causative organism rather than by increasing the frequency of nosocomial infection.

Drug-resistant organisms—whether mutants, transductants containing plasmids, or conjugants containing R factors—selected by the pressure of antibiotic drugs are probably at a disadvantage, however slight, in the absence of the selective pressure. R determinants must represent an energy "load" for the host bacterium. If this were not so, "wild" bacteria in the community would likely be drug-resistant or would at least be a mixture of sensitive and resistant cells. Although R factor–containing bacteria acquired in the hospital persist for a time in the community free of the selection pressure of antibiotics, they generally decay in the absence of the selective pressure. In only 50 percent of infants who acquired enteric organisms containing R factor–mediated resistance to kanamycin, for example, was the original organism present after 1 year [8].

Antibiotics and Host Susceptibility

Antibiotics may affect host susceptibility to infection by either a direct effect on host defense mechanisms or an indirect effect resulting from alteration of the metabolic and immunologic state of the host. Antibiotics additionally exert a profound influence on the nature of host microflora, and although this selection effect may not directly influence host susceptibility to infection, as previously noted, it very directly influences the nature of the organisms that colonize and subsequently infect hospitalized patients.

Direct Effect of Antibiotics on Host Defense Mechanisms

The most obvious and dramatic examples of a direct effect of antibiotics on host defense mechanisms are instances of granulocytopenia or bone marrow aplasia occasionally encountered with the use of several antibiotics, notably chloramphenicol and the sulfonamides. Adverse reactions to penicillins, cephalosporins, sulfonamides and, less frequently, other antibiotics may take the form of a severe dermatitis, including exfoliation; such direct immunologic injury to the skin may, of course, enhance host susceptibility to infection. These adverse effects of antibiotic therapy are well-known and profoundly influence host susceptibility to infection.

Direct effects of individual antibiotics on the components of host defense—that is, polymorphonuclear leukocyte function, immunoglobulin synthesis and function, and cell-mediated immune mechanisms—have not been systematically studied. There is, however, a gradually increasing body of data from which a few conclusions may be drawn [27, 34, 39, 58].

With regard to function of polymorphonuclear leukocytes, neither β-lactam nor aminoglycoside drugs appear to have any deleterious effects on leukocyte function, although there is evidence that tetracycline hydrochloride, chlortetracycline, and doxycycline may inhibit leukocyte chemotaxis and impair phagocytosis. In addition, several sulfonamide drugs, including sulfadiazine, sulfathiazole, and sulfisoxazole, may inhibit leukocyte microbicidal activity. In the case of the tetracyclines, these effects may be seen in clinically attainable concentrations; whether they are of clinical significance has not been established.

Chloramphenicol, in clinically attainable concentrations, can be shown to diminish the antibody response to antigenic stimulation, but this effect has not been shown to be of general clinical significance. Rifampicin can be shown in vitro to inhibit antibody production, but the effects of rifampicin on antibody response in humans are variable.

Modulation of the most immune response to an infectious agent by specific chemotherapy—such as occurs in the treatment of rickettsial infections with chloramphenicol or tetracycline, penicillin treatment of group A streptococcal infections, or ampicillin treatment of *H. influenzae* type B infections—may, over long periods of time, alter the susceptibility of a population to a particular infectious agent, but this phenomenon probably is of little, if any, significance in the context of nosocomial infection.

Neither the β-lactam nor aminoglycoside antibiotics are known to have any significant effect on host cell-mediated immune mechanisms. Rifampicin, the tetracyclines, and trimethoprim have been shown to suppress lymphocyte blastogenesis at concentrations that might been encountered during clinical use. Several other antibiotics, including clindamycin, erythromycin, and nitrofurantoin, can similarly impair lympyhocyte blastogenesis but only at concentrations rarely achieved during clinical use. Rifampicin can also be shown to suppress delayed cutaneous hypersensitivity to purified protein derivative of tuberculin (PPD) in patients with tuberculosis who are receiving the drug. This effect of rifampicin, however, has not been shown to alter host susceptibility to infection in patients being treated for tuberculosis, nor has it been associated with a poor therapeutic result.

Thus there is little evidence that antibiotic therapy has a major, direct effect on host defense mechanisms except in instances of adverse drug reactions precipitating severe dermatitis, bone marrow depression, or other such events. In general, data thus far suggest that antibiotics that are taken up and concentrated within cells (e.g., erythromycin, tetracyclines, rifampicin) or that effect intracellular metabolic processes such as protein synthesis, are more likely than others to alter host defense mechanisms. As noted, however, this area has not been systematically studied, and investigational methods have not been standardized. Interested readers are referred to an excellent recent review [27].

Indirect Effect of Antibiotics due to Alteration of Host Metabolic State

Many antibiotics cause direct toxic or immunologically mediated injury to target organs regulating the metabolic activity of the host,

particularly the liver, kidneys, gastrointestinal tract, and lungs. The resulting dysfunction of these organs may alter host susceptibility to infection. These indirect effects of antibiotics can, in most instances, be minimized or avoided altogether by the rational and careful use of potentially toxic drugs.

Kidneys

Interstitial nephritis has been associated with a number of drugs, notably the penicillins, including the penicillinase-resistant penicillins. Direct toxic injury to renal tublar epithelium is caused by many drugs, notably cephaloridine, all of the aminoglycosides, the polymyxins, and amphotericin B. Also, glomerulonephritis has been noted shortly after rifampicin therapy in persons with previous exposure to the drug. Renal failure and its resulting metabolic consequences have a direct suppressive effect on host defense mechanisms. Clearly, the therapeutic modalities used in the management of renal failure also represent added infection risk factors.

Liver

Minor alterations of hepatic function are found frequently in the course of antibiotic therapy but, in the vast majority of instances, such alterations cannot be shown to influence host susceptibility to infection. Intrahepatic cholestasis, such as may occur during therapy with the sodium lauryl sulfate ester of erythromycin, similarly does not appear to represent a major threat to host defense mechanisms. Overwhelming hepatic injury has been associated with both tetracycline and isoniazid therapy, but the unquestionably reduced host resistance to infection is of lesser importance than the more immediate metabolic threat to the host.

Colon

Necrotizing enterocolitis has been recognized as a complication of therapy with many antibiotic drugs, notably the penicillins, cephalosporins, and clindamycin. Unlike staphylococcal necrotizing enterocolitis associated with tetracycline therapy, frequently seen during the 1950s and 1960s, most necrotizing enterocolitis seen at present is due to an enterotoxin produced by *Clostridium difficile* [2, 3, 46]. This adverse effect appears to be related to the alteration of host gastrointestinal tract flora caused by the administered antibiotic.

Lungs

Immunologically mediated injury to the lungs is an occasional consequence of antibiotic therapy, particularly with penicillins and nitrofurans. It is likely that host susceptibility to infection is only mildly enhanced by such injury.

Influence of Antibiotic Therapy on Host Microflora

Virtually all antibiotics in therapeutic doses produce marked changes in the microflora of the skin, upper respiratory tract, gastrointestinal tract, and genital tract—indeed, any site in the host normally colonized by bacteria. Antibiotic-resistant organisms, if present or acquired, are selected out and multiply freely to replace the susceptible organisms inhibited by antibiotic therapy. In the majority of patients, these changes in host microflora are of no demonstrable consequence. As is well recognized, however, the antibiotic-resistant microflora may, on occasion, result in serious or fatal infection. It is through this mechanism that antibiotic therapy appears to exert its major influence on nosocomial infection— that is, by determining the character, rather than the frequency, of nosocomial infections.

Gastrointestinal Tract

Historically, perhaps the clearest example of alteration of host microflora that led directly to overgrowth and subsequent infection by antibiotic-resistant bacteria was staphylococcal enterocolitis associated with or following tetracycline therapy. This appeared to be a direct result of antibiotic therapy, which suppressed the normal gastrointestinal tract flora and permitted rapid and uninhibited overgrowth of drug-resistant staphylococci. In the necrotizing enterocolitis encountered in re-

cent years, the toxin-producing strains of *C. difficile* may not necessarily demonstrate in vitro resistance to the precipitating antibiotic, but presumably the antibiotic suppresses the more sensitive gastrointestinal tract flora, allowing the less susceptible clostridia to multiply or produce enterotoxin [2, 3, 46].

Colonization of the gastrointestinal tract by multiply drug-resistant gram-negative bacilli, presumably under the influence of antibiotic therapy, has been repeatedly demonstrated [20, 48, 50, 51, 60]. In a study at the Denver Veterans Administration Hospital, Selden and associates [51] found that gastrointestinal tract colonization by multiply drug-resistant *Klebsiella* acquired in the hospital was an important intermediary step in the subsequent development of disease caused by that organism. In recent years, evidence has been presented suggesting that hospital food may frequently be contaminated by multiply drug-resistant gram-negative bacilli and that this may be an important source of nosocomial colonization in patients whose normal gastrointestinal tract flora is suppressed by antibiotic therapy. The sources of multiply drug-resistant gram-negative bacilli in hospital food, including, for example, fresh garden salads, has not been clarified.

It has become apparent that some kinds of antibiotics, particularly those active against many components of the anaerobic flora of the gastrointestinal tract, are more likely to be associated with colonization by multiply drug-resistant organisms than are antibiotics less broadly active against the anaerobic flora of the gastrointestinal tract [60]. This has led to the concept of so-called colonization resistance, suggesting that an intact colonic anaerobic flora is of major importance in decreasing the chance of colonization by new aerobic gram-negative bacilli.

Hooker and DiPiro [19] have published a comprehensive recent review of the effects of antibiotics on gastrointestinal tract flora. Although antibiotics are the most obvious class of drugs that affect bowel flora, other drug classes have some effects as well, including antineoplastic drugs, immunosuppresive drugs, and histamine H$_2$ blockers. In general, the most profound changes in bowel flora are caused by oral antibiotics that are poorly or incompletely absorbed from the gastrointestinal tract or antibiotics given by any route that are secreted or excreted in high concentration into saliva, bile, or intestinal secretions. If the antibiotic in question has intrinsic activity against anaerobic bacteria, the alteration of host bowel microflora is even more profound. This leads directly to selection and overgrowth of antimicrobial-resistant strains.

The most profound effects on bowel flora, and disruption of colonization resistance, have been seen with second- and third-generation cephalosporins and extended-spectrum penicillins. Even within these classes, however, effects are variable among different drugs. Moxalactam, cefoperazone, cefuroxime, cefoxitin, and ceftriaxone profoundly suppress both aerobic and anaerobic bowel flora; ceftazidime and cefotaxime have a lesser effect. Parenterally administered aminoglycosides and monobactams have only minor effects on bowel flora. The quinolones have significant activity against the aerobic gram-negative bacteria in the gut but only limited activity against anaerobes.

The most promising approaches to minimize or prevent the risks of colonization and spread of antibiotic-resistant organisms in the gastrointestinal tract are simple but, unfortunately, are not often given much consideration in antibiotic decision making. These are: (1) avoidance of unnecessary antibiotic therapy; (2) use of the shortest possible duration of treatment; (3) avoidance of drugs that have antianaerobic activity except when necessary; and (4) the preferential use of antibiotics that are well absorbed after oral administration or are minimally excreted via the biliary tract.

Respiratory Tract

The respiratory tract is also highly susceptible to antibiotic-induced changes in microflora. In a thorough study of bacterial colonization and suprainfection of the respiratory tract, Tillotson and Finland [59] showed that colonization and suprainfection were common

following high doses of penicillin and aminoglycosides or broad-spectrum antibiotics alone. They did not, however, find a higher rate of colonization or infection by gram-negative bacilli following treatment with various semisynthetic penicillins, nor did ampicillin therapy appear to confer any additional risk beyond that observed with penicillin G. Louria and Brayton [32] found that the risk of suprainfection following penicillin treatment of pneumonia was related, at least in part, to unnecessarily high doses of penicillin.

It is important to appreciate that antibiotic therapy is by no means the only factor influencing colonization and suprainfection. Johanson and associates [24, 25] were among the first to point out the importance of the severity of the underlying disease, independent of antibiotic therapy, in pharyngeal colonization by gram-negative bacilli. Rose and Babcock [47], studying colonization with gram-negative bacilli of patients in an intensive care unit, observed that colonization in surgical patients appeared to be related more strongly to the presence of indwelling tubes and the consequent colonization of multiple sites in the same patient than to the use of antimicrobial drugs. In medical patients, however, colonization appeared to be related primarily to antibiotic therapy. Tenney and associates [57] at the Denver Veterans Administration Hospital, who also studied pharyngeal colonization in a medical intensive care unit, found that no single risk factor for gram-negative rod colonization, such as antibiotic therapy, was associated with more than two-thirds of colonized patients and that most risk factors were present in fewer than one-third of patients. In addition to antibiotic therapy, the risk factors studied included the severity of the underlying illness, presence of acidosis, steroid therapy, mechanically assisted ventilation, tracheal intubation, nasogastric suction, and others.

Johanson and colleagues [24, 25] suggested that the oropharynx is episodically or continually exposed to gram-negative bacilli and *S. aureus,* perhaps in small numbers, and that patients vary in their ability to clear them. Pharyngeal colonization may occur only in patients (1) whose pharyngeal clearance mechanisms are compromised by underlying disease, metabolic state, mechanically assisted respiration, or foreign bodies; (2) who are exposed to large inocula of gram-negative bacilli (for example, by contaminated nebulizers); or (3) in whom gram-negative bacilli are permitted to multiply more rapidly than they can be cleared, such as when antibiotic therapy suppresses normal flora. The risk of disease occurring after colonization has been established is more likely to be related to the state of host pulmonary defense mechanisms and to the virulence of the specific colonizing species than to the use of antibiotic therapy or other risk factors per se.

Sprunt and colleagues [54, 55] have suggested that α-hemolytic streptococci inhibit the growth of gram-negative bacilli in vitro, and they have furthermore noted the disappearance of inhibitory α-hemolytic streptococci from the oropharynx in patients colonized with gram-negative bacilli. Thus bacterial interference, with α-hemolytic streptococci acting as the inhibitory species, may be one mechanism for maintaining the normal flora of the upper respiratory tract. If these or other inhibitors are eliminated or depressed by antibiotic therapy, other drug-resistant bacteria may be able to multiply to reach detectable levels. This may represent the analogue of colonization resistance within the gastrointestinal tract and may occur in other areas of the body as well, such as the skin.

General Conclusions

In summary, there is abundant evidence that antibiotic therapy is a determinant; and perhaps the *major* determinant, of alterations in host microflora and colonization of the host by drug-resistant organisms. There is also evidence, however, that antibiotic therapy is by no means the only determinant involved and that it may be only one of a number of risk factors commonly encountered by hospitalized patients that facilitate colonization and often subsequent disease by drug-resistant organisms, including both staphylococci and gram-negative bacilli.

Interrelation of Antibiotic Therapy, Resistance to Antibiotics, and Nosocomial Infection

The interrelation of antibiotic therapy, intrinsic or acquired resistance to antibiotics in bacteria, and nosocomial infection in the hospitalized host represent an extraordinarily complex equation. Considering the large numbers of other risk factors that affect patients in hospitals, it is perhaps not surprising that data simply do not exist that would permit satisfactory and valid conclusions concerning the exact role of antibiotic use in determining either the magnitude or the frequency of hospital infection. As in many areas, there are differences of opinion. In 1970 William [61] stated:

I have not referred so far to the factors so often cited as responsible for much of the trouble in hospital infection—abuse of antibiotics—because it seems important to appreciate that the secular changes that we have seen have not been wholly, or even mainly, due to alterations in the use of antibiotics or to the development of staphylococci more resistant to antibiotics.

In the same year, Finland [11] wrote:

The major factor presumed to be responsible for the changing ecology of the serious bacterial infections, and for the marked increase in their occurrence, at least at Boston City Hospital, is the selective pressure of the antibiotics so widely and intensively used in therapy, and especially for prophylaxis. Both the large number of drugs and the large doses of each used in the individual patients within the hospital are elements of this selective pressure.

The use of antimicrobial agents tends to promote the emergence of organisms with intrinsic or acquired resistance to those agents and predisposes patients to colonization by such organisms. With increasing use of instrumentation, immunosuppressive drugs, and other technologic accompaniments of contemporary medical practice, resistant organisms may emerge to cause infection. Infection resulting from multiply drug-resistant bacteria, whether staphylococci or gram-negative bacilli, is notoriously more difficult to treat than infection by drug-susceptible pathogens, and the results of therapy in such compromised hosts are clearly less satisfactory.

Wolff and Bennett [62] stated the issues very succinctly:

> The enhanced risks of acquiring gram-negative rod infections consequent to the proper use of antibiotics for legitimate therapeutic and prophylactic purposes clearly seem outweighed by the anticipated benefits. Such risks represent undesirable but nonetheless acceptable concomitants of medical progress. Use of antibiotics for uncertain or improper indications, however, poses an unacceptable risk.

Evaluation of Antibiotic Use: Approaches to Improvement
Incidence of Antibiotic Abuse

That antimicrobial agents are both widely misused and widely overused is now established beyond reasonable doubt. From 20 to 35 percent of patients in U.S. hospitals receive microbial agents during the course of their hospitalization, and this accounts for approximately one-third of hospital drug costs. In one study, no evidence of infection was found in as many as 70 percent of patients who received antimicrobial therapy [49]. Kunin [29] has estimated that as many as 50 percent of hospitalized adults who receive antibiotic therapy (1) do not require antibiotic therapy for their medical condition, (2) do not receive the most effective and least expensive drug, or (3) do not receive the lowest dose and duration of therapy that is considered effective. Furthermore, approximately 70 percent of antibiotics used in hospitals are in two highly expensive drug categories—cephalosporins and aminoglycosides [28].

It is important, however, as emphasized by Kunin [28], to evaluate the problem of antibiotic use in broader perspective rather than to consider it as an isolated example of inappropriate use of drugs. Included in the causation of the problem, and therefore to be considered in resolving the problem, are the ways in which appropriate use of drugs is taught in medical school, how house staff and practicing physicians receive information and advice about new drugs, the nature of the relationship between the pharmaceutical industry and the medical profession, the steadily increasing reliance of the medical profession on drug and laboratory technology in general, and the apparent lack of significant constraints operating to control the escalating cost of health care.

Viewed in such a context, antibiotic abuse is simply another reflection of what has become known as the *technologic imperative* and is comparable to well-known problems such as the overuse of psychoactive drugs or excessive use of laboratory testing. Nonetheless, there is one major difference between other such problems and antibiotic abuse that is too often ignored or forgotten—that is, the biologic consequences, or ecologic "fallout," of antibiotic therapy. As previously discussed in this chapter, the widespread use of antimicrobial agents in the hospital setting frequently leads to selection of organisms resistant to those antimicrobial agents and thus creates and maintains a population of drug-resistant nosocomial pathogens in the hospital environment. Physicians have been reluctant to recognize that a decision to use an antimicrobial agent in a given patient has ecologic consequences that extend well beyond the patient at hand.

Types of Antibiotic Misuse or Abuse

There are, of course, several different categories of misuse or abuse of antibiotics. For example, antibiotics are widely misused in prophylaxis. A study by the Inter-Society Committee on Antimicrobial Drug Usage organized by the American College of Physicians [52], showed that more than 25 percent of the total of antibiotics used in 20 Pennsylvania hospitals was apparently given for surgical prophylaxis and that almost 80 percent of such prophylactic use was accounted for by administration of antibiotic prophylaxis beyond the 24- to 48-hour postoperative period when prophylaxis can be anticipated to be effective. There was, in fact, a strong correlation between duration of hospital stay and duration of prophylactic therapy [52].

Antibiotic therapy is often used as a diagnostic procedure. Frequently, antibiotics are given as an empiric test for patients with fever or other presumed evidence of infection; if the patient responds to antibiotic therapy, then infection is presumed to have been the cause. There are, unquestionably, legitimate indications for such use of antibiotics, but most such use is clearly inappropriate.

Antibiotics are often used to treat a disease that does not respond to antibiotics. Contributing to abuse in this area are simple physician ignorance [42] and the common use of antibiotics to treat viral respiratory tract infections on the grounds that it is not likely to harm the patient and might prevent subsequent bacterial infection.

There are mistakes in the use of antibiotics, such as incorrect dosage, incorrect route of administration, inappropriate duration of therapy, or inappropriate choice of drug. In addition, physicians frequently fail to look for or recognize adverse reactions; toxic effects are relatively frequent and particularly prominent in aminoglycoside therapy.

The preferential use of newer and more expensive antibiotics, particularly third-generation cephalosporin drugs and carbepenems, in clinical situations in which older and less expensive drugs have proved effective represents another apparent category of misuse. Kunin [28] has referred to many of the antimicrobial agents introduced during the past decade as "drugs of fear," suggesting that the physician is fearful of not giving the best drug for a presumed infection. Fear that an infection may be due to a highly resistant pathogen is a potent stimulus to physicians to use the broadest-spectrum antibiotics available, at least for initial empiric therapy. The use of second- or third-generation cephalosporins for therapy or surgical prophylaxis in situations in which first-generation cephalosporins have been shown to be effective is a clear example of misuse of "drugs of fear."

Methods for Auditing Antibiotic Usage

Increased recognition of the problem of antibiotic abuse has led to recommendations from advisory bodies and demands from the Joint Commission on Accreditation of Healthcare Organizations (JCAHO) that individual hospitals review their own use of antimicrobial agents. Unfortunately, the mandate to audit preceded the development of techniques demonstrated to be effective in performing such an evaluation and was issued in the absence of any convincing evidence that self-examination on such a massive scale would beneficially affect the problem.

Nevertheless, a variety of techniques have been employed for conducting surveillance or monitoring antibiotic use within hospitals. These have been summarized by Kunin [28], as shown in Table 12-3:

1. *Gross utilization data based on pharmacy records* is relatively inexpensive and may be used to track the costs and trends in use of specific drugs. Such information cannot readily be used for interhospital comparisons unless adjusted for case mix and the number of patient-days in the hospital. Its major use may be to identify specific problems requiring more detailed investigation.
2. *Survey of use on individual services* is feasible only if pharmacy records can identify use by specific nursing units or patients assigned to individual services. It is a slight improvement over gross utilization data

Table 12-3. Methods of surveillance of antimicrobial use in hospitals

1. Gross utilization data based on pharmacy records
2. Survey of use on individual services
3. Survey of routine orders for prophylaxis in surgery
4. Survey of antibiotic therapy for specific infectious diseases
5. Individual case review of independent experts
6. Audits of specific clinical problems based on national criteria

Source: Adapted from C.M. Kunin, Evaluation of antibiotic usage: A comprehensive look at alternative approaches. *Rev. Infect. Dis.* 3:745, 1981.

inasmuch as potential problem areas can be pinpointed more closely.

3. *Survey of routine orders for prophylaxis in surgery* is somewhat more labor-intensive and requires individual chart review of all cases for specific operations being surveyed. It does permit interhospital comparison and provides specific data on the practices of individual surgeons; thus such information can be used for educational feedback to the surgical service.

4. *Survey of antibiotic orders for specific infectious diseases* must, of course, be based on the clinical condition being treated, such as community-acquired pneumonia, hospital-acquired pneumonia, or urinary tract infection. The patterns of practice of individual physicians can be identified and compared. Such information is useful for educational feedback.

5. *Individual case review by independent experts* is expensive and labor-intensive. It can be useful only if the standards for review are clearly articulated and agreed on by the physicians under review, whether a subspecialty group or an entire service. Lacking that, the findings are less likely to be accepted by the physicians whose antibiotic use is being reviewed.

6. *Audits for specific clincial problems based on national criteria* represent the most labor-intensive and least documented approach to modifying antibiotic use. Since antibiotic audit is mandated by the JCAHO, it may be assumed that hospital and medical staff will expend many hours carrying out this mandate. It is highly desirable, therefore, that this obligation be approached in a way that is likely to be effective educationally and that might have a significant impact on antibiotic use, rather than simply as a pro forma requirement that must be met.

The following suggestions are offered to help maximize the potential benefit of antibiotic auditing. First, the focus should be on several specific clinical issues rather than making an attempt to audit all antimicrobial use. Questions should be constructed specifically, remembering that the primary reason for an tibiotic audit is to improve medical care and reduce its cost. The purpose is not to introduce conflict among the medical staff or to identify one or more physicians as being "guilty" of antibiotic abuse.

Second, the audit should concentrate on areas of therapy or prophylaxis in which generally accepted national standards exist. Such national standards should be developed by, explained to, and agreed on by that segment of the medical staff involved in a given area of audit. The standards should be agreed on by all concerned as representing appropriate standards of therapy or prophylaxis. Reasonable and nationally acceptable standards of therapy exist or could be developed for a number of medical conditions such as pneumonia, intraabdominal infections, septicemia, endocarditis, and osteomyelitis; in many areas of antibiotic therapy, however, controversy exists; often there are legitimate differences of opinion as to the best approach to therapy. It is important that such areas be avoided as subjects for audit and that efforts be concentrated on areas for which acceptable and reasonable standards do exist.

Third, audits of the prophylactic use of antibiotics in surgery have been emphasized, since this area has been identified as a major contributor to antibiotic cost and misuse. Procedures for which prophylaxis is currently recommended include prosthetic valve and open-heart procedures; coronary artery bypass surgery; insertion of prosthetic joints; colonic surgery; biliary tract surgery in a patient older than 70 years or with acute cholecystitis, obstructive jaundice, or choledocholithiasis; vaginal hysterectomy; cesarean section; and urologic surgery on bacteriuric patients. It is important to emphasize the appropriate preoperative timing of surgical prophylaxis and that prophylaxis should be terminated within 24 hours after surgery is completed. (See Chap. 33.)

Fourth, antibiotic audit should be by peer review rather than review strictly by hospital administration, infection control personnel, or pharmacy personnel. Thus it should be a medical staff responsibility, as specified by the JCAHO, with standards defined and agreed on by infectious disease consultants among the staff and by the medical staff being audited. Infection control personnel and pharmacy personnel may be extraordinarily helpful in the conduct of the audit but should not have a dominant role in identifying the standards to be met. Broader acceptance of the results of an audit will follow if it is seen as a medical staff review rather than an administrative review.

Fifth, few, if any, of the standards to be developed should be so rigid as to prohibit exception. Few absolute standards exist; variation from agreed-on standards should appropriately prompt additional review but should not be automatically construed as indicating error. Reviewers must allow for the variety of clinical circumstances that might dictate some degree of variation from generally accepted standards.

Finally, if problems are identified in a given area of audit, the audit should be used to bring about change. This requires feedback of the information derived to that segment of the medical staff being audited, together with recommendations to improve use. Whether improvement results can be evaluated only by ongoing or repeat audit.

Control of Antimicrobial Agents in Hospitals

A number of additional approaches to controlling the use of antimicrobial agents in hospitals have been described. These have been summarized by Kunin [28] and are outlined in Table 12-4.

Educational programs on the appropriate use of antimicrobial agents have long been a principal approach to minimizing antibiotic abuse. This method has been of particular interest since the dramatic demonstration by Neu and Howrey [42] of major deficiencies in physician knowledge of antibiotic use. On the other hand, evidence that educational programs have been useful in creating change in antibiotic use have been conflicting at best [14, 16, 21, 26, 43, 63]. In fact, several recent reports have suggested that some educational

programs have little, if any, effect on antimicrobial use in hospitals. At other institutions, however, educational programs have made a significant impact in the hospital setting, suggesting that continuing, focused, and scientifically supported recommendations are effective, especially if supplemented by the feedback of audits of antibiotic use within a specific hospital setting [17].

Kunin [28] believes strongly that some control of the nature and frequency of contact between pharmaceutical representatives and medical staff physicians is important. Precise guidelines cannot be easily established, but some attention should be given to the points listed in Table 12-4. Potential conflicts of interest among speakers sponsored by the pharmaceutical industry should be clearly identified, and it behooves each of these representatives to discuss his or her sponsor's product in the perspective of other comparable, and possibly less expensive, products.

The Pharmacy and Therapeutics Committee in a hospital should play a major role in keeping to a minimum the number of agents needed for optimal therapy and in publicizing guidelines for medical staff to select the least expensive effective agents from complex drug classes such as cephalosporins [63].

The potential role of the diagnostic microbiology laboratory in influencing antibiotic use is often overlooked. Use of generic terminology and restrictions on the reporting of sensitivity tests with new and costly drugs, unless specifically requested or indicated, are critically important considerations. Pharmaceutical representatives know only too well that one important way to increase use of their newest product is for the hospital microbiology susceptibility report to contain a specific listing for that drug.

A number of administrative restraints, minor and major, have been effectively used in some hospital settings to modulate antibiotic use, especially the use of new and costly antibiotics [17, 21, 38, 43, 45]. These range from automatic stop orders for specific costly drugs, especially if used for surgical prophylaxis, to the requirement for approval from infectious disease consultants for the use of new and

Table 12-4. Methods for control of antimicrobial use in hospitals

1. Educational programs on use of antimicrobial agents
   a. Staff conferences
   b. Lectures by outside authorities
   c. Audiovisual programs
   d. Consultations with clinical pharmacists
   e. Hospital Pharmacy Committee newsletters
   f. Independent sources of information (*Medical Letter, AMA Drug Evaluations*)
2. Control of contact between pharmaceutical representatives and staff physicians
   a. Registration in the pharmacy
   b. Visits to staff physicians by appointment only
   c. Policy concerning entry of salespersons to patient care areas
   d. Restricted time and place of displays
   e. Policy on free samples, fittings
   f. Policy on sponsoring speakers, distribution
3. Hospital formulary
   a. Restriction of formulary to minimal number of agents needed for most effective therapy
   b. Elimination of duplicative agents
   c. Rules for selection of least expensive, most effective agent from a given class of agents
   d. Requirement for generic terminology for all orders and labels
4. Sensitivity tests from the diagnostic microbiology laboratory
   a. Appropriate selection of antibiotic sensitivity tests for organism and site of infection
   b. Use of generic class disks
   c. Restriction of reports on specialized agents unless specifically requested or indicated
   d. Use of generic terminology on laboratory report forms
5. Automatic stop orders for specific high-cost agents
6. Written justification for high-cost agents in cases in which alternative, equally effective, less expensive, or less toxic agents may be used (e.g., oral cephalosporins, new parenteral aminoglycosides and cephalosporins, lincosamides, chloramphenicol)
7. Required consultation with infectious disease service after administration of first three doses of specific high-cost agents (e.g., aminoglycosides, parenteral cephalosporins, carbenicillin-ticarcillin, lincosamides)
8. Required approval from infectious disease consultants for release of specific agents that may alter ecology of hospital flora (e.g., amikacin, carbenicillin-ticarcillin)
9. Establishment of guidelines and audits of antimicrobial use that permit the hospital staff to set standards of use based on local needs and judgments, guided by independent criteria. Audit is based on voluntary compliance with standards but requires a well-structured channel for authoritative feedback

Source: Adapted from C.M. Kunin, Evaluation of antibiotic usage: A comprehensive look at alternative approaches. *Rev. Infect. Dis.* 3:745, 1981.

costly drugs. The interposition of such administrative restraints must be carefully individualized to the specific hospital setting [28]. For example, the requirement for infectious disease consultation has worked effectively in some academic centers with full-time infectious disease staff and fellows, whereas in community hospital settings, infectious disease consultants on the medical staff have generally rejected the role of policing antibiotic therapy. More broadly applicable is the requirement for written justification, either in the patient's chart or on the order sheet, for costly agents such as new aminoglycosides

or cephalosporins or the requirement for consultation after 24 or 48 hours of use of such agents.

The Infectious Diseases Society of America has long been concerned about the overuse of antibiotics in hospitals and, in 1985, appointed an Antimicrobial Agents Committee to assess this problem and to make recommendations. The Society in 1988 published *Guidelines for Improving the Use of Antimicrobial Agents in Hospitals* [35]. The first step in the recommendation is the creation of a local hospital antimicrobial agents team, to consist of an infectious disease physician, the hospital infection control practitioner, the clinical microbiologist, and the clinical pharmacist. A three-point program was recommended, to include (1) selection of antimicrobial agents for the hospital formulary; (2) development of educational programs; and (3) introduction of one or more methods to improve antimicrobial selection and usage. Possible approaches to effecting improvement include antibiotic order forms, automatic stop orders, limited susceptibility test reporting, concurrent monitoring, specific audits of antimicrobial drug use, regulation of promotional efforts by pharmaceutical representatives within the hospital, and close monitoring and control of clinical trials carried out within the institution. Bryan [5] has summarized the advantages and disadvantages of various strategies for improving antibiotic use, and these are shown in Table 12-5. As the antimicrobial drug resistance of nosocomial pathogens in-

creases and as the cost of new antibiotics mounts, implementation of these sound and sensible recommendations will become even more important.

With a significant number of multiply drug-resistant nosocomial pathogens (e.g., vancomycin-resistant enterococci and multiresistant *Pseudomonas*), we are already dangerously close to having no effective antimicrobial therapy. Resistance to the broad-spectrum cephalosporins is increasing. Carbepenem resistance has been identified in *Enterobacter, Serratia,* and *Pseudomonas* strains. Hospitals will likely continue to be a major breeding ground for the development of multiply drug-resistant pathogens.

Knowledge of resistance mechanisms should guide the pharmaceutical industry in developing new drugs designed to obviate specific resistance genes or gene products or to identify new mechanisms of bacterial kill-

Table 12-5. Strategies for improving antibiotic use

Strategy	Advantages	Disadvantages
Education	Palatable; does not encroach on the "practice of medicine"	Requires continuous reinforcement; effectiveness is difficult to document
Hospital formulary	Immediate impact; enables generic and therapeutic equivalency substitutions	Requires strong Pharmacy and Therapeutics Committee; perception that patient care is being compromised
Ordering policies	Special order sheets have been shown to be effective; automatic stop orders are also useful	Extra paperwork; physicians may be resentful; automatic stop orders may at times compromise patient care
Drug utilization review	Provides feedback to physicians; ongoing, comprehensive review enables intervention	Labor-intensive; requires contact time between reviewers and physicians
Restriction policies	Enables tight control, especially of the newer, more expensive agents	Limits freedom of physicians; may arouse resentment against the "police officers"
Control of laboratory susceptibility testing	Easily accomplished; can influence prescribing habits	May hinder appropriate use, especially of the newer agents
Limitation of contact time between physicians and pharmaceutical representatives	Probably effective in the teaching setting; minimizes confusion among residents	Probably ineffective in the private practice setting

Source: Reprinted with permission from C.S. Bryan, Strategies to improve antibiotic use. *Infect. Dis. Clin. North Am.* 3:723, 1989.

ing. As suggested by Jacoby and Archer [22], it may prove possible for molecular geneticists to create genes capable of inactivating resistance determinants. Meanwhile, until such biotechnologic advances are made, we must continue all efforts to ensure optimal and wise use of antibiotics in hospitals as well as in the community, in order to minimize the selection and spread of antibiotic-resistant nosocomial pathogens.

References

1. Barber, M., et al. Reversal of antibiotic resistance in hospital staphylococcal infection. *Br. Med. J.* 1:11, 1960.
2. Bartlett, J.G., et al. Antibiotic-associated pseudomembranous colitis due to toxin-producing clostridia. *N. Engl. J. Med.* 298:531, 1978.
3. Bartlett, J.G., Onderdonk, A.B., and Cisneros, R.L. Clindamycin-associated colitis in hamsters due to a toxin-producing clostridial species. *J. Infect. Dis.* 136:701, 1977.
4. Bauer, A.W., Perry, D.M., and Kirby, W.M.M. Drug usage and antibiotic susceptibility of staphylococci. *J.A.M.A.* 173:475, 1960.
5. Bryan, C.S. Strategies to improve antibiotic use. *Infect. Dis. Clin. North Am.* 3:723, 1989.
6. Buckwold, F.J., and Ronald, A.R. Antimicrobial misuse: Effects and suggestions for control. *J. Antimicrob. Chemother.* 5:129, 1979.
7. Bulger, R.J., Larson, E., and Sherris, J.C. Decreased incidence of resistance to antimicrobial agents among *Escherichia coli* and *Klebsiella-Enterobacter:* Observations in a university hospital over a 10-year period. *Ann. Intern. Med.* 72:65, 1970.
8. Damato, J.J., Eitzman, D.V., and Baer, H. Persistence and dissemination in the community of R factors of nosocomial origin. *J. Infect. Dis.* 129:205, 1974.
9. Davies, J.E., Resistance to aminoglycosides: Mechanisms and frequency. *Rev. Infect. Dis.* 5:S261, 1983.
10. Finland, M. And the walls come tumbling down. More antibiotic resistance, and now the pneumococcus. *N. Engl. J. Med.* 299:770, 1978.
11. Finland, M. Changing ecology of bacterial infections as related to antibacterial therapy. *J. Infect. Dis.* 122:419, 1970.
12. Finland, M. Changing patterns of susceptibility of common bacterial pathogens to antimicrobial agents. *Ann. Intern. Med.* 76:1009, 1972.
13. Franco, J.A., Eitzman, D.V., and Baer, J. Anti-

biotic usage and microbial resistance in an intensive care nursery. *Am. J. Dis. Child.* 126:318, 1973.
14. Geddes, A.M., and Gully, P.R. Antibiotic use in hospital. *Lancet* 2:532, 1981.
15. Gibson, C.D., Jr. and Thompson, W.C., Jr. The response of burn wound staphylococci to alternating programs of antibiotic therapy. *Antibiot. Annu.* 1955–56:32, 1956.
16. Gilbert, D.N. and Jackson, J. Effect of an education program on the proper use of gentamicin in a community hospital (abstr.). *Clin. Res.* 24:112A, 1976.
17. Hirschman, S.Z., et al. Use of antimicrobial agents in a university teaching hospital: Evolution of a comprehensive control program. *Arch. Intern. Med.* 148:2001, 1988.
18. Holmberg, S.D., Solomon, S.L., and Blake, P.A. Health and economic impacts of antimicrobial resistance. *Rev. Infect. Dis.* 9:1065, 1987.
19. Hooker, K.D., and DiPiro, J.T. Effect of antimicrobial therapy on bowel flora. *Clin. Pharm.* 7:878, 1988.
20. Houang, E.T., Caswell, M.W., Simms, P.A., and Horton, R.A. Hospital-acquired faecal klebsiellae as source of multiple resistance in the community. *Lancet* 1:148, 1980.
21. Jackson, G.G. Antibiotic policies, practices, and pressures. *J. Antimicrob. Chemother.* 5:1, 1979.
22. Jacoby, G.A., and Archer, G.L. New mechanisms of bacterial resistance to antimicrobial agents. *N. Engl. J. Med.* 324:601, 1991.
23. Jessen, O., et al. Changing staphylococci and staphylococcal infections. *N. Engl. J. Med.* 281:627, 1969.
24. Johanson, W.G., Jr., Pierce, A.K., and Sanford, J.P. Changing pharyngeal bacterial flora of hospitalized patients: Emergence of gram-negative bacilli. *N. Engl. J. Med.* 281:1137, 1969.
25. Johanson, W.G., Jr., Pierce, A.K., Sanford, J.P., and Thomas, G.D. Nosocomial respiratory infections with gram-negative bacilli: The significance of colonization of the respiratory tract. *Ann. Intern. Med.* 77:701, 1972.
26. Jones, S.R. The effect of an educational program upon hospital antibiotic use. *Am. J. Med. Sci.* 273:79, 1977.
27. Korzeniowski, O.M. Effects of antibiotics on the mammalian immune system. *Infect. Dis. Clin. North Am.* 3:469, 1989.
28. Kunin, C.M. Evaluation of antibiotic usage: A comprehensive look at alternative approaches. *Rev. Infect. Dis.* 3:745, 1981.
29. Kunin, C.M., Tupasi, T., and Craig, W.A. Use of antibiotics: A brief exposition of the problem and some tentative solutions. *Ann. Intern. Med.* 79:555, 1973.

30. Lepper, M.H., et al. Epidemiology of erythromycin-resistant staphylococci in a hospital population: Effect on therapeutic activity of erythromycin. *Antibiot. Annu.* 1953–54:308, 1954.

31. Liss, R.H., and Batchelor, F.R. Economic evaluations of antibiotic use and resistance—a perspective: Report of Task Force 6. *Rev. Infect. Dis.* 9(Suppl 3):S297, 1987.

32. Louria, D.B., and Brayton, R.G. The efficacy of penicillin regimens: With observations on the frequency of superinfection. *J.A.M.A.* 186:987, 1963.

33. Lowbury, E.J.L., Babb, J.R., and Roe, E. Clearance from a hospital of gram-negative bacilli that transfer carbenicillin resistance to *Pseudomonas aeruginosa*. *Lancet* 2:941, 1972.

34. Mandell, L.A. Effects of antimicrobial and antineoplastic drugs on the phagocytic and microbicidal function of the polymorphonuclear leukocyte. *Rev. Infect. Dis.* 4:683, 1982.

35. Marr, J.J., Moffet, H.L., and Kunin, C.M. Guidelines for improving the use of antimicrobial agents in hospitals: A statement by the Infectious Diseases Society of America. *J. Infect. Dis.* 157:869, 1988.

36. McGowan, J.E., Jr. Antimicrobial resistance in hospital organisms and its relation to antibiotic use. *Rev. Infect. Dis.* 5:1033, 1983.

37. McGowan, J.E., Jr., and Finland, M. Infection and antibiotic usage at Boston City Hospital: Changes in prevalence during the decade 1964–1973. *J. Infect. Dis.* 129:421, 1974.

38. McGowan, J.E., Jr., and Finland, M. Usage of antibiotics in a general hospital: Effect of requiring justification. *J. Infect. Dis.* 130:165, 1974.

39. Milatovic, D. Antibiotics and phagocytosis. *Eur. J. Clin. Microbiol.* 2:414, 1983.

40. Mitsuhashi, S. (Ed.). *Transferable Drug Resistance Factor R.* Baltimore: University Park Press, 1971.

41. Murray, B.E. New aspects of antimicrobial resistance and the resulting therapeutic dilemmas. *J. Infect. Dis.* 163:1185, 1991.

42. Neu, H.C., and Howrey, S.P. Testing the physician's knowledge of antibiotic use: Self-assessment and learning via videotape. *N. Engl. J. Med.* 293:1291, 1975.

43. Noone, P., and Shafi, M.S. Controlling infection in a district general hospital. *J. Clin. Pathol.* 26:140, 1973.

44. Price, D.J.E., and Sleigh, J.D. Control of infection due to *Klebsiella aerogenes* in a neurosurgical unit by withdrawal of all antibiotics. *Lancet* 2:1213, 1970.

45. Recco, R.A., Gladstone, J.L., Friedman, S.A., and Gerken, E.H. Antibiotic control in a municipal hospital. *J.A.M.A.* 241:2283, 1979.

46. Rifkin, G.D., Fekety, F.R., and Silva, J. Antibiotic-induced colitis: Implication of a toxin neutralized by *Clostridium sordellii* antitoxin. *Lancet* 2:1103, 1977.

47. Rose, H.D., and Babcock, J.B. Colonization of intensive care unit patients with gram-negative bacilli. *Am. J. Epidemiol.* 101:495, 1975.

48. Rose, H.D., and Schreier, J. The effect of hospitalization and antibiotic therapy on the gram-negative fecal flora. *Am. J. Med. Sci.* 255:228, 1968.

49. Scheckler, W.E., and Bennett, J.V. Antibiotic usage in seven community hospitals. *J.A.M.A.* 213:264, 1970.

50. Schimpff, S.C., et al. Origin of infection in acute nonlymphocytic leukemia: Significance of hospital acquisition of pathogens. *Ann. Intern. Med.* 77:707, 1972.

51. Selden, R., et al. Nosocomial *Klebsiella* infections: Intestinal colonization as a reservoir. *Ann. Intern. Med.* 74:657, 1971.

52. Shapiro, M., Townsend, T.R., Rosner, B., and Kass, E.H. Use of antimicrobial drugs in general hospitals: Patterns of prophylaxis. *N. Engl. J. Med.* 301:351, 1979.

53. Sogaard, H., Zimmerman-Nielson, C., and Siboni, K. Antibiotic-resistant gram-negative bacilli in a urological ward for male patients during a nine-year period: Relationship to antibiotic consumption. *J. Infect. Dis.* 130:646, 1974.

54. Sprunt, K., Leidy, G.A., and Redman, W. Prevention of bacterial overgrowth. *J. Infect. Dis.* 123:1, 1971.

55. Sprunt, K., and Redman, W. Evidence suggesting importance of role of interbacterial inhibition in maintaining balance of normal flora. *Ann. Intern. Med.* 68:579, 1968.

56. Stevens, G.P., Jacobson, J.A., and Burke, J.P. Changing patterns of hospital infections and antibiotic use: Prevalance surveys in a community hospital. *Arch. Intern. Med.* 141:587, 1981.

57. Tenney, J.H., Hopkins, J.A., LaForce, F.M., and Wang, W.-L.L. Pneumonia and pharyngeal colonization in a medical intensive care unit: Implications for prevention. Presented at the annual Epidemic Intelligence Service Conference, CDC, Atlanta, 1974.

58. Thong, Y.H. Immunomodulation by antimicrobial drugs. *Med. Hypotheses* 8:361, 1982.

59. Tillotson, J.R., and Finland, M. Bacterial colonization and clinical superinfection of the respiratory tract complicating antibiotic treatment of pneumonia. *J. Infect. Dis.* 119:597, 1969.

60. Van der Waaj, D. Colonization resistance of the digestive tract: Clinical consequences and implications. *J. Antimicrob. Chemother.* 10:263, 1982.

61. Williams, R.E.O. Changing Perspectives in Hospital Infection. In: P.S. Brachman and

T.C. Eickhoff (Eds.), *Proceedings of the International Conference on Nosocomial Infections.* Chicago: American Hospital Association, 1971. Pp. 1–10.

62. Wolff, S.M., and Bennett, J.V. Gram-negative-rod bacteremia (edit.). *N. Engl. J. Med.* 291: 733, 1974.

63. Zeman, B.T., Pike, M., and Samet C. The antibiotic utilization committee: An effective tool in the implementation of drug utilization review that monitors the medical justification and cost of antibiotics. *Hospitals* 48:73, 1973.

13

Multiply Drug-Resistant Pathogens: Epidemiology and Control

Robert A. Weinstein

Our antimicrobial pharmacopeia and the organisms that colonize and infect our patients are in continual competition. At times, the lag between introduction of a new antibiotic and increasing prevalence of resistant bacteria (and fungi and viruses) has been very long; for example, ampicillin was in use for many years before the widespread emergence of resistant *Hemophilus influenzae*. At other times, resistance has occurred even before the clinical use of a specific antibiotic; for example, sulfonamide and aminoglycoside resistance can be found in gram-negative bacilli isolated long before our use of these compounds. Such disparities have led to a controversy over whether antibiotic use and abuse or other host and environmental factors are most responsible for the increasing prevalence of antibiotic-resistant microorganisms in the community and in hospitals [83] (see Chap. 12). Nevertheless, it appears to be conventional wisdom that our antibiotic choices seldom remain more than a very few drugs ahead of the resistant strains.

Since the 1960s, reports of antibiotic-resistant bacteria in hospitals have appeared with increasing frequency. For example, before 1965 no hospital outbreaks involving multiply resistant gram-negative bacilli were investigated by the Centers for Disease Control (CDC). During 1965–1975, however, 11 of 15 nosocomial epidemics of Enterobacteriaceae studied involved multiply resistant strains [129]. Among gram-positive bacteria, resistance of *Staphylococcus aureus* to penicillins became epidemic in the early 1960s and ultimately has come to be considered the norm. Since the late 1960s, outbreaks of methicillin-resistant *S. aureus* (MRSA) have been reported, first from Europe and, more recently, from the United States [50] (see Chaps. 12, 37).

In the 1980s, large families of β-lactamases that mediate resistance to newer cephalosporin antibiotics emerged in Enterobacteriaceae; vancomycin resistance in gram-positive cocci was described; and aminoglycoside-resistant, β-lactamase-containing enterococci surfaced. The 1990s have begun to witness staphylococcal and pseudomonal resistance to the new fluoroquinolone antimicrobials.

Bacterial resistance has become a fact of hospital life and is so common that it often goes unnoted until it is either extreme or epidemic. In this chapter, we review the epidemiology of drug-resistant strains in hospitals and discuss prevention and control strategies.

Definition, Mechanisms, and Genetics of Multiple Resistance

Although there is no standard definition for multiple resistance in bacteria, one definition commonly used is resistance to two or more unrelated antibiotics to which the bacteria are normally considered susceptible [83, 141].

Alternatively, resistance to certain key or first-line drugs may be used as a marker for problems, such as aminoglycoside (gentamicin, tobramycin, amikacin, or netilmicin or third-generation cephalosporin (e.g., ceftzazidime, ceftriaxone, etc.) resistance in gram-negative bacilli. Indeed our level of concern often depends on the nature and availability of other agents. Thus penicillin-resistant staphylococci were accepted relatively passively once methicillin became available. However, the therapeutic alternative for methicillin-resistant strains, vancomycin, is a relatively toxic agent, which has heightened our concern about resistant staphylococcal strains.

The most common mechanisms of resistance include production by bacteria of antibiotic-inactivating enzymes, such as β-lactamases or aminoglycoside-modifying enzymes; changes in cell wall permeability or uptake of antibiotics; alteration in target sites, such as ribosomes; changes in susceptible metabolic pathways; or changes in cell wall binding sites, such as the penicillin-binding proteins (see Chap. 14) [61A].

Resistance may be mediated by either the bacterial chromosome or extrachromosomal DNA (plasmids) [34] (see Chaps. 12, 14). Chromosomal resistance occurs by spontaneous mutation and darwinian selection of organisms resistant to single (or closely related) agents. In contrast, bacteria may acquire resistance rapidly by the accrual of resistance plasmids (R factors), which often encode multiple resistances to unrelated drugs. Plasmids may spread across species lines and even between genera. An example of extensive spread is the presence of the same plasmid-mediated TEM-1 β-lactamase—an enzyme that confers resistance to ampicillin—in a variety of gram-negative bacteria, including Enterobacteriaceae, gonococci, and *H. influenzae*. There has also been a recent rekindling of interest in the study of environmentally induced or directed mutagenesis [14].

At the molecular level, portions of plasmids called *transposons* may hitchhike from one plasmid to another or between plasmid and bacterial chromosome. Transposons carrying genes for resistance may align with other elements, such as those encoding virulence or colonization factors, creating R factors with an awesome "one-two punch."

Pathogens and Incidence

The problem of resistance occurs in the community and hospital for both gram-positive and gram-negative bacteria. For example, resistance at the community level has affected *Salmonella, Shigella, Escherichia coli, Neisseria gonorrhoea, H. influenzae* and, most recently, *Streptococcus pneumoniae*. In hospitals, resistance has appeared in a variety of gram-negative bacilli as well as in common skin flora such as coagulase-negative staphylococci and corynebacteria. Although the specific "problem bugs" vary from hospital to hospital and depend on the interaction of a number of factors to be described, there are some general correlations between hospital settings and resistant flora (Table 13-1).

One of the greatest concerns in the 1970s and early 1980s was the emergence of aminoglycoside resistance in nosocomial Enterobac-

Table 13-1. Resistance problems in the 1990s

Setting	Bacteria	Key resistances
General hospitals and intensive care units	Enterobacteriaceae	Newer cephalosporins, aminoglycosides
	Pseudomonas aeruginosa	Aminoglycosides, antipseudomonal penicillins, newer cephalosporins, carbapenems, quinolones
	Acinetobacter species	Aminoglycosides, multiple
	Xanthomonas maltophilia	Multiple
	Staphylococcus aureus	Methicillin, quinolones, multiple
	Streptococcus pneumoniae	Penicillin, multiple
	Enterococci	Gentamicin, ampicillin, vancomycin
Oncology units	Enterobacteriaceae	Trimethoprim-sulfamethoxazole
	JK diphtheroids	Multiple
	Staphylococcus epidermidis	Multiple
Geriatric units	*Proteus, Providencia, Morganella*	Aminoglycosides
	Staphylococcus aureus	Methicillin, quinolones

teriaceae and *Pseudomonas*. In individual hospitals, the prevalence of aminoglycoside-resistant gram-negative bacilli varies considerably, usually being greatest in large hospitals and teaching institutions [23, 57, 60, 94, 106]. Data from the National Nosocomial Infection Surveillance (NNIS) System show that the percentage of *Pseudomonas aeruginosa* resistant to gentamicin increased from 6.6 percent in 1975 to 13.1 percent in 1979 [2] but was still 13.4 percent in 1984 [57] and also in 1990.

More recently, the availability of the second-generation cephalosporins, such as cefamandole, cefoxitin, and cefuroxime, or third-generation agents, such as cefotaxime, cefoperazone, ceftizoxime, ceftriaxone, and ceftazidime, and of the combination agent, ticarcillin-clavulanate, has called attention to an additional set of potential resistances in nosocomial gram-negative bacilli [116]. For instance, *Enterobacter* species were considered initially susceptible to cefamandole but frequently developed resistance during therapy due to spontaneous derepression of intrinsic chromosomal type I β-lactamase [98, 115]. Now that the second- and third-generation drugs have been available for several years, resistance among *Enterobacter* species is widespread. In a recent six-hospital study of 136 cases of *Enterobacter* bacteremia, 32 percent of isolates were resistant to all cephalosporins and penicillins [18]. The extent to which the regional differences and increases in resis-

tance correlate with the use of these agents needs to be assessed.

Families of plasmidborne extended-spectrum β-lactamases, first identified in 1983–1985 in Europe, are also capable of inactivating many of the newer cephalosporins and broad-spectrum penicillins [102A]. These enzymes evolved by point mutations from common older plasmidborne enzymes and are transferable to bacteria that do not have the intrinsic chromosomal genetic material to allow broad-spectrum resistance. These extended-spectrum β-lactamases are now being reported from several centers in the United States [102A].

The broadest-spectrum commercially available parenteral antimicrobial is the carbapenem, imipenem. Preliminary analysis of 1986–1989 NNIS data showed that only 1.4 percent of 1282 *Enterobacter* species isolates were resistant to this agent [39]. However, imipenem resistance in *P. aeruginosa* was already 11 percent in the NNIS hospitals [39].

The prevalence of enteric bacilli resistant to trimethoprim (TMP) and TMP-sulfonamide combinations has been variable [46, 53]. For example, TMP has been in use in Finland since 1973; in 1980–1981, from 8.6 to 38.3 percent of nosocomial urinary isolates (*Pseudomonas* excluded) were resistant, depending on the hospital studied [61]. When TMP-sulfamethoxazole has been used in a variety of settings for prophylaxis, prevalence of resistant strains has varied from 0 to 100 percent. In many U.S. hospitals, however, bacteria resistant to newer cephalosporins are often still susceptible to TMP-sulfamethoxazole [18].

For gram-positive bacteria, methicillin resistance in *S. aureus* and the increasing occurrence of disease caused by multiply resistant coagulase-negative staphylococci have been of concern. In 63 NNIS hospitals during 1974–1981, the percentage of *S. aureus* infections resistant to methicillin rose from a low of 2.4 percent (1975) to a high of only 5 percent (1981) [50]. This increase was due entirely to four large teaching institutions in which the percentages rose from 0 to 5 percent to 15 to 50 percent. However, by 1989, MRSA had become hyperendemic in many of the NNIS hospitals (Table 13-2) [99].

In NNIS hospitals, gentamicin resistance in *S. aureus* increased from 1 to 13 percent during 1975–1979, whereas resistance in coagulase-negative staphylococci increased from 2 to 24 percent [2]. The incidence of infection due to all coagulase-negative staphylococci in leukemia patients increased at one large cancer center from 2 per 1,000 days of hospitalization in 1974 to 15 per 1,000 days in 1979 [136]. Methicillin resistance occurred in 40 percent of 87 strains tested. Multiply resistant coagulase-negative strains have also caused symptomatic bacteremia in 3 percent of newborns in a large referral intensive care unit (ICU) [5] and in increasing numbers of adult patients in some hospitals [19].

The fluoroquinolone antibiotics, such as norfloxacin and ciprofloxacin, offer a new class of broad-spectrum agents that usually do not show cross-resistance with older classes of antimicrobials. Moreover, in vitro emergence of bacterial resistance appears to be less frequent for quinolones than for cephalosporins. However, the widespread community use of the quinolones suggests the need for careful prospective studies of resistance, particularly in *Pseudomonas* and *S. aureus,* two potential problem bacteria for this class. In fact, in some centers more than 50 percent of MRSA strains are now also resistant to ciprofloxacin, an agent to which all the strains were initially susceptible.

Classification and Diagnostic Criteria

Determining whether resistant bacteria are hospital-acquired is often problematic since patients may be colonized asymptomatically when they enter the hospital. For example, in our experience [32, 34, 38, 97, 142] and others' [16], 15 to 25 percent of patients colonized or infected with aminoglycoside-resistant gram-negative bacilli and as many as 50 percent of patients who appear to acquire cefazolin-resistant Enterobacteriaceae after surgery [32, 33] have brought these strains into the hospital. Moreover, the incubation period for many infections caused by resistant bacteria is not clearly delineated.

In addition to the difficulties in defining hospital acquisition, there is often the question of whether the patient is colonized or has clinical disease due to the resistant strain. This is particularly difficult with lower respiratory tract infection (see Chap. 29). Criteria for making this differentiation are discussed in the chapters on site-specific infections; however, we consider colonization an impor-

Table 13-2. Percent of nosocomial *Staphylococcal aureus* isolates resistant to methicillin, oxacillin, or nafcillin, in National Nosocomial Infection Surveillance System hospitals

Hospital size	Hospital's medical school affiliation	Average 1975–1989	1989
≤ 200 Beds	Nonteaching	3.6	3.1
> 200 Beds	Nonteaching	4.9	12.8
≤ 500 Beds	Teaching	5.0	16.0
> 500 Beds	Teaching	8.3	21.6

Source: Adapted from A. Panlilio et al., Prevalence and distribution of methicillin-resistant *Staphylococcus aureus* in the United States. *Infect. Control Hosp. Epidemiol.* 1992 (in press).

tant epidemiologic problem since it increases the reservoir of resistant bacteria and is often a precursor to clinical disease [123].

From a microbiologic standpoint, defining resistance also may have pitfalls (see Chap. 9). In testing by disk diffusion, as a general example, antibiotic-containing disks may be outdated or inadequately tamped onto the agar surface, the bacterial inoculum may be too heavy or too light, the depth or pH of the agar may be incorrect, or the wrong drugs may even be used. Some gram-negative bacilli, such as *Flavobacterium*, are intrinsically resistant to the usual gram-negative panel of antibiotics and, unless the appropriate drugs are tested, such bacteria may appear untreatable. Moreover, some automated systems have difficulty with certain antibiotics against specific bacteria. Problems in testing specific "drug-bug" combinations are cited under the heading Specific Organisms.

Sources of Resistant Strains

The source of most resistant strains in hospitals appears to be patients who are colonized or infected [123, 141]. Because the normal pharyngeal and intestinal flora of hospitalized patients may be displaced by multiply resistant enteric bacteria and *P. aeruginosa* (urine, perineum, and wounds may be similarly affected [43, 86]), there are often many colonized patients for each patient with recognized infection—the so-called iceberg effect. This shift in flora often occurs within a

very few days of admission (Fig. 13-1) and affects the older, generally sicker or more debilitated patients. The importance of various risk factors (e.g., specific exposures versus more hands-on care in general) and the pathophysiology of this shift (e.g., possible changes in membrane receptors or ligands, antibiotic suppression of normal flora) are not well delineated [28]. In our experience, much of this shift results from emergence of low-count community-acquired strains in the face of antibiotic exposure rather than from true nosocomial acquisition (Table 13-3) [33].

Personnel have been documented to dis-

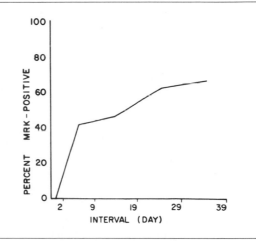

Fig. 13-1. Percentage of 138 patients positive for multiply resistant *Klebsiella* (MRK) on rectal culture, by interval from admission. (Reprinted with permission from R. Selden, et al., Nosocomial *Klebsiella* infections: Intestinal colonization as a reservoir. *Ann. Intern. Med.* 74:657, 1971.)

Table 13-3. Characteristics of cardiac surgery patients colonized with cefazolin-resistant gram-negative bacilli

| *Species* | *Number of patients colonized (n = 87)* | Location at first positive culture (% patients) | | | *Percent of colonization due to horizontal transmission* | *Percent developing clinical infection* |
		At admission	*48–72 hr into CSICU*	*>72 hr into CSICU*		
Enterobacter species	58	50	34	16	16	21
Citrobacter species	37	49	22	29	?	3
Pseudomonas aeruginosa	33	55	12	33	9	27
Serratia marcescens	7	43	57	0	29	29

CSICU = cardiac surgery intensive care unit; ? = unknown (no typing system used).
Source: Adapted from D.M. Flynn, R.A. Weinstein, and S.A. Kabins, Infections with gram-negative bacilli in a cardiac surgery intensive care unit: The relative role of *Enterobacter*. *J. Hosp. Infect.* 11:367, 1988.

seminate resistant gram-positive strains, such as MRSA [21] and even coagulase-negative staphylococci [9]. However, personnel carriage of resistant gram-negative bacilli (other than transient hand carriage described in the following section) appears to be very unusual. Exceptions include outbreaks reportedly traced to carriers of *Acinetobacter, Citrobacter,* and *Proteus. Acinetobacter,* one of the few gram-negative bacilli that may be among normal skin flora, was noted in one outbreak to recur periodically despite disinfection of the apparent environmental reservoirs. The outbreak was ultimately traced to the colonized hands of a respiratory therapy technician who had dermatitis and apparently contaminated respiratory therapy equipment while assembling it [13]. There have also been clusters of *Citrobacter* infections of the central nervous system in neonates, traced to hand carriage by nurses [44, 100], and an outbreak of *Proteus* infections in newborns traced to a nurse who was a chronic carrier [11].

Foodborne contamination with multiply resistant gram-negative bacilli has been cited in several investigations [50, 125] and has been incriminated particularly in oncology units [48]. Despite the potential importance of these observations, however, the overall role of food in introducing resistant strains into the general hospital remains unclear.

Environmental sources and reservoirs of resistant strains have been a recurrent problem, especially when patient care equipment, such as urine-measuring devices, become contaminated with enteric bacilli or *Pseudomonas* [80, 141]. Extensive outbreaks of urinary tract infections (and respiratory tract, perineal, or intestinal colonization) may result when such contaminated equipment is shared by many patients.

Finally, there has been perennial concern about contamination of many areas of the inanimate environment with which patients do not have direct contact, such as flowerpots [143] and sink traps [30, 73, 102]. Despite heavy contamination, these sites usually have not been implicated epidemiologically in the spread of bacteria in hospitals. However, for high-risk immunocompromised patients, es-

pecially those who have the opportunity for environmental exposures (e.g., the debilitated oncology patient who sits at the sink to wash), strains from sink surfaces have been linked to patient colonization and infection [48].

Modes of Transmission

The most important way that resistant bacteria are spread in the hospital is from an infected patient to a susceptible patient via transient carriage on hands of personnel. Such spread contributes to the iceberg of colonized patients and greatly increases the source and reservoir of resistant strains in the hospital (Fig. 13-2). Most of the evidence incriminating hands of personnel is circumstantial [1, 68, 114]. However, the weight of experience, dating back to the successful introduction of hand-washing as a control measure by Semmelweis, strongly supports this concept. Indexes of hands-on exposure to personnel, used in a few studies to quantitate patients' risk, have provided an additional measure.

Common-source spread of resistant strains has been noted primarily in outbreak settings. The attention of the medical community (and journal editors) is often attracted to such epidemics because of striking features, such as large numbers of patients infected with very resistant bacteria, unusual breaks in techniques or protocols, or contaminated commercial products. Perhaps more common than such "extravaganzas" are the ongoing episodes of limited cross-infection due to contamination of shared patient care equipment, such as measuring containers and other environmental reservoirs, which probably account for a significant portion of seemingly endemic infections [142].

Airborne spread of resistant bacteria has been documented rarely. For MRSA, the most recent experience suggests that airborne spread is not a significant problem. For gram-negative bacilli, there was concern in one hospital that contamination in a 16-storey chute-hydropulping waste disposal system

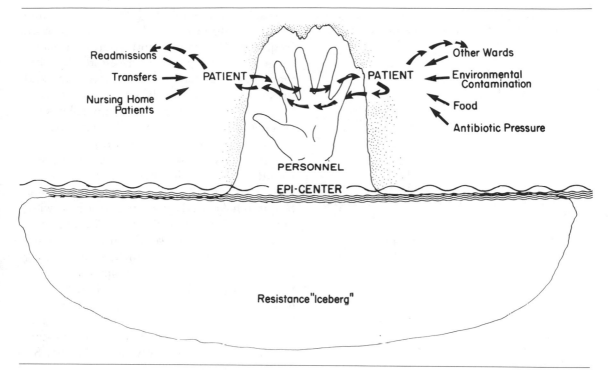

Fig. 13-2. The dynamics of nosocomial resistance: resistance iceberg. (Reprinted with permission from R.A. Weinstein, and S.A. Kabins, Strategies for prevention and control of multiple drug-resistant nosocomial infection. *Am. J. Med.* 70:449, 1981.)

led to airborne dispersal and transmission of *Pseudomonas* and enteric bacilli [47]. Waste pulp in the chute had 10^8 colony-forming units (cfu) per gram; air samples from hallways connecting the chute and nursing units had greater than 150 cfu per cubic foot of air. After closing the chute, air counts fell by more than 75 percent and the incidence of nosocomial gram-negative bacteremias fell by more than 65 percent. However, this experience appears unique.

Various insect vectors, such as flies and cockroaches, are probably unimportant in the transmission of resistant bacteria in most U.S. hospitals.

Predisposing Factors
Patients

A number of host factors have been associated with acquisition of antibiotic-resistant bacteria (Table 13-4). Our epidemiologic understanding of these factors has remained somewhat limited because most work has focused on epidemic and few on endemic situations [35, 65, 106, 142], most studies have been retrospective and therefore limited in ability to gather complete host profiles, some studies have not included control groups and, until recently, relatively few of the studies have used multivariate analyses to control for relatedness of host factors [17, 45]. Indeed many of the factors are undoubtedly linked and are serving as indirect markers of frequency of patient-staff contact (i.e., risk of indirect contact spread by hands of personnel).

The studies from which the information is drawn for Table 13-4 include experience with both gram-negative bacilli and gram-positive bacteria. The host factors for both types of epidemics have been generally similar except that gram-negative bacilli involve the urinary tract and associated factors more often, such as indwelling bladder catheters, whereas gram-positive bacteria affect the skin and related factors somewhat more, such as duration of intravenous catheterization.

Of the many factors, the role of antibiotics

Table 13-4. Examples of host factors associated with epidemic antimicrobial resistance in selected case-control studies

Factor	Reference
Antimicrobial drugs	
Prophylaxis	[45, 107, 136]
Therapy	[7, 17, 21, 40, 44, 45, 49, 69, 90, 117–119, 123, 124, 128, 133, 140, 145]
Apgar score	[45]
Duration of hospital or ICU stay	[13, 17, 19, 40, 45, 117, 123, 145]
Decreased WBC	[128]
Elderly age	[21, 45]
Endotracheal intubation (or tracheostomy)	[13, 45, 92, 145]
Exchange transfusions	[45]
Gastrointestinal colonization	[17, 123]
Gavage feeding	[44]
Genitourinary instrumentation	[119]
Hyperalimentation	[19, 45]
Intravenous therapy	[45]
Low birth weight	[45]
Mucocutaneous defects	[128]
Nasogastric suction	[123]
Proximity to other patients	[17, 77]
Race	[44]
Respiratory therapy	[17, 123]
Severity of underlying disease	[21, 140]
Sex	[128]
Surgery (or number of operations)	[17, 21, 133]
Urinary catheter	
Condom	[86]
Indwelling	[23, 40, 107, 118, 119, 145]
Urinary irrigation	[119]

ICU = intensive care unit; WBC = white blood cell count.

has been the most controversial [83], and several issues warrant emphasis. Many studies document the emergence of aminoglycoside-resistant strains after use of topical aminoglycoside ointments [45], related to nonabsorbable aminoglycosides in enteral regimens for suppression of gut bacteria in oncology patients [37, 46], or after parenteral aminoglycoside therapy [84, 93, 107, 126]. In some studies, resistant strains have occurred more frequently in wound and sputum isolates, suggesting emergence of resistance at sites more likely to have poor penetration, and thus subinhibitory levels, of aminoglycosides [142]. The emergence of resistant isolates has also been correlated with inadequate doses of aminoglycosides [35, 81, 84, 142].

There has been some controversy surrounding the relation between amikacin use and resistance [3, 84, 87, 105, 144]. Some hospitals have used amikacin extensively without noting any increase in resistance [81]. However, the incidence depends to some extent on how prevalent amikacin-inactivating enzymes are in the particular hospital, as well as on the adequacy of dosing. Regardless, cross-resistance to multiple aminoglycosides, including amikacin, occurs in up to 60 percent of gram-negative bacilli resistant to gentamicin or tobramycin [3, 58, 81, 82, 122, 144].

Use of the newer cephalosporin antibiotics has been associated with emergence of cephalosporin-resistant strains, particularly of *Enterobacter, Serratia,* and *Pseudomonas* [116]. For example, as many as 50 percent of *Enterobacter* species may be resistant by the end of treatment [138].

The use of TMP has been associated with the emergence of TMP-resistant strains in a variety of settings, including treatment of urinary tract infections, prophylaxis of traveler's diarrhea, and gut sterilization in oncology patients. Of particular concern, this resistance is often carried on transferable R factors that confer resistance to multiple antimicrobials, emphasizing the way one agent may effect resistance to many others. In one study, 96 percent of 165 TMP-resistant *E. coli* were resistant to at least four drugs, and 25 percent were resistant to seven; TMP resistance was transferable in 40 of 100 strains tested [90].

Regarding gram-positive bacteria, studies in the 1960s suggested that patients were at greater risk of being colonized with *S. aureus* after antibiotic treatment [7]. Methicillin-resistant staphylococci have been found in hospitalized drug addicts who had self-prescribed oral cephalosporins, emphasizing the potential impact of antibiotic use in the community on hospital flora [117].

Epidemics

The events leading to any nosocomial epidemic are probably multifactorial. In most outbreaks of multiply drug-resistant bacteria, precipitating events have not been well elucidated. Factors that could increase person-to-person spread include poor aseptic practices, as in crowded units or when the nurse-to-patient ratio becomes too low. Spread from the environment is facilitated by poor housekeeping practices that lead to reservoirs of resistant organisms within the hospital, as when infected urine is allowed to remain in urine measuring or testing devices. Excessive use of antibiotics may increase the selective pressure for resistant strains [83].

Certain fortuitous events may precipitate outbreaks, such as contamination of a commercial product, admission of a patient who is a heavy shedder of multiply resistant bacteria [37], or acquisition of resistance by a bacterial species that is adept at colonization or unusually resistant to disinfection. Also, advances in medical technology, such as transplantation, dialysis, and new prosthetic devices, create additional epidemic risks.

Particular areas within the hospital, especially intensive care (see Chap. 20), burn (see Chap. 34), neurosurgical, and urology units, are prone to outbreaks. These areas house acutely ill patients who are subjected to many invasive procedures and are often exposed to multiple antibiotics under circumstances in which asepsis may be trampled in the rush of crisis care. We have found that multiply resistant bacteria may breed in such units, which we call *epicenters* (Fig. 13-2) [141]. As colonized patients are transferred to other areas of the hospital, they may leave a trial of resistance.

Plasmid and Transposon Outbreaks

Most reported outbreaks have been due to epidemic spread of single strains. In the past few years, however, several plasmid outbreaks have been described in which a resistance plasmid has caused either simultaneous or sequential resistance to occur in epidemic fashion in different species or genera (Table 13-5) [26, 64, 79, 109, 110, 112, 135]. We are also recognizing that transposition of plasmid segments (or other spatial rearrangements of genetic material) may lead to "transposon outbreaks" involving whole families of related resistance plasmids [109].

The epidemiology of most plasmid outbreaks, specifically the reservoirs for the resistance plasmids, time and place of transfer of plasmids, and pressures involved, has been largely speculative [36, 83, 108]. Transfer can occur in the gut, on skin, in urine, and in the environment (e.g., in urine containers) and may be facilitated by antimicrobial therapy [108]. Moreover, relatively avirulent bacterial strains may serve as reservoirs for resistance. For example, gentamicin resistance in *Staphylococcus epidermidis* or *S. aureus* may be mediated by identical plasmids that can pass between these two species in vitro and on human skin [61].

Plasmid outbreaks may be difficult to detect but should be sought through surveillance for the occurrence of multiple species or genera with identical or very similar multiple drug (or even just key drug) resistance patterns. If available, similar gel electrophoretic patterns of plasmid DNA could facilitate detection (see Chap. 14). Once recognized, plasmid epidemics are at present controlled much like single-strain outbreaks (see under the heading Control). In the future, technologic refinements may facilitate more extensive epidemiologic investigation of plasmid and transposon resistance and allow more specific control measures.

Other Multiple-Strain Outbreaks

Occasionally, common sources may become contaminated with several bacterial species, leading to outbreaks of otherwise unrelated strains. For example, one multiple-strain outbreak of orthopedic wound infections was traced to a common bucket used to mix cast material. The bucket was not routinely disin-

Table 13-5. Examples of plasmid outbreaks

Setting (ref.)	Bacteria (no.)	Predominant infections	Appearance of resistance (duration)	Plasmidborne resistances
Neonatal ICU [79]	*Klebsiella* Serotype 30 (21) Serotype 19 (6)	NS	Sequential (9 mo, 5 mo)	Gm, kn, am, cf, cb
Hospitalwide [135]	*Serratia* (71) *Klebsiella Citrobacter Proteus Enterobacter Providencia* } (68)	UTI	Simultaneous (3 yr)	Gm, tb, kn, am, cf, cb, st, su
Burn unit [26]	*Klebsiella Enterobacter* Three other genera } (NS)	Burn	Simultaneous (11 mo)	Tb, kn, ne
Hospitalwide [112]	*Klebsiella* (69) *Escherichia coli Enterobacter Proteus* } (16)	UTI, wd, resp	Index case admitted with epidemic strain; remainder ~ simultaneous (2 yr)	Gm, tb, kn, am, cf, cb, ch, su

ICU = intensive care unit; NS = not stated; UTI = urinary tract infection; wd = wound infection; resp = respiratory infection; gm = gentamicin; kn = kanamycin; am = ampicillin; cf = cephalothin; cb = carbenicillin; tb = tobramycin; st = streptomycin; su = sulfonamide; ne = neomycin; ch = chloramphenicol.

fected and contained a variety of contaminants that probably were inoculated into wounds during application of casts. Such outbreaks may go unrecognized unless one strain predominates or the strains or epidemiologic circumstances are very unusual.

Control
Control of Epidemic Resistance

Control of resistant bacteria has usually focused on epidemics (Table 13-6) and traditionally has involved efforts to strengthen aseptic practices while an epidemiologic analysis of cases (and controls) is quickly undertaken to exclude common-source exposures [141] (see Chap. 6). Empiric attempts to decrease transmission usually have also included isolating or cohorting infected or colonized patients. Identifying the colonized patients (see Fig. 13-2) often requires culture surveys, which may be facilitated by the use of selective media (see Chap. 9). In some outbreaks, susceptible patients, such as those with indwelling urinary catheters, have been physically separated to decrease the likelihood that personnel would passively carry pathogens

Table 13-6. Traditional control measures

Identify reservoirs
Colonized and infected patients
Environmental contamination; common sources
Halt transmission among patients
Improve hand-washing and asepsis
Barrier precautions (gloves, gown) for colonized and infected patients
Eliminate any common source; disinfect environment
Separate susceptible patients
Close unit to new admissions if necessary
Halt progression from colonization to infection
Discontinue compromising factors (Table 13-4) when possible (e.g., extubate, remove nasogastric tube, discontinue bladder catheters, as clinically indicated); rotate intravenous catheter sites; employ proper respirator care (see Chap. 29)
Modify host risk
Treat underlying disease and complications
Control antibiotic use (rotate, restrict, or cease)

from one patient or drainage bag to the next [77]. In drastic situations, units have been closed to new admissions.

In some instances, antibiotic controls may help restrict the spread of resistant bacteria

[83, 93]. First, in high-density units such as ICUs, restricting antibiotic use may be important [35, 36, 46, 83, 93, 107]. In rare situations, antibiotic use has been totally suspended [104]. Second, antibiotic restrictions may decrease selective pressures in some plasmid outbreaks. Chemicals that "cure" bacterial plasmids in vitro are currently too toxic for use in humans. Safer agents such as nalidixic acid, which may prevent transfer of plasmids [41], have yet to be used for this purpose in clinical situations. Third, more careful dosing with aminoglycosides may decrease the chance that subinhibitory levels will select resistant subpopulations (due to spontaneous chromosomal mutations), particularly in sites that have large bacterial populations, such as wounds or the respiratory tract. Finally, the control of antibiotics that select for sensitive precursors of resistant organisms (e.g., cephalosporins selecting for *Pseudomonas*) may be necessary.

Experimental Approaches to Epidemic Control

Table 13-7 lists several epidemic control methods that have been tried. Topical and nonabsorbable antimicrobials have been used for prophylaxis in several settings, including epidemics of resistant bacteria. For example, polymyxin spray was used experimentally in one ICU to forestall pharyngeal colonization and pneumonia with *Pseudomonas* (see Chap. 29). In limited studies, this approach appeared to work but, when applied in the ICU in a continuous fashion, the consequence was a compensatory increase in pneumonias caused by polymyxin-resistant bacilli [30]. More recently, use of combinations of topical agents (see later) has been successful in European ICUs in controlling outbreaks of multiply resistant gram-negative bacilli [10, 139].

In the 1960s, attempts were made to use avirulent staphylococci to reduce colonization with epidemic strains. This form of bacterial interference has been reexplored recently. In one study, pharyngeal implantation of α-hemolytic streptococci successfully displaced resistant enteric organisms in infants in a neonatal ICU [127]. In an outbreak, this ap-

Table 13-7. Experimental approaches for controlling resistance

Prevention of acquisition by use of topical antimicrobials
    Respiratory spray
    Oral nonabsorbables
Disinfectants in devices and in environmental reservoirs
Bacterial interference
Treatment of colonized patients
    Topical or systemic antimicrobials
Immune enhancement

proach was used with other measures to control successfully colonization of neonates by amikacin-resistant *Serratia* and *Klebsiella* [20]. However, this work needs to be confirmed and studies extended to adults before any conclusions can be made about its general applicability.

Another control measure from the past that is being reinvestigated is disinfection of urinary catheter drainage bags. Earlier use of this method, with formalin in drainage bottles, ended when closed systems were widely adopted. Unfortunately, closed drainage cannot prevent contamination of collection bags indefinitely; in as many as 30 percent of patients with initially sterile urine, contamination of the bag may precede bladder infection [86]. In one study, disinfection of drainage bags with hydrogen peroxide forestalled urinary infections in a small number of patients with acute spinal injury [75]. Organisms may still ascend from the perineum around the catheter, however, and in a controlled study in a large teaching hospital, bag decontamination did not appear to reduce infection rates [134]. Nevertheless, bag disinfection may reduce reservoirs of contaminated urine in the hospital environment [86] and warrants additional controlled study.

Attempts to decontaminate relatively remote environmental reservoirs of resistant bacteria, such as sink traps, have been innovative [76]. However, based on the failure of such efforts to decrease infection rates [30] and on the lack of any epidemiologic link between sink traps and patients [73, 102], these extraordinary measures do not appear routinely warranted except, perhaps, in units housing oncology patients [48].

Finally, in drastic situations systemic antibiotics have at times been administered to patients who are only colonized with multiply resistant bacteria (e.g., multiply resistant pneumococci) [69].

Control of Endemic Resistance

A variety of epidemic control measures may be applied to endemic situations. For ex-

ample, we have used antibiotic resistance precautions (Fig. 13-3) for all patients who are colonized or infected with resistant gram-negative bacilli [141]. In our experience, such barrier-type precautions have markedly decreased the incidence of aminoglycoside-resistant *E. coli, Klebsiella,* and *Enterobacter,* and probably have limited the extent of recurrent miniepidemics of resistant *Serratia* (Fig. 13-4) [142]. In sharp contrast, the incidence of aminoglycoside-resistant *Pseudo-*

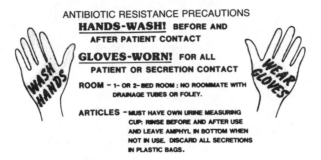

Fig. 13-3. Placard stating barrier-type antibiotic resistance precautions to be placed on door to patient's room and above bed; stickers with similar precautions may be affixed to urinary drainage bag or other items to alert personnel that patient is colonized or infected with resistant bacteria.

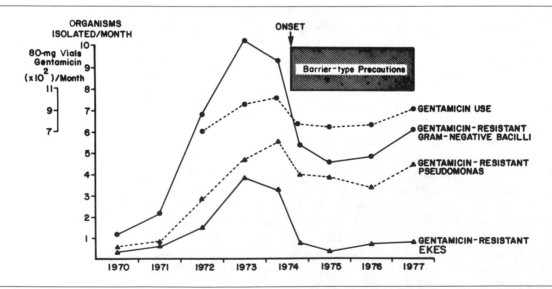

Fig. 13-4. Gentamicin use and gram-negative bacilli resistant to gentamicin at Michael Reese Medical Center, 1970–1977. Data are plotted as the monthly average, and averages for the first 7 and last 5 months of 1974 are plotted separately to demonstrate the effect of barrier precautions, which began in August 1974. EKES = *Escherichia coli, Klebsiella, Enterobacter,* and *Serratia.* (Reprinted with permission from R.A. Weinstein, et al., Endemic aminoglycoside resistance in gram-negative bacilli: Epidemiology and mechanisms. *J. Infect. Dis.* 141:338, 1980.)

monas infections appears to a greater extent to have paralleled antibiotic use rather than to have been affected appreciably by barrier-type precautions. In fact, we have frequently found that in individual patients *P. aeruginosa* became resistant in the face of aminoglycoside therapy [96, 97, 142].

An update of our experience has confirmed these findings [37]. However, we have found that as barrier-type precautions diminished the incidence of plasmid-mediated resistance in Enterobacteriaceae, the remaining resistant isolates followed a pattern like that of *Pseudomonas,* with broad cross-resistant strains emerging from endogenous flora after antibiotic therapy. It is unlikely that the incidence of such strains will be reduced additionally by barrier-type precautions alone. This emphasizes the need to develop better control strategies. For example, recent studies of topical antimicrobials for selective decontamination have focused on the use of combinations of agents (e.g., polymyxin with tobramycin [or gentamicin] and amphotericin B [or nystatin]) applied to the oropharyngeal and gastrointestinal reservoir of endogenous gram-negative bacilli [139]. Such an approach has reduced ICU-related infections in several studies by more than 50 percent compared to historical controls [72, 130], without emergence of resistant strains to date [131]. Certain high-risk patient populations in the United States may also benefit from this strategy [31].

Based on our studies, we suggest a multifaceted approach to control of endemic antibiotic-resistant gram-negative bacilli and MRSA in large acute-care hospitals [141]:

1. Antibiotic resistance precautions (see Fig. 13-3) should be used for all patients who are colonized or infected with aminoglycoside-resistant or broad-spectrum cephalosporin–resistant Enterobacteriaceae. These precautions should be extended to any patient who is a persistent shedder of other multiply resistant bacteria, especially if the patient has draining wounds, receives repeated courses of antibiotics, or requires intensive nursing care.

   The use of universal precautions should reduce the need for such additional measures (see Chap. 11). However, antibiotic resistance precautions also focus on the environment. Moreover, control of epidemics of resistant gram-negative bacilli or staphylococci by increased attention to gloving and cohorting suggest that universal precautions are frequently breached.

2. Such precautions should be used while appropriate cultures are being processed from patients who are admitted (or readmitted) with a history of colonization or infection with resistant organisms.

3. Patients transferred from nursing homes or other hospitals should be evaluated for carriage of resistant bacteria [37, 49, 142]. Certain patients, such as those who are incontinent, have recently received antibiotics, have indwelling urinary catheters or percutaneous feeding tubes, or come from large nursing homes or hospitals, may warrant precautions while appropriate cultures are processed.

4. Appropriate aminoglycoside usage and dosage should be ensured to decrease selection of spontaneous mutations among *P. aeruginosa* and, to a lesser extent, among Enterobacteriaceae.

5. Surveillance of patients and clinical laboratory results should be maintained to detect miniepidemics (2 or more patients with similarly resistant organisms) so that cross-infection or significant environmental reservoirs can be identified and controlled (see Chap. 5).

6. When patients who are colonized or infected with resistant bacteria are transferred to another hospital or nursing home, the receiving institution should be notified of the isolation status.

7. Compromising factors (see Table 13-4) in high-risk patients should be eliminated whenever possible. In certain specialty units, such as ICUs, control of antibiotic usage as discussed previously may also help to control endemic resistance. However, several factors may limit the efficacy of this measure. First, use of one antibiotic may lead to cross-resistance to others, as seen with aminoglycoside cross-resistance

as well as with plasmid colinkage of resistance. Next, sequential acquisition of bacterial resistance when antibiotics are rotated has been well described [45]. Finally, if and when controls are lifted, resistant organisms that have remained in low numbers in colonized patients may reemerge [93].

8. In settings where careful prospective microbiologic and epidemiologic monitoring is available, selective decontamination, as described earlier, may be used as an interim epidemic control measure [139].

Threshold for Investigation and Control

In certain situations, ongoing control measures are appropriate. First, some organisms always warrant prompt attention because of key resistances. Such bacteria include MRSA, high-level penicillin-resistant *S. pneumoniae,* and carbenicillin-aminoglycoside-resistant *P. aeruginosa.* Second, in units such as ICUs, which may serve as epicenters, aggressive containment of multiply resistant strains can be justified. Third, certain types of patients warrant antibiotic resistance precautions. These include patients who are colonized with multiply resistant strains at several sites and whose severity of illness requires frequent physical attention by physicians, nurses, respiratory therapists and so forth, and thus higher risk for spread of resistant bacteria to other patients.

In other situations, the individual hospital must rely on local surveillance and experience to help set formal or intuitive epidemic thresholds for instituting aggressive containment measures and epidemiologic investigations. The thresholds will probably differ for each hospital and for specific multiply resistant strains. For example, with *Serratia* a low threshold may trigger an investigation because of the iceberg effect often seen in patients with urinary catheters or on respirators. In some hospitals, ongoing laboratory studies, such as serotyping or biotyping, may be used to help evaluate possible single-strain outbreaks [29] (see Chap. 9). Plasmid outbreaks and multiple-strain outbreaks may be more difficult to identify even with ongoing surveillance, and the mere suspicion of clustering of similarly resistant Enterobacteriaceae may warrant an investigation. Finally, if clusters of resistant organisms occur in the face of barrier precautions, our experience suggests that a chronically colonized patient or an environmental source should be sought vigorously [37].

Specific Organisms
Enterobacteriaceae

Antibiotic-resistant Enterobacteriaceae are common in hospitals, especially resistant *Klebsiella, Serratia,* and *Enterobacter* [143]. Drug-resistant *Proteus, Providencia,* and *Morganella* are also very common, particularly in geriatric wards and in patients transferred from nursing homes [37, 38, 142]. The clinical aspects of infections caused by Enterobacteriaceae are described in chapters on urinary tract infection (see Chap. 28), pneumonia (see Chap. 29), wound infection (see Chap. 33), and bacteremia (see Chap. 40). Microbiologic diagnosis of these infections usually poses no problem for the modern laboratory, particularly with the availability of newer diagnostic kits (see Chap. 9).

Predisposing factors for, and the epidemiology of, resistant Enterobacteriaceae have differed somewhat from genus to genus (Table 13-8) [119]. Some organisms, such as *Klebsiella,* may be more viable on human skin and thus may have a greater potential for person-to-person spread on the hands of hospital personnel [52, 53]. *Serratia* commonly causes asymptomatic colonization of urinary tract and respiratory tract, and chronically colonized patients are often a source for large numbers of cross-infections [37, 118]. There have also been several outbreaks described in which environmental contamination with *Serratia,* notably of graduated cylinders and ventilators, led to epidemics of urinary tract infection, peritonitis, or pneumonia [37]. *Enterobacter,* as well as *Serratia, Citrobacter, Pseudomonas,* and some *Proteus* and *Providencia,* strains often become resistant to second- and third-generation cephalosporins during therapy [98, 115, 116]. This genetic predilection

Table 13-8. Epidemiologic patterns in outbreaks of urinary tract infection by multiply resistant organisms

| Factor | Organism[a] | | |
	Klebsiella pneumoniae	Serratia marcescens	Proteus rettgeri
Reservoir			
Symptomatic GU infection	++++	±	++
Asymptomatic GU infection	++	++++	+++
Gastrointestinal colonization	++	0	0
Mode of transmission	Hands[b]	Hands	Hands
Spatial clustering of cases prominent	++	++++	++++
Risk factors			
Urinary catheterization	Yes	Yes	Yes
Broad-spectrum antimicrobial			
exposure	Yes	Yes	Yes
Urinary catheter irrigation	Yes	No	No
GU instrumentation	No	No	Yes

GU = genitourinary.
[a]Scale: 0 (no contribution) to ++++ (maximal contribution).
[b]Contact spread on hands of personnel.
Source: Adapted from D.R. Schaberg, R.A. Weinstein, and W.E. Stamm, Epidemics of nosocomial urinary tract infection caused by multiply resistant gram-negative bacilli: Epidemiology and control. *J. Infect. Dis.* 133:363, 1976.

and the ubiquity of *Enterobacter* may explain in part why *Enterobacter* species are a relatively common cause of mediastinitis after open-heart surgery despite cephalosporin prophylaxis [32, 33, 98].

As noted earlier, in some hospitals 15 to 25 percent or more of all antibiotic-resistant Enterobacteriaceae are cultured from patients at the time of admission. Patients with chronic respiratory or urinary tract infections, those who have frequent admissions, and patients transferred from nursing homes or other hospitals are particularly likely to bring resistant strains into the hospital [37, 142]. In several instances, such patients have been the index cases in outbreaks [16, 24, 40, 44].

Since drug-resistant Enterobacteriaceae appear to spread largely from patient to patient on the hands of hospital personnel (Table 13-9), and since colonized or infected patients are usually the major reservoir in the hospital, it has generally been possible in the past to contain resistant Enterobacteriaceae using the precautions described previously [37, 141]. However, the more recent problems with emergence of chromosomal mutations that encode resistance to newer cephalosporins and with plasmids that encode novel

Table 13-9. Epidemiology of endemic antibiotic resistance in nosocomial gram-negative bacilli

Factor	Relative contribution (%)
Cross-infection	30–40
Antibiotic pressures	20–25
Community acquisition	20–25
Other (environment, food, personnel, air, unknown)	20

β-lactamases [63, 70] suggest the need to heighten surveillance for such strains, tighten precautions for colonized patients, and consider selective decontamination, as noted previously, in some settings [139].

Pseudomonas aeruginosa

P. aeruginosa has intrinsic resistance to most available antibiotics, leaving aminoglycosides, antipseudomonal penicillins, newer cephalosporins, imipenem, and fluoroquinolones as treatment options for systemic infection. *Pseudomonas* is ubiquitous in the hospital, frequently colonizing patients before admission and contaminating water and various foods, particularly salads and fresh vegetables [48, 74, 96, 97, 125]. Laboratory identification is not difficult, although aminoglycoside susceptibility testing was confounded until the recognition that the divalent cation content of media needs to be carefully controlled.

There has been considerable controversy over whether resistant gram-negative bacilli are less virulent than sensitive strains. In a number of studies using a variety of measures of virulence, such as chills, fever, elevated white cell count, pyuria, and other local findings of infection, there have been no differences detected [85, 107]. In a few studies, however, particularly in oncology patients, aminoglycoside-resistant *Pseudomonas* strains have been less prone to cause bacteremia than sensitive strains [46, 67].

Several studies have shown that aminoglycoside-resistant *Pseudomonas* may emerge from sensitive populations of the same serotype during treatment [3, 35, 48, 96, 97, 142]. In fact, some institutions have found that despite isolating patients with antibiotic-resistant *P. aeruginosa,* the incidence of colonization with these strains has continued to increase [37, 74, 92, 96, 97, 142], in part paralleling the increasing use of aminoglycoside antibiotics.

In epidemic situations, *P. aeruginosa* has been noted to spread from contaminated common sources to persons as well as from person to person [23, 29, 48, 80]. Such transmission may be more amenable to the control measures outlined previously. However, control of endemic *P. aeruginosa* infections is problematic and may well require more innovative strategies that interfere with the ability of *Pseudomonas* to colonize or invade.

Staphylococcus aureus

Resistance of *S. aureus* to methicillin (aminoglycosides, or clindamycin) has been reported with increasing frequency in the United States over the past few years [21, 50, 99, 117, 124] (see Table 13-2).

Microbiologic diagnosis is facilitated when the potential causes of false-negative tests for methicillin resistance are recognized [50]. MRSA may be erroneously reported when colonies from mixed cultures of resistant coagulase-negative and sensitive *S. aureus* are

not picked carefully. Enterococcal colonies, if picked from blood agar, can give false-positive catalase tests and the impression that the enterococci, which can give positive coagulase tests, are MRSA.

The epidemiology of drug-resistant isolates of *S. aureus* appears to be similar to that of susceptible strains (see Chap. 37). In addition, particular reservoirs for methicillin-resistant staphylococci include intravenous drug addicts, burn-unit patients, nursing-home patients, and hospital personnel with dermatitis. In Detroit, MRSA arose as a major community problem in drug addicts who frequently self-prescribed antibiotics to forestall or treat infections related to the illicit use of contaminated needles. When these addicts were admitted to hospitals, waves of nosocomial methicillin-resistant infections followed [117]. In some areas, the growing prevalence of methicillin-resistant staphylococci in hospitals can be traced in part to admission to hospital of colonized patients from nursing homes [59].

The newest antibiotic resistance problem in staphylococci, the emergence of ciprofloxacin resistance [103, 120], warrants close monitoring.

Once drug-resistant staphylococci have become entrenched in the hospital, eradication is difficult. Control has required accurate laboratory identification, prospective surveillance for colonized and infected patients (including, in some hospitals, periodic culture surveys of high-risk patients), identification of previously colonized patients at readmission, appropriate isolation of all identified patients, search for environmental and personnel sources, and aggressive antibiotic therapy of infected patients (vancomycin with or without rifampicin) [21, 50, 133]. Aggressive attempts to eradicate specific strains from colonized patients or personnel have been variably successful (see Chap. 37). Commonly recommended regimens include combinations of rifampicin, TMP-sulfamethoxazole, and ciprofloxacin [25, 103, 137] with the caveat that use of a single agent may heighten risk of further resistance; topical mupirocin, vancomycin, or antiseptics have also been used, with mupirocen appearing particularly promising [4, 8, 22, 54]. These efforts are indicated for personnel who have been epidemiologically linked to spread of resistant strains, for patients whose nursing homes refuse to take them back while positive cultures persist, for patients with recurrent infections, and in some outbreaks.

Coagulase-Negative Staphylococci

Coagulase-negative staphylococci, formerly believed to be an avirulent part of our normal flora, have become a problem pathogen in patients with implanted prosthetic joints (see Chap. 36), heart valves (see Chap. 35), or neurosurgical shunts (see Chaps. 32, 42); in patients with intravascular catheters [5], particularly long-duration central lines [19] such as Hickman catheters (see Chap. 40); and in immunosuppressed patients, particularly those who have received broad-spectrum antibiotics to treat or prevent infection with gram-negative bacilli.

Methicillin-resistant coagulase-negative staphylococci may be present in low numbers on the skin of patients and emerge in hospital as predominant flora and potential pathogens, especially after surgical antimicrobial prophylaxis [66], which is very similar to the epidemiology of *Enterobacter* infection [32, 33]. Using gentamicin resistance as a marker, we found that resistant coagulase-negative staphylococci are relatively uncommon in healthy nonhospitalized persons but are rapidly acquired in the hospital, related to either previous antibiotic exposure or ubiquitous environmental contamination [140]. The resistance was plasmid-mediated and could be transferred in vitro or on skin to *S. aureus* [62]. In one study, most nosocomial isolates of gentamicin-resistant *S. aureus* appeared to result from in vivo plasmid spread from resistant coagulase-negative staphylococci rather than from person-to-person transfer of resistant strains [140].

Since drug-resistant coagulase-negative staphylococci often become part of the patient's normal flora and are so ubiquitous [6, 140], control is difficult. In patients with indwelling intravascular catheters or patients undergoing implantation of foreign bodies, preventing infections with coagulase-negative staphylococci at present depends on strict attention to asepsis and, in some situations, antibiotic prophylaxis. More recent observations of wound infection due to dissemination of coagulase-negative strains by colonized surgeons [9] suggest the need to consider this mode of transmission when wound infection rates exceed expected norms.

Finally, the potential impact on hospitals of the recently described vancomycin-resistant coagulase-negative staphylococci remains undetermined [121].

Penicillin-Resistant Pneumococci

Although multiply resistant *S. pneumoniae* infections have not been a significant nosocomial problem in the United States, they reached epidemic proportions on crowded pediatric wards in South African hospitals in 1977–1978 [69]. During that time, 48 patients, almost all younger than 3 years, had positive blood or cerebrospinal fluid cultures, representing 8.5 percent of all pneumococcal isolates from these two sites. In addition, more than 300 carriers of resistant pneumococci were found. Successful control measures included restriction of unnecessary antibiotic use (since antibiotic exposure increased the risk of colonization), susceptibility testing of all pneumococci, nasopharyngeal culture surveys, respiratory isolation of all infected and colonized patients, and aggressive use of antimicrobials to eradicate carriage.

JK Diphtheroids

The JK strain of *Corynebacterium*, often susceptible only to vancomycin, has been noted in the past few years to be an increasingly common pathogen in immunocompromised oncology patients, mostly causing bacteremia or wound infections at bone marrow aspiration and intravenous catheter sites [42, 51, 128]. JK diphtheroids appear commonly to colonize the skin of hospitalized patients [42, 128] but, interestingly, are found more often in men and postmenopausal women, suggesting a possible relation between colonization and sebum content of skin. Because of extensive skin colonization, control of endemic infections with JK diphtheroids, like control of coagulase-negative staphylococci, may depend in large part on good aseptic technique. In addition, at least one outbreak of JK diphtheroids has been described in which evidence suggested possible person-to-person spread and a role for careful hand-washing in preventing infections.

Enterococci

High-level resistance of enterococci to aminoglycosides, including streptomycin, gentamicin, and amikacin, is well described [88] and has recently become a problem in nosocomial infections. Transmissible penicillin resistance and β-lactamase activity also have been demonstrated in clinical isolates of enterococci [89, 101] and plasmid-mediated vancomycin and teicoplanin resistance have been described in enterococci [71, 113].

In one set of studies, the reservoir for gentamicin-resistant enterococci appeared to be the gastrointestinal tract of asymptomatic patients and nursing-home transfers and spread was from person to person on hands of hospital personnel [146, 147]. It has been suggested that in response to this problem, hospitals should conduct systematic screening for enterococci that have high-level resistance to gentamicin and that antimicrobial use policies and infection control practices should be directed at control of these strains [55].

In institutions where clinically significant and difficult-to-treat disease [12, 91] is caused by antibiotic-resistant enterococci, the extent of the patient and environmental reservoir should be determined, and barrier precautions should be considered for colonized and infected patients.

Other Resistant Organisms

A variety of vancomycin-resistant gram-positive bacteria, such as *Leuconostoc*, *Pediococcus*, and *Lactobacillus* species, have been described recently [56, 111]. Whether the increased use of vancomycin in hospitals will create enough pressure to allow these uncommon, usually avirulent strains to emerge as pathogens, particularly in the highly susceptible, heavily vancomycin-exposed populations such as oncology patients, remains to be seen.

Clindamycin resistance in the *Bacteroides fragilis* group has been a sporadic, relatively unusual problem that is plasmid-mediated and has occurred in 0 to 10 percent of strains in various medical centers [132]. One group described an outbreak of clindamycin-resistant *B. fragilis* on a surgical ward in which 7 (13 percent) of 52 isolates were affected [27]; 85 percent of involved patients had received clindamycin or erythromycin before recovery of a resistant strain. The epidemiology of this outbreak is not entirely clear.

Resistance of fungi to amphotericin B, 5-flucytosine, and newer antifungal agents such as fluconazole, has been described. Little is known about the epidemiology, impact, or potential for control of these strains in hospitals. However, as the number of broad-spectrum antibacterial agents available in hospitals increases, and with the recent availability of oral fluconazole, we may see more overgrowth by resistant fungal organisms, and a new chapter in nosocomial drug resistance may unfold. Similarly, the increasing availability of antiviral agents such as acyclovir presents the problem of acquired drug resistance in herpes virus and other viruses, a problem already arising in acquired immunodeficiency syndrome (AIDS) patients.

Future Challenges

The ingenious ways in which microorganisms learn to evade our antimicrobial pharmacopeia will no doubt continue to astound, and at times confound, and perplex us. As the pressures on our antimicrobial armamentarium increase, and as our patients are subjected to more invasive procedures and immunosuppressive regimens, we can look forward to greater resistance and more problems with the traditionally avirulent normal flora.

Unfortunately, our control of resistant strains has advanced little since the singular contribution of Semmelweis. Moreover, we still have trouble encouraging and motivating personnel to follow the most basic concepts in asepsis. In fact, our most successful advances are attributable to the development of newer antimicrobials and less infection-prone devices rather than to improvements in application of basic aseptic principles.

At the same time, we need to use advances in microbiologic techniques to obtain a better understanding of the epidemiology of nosocomial resistance, not only in single-strain outbreaks but also in the endemic setting and in plasmid and even transposon outbreaks. As we increase our understanding of bacterial [15] and host factors that control colonization with normal flora and lead to overgrowth of resistant bacteria, new approaches may emerge for preventing colonization with nosocomial pathogens, blocking adherence of unwanted resistant strains, or halting progression from colonization to infection.

In the meantime, I believe the key is not to delay in applying the strategies available to us and not to apply measures in too piecemeal a fashion lest control always lag behind resistance. The growing interchange of resistant bacteria among nursing homes, community hospitals, tertiary care centers, and high-risk outpatient populations emphasizes the need for concerted control efforts.

References

1. Adams, B. G., and Marrie, T. J. Hand carriage of aerobic gram-negative rods may not be transient. *J. Hyg.* (Camb.) 89:33, 1982.
2. Allen, J. R., Hightower, A. W., Martin, S. M., and Dixon, R. E. Secular trends in nosocomial infections: 1970–1979. *Am. J. Med.* 70:389, 1981.
3. Amirak, I. D., Williams, R. J., Noone, P., and Wills, M. R. Amikacin resistance developing in patient with *Pseudomonas aeruginosa* bronchopneumonia. *Lancet* 1:537, 1977.
4. Bartzokas, C. A., et al. Control and eradication of methicillin-resistant *Staphylococcus aureus* on a surgical unit. *N. Engl. J. Med.* 311:1422, 1984.
5. Baumgart, S., Hall, S. E., Campos, J. M., and Polin, R. A. Sepsis with coagulase-negative staphylococci in critically ill newborns. *Am. J. Dis. Child.* 137:461, 1983.
6. Bentley, D. W., Hahn, J. J., and Lepper,

M. H. Transmission of chloramphenicol-resistant *Staphylococcus epidermidis:* Epidemiologic and laboratory studies. *J. Infect. Dis.* 122:365, 1970.
7. Berntsen, C. A., and McDermott, W. Increased transmissibility of staphylococci to patients receiving an antimicrobial drug. *N. Engl. J. Med.* 262:637, 1960.
8. Bitar, C. M., et al. Outbreak due to methicillin- and rifampin-resistant *Staphylococcus aureus:* Epidemiology and eradication of the resistant strain from the hospital. *Infect. Control* 8:15, 1987.
9. Boyce, J. M., et al. A common-source outbreak of *Staphylococcus epidermidis* infections among patients undergoing cardiac surgery. *J. Infect. Dis.* 161:493, 1990.
10. Brun-Buisson, C., et al. Intestinal decontamination for control of nosocomial multiresistant gram-negative bacilli. Study of an outbreak in an intensive care unit. *Ann. Intern. Med.* 110:873, 1989.
11. Burke, J. P., et al. *Proteus mirabilis* infections in a hospital nursery traced to a human carrier. *N. Engl. J. Med.* 284:115, 1971.
12. Bush, L. M., et al. High-level penicillin resistance among isolates of enterococci. Implications for treatment of enterococcal infections. *Ann Intern. Med.* 110.515, 1989.
13. Buxton, A. E., Anderson, R. L., Werdegar, D., and Atlas, E. Nosocomial respiratory tract infection and colonization with *Acinetobacter calcoaceticus:* Epidemiologic characteristics. *Am. J. Med.* 65:507, 1978.
14. Cairns, J., Overbaugh, J., and Miller, S. The origin of mutants. *Nature* 335:142, 1988.
15. Casewell, M. S. The Different Characteristics of Antibiotic-Resistant and Sensitive Bacteria. In C.H. Stuart-Harris and D.M. Harris (Eds.), *The Control of Antibiotic-Resistant Bacteria.* London: Academic, 1982. P. 77.
16. Casewell, M.W., Dalton, M.T., Webster, M., and Phillips, I. Gentamicin-resistant *Klebsiella aerogenes* in a urological ward. *Lancet* 2:444, 1977.
17. Chow, A.W., Taylor, P.R., Yoshikawa, T.T., and Guze, L. B. A nosocomial outbreak of infections due to multiply resistant *Proteus mirabilis:* Role of intestinal colonization as a major reservoir. *J. Infect. Dis.* 139:621, 1979.
18. Chow, J.W., et al. *Enterobacter* bacteremia: Clinical features and emergence of antibiotic resistance during therapy. *Ann. Intern. Med.* 115:585, 1991.
19. Christensen, G.D., et al. Nosocomial septicemia due to multiply antibiotic-resistant *Staphylococcus epidermidis. Ann. Intern. Med.* 96:1, 1982.
20. Cook, L.N., Davis, R.S., and Stover, B.H. Outbreak of amikacin-resistant Enterobacte-

riaceae in an intensive care nursery. *Pediatrics* 65:264, 1980.

21. Craven, D.E., et al. A large outbreak of infections caused by a strain of *Staphylococcus aureus* resistant to oxacillin and aminoglycosides. *Am. J. Med.* 71:53, 1981.

22. Denning, D.W., and Haiduven-Griffiths, D. Eradication of low-level methicillin-resistant *Staphylococcus aureus* skin colonization with topical mupirocin. *Infect. Control Hosp. Epidemiol.* 9:261, 1988.

23. Duncan, I.B.R., Rennie, R.P., and Duncan, N.H. A long-term study of gentamicin-resistant *Pseudomonas aeruginosa* in a general hospital. *J. Antimicrob. Chemother.* 7:147, 1981.

24. Edwards, L.D., Cross, A., Levin, S. and Landau, W. Outbreak of a nosocomial infection with a strain of *Proteus rettgeri* resistant to many antimicrobials. *Am. J. Clin. Pathol.* 61:41, 1974.

25. Ellison, R.T., et al. Oral rifampin and trimethoprim/sulfamethoxazole therapy in asymptomatic carriers of methicillin-resistant *Staphylococcus aureus* infections. *West. J. Med.* 140:735, 1984.

26. Elwell, L.P., Inamine, J.M., and Minshew, B.H. Common plasmid specifying tobramycin resistance found in two enteric bacteria isolated from burn patients. *Antimicrob. Agents Chemother.* 13:312, 1978.

27. England, A.C., III, Bond, E.J., Livingston, H., and Nelson, K.E. Epidemiology of clindamycin-resistant *Bacteroides fragilis*. In: *Programs and Abstracts of the Annual Meeting of the American Society for Microbiology*, Atlanta, GA, March 7–12, 1982. Washington, DC: American Society for Microbiology, 1982. P. 87, abstract L27.

28. Fainstein, V., et al. Patterns of oropharyngeal and fecal flora in patients with acute leukemia. *J. Infect. Dis.* 144:10, 1981.

29. Farmer, J.J., Weinstein, R.A., Zierdt, C.H., and Brokopp, C.D. Hospital outbreaks caused by *Pseudomonas aeruginosa:* Importance of serogroup 011. *J. Clin. Microbiol.* 16:266, 1982.

30. Feeley, T.W., et al. Aerosol polymyxin and pneumonia in seriously ill patients. *N. Engl. J. Med.* 293:471, 1975.

31. Flaherty, J., Nathan, C., Kabins, S.A., and Weinstein, R.A. Pilot trial of selective decontamination for prevention of bacterial infection in an intensive care unit. *J. Infect. Dis.* 162:1393, 1990.

32. Flynn, D.M., et al. Patients' endogenous flora as the source of "nosocomial" *Enterobacter* in cardiac surgery. *J. Infect. Dis.* 156:363, 1987.

33. Flynn, D.M., Weinstein, R.A., and Kabins, S.A. Infections with gram-negative bacilli in

a cardiac surgery intensive care unit: The relative role of *Enterobacter. J. Hosp. Infect.* 11:367, 1988.

34. Foster, T.J. Plasmid-determined resistance to antimicrobial drugs and toxic metal ions in bacteria. *Microbiol. Rev.* 47:361, 1983.

35. Gaman, W., et al. Emergence of gentamicin- and carbenicillin-resistant *Pseudomonas aeruginosa* in a hospital environment. *Antimicrob. Agents Chemother.* 9:474, 1976.

36. Gardner, P., and Smith, D.H. Studies on the epidemiology of resistance (R) factors. I. Analysis of *Klebsiella* isolates in a general hospital. II. A prospective study of R-factor transfer in the host. *Ann. Intern Med.* 71:1, 1969.

37. Gaynes, R.P., et al. Control of aminoglycoside resistance by barrier precautions. *Infect. Control* 4:221, 1983.

38. Gaynes, R.P., Weinstein, R.A., Chamberlin, W., and Kabins, S.A. Antibiotic-resistant flora in nursing home patients admitted to the hospital. *Arch. Intern. Med.* 145:1804, 1985.

39. Gaynes, R., Culver, D., and the National Nosocomial Infection Surveillance (NNIS) System. Resistance to imipenem among selected gram-negative bacilli (GNB) in the United States. In: *Abstracts from the Thirteenth Interscience Conference on Antimicrobial Agents and Chemotherapy, 1990*. Washington, DC: American Society for Microbiology, 1990.

40. Gerding, D.N., et al. Nosocomial multiply resistant *Klebsiella pneumoniae:* Epidemiology of an outbreak of apparent index case origin. *Antimicrob. Agents Chemother.* 15:608, 1979.

41. Gill, S., and Iyer, V.N. Nalidixic acid inhibits the conjugal transfer of conjugative N incompatibility group plasmids. *Can J. Microbiol.* 28:256, 1982.

42. Gill, V.J., et al. Antibiotic-resistant group JK bacteria in hospitals. *J. Clin. Microbiol.* 13:472, 1981.

43. Gilmore, D.S., Schick, D.G., and Montgomerie, J.Z. *Pseudomonas aeruginosa* and *Klebsiella pneumoniae* on the perinea of males with spinal cord injuries. *J. Clin. Microbiol.* 16:865, 1982.

44. Graham, D.R., et al. Epidemic nosocomial meningitis due to *Citrobacter diversus* in neonates. *J. Infect. Dis.* 144:203, 1981.

45. Graham, D.R., et al. Epidemic neonatal gentamicin-methicillin-resistant *Staphylococcus aureus* infection associated with nonspecific topical use of gentamicin. *J. Pediatr.* 97:972, 1980.

46. Greene, W.H., et al. *Pseudomonas aeruginosa* resistant to carbenicillin and gentamicin. *Ann. Intern. Med.* 79:684, 1973.

47. Grieble, H.G., Bird, T.J., Nidea, H.M., and Miller, C.A. Chute-hydropulping waste dis-

posal system: A reservoir of enteric bacilli and *Pseudomonas* in a modern hospital. *J. Infect. Dis.* 130:602, 1974.

48. Griffith, S.J., et al. The epidemiology of *Pseudomonas aeruginosa* in oncology patients in a general hospital. *J. Infect. Dis.* 160:1030, 1989.

50. Halcy, R.W., et al. The emergence of methicillin-resistant *Staphylococcus aureus* infections in United States hospitals. *Ann. Intern. Med.* 97:297, 1982.

51. Hande, K.R., et al. Sepsis with a new species of *Corynebacterium. Ann. Intern. Med.* 85:423, 1976.

52. Hart, C.A., and Gibson, M.F. Comparative epidemiology of gentamicin-resistant enterobacteria: Persistence of carriage and infection. *J. Clin. Pathol.* 35:452, 1982.

53. Hart, C.A., Gibson, M.F., and Buckles, A.M. Variation in skin and environmental survival of hospital gentamicin-resistant enterobacteria. *J. Hyg.* (Camb.) 87:277, 1981.

54. Hill, R.L.R., Duckworth, D.J., and Casewell, M.W. Elimination of nasal carriage of methicillin-resistant *Staphylococcus aureus* with mupirocin during a hospital outbreak. *J. Antimicrob. Chemother.* 22:377, 1988.

55. Hoffmann, S.A., and Moellering, R.C. The enterococcus: "Putting the bug in our ears." *Ann. Intern. Med.* 106:757, 1987.

56. Hoi, A.B., Branger, C., and Acar, J.F. Vancomycin-resistant streptococci or *Leuconostoc* sp. *Antimicrob. Agents Chemother.* 28:458, 1985.

57. Horan, T., et al. Nosocomial infection surveillance, 1984. *M.M.W.R.* 35:17SS, 1986.

58. Houang, E.T., and Greenwood, D. Aminoglycoside cross-resistance patterns of gentamicin-resistant bacteria. *J. Clin. Pathol.* 30:738, 1977.

59. Hsu, C.C.S., Macaluso, C.P., Special, L., and Hubble, R.H. High rate of methicillin resistance of *Staphylococcus aureus* isolated from hospitalized nursing home patients. *Arch. Intern. Med.* 148:569, 1988.

60. Hughes, J., et al. Nosocomial aminoglycoside-resistant gram-negative bacillary infections in the United States, 1975–1982. In: *Programs and Abstracts of the Twenty-Third Interscience Conference on Antimicrobial Agents and Chemotherapy.* Las Vegas, October 24–26, 1983. Washington, DC: American Society for Microbiology, 1983. P. 248, abstract 893.

61. Huovinen, P., Mantyjarvi, R., and Toivanen, P. Trimethoprim resistance in hospitals. *Br. Med. J.* 284:782, 1982.

61A. Jacoby, G.A., and Archer, G.L. New mechanisms of bacterial resistance to antimicrobial agents. *N. Engl. J. Med.* 324:601, 1991.

62. Jaffe, H.W., et al. Identity and interspecific transfer of gentamicin-resistant plasmids in *Staphylococcus aureus* and *Staphylococcus epidermidis. J. Infect. Dis.* 141:738, 1980.

63. Jarlier, V., Nicolas, M.H., Fournier, G., and Philippon, A. Extended broad-spectrum beta-lactamases conferring transferrable resistance to newer beta-lactam agents in Enterobacteriaceae: Hospital prevalence and susceptibility patterns. *Rev. Infect. Dis.* 10:867, 1988.

64. John, J.F., McKee, K.T., Twitty, J.A., and Schaffner, W. Molecular epidemiology of sequential nursery epidemics caused by multiresistant *Klebsiella pneumoniae. J. Pediatr.* 102:825, 1983.

65. Kauffman, C.A., et al. Surveillance of gentamicin-resistant gram-negative bacilli in a general hospital. *Antimicrob. Agents Chemother.* 13:918, 1978.

66. Kernodle, D.S., Barg, N.L., and Kaiser, A.B. Low-level colonization of hospitalized patients with methicillin-resistant coagulase-negative staphylococci and emergence of the organisms during surgical antimicrobial prophylaxis. *Antimicrob. Agents Chemother.* 32:202, 1988.

67. Keys, T.F., and Washington, J.A. Gentamicin-resistant *Pseudomonas aeruginosa:* Mayo Clinic experience, 1970–1976. *Mayo Clin. Proc.* 52:797, 1977.

68. Knittle, M.A., Eitzman, D.V., and Baer, H. Role of hand contamination of personnel in the epidemiology of gram-negative nosocomial infections. *J. Pediatr.* 86:433, 1975.

69. Koornhof, H.J., et al. Therapy and Control of Antibiotic-Resistant Pneumococcal Disease. In: *Microbiology 1979.* Washington, DC: American Society for Microbiology, 1979. P. 286.

70. Labia, R., et al. Interactions of new plasmid-mediated beta-lactamases with third-generation cephalosporins. *Rev. Infect. Dis.* 10:885, 1988.

71. Leclercq, R., Derlot, E., Duval, J., and Courvalin, P. Plasmid-mediated resistance to vancomycin and teicoplanin in *Enterococcus faecium. N. Engl. J. Med.* 319:157, 1988.

72. Ledingham, I.M., et al. Triple regimen of selective decontamination of the digestive tract, systemic cefotaxime, and microbiological surveillance for prevention of acquired infection in intensive care. *Lancet* 1:785, 1988.

73. Levin, M., et al. Pseudomonas in ICU sinks: Relation to patients. *J. Clin. Pathol.* 37:424, 1984.

74. Lowbury, E.J.L., et al. Sources of infection with *Pseudomonas aeruginosa* in patients with tracheostomy. *J. Med. Microbiol.* 3:39, 1970.

75. Maizels, M., and Schaeffer, A.J. Decreased

incidence of bacteriuria associated with periodic instillations of hydrogen peroxide into the urethral catheter drainage bag. *J. Urol.* 123:841, 1980.

76. Makela, P., Ojajarvi, J., and Salminen, E. Decontaminating waste-trap. *Lancet* 1:1216, 1972.

77. Maki, D.G., et al. Nosocomial urinary tract infection with *Serratia marcescens:* An epidemiologic study. *J. Infect. Dis.* 128:579, 1973.

78. Maliwan, N., Grieble, H.G., and Bird, T.J. Hospital *Pseudomonas aeruginosa:* Surveillance of resistance to gentamicin and transfer of aminoglycoside R factor. *Antimicrob. Agents Chemother.* 8:415, 1975.

79. Markowitz, S.M., et al. Sequential outbreaks of infection due to *Klebsiella pneumoniae* in a neonatal intensive care unit: Implication of a conjugative R plasmid. *J. Infect. Dis.* 142:106, 1980.

80. Marrie, T.J., et al. Prolonged outbreak of nosocomial urinary tract infection with a single strain of *Pseudomonas aeruginosa. Can. Med. Assoc. J.* 119:593, 1978.

81. Mathias, R.G., et al. Clinical evaluation of amikacin in treatment of infections due to gram-negative aerobic bacilli. *J. Infect. Dis.* 134:S394, 1976.

82. Mawer, S.L., and Greenwood, D. Aminoglycoside resistance emerging during therapy. *Lancet* 1:749, 1977.

83. McGowan, J.E. Antimicrobial resistance in hospital organisms and its relation to antibiotic use. *Rev. Infect. Dis.* 5:1033, 1983.

84. Meyer, R.D. Patterns and mechanisms of emergence of resistance to amikacin. *J. Infect. Dis.* 136:449, 1977.

85. Meyer, R.D., Lewis, R.P., Halter, J., and White, M. Gentamicin-resistant *Pseudomonas aeruginosa* and *Serratia marcescens* in a general hospital. *Lancet* 1:580, 1976.

86. Montgomerie, J.Z., and Morrow, J.W. *Pseudomonas* colonization in patients with spinal cord injury. *Am. J. Epidemiol.* 108:328, 1978.

87. Moody, M.M., deJongh, C.A., Schimpff, S.C., and Tilman, G.L. Long-term amikacin use: Effects on aminoglycoside susceptibility patterns of gram-negative bacilli. *J.A.M.A.* 248:1199, 1982.

88. Murray, B.A. The life and times of the enterococcus. *Clin. Microbiol. Rev.* 3:46, 1990.

89. Murray, B.E., and Mederski-Samaroj, B. Transferable beta-lactamase: A new mechanism for in vitro penicillin resistance in *Streptococcus faecalis. J. Clin. Invest.* 72:1168, 1983.

90. Murray, B.E., Rensimer, E.R., and DuPont, H.L. Emergence of high-level trimethoprim resistance in fecal *Escherichia coli* during oral administration of trimethoprim or trimetho-prim-sulfamethoxazole. *N. Engl. J. Med.* 306:130, 1982.

91. Nachamkin, I., et al. Multiply high-level-aminoglycoside-resistant *Enterococci* isolated from patients in a university hospital. *J. Clin. Microbiol.* 26:1287, 1988.

92. Noone, M.R., et al. *Pseudomonas aeruginosa* colonisation in an intensive therapy unit: Role of cross-infection and host factors. *Br. Med. J.* 286:341, 1983.

93. Noriega, E.R., et al. Nosocomial infection caused by gentamicin-resistant, streptomycin-sensitive *Klebsiella. J. Infect. Dis.* 131:S45, 1975.

94. O'Brien, T.F., et al. International comparison of prevalence of resistance to antibiotics. *J.A.M.A.* 239:1518, 1978.

95. O'Callaghan, R.J., et al. Analysis of increasing antibiotic resistance of *Klebsiella pneumoniae* relative to changes in chemotherapy. *J. Infect. Dis.* 138:293, 1978.

96. Olson, B., et al. Epidemiology of endemic *Pseudomonas aeruginosa:* Why infection control efforts have failed. *J. Infect. Dis.* 150:808, 1984.

97. Olson, B., et al. Occult aminoglycoside resistance in *Pseudomonas aeruginosa:* Epidemiology and implications for therapy and control. *J. Infect. Dis.* 152:769, 1985.

98. Olson, B., Weinstein, R.A., Nathan, C., and Kabins S.A. Broad-spectrum beta-lactum resistance in *Enterobacter:* Emergence during treatment and mechanisms of resistance. *J. Antimicrob. Chemother.* 11:299, 1983.

99. Panlilio, A., et al. Prevalence and distribution of methicillin-resistant *Staphylococcus aureus* in the United States. *Infect. Control Hosp. Epidemiol.* 1992 (in press).

100. Parry, M.F., et al. Gram-negative sepsis in neonates: A nursery outbreak due to hand carriage of *Citrobacter diversus. Pediatrics* 65:1105, 1980.

101. Patterson, J.E., et al. Molecular epidemiology of beta-lactamase-producing *Enterococci. Antimicrob. Agents Chemother.* 34:302, 1990.

102. Perryman, F.A., and Flournoy, D.J. Prevalence of gentamicin- and amikacin-resistant bacteria in sink drains. *J. Clin. Microbiol.* 12:79, 1980.

102A. A. Philippon, A., Labia, R., and Jacoby, G. Extended spectrum β-lactamases. *Antimicrob. Agents Chemother.* 33:1131, 1989.

103. Piercy, E.Z., Barbaro, D., Luby, J.P., and Mackowiak, P.A. Ciprofloxacin for methicillin-resistant *Staphylococcus aureus* infections. *Antimicrob. Agents Chemother.* 33:128, 1989.

104. Price, D.J.E., and Sleigh, J.D. Control of infection due to *Klebsiella aerogenes* in a neurosurgical unit by withdrawal of all antibiotics. *Lancet* 2:1213, 1970.

105. Price, K.E., et al. Epidemiological studies of aminoglycoside resistance in the U.S.A. *J. Antimicrob. Chemother.* 8:89, 1981.

106. Rennie, R.P., and Duncan, I.B.R. Emergence of gentamicin-resistant *Klebsiella* in a general hospital. *Antimicrob. Agents Chemother.* 11:179, 1977.

107. Roberts, N.J., and Douglas, R.G. Gentamicin use and *Pseudomonas* and *Serratia* resistance: Effect of a surgical prophylaxis regimen. *Antimicrob. Agents Chemother.* 13:214, 1978.

108. Roe, E., Jones, R.J., and Lowbury, E.J.L. Transfer of antibiotic resistance between *Pseudomonas aeruginosa, Escherichia coli,* and other gram-negative bacilli in burns. *Lancet* 1:149, 1971.

109. Rubens, C.E., Farrar, W.E., McGee, Z.A., and Schaffner, W. Evolution of a plasmid-mediating resistance to multiple antimicrobial agents during a prolonged epidemic of nosocomial infections. *J. Infect. Dis.* 143:170, 1981.

110. Rubens, C.E., McNeill, W.F., and Farrar, W.E. Evolution of multiple-antibiotic-resistance plasmids mediated by transposable plasmid deoxyribonucleic acid sequences. *J. Bacteriol.* 140:713, 1979.

111. Ruoff, K.L., Kuritzkes, D.R., Wolfson, J.S., and Ferraro, M.J. Vancomycin-resistant gram-positive bacteria isolated from human sources. *J. Clin. Microbiol.* 26:2064, 1988.

112. Sadowski, P.L., Peterson, B.V., Gerding, D.N., and Cleary, P.P. Physical characterization of ten R plasmids obtained from an outbreak of nosocomial *Klebsiella pneumoniae* infections. *Antimicrob. Agents Chemother.* 15:616, 1979.

113. Sahm, D.F., et al. In vitro susceptibility studies of vancomycin-resistant *Enterococcus faecalis. Antimicrob. Agents Chemother.* 33:1588, 1989.

114. Salzman, T.C., Clark, J.J., and Klemm, L. Hand contamination of personnel as a mechanism of cross-infection in nosocomial infections with antibiotic-resistant *Escherichia coli* and *Klebsiella aerobacter. Antimicrob. Agents Chemother.* 1967:97, 1968.

115. Sanders, C.C., et al. Resistance to cefamandole: A collaborative study of emerging clinical problems. *J. Infect. Dis.* 145:118, 1982.

116. Sanders, W.E., and Sanders C.C. Inducible beta-lactamases: Clinical and epidemiologic implications for use of newer cephalosporins. *Rev. Infect. Dis.* 10:830, 1988.

117. Saravolatz, L.D., et al. Methicillin-resistant *Staphylococcus aureus.* Epidemiologic observations during a community-acquired outbreak. *Ann. Intern. Med.* 96:11, 1982.

118. Schaberg, D.R., et al. An outbreak of nosocomial infection due to multiply resistant *Serratia marcescens:* Evidence of interhospital spread. *J. Infect. Dis.* 134:181, 1976.

119. Schaberg, D.R., Weinstein, R.A., and Stamm, W.E. Epidemics of nosocomial urinary tract infection caused by multiply resistant gram-negative bacilli: Epidemiology and control. *J. Infect. Dis.* 133:363, 1976.

120. Schaefler, S. Methicillin-resistant strains of *Staphylococcus aureus* resistant to quinolones. *J. Clin. Microbiol.* 27:335, 1989.

121. Schwalbe, R.S., Stapleton, J.T., and Gilligan, P.H. Emergence of vancomycin resistance in coagulase-negative staphylococci. *N. Engl. J. Med.* 316:927, 1987.

122. Seal, D.V., and Strangeways, J.E.M. Aminoglycoside resistance due to mutation. *Lancet* 1:856, 1977.

123. Selden, R., et al. Nosocomial *Klebsiella* infections: Intestinal colonization as a reservoir. *Ann. Intern. Med.* 74:657, 1971.

124. Semel, J.D., Trenholme, G.M., and Levin, S. Gentamicin- and clindamycin-resistant *Staphylococcus aureus. Am. J. Med. Sc.* 280:4, 1980.

125. Shooter, R.A. Bowel colonization of hospital patients by *Pseudomonas aeruginosa* and *Escherichia coli. Proc. R. Soc. Med.* 64:27, 1971.

126. Shulman, J.A., Terry, P.M., and Hough, C.E. Colonization with gentamicin-resistant *Pseudomonas aeruginosa,* pyocine type 5, in a burn unit. *J. Infect. Dis.* 124:S18, 1971.

127. Sprunt, K., Leidy, G., and Redman, W. Abnormal colonization of neonates in an ICU: Conversion to normal colonization by pharyngeal implantation of alpha-hemolytic *Streptococcus* strain 215. *Pediatr. Res.* 14:308, 1980.

128. Stamm, W.E., et al. Infection due to *Corynebacterium* species in marrow transplant patients. *Ann. Intern. Med.* 91:167, 1979.

129. Stamm, W.E., Weinstein, R.A., and Dixon, R.E. Comparison of endemic and epidemic nosocomial infections. *Am. J. Med.* 70:393, 1981.

130. Stoutenbeek, C.P., et al. Nosocomial gram-negative pneumonia in critically ill patients. A 3-year experience with a novel therapeutic regimen. *Intensive Care Med.* 12:419, 1986.

131. Stoutenbeek, C.P., van Saene, H.K., and Zandstra, D.F. The effect of oral nonabsorbable antibiotics on the emergence of resistant bacteria in patients in an intensive care unit. *J. Antimicrob. Chemother.* 19:513, 1987.

132. Tally, F.P., et al. Susceptibility of the *Bacteriodes fragilis* group in the United States in 1981. *Antimicrob. Agents Chemother.* 23:536, 1983.

133. Thompson, R.L., Cabezudo, I., and Wenzel, R.P. Epidemiology of nosocomial infections caused by methicillin-resistant *Staphylococcus aureus. Ann. Intern. Med.* 97:309, 1982.

134. Thompson, R.L., et al. Effect of periodic instillation of hydrogen peroxide (H_2O_2) into urinary drainage systems in the prevention

of catheter-associated bacteriuria (CAB). In: *Programs and Abstracts of the Twenty-Second Interscience Conference on Antimicrobial Agents and Chemotherapy,* Miami Beach, FL, Washington, DC: American Society for Microbiology, 1982. October 4–6, 1982. P. 201, abstract 769.

135. Tompkins, L.S., Plorde, J.J., and Falkow, S. Molecular analysis of R-factors from multiresistant nosocomial isolates. *J. Infect. Dis.* 141:625, 1980.

136. Wade, J.C., Schimpff, S.C., Newman, K.A., and Wiernik, P.H. *Staphylococcus epidermidis:* An increasing cause of infection in patients with granulocytopenia. *Ann. Intern. Med.* 97:503, 1982.

137. Ward, T., Winn, R.E., Hartstein, A.I., and Sewell, D.L. Observations relating to an inter-hospital outbreak of methicillin-resistant *Staphylococcus aureus:* Role of antimicrobial therapy in infection control. *Infect. Control* 2:453, 1981.

138. Weinstein, R.A. Endemic emergence of cephalosporin-resistant *Enterobacter:* Relation to prior therapy. *Infect. Control* 7:120, 1986.

139. Weinstein, R.A. Selective intestinal decontamination—an infection control measure whose time has come. *Ann. Intern. Med.* 110:853, 1989.

140. Weinstein, R.A., et al. Gentamicin-resistant staphylococci as hospital flora: Epidemiology and resistance plasmids. *J. Infect. Dis.* 145:374, 1982.

141. Weinstein, R.A., and Kabins, S.A. Strategies for prevention and control of multiple drug-resistant nosocomial infection. *Am. J. Med.* 70:449, 1981.

142. Weinstein, R.A., Nathan, C., Gruensfelder, R., and Kabins, S.A. Endemic aminoglycoside resistance in gram-negative bacilli: Epidemiology and mechanisms. *J. Infect. Dis.* 141:338, 1980.

143. Wenzel R.P., Veazey, J.M., and Townsend, T.R. Role of the Inanimate Environment in Hospital-Acquired Infections. In K.R. Cundy and W. Ball (Eds.), *Infection Control in Health Care Facilities: Microbiological Surveillance.* Baltimore: University Park Press, 1977. P. 71.

144. Wormser, G.P., Tatz, J., and Donath, J. Endemic resistance to amikacin among hospital isolates of gram-negative bacilli: Implications for therapy. *Infect. Control* 4:93, 1983.

145. Yu, V.L., Oakes, C.A., Axnick, K.J., and Merigan, T.C. Patient factors contributing to the emergence of gentamicin-resistant *Serratia marcescens. Am. J. Med.* 66:468, 1979.

146. Zervos, M.J., et al. Nosocomial infection by gentamicin-resistant *Streptococcus faecalis. Ann. Intern. Med.* 106:687, 1987.

147. Zervos, M.J., et al. High-level aminoglycoside-resistant enterococci. Colonization of nursing home and acute care hospital patients. *Arch. Intern. Med.* 147:1591, 1987.

R Plasmids and Their Molecular Biology

Dennis R. Schaberg

The development of effective antimicrobial agents has been a significant advance in the treatment of infectious diseases. Based on the idea that mutation would be the primary mechanism for resistance, the development of resistance to antimicrobials was not anticipated as a serious problem. As each new antimicrobial has been introduced, however, bacterial pathogens resistant to that drug have been encountered. The experience with nosocomial *Staphylococcus aureus* infections, summarized in Chapter 12, is one example of this phenomenon.

The unexpected explanation for much of the resistance encountered was found in the recognition of resistance plasmids, which could be transferred from one bacterial cell to another, carrying genes coding for antimicrobial resistance. These *R plasmids* were first recognized in gram-negative organisms in the enteric pathogen *Shigella* but since have been found in virtually all clinically important nosocomial pathogens.

The hospital presents an environment in which circumstances conspire to accelerate the evolution of antimicrobial resistance. The most frequently encountered nosocomial pathogens—the aerobic gram-negative bacilli, staphylococci, and enterococci—all have the ability to acquire resistance rapidly. Intensive use of antimicrobials exerts extensive selection pressure favoring those organisms that have acquired resistance. In addition, therapy with antimicrobials alters normal flora, which appears to be an important contributor to R plasmid transfer in vivo in the human gastrointestinal tract. Transfer also can be readily observed in aqueous reservoirs peculiar to the hospital environment, such as urinary catheter collection bags. Compromised patients receiving antimicrobials who are hospitalized for prolonged periods of time provide an animate reservoir for resistant organisms once selected. In addition, antimicrobials find their way into the general inanimate environment, also contributing to the selective advantage obtained by R plasmid–containing organisms.

General Properties of Plasmids

Plasmids are self-replicating extrachromosomal genetic elements of bacteria (see Chaps. 12, 13). The genetic information necessary for metabolism and growth of the bacterial cell is on the bacterial chromosome. Because this is usually unaltered by plasmid acquisition, plasmids can be acquired or lost without affecting basic cellular function. However, plasmids carry additional genes that often assist the bacterial cell in surviving or competing in adverse environments. This is in contrast to chromosomal mutation, which results in structural changes in cellular function and metabolism.

Plasmids are isolated from bacterial cells as circular or supercoiled DNA molecules of a mass ranging from 0.5 to 300×10^6 daltons. The mass of the average bacterial chromosome is approximately 2×10^9 daltons. The coding capacity of such plasmids can be substantial, with larger plasmids carrying sufficient DNA to code for hundreds of new proteins, if all the plasmid DNA is expressed. For many plasmids, known functions can be ascribed, including antimicrobial resistance and sometimes virulence factors such as mucosal attachment properties or the ability to scavenge iron from the host. For some plasmids, no phenotypic properties are known. Plasmids with no detectable phenotype are common in many nosocomial isolates and are termed *cryptic plasmids*.

Plasmids are often classified into two general categories based on transmissibility: conjugative and nonconjugative. A plasmid is *conjugative* if it is self-transmissible from one bacterial cell to another. The classic example of a conjugative plasmid is the sex factor F. When a bacterial cell contains this conjugative plasmid, a proteinaceous appendage called a *sex pilus* is found on the outside of the cell; this together with other plasmid-mediated proteins provides for cell-to-cell transmission of the plasmid DNA. Conjugative plasmids of gram-positive bacteria do not utilize pili for conjugation. Cell-to-cell contact is required, in some cases facilitated by plasmid-coded proteins that enhance clumping of donor and recipient cells. The genes of a conjugative plasmid are usually found in functional clusters, with part of the genes encoding for transfer functions and part devoted to replication; the function of the remaining DNA is often unknown or is concerned with other identifiable functions such as antibiotic resistance.

Nonconjugative plasmids are not self-transmissible and do not encode for transfer-specific proteins or a sex pilus. They are usually smaller in mass than conjugative plasmids. Nonconjugative plasmids can be transferred from cell to cell by a process called *mobilization*, in which a coresident nonconjugative plasmid takes advantage of the transfer of a coexisting conjugative one. In addition, nonconjugative and conjugative plasmids may also be transmitted by bacterial virus vectors called *bacteriophages*, a process termed *transduction*. In this process, plasmid DNA instead of phage DNA is packaged within the viral protein coat and, on infection of a suitable recipient cell, the plasmid DNA is released and begins replication within the new host.

Since transduction requires that the plasmid DNA be packaged within the protein coat of a bacteriophage, the amount of plasmid DNA that can be transduced is limited to approximately the size of the phage genome. This process operates much more efficiently for the smaller nonconjugative plasmids and appears to be an important mechanism of plasmid exchange in *S. aureus*. In gram-negative bacilli and streptococci, on the other hand, conjugation and mobilization seem to be the most common means of transfer. Conjugative transfer of resistance has been described in *S. aureus*, and it may be an important mechanism of gene exchange in more recent nosocomial staphylococcal isolates [8, 12].

Direct uptake of both conjugative and nonconjugative plasmid DNA by a recipient cell can also occur, a process termed *transformation*. To induce transformation in the laboratory, bacteria are usually treated with calcium chloride to render them able to take up the plasmid DNA, a state referred to as *competence*. The ability to render *Escherichia coli* competent was important in the development of recombinant DNA technology, since fragments of DNA to be "cloned" are usually inserted into nonconjugative plasmids, which are then transformed into *E. coli* for expression of the cloned DNA. The amount of DNA that can be picked up by a recipient cell is limited, and it is unlikely that transformation plays a significant role in plasmid transfer in the hospital.

In addition to transferability, another important feature of plasmids is *compatibility*. Compatibility refers to the ability of two plasmids to coexist within the same bacterial cell. If two plasmids cannot coexist, they are said to be of the same compatibility class. Compatibility classifications have been applied to plasmids isolated from the various enteric gram-negative bacilli as well as from *Pseudomonas aeruginosa* and to plasmids from *S. aureus*. Compatibility testing has proved useful in several epidemiologic investigations [4]. For example, when R plasmids encoding for chloramphenicol resistance were isolated from both *Salmonella typhi* and *Shigella dysenteriae* in Mexico, many investigators believed that these were closely related R plasmids. Since these R plasmids could coexist in the same cell and were of differing compatibility classes, they were not closely related. Plasmids that are not compatible generally share many genes in common, especially those required for replication.

Transmissibility and compatibility are properties of an entire plasmid. Our understanding of the evolution and diversity of bacterial plasmids has been expanded by the discovery of the process of transposition, whereby plasmid subunits can disperse separately from the entire plasmid. The rapidity with which antimicrobial resistance has been encountered in some organisms is in part related to this process.

A transposition sequence is a well-defined genetic segment, usually of constant size, that can move as an intact unit from one replicating DNA unit to another. These sequences can "jump" from plasmid to plasmid, plasmid to bacteriophage, plasmid to chromosome, or the reverse. Transposition elements specifying resistance, or *transposons*, have been described for most of the widely used antimicrobial agents, including the newer aminoglycosides [7]. In theory, any plasmid could gain these elements; it would only be necessary for the DNA containing the transposon to coexist in a cell long enough for transposition to occur.

Mechanisms of Resistance

The resistance genes carried by R plasmids code for the synthesis of new proteins. These proteins frequently provide the bacterial cell with new enzymatic capabilities allowing for resistance. This is in contrast to chromosomal mutations resulting in resistance, which often alter subcellular structures. These changes in essential cellular components, although resulting in antimicrobial resistance, are also often a disadvantage to the bacterial cell because the function of the component of the cell that is affected is compromised. R plasmids provide an advantage since essential bacterial cell functions are uncompromised. The known modes of R plasmid–coded resistance have several mechanisms and involve proteins that (1) enzymatically inactivate the antibiotic, (2) alter the target sites for the antibiotic, (3) block the transport of the antibiotic into the bacterial cell, or (4) bypass the metabolic steps inhibited by the antibiotic.

Plasmid-mediated resistance to ampicillin is an example of enzymatic inactivation. The penicillins and cephalosporins are β-lactam antibiotics, which are important as components of modern antimicrobial therapy. Resistance to these agents stems most often from β-lactamases, enzymes that hydrolyze the β-lactam ring and detoxify the drugs. The β-lactamase can be chromosome- or plasmid-mediated.

An example of plasmid-mediated alteration of an antibiotic-sensitive target is erythromycin resistance in gram-positive bacteria, typically staphylococci and streptococci. In this instance, the 23 S RNA of the 50 S ribosome unit is methylated by a plasmid-mediated enzyme. Methylation of specific adenine residues on the RNA prevents binding of the erythromycin and lincomycin classes of antimicrobials, and bacteria containing this plasmid gene exhibit high-level resistance.

A common example of blocking antimicrobial uptake is resistance to aminoglycoside antibiotics. R plasmid–mediated resistance to aminoglycosides does not show large inoculum effects, and the active antibiotic does not disappear from the culture medium after the plasmid-containing organisms are grown. This is true although the mechanism of resistance is due to the presence of plasmid-coded aminoglycoside-modifying enzymes.

These enzymes are at the inner membrane of bacterial cells, and the modified aminoglycoside blocks transport of the antibiotic into the cell. The phenotypic expression of aminoglycoside resistance will depend on the site at which the enzyme acts and on whether that site is present or available for enzymatic inactivation on a given aminoglycoside.

Bypass of inhibited metabolism is exemplified by the resistance to sulfonamides and trimethoprim. This is based on a plasmid-coded enzyme that substitutes for a chromosomal enzyme normally inhibited by these drugs. Sulfonamides work through competitive inhibition of the enzyme dihydropteroate synthetase. The plasmid-coded enzyme is smaller and more heat-sensitive and requires a thousand times as much sulfonamide to inhibit it as does the chromosomal enzyme [24]. Similarly, some strains resistant to high levels of trimethoprim, an agent that inhibits dihydrofolate reductase, contain a plasmid-mediated gene coding for a new trimethoprim-resistant dihydrofolate reductase. In each of these instances, the plasmids provide a mechanism whereby products vital to the bacterial cell can be synthesized and the inhibiting effect of the drug is bypassed.

Recent developments have led to the recognition that mutation and R plasmid exchange can interact in the evolution of resistance. Clinical isolates were encountered that were resistant to newer β-lactams. These drugs had been developed to resist hydrolysis by common R plasmid β-lactamases, the TEM enzymes. Mutations in the preexisting TEM enzymes resulted in new substrate affinities such that the drugs were now readily inactivated [14].

Molecular Analysis of Resistance

Simplified techniques for isolating and characterizing bacterial plasmids have been developed in recent years [3, 10, 21]. Application of this technology to clinical situations involving antimicrobial resistance has improved our understanding of the evolution of resistance within hospitals. We are aware now that the development of resistance operates at three levels of genetic organization. The first level is dissemination within the hospital of an R plasmid–containing strain. The next level occurs with plasmid spread, in which an R plasmid is moved from strain to strain or from one species to another. The third level involves transposition of individual resistance determinants from one plasmid to another or from chromosome to plasmid. The latter process may be one way that R plasmids gradually accumulate multiple resistances.

Numerous examples of epidemics due to resistant microorganisms have been reported. A common feature of most of the outbreaks is the emergence of a strain able to resist the action of agents preferred for treating serious infections in hospitalized patients. Most commonly for the gram-negative pathogens, the antimicrobials concerned are newer aminoglycosides, such as gentamicin and tobramycin, or β-lactams, such as carbenicillin and ticarcillin. One such outbreak occurred in Nashville, Tennessee, where resistance to gentamicin was uncommon before 1973. Isolates of *Serratia marcescens* with high-level resistance to gentamicin were first discovered in that year and, over the next 2 years, caused a large number of infections. These isolates were of an identical phagetype and serotype and thus represented clonal dissemination of a single strain [22]. Similar hospital outbreaks involving *Klebsiella pneumoniae, P. aeruginosa,* and other gram-negative bacilli have been described.

When strain dissemination is suspected, various techniques can be applied to determine the probable identical nature of strains. The easiest and most available are those used in the routine evaluation of the isolates in the clinical laboratory. Species identification, biotype, and antimicrobial susceptibility pattern all provide useful clues to strain identity. More information is often necessary, however, because many common nosocomial pathogens provide little variability in biotype or susceptibility pattern. This makes accurate determination of the sameness of isolates difficult using the readily available data; additional laboratory study of the strains becomes necessary.

Additional typing information is obtained from referral centers and is usually dependent on the species to be examined [1]. Serotyping, phage typing, bacteriocin production, and bacteriocin susceptibility can be useful, depending on the organism (see Chap. 9). Additional procedures that have provided information useful for typing isolates are analysis of the total plasmid content of bacterial cells by agarose gel electrophoresis (AGE) [18] or analysis of total DNA content by field inversion gel electrophoresis (FIGE). The electrophoretic analysis of plasmid DNA is extended to whole-cell DNA and used for typing as well. Whole-cell DNA is digested by restriction endonucleases and electrophoresed using pulsed-field electrophoresis. Similar to plasmid analysis, a "fingerprint" of the strain is created by the resulting digest pattern [2, 20]. Recent technical advances now allow such analyses to be completed within 1 day of isolation of an organism in pure culture. The information generated by AGE or FIGE is especially important in organisms such as *Citrobacter* species, *Enterobacter,* non-*aeruginosa Pseudomonas* species, and *Staphylococcus epidermidis,* when other typing systems are not available. The presence of cryptic plasmids along with R plasmids in nosocomial isolates often provides a characteristic electrophoretic pattern useful to fingerprint a strain. When an outbreak is suspected or an infection problem occurs, such as serial *S. epidermidis* infections in cardiac surgery, in which knowledge of the sameness of multiple isolates would assist in evaluation, AGE can provide useful information rapidly. It also provides information about plasmid content should plasmid spread be suspected. Most large referral hospitals should be able to establish these techniques. Smaller institutions can seek assistance from most university centers, especially those involved in recombinant DNA research, where these techniques are applied virtually every day.

Intergeneric R plasmid exchange can and has contributed to problems encountered with resistant pathogens in a number of hospitals (Table 14-1). Common features of all these reports have been their occurrence in large referral hospitals, involvement of special care units, and simultaneous acquisition by the recipient of the "epidemic" R plasmid of resistance to multiple antimicrobials.

To find out whether there has been possible plasmid spread, comparison of patterns of resistance is coupled with observation of the ability of the natural isolates to transfer similar resistances into reference host strains. *E. coli* strain K-12, onto which resistance to selected antimicrobials such as nalidixic acid or streptomycin has been introduced by mutation, is often chosen to serve as recipient. Similar laboratory strains for use as recipients in *Pseudomonas* transfers also have been developed. The potential donor and recipient are grown in mixed culture and, through use of selective media, the ability of the resistance to be transferred can be documented. Strains transferring resistances can then be analyzed by AGE, along with their transconjugants, for total plasmid content. This technique allows the visualization of plasmids and an approximation of their molecular mass. Bacterial lysates are prepared, placed in slots of an agarose slab gel, and separated by electrophoresis. After staining with ethidium bromide, which binds to DNA by inserting between

Table 14-1. Studies demonstrating intergeneric R plasmid transfer within the hospital

Investigator	Geographic location	Species involved	Clinical setting	Molecular mass (md)	Resistances conferred by plasmid
Thomas et al. [22] Rubens et al. [15]	Nashville	*Klebsiella pneumoniae* *Pseudomonas aeruginosa* *Serratia marcescens*	Hospitalwide	105	Gm, tm, km, sm, su, tc, cb, ap, cm
Elwell et al. [6]	Dallas	*Klebsiella pneumoniae* *Enterobacter cloacae*	Burn unit	60	Tm, km, sm, ap, cb
Schaberg et al. [19]	Dallas	*Klebsiella pneumoniae* *Enterobacter cloacae*	Neonatal intensive care	80	Gm, tm, km, cm, ap, cb
Tompkins et al. [23]	Seattle	*Serratia marcescens* *Klebsiella pneumoniae* *Enterobacter aerogenes* *Citrobacter freundii* *Klebsiella oxytoca* *Providencia rettgeri*	Hospitalwide	45	Gm, tm, km, ap, cb, cf, sm, su
Gerding et al. [9] Sadowski et al. [17]	Minneapolis	*Klebsiella pneumoniae* *Escherichia coli* *Enterobacter cloacae* *Morganella morganii*	ICU and hospitalwide	58	Gm, tm, km, ap, cb, cf, cm, su
O'Brien et al. [13]	Unknown	*Klebsiella pneumoniae* *Enterobacter aerogenes* *Serratia marcescens* *Escherichia coli* *Citrobacter freundii* *Morganella morganii*	ICU and hospitalwide	56.5	Gm, tm, su, cm, ap, cb
Knight et al. [11]	London	*Klebsiella pneumoniae* *Escherichia coli* *Citrobacter freundii* *Enterobacter cloacae*	Hospitalwide	110	Gm, tm, km, sm, su, tc, cb, ap, cm

Gm = gentamicin; tm = tobramycin; km = kanamycin; sm = streptomycin; su = sulfonamide; tc = tetracycline; cb = carbenicillin; ap = ampicillin; cm = chloramphenicol; cf = cephalothin; ICU = intensive care unit.

bases, the plasmids can be visualized as discrete bands using ultraviolet light. Photography using special filters provides a permanent record of the gel. R plasmids from a single hospital carrying identical resistances and of similar molecular mass suggest R plasmid exchange has occurred.

Plasmids encoding similar resistances and of approximately the same size can be additionally explored for identity by endonuclease restriction analysis. The plasmids are subjected to digestion with endonuclease restriction enzymes, which generates a characteristic DNA fragment pattern depending on the plasmid and particular enzyme used (Fig. 14-1). There are a large number of enzymes available, and each one recognizes discrete nucleotide sequences on a plasmid. Demonstration of identically sized plasmids encoding for identical resistances with identical restriction endonuclease fragment patterns is strong evidence that two plasmids are identical. The finding that they come from multiple genera in the same hospital provides support that intergeneric R plasmid exchange within the hospital environment is happening. How important R plasmid exchange is in the overall picture of resistance remains uncertain, but this mechanism does operate in special care areas of large hospitals where selective pressure of therapy is greatest.

It is not clear from where antimicrobial resistance genes have originated and how multiple determinants for antimicrobial resis-

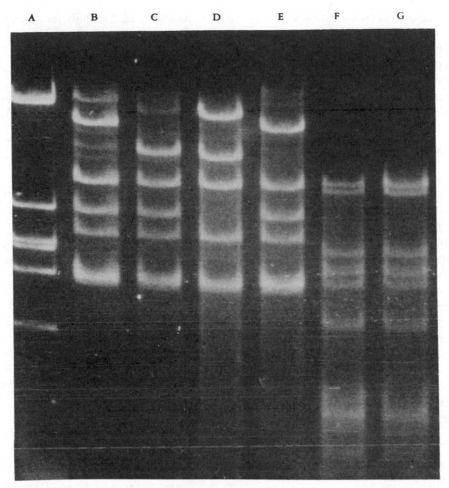

Fig. 14-1.   Agarose gel electrophoresis of restriction endonuclease–digested plasmid DNA. Lane A contains bacteriophage lambda DNA digested with EcoR1. Lanes B through E contain gentamicin R plasmids of similar size on screening and are believed to be identical. Lanes B and E did give identical patterns, as confirmed by digestion with enzyme HindIII, shown in F and G. The plasmids in lanes C and D gave different enzyme digestion patterns.

tance accumulate on a given R plasmid. The movement of resistance genes from plasmid to plasmid or from chromosome to plasmid via transposition may play a role in the "building" of R plasmids. Several studies have shown that this process has worked in the hospital environment [5, 15, 16]. In the studies by Rubens and co-workers [15, 16], a gentamicin-resistance determinant originally present on a small nonconjugative plasmid was transposed onto a larger, self-transferable plasmid. Once on the conjugative element, the resistance was efficiently transferred among genera within the hospital. This process provided a mechanism to stack new resistance determinants on a preexisting plasmid and appears to be one way that R plasmid development can take place. Unfortunately, the techniques for studying transposition remain cumbersome and available only in research laboratories.

Approach to Control

In theory, one approach to control of antimicrobial resistance is to prevent the exchange of R plasmids and interrupt the transposition process in the development of R plasmids.

Unfortunately, no agents are available that allow us to do this selectively and efficiently. Rather, we are forced to contend as best we can with the first level of organization, resistant strains, and await modalities to attack the R plasmids specifically.

Adding to the problem is the fact that as many as 10 to 12 resistances may be present on a single R plasmid. The linkage of these resistance determinants makes it possible for therapy with a single antimicrobial to select for resistance to various unrelated antibiotics. Rotation of antibiotics and restricting certain ones may not be as effective as hoped in decreasing resistance. Use of a totally different antimicrobial, if the plasmid encodes for resistance to both, will continue to select for persistence of the resistant strains.

Measures have been developed that can be successful in controlling dissemination of resistant strains and are based on an understanding of the epidemiology of each circumstance. Strategies of use to many hospitals are summarized in Chapter 13. As we acquire a clearer understanding of the factors in R plasmid exchange, we hope to be able to intervene in the fundamental processes involved in the evolution of R plasmids and to prevent the development of multiple resistant strains.

References

1. Aber, R.C., and Mackel, D.C. Epidemiologic typing of nosocomial microorganisms. *Am. J. Med.* 70:899, 1981.
2. Arbeit, R.D., et al. Resolution of recent evolutionary divergence among *Escherichia coli* from related lineages: The application of pulsed field electrophoresis to molecular epidemiology. *J. Infect. Dis.* 161:230, 1990.
3. Bidwell, J.L., Lewis, D.A., and Reeves, D.S. A rapid single-colony lysate method for the selective visualization of plasmids in Enterobacteriaceae, including *Serratia marcescens*. *J. Antimicrob. Chemother.* 8:481, 1981.
4. Datta, N. Plasmid Classification: Incompatibility Grouping. In K.N. Timmis and A. Pichler (Eds.), *Plasmids of Medical, Environmental, and Commercial Importance*. Amsterdam: Elsevier/North-Holland Biomedical Press, 1979. Pp. 47–53.
5. Datta, N., Hughes, V.M., Nugents, M.E., and

Richards, H. Plasmids and transposons and their stability and mutability in bacteria isolated during an outbreak of hospital infection. *Plasmid* 2:182, 1979.
6. Elwell, L.P., Inamine, J.M., and Minshew, B.H. Common plasmid specifying tobramycin resistance found in two enteric bacteria isolated from burn patients. *Antimicrob. Agents Chemother.* 13:312, 1978.
7. Farrar, W.E. Gentamicin transposons. *J. Antimicrob. Chemother.* 6:4, 1980.
8. Forbes, B.A., and Schaberg, D.R. Transfer of resistance plasmids from *Staphylococcus epidermidis* to *Staphylococcus aureus:* Evidence for conjugative exchange of resistance. *J. Bacteriol.* 153:627, 1983.
9. Gerding, D.N., et al. Nosocomial multiply-resistant *Klebsiella pneumoniae:* Epidemiology of an outbreak apparent index case origin. *Antimicrob. Agents Chemother.* 15:608, 1979.
10. Kado, C.I., and Liu, S.T. Rapid procedure for detection and isolation of large and small plasmids. *J. Bacteriol.* 145:1365, 1981.
11. Knight, S., and Casewell, M.W. Dissemination of resistance plasmids among gentamicin-resistant enterobacteria from hospital patients. *Br. Med. J.* 283:755, 1981.
12. McDonnell, R.W., Sweeney, H.M., and Cohen, S. Conjugational transfer of gentamicin resistance plasmids intra- and interspecifically in *Staphylococcus aureus* and *Staphylococcus epidermidis*. *Antimicrob. Agents Chemother.* 23:151, 1983.
13. O'Brien, T.F., et al. Dissemination of an antibiotic resistance plasmid in hospital patient flora. *Antimicrob. Agents Chemother.* 17:537, 1980.
14. Philippon, A., Labia, R., and Jacoby, G. Extended-spectrum β-lactamases. *Antimicrob. Agents Chemother.* 33:1131, 1989.
15. Rubens, C.E., Farrar, W.E., McGee, Z.A., and Schaffner, W. Evolution of a plasmid mediating resistance to multiple antimicrobial agents during a prolonged epidemic of nosocomial infections: A molecular biological investigation. *J. Infect. Dis.* 143:170, 1981.
16. Rubens, C.E., McNeill, W.F., and Farrar, W.E. Evolution of multiple antibiotic-resistance plasmids mediated by transposable deoxyribonucleic acid sequences. *J. Bacteriol.* 140:713, 1979.
17. Sadowski, P.L., Peterson, B.C., Gerding, D., and Cleary, P.P. Physical characterization of ten R plasmids obtained from an outbreak of nosocomial *Klebsiella pneumoniae* infections. *Antimicrob. Agents Chemother.* 15:616, 1979.
18. Schaberg, D.R., Tompkins, L.S., and Falkow, S. Use of agarose gel electrophoresis of plasmid deoxyribonucleic acid to fingerprint gram-negative bacilli. *J. Clin. Microbiol.* 13:1105, 1981.

19. Schaberg, D.R., Tompkins, L.S., Rubens, C.E., and Falkow, S. R plasmids and Nosocomial Infection. In C. Stuttard, and K.R. Royce (Eds.), *Plasmids and Transposons: Environmental Effects and Maintenance Mechanisms.* New York: Academic, 1980. Pp. 43–55.

20. Stevens, D.S., Odds, F.C., and Scherer, S. Application of DNA typing methods to *Candida albicans* epidemiology and correlations with phenotype. *Rev. Infect. Dis.* 12:258, 1990.

21. Takahashi, S., and Nagano, Y. Rapid procedure for isolation of plasmid DNA and application to epidemiological analysis. *J. Clin. Microbiol.* 4:608, 1984.

22. Thomas, F.E., Jackson, R.T., Melly, M.A., and Alford, R.H. Sequential hospital-wide outbreaks of resistant *Serratia* and *Klebsiella* infections. *Arch. Intern. Med.* 137:581, 1977.

23. Tompkins, L.S., Plorde, J.J., and Falkow, S. Molecular analysis of R factors from multiresistant nosocomial isolates. *J. Infect. Dis.* 141:625, 1980.

24. Wise, E.M., and Abou-Donia, M.M. Sulfonamide resistance mechanism in *Escherichia coli:* R plasmids can determine sulfonamide-resistant dihydropteroate synthetases. *Proc. Natl. Acad. Sci. U.S.A.* 72:2621, 1975.

The Inanimate Environment

Frank S. Rhame

The hypothesis that environmental microorganisms cause human disease readily arises from two incontestable observations: (1) Our interaction with the inanimate environment is constant and close, and (2) environmental objects are usually contaminated, often with important human pathogens. Microbes are remarkably efficient at becoming dispersed to virtually all unprotected niches. Where there is moisture and at least small amounts of organic material, proliferation to large numbers occurs. Even on dry, infertile surfaces, microbes survive in various relatively inactive states. Unfortunately, though it is fairly easy to assess the prevalence of microorganisms in the environment, it is relatively difficult to establish the role the organisms in these environments play in causing human disease. Evaluating the evidence in this matter is the fundamental task of this chapter.

The scope of this chapter is determined partly by logic and partly by tradition. The title itself is a misnomer: If the environment were inanimate, it would not require discussion. The major focus is on those normally nonsterile items that may serve as *fomites,** or vectors of infection. Some of these items—for example, internal surfaces of respirator and anesthesia breathing circuits, water in humidifier reservoirs [37], endoscopes passed through nonsterile cavities, and reusable pressure transducer heads [20]—can be kept sterile, though the need to do so is arguable. Some distinctions are quite arbitrary: Pus, while in a patient's wound or on the unwashed

---

*The word *fomite,* although sometimes in disfavor, remains quite useful. A fomite is an inanimate object that may be contaminated with microorganisms and serve in their transmission. The origin of the term *fomites* is the Latin plural of *Fomes,* the genus of fungus that was used as tinder. The dried fungus is porous and thus was considered "capable of absorbing and retaining contagious effluvia" [12].

hands of a hospital worker, would not be considered part of the inanimate environment, but as soon as it is deposited on a surface it would. Skin is not considered in this chapter, but airborne squames are. The traditional items include a variety of living things—potted plants, cut flowers, and fresh fruits, insect infestation, and problems associated with animal visitation in the hospital.

The fomites to be discussed in this chapter include items for which no infection-causing potential has been established. Questions concerning the proper management of these items frequently confront infection control personnel. Even those skeptical of the infection-causing potential of ordinary patient care objects and environmental surfaces advocate processing and cleaning methods that may have considerable financial impact [175]. Concerns cannot be dismissed simply because no infection hazard has been demonstrated. Environmental objects heavily contaminated with recognized human pathogens may come in close approximation to potential portals of entry.

The simplistic dichotomous view (i.e., an item is sterile or not) that we generally apply to sterilization is not applicable to the items being discussed here. Rather, we must contend with the difficulty of determining the appropriate degree of contamination. Rigorous research is hampered in this context because speciation of contaminating organisms becomes relevant. Unfortunately, methods for microbiologic classification of environmental organisms are not nearly so well worked out as for organisms from clinical specimens. In some cases (e.g., dialysis water) standards exist but, for the most part, no standards have been set and there is little rational basis for setting them.

Some objects may be sterile as a by-product of manufacture. For instance, the protected outside surfaces of intravenous bottle stoppers are usually sterile, although manufacturers do not make the claim of sterility because it is burdensome to prove it to regulatory agencies. There are items that are not marketed as sterile but that usually are and ar-

guably should be. When contaminated, these items have been responsible for outbreaks: Elastic bandages have caused *Rhizopus* [133] and *Clostridium perfringens* [149] skin infections; contaminated blood collection tubes have caused pseudobacteremias [101] and true bacteremias [171]; contaminated handcare products have also been implicated as a cause of infection [148]. Clinicians often perceive products that come in closed containers as sterile and use them as such even when they are not so marketed [50]. Most would find surprising the frequency of contamination of oral medications (especially those of animal origin), ointments, nasal sprays, and lotions [105].

We must also recognize that procedures for processing environmental items rest in part on aesthetic and achievability considerations. Carpets may not usually constitute an infection hazard, but fecal stains are unacceptable. Health care professionals may be convinced that microorganisms on the walls and floors play no role in causing human disease, but the lay public's perception is exactly the contrary: In an era of increasing attention to marketing, visible dirt is undesirable. When standards have been set, formally or informally, they are often based on recognition of what reductions in microbial content can be consistently achieved with moderate effort rather than what levels are required to prevent infection.

The occurrence of outbreaks of nosocomial infection due to contaminated inanimate objects is often invoked as a basis for concern about endemic nosocomial infection attributable to the inanimate environment. In fact, most outbreaks of nosocomial infection are associated with person-to-person spread or due to contamination of an item that should be sterile [124, 182]. Such outbreaks contribute to our understanding of the causation of nosocomial infection, but they do not constitute a significant contribution to the problem. These outbreaks stimulate us to seek improved methods of achieving or maintaining sterility of objects that should be sterile, but they are not a sufficient basis for concern about environmental contamination.

Environmentally Altered Microorganisms

It seems paradoxical that environmental objects can frequently be contaminated by human pathogens while only rarely contributing to human infection. A potential explanation lies in the concept of environmentally damaged organisms. This concept has been rigorously demonstrated for *Streptococcus pyogenes* by Rammelkamp, Perry, and their colleagues [150, 151, 157]. In a classic series of experiments, they studied streptococcal transmission in army barracks. Air, dust, and personal effects such as blankets were more often contaminated by streptococci when recruits had streptococcal illness or pharyngeal colonization. However, recruits who had been issued freshly laundered, *Streptococcus*-free blankets acquired streptococcal infection or pharyngeal colonization just as often as barracksmates issued highly contaminated blankets [150]. These authors directly assessed the infectious potential of naturally contaminated barracks dust. Dust samples were repeatedly dispersed in small enclosures (air samples showed between 100 and 1,600 streptococci per cubic foot) without producing pharyngeal colonizations or infection in volunteers within the enclosures. Six volunteers had 17 direct inoculations of dust containing 1,800 to 42,000 streptococci onto the posterior pharynx. There resulted only transient colonization lasting no more than 30 minutes [151]. Hypothesizing that dryness was responsible for the inability of the streptococci to produce colonization, the investigators assessed the infectious potential of oropharyngeal secretions that were mixed with sterile dust. When the inoculated dust was permitted to dry for 4 to 8 hours, 2 of 8 volunteers developed streptococcal pharyngitis. Two of the remaining 6 volunteers developed pharyngitis on subsequent inoculation of smaller numbers of streptococci transferred on swabs of nosopharyngeal sections [157]. The designation of this phenomenon as *environmental damage* reflects a rather anthropocentric perspective. Streptococci presumably shift their metabolism to meet their current needs. The physiologic basis of bacterial adaptation to desiccation has been explored [119] and involves substantial changes in internal constituents.

The loss of human pathogenicity associated with adaptation to the environment has been established for desiccated *Streptococcus pyogenes*. It seems plausible that other species have different adaptations to various environmental situations that would also reduce their pathogenicity for humans. For some organisms, however, it is reasonable to speculate that the required adaptations are less debilitating. "Water bacteria" in moist environments might be in metabolic states less different from their most pathogenic state. Viruses are either viable or not. *Clostridium difficile* as an environmental spore is more durable; if the spore is an infectious form for humans, environmental damage would not be relevant. These matters are, at present, largely unexplored.

Epistemology

With the foregoing generalities in mind, we confront the methodologic inadequacies that characterize most published studies asserting a causative role of inanimate objects in human disease. There are six classes of evidence suggesting that a fomite has a role in causing disease due to a particular pathogen. They are ordered here by the rigor with which they establish the point. Each argument is strengthened when subspecies or strain analysis of the implicated pathogen shows similarity between human and environmental isolates.

1. *The organism can survive after inoculation onto the fomite.* This is the weakest form of evidence, yet good journals allocate space to these studies, which sometimes achieve widespread attention from the press. A case in point is a demonstration that herpes simplex virus can survive when inoculated on hot-tub seats [143]. The finding was published despite the cogent words of the accompanying editorial [68], which pointed out the incon-

clusiveness of the observation. At present, it is not possible to provide firm generalizations on the duration of survival required for significance.

2. *The pathogen can be cultured from in-use fomites.* A vast set of publications report the recovery of human pathogens from health care items. These demonstrations are an important element in the assertion that a fomite causes infection, but they are only a first step. When the pathogen is present more frequently or in higher concentration in association with infected humans, this element is marginally strengthened. However, this association is as likely to arise from the patient infecting the environment as vice versa [125]. When the pathogen cannot be cultured, other markers may be used (e.g., hepatitis B surface antigen in the case of hepatitis B [118]). When it is suspected that environmental adaptation may reduce pathogenicity, it is desirable that the detection method simulate the natural infection (e.g., animal inoculation).

3. *The pathogen can proliferate in the fomite.* Whether proliferation must be demonstrated is largely a function of the size of the inoculum required to cause infection. For instance, this element is important in the case of contaminated intravenous solution: Most intravenous fluid contamination is at low concentrations, and humans ordinarily tolerate a few organisms given intravenously. For intravenous fluid contamination to be a hazard, the organisms must have the ability and time to proliferate. In general, contaminated objects do not cause infection unless the contaminating organism can proliferate in the contaminated environment or the contamination is heavy and occurs shortly before exposure.

4. *Some fraction of acquisition cannot be accounted for by other recognized methods of transmission.* An example of this type of evidence is found in the last of a series of studies that began with the classic demonstration of the importance of hands and contact in nursery acquisition by newborns of *Staphylococcus aureus*. In the final study of the series, Mortimer and colleagues [137] went to great lengths to eliminate contact transmission in a nursery

in which index babies were colonized by *S. aureus*. At least 9 of 158 contact-protected babies became colonized. This (along with other observations) was taken as evidence that air was the vector of transmission. A more recent example occurred during a nursing-home outbreak of Norwalk diarrhea. Thirteen ill employees were very unlikely to have had stool contact. The authors suggested that airborne spread had occurred [82].

This element may appear to be present simply because of the vicissitudes of biologic systems. It is inevitable that it will be difficult to account for all transmissions by any given mechanism. Implication of a fomite by exclusion of alternatives should be considered weak evidence unless a large fraction of transmissions cannot otherwise be explained. This line of logic can also lead to false exoneration of important mechanisms, when several are operating at the steep portion of the dose-infection curve [35].

5. *Case-control studies show an association between exposure to the contaminated fomite and infection.* Most well-studied epidemics implicating fomites include this element. One must always be cautious about projecting from epidemics to endemic infections. Case-control methodology is discussed in Chapters 1 and 6.

6. *Prospective studies allocating exposure to the contaminated fomite to a subset of patients show an association between the exposure and infection.* Ideally, the exposed group is selected randomly.

Only evidence from categories 5 and 6 should be considered strong enough to implicate a fomite. Unfortunately, most published studies of fomite transmission present evidence of types 1 or 2. Accordingly, chapters such as this one often appear to be a litany of inconclusiveness. Whenever possible in this chapter, we eschew data of type 1 or 2 in favor of higher levels of evidence. We continue with an analysis of a variety of potential fomites that are usually nonsterile but are plausible enough causes of nosocomial infection to warrant discussion. The ultimate extension of concern about the inanimate environment, ultraclean protective environments for immunosuppressed patients, is also discussed. We conclude with sections on disinfection and sterilization and routine microbiologic monitoring of inanimate objects in the hospital.

Air

There has probably been concern about air as a vehicle for transmission of infection for as long as there has been recognition of the transmissibility of disease. Surely more data have been generated for this fomite than for any other. Entire books have been devoted to the subject [72, 115], suggesting that concise summarization is difficult. As an indication of trends in this area, there were six articles dealing with airborne spread presented at the initial International Conference on Nosocomial Infections in 1970 and an estimate in 1970 by Brachman [32] that between 10 and 20 percent of endemic nosocomial infections resulted from the airborne route. At the Second International Conference on Nosocomial Infections in 1982, however, there was only one presentation about airborne organisms [121], and it dealt with the operating room. At the Third International Conference in 1990, except for measles virus transmission, the topic was not discussed.

Despite concern about air as a vector of disease, there are surprisingly few general surveys of the microbial content of hospital air, with complete identification of the organisms recovered. This lack no doubt results from the formidable obstacles to such an undertaking. There is not yet a consensus on the optimal sampling method. (For a concise discussion of the available methods, see Chapter 9 and Groschell [91].) It is not even clear whether volumetric sampling or settling techniques are better. Volumetric sampling produces quantitative data that are more readily conceptualized; this technique is probably more relevant to situations in which a pathogen is inhaled. Settling techniques may be more relevant to infections that result from settling organisms (e.g., wound infections). Because the concentration of certain organ-

isms in the air is small compared to the volumes that can be conveniently assessed, culturing air is often subject to considerable sampling error. Furthermore, there is tremendous variation in the microbial content of air, depending on location in the hospital, ventilation systems, concurrent human activity, and proximity to sources of organisms. Finally, the broadest survey available was performed more than 30 years ago, which raises questions about its current applicability [87, 88].

In the previously mentioned general survey, Greene and colleagues [87, 88] found a mean organism count of roughly 10 to 20 organisms per cubic foot.* The highest counts were in laundry handling areas, followed closely by other storage and disposal areas. The lowest counts were in operating and delivery rooms. Roughly one-third of the organisms recovered were gram-positive cocci, roughly one-third gram-positive bacilli, and the remainder gram-negative bacilli or fungi. Gram-positive cocci constituted a higher proportion of the organisms in operating rooms; gram-positive bacilli (presumably mostly *Bacillus* species) constituted a higher proportion of the organisms in the laundry and waste storage areas; and gram-negative bacilli were relatively high in corridors.

More detailed consideration of air as a fomite is best made by specific organism. Airborne[†] transmission of *Mycobacterium tuberculosis,* varicella-zoster virus, smallpox, influenza, and measles has been convincingly established and probably constitutes the major mechanism of spread within the hospital. The epidemiology of rubella and mumps suggests they have similar transmission mechanisms. Except in the case of two pathogens, control of airborne transmission in hospitals consists mainly of identifying patients with

---

*The units used will be those of the original article: (1 cubic foot = 28.3 liters = 0.283 cubic meters; 1 cubic meter = 1,000 liters = 34.9 cubic feet.)

[†] In the context of infection transmission, *airborne* means "borne on the air," rather than "transported through the air." Large droplets travel up to 1 to 2 m through the air but are not borne on it. Large-droplet transmission is considered a type of contact spread (see Chap. 1).

active infection and promptly placing them in isolation rooms with proper air control. Tuberculosis control in the acquired immunodeficiency syndrome [AIDS] era requires special air control measures in sites where inhalational pentamidine is administered and where sputum induction is performed [45]. Influenza control during community outbreaks is a bit more complicated because of the high prevalence of infectious patients and personnel and because infectious persons may have subtle or no respiratory symptoms [19]. Preventing nosocomial influenza during community influenza outbreaks is one of the few solid rationales for human traffic control within hospitals.

Staphylococcus aureus

There is a solid theoretic basis for concern about the importance of airborne transmission of *S. aureus* (see Chap. 37). Noble [145], probably the most avid student of this matter, summarizes information bearing on the origin of airborne *S. aureus* as follows: Humans liberate approximately 3×10^8 squames per day. Because the size distribution of airborne particles containing *S. aureus* (approximately 4 to 25 μm in diameter) is nearly that of squames and well above the diameter of naked, single *S. aureus* cells (approximately 1 μm in diameter), it is presumed that most or all airborne *S. aureus* organisms are carried on these skin flakes. Since particles of this size become impacted on the nasal turbinates, a closed loop may occur: proliferation of *S. aureus* on the nasal mucosa, hand transfer of *S. aureus* to the skin, liberation on squames, airborne transport of squames, and impaction on the nasal mucosa. Hospital air contains approximately 0.02 colony-forming units (cfu) of *S. aureus* per cubic foot of air [173].

Outbreaks of *S. aureus* (and *S. pyogenes*) surgical wound infection have been solidly linked to airborne spread from dispersers in the operating room (see Chap. 33). In this context, surgical gowns make direct contact improbable and masks make droplet spread improbable. However, the importance of air for endemic *S. aureus* transmission in other

settings is less clear. The strongest positive evidence is that of Mortimer and co-workers [137], who studied acquisition of staphylococcal colonization in newborn infants housed in a special nursery that was also used for the care of known colonized infants. Extraordinary measures were undertaken to eliminate contact transfer of *S. aureus* from the index babies to the study babies. Nevertheless, at least 9 of 158 newborns became colonized. The authors offered as evidence that these acquisitions were airborne the following points: Contact transmission did not occur; index strains of *S. aureus* were recovered on settling plates throughout the nursery; the infants were at least 2.1 m apart, making large-droplet transmission unlikely; and the study infants tended to be colonized in the nose first, whereas in previous studies infants acquiring *S. aureus* by physical transfer tended to be colonized at the umbilicus first. Wenzel and colleagues [191] have critically analyzed nine additional articles published between 1966 and 1976 purporting to show airborne transmission of *S. aureus*. None of these additional studies provides even strongly suggestive evidence of airborne spread. A bit of negative evidence with respect to endemic operating room acquisition of *S. aureus* came from the National Academy of Sciences–National Research Council study [56] of the influence of ultraviolet radiation on postoperative wound infection (see Chap. 22). In the study, high-intensity ultraviolet light in the operating room reduced airborne bacterial counts, as measured on settling plates, by 52 or 63 percent, depending on the ultraviolet intensity used. At neither intensity was there a similar reduction in postoperative wound infection rates.

Gram-Negative Bacilli

Volumetric sampling of ordinary hospital air with identification of Enterobacteriaceae and nonfermenters has been rare. Available studies tend to focus on specialized areas of the hospital (especially operating rooms), use settling-plate methods, assess outbreak situations, or provide incomplete microbiologic identification. *Klebsiella* [185], *Pseudomonas* [64], and other gram-negative organisms can be recovered from hospital areas, but the best correlation with patient acquisition is handborne rather than airborne organisms [17].

Clinicians have been particularly concerned about the spread of *Pseudomonas aeruginosa* from or to hospitalized patients with cystic fibrosis. In one study, the organism was recovered on settling plates near the patients with cystic fibrosis [26]. A more definitive result, however, arose from study of 1,740 children hospitalized during 1981 on a university hospital pediatrics ward [126]. During this interval, 28 cystic fibrosis patients with gentamicin-resistant *P. aeruginosa* were hospitalized. Only one acqusition of a gentamicin-resistant *P. aeruginosa* infection occurred among the noncystic patients. Nor has cross-infection been demonstrated in the community [106, 181]. The ultimate source of *P. aeruginosa* must be environmental but not immediately from other patients. Ribotype analysis has suggested a single *Pseudomonas cepacia* transmission between cystic fibrosis patients [122], so the issue must remain under consideration.

Two studies have described an association between airborne gram-negative bacilli and endemic nosocomial infection. The first and more convincing situation resulted from a very unusual circumstance. The newly constructed Hines Veterans Administration Hospital had a novel chute hydropulping waste disposal system that introduced malodorous bacteria-laden air throughout the hospital. Air sampling near the system demonstrated more than 160 cfu of *Pseudomonas* organisms and Enterobacteriaceae (unfortunately, the relative amounts were unspecified) per cubic foot [89]. Concurrent continuous infection surveillance indicated that the nosocomial bacteremia rate approximately doubled coincident with moving to the new hospital and fell to the baseline level after the chute hydropulping system was closed down. In a second study, carried out over a 5-year interval by Kelsen and McGuckin [108], there was a significant positive correlation between the monthly rate of nosocomial respiratory tract infection in patients hospitalized in an intensive care unit (ICU) and the average bacterial content of the ICU air. During periods of heavy air contamination, the authors found an unusually high concentration of airborne gram-negative bacilli ranging up to a *P. aeruginosa* content of 30 cfu per cubic foot and *Klebsiella* content of 9 cfu per cubic foot. As the authors point out, the association may not imply that airborne gram-negative rods directly cause nosocomial respiratory tract disease: It is possible that airborne bacteria seeded nebulizers [109] or another intermediate reservoir. The association may have resulted from a third factor affecting both bacterial content of the air and the nosocomial infection rate. Finally, it is possible that the air may reflect patient illness rather than vice versa.

Ultimately, the best evidence that endemic nosocomial infection does not often result from airborne gram-negative bacilli probably arises from the repeated failure to recover such organisms in air cultures obtained during epidemic investigations. Although these situations may be atypical, as negative evidence they are convincing, since this may be expected to be the situation most likely to produce positive air cultures. The widespread belief that gram-negative bacilli do not survive for prolonged periods when airborne, if true, may provide additional evidence. Here the experimental support is more tenuous than one might wish. Under certain conditions of humidity, temperature, and physiologic state, *Escherichia coli* can sustain up to 100 percent survival for ½ hour in microaerosols [59, 127a]. In general, *E. coli* survives better when aerosols are generated using broth cultures of organisms in relatively inactive states.

In summary, although there is insufficient evidence that airborne gram-negative bacilli constitute a source of endemic nosocomial infection to warrant changes in our current practices, situations that lead to high airborne concentrations of gram-negative bacilli should be avoided. This includes the use of aerosol-generating room humidifiers, which have been shown to cause considerable dissemination of *Pseudomonas* [90] and *Acinetobacter* [178].

Legionella

In at least some outbreaks, *Legionella pneumophila* transmission by the airborne route has occurred. For nosocomial legionellosis, however, emphasis has been on control of contamination in the potable water supply, as discussed in the next section.

Aspergillus

Several lines of evidence strongly suggest that airborne *Aspergillus fumigatus* spores cause aspergillosis in immunosuppressed patients [162]:

1. *Aspergillus* spores are always present in unfiltered air and the organism is highly adapted to airborne spread.
2. Most nosocomial aspergillosis appears first as pneumonia—even if there is an intermediate step of nasopharyngeal colonization, airborne spores would be the ultimate source.
3. Two hospitals have reported a decrease in endemic nosocomial aspergillosis coincident with moving to new facilities with improved air filtration systems.
4. In all reported outbreaks of nosocomial aspergillosis, there has been an implicated airborne source.
5. Nosocomial aspergillosis arising in a patient cared for in a high-efficiency particulate air (HEPA) air-filtered room has not been described in print [16].
6. In one hospital, reductions in airborne *Aspergillus* spores coincided with a lowered rate of nosocomial aspergillosis in bone marrow transplant recipients.

It is likely that many other fungal organisms, such as *Mucor*, *Fusarium*, and *Pseudoallescheria* (formerly known as *Petriellidium*), also are transmitted to patients through the air. Hospitals caring for highly immunosuppressed patients should probably strive to maintain air free from fungal spores. Wet organic materials used in hospital construction,

such as fire proofing, should be treated with a fungicide [162].

Human Immunodeficiency Virus

There has been anxiety about airborne human immunodeficiency virus (HIV) transmission, especially in the operating room and the autopsy suite (see Chap. 39). This anxiety persists even in the absence of any evidence for community airborne HIV transmission (or, to date, operating room percutaneous HIV transmission) because of the potential for blood, tissue, and bone dust aerosol generation by mechanical saws [86] or other activities special to the operating room. Clearly, splatter of blood and tissue occurs in these locations, and scrupulous attention to barriers for the surgeon or prosector are warranted. The available studies do not, unfortunately, adequately distinguish between those droplets and tissue fragments that travel in smooth arcs to the ground and aerosols that remain airborne and threaten persons at a greater distance from the aerosol generation point. The hepatitis B precedent would suggest that only operating room or autopsy personnel in direct contact with blood are at risk. At this time, special devices to protect against airborne HIV transmission are not warranted.

Water
Potable Water

Achievement of potability of water is a major public health activity and beyond the scope of this book. Standard works may be consulted for details of water treatment and examination [10]. Verification of ordinary potability is of importance to infection control personnel only in hospitals with private water supplies in which verification of water quality is a hospital responsibility. It should be noted that federal drinking water regulations call for only one microbiologic assessment [188]: a coliform count (acceptable levels depend on sampling frequency but must average less than 1 per 100 ml). Even for community water, this sole criterion is probably inadequate considering the variety of water sources, potential contaminants, and uses of water

[81]. The European Community standards also include a limit on the total viable count [74]. Except for legionellosis (see later), there is only one report of nosocomial infection arising from drinking water [152]; thus further consideration of water will focus on specialized uses in the hospital.

Potable water supply systems must be protected by vacuum breakers or other devices to keep water from being sucked back into the system during unusual events. To save expense, some building designers plan separate potable and nonpotable water systems. These systems must not be interconnected. Common sense requires that the potable water system be used for all hand-washing, patient bathing, cooking, washing of foods and utensils for cooking and eating, food preparation or processing, and laundry. Given the few valid uses for nonpotable water in the hospital and the difficulty in forever preventing cross-connection, the value of designing hospitals with separate nonpotable water systems is questionable.

Dialysis Water

Detailed standards for hemodialysis water have been prepared by the Association for the Advancement of Medical Instrumentation (AAMI) and accepted by the American National Standards Institution [14]. The standard specifies that water used to prepare dialysate shall have a total microbial count of less than 200 per milliliter and the dialysate itself shall have fewer than 2,000 microbes per milliliter (see Chap. 19). The rationale for the AAMI standard lies in studies carried out in the 1970s indicating that pyrogenic reactions did not occur when dialysate had fewer than 2,000 organisms per milliliter [61, 76]. Bacteria do not cross an intact dialysis membrane, but endotoxin may. The viable bacterial concentration is a rough measure of the endotoxin concentration. The rationale for the stricter (fewer than 200 organisms per milliliter) standard for water used to prepare dialysate is that organism multiplication may occur within the dialyzer. This is a more important problem for recirculating systems than for single-pass systems [117], a distinc-

tion not recognized in the AAMI standard. In recirculating systems, dialyzed materials can provide nutrition to contaminating bacteria.

There are many types of water treatment devices for use in preparing dialysate. A brief discussion is available in Appendix B to the AAMI standard [14]. A more detailed discussion is available in a Food and Drug Administration (FDA) Technical Report [110].

Hydrotherapy Pools and Tanks

A number of features of hydrotherapy tanks produce a concern that they may have been causes of infection: Patients using them may have active infection, which may introduce hazardous bacteria and organic debris, or patients may be incontinent of feces; warm temperature, water agitation, and a high number of successive patients per unit volume of water reduce available chlorine; the internal channels of agitators are difficult to disinfect; and highly contaminated water may be brought into close contact with potential portals of entry such as pressure sores, Foley catheters, or percutaneous devices (see Chap. 40). An outbreak of *P. aeruginosa* wound infections has been reliably linked to these tanks [132]. Since a wide variety of other human pathogens such as coliforms, staphylococci, and fungi have been isolated from immersion tanks [186], there is a broader potential of transmission. Indeed, in a burn center, where the infection potential of hydrotherapy tanks may be most severe, Mayhall and colleagues [129] have reported a bacteremia outbreak due to *Enterobacter cloacae*, which may have been associated with hydrotherapy transmission. To the extent that hydrotransmission tanks are similar to hot tubs and whirlpool spas, there is a more ominous possibility. Contamination of these water sources has resulted in *P. aeruginosa* folliculitis [93], urinary tract infections [168], and even pneumonia [164]. The danger from in-hospital hydrotherapy tanks is probably mitigated by higher standards of disinfection: In the outbreaks of community-acquired *P. aeruginosa* skin infections, even rudimentary standards of water maintenance were not in effect [93].

The Centers for Disease Control (CDC)

published recommendations for disinfection of hydrotherapy pools and tanks in 1974 [43]. For immersion tanks, the CDC recommended maintaining a free chlorine residual of 15 mg/L with a pH of 7.2 to 7.6, draining tanks between each patient use, scrubbing out the tank with a germicidal detergent, and circulating chlorine solution through the agitator of the tank for at least 15 minutes at the end of each treatment day. For hydrotherapy pools, the CDC favored continuous filtration and the maintenance of free chlorine residuals of 0.4 to 0.6 mg/L. In the absence of continuous filtration, the CDC recommended potassium iodide and chloramine.

High-Purity Water

Distillation apparatus, reverse osmosis devices, and ion-exchange resin beds are all subject to contamination. Some hospital personnel erroneously presume this type of water is sterile. Distilled water, even if subsequently sterilized, may contain endotoxin. Febrile reactions caused by exposure to items rinsed in endotoxin containing distilled water have occurred [44].

Water Bacteria

So-called water bacteria are organisms that proliferate in relatively pure water. The most adept species is *P. cepacia*. Carson and colleagues [40] found *P. cepacia* strains that could multiply to the levels of 10^7 per milliliter and remain at these high levels for weeks in distilled water of very high resistivity. *P. aeruginosa* follows closely behind in this ability [75]. Furthermore, *P. aeruginosa* strains adapted to distilled water are relatively resistant to disinfectants [39]. *Acinetobacter calcoaceticus* seems particularly well adapted to highly aerated water sources. An enrichment technique for isolation of *Acinetobacter* from environmental samples using vigorous aeration has been described [18]. This feature of *Acinetobacter* presumably accounts for its increased relative frequency as a cause of humidifier or other respiratory device contamination [57, 83]. Other water bacteria include *Flavobacterium meningosepticum* [158], other *Pseudomonas* species, *Acromobacter* species, *Aeromonas*

hydrophila, Flavimonas [62], and certain nontuberculous mycobacteria [70]. The last are also relatively resistant to various disinfectants [41], including formaldehyde [98]. Among the water bacteria, *P. aeruginosa* and *Acinetobacter* [21] are unusual in that they also are frequent colonizers of healthy humans. Virtually every unprotected wet area in a hospital should be considered contaminated at high levels with one or more water bacteria. These sources include tap water, drains and sinks, water baths, shower heads; flower water, ice machines, and water carafes.

Legionella

Among the important nosocomial pathogens, Legionellaceae are the agents for which environmental sources are the most securely established. Person-to-person transmission of *Legionella pneumophila* is either very rare or nonexistent [196]. Nosocomial *L. pneumophila* pneumonia has been strongly associated with hot-water distribution systems and, perhaps, cooling towers (see Chap. 29). *L. micdadei* appears to have a similar epidemiology [66]. An outbreak of *L. dumoffii* surgical wound infections due to tap water contamination of fresh wounds appears to be a more atypical problem [123].

Muder and co-workers [139] have critically reviewed the mechanisms of transmission of *L. pneumophila*. Most of the initial outbreak reports, particularly those occurring in nonhospital settings, were associated with adjacent excavation or contaminated air-handling system cooling towers. However, more recent hospital outbreaks have securely been linked to contamination of hot-water systems. At the Wadsworth Veterans Administration Hospital in Los Angeles, where a large outbreak of nosocomial legionellosis occurred over a period of several years, improvements in the air-handling system preceded efforts to eliminate *Legionella* from the water system. Only the latter was followed by a reduction in the number of cases [174]. Many additional reports have attributed cessation of nosocomial cases to reductions in hot-water system *L. pneumophila*. Unfortunately, with few exceptions [100], follow-up has been of less than 1 year's duration and case ascertainment insecure.

The mechanism by which hot-water system *L. pneumophila* contamination produces nosocomial pneumonia is not established. Presumably, inhalation of freshly aerosolized droplets predominates, although inhalation of particles airborne from distant sources, aspiration of colonizing pharyngeal organisms, ingestion of drinking water, or contaminated respiratory therapy devices all remain possibilities [139]. An association of cases with the use of contaminated shower heads has been found in some [33, 34], but not the majority, of investigations.

Hot-water distribution system *L. pneumophila* contamination is variably present in hospitals. Vickers [190] found it in 9 of 15 Pennsylvania hospitals. Systems more likely to be contaminated were older and tended to be in a vertical configuration, perhaps because of a greater tendency to have accumulated scale. Systems at greater than 60°C were less likely to be contaminated. Given the exacting nutritional requirements of the Legionellaceae, it might be unexpected for this contamination to be present. A potential explanation is the promotion of *Legionella* growth by other bacteria [140] or their ability to survive within amebae [15]. In one investigation, shower heads contaminated with *L. pneumophila* were more likely to harbor amebae [34]. These associations may ultimately permit indirect *Legionella* decontamination methods.

The need to keep hospital hot-water systems free of Legionellaceae and the role of routine culture confirmation are unresolved. CDC personnel have opposed culturing hospital water not associated with patient cases [53], but nosocomial *Legionella* pneumonia often goes unrecognized unless avidly sought [138], making it difficult for any hospital to be comfortable with its *Legionella* situation. There is at least one demonstration of a hospital with a contaminated potable water system and a fairly secure demonstration of the absence of nosocomial legionellosis [154], but such reports are rare. Yu [195], the foremost student of nosocomial legionellosis, has advocated a 1-year quarterly cycle of hospital

water cultures in hospitals where identification of nosocomial *Legionella* pneumonia cases is insecure. The availability of commercial media for *Legionella* cultivation makes such surveillance relatively simple, although some expertise is required for confirmation of recovered isolates. Detailed protocols for routine culture programs are lacking. Presumably shower head water and water from the base of hot-water storage tanks should be included. Hospitals recovering *L. pneumophila* and, perhaps, *L. micdadei* should strengthen clinical case ascertainment methods.

Hospitals with nosocomial *Legionella* pneumonia cases and contaminated hot-water systems must strive to eliminate the latter. Superheating the water (to as high as 77°C [170°F]) provides an immediate solution but may cause scalding of patients or personnel. Long-term solutions are more difficult. Persistent colonization of hospital potable water systems by *L. pneumophila* arises, at least in part, because the organism can tolerate low levels of chlorine for relatively long periods of time [114]. Hyperchlorination damages some plumbing system components. Raising the pH aggravates scale formation [183]. Other possibilities include instantaneous steam water heaters, ultraviolet light, and ozonation [140].

Eyewash Stations

Clinical laboratories have eyewash stations for emergency eye flushing. These often go unused for months. There have been recent demonstrations that water in these stations becomes contaminated with *Acanthamoeba* and other amebae [23] capable of causing chronic destructive keratitis. Although no such infections have been reported, a weekly flush reduces the contamination.

Walls, Floors, and Other Smooth Surfaces

Maki and his infection control group [125] performed a landmark study assessing the relation between organisms on environmental surfaces and nosocomial infection. During 1979, the University of Wisconsin Hospital moved to a new facility. There was no change in the rate of nosocomial infection at any patient site or due to any pathogen associated with this change. Cultures of floors, walls, and other surfaces (as well as air, water, faucets, and sink drains) showed very similar organism profiles in the old facility and, after 6 to 12 months of occupancy, in the new facility. In contrast, corresponding cultures taken in the new facility before occupancy were relatively devoid of common nosocomial pathogens. The constancy of infection rates provides strong evidence that the association between hospital environmental organism content and nosocomial infection arises because patients infect the environment, not vice versa. It is important to realize some limitations of the Maki study: The two pathogens for which environmental content is of primary importance (*Aspergillus* and *Legionella*) were not assessed; neither were the environmental cultures processed for anaerobes (e.g., *Clostridium difficile*) or viruses.

This study virtually rules out the environment as a significant vector for the assessed organism-object combinations and severely undercuts the rationale for concern about other combinations in the absence of specific data to the contrary. In fact, one is forced to question seriously even such relatively modest recommendations as the use of antimicrobial detergents in hospital cleaning, terminal disinfection of isolation rooms, special cleaning of objects removed from isolation rooms, and the wearing of gowns and gloves when entering the room of patients in isolation when no patient contact is anticipated.

Respiratory Syncytial Virus

One pathogen clearly transmissible in the hospital by fomites is respiratory syncytial virus (RSV) (see Chap. 29). Indirect evidence suggests that RSV transmission occurs by contact: Inoculation of the RSV onto nasal or eye membranes causes infection quite efficiently [96]. RSV survives for several hours on smooth surfaces [95]. Direct evidence of fomite transmission is now available [94]: Volunteers entering a hospital room recently vacated by an RSV-infected patient, after handling objects

in the room and touching their eyes and nose, became infected with RSV more than half as often as volunteers who cuddled RSV-infected babies. Volunteers sitting in the room with an RSV-infected baby did not contract the illness. The relative importance of hand and fomite transmission is unknown, but it is of interest that RSV survives approximately ten times better on smooth surfaces than on skin [95].

Clostridium difficile

Sophisticated strain analysis techniques have unequivocally established that in-hospital transmission of *C. difficile* can occur (see Chap. 30) [193]. Variation in hospital *C. difficile* transmission would provide a satisfactory explanation for the apparent wide variation in rates of *C. difficile* colitis in different hospitals. As is the case for many nosocomial pathogens, increased environmental presence of *C. difficile* is associated with infected patients. In their excellent review, McFarland and Stamm [130] found five supportive studies. Regarding environmental concerns, what distinguishes *C. difficile* is its ability to form spores, with the consequent prolonged survival of the organism in the environment and the plausibility that the spores retain full infectiousness. However, a controlled study of glove use suggested that most *C. difficile* transmissions arise from hand carriage [103]. The same group has used restriction endonuclease strain analysis to establish that *C. difficile* acquisition does not geographically cluster within wards and is not more likely to be transmitted to a subsequent bed occupant [102]. No special environmental cleaning techniques for *C. difficile* contamination have been formally advocated.

Hepatitis B Virus

Concern about environmental hepatitis B virus (HBV) transmission arises from several lines of evidence. Clinical laboratories and hemodialysis units, areas with frequent contamination of the environment by blood, were foci of HBV transmission throughout the 1970s (see Chaps. 18, 19). Many of the ward-acquired, and an even larger fraction of the laboratory-acquired, HBV cases occurred without recognized percutaneous inoculation of blood. A decline in the incidence of health care worker hepatitis began in the mid-1970s (before the introduction of HBV vaccine) when concern about blood contact became widespread [147]. Approximately 30 to 40 percent of community HBV acquisitions cannot be ascribed to sexual contact, needle sharing, or therapeutic blood component exposure [4]. Hepatitis B surface antigen (HBsAg) may be antigenically detected on surfaces in hospital areas likely to have been blood-contaminated [118]. Surfaces not visibly contaminated with blood may also yield HBsAg. Even today, blood contamination can frequently be found on patient care items [78]. HBV in blood remains viable after desiccation at room temperature up to 1 week [30], although it is not hard to inactivate with disinfectant [31]. Very high dilutions of HBV-containing blood can transmit hepatitis B.

These lines of evidence do not establish a role of the environment in HBV transmission. Coincident with efforts to eliminate or decontaminate environmental blood was adoption of segregation of HBsAg-positive patients in dialysis and more widespread recognition of the hazard of needle stick. Nevertheless, when contaminated objects will be in close approximation to a portal of entry, such as the finger platform of an automatic finger stick device, HBV transmission by inanimate objects has been demonstrated [69].

To clean blood spills, the CDC most recently recommended the use of any chemical germicide that is approved by the U.S. Environmental Protection Agency (EPA) as a "hospital disinfectant" and is tuberculocidal [52]. Since no contact time was specified, this recommendation is not quite intermediate or high-level disinfection. With large spills of cultured or concentrated agents in the laboratory, the contaminated area should be flooded with the germicide before cleaning. Otherwise, the area should be cleaned and then decontaminated.

Viral Hemorrhagic Fever
In 1980, the CDC issued recommendations for the management of patients with Lassa fever [51]. Because fatal nosocomial transmission had occurred in several instances and the mechanisms of transmission were incompletely understood, the recommendations were rigorous. They included special isolation units with exhaust air filtration, use of a chemical toilet, disinfection of all items taken from the patient room, and disinfection of the vacated patient room with gaseous formalin or paraldehyde. Other acute viral hemorrhagic fevers were included because of suggestive but limited epidemiologic similarities and because these illnesses also produce high viral titers in blood.

In 1988, after additional experience indicated the risks of nosocomial transmission of these agents were more limited, the CDC issued revised recommendations for management of affected patients [47]. The guidelines were restricted to patients with confirmed or suspected hemorrhagic fever due to the agents of Lassa, Marburg, Ebola, and Crimean-Congo hemorrhagic fever. The revised recommendations still include a chemical toilet; double bagging of linen, bedclothes, and other patient contact items; sponging with disinfectant the outside of containers leaving the patient's room; and special procedures for handling specimens.

Other Environmental Objects
Carpets
Carpeting a floor increases the microbiologic content per unit of floor surface by approximately four orders of magnitude [11]. Contaminating organisms include *S. aureus, E. coli* and, more rarely, *Pseudomonas*. After removal from hospital environments, carpet content of *S. aureus* remains stable for more than a month, and of other organisms for up to 6 months. In the best-controlled study, however, the total bacterial content of air is apparently unaffected by the presence or absence of carpet in the sampled area [172]. For areas with carpets, air content was also not significantly influenced by vacuuming frequency (daily, every other day, or every third day) [172]. The infection hazard of carpets may be more important when there is direct contact

of patients with carpeting (e.g., in pediatric areas) or when patients use wheelchairs. Wet machine cleaning has been associated with *Aspergillus flavus* proliferation. However, there has yet to be a demonstration that any nosocomial infection has arisen from a carpet. In recent years, manufacturers have marketed carpets with antimicrobial substances. As yet, these have not been rigorously assessed in independent studies.

Air-Fluidized Beds

Designed to prevent pressure sores by "flotation," air-fluidized beds have a number of unprecedented design features posing novel questions with respect to infection transmission. Flotation is accomplished by driving air up through a 25-cm-deep layer of silicon-coated, soda lime glass microspheres 50 to 150 μm in diameter. The microspheres are held in the bed by a monofilament polyester filter sheet with openings of approximately 37 μm, through which the microspheres cannot pass. Disinfection of the beds is accomplished by sieving out clumps of beads and organic debris, then operating the bed at high temperature and air flow to inactivate organisms by heat, abrasion [192], and desiccation.

Initial anxieties about the infection hazard from air-fluidized beds have largely dissipated. Beds spiked with *Staphylococcus epidermidis, P. aeruginosa,* and *Bacillus subtilis* did not cause airborne dissemination of these organisms, even shortly after inoculation [189]. Air over beds contaminated by use did not contain more organisms than control air over ordinary beds [29]. Reports of infection transmission have not appeared. There remains the theoretic possibility that the air fluidization process renders airborne organisms that usually remain harmlessly attached to surfaces (e.g., *Mycobacterium tuberculosis*), and a study of the beds in the most heavily contaminated contexts has not been undertaken.

Soap

Given the emphasis on hand-washing, it is surprising that the problem of soap contamination is not better studied. That the problem is largely theoretic is suggested by the paucity

of reported outbreaks attributed to contaminated soap. The outbreak most often cited [136] is relatively unconvincing. Recently, however, clinical illness has been securely attributed to an antiseptic soap [148]. It is reasonable to postulate that it is advantageous to hand-wash with sterile soap (liquid or leaf) dispensed from forearm or leg-operated dispensers that are resistant to contamination.

Data confirming the expected contamination of in-use bar soap have been widely disseminated in the promotion of dispensed liquid soap [99]. However, data comparing the microbial burden on hands washed using a contaminated soap bar with that using uncontaminated nonmedicated soap are unavailable. At the least, it seems prudent to reduce the microbial content of soaps by using disposable liquid soap containers, thoroughly cleaning reusable liquid soap containers or, if bar soap is used, purchasing small bars and providing soap racks that permit water drainage. The relative merits of these alternatives await additional study.

Flowers

Flowers pose two theoretic infection hazards: Vase water inevitably contains large concentrations of potential nosocomial pathogens [105a], and any decaying organic matter may provide a substrate for fungal growth. Although there are no convincing data establishing vase water as a cause of nosocomial infections, many hospitals bar flowers from the rooms of immunosuppressed patients and intensive care units. If vase water were to be disposed of gently and patients, personnel, and visitors washed their hands after touching the water, little danger should arise. Unfortunately, achieving uniform compliance with these precautions is improbable.

Animal Visitation

Sanctioned animal contact with hospital patients is of several types: blind patients or personnel may be accompanied by seeing eye dogs, family members may bring pets to visit sick children, volunteer groups may use animal acts to entertain patients, and research animals may be housed in areas near patient care units. Although Q fever is the only zoonosis shown to have caused epidemics in health care facilities, more than 100 organisms infect both humans and other animals [2]. Knowledge of transmission mechanisms of these organisms suggests several prudent measures.

Seeing eye dogs may be used by personnel, visitors, or patients. Patient use should occur infrequently since patients are usually escorted to places within the hospital. However, some blind patients may desire the companionship of their animal or may be physically capable of walking outside the hospital even though they need hospitalization. Minimum reasonable requests in these situations include assurance that the dog is vaccinated against rabies, is regularly treated for and appears free of ectoparasites, and healthy (in particular, ringworm should not be present). The patient should make arrangements for someone to walk the dog and assume responsibility for disposal of animal excreta. There are effective vaccines for dog leptospirosis, although it seems unlikely that patient contact with dog urine would occur. The remaining dog vaccines are for pathogens that are not transmitted to humans. There are numerous enteric pathogens that may spread from dogs to humans, but attention to proper disposal of dog feces should eliminate this hazard.

Several outbreaks of Q fever have been reported resulting from exposure to pregnant ewes used in research centers [97]. Hospitalized patients have not been affected in these outbreaks. However, airborne transmission to personnel having no direct contact with pregnant ewes has occurred. The hazard appears to be most severe at or near parturition [1]. The magnitude of this phenomenon is unclear because Q fever is not clinically distinctive, and Coxiella burnetii serologic studies are infrequently performed. It seems prudent to bar all contact between patients and pregnant ewes and to ensure that pregnant ewes used for research are never, even during transportation, in areas from which airborne spread to patients can occur. More stringent recommendations for protection of

personnel working with pregnant ewes have been published [22].

Certain animal contacts with children seem inadvisable in any circumstance: Turtles cannot be reliably certified to be free of salmonellosis; wild carnivores (e.g., skunks, raccoons) and bats pose an unacceptably high risk of rabies; and sick birds of virtually any species may transmit Chlamydia psittaci. Any contact with animal urine should be followed by handwashing and, if appropriate, more extensive disinfection procedures because of the possibility of leptospirosis. Contact with mouse or hamster urine is also hazardous to the immunocompromised patient because of the possibility of transmission of lymphocytic choriomeningitis virus.

Linen

Laundry processing and the protection of laundry workers is discussed in Chapter 16. This section will highlight hazards to patients. Considering how heavily contaminated soiled linen is [25], it is remarkable how rarely it causes infection. Laundry workers, who have prolonged close contact with soiled linen, seem at risk only due to blood-contaminated sharps, hepatitis A [49] and other enteric pathogens, or unusually infectious organisms, such as C. burnetii [13]. None of these dangers represent a meaningful hazard to patients. It seems prudent to handle soiled linen gently to reduce the dispersal of microorganisms in patient care areas. Beyond that, there is little basis for special procedures. Given the improbability that soiled laundry reposing in a partially filled hamper causes infection (or even adds organisms to the environment), it is difficult to understand the emphasis that hospital inspection agencies have previously placed on closing soiled-linen hampers. The current Joint Commission on Accreditation of Healthcare Organizations (JCAHO) standard is more rational [104]: The 1992 version requires that soiled linen be "collected in such a manner as to minimize microbial dissemination into the environment" (Standard IC.5.2.2). Unfortunately, state hospital licensing agencies and agencies establishing that hospitals meet the conditions of participation in federal Medicare programs still sometimes cite hospitals for uncovered soiled laundry hampers.

Clean laundry, even after cold-water processing, contains few pathogenic organisms. Sheets have a total aerobic colony-forming unit count of approximately 0.2 cfu/cu cm, and terry cloth items approximately 2 cfu/cu cm. The profile of contaminating organisms (*Bacillus* species, 58 percent; coagulase-negative staphylococci, 25 percent; *Corynebacterium* species, 18 percent) is markedly changed from the prewash profile. Pathogenic species are rare. The proper handling of clean linen during transportation and storage is probably the most important determinant of the microbial content at the time of patient use. Meyer and colleagues [134] studied newborn intensive care laundry that had been washed at 75°C (167°F), dried at 96°C (205°F), and carefully handled. Rodac contact plates showed no organisms one-third of the time and greater than ten colonies per contact plate only 9 percent of the time. Linen near the top of the stack had a higher incidence of positivity and a greater number of colonies per plate than linen in the middle of the stack, suggesting that handling was the source of organisms.

Nosocomial *Bacillus cereus* infection has been attributed to cleaned linen [24, 156]. The reported outbreak consisted of *B. cereus* umbilical colonization without clinical signs of infections in normal neonates and neonates in a special baby care unit. The source was considered to be contaminated cleaned diapers because the implicated *B. cereus* type was found in washed diapers and the laundry machine. Since the implicated *B. cereus* type was also recovered from the hands of nursing staff, this attribution is unconvincing. Other reports of nosocomial infection due to cleaned linen—tinea pedis in a nursing home [73], staphylococcal disease in newborns [84], and urinary tract infection [111]—are likewise unpersuasive.

The last revision of the American Hospital Association's *Infection Control in the Hospital* [8] recommended autoclaving linen for pa-

tients "particularly susceptible to infections," such as burned patients, and for the nursery (p. 67). The American Academy of Pediatrics [6 (pp. 118–119)] supported this recommendation until they softened their stand in 1983 [7 (p. 116)]. No consensus body has such a recommendation extant. One line of argument against autoclaving linen arises after consideration of the panoply of techniques required to maintain sterility until point of use. Applying these procedures to autoclaved linen would be burdensome and costly. Only one rationale for autoclaving laundry seems plausible: Laundry dried in unfiltered air becomes contaminated by *Aspergillus fumigatus*, and in specialized patient care units with very low fungal spore content and low air change rates, a few introduced spores can contribute a substantial portion of the ambient spores [159].

Ultraclean Protective Environments

The ultimate expression of concern that environmental organisms pose an infection hazard is the ultraclean protective environment. When fully developed, these environments include HEPA air filtration with horizontal or vertical laminar airflow; sterile or low-organism-content food; frequent disinfection of walls, floors, and other environmental surfaces; sterile linen and drinking water; toilet water disinfection; use of sterile booties, gowns, caps, and gloves for personnel and visitors entering the room; and elaborate protective garb when patients leave the room. Patients placed in such an environment are generally given oral nonabsorbable, topical, or systemic antimicrobials. This package of protective measures has been termed the *total protective environment, life island, protected environment,* or *barrier isolation.*

It has long been recognized that these special efforts can produce environmental surfaces and ambient air with markedly reduced organism content [180]. More importantly, a meta-analysis [161] of random allocation trials of various forms of ultraclean protective environments suggested that this package of patient care techniques produces a statistically significant reduction in the incidence of infection. Of ten trials [28, 36, 65, 112, 120, 163, 169, 170, 184, 194], five showed a statistically significant reduction in overall, severe, or fatal infections. Of the remaining studies, three showed a trend to fewer infections in the protected patients, and one did not report infection rates. This infection prevention effect generally occurred after the second week, consistent with the view that there is a lag between becoming colonized with a nosocomial pathogen and subsequent infection.

However, the use of ultraprotective environments remains controversial for a number of reasons:

1. *Expense.* In new hospital construction, the capital cost of laminar airflow rooms is not great, especially when amortized over the life of a building. Modular units are commercially available. However, depending on what additional features are incorporated into the protective package, substantial ongoing expenses may be incurred.

2. *Deleterious effects.* During periods of severe illness, seeing only masked, gowned people, being served relatively unpalatable food, remaining confined to a small room, and consuming foul-tasting, diarrheogenic antibiotics aggravates the psychologic stress of having a potentially fatal condition. Premature withdrawal from protected environments may predispose to gut colonization and subsequent disease caused by environmental pathogens.

3. *Difficulty in apportioning benefit* among the various features of protected environments. With few exceptions [170], the available studies deal with the impact of the total package versus conventional patient management. If infections are prevented, it is difficult to factor out which component is responsible. It is even possible that the beneficial effect results from enhanced adherence to standard infection control procedures (e.g., cannula or Foley catheter management) rather than the protected environment per se.

4. *Doubts about study design.* Diagnosis of infection in highly complicated, very immunosuppressed patients is problematic. The physicians providing direct care of the patients, who are in the best position to make the assessment, are also the least blinded with respect to study group. All of these studies are described as using random allocation. However, the vicissitudes of room availability at the time of patient admission and the many factors involved in assignment of patients to rooms make true randomization awkward. Only six of the studies provide detailed information about comparability of the patient groups. The studies from the M.D. Anderson Hospital [28, 163] have a troublesome design feature: The protected patients received more intensive chemothcrapy. The investigators proceeded on the unproved but logical presumption that subsequent courses of induction could be more intensive in patients with no previous infection. The improved survival may have resulted from the more intensive therapy, which may have been administrable to the more often previously infected control patients.

5. *Doubts about the larger significance of a real difference in infection rates.* In many of the studies, the lower infection rate provided only a brief postponement of death; longevity was most strongly influenced by severity of underlying illness. The reduction in infection, if real, may be most meaningful for patients undergoing potentially curative therapies, such as children with acute lymphocytic leukemia or patients undergoing bone marrow transplantation.

Clearly, special efforts are warranted to reduce fungal spore concentration in the rooms of highly immunosuppressed patients [160]. It is important to consider separately several features of air purification systems: filter efficiency, location of filters, air change rate, and laminar airflow. Top-of-the-line bag filters probably remove nearly all fungal spores, but many hospitals prefer HEPA filters because they add relatively little capital expense and meet standards more directly related to microbial filtration. It may be desirable to place duct insulation outside the ducts [79]. Placing filters at the point of entrance of air into the patient's room permits safe maintenance while the room is otherwise unoccupied by patients. Malfunction or maintenance of central systems may cause patient exposure to unfiltered air unless the entire unit can be freed of patients. Increasing the air change rate reduces potential patient exposure to infiltrating spores (e.g., through incompletely sealed windows or brought into the rooms by personnel or on objects) [159]. Laminar airflow is a misnomer in this context, since objects in the room cause considerable turbulence. These units are best thought of as ultrahigh air change rate rooms. Air change rates of 100 to 400 changes per hour can be achieved.

There are problems associated with other efforts to eliminate patient exposure to environmental organisms. Even low-organism-content food is unpalatable. Organisms on surfaces that do not come in contact with the patient probably are harmless. Elimination of environmental organisms can be very difficult. In one ultraprotective unit, there was a prolonged struggle to eliminate an unusual *Pseudomonas* species from toilet bowl water. Notably, although the organism was present for 20 months, no instance of infection or colonization due to the organism was recognized [144].

Except for fungal spore control, ultraprotective environments are not yet an established infection control measure. Even their advocates do not believe they are truly indicated except for patients undergoing bone marrow transplantation or intensive chemotherapy likely to produce more than 25 days of granulocytopenia [153]. What is critically needed is analysis of the relative benefit of the components of the protective package.

Disinfection and Sterilization
Definitions
Sterilization means the complete elimination of all viable microorganisms including all spores. Nonviable is best taken to mean the

irreversible loss of the ability to propagate indefinitely [60]. Ultraviolet light, although lethal, does not interrupt germination and temporary growth and, conversely, seemingly killed, mercury-treated microorganisms can be resurrected by compounds that displace mercury from sulfhydryl groups. Disinfection is divided into three levels [74a]. *High-level disinfection* means the elimination of all viruses and vegetative microorganisms and most but not necessarily all bacterial or fungal spores. *Intermediate disinfection* means the elimination of all vegetative pathogenic bacteria, including *Mycobacterium tuberculosis*, but not necessarily all viruses (nonenveloped and smaller viruses are more resistant to disinfection). Inactivation of *M. tuberculosis* is used in this definition not primarily because of concern about *M. tuberculosis* contamination. Mycobactericidal capacity is used because the organism is relatively resistant to disinfection compared to other vegetative bacteria and a procedure to assess mycobactericidal activity has been established by the Association of Official Analytical Chemists (AOAC) [14a]. Unfortunately, even the AOAC procedure has been questioned recently [55]. Whether the AOAC procedure should be made more stringent or whether the original procedure suffices (since it was used as a surrogate indication of increased disinfectant capacity) is unresolved. *Low-level disinfection,* roughly equivalent to *sanitization,* means the elimination of most pathogenic bacteria. *Cleaning* means the removal of all visible debris. All items should be scrupulously cleaned before disinfection since disinfecting modalities may not penetrate debris. *Antisepsis* is the application of compounds to skins or mucous membranes to reduce microorganism content substantially.

Although the foregoing definitions correspond best to practical use requirements, the federal EPA uses a noncongruent classification of chemical germicides. *Sporicides* meet an AOAC standard for spore distinction [14a]. They achieve sterilization or high-level disinfection depending on contact time. *Hospital disinfectants* inactivate *Salmonella choleraesuis, S. aureus,* and *P. aeruginosa* in highly specified

AOAC tests [14a]. *Disinfectants* and *sanitizers* meet other tests. The EPA registration categories make no reference to effectiveness against *M. tuberculosis,* the critical distinction between intermediate- and low-level disinfectants, or to effectiveness in inactivating all viruses, the critical distinction between high- and intermediate-level disinfection.

Kinetics of Microbial Killing

It is generally presumed, although not always supported by experimental evidence, that most microbial inactivation processes follow a "one-hit" killing curve. This presumption is equivalent to asserting that all the organisms in the population are equally susceptible to the process. These presumptions can be restated mathematically as follows: The number of microorganisms killed is proportional to the number present, and the proportion does not change as the population of remaining organisms decreases. When the logarithm of the concentration of organisms is displayed on the vertical scale and time on the horizontal scale, this relation results in the familiar straight-line killing curve. The steepness of the killing curve is the measure of the rapidity of organism destruction. It is most often expressed as the *decimal reduction time,* the time interval required to bring the concentration of organisms to one-tenth its previous concentration (i.e., 90 percent destruction). The difficulty in validating one-hit kinetics arises because of technical obstacles to ruling out experimentally the possibility that a very small fraction of the starting population of organisms is more resistant to killing. The potential difficulty in killing the last few (possibly more resistant) contaminating organisms is one basis for the overkill prescribed in most sterility standards.

The preceding kinetics analysis establishes the importance of exposure time in accomplishing microbial destruction. A perfectly acceptable disinfection process will fail if not applied for sufficient time. If extremely high numbers of organisms must be inactivated with a very high probability that no survivors remain (e.g., vaccine manufacture), prolonged exposure times may be required. Furthermore, a given process may be sanitizing, disinfecting, or sterilizing, depending on the length of time it is applied.

Microbial Safety Index

The kinetics analysis additionally establishes the inescapable reality that sterility is a probabilistic assertion, not an all-or-nothing phenomenon [107]. This fact has led to the recommendation that the label *sterile* be supplemented by a microbial safety index (MSI) [38], defined as "the absolute value of the logarithm of the probability that the item is contaminated." For example, an item with an MSI of 3 would have a probability of 1 in 1,000 of containing a viable microorganism. As a practical matter, establishment that an item in a lot has an MSI in excess of 3 is extremely difficult by direct microbiologic assessment. With even the most rigorous culture technique, it is difficult to avoid introducing contamination at a level less than 1 per 1,000 cultured items. Furthermore, the mathematics of sterility testing are unfavorable. For instance, to establish with 95 percent confidence that a lot containing 10,000 items is contaminated at a rate of less than 1 per 1,000, almost 3000 of the items must be cultured and found sterile.

Administrative Issues

The Food and Drug Administration requires that reusable medical devices be sold with specific instructions regarding reprocessing methods [74a]. The use of alternate methods may invalidate a warranty or create a medicolegal exposure. The latter problem arises if a product failure damages a patient. The manufacturer may try to shift liability to the hospital because the product was not used according to instructions. Manufacturers may thus escape the stringency of strict liability for product failure.

These same considerations apply to reprocessing disposable items. Through the early 1980s, relevant standard-setting organizations lined up fairly solidly against reprocessing disposable items. The CDC recommended in 1982 that "no disposable object designed for sterile, single use should be resterilized"

[175]. This restriction was rescinded in 1985 [80]. Through 1984, the JCAHO flatly opposed any reprocessing. However, the current JCAHO standards are less restrictive, merely requiring hospitals to have written policies that address reprocessing methods [104 (Standard IC.5.1.3)]. A 1977 FDA policy guide assigned full responsibility to the hospital when disposable medical devices are reused [77]. However, the FDA guide explicitly sanctioned the reuse of disposable items when the facility can establish that the item can be cleaned and sterilized adequately, its "physical characteristics or quality are not adversely affected by their reprocessing" and, somewhat redundantly, the product remains safe and effective for its intended use.

None of these statements address the resterilization of an unused item. Occasionally, an item is removed from its package or the package is damaged, but the item has not been used. Consistency requires similar considerations regarding resterilization of used items.

A key question, begged by all the aforementioned bodies, is: "How does one determine whether an item is disposable?" Currently, the manufacturer makes the determination: An item is disposable if it comes in a package labeled with the words *disposable, single-use only*, or the like. Some manufacturers have added such language to packages of products previously marketed with resterilization instructions. Indeed, manufacturers have little incentive, at least in the short run, to do otherwise. Labeling an item as disposable minimizes liability and maximizes sales volume.

The most compelling case for reuse of disposable items has been made for dialyzers [3, 85, 155]. First use of hollow-fiber dialyzers may be more often associated with mechanical failure and systemic reactions (fever, chest pain, transient fall in white blood cell count) due to chemicals leaching out of the membrane or increased complement activation by new dialysis membranes. Some first-use-type reactions continue to occur, however, with reused dialyzers [54]. Other items may be very expensive and capable of withstanding reprocessing methods. Since resterilization of

an item costs a hospital between $10 and $20, depending on the time required to clean and package it and the sterilization method used, the impetus to reuse exists only for such expensive items. A detailed protocol for reuse of specific items has been successfully employed [71].

The JCAHO requires written hospital policies regarding decontamination and sterilization activities, the performance of sterilizing equipment, and the shelf life of all stored sterile items [104 (Standard IC.5.1)]. The CDC guidelines recommend weekly biologic monitoring of all sterilizers [80]. When an implantable device is sterilized, a biologic indicator should be used and found sterile before the device is implanted. A chemical indicator should be visible on the outside of all sterilized packages. Careful follow-up of unconverted indicators should be undertaken, as investigation often reveals significant problems [5].

Choice of Sterilization or Disinfection Level

Support continues for Spaulding's classification scheme indicating the level of sterilization or disinfection required for various items [74a, 80, 166]. *Critical* items enter tissue or the vascular space. *Semicritical* items contact mucous membranes or nonintact skin. *Noncritical* items contact intact skin. Critical items are generally held to require sterilization, semicritical items to require high-level disinfection, and noncritical items to require intermediate- or low-level disinfection [74a, 80, 166]. Virtually all germicides are effective against HIV [168a].

High-level disinfection is, in fact, rather difficult to achieve. Since the definition includes tuberculocidal capability, it seems reasonable to use conditions that are necessary to achieve the AOAC standard for this activity. But most germicides require 20 to 45 minutes to achieve tuberculobactericidal activity, exposure times well in excess of common usage [166b]. Furthermore, if the device really had to be at a state of high-level disinfection at the time of subsequent patient use, it would have to be subject to sterile water rinsing, manipulation using sterile technique, air drying with filtered air, and protective wrapping. Such precautions are practically never used in hospital practice [166b]. Nor are they called for in many specialty societies published guidelines for the reprocessing of semicritical items [179]. This amounts to an acknowledgment that organisms carried over from the previous patient are the primary target of reprocessing techniques. This is a rational emphasis provided that the disinfected device is protected from "water bacteria" by complete drying and gross recontamination or hand contact prior to subsequent usage.

The assertion that all semicritical items must be processed by high-level disinfection is difficult to justify. This amounts to saying that items contacting mucous membranes can be contaminated with no more than a few bacterial or fungal spores. This seems unwarranted for items that will contact normally contaminated mucous membranes such as the mouth or the colon. The distinction between mouthpieces, for which some authorities have recommended high-level disinfection [165], and silverware is difficult to understand. For items in contact with the gut, elimination of carry-over enteric pathogens is the goal. Unfortunately, assessment of the ability to inactivate small nonenveloped viruses, which are the most resistant enteric pathogens, is not routinely available.

The evolution of the category of intermediate-level disinfection is intriguing. It was not included in the CDC guidelines published through 1983 [174a]. The category was defined in the 1985 CDC revision [80], although there were no specific recommendations for how to achieve it nor distinctions made between items requiring low- versus intermediate-level disinfection. In 1987, Rutala's table combined low- and intermediate-level disinfection [167b]. In the APIC [166] guideline, the categories were separated with specific indications for each. Both were described with *maximum* exposure times, suggesting any contact with the disinfectant sufficed and, further, that intermediate-level disinfection was not well thought out. Unfortunately, although the difficulty in achieving and maintaining high-level disinfection suggests a need for de-

velopment of a less intensive disinfection level, there remains practically no rigorous study or evidentiary basis providing a foundation for the category of intermediate-level disinfection.

Special issues regarding certain devices should be recognized. Nebulizers produce, by design, particles that become deposited in the alveoli. Accordingly, nebulizer cups and solutions intended for nebulization must be sterile. Endoscopic retrograde cholangiopancreatography (ERCP) is potentially much more hazardous than all other forms of endoscopy. This results from the vulnerability of partially obstructed biliary tracts to infection and the severe nature of acute cholangitis. Contamination of the biliary tract can arise if the water channel in an endoscope used for ERCP has contaminated water. When water is expelled from the catheter, then drawn back into the suction channel, organisms introduced into the suction channel can be picked up by the cannula before entrance into the ampulla of Vater. Tonometers pose special problems. Numerous adenovirus outbreaks have resulted from inadequate disinfection procedures [44a, 113]. Adenoviruses, which are small with nonlipid envelopes, are relatively difficult to disinfect. Furthermore, tonometer tips are expensive, harmed by many disinfectants, and used frequently. In addition, pneumotonometer tips have a cavity that can retain germicides with the potential for subsequent damage of a patient's cornea. The American Academy of Ophthalmology recommendations for simple alcohol wiping do not achieve even intermediate-level disinfection [5a]. The CDC, in turn, has recommended disinfection procedures in excess of those ordinarily associated with intermediate-level disinfection [44a]. Automated reprocessing machines have also produced disinfection failures [48a]. Standards for evaluating these machines have been published [158a].

Table 15-1 presents the sterilization and disinfection levels used at the University of Minnesota Hospital and Clinic. Our requirements are less stringent than many have advocated but, we believe, more rigorous than actually practiced in many institutions. The

Table 15-1. Minimum sterilization or disinfection level requirements for various devices at the University of Minnesota Hospital and Clinic

Sterilization

Arthroscope
Cardiac catheter
Culdoscope
Cytoscope
Dermabrasion wheel
Dialysis and pheresis machine surfaces in contact in blood
Endoscopic biopsy forceps, cannulas, papillotomes, guidewires
Endoscope, rigid
Implantable device
Intravascular device
Needle
Peritoneoscope
Surgical and dental instruments
Transducer head
Ureteroscope
Urinary catheter
Urologic laser
Vaginal speculum (for use after rupture of membranes)

High-level disinfection

Bronchoscope
Cryoprobe
Dialysis machine surfaces in contact with dialysate
Endoscope, flexible fiberoptic or video
Endotracheal tube
Laryngeal blades
Maschiadscope
Prostate ultrasound probe
Sinuscope
Tonometer

Intermediate disinfection

Anoscope
Breathing circuit
Dental hand piece
Ear speculum and ear-examining instruments
Electroencephalographic or electrocardiographic electrode
Electric razor head
Laryngeal mirror
Mouthpiece, anesthesia or pulmonary function
Nasal speculum
Thermometer (between patients)
Vaginal speculum (except after rupture of membranes)
Vaginal ultrasound probe
Ventilation bag connector

Low-level disinfection

Bathtub, infant
Bite block, radiation therapy (between uses on a single patient)
Hydrotherapy tank
Infant furniture and toys
Thermometer (between uses on a single patient)

Cleaning

Bathtub, ceramic
Bedpan
Bed rails
Blood pressure cuff
Earphones
Electric razor body
Examination table
Food utensil
Shampoo tray
Sliding board
Ventilation bag

major variation from standard practice is the use of intermediate-level disinfection for many devices that contact normally nonsterile membranes. We have also defined intermediate-level disinfection (see below) more rigorously than other authorities [166]. Many of these distinctions are arbitrary and reflect what can be practically accomplished. Our rigid endoscopes can be steam autoclaved, so we sterilize them. A laryngeal blade passes the epiglottis and is subjected to high-level disinfection, while a laryngeal mirror is only subjected to intermediate-level disinfection.

Steam Sterilization

Steam sterilization is highly reliable and is the sterilization method of choice when the device can tolerate the procedure. Nevertheless, there are subtleties to its use that sometimes go unrecognized. Steam is more than an efficient conveyor of heat. The water molecules participate in the denaturation of proteins and the disruption of other complex molecules. Accordingly, it is essential that steam reach all the surfaces to be sterilized. In gravity displacement autoclaves, the introduced steam, which is less dense than air, forces air down and out through the autoclave drain. Devices with depressions that are not placed on their side or that have curved lumens will not be completely exposed to steam. The AAMI standard for 132°C (270°F) sterilization presumes that this problem can be overcome by extending the cycle to 10 minutes [13a]. Unfortunately, if steam does not reach the surface, this is equivalent to dry heat, a process that is generally held to require 2 hours of exposure. The penetration of steam into wrapped packages, porous materials, or in overpacked chambers is also not secure in gravity displacement autoclaves. These problems are mitigated in vacuum displacement autoclaves, which are evacuated prior to the introduction of steam. Pulsed vacuum autoclaves are even more efficient since they go through several cycles of vacuum and steam replacement, more reliably eliminating air.

Flash autoclaving is also problematic. The term itself is used variably to refer to short-duration, high-temperature steam autoclaving, autoclaving devices without wrapping, gravity displacement autoclaving, or some combination of the foregoing. There is doubtlessly a need for rapid sterilization of low-inventory instruments that inadvertently become contaminated during surgery or highly tailored implantable items for which it is difficult to maintain a complete inventory. Recent evidence suggests that the widely accepted 3-minute standard for 132°C (270°F) autoclaving should be extended to 4 minutes [189a]. Anxieties about the low margin of safety from the 3-minute autoclaving underlie the CDC's recommendation [80] that the 3-minute cycle is not sufficient for implantable objects. The CDC did not specify any minimum duration for implantable objects, although AAMI suggests 10 minutes suffices [13a].

The duration of sterilization cycles at standard (121°C [250°F]) sterilization temperatures for liquids is also somewhat arbitrary. In this situation steam is only conveying heat, so by extension from the standard 30-minute cycle for solid objects, greater times should be required for large volumes of liquids. The fact that most standards recommend less than 30 minutes or, for volumes in excess of 1 liter, only 45 minutes, probably reflects the low organism burden most such materials contain prior to sterilization.

Selection and Use of Germicides
There are many physical modalities and chemical agents that are useful in various contexts for disinfection or sterilization [27].

A tabular summary of methods appropriate for various uses was updated periodically and last published by the CDC in June 1983 [174a, 175]. Unfortunately, the CDC was forced to refrain from tying recommendations so closely to particular products. The substituted CDC environmental guideline [80] discussed disinfectants and sterilants in a more general way. Revisions of the initial CDC tabular summary have appeared [161, 166a]. The most recent is presented in the *Association for Practitioners in Infection Control* (APIC) *Guideline for Selection and Use of Disinfectants,* authored by Rutala [166]. Given the increase in type and composition of medical devices and the great variety of disinfection methods, this tabular approach has become an oversimplification. The object categories are overlapping and not comprehensive. The methods descriptions are largely references to manufacturers' recommendations for germicide concentrations, temperatures, and exposure times. We at the University of Minnesota Hospital and Clinic have found it more useful to specify the level of disinfection or sterilization required for each device (Table 15-1) and specify how those levels may be achieved.

The APIC guideline [166] contains an excellent discussion of the mechanism of action, advantages and disadvantages, and tips on use of various modalities. Besides the level of sterilization or disinfection indicated, selection of a method involves its impact on the integrity of the device to be reprocessed, impact on the warranty and liability exposure, and occupational safety. Ethylene oxide, formaldehyde, and glutaraldehyde all pose potential risk to personnel. A recently proposed federal glutaraldehyde exposure standard, 0.2 parts per million ceiling, will preclude glutaraldehyde use without evacuation hoods, personnel protection devices, or special enclosed reprocessors [146]. Whatever modality is selected, manufacturer's instructions should be used to determine contact times and other use parameters. The modality must be in contact with all relevant surfaces for the entire specified contact time.

It is commonly recommended that a particular product be purchased based on reference to standard guidelines, scientific literature, and manufacturers' recommendations. At a practical level, however, it is very difficult to use the first two. There is such a profusion of products that the standard recommendations [80, 166] do not have enough specificity. Furthermore, manufacturers regularly modify their formulations so that standard recommendations may be out of date and flaws described in scientific publications [55, 167] may be corrected. Thus, users are forced to rely on manufacturers' information. The only intensely regulated statement from manufacturers is that on the label applied to the actual product. The EPA requires that companies generate data underlying a claim that a product is a sporicide, hospital disinfectant (i.e., meets AOAC standards for disinfection of *S. aureus, P. aeruginosa,* and *S. choleraesius*), or a tuberculocide. The label must also specify the dilution, exposure time, and any other conditions required to achieve these activities. Reliance on the label is problematic for several reasons: the EPA does not independently verify manufacturers' claims [80, 92, 188a], independent testing reveals failures to meet standards [167a], some disinfectant types may be inherently deficient [166], translating the EPA categories into the high-, intermediate-, and low-level disinfection system is somewhat arbitrary, and manufacturers do not always put all the relevant information on the label. For instance, some manufacturers make a label claim of "hospital strength disinfectant," a term not sanctioned by the EPA. This is probably a technical violation of the Federal Insecticide, Fungicide, and Rodenticide Act but probably also means the germicide meets criteria for a hospital disinfectant. Likewise, a manufacturer's written statement that a given product passes certain AOAC tests probably can be relied upon even if it is not asserted on the label.

Notwithstanding all the difficulties relying on the EPA-registered product label and other written statements by manufacturers, most users must rely on them in product selection. At the University of Minnesota Hospital and Clinic, we consider that sterilization can be achieved by any germicide that has EPA registration as a sporicide when used at the dilution, temperature, and exposure time required for sporicidal activity. In addition, steam, ethylene oxide, and dry heat are accepted as producing sterilization. When a liquid germicide is used for sterilization, we require that it be rinsed in sterile water, thoroughly dried, and packaged sterilely. We consider that high-level disinfection can be achieved by any germicide registered as a sporicide and a tuberculocide when used at a dilution, temperature, and time required to produce tuberculocidal activity. We allow rinsing in tap water, thorough drying, and handling of endoscopes. In addition, we have accepted sodium hypochlorite at 10,000 parts per million (ppm) for 5 minutes and 1,000 ppm for 20 minutes, and pasteurization at 75° C (170° F) for 30 minutes or 90° C (195° F) for 10 minutes [22a]. We consider that intermediate-level disinfection can be achieved by any germicide with EPA registration as a hospital disinfectant and a tuberculocide when used at the concentration and temperature required to produce tuberculocidal activity with an exposure time of at least 10 minutes. We have also accepted sodium hypochlorite at 1,000 ppm and ethanol or isopropyl alcohol at 70 to 90 percent at an exposure time of 10 minutes. We have no better basis for the 10-minute exposure time than practicality. Finally, we have accepted as establishing low-level disinfectant any germicide registered as a hospital disinfectant when used at the label concentration and temperature required to produce hospital disinfection, sodium hypochlorite at 100 ppm, and ethanol or isopropyl alcohol at 70 to 90 percent. We have not specified any minimum exposure time for low-level disinfection and, thus, accept merely wiping with the disinfectant.

Creutzfeldt-Jakob Agent

The Creutzfeldt-Jakob agent, apparently a transmissible agent composed of protein without nucleic acid [128], is unusually resistant to inactivation. Human transmissions have occurred from stereotactic instruments, pituitary-derived growth hormone, corneal transplants, and dura mater grafts. Sporadic cases in histopathology technicians raise anxiety about transmission to health care workers [135, 177]. Critical and semicritical items previously in contact with brain tissue from Creutzfeldt-Jakob patients should be autoclaved for 1 hour at 132° C (270° F) or immersed for 1 hour in 1 N sodium hydroxide [55a, 166]. Given the frequency with which Creutzfeldt-Jakob disease remains undiagnosed, the potential for transmission by other tissues than brain, and the paucity of adequate disinfection methods, there is currently no practical way to accommodate fully the potential for transmission of this agent.

Routine Microbiologic Surveillance of Inanimate Objects

Environmental sampling accounted for a large fraction of nosocomial infection control efforts in the United States through 1970. As late as 1976, 74 percent of hospitals with 50 beds or more conducted routine environmental culturing [127]. This activity was under way despite explicit statements by the CDC in 1970 [48] and the American Hospital Association in 1973 [9] recommending sharp circumscription of routine environmental culturing. These statements advocated abandonment of routinely culturing floors, walls, linens, and air, but left open the possibility of epidemiologically indicated cultures, spotchecking of critical hospital equipment items (e.g., respiratory care equipment), routine microbial evaluation of hospital-prepared infant formula, and verification of sterilization procedures. Only the last, however, was deemed necessary (see Chap. 9).

Possible grounds for routine culturing of inanimate objects include prevention of infection, education of personnel, and response to statements from a welter of organizational and government agencies. To contribute to the prevention of infection, the culture must at least have an interpretable result. When sterility is the goal, interpretation is possible. Culturing may also be of value, however, when the need for sterility is not established

(e.g., infant formula, dialysis water). Perhaps the best operational definition of interpretability is that certain results lead to specific actions. An additional, less commonly articulated criterion is that the cultured object have a high enough probability of contamination, with a severe enough consequence if contaminated, to justify the culture. Routine culturing of purchased sterile supplies is not justified because of the very low chance of a positive culture.

The educational value of culturing inanimate objects is limited but may be a valid adjunct to other teaching efforts. Care must be taken to prevent such efforts from growing beyond the bounds of a specific educational objective.

Responding to the statements of various organizations quickly becomes an arcane and talmudistic exercise. First, these bodies have considerably varied standings. One *must* comply with the rules of regulatory agencies such as the FDA, the federal and state Occupational Health and Safety Administration (OSHA), or the Federal End Stage Renal Dialysis (ESRD) program. Any hospital with a training program must meet the standards of the JCAHO. However, the degree of compulsion diminishes for the recommendations of the many respected government (e.g., CDC) and nongovernment (e.g., AAMI) agencies.

A second problem in formulating a hospital's response to these various statements is that statements themselves are sometimes frankly inconsistent. For instance, the CDC's *Guideline for Prevention of Intravascular Infection* [46] makes no mention of culturing hospital-compounded infusion solutions. In contrast, the JCAHO seems to require such culturing.

A third problem, ambiguity, is illustrated by the JCAHO statement on monitoring parenteral medication. Through 1991 (but not in 1992), solutions "manufactured" in the hospital "should be examined on a sampling basis" [104a (Standard PH.3.3.4.2)]. We can only presume that the intent was for microbiologic examination.

A fourth problem is lack of regular updating. Although some agencies, such as the

JCAHO and AAMI, have formal updating mechanisms that include specific rescission of previous statements, others have actually disbanded (e.g., the USP-FDA-sponsored National Coordinating Committee on Large-Volume Parenterals [NCCLVP]).

A fifth complexity involves interlocking use of these dicta. The AAMI dialysis water–culturing protocol is explicitly intended to be flexible. However, the federal ESRD program requires exact compliance [63]. The American Society of Hospital Pharmacists has formally accepted the NCCLVP recommendations, giving them a longevity beyond their creator [141]. Despite these complexities, infection control personnel must consider the statements of these bodies in making decisions about culturing inanimate objects. If nothing else, these statements can assume substantial medicolegal importance.

A general problem that arises in considering culturing protocols for any product is determining when in the preparation-use sequence to perform the culture. It is logistically simpler to obtain the culture at the point of preparation, and the impetus to culture patient care items often comes from the quality control effort of the department preparing them. However, more relevant to any patient care implication is the status of the item at the time of patient use. If cultures are positive at the end of the preparation-use sequence, efforts may be undertaken to determine the sources of contamination.

Some unusual biologic items probably should be routinely cultured. Organs, including corneas, bone, kidneys, livers, hearts, pancreases, and bone marrow for transplantation, may become contaminated in procurement, transportation, or storage. Positive cultures can have therapeutic implications in addition to suggesting the need for improved sterile technique. A biologic product that probably does not need routine culture is banked, expressed human milk: It is administered orally and inevitably is frequently contaminated [116]. Consensus on two possible recommendations—routine culturing of hospital water for *Legionella* and of air for fungi—may soon

emerge. Routine culturing of air should be relevant only in hospitals with highly immunosuppressed patients. Specific items are discussed in the following sections.

Dialysis Water

The AAMI standard for culturing dialysis water (presented earlier) has been endorsed by the CDC [80]. Sampling frequency should be at least monthly. It is preferable to sample system water just before a disinfection cycle. Machine water should be taken from different machines to ensure that all defects are identified.

Hospital-Compounded Pharmacy Products

There is currently confusion regarding whether the production, mixing, or aliquoting of sterile materials by hospital pharmacies should be considered compounding or manufacturing. Preparations for individual patients are clearly the former. Batches made in advance for multiple patients may be interpreted as the latter. The implications are considerable. Compounding is governed by state boards of pharmacy and is subject to less stringent requirements. Manufacturing is governed by the FDA and, thus, must comply with Good Manufacturing Practice (GMP) [187 (General Chapter 1077)]. GMP standards, like JCAHO standards, are broadly phrased but are taken to require detailed compliance. With respect to sterility, these requirements include (1) culturing 2 items from batches of fewer than 20 items, 10 percent of lots of 20 to 200 items, and 20 units of larger lots [187 (General Chapter 1211)]; (2) detailed culturing procedures that include 14 days of observation for most items [187 (General Chapter 71)]; and (3) quarantine of the entire batch until the sterility testing is completed [187 (General Chapter 1077)]. These requirements would be burdensome for hospital pharmacies.

Additional considerations apply to infusion solutions. A 1980 NCCLVP statement "endorses the concept of hospital pharmacies using sterility testing of IV admixtures as a method for monitoring the performances of pharmacy equipment and personnel" [141]. The rationale is included to avoid the requirement that sterility testing be completed before administering the solutions. The JCAHO eliminated an apparent requirement for culturing of parenteral medications and solutions in 1992.

These recommendations may be challenged on several grounds. Currently, the bulk of infusion-caused infection arises from organisms ascending along the tissue-cannula interface rather than by fluid contamination (see Chap. 40). Much of the contamination of in-use infusion fluid probably arises during administration rather than compounding. Even the need for sterility of infusion fluid is arguable. Most in-use fluid contamination is at very low concentrations, is due to relatively nonpathogenic strains, and is not associated with patient illness.

The least irrational program of infusion fluid culturing would focus on the in-use product, would use culture methods that do not yield positive cultures with very low levels of contamination, and would involve organism speciation to identify properly the few hazardous species capable of proliferating in the product.

Respiratory Therapy and Anesthesia Equipment

Although the CDC and American Hospital Association view culturing respiratory therapy equipment as potentially rational, there appears to be no organizational statement that actually favors it. Advocates of routine culturing of breathing circuits must surmount two counterarguments: first, that there is not secure demonstration that small numbers of organisms on internal surfaces of breathing circuits cause patient disease and, second, that in-use breathing circuits frequently become contaminated with the patient's organisms even if the circuits start out sterile [58]. Most reports of infection caused by contamination of breathing circuits are not convincing. In others, it is not possible to be sure the contamination was of tubing rather than a nebulizer or that the tubing was thoroughly

dried after reprocessing [42]. The ideal program of routine culturing of these items should cope with the logistic problem of examining the most relevant specimens—those actually in patient use.

Laminar Airflow Hoods

Since HEPA filters do develop leaks, routine periodic evaluation is indicated. However, dioctyl phthalate testing is more reliable than settling plates or other microbiologic assessments [142]. Through 1991 the JCAHO required microbiologic monitoring [104a (Standard PH.2.3.1)], but in 1992 the requirement was abridged to "a suitable area for manipulation of parenteral medications" [104 (Standard PH.2.3)].

Formula

Through 1977, successive editions of *Standards and Recommendations for Hospital Care of Newborn Infants,* published by the American Academy of Pediatrics [6], recommended routine culturing of hospital-manufactured formula obtained from nursing units. Plate counts exceeding 25 organisms per milliliter were deemed to indicate that technique was faulty and immediate corrective action required. The CDC supported this measure in 1982 [175]. A 1983 American Academy of Pediatrics and American College of Obstetricians and Gynecologists publication, *Guidelines for Perinatal Care* [7], has superseded the former series, and it is silent with respect to culturing hospital-manufactured formula. Similarly, recent relevant statements by the American Hospital Association [8] and the JCAHO [104] contain no reference to this issue. Abandonment of this widely accepted practice—even by those skeptical of environmental culturing [131]—probably reflects a perception that most hospitals have switched to commercially prepared formulas. Though this is true of routine infant care, there is an increase in the development of hospital-prepared specialized enteral feedings for which specific guidelines may need to be developed.

Clearly, it is necessary for infant formula

and adult enteral supplements to be free of enteric pathogens and organisms capable of generating enterotoxins (e.g., *S. aureus*). It seems desirable that formula be free of high concentrations of potent nosocomial pathogens. Neonatal *Klebsiella* bacteremia has followed oral ingestion of *Klebsiella*-contaminated breast milk [67]. *Enterobacter sakazakii* diarrhea with bacteria in neonates has resulted from contaminated powdered milk [176]. Freedom from *Aspergillus flavus* is probably desirable for all foodstuffs because of the potential of aflatoxin production. Nonetheless, previous recommendations call for no organism identification, and it is unclear that even large numbers of organisms, excluding those mentioned previously, constitute any hazard.

Establishing protocols for culturing formula leads to many questions:

1. *Which of the many formulas hospitals now make must meet the standard?* The usual age break point for infants is 1 year, but it is likely that a contaminated enteral formula poses a greater hazard to an immunocompromised adult than to a relatively healthy 11-month-old baby.
2. *What culture methods should be used?* Since dry formula powder may contain high concentrations of spores, culture techniques that promote thermophilic organism growth frequently produce excessive counts from nonhazardous formulas.
3. *If counts exceed 25 cfu per milliliter, what actions should be taken?* Hospitals producing many small batches of highly individualized enteral formulas find it very burdensome to use sterile blenders and, when possible, sterile formula components. Blenders are often difficult to sanitize because of the crevices in the blade housing. Many specialized supplements rapidly lose nutritional value at $100°C$ ($212°F$), precluding postpreparation treatment.

The least irrational routine culturing program would focus on formula to be given to the most debilitated neonates or other patients, would use culturing methods yielding only human pathogens—perhaps only enteric pathogens—and would be considered only a marginal supplement to general sanitary measures.

References

1. Abinanit, F.R., Welsh, H.H., Lennette, E.H., and Brunetti, O. Q fever studies: XVI. Some aspects of the experimental infection induced in sheep by the intratracheal route of inoculation. *Am. J. Hyg.* 57:170, 1953.
2. Acha, P.N., and Szyfres, B. *Zoonoses and Communicable Diseases Common to Man and Animals.* Scientific Publication No. 354. Washington, DC: Pan American Health Organization, 1980.
3. Alter, M.J., et al. Reuse of hemodialyzers: Results of nationwide surveillance for adverse effects. *J.A.M.A.* 260:2073, 1988.
4. Alter, M.J., et al. The changing epidemiology of hepatitis B in the United States: Need for alternative vaccination strategies. *J.A.M.A.* 263:9, 1990.
5. Alvarado, C.J., Stolz, S.M., and Maki, D.G. Nosocomial *P. aeruginosa* Infections from Contaminated Endoscopes. In: *ASM International Symposium on Chemical Germicides*, Atlanta, GA, July 27–29, 1990 (abstr. 39). Madison, WI: University of Wisconsin, 1990.
5a. American Academy of Ophthalmology. *Updated Recommendations for Ophthalmic Practice in Relation to the Human Immunodeficiency Virus.* San Francisco: American Academy of Ophthalmology, 1988.
6. American Academy of Pediatrics. *Standards and Recommendations for Hospital Care of Newborn Infants* (6th ed.). Evanston, IL: American Academy of Pediatrics, 1977.
7. American Academy of Pediatrics and American College of Obstetricians and Gynecologists. *Guidelines for Perinatal Care.* Evanston, IL: American Academy of Pediatrics, 1983.
8. American Hospital Association. *Infection Control in the Hospital* (4th ed.). Chicago: American Hospital Association, 1979.
9. American Hospital Association. Statement on microbiological sampling in the hospital. *Hospitals* 48:125, 1974.
10. American Public Health Association. *Standard Methods for the Examination of Water and Wastewater* (17th ed.). Washington, DC: American Public Health Association, 1989.
11. Anderson, R.L. Biological evaluation of carpeting. *Appl. Microbiol.* 18:180, 1969.
12. Anonymous. *Oxford English Dictionary.* Glasgow: Oxford University Press, 1971.

13. Anonymous. Smallpox (edit.). *Br. Med. J.* 1: 288, 1951.

13a. Association for the Advancement of Medical Instrumentation. *Standards and Recommended Practices. Vol. 2: Sterilization.* Arlington, VA: Association for the Advancement of Medical Instrumentation, 1990.

14. Association for the Advancement of Medical Instrumentation. *American National Standard for Hemodialysis Systems.* Arlington, VA: Association for the Advancement of Medical Instrumentation, 1981.

14a. Association of Official Analytical Chemists. (K. Helrich, Ed.). *Official Methods of Analysis of the Association of Official Analytical Chemists* (15th ed.). Arlington, VA: Association of Official Analytical Chemists, 1990.

15. Barbaree, J.M., et al. Isolation of protozoa from water associated with a legionellosis outbreak and demonstration of intracellular multiplication of *Legionella pneumophila. Appl. Environ. Microbiol.* 51:422, 1986.

16. Barnes, R.A., and Rogers, T.R. Control of an outbreak of nosocomial aspergillosis by laminar air-flow isolation. *J. Hosp. Infect.* 14:89, 1989.

17. Bauer, T.M., et al. An epidemiological study assessing the relative importance of airborne and direct contact transmission of microorganisms in a medical intensive care unit. *J. Hosp. Infect.* 15:301, 1990.

18. Baumann, P. Isolation of *Acinetobacter* from soil and water. *J. Bacteriol.* 96:39, 1968.

19. Bean, B., et al. Influenza B: Hospital activity during a community epidemic. *Diagn. Microbiol. Infect. Dis.* 1:177, 1983.

20. Beck-Sague, C.M., and Jarvis, W.R. Epidemic bloodstream infections associated with pressure transducers: A persistent problem. *Infect. Control Hosp. Epidemiol.* 10:54, 1989.

21. Bergogne-Baérézin, E., Joly-Guillou, M.L., and Vieu, J.F. Epidemiology of nosocomial infections due to *Acinetobacter calcoaceticus. J. Hosp. Infect.* 10:105, 1987.

22. Bernard, K.W., Parham, G.L., Winkler, W.G., and Melmick, C.G. Q fever control measures: Recommendations for research facilities using sheep. *Infect. Control* 3:461, 1982.

22a. Best, M., Sattar, S.A., Springthorpe, V.S., and Kennedy, M.E. Efficacies of selected disinfectant against *Mycobacterium tuberculosis. J. Clin. Microbiol.* 28:2234, 1990.

23. Bier, J.W., and Sawyer, T.K. Amoebae isolated from laboratory eyewash stations. *Curr. Microbiol.* 20:349, 1990.

24. Birch, B.R., et al. *Bacillus cereus* cross-infection in a maternity unit. *J. Hosp. Infect.* 2:349, 1981.

25. Blaser, M.J., et al. Killing of fabric-associated bacteria in hospital laundry by low-temperature washing. *J. Infect. Dis.* 149:48, 1984.

26. Blessing-Moore, J., Maybury, B., Lewiston, N., and Yeager, A. Mucosal droplet spread of *Pseudomonas aeruginosa* from cough of patients with cystic fibrosis. *Thorax* 34:429, 1979.

27. Block, S.S. (Ed.). *Disinfection, Sterilization and Preservation* (3rd ed.). Philadelphia: Lea & Febiger, 1983.

28. Bodey, G.P., Rodriguez, V., Cabanillas, F., and Freireich, E.J. Protected environment–prophylactic antibiotic program for malignant lymphoma: Randomized trial during chemotherapy to induce remission. *Am. J. Med.* 66:74, 1979.

29. Bolyard, E.A., Townsend, T.R., and Horan, T. Airborne contamination associated with in-use air-fluidized beds: A descriptive study. *Am. J. Infect. Control* 15:75, 1987.

30. Bond, W.W., et al. Survival of hepatitis B virus after drying and storage for one week. *Lancet* 1:550, 1981.

31. Bond, W.W., Favero, M.S., Petersen, N.J., and Ebert, J.W. Inactivation of hepatitis B virus by intermediate-to-high-level disinfectant chemicals. *J. Clin. Microbiol.* 18:535, 1983.

32. Brachman, P.S. Nosocomial Infection—Airborne or Not? In: *Proceedings of the International Conference on Nosocomial Infections,* Centers for Disease Control, Atlanta, GA, August 3–6, 1970. Chicago: American Hospital Association, 1970. Pp. 189–192.

33. Brady, M.T. Nosocomial Legionnaires' disease in a children's hospital. *J. Pediatr.* 115:46, 1989.

34. Breiman, R.F., et al. Association of shower use with Legionnaires' disease. *J.A.M.A.* 263:2924, 1990.

35. Brisco, J. Intervention studies and the definition of dominant transmission routes. *Am. J. Epidemiol.* 120:449, 1984.

36. Buckner, C.D., et al. Protective environment for marrow transplant recipients: A prospective study. *Ann. Intern. Med.* 89:893, 1978.

37. Cahill, C.K., and Heath, J. Sterile water used for humidification in low-flow oxygen therapy: Is it necessary? *Am. J. Infect. Control* 18:13, 1990.

38. Campbell, R.W. Sterile is a sterile word. *Radiat. Phys. Chem.* 15:121, 1980.

39. Carson, L.A., Favero, M.S., Bond, W.W., and Petersen, N.J. Factors affecting comparative resistance of naturally occurring and subcultured *Pseudomonas aeruginosa* to disinfectants. *App. Microbiol.* 23:863, 1972.

40. Carson, L.A., Favero, M.S., Bond, W.W., and Petersen, N.J. Morphological, biochemical, and growth characteristics of *Pseudomonas*

cepacia from distilled water. *Appl. Microbiol.* 25:476, 1973.

41. Carson, L.A., Petersen, N.J., Favero, M.S., and Aguero, S.M. Growth characteristics of atypical mycobacteria in water and their comparative resistance to disinfectants. *Appl. Environ. Microbiol.* 36:839, 1978.

42. Cefai, C., Richards, J., Gould, F.K., and McPeake, P. An outbreak of *Acinetobacter* respiratory tract infection from incomplete disinfection of ventilatory equipment. *J. Hosp. Infect.* 15:177, 1990.

43. Centers for Disease Control. *Disinfection of Hydrotherapy Pools and Tanks.* Atlanta: Hospital Infections Program, Center for Infectious Diseases, Centers for Disease Control, 1974 (reprinted 1982).

44. Centers for Disease Control. Endotoxic reactions associated with the reuse of cardiac catheters—Massachusetts. *M.M.W.R.* 28:25, 1979.

44a. Centers for Disease Control. Epidemic keratoconjunctivitis in an ophthalmology clinic—California. *M.M.W.R.* 39:598, 1990.

45. Centers for Disease Control. Guidelines for preventing the transmission of tuberculosis in health-care settings, with special focus on HIV-related issues. *M.M.W.R.* 39(RR-17):1, 1990.

46. Centers for Disease Control. Guidelines for prevention of intravascular infections. *Infect. Control* 3:61, 1982.

47. Centers for Disease Control. Management of patients with suspected viral hemorrhagic fever. *M.M.W.R.* 37(No. S-3):1, 1988.

48. Centers for Disease Control. *Microbial Environmental Surveillance in the Hospital.* National Nosocomial Infections Study Report. Atlanta: Centers for Disease Control, June 1970.

48a. Centers for Disease Control. Nosocomial infection and pseudoinfection from contaminated endoscopes and bronchoscopes—Wisconsin and Missouri. *M.M.W.R.* 40:675, 1991.

49. Centers for Disease Control. Outbreak of viral hepatitis in the staff of a pediatric ward—California. *M.M.W.R.* 26:77, 1977.

50. Centers for Disease Control. *Pseudomonas cepacia* colonization—Minnesota. *M.M.W.R.* 30:610, 1981.

51. Centers for Disease Control. Recommendations for initial management of suspected or confirmed cases of Lassa fever. *M.M.W.R.* 28(Suppl):52, 1980.

52. Centers for Disease Control. Recommendations for prevention of HIV transmission in health-care settings. *M.M.W.R.* 36(No. 2S):1S, 1987.

53. Centers for Disease Control. Should hospital water be checked for *Legionella? Hosp. Infect. Control* 10:125, 1983.

54. Centers for Disease Control. Update: Acute allergic reactions associated with reprocessed hemodialyzers—United States, 1989–1990. *M.M.W.R.* 40:147, 1991.

55. Cole, E.C., et al. Effect of methodology, dilution, and exposure time on the tuberculocidal activity of glutaraldehyde-based disinfectants. *Appl. Environ. Microbiol.* 56:1813, 1990.

55a. Committee on Health Care Issues, American Neurological Association. Precautions in handling tissues, fluids, and other contaminated materials from patients with documented or suspected Creutzfeldt-Jakob disease. *Ann. Neurol.* 19:75, 1986.

56. Committee on Trauma, Division of Medical Sciences, National Academy of Sciences—National Research Council. Postoperative wound infections: The influence of ultraviolet irradiation of the operating room and of various other factors. *Ann. Surg.* 160(Suppl):1, 1964.

57. Contant, J., et al. Investigation of an outbreak of *Acinetobacter calcoaceticus* var. *anitratus* infections in an adult intensive care unit. *Am. J. Infect. Control* 18:288, 1990.

58. Craven, D.E., Goularte, T.A., and Make, B.J. Contaminated condensate in mechanical ventilation circuits: A risk factor for nosocomial pneumonia? *Am. Rev. Respir. Dis.* 129:625, 1984.

59. Dark, F.A., and Callow, D.S. The Effect of Growth Conditions on the Survival of Airborne *E. coli.* In: J.F. Hers and K.C. Winkler (Eds.), *Airborne Transmission and Airborne Infection.* New York: Wiley, 1973. Pp. 97–99.

60. Davis, B.D. Growth and Death of Bacteria. In: B.D. Davis, R. Dulbecco, H.N. Eisen, and H.S. Ginsberg (Eds.), *Microbiology* (4th ed.). Philadelphia: Lippincott, 1990. Pp. 57–63.

61. Dawids, S.G., and Vejlsgaard, R. Bacteriological and clinical evaluation of different dialysate delivery systems. *Acta Med. Scand.* 199:151, 1976.

62. Decker, C.F., Simon, G.L., and Keiser, J.F. *Flavimonas oryzihabitans* (*Pseudomonas oryzihabitans;* CDC Group Ve-2) bacteremia in the immunocompromised host. *Arch. Intern. Med.* 151:603, 1991.

63. Department of Health and Human Services. Standards for the reuse of hemodialysis filters and other dialysis supplies. *Fed. Reg.* 52:36926, 1987.

64. Dexter, F. *Pseudomonas aeruginosa* in a regional burn center. *J. Hyg.* 69:179, 1971.

65. Dietrich, M., et al. Protective isolation and antimicrobial decontamination in patients with high susceptibility to infection: A prospective cooperative study of gnotobiotic care in acute leukemia patients. I. Clinical results. *Infection* 5:107, 1977.

66. Doebbeling, B.N., et al. Nosocomial *Legionella micdadei* pneumonia: 10 years experience and a case-control study. *J. Hosp. Infect.* 13:289, 1989.

67. Donowitz, L.G., Marsik, F.J., Fisher, K.A., and Wenzel, R.P. Contaminated breast milk: A source of *Klebsiella* bacteremia in a newborn intensive care unit. *Rev. Infect. Dis.* 3:716, 1981.

68. Douglas, J.M., and Corey, L. Fomites and herpes simplex viruses: A case for nonvenereal transmission? *J.A.M.A.* 250:3093, 1983.

69. Douvin, C., et al. An outbreak of hepatitis B in an endocrinology unit traced to a capillary-blood-sampling device. *N. Engl. J. Med.* 322:57, 1990.

70. DuMoulin, G.C., and Stottmeier, K.D. Waterborne mycobacteria: An increasing threat to health. *A.S.M. News* 52:525, 1986.

71. Dunnigan, A., et al. Success of re-use of cardiac electrode catheters. *Am. J. Cardiol.* 60:807, 1987.

72. Edmonds, R.L. (Ed.). *Aerobiology: The Ecological Systems Approach.* Stroudsburg, PA: Dowden, Hutchinson & Ross, 1979.

73. English, M.P., Wethered, R.R., and Duncan, E.H.L. Studies in the epidemiology of tinea pedis: VIII. Fungal infection in a long-stay hospital. *Br. Med. J.* 3:136, 1967.

74. European Community Council Directive No. 80/778/EEC of 15 July 1980 relating to the quality of water intended for human consumption. *Off. J. European Communities* L229:11, 1980.

74a. Favero, M.S., and Bond, W.W. Chemical Disinfection of Medical and Surgical Materials. In: S.S. Block (Ed.), *Sterilization, and Preservation* (4th ed.). Philadelphia: Lea & Febiger, 1991. Pp. 617–641.

75. Favero, M.S., Carson, L.A., Bond, W.W., and Petersen, N.J. *Pseudomonas aeroginosa:* Growth in distilled water from hospitals. *Science* 173:836, 1971.

76. Favero, M.S., et al. Gram-negative bacteria in hemodialysis systems. *Health Lab. Sci.* 12:321, 1975.

77. Food and Drug Administration. Devices: Reuse of Medical Disposal Devices. In: *Food and Drug Administration Compliance Policy Guide #7124.23.* Washington, DC: Executive Director of Field Operations, Division of Field Operations, 1977. Chap. 24.

78. Forester, G., Joline, C., Wormser, G.P. Blood contamination of tourniquets used in routine phlebotomy. *Am. J. Infect. Control* 18:386, 1990.

79. Fox, B.C., et al. Heavy contamination of operating room air by *Penicillium* species: Identification of the source and attempts at decontamination. *Am. J. Infect. Control* 18:300, 1990.

80. Garner, J.S., and Favero, M.S. CDC guidelines for the prevention and control of nosocomial infections. Guideline for handwashing and hospital environmental control, 1985. *Am. J. Infect. Control* 14:110, 1986. (Also available as HHS Publication No. 99-1117.)

81. Geldreich, E.E. Current status of microbiological water quality criteria. *A.S.M. News* 47:23, 1981.

82. Gellert, G.A., et al. An outbreak of acute gastroenteritis caused by a small round structured virus in a geriatric convalescent facility. *Infect. Control Hosp. Epidemiol.* 11:459, 1990.

83. Gervich, D.H., and Grout, C.S. An outbreak of nosocomial *Acinetobacter* infections from humidifiers. *Am. J. Infect. Control* 13:210, 1985.

84. Gonzaga, A.J., Mortimer, E.A., Jr., Wolinsky, E., and Rammelkamp, C.H., Jr. Transmission of staphylococci by fomites. *J.A.M.A.* 189:711, 1964.

85. Gordon, S.M., Tipple, M., Bland, L.A., and Jarvis, W.R. Pyrogenic reactions associated with the reuse of disposable hollow-fiber hemodialyzers. *J.A.M.A.* 260:2077, 1988.

86. Green, F.H.Y., and Yoshida, K. Characteristics of aerosols generated during autopsy procedures and their potential role as carriers of infectious agents. *Appl. Occup. Environ. Hyg.* 5:853, 1990.

87. Greene, V.W., Vesley, D., Bond, R.G., and Michaelsen, G.S. Microbiological contamination of hospital air: I. Quantitative studies. *Appl. Microbiol.* 10:561, 1962.

88. Greene, V.W., Vesley, D., Bond, R.G., and Michaelsen, G.S. Microbiological studies of hospital air: II. Qualitative studies. *Appl. Microbiol.* 10:567, 1962.

89. Grieble, H.G., Bird, T.J., Nidea, H.M., and Miller, C.A. Chute-hydropulping waste disposal system: A reservoir of enteric bacilli and *pseudomonas* in a modern hospital. *J. Infect. Dis.* 130:602, 1974.

90. Grieble, H.G., et al. Fine-particle humidifiers: Source of *Pseudomonas aeruginosa* infections in a respiratory-disease unit. *N. Engl. J. Med.* 282:531, 1970.

91. Groschell, D.H.M. Air sampling in hospitals. *Ann. N.Y. Acad. Sci.* 353:230, 1980.

92. Groschell, D.H.M. Caveat emptor—do your

disinfectants work? *Infect. Control* 4:144, 1983.

93. Gustafson, T.L., Bank, J.D., Hutcheson, R.H., Jr., and Schaffner, W. *Pseudomonas* folliculitis: An outbreak and review. *Rev. Infect. Dis.* 5:1, 1983.

94. Hall, C.B., and Douglas, R.G., Jr. Modes of transmission of respiratory syncytial virus. *J. Pediatr.* 99:100, 1981.

95. Hall, C.B., Douglas, R.G., Jr., and Geiman, J.M. Possible transmission by fomites of respiratory snycytial virus. *J. Infect. Dis.* 141:98, 1980.

96. Hall, C.B., Douglas, R.G., Jr., Schnabel, K.C., and Geiman, J.M. Infectivity of respiratory syncytial virus by various routes of inoculation. *Infect. Immun.* 33:779, 1981.

97. Hall, C.J., et al. Laboratory outbreak of Q fever acquired from sheep. *Lancet* 1:1004, 1982.

98. Hays, P.S., McGiboney, D.L., Band, J.D., and Feeley, J.C. Resistance of *Mycobacterium chelonei*-like organisms to formaldehyde. *Appl. Environ. Microbiol.* 43:722, 1982.

99. Heinze, J.E. Bar soap and liquid soap (lett.). *J.A.M.A.* 251:3222, 1984.

100. Helms, C.M., et al. Legionnaires' disease associated with a hospital water system: A five-year progress report on continuous hyperchlorination. *J.A.M.A.* 259:2423, 1988.

101. Hoffman, P.C., et al. False positive blood cultures: Association with non-sterile blood collection tubes. *J.A.M.A.* 236:2073, 1976.

102. Johnson, S., et al. Nosocomial *Clostridium difficile* colonisation and disease. *Lancet* 336:97, 1990.

103. Johnson, S., et al. Prospective, controlled study of vinyl glove use to interrupt *Clostridium difficile* nosocomial transmission. *Am. J. Med.* 88:137, 1990.

104. Joint Commission on Accreditation of Healthcare Organizations. *Accreditation Manual for Hospitals, 1992.* Oakbrook Terrace, IL: Joint Commission on Accreditation of Healthcare Organizations, 1991.

104a. Joint Commission on Accreditation of Healthcare Organizations. *Accreditation Manual for Hospitals, 1991.* Oakbrook Terrace, IL: Joint Commission on Accreditation of Healthcare Organizations, 1990.

105. Kallings, L.O. Contamination of Therapeutic Agents. In: *Proceedings of the International Conference of Nosocomial Infections,* Atlanta, GA, August 3–6, 1970. Pp. 241–245.

105a. Kates, S.G., McGinley, K.J., Larson, E.L., and Leyden, J.J. Indigenous multiresistant bacteria from flowers in hospital and nonhospital environments. *Am. J. Infect. Control* 19:156, 1991.

106. Kelly, N.M., et al. Does *Pseudomonas* cross-infection occur between cystic fibrosis patients? *Lancet* 2:688, 1982.

107. Kelsen, J.C. The myth of surgical sterility. *Lancet* 2:1301, 1972.

108. Kelsen, S.G., and McGuckin, M. The role of airborne bacteria in the contamination of fine-particle nebulizers and the development of nosocomial pneumonia. *Ann. N.Y. Acad. Sci.* 353:218, 1980.

109. Kelsen, S.G., McGuckin, M., Kelsen, D.P., and Cherniak, N.S. Airborne contamination of fine-particle nebulizers. *J.A.M.A.* 237:2311, 1977.

110. Kesmaviam, P., Luehmann, D., Shapiro, F.. and Comty, C. *Investigation of the Risks and Hazards Associated with Hemodialysis Systems.* (Technical report, Contract #223-78-5046). Washington, DC: FDA Bureau of Medical Devices, June 1980.

111. Kirby, W.M.M., Corpron, D.O., and Tanner, D.C. Urinary tract infections caused by antibiotic-resistant coliform bacilli. *J.A.M.A.* 162:1, 1956.

112. Klastersky, J., Debusscher, L., Weerts, D., and Daneau, D. Use of oral antibiotics in protected environment units: Clinical effectiveness and role in the emergence of antibiotic-resistant strains. *Pathol. Biol.* (Paris) 22:5, 1974.

113. Koo, D., et al. Epidemic keratoconjunctivitis in a university medical center ophthalmology clinic; need for re-evaluation of the design and disinfection of instruments. *Infect. Control Hosp. Epidemiol.* 10:547, 1989.

114. Kuchta, J.M., et al. Susceptibility of *Legionella pneumophila* to chlorine in tap water. *Appl. Environ. Microbiol.* 46:1134, 1983.

115. Kundsin, R.B. (Ed.). Airborne contagion. *Ann. N.Y. Acad. Sci.* 353:1, 1980.

116. Larson, E., Zuill, R., Zier, V., and Berg, B. Storage of human breast milk. *Infect. Control* 5:127, 1984.

117. Lauer, J.L., et al. The bacteriological quality of hemodialysis solution as related to several environmental factors. *Nephron* 15:87, 1975.

118. Lauer, J.L., Van Drunen, N.A., Washburn, J.W., and Balfour, H.H., Jr. Transmission of hepatitis B virus in clinical laboratory areas. *J. Infect. Dis.* 140:512, 1979.

119. LeRudulier, D., et al. Molecular biology of osmoregulation. *Science* 224:1064, 1984.

120. Levine, A.S., et al. Protected environments and prophylactic antibiotics: A prospective controlled study of their utility in the therapy of acute leukemia. *N. Engl. J. Med.* 288:477, 1973.

121. Lidwell, O.M. Airborne bacteria and surgical infection. *Am. J. Med.* 70:693, 1981.

122. LiPuma, J.J., et al. Person-to-person transmission of *Pseudomonas cepacia* between patients with cystic fibrosis. *Lancet* 336:1094, 1990.

123. Lowry, P.W., et al. A cluster of *Legionella* sternal-wound infections due to postoperative topical exposure to contaminated tap water. *N. Engl. J. Med.* 324:109, 1991.

124. Maki, D.G. Epidemic Nosocomial Bacteremias. In: R.P. Wenzel (Ed.), *CRC Handbook of Hospital Acquired Infections.* Boca Raton, FL: CRC Press, 1981. Pp. 371–512.

125. Maki, D.G., Alvarado, C.J., Hassemer, C.A., and Zilz, M.A. Relation of the inanimate hospital environment to endemic nosocomial infections. *N. Engl. J. Med.* 307:1562, 1982.

126. Maki, D.G., and Zilz, M. Minimal transmissibility of gentamicin-resistant *Pseudomonas aeruginosa* from cystic fibrosis patients. Presented at the Ninth Annual Conference of the Association of Practitioners in Infection Control, New Orleans, May 1982.

127. Mallison, G.F., and Haley, R.W. Microbiological sampling of the inanimate environment in U.S. hospitals, 1976–1977. *Am. J. Med.* 70:941, 1980.

127a. Marthi, B., Fieland, V.P., Walter, M., and Seidler, R.J. Survival of bacteria during aerosolization. *Appl. Environ. Microbiol.* 56:3463, 1990.

128. Marx, J. Prion proposal proved? *Science* 251:1022, 1991.

129. Mayhall, C.G., Lamb, V.A., Gayle, W.E., Jr., and Haynes, B.W., Jr. *Enterobacter cloacae* septicemia in a burn center: Epidemiology and control of an outbreak. *J. Infect. Dis.* 139:166, 1979.

130. McFarland, L.V., and Stamm, W.E. Review of *Clostridium difficile*–associated diseases. *Am. J. Infect. Control* 14:99, 1986.

131. McGowan, J.E., Jr. Environmental factors in nosocomial infection: A selective focus. *Rev. Infect. Dis.* 3:760, 1981.

132. McGuckin, M.B., Thorpe, R.J., and Abrutyn, E. An outbreak of *Pseudomonas aeruginosa* wound infections related to Hubbard tank treatments. *Arch. Phys. Med. Rehabil.* 62:283, 1981.

133. Mead, J.H., Lupton, G.P., Dillavon, C.L., and Odom, R.B. Cutaneous *Rhizopus* infection. Occurrence as a postoperative complication associated with an elasticized adhesive dressing. *J.A.M.A.* 242:272, 1979.

134. Meyer, C.L., et al. Should linen in new born intensive care units be autoclaved? *Pediatrics* 67:362, 1981.

135. Miller, D.C. Creutzfeldt-Jakob disease in histopathology technicians. *N. Engl. J. Med.* 318:853, 1988.

136. Morse, L.J., et al. Septicemia due to *Klebsiella pneumoniae* originating from a hand-cream dispenser. *N. Engl. J. Med.* 277:472, 1967.

137. Mortimer, E.A., Jr., Wolinsky, E., Gonzaga, A.J., and Rammelkamp, C.H., Jr. Role of airborne transmission in staphylococcal infections. *Br. Med. J.* 1:319, 1966.

138. Muder, R.R., et al. Nosocomial Legionnaire's disease uncovered in a prospective study: Implications for underdiagnosis. *J.A.M.A.* 249:3184, 1983.

139. Muder, R.R., Yu, V.L., and Woo, A.H. Mode of transmission of *Legionella pneumophila:* A critical review. *Arch. Intern. Med.* 146:1607, 1986.

140. Muraca, P.W., Yu, V.L., and Stout, J.E. Environmental aspects of Legionnaires' disease. *J. Am. Water Works Assoc.* 80:78, 1988.

141. National Coordinating Committee on Large-Volume Parenterals. Recommended guidelines for quality assurance in hospital centralized intravenous admixture services. *Am. J. Hosp. Pharm.* 37:645, 1980.

142. National Sanitation Foundation. *Standard No. 49 for Class II (Laminar Flow) Biohazard Cabinetry.* Ann Arbor, MI: National Sanitation Foundation, 1976. P. B4.

143. Nerurkar, L.S., West, F., Madden, D.L., and Sever, J.L. Survival of herpes simplex virus in water specimens collected from hot tubs in spa facilities and on plastic surfaces. *J.A.M.A.* 250:3081, 1983.

144. Newman, K.A., et al. Persistent isolation of an unusual *Pseudomonas* species from a phenolic disinfectant system. *Infect. Control* 5:219, 1984.

145. Noble, W.C. Dispersal of Microorganisms from Skin. In *Microbiology of Human Skin* (2nd ed.). London: Lloyd-Luke Ltd., 1981. Pp. 79–85.

146. Occupational Health and Safety Agency. Glutaraldehyde. *Fed. Reg.* 54:2464, 1989.

147. Osterholm, M.T., and Garayalde, S.M. Clinical viral hepatitis B among Minnesota hospital personnel. *J.A.M.A.* 254:3207, 1985.

148. Parrott, P.L., et al. *Pseudomonas aeruginosa* peritonitis associated with contaminated poloxamer-iodine solution. *Lancet* 2:683, 1982.

149. Pearson, R.D., Valenti, W.M., and Steigbigel, R.T. *Clostridium perfringens* wound infection associated with elastic bandages. *J.A.M.A.* 244:1128, 1980.

150. Perry, W.D., et al. Transmission of group-A streptococci: I. The role of contaminated bedding. *Am. J. Hyg.* 66:85, 1957.

151. Perry, W.D., Siegel, A.C., and Rammelkamp, C.H., Jr. Transmission of group-A streptococci: II. The role of contaminated dust. *Am. J. Hyg.* 66:96, 1957.

152. Picard, B., and Goullet, P. Seasonal prevalence of nosocomial *Aeromonas hydrophila* infection related to aeromonas in hospital water. *J. Hosp. Infect.* 10:152, 1987.

153. Pizzo, P.A. The value of protective isolation in preventing nosocomial infections in high risk patients. *Am. J. Med.* 70:631, 1981.

154. Plouffe, J.F., et al. Subtypes of *Legionella pneumophila* serogroup 1 associated with different attack rates. *Lancet* 2:649, 1983.

155. Pollak, V.E. Adverse effects and pyrogenic reactions during hemodialysis. *J.A.M.A.* 260:2106, 1988.

156. Public Health Laboratory Service. *Bacillus cereus* infections in hospitals. *Communicable Dis. Rep.* 44:3, 1990.

157. Rammelkamp, C.H., Jr., et al. Transmission of group-A streptococci: III. The effect of drying on the infectivity of the organism for man. *J. Hyg.* (Lond.) 56:280, 1958.

158. Ratner, H. *Flavobacterium meningosepticum. Infect. Control.* 5:237, 1984.

158a. Reichert, M. Automatic washers/disinfectors for flexible endoscopes. *Infect. Control Hosp. Epidemiol.* 12:497, 1991.

159. Rhame, F.S. Endemic nosocomial filamentous fungal disease: A proposed structure for conceptualizing and studying the environmental hazard. *Infect. Control* 7(Suppl):124, 1986.

160. Rhame, F.S. Nosocomial aspergillosis: How much protection for which patients? *Infect. Control Hosp. Epidemiol.* 10:296, 1989.

161. Rhame, F.S. The Inanimate Environment. In: J.V. Bennett and P.S. Brachman (Eds.), *Hospital Infections* (2nd ed.). Boston: Little, Brown, 1986. Pp. 223–249.

162. Rhame, F.S., Streifel, A.J., Kersey, J.H., Jr., and McGlave, P.B. Extrinsic risk factors for pneumonia in the patient at risk. *Am. J. Med.* 76(5A):42, 1984.

163. Rodriguez, V., et al. Randomized trial of protected environment—prophylactic antibiotics in 145 adults with acute leukemia. *Medicine* 57:253, 1978.

164. Rose, H.D., et al. *Pseudomonas* pneumonia associated with use of a home whirlpool spa. *J.A.M.A.* 250:2027, 1983.

165. Rutala, D.R., Rutala, W.A., Weber, D.J., and Thomman, C.A. Infection risks associated with spirometry. *Infect. Control Hosp. Epidemiol.* 12:89, 1991.

166. Rutala, W.A. APIC guideline for selection and use of disinfectants. *Am. J. Infect. Control* 18:99, 1990.

166a. Rutala, W.A. Disinfection, Sterilization, and Waste Disposal. In: R.P. Wenzel (Ed.), *Prevention and Control of Nosocomial Infections.* Baltimore: Williams & Wilkins, 1987. Pp. 257–282.

166b. Rutala, W.A., Clontz, E.P., Weber, D.J., and Hoffmann, K.K. Disinfection practices for endoscopes and other semicritical items. *Infect. Control Hosp. Epidemiol.* 12:282, 1991.

167. Rutala, W.A., and Cole, E.C. Ineffectiveness of hospital disinfectants against bacteria: A collaborative study. *Infect. Control* 8:501, 1987.

167a. Rutala, W.A., Cole, E.C., Wannamaker, N.S., and Weber, D.J. Inactivation of *Mycobacterium tuberculosis* and *Mycobacterium bovis* by 14 hospital disinfectants. *Am. J. Med.* 91(Suppl 3B):3B–267S, 1991.

167b. Rutala, W.A., and Weber, D.J. Environmental Issues and Nosocomial Infections. In: B.F. Farber (Ed.), *Infection Control in Intensive Care.* New York: Churchill Livingstone, 1987. Pp. 131–171.

168. Salmen, P., Dwyer, D.M., Vorse, H., and Kruse, W. Whirlpool-associated *Pseudomonas aeruginosa* urinary tract infections. *J.A.M.A.* 260:2025, 1983.

168a. Sattar, S.A. and Springthorpe, V.S. Survival and disinfectant inactivation of the human immunodeficiency virus: a critical review. *Rev. Infect. Dis.* 13:430, 1991.

169. Schimpff, S.C., et al. Infection prevention in nonlymphocytic leukemia: Laminar air flow room reverse isolation with oral, nonabsorbable antibiotic prophylaxis. *Ann. Intern. Med.* 82:351, 1975.

170. Schimpff, S.C., et al. Comparison of basic infection prevention techniques with standard room reverse isolation or with reverse isolation plus added air filtration. *Leuk. Res.* 2:231, 1978.

171. Semel, J.D., et al. *Pseudomonas maltophilia* pseudosepticemia. *Am. J. Med.* 64:403, 1978.

172. Shaffer, J.G. Microbiology of hospital carpeting. *Health Lab. Sci.* 3:73, 1966.

173. Shaffer, J.G., and Key, I.D. A three-year study of carpeting in a general hospital. *Health Lab. Sci.* 6:215, 1969.

174. Shands, K.N., et al. Potable water as a source of Legionnaires' disease. *J.A.M.A.* 253:1412, 1985.

174a. Simmons, B.P. CDC guidelines for the prevention and control of nosocomial infections. *Am. J. Infect. Control* 11:97, 1983.

175. Simmons, B.P. Guideline for hospital environmental control. *Infect. Control* 2:131, 1981. (Revision of July 1982, available from CDC, Atlanta, GA 30333.)

176. Simmons, B.P., et al. *Enterobacter sakazakii* infections in neonates associated with intrinsic contamination of a powdered infant formula. *Infect. Control Hosp. Epidemiol.* 10:398, 1989.

177. Sitwell, L., et al. Creutzfeldt-Jakob disease in

histopathology technicians. *N. Engl. J. Med.* 318:854, 1988.

178. Smith, P.W., and Massanari, R.M. Room humidifiers as the source of *Acinetobacter* infections. *J.A.M.A.* 237:795, 1977.

179. Society of Gastroenterology Nurses and Associates. *Recommended Guidelines for Infection Control in Gastrointestinal Endoscopy Settings.* Rochester, NY: Society of Gastroenterology Nurses and Associates, 1990.

180. Solberg, C.O., et al. Laminar airflow protection in bone marrow transplantation. *Appl. Microbiol.* 21:209, 1971.

181. Speert, D.P., Lawton, D., and Damm, S. Communicability of *Pseudomonas aeruginosa* in a cystic fibrosis summer camp. *J. Pediatr.* 101:227, 1982.

182. Stamm, W.E., Weinstein, R.A., and Dixon, R.E. Comparison of endemic and epidemic nosocomial infections. *Am J. Med.* 70:393, 1981.

183. States, S.J., et al. Chlorine, pH, and control of *Legionella* in hospital plumbing systems. *J.A.M.A.* 261:1882, 1989.

184. Storb, R., et al. Graft-versus-host disease and survival in patients with aplastic anemia treated by marrow grafts from HLA-identical siblings: Beneficial effect of a protective environment. *N. Engl. J. Med.* 308:302, 1983.

185. Turner, A.G., and Craddock, J.G. *Klebsiella* in a thoracic ICU. *Hospitals* 47:79, 1973.

186. Turner, A.G., Higgins, M.M., and Craddock, J.G. Disinfection of immersion tanks (Hubbard) in a hospital burn unit. *Arch. Environ. Health* 28:101, 1974.

187. United States Pharmacopeial Convention, Inc. *The United States Pharmacopeia XXII, The National Formulary XVII.* Rockville, MD: USP, 1989.

188 U.S. Environmental Protection Agency. National interim primary drinking water regulations. *Fed. Reg.* 40:59566, 1975.

188a. United States General Accounting Office. *Disinfectants: EPA Lacks Assurance They Work.* Gaithersburg, MD: GAO, 1990.

189. Vesley, D., Hankinson, S.E., and Lauer, J.L. Microbial survival and dissemination associated with an air-fluidized therapy unit. *Am. J. Infect. Control* 14:35, 1986.

189a. Vesley, D., Langholz, A.C., Rohlfing, S.R., and Foltz, W.E. Fluorimetric detection of a *Bacillus stearothermophilus* spore-bound enzyme, alpha-D-glucosidase, for rapid indication of flash sterilization failure. *J. Environ. Microbiol.* (In press.)

190. Vickers, R.M., et al. Determinants of *Legionella pneumophila* contamination of water distribution systems: 15-hospital prospective study. *Infect. Control* 8:357, 1987.

191. Wenzel, R.P., Veazey, J.M., Jr., and Townsend, T.R. Role of the Inanimate Environment in Hospital-Acquired Infections. In: K.R. Cundy and W. Ball (Eds.), *Infection Control in Health Care Facilities: Microbiological Surveillance.* Baltimore: University Park Press, 1977. Pp. 71–98.

192. Winters, W.D. A new perspective of microbial survival and dissemination in a prospectively contaminated air-fluidized bed model. *Am. J. Infect. Control* 18:307, 1990.

193. Wust, J., Sullivan, N.M., Hardegger, U., and Wilkins, T.D. Investigation of an outbreak of antibiotic-associated colitis by various typing methods. *J. Clin. Microbiol.* 16:1096, 1982.

194. Yates, J.W., and Holland, J.F. A controlled study of isolation and endogenous microbial suppression in acute myelocytic leukemia patients. *Cancer* 32:1490, 1973.

195. Yu, V.L. Nosocomial Legionellosis: Current Epidemiological Issues. In: J.S. Remington and M.N. Swartz (Eds.), *Current Clinical Topics in Infectious Disease* (7th ed.). New York: McGraw-Hill, 1986. Pp. 239–253.

196. Yu, V.L., Zuravleff, J.J., Gavlik, L., and Magnussen, M.H. Lack of evidence for person-to-person transmission of Legionnaires' disease. *J. Infect. Dis.* 147:362, 1983.

16

Central Services, Linens, and Laundry

Gina Pugliese
Cynthia A. Hunstiger

Central Services

The *central service department* (CSD), also referred to as the *processing* or *central supply department,* is responsible for preparing, processing, storing, and distributing medical and surgical supplies and equipment, both sterile and nonsterile, required for patient diagnosis, treatment, and care. In carrying out these functions, the CSD staff is responsible for removing or destroying potentially infectious contamination on reusable devices and distributing both reusable and single-use items to the various sites where patient activities occur.

The importance of this role in the prevention of nosocomial infections is clear: reusable medical devices improperly handled, disinfected, or sterilized provide a source of contamination and increase the risk of transmission of infection to both patients and the staff involved in reprocessing procedures [23]. As such, all reusable equipment and devices that have come in contact with a patient's blood or body fluids should be considered potentially infectious and must be decontaminated and reprocessed prior to being used again [18, 19, 23].

Hospitals have found it preferable to handle the cleaning, disinfection, and sterilization procedures for all reusable supplies and equipment in a central, specially designed and equipped location for efficiency of operations and economic reasons and to maintain high quality control standards [34]. There must be specific written policies and procedures for all aspects of reprocessing, storage, and distribution activities, and these must be followed consistently throughout the facility [27, 28]. These policies and procedures should also specify methods for monitoring the disinfection and sterilization activities, assuring continued sterility of both hospital-sterilized and commercially prepared sterile items, recalling items that are potentially contaminated and for which removal from patient use is indicated, and reprocessing disposable items that are reused when clinically necessary [27, 28].

Collection and Transport of Contaminated Devices

Precleaning reusable supplies and equipment in patient care areas, other than for removal of gross soil, is difficult to accomplish in a safe manner with personnel not attired or equipped for this procedure. It is often more efficient and cost-effective to utilize the CSD when available. Therefore, items for reprocessing should be removed from the area of use and placed in a designated holding area for pickup and timely return to the CSD. Soiled instruments and devices from the operating room may be precleaned and decontaminated in designated and specially equipped areas by trained and experienced personnel, to remove gross soil and to render them safe for handling prior to transport to a central processing area, where they will be prepared and packaged prior to sterilization [9, 12].

All soiled reusable supplies and equipment should be collected, contained, and transported to the CSD in a manner that reduces risk of contamination of personnel and the environment. Containers or bags used for holding and transporting soiled items should be clearly marked to indicate that the items are contaminated. Sharp items should be handled with caution and collected and transported in specially labeled, puncture-resistant containers. Transport of bulk soiled supplies should be made on dedicated carts or mechanical conveyances. A dedicated soiled cart lift from the operating room to the CSD is recommended when architecturally feasible [4]

Design of the CSD

The CSD should incorporate adequate space to carry out its responsibilities and process the needed inventories. Soiled and contaminated supplies and procedures must be physically separated from those that are clean or sterile.

This is accomplished by a facility design (walls or partitions) that separates the functional work areas and management of work flow and controls traffic [9, 27, 28]. The ideal design provides four separate functional areas: (1) soiled receiving and decontamination, (2) sterile assembly and processing, (3) clean or sterile supply and equipment storage, and (4) distribution [3]. Additional functional areas may be required for surgical linen pack preparation and staging of surgical case carts or supply exchange carts. Administrative areas, janitors' closets, conveniently located hand-washing facilities, and appropriate staff space (lockers, changing areas) are also necessary [4].

Proper ventilation, humidity, and temperature control is necessary to control the bioburden and environmental contamination, to provide appropriate hydration for packaging materials, and to ensure comfortable working conditions. The ventilation system should be designed so that air flows into relatively soiled areas from clean adjoining spaces, with the appropriate number of air exchanges per hour [3, 9]. Air movement in the soiled areas should be under negative pressure in relation to adjacent areas [3]. Air movement in the sterile processing areas and the clean and/or sterile supply storage areas should be under positive pressure in relation to adjacent areas [3, 9]. All air from soiled processing areas should be exhausted to the outside or to a partial recirculating system [3, 9].

New hospital and facility renovation designs should provide efficient adjacencies between the CSD and the receiving dock, general stores, laundry, operating rooms, emergency rooms, and major patient care areas. Location, type, and number of elevators and other materials-handling conveyances, as well as traffic patterns, should be considered to maintain separation of supply transport from patients, staff, and visitors [3].

Manual transport of supplies by hospital personnel is the most frequently used method of transferring supplies to and from the CSD. Depending on the type, size, and design of the health care facility, automated materials-handling systems (pneumatic tubes, automated box conveyors, or automated guided vehicle systems) may be indicated for efficient material handling. However, automated or semiautomated systems must be properly sized, designed, and managed to be effective.

Decontamination

The decontamination process should take place in an environment designed, maintained, and controlled to ensure the safety and efficacy of the process and to protect staff from exposure to infectious materials or toxic and hazardous substances.

All CSD personnel assigned to the decontaminated area must be properly trained to carry out carefully the decontamination procedures designed to render items safe for subsequent handling and further processing. To reduce the risk of exposure to potentially infectious blood and body fluids during decontamination procedures, personnel should wear protective apparel, such as gowns, gloves, masks, protective eyewear, or face shields. The criteria for selection of the appropriate type of protective apparel should address the probability of splashing, splattering, and soiling of clothing and exposed skin or mucous membranes.

Reprocessing procedures for reusable items include cleaning, decontamination, low-level, intermediate, or high-level disinfection, and sterilization. The specific processes indicated for an item will depend on its intended use.

The process begins with removal of items from their protective packaging or containers and sorting as to the type of reprocessing procedures required. The cleaning recommendations, selection and use of cleaning equipment, chemicals, and exposure times suggested by the device manufacturers should be followed to prevent damage to the items or risk to the staff during the process [18, 23].

Reusable items must first be thoroughly cleaned. Organic materials, such as blood, may contain high concentrations of microorganisms, may inactivate some chemical germicides, and may protect microorganisms from the disinfection or sterilization process [23]. For most noncritical items that either do not ordinarily touch patients or touch only

intact skin, such as blood pressure cuffs, a thorough washing with a detergent or disinfectant-detergent, rinsing, and thorough drying is all that is necessary [23].

The cleaning process may be accomplished manually or mechanically and depends on the characteristics of the device being cleaned. Presoaking or prerinsing of items requiring further reprocessing may be indicated if protein residues have been allowed to dry on the items. All jointed instruments should be opened and equipment that is easily disassembled should be taken apart to facilitate the cleaning and decontamination process. Presoaking is accomplished in cool water or exposure to a protein and blood–dissolving enzyme solution. Care must be taken to avoid splashing or aerosolization of solutions, and personnel should be properly attired [6].

Manual cleaning is indicated for many noncritical reusable items, such as bulky or electric equipment and some delicate or complex devices or instruments. Manual cleaning requires multiple sinks and adequate counter space. Care should be taken during handling and manual cleaning of all sharp items to avoid injury. Mechanical cleaning is an efficient and effective process and should be used for all items that will not be damaged by this process and, whenever possible, for cleaning of sharp items. Equipment used for mechanical cleaning, decontamination, disinfection, or sterilization includes ultrasonic cleaners, washer disinfectors, washer sterilizers, cart washers, and scope disinfectors. The specific equipment used will depend on the type, volume, and material specifications of the devices and the processing outcomes desired [6].

Following the cleaning and decontamination procedures, semicritical and critical items require further disinfection or sterilization processing. Semicritical items, such as endoscopes or endotracheal tubes, that touch mucous membranes and do not penetrate body surfaces, should receive high-level disinfection. Critical items, such as surgical instruments, that enter normally sterile tissue or the vascular system or through which blood flows should be subjected to a sterilization procedure before each use [23]. Specific guidelines for disinfection and sterilization methods are described in Chapter 15 and by Garner and Favero [23].

Assembly and Sterile Processing

Department designs that incorporate pass-through equipment and prevent staff access from decontamination to clean areas of the CSD are preferred. Devices that have been cleaned in the decontamination area are inspected and tested prior to packaging or sterilization to ensure that cleanliness and proper functioning exist. The CSD should be equipped to test routinely prior to reuse the function of clean patient care equipment, such as suction machines. Routine preventive maintenance and equipment repair should be designated to the appropriate department [43].

The packaging of items requiring sterilization should be selected according to the size, shape, and weight of the device and should be appropriate for the sterilization process used [9, 10, 12]. Only materials that provide penetration and removal of the sterilant, maintain a barrier to microorganisms, and allow sterile presentation of package contents should be used. Appropriate materials include 180– to 240–thread count woven textiles, sterilization containers, and nonwoven, disposable materials [4].

Reliable sterilization depends on the contact of the sterilant with all surfaces of the device. Therefore, disassembly and arrangement of instruments in a tray, packaging, sterilizer loading, and air evacuation are important considerations in the sterilization process and should be monitored [5, 9, 10, 12].

Sterilizers should be validated on installation and their performance reassessed by engineering studies on a yearly basis. All sterilizers should be tested with live bacterial spores at least weekly or with each load; if sterilization activities are performed less frequently, such tests should be performed daily [27, 28]. Sterilizers should be monitored with commercial preparations of live bacterial spore monitors specifically intended for each type of sterilizer (i.e., *Bacillus stearothermophilus* for steam sterilizers and *Bacillus subtilis* for

ethylene oxide and dry-heat sterilizers) [23]. Chemical indicators should be used with each package sterilized. When implantable or intravascular materials undergo sterilization, live spore controls should be used with each load, and the results of the spore tests should be obtained before the items are used [27, 28].

The use of flash sterilizers should be limited to those urgent situations in which patient care requirements preclude the use of other sterilization methods [12, 28].

Records must be kept of all sterilizer preventive maintenance and performance verification procedures. If bacterial spores are not killed during routine spore testing, the sterilizer should be checked for proper use and function and the spore test repeated. Items other than implantable objects do not need to be recalled because of a single positive spore test unless the sterilizer or sterilization procedure is defective, as indicated by the other mechanical or chemical sterilization monitors [23]. If the spore test remains positive, use of the sterilizer should be discontinued until it is serviced, and all items from the load should be recalled and reprocessed. Recall is expedited when each package is labeled with a control number that indicates the sterilizer used, the cycle, date of sterilization, and expiration information [12].

Surgical Textile Packs

Textile packs used as gowning and draping material during sterile procedures should be prepared under controlled conditions to minimize the lint in the environment and within the pack [11]. Many hospitals transport clean textiles to the CSD where they are inspected, packaged, and then sterilized. Pack construction must not inhibit steam penetration, and the recommended size and weight of packs should be no larger than $30 \times 30 \times 50$ cm (12 $\times$ 20 in.), and 12 lb. Maximum density must not exceed 7.2 lb/cu ft [9].

Storage of Sterile Supplies

All sterile packs should be handled as little as possible to reduce the opportunity for microbial contamination of the contents. Storage areas for clean and sterile items should be designed and maintained to limit traffic, encourage easy identification of items, facilitate stock rotation, promote cleanliness, and protect the packages. Three conditions can directly compromise the ability of a package to maintain its sterile integrity: moisture, soil, and physical damage by penetration. As such, proper humidity and temperature control are essential to maintain package integrity [3–5].

Storage of clean and sterile supplies is generally on carts or fixed wall shelving. Both open and closed shelving systems are used. The system design should facilitate routine cleaning of the storage units and the environment without compromising the sterile integrity of the packages. Sterile supplies should not be stored in outside shipping cartons; rather, they should be removed from these cartons and stored in washable storage containers. Shelving systems should be designed so that packages are placed at least 8 in. from the floor, 2 in. from outside walls, and 18 in. from ceiling fixtures, such as sprinklers. Sterile items should always be stored away from sources of water, windows, doors, exposed pipes, and vents. Items on the top shelf should also be protected from contaminants that may fall from the ceiling, ceiling fixtures, or ventilation system [4].

Safe Storage Times for Sterile Items
Shelf-life policies for CSD-sterilized items and other devices commercially sterilized should be determined by the health care facility's infection control program. Considerations must be given to the type of packaging materials used, storage conditions, and handling practices of the staff.

Storage of hospital-sterilized packages without contamination (under open and closed clean-storage conditions) has been documented for periods of up to 50 weeks [31]. The packaging materials in this study included nonbarrier woven textiles, barrier nonwovens, and polypropylene peel pouches. Dust covers provided no advantage in extending the shelf life of sterile packs. Thus, shelf life may be considered to depend on events rather than on time.

Some hospitals still prefer to designate specific times when sterile packs are outdated. Policies and procedures should indicate the method to be used for designation of shelf life and methods for stock rotation. Inventory levels should be kept low so that packages are not damaged by overcrowding or do not become obsolete. If an event-related designation is used, procedures should specify those events that would indicate an item should not be used—for example, package wrappings that are torn, punctured, or wet [23].

Reuse of Single-Use Items
The reuse of devices intended by the manufacturer to be for single patient use only (disposable) is a controversial topic. Each facility must address this issue in view of the needs of its patient population, information about risks associated with reprocessing of specific devices, manufacturers' warnings, and liability from equipment malfunction from the reprocessing procedure. Policies and procedures should address the facility's position on reprocessing of disposable items and should detail protocols for reprocessing of such items [2]. Additional information on the reuse of single-use items is described in Chapter 15.

Quality Control
Infection prevention and control education must be provided for all CSD staff. Compliance with the policies and procedures should be verified by ongoing quality audits. Appropriate follow-up and corrective action should be taken when monitoring reveals a failure to follow recommended practices. All quality control and monitoring activities should be documented.

Linens and Laundry

Soiled health care linens, like other used patient care items, can be a potential source of human pathogens and require appropriate handling and processing to reduce the risk of cross-transmission of potentially infectious organisms. Appropriate procedures are also necessary to minimize risk of dermal irritation or related illness from exposure to residual chemicals used in the laundering process [8, 36].

Although soiled linen has been found to contain large numbers of pathogenic microorganisms, reports of transmission of infections to patients are rare. Reports suggesting linen as a source of patient infections have been limited to staphylococcal and *Bacillus cereus* colonization and infections of newborns [15, 25] and antibiotic-resistant organisms causing urinary tract infections in catheterized patients [30]. It is unlikely that the linen was the actual source of the infection in these reports because the organisms causing infections were also found on other patient care items and the hands of health care personnel. Rather, the linen may have become contaminated from contact with the infected patient or contaminated hands of the health care worker. This lack of risk from contaminated inanimate items, such as linen, is consistent with the results of numerous epidemiologic studies that have shown the source of organisms causing nosocomial infections is most frequently animate (human). Additional information on the inanimate environment as a source of nosocomial pathogens is described in Chapter 15.

One additional report in the literature suggesting patient infection from linen involved an outbreak of tinea pedis (ringworm of the feet) in a residential care hospital. However, improperly washed patient care linens, including socks, and communal ownership of socks and towels were more likely to have contributed to this outbreak [22].

Infections in workers handling soiled linen are also rarely reported and are frequently the result of improper handling. Reports of worker infections related to these type of incidents over the past 30 years have included Q fever [33], salmonellosis [21, 37, 40], fungal infections [38], scabies [41], hepatitis A [17], and smallpox [7].

Although other episodes of infections related to linens may have occurred and not been recognized or reported in the scientific literature, the paucity of such reports suggests that risk of actual disease transmission is rare, even among workers who have direct and frequent contact with soiled linens as part of their daily routine.

The low risk of infection may be related to adherence to appropriate handling and processing procedures designed to reduce the risk of transmission of infectious agents to patients and workers handling soiled linen [27–29].

The Centers for Disease Control (CDC) has recognized that the risk of disease transmission associated with soiled linen is negligible and has published guidelines recommending hygienic and common-sense handling, storage, and processing rather than rigid rules and regulations [18, 23]. These guidelines were reemphasized in the CDC's universal precautions guidelines for prevention of transmission of bloodborne pathogens [18, 19]. The most practical application of universal precautions is to handle and process any patient care linen soiled with blood, body fluids, secretions, or excretions in the same manner, regardless of the patient source.

Collection

Soiled patient care linen should be collected and handled with minimum agitation to prevent contamination of the air and persons handling the linen. Special care should be taken with those items visibly soiled with blood or body fluids to prevent contamination of workers handling them. If the linen is heavily soiled, protective barriers (such as gloves) may be necessary. However, in some situations, a relatively clean or lightly soiled item can serve as a barrier by using it to collect a heavily soiled item or portion of an item in such a way—either by folding or rolling—as to keep the visibly or heavily soiled areas contained in the center of the bundle. This technique can also serve to prevent contamination of the worker and soaking through of the laundry bag. All soiled linen should be bagged at the location where it was used. The collection bag should be of sufficient quality to contain the wet or soiled linen and prevent leakage during transport. Both cloth and plastic laundry bags are available. However, the type of bag used should depend on the amount and type of soil present. Cloth laundry bags are adequate for the majority of patient care linens. For linen soaked with blood or body fluids, such as linen from some surgical or trauma cases, some facilities prefer the use of plastic bags. However, the use of cloth bags, which can be washed and reused, will reduce the cost associated with single-use plastic bags and reduce the unnecessary generation of disposable waste.

In the past, linen from isolation patients was handled differently from linen of other patients [24]. This involved double bagging of isolation linen, with the inner bag made of a water-soluble material that could be placed directly into the washer, eliminating presorting of the contents and minimizing handling by laundry workers. This practice was based on the belief that all isolation linen posed a greater risk of disease transmission than linen coming from other areas. Two recent studies comparing double-bagged isolation linen with single-bagged linen from nonisolation patients found no significant difference in the level of bacterial contamination of either the outside of the bags or the linen inside the bag [32, 44]. In fact, it was noted in one of these studies that nonisolation linen was more often grossly soiled with feces, urine, and blood, and that the degree of soiling was more closely related to whether the patient was incontinent or the type of procedures being performed rather than to the patient's isolation status [44]. As such, there is no infection control advantage to double bagging linen unless the primary bag leaks. In addition, the use of water-soluble bags is generally not necessary for a number of reasons [35]. First, it adds to the cost of bagging and processing. Second, water-soluble bags only dissolve in hot water, which cannot be used in the initial flush of the laundry cycle if one is to achieve effective stain removal. Third, if the stains are not properly removed, they can render the item unsuitable for further use. Finally, because laundry in water-soluble bags is not sorted before washing, instruments and other items inadvertently left in the laundry can cause damage to the laundry equipment, the linen itself, and also the laundry workers sorting the linen after washing.

Care should be taken during collection and bagging to ensure that all nonlinen items such as instruments, needles, or plastic underpads are removed. The greatest risk to health care workers for acquiring bloodborne infections such as hepatitis B virus and human immuodeficiency virus infections is from accidental punctures or injuries from sharp items that are contaminated with blood of infected patients [18, 19]. All personnel should be trained in the proper procedures for handling and disposing of needles and other sharp items.

Soiled linen should be contained (bagged) in such a manner that all those involved in collecting, transporting, and processing can easily identify it. All personnel should be trained in the proper procedures for handling soiled linen.

Transportation and Storage

Clean and soiled linen should be functionally separated during storage and transport. Separation may be maintained if the container used to transport soiled linen is properly cleaned before its use to transport clean linen, the clean linen is wrapped properly, or transportation of clean and soiled linen is done in separate containers [29].

The precise length of time that soiled linen can remain bagged and stored prior to washing is not based on a risk of disease transmission but rather on concerns for stain removal and aesthetics. After the soiled linen is properly collected, reasonable schedules should be developed for transport and processing. Laundry carts or hampers used to collect or transport soiled linen need not be covered. The Joint Commission on Accreditation of Healthcare Organizations no longer requires that individual laundry hampers be covered [27, 28].

The linings of hard-surfaced carts should be cleaned frequently. If soiled linen is transported in carts with cloth liners or in cloth bags on rolling hampers, the cloth liners and bags should be washed daily. The individual cloth bags used to bag soiled linen require the same processing as their contents each time the bags are used. If laundry chutes are used, all soiled linen should be bagged and the laundry chute should discharge into the soiled linen collection area [3, 23, 26].

Clean linen should be properly protected during storage and transport to prevent contamination. Although protection is recommended during transport and storage of bulk supplies on clean linen carts, once clean linen is distributed for individual patient use, additional protection is not necessary [27, 28].

Sorting and Handling

All workers involved in sorting and handling soiled linen should wear protective apparel to reduce the risk of contamination of exposed areas of the skin and soiling of clothing. Appropriate protective apparel may include gloves and gowns or aprons. Protective eyewear is generally not necessary because splashing of blood or body fluids is unlikely in the laundry setting. Hands should be washed after gloves are removed, and reusable protective apparel, such as gowns, should be washed after use. Personnel should also be instructed in the principles of personal hygiene, including frequent hand-washing; thus hand-washing facilities must be conveniently located. Because all linen is handled and sorted in a similar manner with appropriate protective apparel, prewashing of linen to reduce microbial contamination prior to handling is unnecessary for prevention of infections.

Plant Facilities

A separate room should be provided for receiving and holding soiled linen until ready for pickup. Processing of linen may be done within the facility, in a separate building on or off site, or in a commercial or shared laundry. The soiled linen processing facility, when located in the hospital, should be separated from the clean linen storage and processing areas, from patient rooms, from food preparation and storage areas, and from areas where clean supplies or equipment is stored [3, 27, 28]. The laundry facility should also be designed, equipped, and ventilated to minimize mixing of air from clean and soiled operations. Functional separation of clean and soiled areas may be achieved by a physical barrier, negative pressure system in the soiled area, or positive airflow from the clean to soiled area [29]. Hand-washing facilities

should be available in each area where clean or soiled linen is handled or processed [3].

Processing and Laundering

There are no standards on acceptable levels of microbial contamination of clean linen. This is in part due to the variability of microbial survival depending on the degree of soiling, laundering techniques, and ability of the microbes to adhere to various fabrics [39]. Significant reduction in microbial counts occur during the laundering process as part of the mechanical action and dilution of washing and rinsing [16, 42]. Detergents, which act as surfactants, loosen and lift the soil from the laundry and enhance the penetration of the textile fiber by water, which assists with the removal of foreign substances, including microbes [36]. Hot water also destroys microorganisms, and a temperature of at least 71°C (160°F) for a minimum of 25 minutes is recommended for hot-water washing [18, 23]. The addition of other chemicals, such as chlorine bleach, reduces bacterial counts further [16].

One of the last steps in the washing process is the addition of a mild acidic agent, referred to as a *sour,* to neutralize the alkalinity from the fabrics, water, and detergent. This shift in pH from approximately 12 to 5 inactivates some microorganisms and reduces the risk of skin irritation [16]. Also, the addition of fabric softeners or bacteriostats in the final rinse leaves a residual on the fabric that inhibits bacterial growth.

Recent studies have shown that a satisfactory reduction of microbial contamination can be achieved at lower water temperatures (less than 70°C) when washing formulations, wash cycles and, in particular, the use of bleach is carefully controlled [14, 16, 20, 39]. Although some recontamination of washed linens may occur during removal from the washing machine, the high temperatures achieved during drying and ironing are also effective mechanisms in reducing any microbial contamination.

The CDC guidelines recommend that soiled linen not be sorted or rinsed in patient care areas [18, 23]. These recommendations were intended for processing of patient care linens that are routinely soiled with blood, body fluids, and substances. In some health care settings, patient linens and clothing are not routinely soiled with blood or body fluids. For example, in ambulatory care settings, such as psychiatric units, patient clothing is often washed in designated locations near patient care areas by the staff or even by the patients themselves as part of their activities of daily living. In these situations, guidelines should be developed to ensure that staff and patients are instructed on appropriate processing procedures.

Sterilization of Linens

It is recommended that surgical gowns and drapes that come in contact with the operative field be rendered sterile [11]. Reusable gowns and linens are sterilized by steam autoclaving after laundering. The need for sterile nursery linens to prevent infections has never been established and is no longer recommended [1]. However, the need for thorough rinsing after washing nursery linens is essential to reduce the risk of skin irritation from residual chemicals.

Disposable Linens

Both disposable and reusable patient care linens are available in the health care setting. Certain disposable items are considered more cost-effective by some hospitals. These include small items that carry a proportionately higher handling charge when recycled, such as caps, masks, shoe covers, washcloths, diapers, underpads, and some wrappers [13]. In choosing between disposable and reusable patient care items, necessary considerations include not only cost but also accessibility, life expectancy of a reusable, availability of laundering facilities, storage space for disposables, delivery capabilities, size and type of hospital, and cost of disposal.

References

1. American Academy of Pediatrics and American College of Obstetricians and Gynecologists. *Guidelines for Perinatal Care.* Elk Grove Village, IL: American Academy of Pediatrics, 1988.

2. American Hospital Association. *Technical Advisory Bulletin on Reuse of Disposable Medical Devices.* Chicago: American Hospital Association, 1986.

3. American Institute of Architects and U.S. Department of Health and Human Services. *Guidelines for Construction and Equipment of Hospital and Medical Facilities.* Washington, DC: The American Institute of Architects Press, 1987.

4. American Society for Healthcare Central Services. *Training Manual for Central Service Technicians.* Chicago: American Hospital Association, 1986.

5. American Society for Healthcare Central Services. *Recommended Practices for Central Service: Sterilization.* Chicago: American Hospital Association, 1988.

6. American Society for Healthcare Central Services. *Recommended Practices for Central Service: Decontamination.* Chicago: American Hospital Association, 1990.

7. Anonymous. Smallpox (edit.). *Br. Med. J.* 1: 288, 1951.

8. Armstrong, R.W., et al. Pentachlorophenol poisoning in a nursery for newborn infants: II. Epidemiologic and toxicologic studies. *J. Pediatr.* 75:317, 1969.

9. Association for the Advancement of Medical Instrumentation. *American National Standards and Recommended Practices for Sterilization.* Arlington, VA: Association for the Advancement of Medical Instrumentation, 1988.

10. Association of Operating Room Nurses. Recommended practices: Selection and use of packaging material. *A.O.R.N. J.* 48:961, 1988.

11. Association of Operating Room Nurses. Recommended practices: Aseptic barrier materials for surgical gowns and drapes. *A.O.R.N. J.* 47:572, 1988.

12. Association of Operating Room Nurses. Recommended practices: Sterilization and disinfection. *A.O.R.N. J.* 45:440, 1987.

13. Badner, B., Zelner, L., Merchant, R., and Laufman, H. Costs of linen vs. disposable OR packs. *Hospitals* 47:76, 1973.

14. Battles, D.R., and Vesley, D. Wash water temperature and sanitation in the hospital laundry. *J. Environ. Health* 43:244, 1981.

15. Birch, B.R., et al. *Bacillus cereus* cross infection in a maternity unit. *J. Hosp. Infect.* 2:349, 1981.

16. Blaser, M.J., et al. Killing of fabric-associated bacteria in hospital laundry by low temperature washing. *J. Infect. Dis.* 149:48, 1984.

17. Centers for Disease Control. Outbreak of viral hepatitis in the staff of a pediatric ward—California. *M.M.W.R.* 28:77, 1977.

18. Centers for Disease Control. Recommendations for prevention of HIV transmission in

health care settings. *M.M.W.R.* 36 (Suppl. 2S): 3S 1987.

19. Centers for Disease Control. Update: Universal precautions for prevention of transmission of HIV, HBV, and other bloodborne pathogens in the health setting. *M.M.W.R.* 37:377, 1988.

20. Christian, R.R., Manchester, J.T., and Mellor, M.T. Bacteriologic quality of fabrics washed at lower-than-standard temperatures in a hospital laundry facility. *Appl. Environ. Microbiol.* 45:591, 1983.

21. Datta, N., Pridie, R.B., and Anderson, E.S. An outbreak of infection with *Salmonella typhimurium* in a general hospital. *J. Hyg.* (Camb.) 58:229, 1960.

22. English, M.P., Wethered, R.R., and Duncan, E.H.L. Studies of the epidemiology of tinea pedis: VIII. Fungal infection in a long-stay hospital. *Br. Med. J.* 3:136, 1967.

23. Garner, J.S., and Favero, M.S. *Guideline for Handwashing and Hospital Environmental Control.* Washington, DC: U.S. Government Printing Office (No. 544-436/24441), 1985.

24. Garner, J.S., and Simmons, B.P. CDC guideline for isolation precautions in hospitals. *Infect. Control* 4 (Suppl.): 245, 1983.

25. Gonzaga, A.J., Mortimer, E.A., Jr., Wolinsky, E., and Rammelkamp, C.H., Jr. Transmission of staphylococci by fomites. *J.A.M.A.* 189:711, 1964.

26. Hughes, H.G. Chutes in hospitals. *J. Can. Hosp. Assoc.* 41:56, 1964.

27. Joint Commission on Accreditation of Healthcare Organizations. *Accreditation Manual for Hospitals.* Chicago: Joint Commission on Accreditation of Healthcare Organizations, 1990.

28. Joint Commission on Accreditation of Healthcare Organizations. *Hospital Accreditation Program Scoring Guidelines.* Chicago: Joint Commission on Accreditation of Healthcare Organizations, 1990.

29. Joint Committee on Healthcare Laundry Guidelines. *1988 Guidelines for Healthcare Linen Service.* Hallandale, FL: Textile Rental Services Association of America, 1988.

30. Kirby, W.M.M., Corpron, D.O., and Tanner, D.C. Urinary tract infections caused by antibiotic-resistant coliform bacilli. *J.A.M.A.* 162:1, 1956.

31. Klapes, N.A., Greene, V.W., Langholz, A.C., and Hunstiger, C.A. Effect of long-term stor-

age on sterile status of devices in surgical packs. *Infect. Control* 8:7, 1987.

32. Maki, D.G., Alvarado, C., and Hassemen, B.S. Double-bagging of items from isolation rooms is unnecessary as infection control measure: A comparative study of surface contamination with single and double-bagging. *Infect. Control* 7:535, 1986.

33. Oliphant, J.W., Gordon, D.A., Meis, A., and Parker, R.R. Q fever in laundry workers, presumably transmitted from contaminated clothing. *Am. J. Hyg.* 49:76, 1949.

34. Perkins, J.J. *Principles and Methods of Sterilization in Health Sciences* (3rd ed.). Springfield, IL: Charles C Thomas, 1983.

35. Pugliese, G. Isolating and double-bagging laundry: Is it really necessary? *Health Facilities Manage.* 2:16, 1989.

36. Riggs, C.L., and Sherrill, J.C. *Textile Laundering Technology.* Hallandale, FL: Textile Rental Services Association of America, 1979.

37. *Salmonella typhi. Can. Epidemiol. Bull.* 16:128, 1972.

38. Shah, P.C., Krajden, S., Kane, J., and Summerbell, R.C. Tinea corporis caused by *Microsporum canis:* Report of a nosocomial outbreak. *Eur. J. Epidemiol.* 4:33, 1988.

39. Smith, J.A., Neil, K.R., Davidson, C.G., and Davidson, R.W. Effect of water temperature on bacterial killing in laundry. *Infect. Control* 8:204, 1987.

40. Steere, A.C., et al. Person-to-person spread of *Salmonella typhimurium* after a hospital common source outbreak. *Lancet* 1:319, 1975.

41. Thomas, M.C., Giedinghagen, D.H., and Hoff, G.L. Brief report: An outbreak of scabies among employees in a hospital-associated commercial laundry. *Infect. Control* 8:427, 1987.

42. Walter, W.G., and Schillinger, J.E. Bacterial survival in laundered fabrics. *Appl. Microbiol.* 29:368, 1975.

43. Webb, S.B. *Central Service Technical Manual* (3rd ed.). Chicago: International Association of Hospital Central Service Management, 1986.

44. Weinstein, S.A., Gantz, N.M., Pelletier, C., and Hilbert, D. Bacterial surface contamination of patients' linen: Isolation precautions versus standard care. *Am. J. Infect. Control* 17:264, 1989.

17

Foodborne Disease Prevention in Health Care Facilities

Margarita E. Villarino
Duc J. Vugia
Nancy H. Bean
William R. Jarvis
James M. Hughes

For a foodborne disease outbreak to occur, food must first become contaminated with pathogenic organisms or toxins. In the case of bacterial foodborne pathogens, food must then be mishandled in a way that permits the organisms to proliferate. Finally, the food must be ingested by susceptible persons. Food service departments at hospitals and other health care facilities, such as nursing homes, must cope with problems associated with handling large amounts of raw food, serving large quantities of food throughout the day, preparing food for many different diets, preparing and handling food before serving, delays in serving, and budgetary constraints. In addition, food service departments in health care facilities serve many patients who are at high risk for contracting foodborne disease. Because of these problems, prevention of foodborne disease should be a high priority in health care facilities.

Foodborne disease outbreaks related to food service in health care facilities may affect patients [10, 28, 52, 59, 63], personnel [17], and visitors [14, 43], and may involve food prepared in the health care facility [59] or food prepared elsewhere but served in the health care facility [15, 54]. Hospitalized patients are generally at increased risk for diseases transmitted by food because of host factors (e.g., malignancy, achlorhydria, advanced age, and acquired immunodeficiency syndrome [AIDS]) or iatrogenic factors (e.g., antibiotics, immunosuppressive agents, antacids, and gastric surgery). Hospitalized persons are more likely than nonhospitalized persons to acquire disease when exposed to foodborne agents and to develop serious sequelae associated with such diseases. Small inocula of enteric pathogens that might be innocuous to most healthy people can cause disease and even death in highly susceptible patients.

Secondary transmission of foodborne pathogens may also occur when patients or health care facility personnel become infected and, in turn, expose other patients or personnel as a consequence of poor personal hygiene or faulty patient care technique (see Chap. 30). Epidemics resulting from person-to-person transmission occur most often in nurseries, pediatric wards, and nursing homes, where fecal-oral spread may be facilitated by difficulties in maintaining good hygiene (see Chaps. 21, 24) [41]. Secondary transmission may extend to other patients in the health care facility, to other health care facility personnel, to visitors, or to others (such as family members) outside the hospital setting. Foodborne disease outbreaks affecting large numbers of hospital personnel have led to staffing problems and may hinder delivery of optimal patient care [14, 17]. With assumptions made about the values of indirect costs, the cost of a hospital-based outbreak has been estimated to be as high as $400,000 [64].

The problems of food or dietetic services in health care facilities generally parallel those of large restaurants and catering firms but are even more complex [25]. Health care facilities' food services typically operate 12 to 18 hours daily, 7 days per week. They purchase and rapidly process quantities of food that require large working surfaces, numerous utensils, and many working hands. They must also adhere to tight schedules and ensure rapid preparation and safe storage of a variety of foods. Besides these common issues, food services in health care facilities have additional, unique problems created by the need for a wide variety of special diets, including enteral feedings. Meals and supplemental feedings must be provided from a central kitchen and sometimes from decentralized kitchens on wards. Finally, food must often be transported from a central preparation area throughout the health care facility. Delays between preparation and service present opportunities for proliferation of foodborne pathogens if food is not held at appropriate temperatures.

Epidemiologic Aspects of Foodborne Diseases

The epidemiology of foodborne disease outbreaks has been reviewed extensively elsewhere [5, 7, 32]. During 1978–1987, 48 foodborne outbreaks were reported from hospitals in Scotland, compared with 50 outbreaks during 1973–1977 [20]. Although the incidence of reported outbreaks decreased, the average number of persons affected in outbreaks increased. A marked reduction was seen in the number of outbreaks caused by *Clostridium perfringens* and staphylococcal food poisoning, in contrast with foodborne salmonellosis, which remained a problem. In hospitals in Scotland, the decline in the incidence of food poisoning reflects an increased appreciation by dietary departments of the principles of food temperature control. Salmonellosis outbreaks, however, did not decline, and the average number of persons affected per outbreak increased from 36 in 1973 to 81 in 1987. In England and Wales during 1978–1987, 248 outbreaks of salmonellosis were reported in hospitals, compared with 522 outbreaks of salmonellosis reported during 1968–1977 [36]. This reduction might be a result of improved food-handling practices; environmental health officers from the British department of health have increased the monitoring of hospital food service departments since 1977.

In the United States, from all foodborne outbreaks reported to the Centers for Disease Control (CDC) during 1975–1987, the bacterial agents most frequently identified were *Salmonella* species, *Staphylococcus aureus*, *Clostridium botulinum*, and *C. perfringens* (Table 17-1). Pathogens such as *Salmonella* species and *C. perfringens* are more important in the health care facility setting than *C. botulinum* and *S. aureus*. Transmission of all four of the common foodborne bacterial pathogens was typically associated with certain food vehicles; the sources of contamination varied for the different pathogens (see Table 17-1). Of reported outbreaks during 1975–1987 for which the location was known, hospitals and nursing homes accounted for 3.1 percent of

Table 17-1. Foods commonly involved and reported cause of contamination in foodborne outbreaks of bacterial etiology, United States, 1975–1987

Cause	Numbers of outbreaks	Typical foods	Usual reported cause of contamination			
			Improper holding	Inadequate cooling	Poor hygiene	Contaminated equipment
Salmonella species	721	Beef, poultry, pork, eggs, ice cream	+ +	+	+	+
Staphylococcus aureus	305	Ham, poultry, pastries, beef	+	–	+ +	–
Clostridium botulinum	200	Vegetables, fish	+	+ +	–	–
Clostridium perfringens	166	Beef, poultry, Mexican food	+ +	+	–	–
Shigella species	93	Salad	+	–	+ +	–
Bacillus cereus	56	Fried rice	+ +	+	+	–
Campylobacter jejuni	53	Raw milk	+	+	–	–
Vibrio parahaemolyticus	22	Shellfish	+	+ +	–	–

– indicates less frequent cause; +, frequent cause; + +, most frequent cause.
Source: Centers for Disease Control, Foodborne Disease Surveillance.

347

the outbreaks, 5.1 percent of the cases, and 24.1 percent of the deaths (Table 17-2). Only 89 foodborne disease outbreaks in hospitals were reported during this 12-year period; however, because a foodborne disease outbreak must be recognized, investigated, and reported to the state health department before it can be reported to the CDC, the number of foodborne outbreaks is almost certainly greater than reported. During 1975–1987, reported outbreaks in hospitals and nursing homes were significantly more likely to be caused by bacterial agents than by viruses, parasites, or chemicals (Table 17-3). Nonetheless, a foodborne outbreak of hepatitis A has been reported from a hospital [43], and a parasitic disease outbreak caused by *Giardia lamblia* has been reported from a nursing home [38].

Although foodborne disease outbreaks account for a small proportion of preventable infections acquired in hospitals, investigating them is important in defining sources, modes of spread, and methods for prevention and control of nosocomial disease. Of 233 hospital-based outbreaks investigated by the CDC from 1956 to 1979, the most common type were outbreaks of gastroenteritis, almost all of which were caused by *Salmonella* species and enteropathogenic *Escherichia coli* [55]. Contaminated food vehicles were frequently identified in outbreaks of salmonellosis in adult patients. Outbreaks attributed to cross-infection (e.g., gastroenteritis outbreaks in the nursery caused by *E. coli* or Salmonella) were more difficult to recognize and control than were outbreaks attributed to contaminated food vehicles. Most cross-infection outbreaks were recognized because the infecting microorganism was either unusual or distinctively marked, often by unique antimicrobial resistance. In England and Wales, 71 (30 percent) of 235 reported outbreaks of salmonellosis occurring in hospitals during a 10-year period were attributed to cross-infection, which was slightly more than the 57 (24 percent) outbreaks attributed to foodborne transmission [36]. However, foodborne outbreaks affected more persons (1,862) than did cross-infection outbreaks (558) [36].

In the United States during 1975–1987, there were 257 reported deaths associated with foodborne disease outbreaks of known place of preparation (Table 17-4). Fifty-one (20 percent) occurred in nursing home outbreaks, and 11 (4 percent) deaths occurred in hospital outbreaks. *Salmonella* species accounted for more than half the nursing home and hospital deaths.

Isolation rates of *Salmonella enteritidis* in the United States have been increasing since 1976 [18]. During 1985–1989, 244 *S. enteritidis* outbreaks were reported to the CDC, accounting for 8,607 cases of illness, 1,094 hospitalizations, and 44 deaths. Of these 244 outbreaks, 45 (18 percent) occurred in nursing homes or hospitals, accounting for 15 percent of cases of illness and more than 90 percent of deaths [58]. In 13 outbreaks in which a food vehicle was identified, 10 implicated shell eggs. Four (8 percent) of the 49 *S. enteritidis* outbreaks reported from January 1 to October 31, 1990, occurred in hospitals or nursing homes, compared with 20 (26 percent) of 77 *S. enteritidis* outbreaks in 1989 [18]. The decrease in hospital- and nursing home-associated *S. enteritidis* outbreaks may reflect efforts to improve food safety in these settings (e.g., using pasteurized eggs).

Reported data can help elucidate the relative importance of various factors that contribute to the occurrence of foodborne disease outbreaks. During 1975–1987, food-handling errors of 162 foodborne outbreaks in hospitals or nursing homes were reported (Table 17-5). Holding food at improper temperatures was the most common food-handling error that caused foodborne disease. Other important errors included inadequate cooking, poor personal hygiene of food handlers, using food from unsafe sources, and using contaminated equipment. Training personnel in proper food-handling practices can eliminate these errors and prevent outbreaks.

Food served from a health care facility kitchen can be contaminated before, during, or after preparation. Raw poultry and red meat might be contaminated with organisms (e.g., *Salmonella* species, *C. perfringens, Campy-*

Table 17-2. Reported foodborne outbreaks, cases, and deaths in hospitals, nursing homes, and other known locations, United States, 1975–1987

	Hospitals		Nursing homes		Other known locations	
	Total	Confirmed etiology	Total	Confirmed etiology	Total	Confirmed etiology
No. of outbreaks	89	52	115	52	6,295	2,279
No. of cases	5,477	3,244	4,944	2,270	193,636	100,237
No. of deaths	11	7	51	47	195	179
Deaths/1,000 cases	2.2	2.3	11.4	22.5	1.1	2.1

Source: Centers for Disease Control, Foodborne Disease Surveillance.

Table 17-3. Causes of reported foodborne outbreaks of confirmed etiology related to hospitals, nursing homes, and other known locations, United States, 1975–1987

	Hospitals		Nursing homes		Other known locations	
Cause	Number of outbreaks	% of total	Number of outbreaks	% of total	Number of outbreaks	% of total
Bacterial						
Salmonella species	24	46	27	52	653	29
Staphylococcus aureus	4	8	12	23	285	12
Clostridium perfringens	6	11	6	11	165	7
Shigella species	3	6	1	2	87	4
Bacillus cereus	1	2	1	2	54	2
Campylobacter jejuni	1	2	2	4	48	2
Other bacteria	1	2	1	2	220	10
Subtotal	40	77	50	96	1,512	66
Viral	1	2	0	0	121	5
Parasitic	0	0	1	2	100	4
Chemical						
Scombroid	7	13	0	0	169	7
Ciguatera	0	0	0	0	169	7
Other	4	8	1	2	208	9
Subtotal	11	21	1	2	546	23
Total	52	100	52	100	2,279	98

Source: Centers for Disease Control, Foodborne Disease Surveillance.

Table 17-4. Causes of deaths associated with foodborne disease outbreaks in hospitals, nursing homes, and other known locations, United States, 1975–1987

Cause	Total deaths	Deaths in hospital outbreaks		Deaths in nursing home outbreaks		Deaths in other known locations	
		No.	% of total	No.	% of total	No.	% of total
Salmonella species	77	2	3	38	49	37	40
Clostridium perfringens	10	5	50	2	20	3	30
Staphylococcus aureus	4	0	0	2	50	2	50
Escherichia coli	4	0	0	4	100	0	0
Other known cause	138	0	0	1	1	137	99
Unknown cause	24	4	17	4	17	16	67
Total	257	11	4	51	20	195	76

Source: Centers for Disease Control, Foodborne Disease Surveillance.

Table 17-5. Food-handling errors in reported foodborne outbreaks with known errors, United States, 1975–1987

Type of error	Hospitals (N = 71)		Nursing homes (N = 91)		Other known locations (N = 4,956)	
	No.	%	No.	%	No.	%
Improper holding temperatures	30	42	35	39	1,940	39
Inadequate cooking	12	17	11	12	635	13
Poor personal hygiene	9	13	21	23	932	19
Contaminated equipment	9	13	13	14	675	14
Unsafe source	6	8	2	2	311	6
Other	5	7	9	10	463	9

Source: Centers for Disease Control, Foodborne Disease Surveillance.

lobacter jejuni or, more rarely, *E. coli* 0157 : H7) when purchased. In a 1979 survey of young whole chicken carcasses collected from 15 poultry-processing plants, the frequency of *Salmonella* species contamination was from 2.5 percent to 87.5 percent [29]. *C. jejuni* has been isolated from intestinal contents of up to 100 percent of poultry flock birds [56]. Raw fish and shellfish can be contaminated with such pathogens as *Vibrio parahaemolyticus, C. perfringens,* and *Vibrio vulnificus.* Fecal matter on the surface of unprocessed eggs is often contaminated with *Salmonella* species. Also, current reports of transovarian *S. enteritidis* infection of eggs suggest that vertical transmission may be an even more important factor in eggborne *S. enteritidis* transmission [26, 50]. For the 140 *S. enteritidis* outbreaks reported to the CDC from 1985 through 1988, contaminated food was implicated in 89 (64 percent); of these, grade A shell eggs were implicated in 65 (73 percent) [57]. Food can also become contaminated while being processed: Organisms can originate from hands, coughing, sneezing, and from contaminated equipment such as meat slicers or working surfaces [35]. Finally, bacteria may grow while food is in storage (e.g., when cooked foods are stored in direct contact with raw foods or when foods are held at inadequate temperatures). *Listeria monocytogenes* can survive and grow in food even with adequate refrigeration [27].

Foods and the Immunocompromised Host

Patients in health care facilities are more susceptible to certain foodborne infections than the general population. The elderly, the immunosuppressed, and persons with chronic underlying diseases are generally at increased risk for infections associated with higher morbidity and mortality. Because outbreaks of foodborne disease in nursing homes can be associated with serious morbidity and mortality, efforts to provide the safest possible food to the elderly in nursing homes should be maximized.

Increased susceptibility to foodborne infections in these populations may be caused by associated physiologic changes or therapies of their diseases. Although the gastrointestinal tract is normally resistant to colonization, this resistance can be substantially diminished by antimicrobial therapy, mucositis from cancer treatments, decreased stomach acidity, decreased intestinal motility, and decreased mucosal, humoral, and cellular immunity. Even in numbers smaller than the usual infective dose, ingested microorganisms may cause systemic infection in these patients.

Because *E. coli, Klebsiella* species, and *Pseudomonas aeruginosa* can contaminate fresh fruits, salads, and vegetables [21, 51], these foods should not be served to neutropenic patients [45]. Kominos and colleagues [37] found *P. aeruginosa* of the same pyocin type in clinical specimens and on raw vegetables from a kitchen in a general hospital and concluded that the vegetables were the source of the pathogens for the patients. Another potential contaminant of fresh vegetables is *L. monocytogenes,* a gram-positive bacterium that particularly affects the elderly, pregnant women, and the severely immunosuppressed [27].

Ho and associates [31] investigated an *L. monocytogenes* outbreak involving 20 patients from eight hospitals and concluded that raw vegetables served in hospital meals may have been contaminated. Ten (50 percent) of these patients were immunosuppressed. Dairy products and any raw food of animal origin can also be contaminated with *Listeria* species, *Salmonella* species, and, rarely, *E. coli* 0157 : H7. Ryan and co-workers [46] described an outbreak of *E. coli* 0157 : H7 affecting 34 patients and causing 4 deaths in a nursing home in which hamburger was implicated as the vehicle of infection. Recent studies show that men with AIDS have twenty times the incidence of *Salmonella* species infection compared with men without AIDS [13]. Ingestion of contaminated foods is believed to be an important cause of illness in these patients. All immunocompromised persons should cook raw food of animal origin thoroughly and avoid eating raw shellfish, raw milk, raw meat, and raw eggs [4, 30]. Similarly, dietary departments in health care facilities should follow these recommendations for all hospitalized patients, especially immunocompromised patients.

The potential severity of foodborne salmonellosis in the elderly is underscored by an outbreak caused by *S. enteritidis* in a nursing home; in this outbreak, 25 of 104 affected patients died, constituting an unusually high case-fatality ratio of 24 percent [16]. In a review of foodborne disease outbreaks occurring in nursing homes from 1975 through 1987, Levine and colleagues [38] found that nursing home outbreaks represented 2 percent of all foodborne disease outbreaks reported to the CDC and 20 percent of outbreak-associated deaths. Of 52 outbreaks with known etiology, *Salmonella* species were the most frequently reported pathogens, accounting for 52 percent of outbreaks and 81 percent of associated deaths.

Enteral feeding solutions are being used with increasing frequency to provide nutritional support to seriously ill patients with a functional digestive tract. Such solutions are often prepared in food service departments. Enteral feedings contaminated by bacteria can cause severe nosocomial infections [11, 12, 24, 47, 49]; therefore, infection control practices for their preparation and administration should be reviewed and implemented [39]. A high frequency of microbial contamination of enteral nutrition has been described [1, 40, 48, 52]. Powdered feeds requiring reconstitution might be contaminated with bacteria [2, 44, 53, 61]. Contamination can also occur during assembly of a delivery system on the ward [3] or by bacteria colonizing the nasogastric tube or ascending from the patient's gut [23].

Factors that contribute to the microbial contamination of enteral feeding solutions include (1) the composition of the feeding solution, (2) the lack of preservatives, (3) the number of manipulations involved in the feeding process, (4) the mode and duration of administration, and (5) the timing of sampling [39]. Although most instances of contamination are secondary to manipulation during preparation, adherence to appropri-ate food-handling practices to minimize bacterial contamination during preparation *and* administration and to minimize bacterial growth during storage of these solutions is essential. Monitoring by public health authorities of recommended manufacturing procedures as well as of the regulations on the bacterial content of powdered feeds has been recommended [39].

Prevention of Foodborne Transmission

Requirements and recommendations concerning food services are provided to hospitals and other health care facilities from the Joint Commission on Accreditation of Healthcare Organizations (JCAHO) and the Association for Practitioners in Infection Control (APIC) (Table 17-6). Responsibilities for inspection and certification of food service facilities in health care organizations vary by state. Accreditation by the JCAHO does not guarantee regular food service inspection nor food handler training. The Infection Control Committee of each health care facility has an important responsibility in the prevention of foodborne disease (see Chap. 4). The Infection Control Committee is responsible for cooperating with the food services department in developing written policies and procedures and for reviewing these policies at least annually [34].

To prevent foodborne disease, both the JCAHO requirements and the APIC recommendations focus prevention efforts by hospitals and other health care facilities in two directions: (1) food hygiene (i.e., food preparation, storage, and distribution) and (2) personal health and hygiene of food service personnel. Prevention—limiting contamination and destroying or inhibiting the growth of potential pathogens—is simple in principle but may be difficult in practice; approaches to preventing foodborne disease have been reviewed elsewhere [8, 9, 19]. Health care facilities should consult a dietitian with special training in food service sanitation, a sanitarian, or both about formulating and monitoring

Table 17-6. Summary of requirements and recommendations of the Joint Commission on Accreditation of Healthcare Organizations (JCAHO) and the Association for Practitioners in Infection Control (APIC) for food (dietetic) services

JCAHO	*APIC*
Principle: Dietetic services shall meet the nutritional needs of patients Standards: 1. Organized to provide optimal nutritional care and quality food service. 2. Appropriate training of personnel. 3. Written policies and procedures. 4. Safe, sanitary, and timely provision of food to meet nutritional needs. 5. Diet in accord with care provider's order and appropriate dietetic information recorded in the patient's medical record. 6. Appropriate quality control mechanisms. 7. Quality and appropriateness regularly evaluated in accordance with JCAHO quality assurance characteristics.	Infection control activities of the food service department: 1. Develop purchasing specifications that meet standards of safety and sanitation for food, equipment, and cleaning supplies. 2. Maintain and clean work areas, storage areas, and equipment in accordance with state and local health department standards. 3. Develop written standards for safe food handling; cleaning and sanitizing of trays, utensils, and tableware; and disposing of dietary waste. 4. Comply with local health department regulations for storage, handling, and disposal of garbage. 5. Conduct educational programs for personnel in food preparation and personal hygiene.

Source: From Joint Commission on Accreditation of Healthcare Organizations, *Accreditation Manual for Hospitals, 1991.* Chicago: JCAHO, 1990; and Association for Practitioners in Infection Control, *The APIC Curriculum for Infection Control Practice*, Vol. 2. Dubuque, IA: Kendall/Hunt, 1983. Pp. 816–828.

food-handling operations and procedures. In addition, local or state health departments should be consulted about state and local regulations and standards concerning food service personnel, food sanitation, and waste disposal.

Food Hygiene

Two factors are critical in preventing bacterial foodborne disease: (1) holding food at appropriate temperatures—that is, either above 60°C (140°F) or below 7°C (45°F), and (2) avoiding cross-contamination of cooked food by raw food or by food-handling personnel with overt or silent infection. In addition, pasteurized milk and pasteurized egg products should be used instead of shell eggs and raw milk. Food must be purchased from reliable sources, and commercially filled unopened packages should be used when possible. Microbial contaminants on some raw foods may be kept from multiplying during processing by proper storage, thawing meat products in refrigerators (1°C [34°F] to 7.2°C [45°F]), or adequate heat treatment. Because

work surfaces, knives, slicers, pots, pans, and other kitchen equipment can convey bacteria from contaminated food to other foods, food-contact surfaces of equipment and utensils must be cleaned and decontaminated between preparation of food items. Items such as slicers must be easy to disassemble to ensure proper cleaning. Workers should be trained to operate and maintain equipment properly. All workers must thoroughly wash their hands after handling raw poultry, meat, fish, fruits, and vegetables; after contact with unclean equipment and work surfaces, soiled clothing, washrags, and other items; and, most importantly, after using the bathroom. Spilled food should be cleaned up immediately. Equipment and kitchen layout should be designed to promote rapid processing to minimize chances for cross-contamination; to avoid producing aerosols, sprays, or splashing during processing; and to facilitate cleaning and sanitizing operations [60]. Contamination by insects, rodents, sewage back flow, or drips must be prevented by screening, proper storage (including separating raw meats from processed foods), and adequate plumbing. When storage facilities are limited, paper products may be stored with food supplies. Garbage from hospital kitchens and wards should be enclosed, protected from insects and rodents, and transported or disposed of in a sanitary manner according to state and local regulations.

Cross-contamination can be minimized by adopting standard techniques for cleaning work surfaces and kitchen utensils and by ensuring that raw foods are processed in areas of the kitchen and on work surfaces that are not subsequently used for cooked foods. Separate cutting boards may not be required when the boards in use are nonabsorbent and can be cleaned and sanitized adequately between usage for different food categories. Dishwashing and utensil-washing equipment and techniques that sanitize serviceware and prevent recontamination should be used to ensure sanitary provision of food service. Disposable containers and utensils should be properly discarded after one use. All food hygiene procedures should be reviewed periodically and whenever physical changes are made in the kitchen or new equipment is put into use. New personnel should receive prompt training in good food-handling practices. Food service personnel from all work shifts should receive regular inservice training stressing the epidemiology of foodborne diseases and appropriate food-handling practices.

Foodborne diseases have resulted from poor planning and a lack of understanding of appropriate food-handling practices (e.g., not allowing enough time for poultry to thaw, or assuming that thawing is complete, before cooking). This problem can result in undercooking and can be compounded by keeping undercooked food in the oven after the heat has been shut off, providing ideal incubation conditions for bacteria that survived the initial cooking. Potentially harmful bacteria in foods must be destroyed by thorough cooking or reheating to internal temperatures that reach 74°C (165°F); internal meat temperatures should be measured by bayonet-type thermometers. Periodically, the internal tem-

perature of foods in serving lines should be checked.

The most common error resulting in foodborne disease is storage of food at inappropriate temperatures; this error is most often identified in staphylococcal food poisoning and in short- and long-incubation *Bacillus cereus, C. perfringens,* and *Salmonella* outbreaks. In some outbreaks, even when refrigerator temperatures were adequate, the center temperature of perishable foods was warm enough to permit bacteria to grow or toxin to be produced because the foods were in inadequate holding containers. When cooked foods are kept at room temperature (or are refrigerated in large quantities) for a period of 4 hours or more, certain pathogens remaining in the food may be able to multiply to a high enough level or produce enough toxin to cause disease. Cooked foods have been kept too long at room temperature because of inadequate refrigerator space and failure to perceive the importance of refrigeration. In general, food that requires refrigeration should be stored at no higher than 7°C (45°F) in shallow containers so the food is no more than 4 in. deep.

Storage is a particular problem when food must be delivered from a central kitchen to peripheral areas of the health care facility or other buildings by either truck or food carts. A *C. perfringens* foodborne outbreak affecting 49 patients related to a meals-on-wheels operation in England illustrates the kind of problem that can result when food is not held at appropriate temperatures before serving [33]. Procedures for transporting food must include facilities for keeping hot foods hot and cold foods cold. Thermometers used to measure holding temperatures should be standard equipment in such conveyances. Standby equipment should be on hand or alternative plans formulated to handle emergency conditions arising from equipment failure. Food delivered to a kitchen or ward should be properly stored to prevent growth of bacteria, and it should be distributed with minimum handling by ward personnel. In the event that ward personnel must handle food, they should be carefully supervised to ensure that the same high standards required of kitchen personnel are maintained.

In the past, problems have arisen because of preferences for raw or undercooked foods, such as eggnog. Eggnog prepared from undercooked or raw eggs was an important cause of foodborne salmonellosis before the regulation requiring pasteurization of eggs that are to be dried or frozen. Substitution of pasteurized egg products for fresh eggs in nursing homes and hospitals is strongly recommended. Several outbreaks have been traced to blenders used for both raw eggs and pureed foods. Requiring use of separate blenders to scramble eggs and to puree cooked foods would reduce the risk of cross-contamination. Routine disassembly and sanitation of blenders after blending raw eggs is also important. Avoiding consumption of raw milk is important in preventing *Salmonella* species and *C. jejuni* outbreaks.

Personnel Health and Hygiene

Supervision of food service personnel requires attention to work habits, personal hygiene, and health. Hands of food service personnel may be colonized or infected with microorganisms, such as *S. aureus,* or may become contaminated by organisms from raw foods (*Salmonella* species, *C. jejuni,* and *C. perfringens*) and human excreta (*Salmonella* species, *Shigella* species, Norwalk and Norwalk-like agents, and hepatitis A virus). These organisms may then contaminate previously uncontaminated food. Although thorough cooking of food just before consumption will eliminate the risk of many illnesses, staphylococcal food poisoning will not be eliminated because the staphylococcal enterotoxins are heat-stable.

Hand-washing facilities should be conveniently located to permit use by employees in food preparation and utensil-washing areas and should be located in, or immediately adjacent to, toilet facilities. Each hand-washing facility should be provided with (1) a continuous supply of clear water; (2) a supply of hand-cleaning liquid, powder, or bar soap; and (3) individual sanitary towels, a continuous towel system supplied with a clean towel, or a heated-air hand-drying device. Common hand-drying towels are prohibited. If disposable towels are used, a waste receptacle should be located next to the hand-washing facility.

Various strategies have been used in an attempt to monitor the health of food service personnel, including stool examinations for ova and parasites, for certain enteric bacterial pathogens, or for both. However, these measures are not cost-effective. Further, one stool culture is often not sufficient to detect the small number of organisms in the stool of a person who does not have diarrhea but is infected with enteric pathogens. McCall and co-workers [42] found, for example, that one rectal swab detected only 47 percent of chronic *S. derby* carriers and that seven consecutive daily swabs were needed to detect 95 percent of known carriers. Such extensive culturing is impractical and costly. Furthermore, a person may not be infected on the day the culture specimen is taken, but the same person may later acquire infection. Also, because a carrier may excrete organisms intermittently, sporadic sampling for culture tests may never reveal the true carriage status. Finally, cultures of nose and throat secretions and feces may reveal potential foodborne pathogens, such as *S. aureus,* but this carriage may be of no danger to others; that is, the carrier is usually not disseminating the organisms. Laboratory monitoring of food handlers may actually be counterproductive by giving the food handler and the supervisory staff a false sense of security. Negative culture reports are likely to be interpreted by the employee to mean that he or she is not capable of contaminating food with potential foodborne pathogens. From the management standpoint, laboratory monitoring of food handlers may convey the false impression that food safety is being enhanced. Thus, routine laboratory testing should not be performed because there is no scientific justification [22].

The proper approach to managing the personal aspects of hygiene is to establish and pursue a policy of training food service managers and workers. The health care facility Infection Control Committee should ensure a

program comprising a comprehensive training course in the appropriate languages for
all new employees at the onset of employment, as well as inservice training at regular
intervals for all food service personnel. As appropriate to their level of responsibility, such
courses should include (1) the basic principles
of personal hygiene, emphasizing the need
for good hand-washing practices; (2) the importance of informing supervisors of acute
intestinal diseases, boils, and any skin infection, particularly on the fingers and hands;
(3) the proper inspection, handling, preparation, serving, and storing of food; (4) the
proper cleaning and safe operation of equipment; (5) general food service sanitation
safety; (6) the proper method of waste disposal; (7) portion control; (8) the writing of
modified diets using the diet manual or handbook; (9) diet instruction; and (10) the recording of pertinent dietetic information in
the patient's medical record [6].

Surveillance

Responsibility for preventing, detecting, and
investigating foodborne disease outbreaks
rests with the health care facility Infection
Control Committee and the infection control
practitioner (see Chaps. 4, 6). They should
maintain a monitoring procedure to ensure
that dietetic staff are free from infections
and open skin lesions and should be informed of acute illnesses among food service
workers that could potentially be transmitted
by food. It is important that an atmosphere
be created that does not penalize food handlers for reporting illness. Any work restriction policy should encourage personnel to
report their illnesses or exposures and not
penalize them with loss of wages, benefits, or
job status [62].

Appropriate culture specimens should be
taken and processed during such illnesses
(see Chaps. 3, 9). In cases of acute diarrhea,
rectal swab or fecal specimens promptly inoculated onto appropriate laboratory media are
recommended. Workers should not be permitted to return to their assigned jobs until
their diarrhea has resolved and two stool cultures obtained at least 24 hours apart are neg-

ative (see Chap. 30). If antimicrobial agents
are used, follow-up cultures should be obtained after treatment has been completed.
Personnel with boils, open sores, or cellulitis
of the fingers, hands, and face should be excluded until they are adequately treated. The
infection control practitioner's judgment
should prevail in deciding when the worker
can return to work.

Routine surveillance of patients and employees should detect any cases of gastrointestinal disease related to the health care
facility's food service. Temporal clustering of
such cases should alert the infection control
personnel to the possibility of an outbreak.
Prompt investigation and reporting of outbreaks to the appropriate health authorities is
essential to (1) conduct investigations to identify and correct food-handling error(s), (2)
prevent additional primary and secondary
transmission of disease, and (3) limit outbreaks caused by commercially distributed
foods.

References

1. Anderson, K. R., et al. Bacterial contamination of tube feeding formula. *J. Parenter. Enter.
   Nutr.* 8:673, 1984.
2. Anderton, A. Microbiological quality of products used in enteral feeds. *J. Hosp. Infect.* 7:68,
   1986.
3. Anderton, A., and Aidov, K. E. The effect of
   handling procedures on microbial contamination of enteral feeds. *J. Hosp. Infect.* 11:364,
   1988.
4. Archer, D. L. Food counseling for persons infected with HIV: Strategy for defensive living.
   Public Health Rep. 104:196, 1989.
5. Archer, D. L., and Young, F. K. Contemporary issues: Diseases with a food vector. *Clin.
   Microbiol. Rev.* 1:377, 1988.
6. Association for Practitioners in Infection Control. *The APIC Curriculum for Infection Control
   Practice.* Dubuque, IA: Kendall/Hunt Publishing, 1983.
7. Bean, N. H., Griffin, P. M., Goulding, J. S., and
   Ivey, C. B. Foodborne disease outbreaks, 5-
   year summary, 1983–1987. *J. Food Protect.* 53:
   711, 1990.
8. Bryan, F. L. Prevention of foodborne diseases
   in food-service establishments. *J. Environ.
   Health* 41:198, 1979.

9. Bryan, F. L. Factors that contribute to outbreaks of foodborne disease. *J. Food Protect.* 41:816, 1978.

10. Carter, A. O., et al. A severe outbreak of *Escherichia coli* O157:H7-associated hemorrhagic colitis in a nursing home. *N. Engl. J. Med.* 317:1496, 1987.

11. Caswell, M. W. Bacteriological hazards of contaminated enteral feeds. *J. Hosp. Infect.* 3:329, 1982.

12. Caswell, M. W., Cooper, J. E., and Webster, M. Enteral feeds contaminated with *Enterobacter cloacae* as a cause of septicemia. *Br. Med. J.* 282:973, 1981.

13. Celum, C. L., et al. Incidence of salmonellosis in patients with AIDS. *J. Infect. Dis.* 156:998, 1987.

14. Centers for Disease Control. Hospital-associated outbreak of *Shigella dysenteriae* type 2: Maryland. *M.M.W.R.* 32:250, 1983.

15. Centers for Disease Control. Multistate outbreak of salmonellosis caused by precooked roast beef. *M.M.W.R.* 30:391, 1981.

16. Centers for Disease Control. Salmonellosis: Baltimore, Maryland. *M.M.W.R.* 19:314, 1970.

17. Centers for Disease Control. Shigellosis in children's hospital: Pennsylvania. *M.M.W.R.* 28:498, 1979.

18. Centers for Disease Control. Update: *Salmonella enteritidis* infections and shell eggs—United States, 1990. *M.M.W.R.* 39:909, 1990.

19. Charles, R. H. G. *Mass Catering.* Copenhagen: World Health Organization, 1983.

20. Collier, P. W., et al. Food poisoning in hospitals in Scotland, 1978–87. *Epidemiol. Infect.* 101:661, 1988.

21. Cooke, E. M., et al. *Klebsiella* species in hospital food and kitchens: A source of organisms in the bowel of patients. *J. Hyg.* 84:97, 1980.

22. Cruickshank, J. G., and Humprey, T. J. The carrier food-handler and non-typhoid salmonellosis. *Epidemiol. Infect.* 98:223, 1987.

23. DeLeeuw, I., and Van Alsenoy, L. Bacterial contamination of the feeding bag during catheter jejunostomy. Exogenous or endogenous origin? *J. Parenter. Enter. Nutr.* 9:378, 1985.

24. de Vries, E. G. E., Mulder, N. H., Houwen, B., and de Vries-Hospers, H. G. Enteral nutrition by nasogastric tube in adult patients treated with intensive chemotherapy for acute leukemia. *Am. J. Clin. Nutr.* 35:1490, 1982.

25. Food poisoning in hospitals (edit.). *Lancet* 1:576, 1980.

26. Gast, R. K., and Beard, C. W. Production of *Salmonella enteritidis*–contaminated eggs by experimentally infected hens. *Avian Dis.* 34:438, 1990.

27. Gellin, B. G., and Broome, C. V. Listeriosis. *J.A.M.A.* 261:1313, 1989.

28. Giannella, R. A., and Brasile, L. A hospital foodborne outbreak of diarrhea caused by *Bacillus cereus.* Clinical, epidemiologic, and microbiologic studies. *J. Infect. Dis.* 139:366, 1979.

29. Green, S. S., et al. The incidence of *Salmonella* species and serotypes in young whole chicken carcasses in 1979 as compared with 1967. *Poult. Sci.* 61:288, 1982.

30. Griffin, P. M., and Tauxe, R. V. Food counseling for patients with AIDS (lett.). *J. Infect. Dis.* 158:668, 1988.

31. Ho, J. L., et al. An outbreak of type 4b *Listeria monocytogenes* infection involving patients from eight Boston hospitals. *Arch. Intern. Med.* 1946:520, 1986.

32. Hughes, J. M., and Tauxe, R. V. Food-borne Disease. In: G. L. Mandell, R. G. Douglas, Jr., and J. E. Bennett (Eds.), *Principles and Practice of Infectious Diseases* (3rd ed.). New York: Churchill Livingstone, 1990. Pp. 893–904.

33. Jephcott, A. E., Barton, B. W., Gilbert, R. J., and Shearer, C. W. An unusual outbreak of food-poisoning associated with meals-on-wheels. *Lancet* 2:219, 1977.

34. Joint Commission on Accreditation of Healthcare Organizations. *Accreditation Manual for Hospitals, 1991.* Chicago: Joint Commission on Accreditation of Healthcare Organizations, 1990.

35. Jordan, M. C., Powell, K. E., Corothers, T. E., and Murray, R. J. Salmonellosis among restaurant patrons: The incisive role of a meat slicer. *Am. J. Public Health* 63:982, 1973.

36. Joseph, C. A., and Palmer, S. R. Outbreaks of *Salmonella* infection in hospitals in England and Wales, 1978–87. *Br. Med. J.* 298:1161, 1989.

37. Kominos, S. D., Copeland, C. E., Grosiak, B., and Postic, B. Introduction of *Pseudomonas aeruginosa* into a hospital via vegetables. *Appl. Microbiol.* 24:567, 1972.

38. Levine, W. C., et al. Foodborne disease outbreaks in nursing homes, 1975 to 1987. *J.A.M.A.* 266:2105, 1991.

39. Levy, J. Enteral nutrition: An increasingly recognized cause of nosocomial bloodstream infection. *Infect. Control Hosp. Epidemiol.* 10:395, 1989.

40. Levy, J. et al. Contaminated enteral nutrition as a cause of nosocomial bloodstream infection: A study using plasmid fingerprinting. *J. Parenter. Enter. Nutr.* 10:228, 1989.

41. Linnemann, C. C., Jr., Cannon, C. G., Staneck, J. L., and McNeely, B. L. Prolonged hospital epidemic of salmonellosis: Use of trimethoprim-sulfamethoxazole for control. *Infect. Control* 6:221, 1985.

42. McCall, C. E., Martin, W. T., and Boring, J. R. Efficiency of cultures of rectal swabs and faecal specimens in detecting *Salmonella* carriers:

Correlation with number of salmonellas excreted. *J. Hyg.* (Lond.) 64:261, 1966.

43. Meyers, J. D., Frederic, J. R., Tihen, W. S., and Bryan, J. A. Foodborne hepatitis A in a general hospital: Epidemiologic study of an outbreak attributed to sandwiches. *J.A.M.A.* 231: 1049, 1975.

44. Muytjens, H. L. Roelofs-Willemse, H., and Jaspar, G. H. Quality of powdered substitutes for breast milk with regards to members of the family Enterobacteriaceae. *J. Clin. Microbiol.* 26:743, 1988.

45. Remington, J. S., and Schimpff, S. C. Please don't eat the salads. *N. Engl. J. Med.* 304:433, ≤ 1981

46. Ryan, C. A., et al. *Escherichia coli* 0157:H7 diarrhea in a nursing home: Clinical, epidemiological, and pathological findings. *J. Infect. Dis.* 154:631, 1986.

47. Schimpff, S. C., et al. Origin of infection in acute nonlymphocytic leukemia: Significance of hospital acquisition of potential pathogens. *Ann. Intern. Med.* 77:707, 1972.

48. Schroeder, P., Fisher, D., Volz, M., and Paloucek, J. Microbial contamination of enteral feeding solutions in a community hospital. *J. Parenter. Enter. Nutr.* 7:364, 1983.

49. Selden, R., et al. Nosocomial infections: Intestinal colonization as a reservoir. *Ann. Intern. Med.* 74:657, 1971.

50. Shivasprasad, H. L., et al. Pathogenesis of *Salmonella enteritidis* infection in laying chickens: I. Studies on egg tranmission, clinical signs, fecal shedding, and serologic responses. *Avian Dis.* 34:548, 1990.

51. Shooter, R. A., et al. Isolation of *Escherichia coli, Pseudomonas aeruginosa,* and *Klebsiella* from food in hospitals, canteens, and schools. *Lancet* 2:390, 1971.

52. Shreiner, R. L., et al. Environmental contamination of continuous drip feedings. *Pediatrics* 63:232, 1979.

53. Simmons, B. P., et al. *Enterobacter sakazakii* infections in neonates associated with intrinsic contamination of a powdered infant formula. *Infect. Control Hosp. Epidemiol.* 10:398, 1989.

54. Spitalny, K. C., Okowitz, E. N., and Vogt, R. L. Salmonellosis outbreak at a Vermont hospital. *South Med. J.* 77:168, 1984.

55. Stamm, W. E., Weinstein, R. A., and Dixon, R. E. Comparison of endemic and epidemic nosocomial infections. *Am. J. Med.* 70:393, 1981.

56. Stern, N. J., and Kazmi, S. U. *Campylobacter jejuni.* In: M. P. Doyle (Ed.), *Foodborne Bacterial Pathogens.* New York: Marcel Dekker, 1989.

57. St. Louis, M., et al. The emergence of grade A eggs as a major source of *Salmonella enteritidis* infections. *J.A.M.A.* 259:2103, 1988.

58. Tauxe, R. V., et al. *Salmonella enteritidis* outbreaks in the United States, 1985–1989: The epidemic expands. In: *Proceedings of the Thirtieth Interscience Conference on Antimicrobial Agents and Chemotherapy.* Atlanta, GA: American Society for Microbiology, 1990. P. 238.

59. Thomas, M., et al. Hospital outbreak of *Clostridium perfringens* food poisoning. *Lancet* 1: 1046, 1977.

60. U.S. Department of Health, Education, and Welfare. *Food Service Sanitation Manual.* Washington, DC: Public Health Service, Food and Drug Administration, 1976.

61. U.S. Food and Drug Administration. *Bacterial Contamination of Enteral Formula Products.* Washington, DC: Public Health Service, Food and Drug Administration Bulletin, 1988.

62. Williams, W. W. Guideline for infection control in hospital personnel. *Infect. Control* 4: 326, 1983.

63. Yamagishi, T., et al. A nosocomial outbreak of food poisoning caused by enterotoxigenic *Clostridium perfringens. Microbiol. Immunol.* 27: 291, 1983.

64. Yule, B. F., Macleod, A. F., Sharp, J. C. M., and Forbes, G. I. Costing of a hospital-based outbreak of poultry-borne salmonellosis. *Epidemiol. Infect.* 100:35, 1988.

Clinical Laboratory-Acquired Infections

Michael L. Wilson
L. Barth Reller

Clinical laboratories are an area of special concern in hospital infection control. Laboratory workers may be exposed to infectious agents during all steps of collection, transport, processing, and analysis of patient specimens. Workers in clinical microbiology laboratories in particular are at risk for occupational infection, since the clinical specimens submitted for culture are more likely to contain infectious agents. Moreover, isolation and culture of infectious agents generates large numbers of pathogenic agents which, under certain circumstances, can pose a major hazard to clinical microbiology personnel.

The goals of this chapter are to provide an overview of the epidemiology of laboratory-acquired infections, to highlight those infections of special concern to clinical laboratories, and to make specific recommendations for the prevention and control of laboratory-acquired infections. Not discussed in this chapter are the special problems of clinical virology, research, anatomic pathology, and commercial reference laboratories or laboratories involved in the production or processing of large volumes of pathogenic microorganisms. The reader is referred to Collins's recent monograph [20] for an extensive review of the subject of laboratory-acquired infections. In this text, the role of the clinical microbiology laboratory in infection surveillance, investigation of endemic and epidemic hospital infections, and the control of nosocomial infections is discussed in Chapters 5, 6, and 9, respectively.

Incidence, Causative Agents, and Cost

The exact incidence of laboratory-acquired infections is unknown. Early data [66–69, 78] were derived from surveys, personal communications, and literature reports; hence, they cannot be used to calculate incidence. One recent survey [40] reported an annual incidence of 3 laboratory-acquired infections per 1,000 employees, and another [81] an annual incidence of 3.5 and 1.4 per 1,000 employees among laboratory workers in hospital-based and public health laboratories, respectively. Therefore, it seems reasonable that the annual incidence of laboratory-acquired infections is between 1 and 5 per 1,000 employees. There is some evidence, however, that the overall annual incidence is decreasing [66], particularly for hepatitis B virus (HBV) infections [1], owing to hepatitis B immunization and adoption of universal precautions [27] (see Chap. 38).

Pike's data [67, 68] show that, historically, the most common laboratory-acquired infections have been brucellosis, Q fever, typhoid fever, hepatitis B, tularemia, and tuberculosis. More recent data, however, suggest that the infections most commonly acquired in the clinical laboratory are hepatitis B, shigellosis, and tuberculosis [29–31, 34, 40]. Other agents continue to pose a hazard to laboratory workers, however, as demonstrated by continuing reports of laboratory-acquired brucellosis [30, 34, 75], salmonellosis [5, 6, 31, 39, 76], and meningococcemia [4, 12].

Because the exact incidence of laboratory-acquired infections is unknown, the cost to society for these infections is also unknown. In one report [81], each laboratory-acquired infection resulted in an average of 1.2 lost workdays for hospital-based laboratories and 1.3 lost workdays for public health laboratories. The latter figure, however, does not include the 48 workdays lost when one employee was hospitalized for a laboratory-acquired infection.

An accurate estimate of the cost to society may not be possible without additional data or further studies, but it is clear that the cost to an infected individual can be high. Fatal laboratory-acquired infections still occur [6, 12]. It is estimated that 200 to 300 health care workers die each year as a consequence of chronic HBV infection [85] (see Chap. 38). Since the risk to laboratorians for acquiring HBV is as great as that to any other health care worker [53, 65], it seems reasonable that a substantial proportion of these deaths occurs among laboratorians. Moreover, many workers acquiring HBV infections will become chronic carriers. Finally, laboratory-acquired infection with human immunodeficiency virus (HIV), the causative agent of the acquired immunodeficiency syndrome (AIDS), has been reported in laboratory workers [8, 10, 17, 58] (see Chap. 39). The subsequent effects on the infected individual and his or her family are grave, and the medical costs to society great.

Sources of Infection

Pike [66, 67] and others [26, 40, 60, 81] have attempted to determine which laboratory procedures, accidents, or other exposures to infectious agents are the source of laboratory-acquired infections (Table 18-1). These data indicate that the source of infection is unknown in up to 20 percent of cases, and the infected individual was known only to have worked with the agent in the past in another 21 percent of cases [67]. Thus, the exact source, procedure, or breach in technique can be identified in just over half of cases. Among the recognized sources are accidents, which account for 18 percent of cases. The kinds of accidents that lead to laboratory-acquired infections are listed in Table 18-2.

Laboratory accidents associated with expo-

Table 18-1. Sources of laboratory-acquired infections in the United States and abroad

Proved or probable source	No. of infections	Percentage of total
Working with agent	827	21.1
Unknown and other	783	20.0
Known accident	703	17.9
Animal or arthropod	659	16.8
Aerosol	522	13.3
Patient specimen	287	7.3
Human autopsy	75	1.9
Discarded glassware	46	1.2
Intentional infection	19	0.5
Total	3,921	100.0

Source: Adapted from R.M. Pike, Laboratory-associated infections: Summary and analysis of 3,921 cases. *Health Lab. Sci.* 13:105, 1976.

sure to infectious materials include creation of aerosols from spatters or spills; exposure of skin defects (cuts, abrasions, ulcers, dermatitis, etc.), conjunctivae, or mucosal surfaces; accidental aspiration or ingestion; and traumatic implantation [67]. Needle-stick injuries and cuts with broken glass and other sharps account for up to half of accidents associated with laboratory-acquired infections [26, 60, 66, 67]. The microbiologic hazards associated with needle-stick and sharps injuries have recently been reviewed [21, 59]. Surprisingly, accidental ingestion or aspiration of infectious materials via mouth pipetting continues to be a source of laboratory-acquired infections [26, 60], despite the fact that such behavior is expressly forbidden, or should be, in all laboratories [19, 61, 80].

Aerosol droplets vary in size, with larger droplets rapidly settling onto exposed surfaces. These droplets may carry infectious agents and can thus contaminate environmental surfaces. Smaller droplets remain suspended in the air for a longer period of time and, under the appropriate environmental conditions, can remain suspended indefinitely (see Chap. 1). Aerosols with droplets measuring less than 5 μm in diameter can be inhaled directly into alveoli; those measuring approximately 1 μm are the most likely to be retained within alveoli [7]. Many common laboratory procedures have been shown to produce aerosols in this size range [46, 77, 79, 83]. Both *Mycobacterium tuberculosis* and atypical mycobacteria may be transmitted by the aerosol route [55].

Table 18-2. Kinds of laboratory accidents resulting in infection

Known accident	No. of infections	Percentage of total
Spill or spatter	188	26.7
Needle stick	177	25.2
Broken-glass injury	112	15.9
Bite or scratch	95	13.5
Mouth pipetting	92	13.1
Other	39	5.5
Total	703	99.9

Source: Adapted from R.M. Pike, Laboratory-associated infections: Summary and analysis of 3,921 cases. *Health Lab. Sci.* 13:105, 1976.

Laboratory personnel have among the highest rates of needle-stick injuries [41, 59]. Most needle-stick injuries occur during disposal of used needles, assembly or disassembly of intravenous infusion sets, administration of parenteral injections or infusion therapy, drawing blood, recapping needles, or handling waste containing needles [41, 59]. Recapping, a major problem, causes between 12 and 30 percent of needle-stick injuries [41, 59] (see Chap. 11). It should be noted, however, that *not* recapping needles may also pose a risk to health care workers [42]. The epidemiology of needle-stick injuries in laboratory personnel has not been studied but, since activities such as intravenous infusion and handling infusion sets do not occur in laboratories, it seems likely that recapping and handling waste are the two major activities associated with these injuries in clinical laboratories. Therefore, laboratory personnel should avoid recapping needles whenever possible and should immediately dispose of used needles in sharps containers [59]. Rigid adherence to such a procedure should greatly reduce the incidence of needle-stick injuries from both activities.

Infectious Agents of Special Concern in Clinical Laboratories

The risk of acquiring infections in a clinical laboratory is dependent on several factors [49]. The most important factor is the likelihood of exposure to an infectious agent, which is dependent on the prevalence of that agent in patient specimens received in the laboratory and the occurrence of exposures that can transmit the agent. The probability that such an exposure will result in an infection depends on inoculum size, viability of the infectious agent, the immune status of the exposed individual, and the availability and use of effective postexposure prophylactic therapy.

Human Immunodeficiency Virus

It is estimated that 1 million Americans are infected with HIV and that at least another 40,000 adolescents and adults and 1,500 to 2,000 newborns acquire the infection each year [11]. Of those infected, increasing numbers will develop and die of AIDS [11]. These data indicate that the number of hospitalized patients seropositive for HIV will increase in the foreseeable future as HIV-infected patients seek medical care (see Chap. 39).

The prevalence of HIV-infected patients varies between regions, cities, and even hospitals within a given city. Seropositivity rates also vary widely according to age, sex, race, and socioeconomic group. Seropositivity rates can be as high as 22 percent or as low as 0.9 percent in different patient populations [38, 44, 45, 73]. HIV-positive patients have been reported from all 50 states, and the incidence of HIV infection is increasing in areas previously known to have a low incidence [28]. A recent survey from Seattle showed that HIV antibody was present in 3 percent of all serum or plasma specimens submitted to the clinical chemistry laboratory at an urban teaching hospital [33]. Thus, a significant proportion of clinical specimens may be infected with HIV, and all clinical laboratory personnel can be expected to work eventually with HIV-infected clinical specimens.

Transmission of HIV during an occupational exposure occurs as a result of contact of infected material with nonintact skin or mucosal surfaces or as a result of traumatic implantation of infectious material [10, 17]. It is estimated that the risk of acquiring HIV infection following a single cutaneous exposure to infected blood is no more than 0.05 percent [15] and that the risk of infection from a needle-stick injury is approximately 0.3 to 0.5 percent [15, 36, 58, 87]. Although both types of exposure are common among some health care workers [57], the frequency of such exposures among laboratory personnel has not been reported. Based on knowledge of the rates of acquisition of HBV infection among laboratory personnel [21, 65], however, it is likely that laboratory personnel are among those health care workers most commonly exposed to HIV-infected specimens. The prevalence of HBV serologic markers among clinical laboratory workers who handle blood or serum matches or exceeds that of other health care workers, including nurses and surgeons [84].

The consequences of exposure to HIV are potentially grave. Neither an effective vaccine nor proved postexposure treatment protocols exist [15]. Acquisition of HIV infection is obviously devastating to the affected individual, since the progression to AIDS appears to be inevitable and the disease is uniformly fatal. Moreover, HIV-infected individuals can transmit the infection to others via sexual contact. Since infected individuals may remain asymptomatic for years, the potential for additional exposures is real. Finally, the emotional impact on the infected individual and his or her family is devastating.

Guidelines for the prevention of transmission of HIV infection in the workplace have been published [10, 16, 18]. These guidelines for universal precautions are also useful in preventing occupational exposure to other bloodborne pathogens, particularly HBV (see Chap. 38). These recommendations are based on a common-sense approach to infection control and are relatively easy to follow. Although direct evidence that use of universal precautions has prevented cases of HIV or HBV infection are not available, there is evidence that such precautions reduce occupational exposures to HIV in patient specimens [27, 49, 86]. The cost to implement universal precautions is substantial (an estimated $336 million in the United States for fiscal year 1989) and may have been significantly underestimated heretofore [3, 25]. Universal precautions, however, currently provide the most rational approach to decreasing the risk of acquiring HIV infection and other bloodborne pathogens in the laboratory [33, 49, 86] and are, therefore, a prudent expense.

Hepatitis B Virus

Despite the availability of safe and effective vaccines and effective postexposure treatment regimens, HBV infection remains one of the most common hospital-acquired infections [26, 34, 40]. Surveys have repeatedly shown that laboratorians are among the most frequently infected health care workers [30, 40, 53, 72], with seropositivity rates between two and twenty-seven times that of the general population [37, 54, 62, 63, 72, 84]. It is estimated that of the 300,000 new cases of

HBV infection in the United States each year, 1 to 6 percent (6,000 to 18,000) occur in health care workers [1, 43]. One report estimates that 12 percent of HBV-infected patients require hospitalization, indicating that each year 720 to 2,160 health care workers may require hospitalization for HBV infections [1]. Although it is reported that the incidence of laboratory-acquired HBV infection has decreased by 75 percent since the early 1980s, primarily because of vaccination [1], only 30 to 40 percent of health care workers have been vaccinated [43]. Therefore, programs to ensure vaccination of all laboratorians should be undertaken, which could eliminate HBV infection as an occupational hazard (see Chaps. 3, 38).

Most laboratory-acquired HBV infections probably are not acquired via needle sticks or cuts with infected instruments but rather by clinically inapparent cutaneous or mucosal exposure to blood or blood products [52–54, 63]. Therefore, rigid adherence to published guidelines for prevention of HIV and HBV infection via universal precautions should be followed by all laboratory personnel. Percutaneous exposure is not limited to those employees working directly with body fluids. One outbreak of laboratory-acquired HBV infection occurred among clerical employees whose only risk factor was exposure to HBV-contaminated computer requisitions [64] and, in another study, the highest prevalence of seropositivity in a laboratory was among persons employed as glassware washers [2].

Since the epidemiology of hepatitis C virus (HCV) resembles that of HBV, it is likely that HCV will be documented more frequently as a cause of laboratory-acquired infection now that accurate diagnosis is possible and the frequency of HBV is reduced by administration of vaccine. At present, use of universal precautions is the mainstay of prevention of acquisition of HCV in the laboratory.

Mycobacterium tuberculosis

Employees involved in the processing of clinical specimens or cultures from patients with tuberculosis are at a much greater risk of acquiring tuberculosis than the general population [29, 30, 34, 70]. Although the incidence of tuberculosis was once believed to be waning, the emergence of tuberculosis and other mycobacterial infections as major infectious diseases in patients with AIDS, especially as a consequence of intravenous drug abuse, has once again brought mycobacteria to the forefront of clinical microbiology [9] (see Chap. 29).

Bacteria and Fungi

Bacterial infections of special concern to laboratory personnel are primarily those caused by highly virulent pathogens such as *Brucella* species and *Francisella tularensis* [67, 75]. Other bacteria of special concern include *Shigella* and *Salmonella* species [5, 6, 39]. Enteric bacterial pathogens are important because they are relatively common. Indeed, infections caused by *Shigella* are currently the most common laboratory-acquired bacterial infections in both the United States and Great Britain [34, 40]. Fungal infections of special concern to laboratory personnel are primarily the thermally dimorphic fungi *Coccidioides immitis, Blastomyces dermititidis,* and *Histoplasma capsulatum* [74]. Recommendations for the safe processing of clinical specimens and cultures suspected of containing any of these agents are provided in the next section.

Prevention of Laboratory-Acquired Infections

Each clinical laboratory must develop policies and procedures to prevent, document, and treat laboratory-acquired infections. The laboratory director, in conjunction with a designated laboratory safety officer, should take the lead role in developing and implementing these and should integrate them into the laboratory procedure manual [20, 32, 35, 47, 61, 80]. All employees should receive the appropriate education and training necessary to perform their job safely. They should be explicitly aware of hazards associated with various infectious agents, how to prevent the risk of exposure to each agent, and exactly what should be done should such an exposure occur. Immunization against hepatitis B should be emphasized for all laboratory workers

[1, 13, 14, 84, 85]. Initial and follow-up tuberculin skin tests should be given in accord with current guidelines [9, 47, 48]. Finally, a mechanism for maintaining compliance with these policies and procedures must be implemented, along with the appropriate documentation, counseling and, if necessary, disciplinary action to ensure that employees work in the safest possible manner.

Biosafety Levels

The Centers for Disease Control (CDC) and National Institutes of Health (NIH) have defined four biosafety levels based on "the potential hazard of the agent and the laboratory function or activity" [19]. This document also provides a summary statement of the biosafety level recommended for the safe handling of various infectious agents. In general, most common pathogens may be handled as biosafety level 2. Cultures suspected of containing *Brucella* species, *F. tularensis*, *M. tuberculosis*, *C. immitis*, *B. dermatitidis*, or *H. capsulatum* should be processed only by experienced personnel working in a biologic safety cabinet under biosafety level 3 condi-

tions. Laboratory design, equipment, and procedures necessary to achieve each biosafety level have been formulated jointly by the CDC and NIH [19].

Universal Precautions

Special policies and procedures are necessary for the safe handling and disposal of certain highly virulent pathogens. Rigorous adherence to universal precautions is sufficient to decrease or eliminate the risk of acquiring an infection from most patient specimens processed in clinical laboratories. Implementation of universal precautions is successful only if laboratory administrators and workers integrate CDC recommendations into routine laboratory operations and make every reasonable attempt to maintain and enforce such policies (see Chap. 11). Universal precautions have been shown to decrease the number of occupational exposures to blood and other body fluids among one group of health care workers (27, 86). CDC recommendations for universal precautions for all health care workers are discussed in Chapter 11, and those specific to clinical laboratorians are given in Table 18-3.

Table 18-3. Universal precautions for workers in diagnostic pathology laboratories

1. All specimens of blood and body fluids should be put in a well-constructed container with a secure lid to prevent leaking during transport. Care should be taken when collecting each specimen to avoid contaminating the outside of the container and the laboratory form accompanying the specimen.

2. All persons processing blood and body fluid specimens (e.g., removing tops from vacuum tubes) should wear gloves. Masks and protective eyewear should be worn if mucous-membrane contact with blood or body fluids is anticipated. Gloves should be changed and hands washed after completion of specimen processing.

3. For routine procedures, such as histologic and pathologic studies or microbiologic culturing, a biologic safety cabinet is not necessary. However, biologic safety cabinets (class I or II) should be used whenever procedures are conducted that have a high potential for generating droplets. These include activities such as blending, sonicating, and vigorous mixing.

4. Mechanical pipetting devices should be used for manipulating all liquids in the laboratory. *Mouth pipetting must not be done.*

5. Use of needles and syringes should be limited to situations in which there is no alternative, and the recommendations for preventing injuries with needles (outlined in Chap. 11) should be followed.

6. Laboratory work surfaces should be decontaminated with an appropriate chemical germicide after a spill of blood or other body fluids and when work activities are completed.

7. Contaminated materials used in laboratory tests should be decontaminated before reprocessing or be placed in bags and disposed of in accordance with institutional policies for disposal of infectious waste.

8. Scientific equipment that has been contaminated with blood or other body fluids should be decontaminated and cleaned before being repaired in the laboratory or transported to the manufacturer.

9. All persons should wash their hands after completing laboratory activities and should remove protective clothing before leaving the laboratory.

Standard Microbiologic Practices

When used in conjunction with universal precautions, the following practices should be effective in preventing most laboratory-acquired infections. These or equivalent procedures should be routine practice in all clinical laboratories [16, 18, 22–24, 32, 49–51, 56, 61, 71, 80, 82, 86].

1. Laboratory access
   a. Only trained laboratory personnel should be allowed in a laboratory under ordinary circumstances.
   b. Maintenance personnel, delivery persons, and other visitors with a legitimate reason for being in the laboratory should be either escorted or closely supervised to prevent unnecessary exposure to infectious agents.
   c. Laboratory trainees, house staff, and other students should be supervised closely.
   d. Children should not be allowed in laboratories.
2. Personnel policies
   a. All personnel should have training commensurate with the level of expertise needed to perform all necessary procedures safely. Suggested topics for such training are given in Table 18-4.

Table 18-4. A 10-step program for training laboratory workers in biohazard safety

1. Universal precautions for handling blood and body fluids
2. Aseptic technique and procedures
3. Personal hygiene and protective equipment
4. Criteria for biosafety levels 1–4
5. Effective use of biologic safety cabinets I–III
6. Safe use of centrifuges and autoclaves
7. Decontamination, disinfection, and sterilization
8. Handling, packaging, and disposal of biohazardous waste
9. Packaging, transporting, and shipping of biohazardous waste
10. Reporting incidents and accidents

Source: Modified from the U.S. National Research Council, Committee on Hazardous Biological Substances in the Laboratory, *Biosafety in the Laboratory: Prudent Practices for the Handling and Disposal of Infectious Materials.* Washington, DC: National Academy of Sciences, 1989.

b. All personnel should receive the necessary continuing education and training to ensure job safety.
   c. Employee job appraisals should include documented lapses in safety, techniques, or other behaviors that could result in occupational exposure to infectious agents. Persons exhibiting such behavior should be counseled or retrained.
3. Laboratory facility
   a. Laboratories should be designed to minimize traffic and unnecessary access to work areas.
   b. Laboratory furniture should be sturdy and easy to clean.
   c. Laboratories should be uncluttered and easy to clean.
   d. Foot-, knee-, or elbow-operated hand-washing sinks should be available and located near laboratory exits.
   e. The laboratory facility should be designed and constructed to meet criteria recommended for the appropriate biosafety level [29].
4. Hygiene for workers
   a. Eating, drinking, smoking, and applying cosmetics should be strictly prohibited within the laboratory [29].
   b. All personnel should wear and button full-length white laboratory coats while in the laboratory. Laboratory coats should not be worn outside the laboratory.
   c. Personnel and visitors should wash their hands before leaving the laboratory.
   d. Food and other personal items should not be stored in refrigerators or freezers used to store clinical specimens or cultures. Refrigerators, freezers, and microwave ovens used to store or prepare food must be located outside the laboratory.
5. Clinical specimens
   a. Specimens must be labeled with the patient's full name, hospital identification number, and the date drawn.
   b. Specimens received in damaged, leaking, or contaminated containers should not be processed; the person who collected the specimen should be notified and the specimen recollected.

6. Microbiologic techniques [19]
   a. Mouth pipetting should be *strictly* prohibited. Mechanical pipetting devices should be immediately available within the laboratory.
   b. All procedures should be carefully performed to prevent the formation of aerosols; procedures that generate aerosols should be performed in a biologic safety cabinet.
   c. Cylindric electric burners are preferable to flame burners for sterilizing inoculating loops or needles and the tips of other small instruments.
   d. If flame burners are used, care should be taken to avoid spattering. This can be achieved by slowly drawing loops or needles through the flame, with the loop entering the flame last.
   e. Cool inoculating loops and needles should be used when touching plates, colonies, or broth cultures.
   f. Work surfaces should be decontaminated at least once daily with an acceptable germicide. Work surfaces should also be decontaminated after spills (see under the heading Safety in Handling Accidents, Using Equipment, and Disposing of Wastes).
   g. Infectious wastes and patient specimens should be disinfected before disposal (see under the heading Safety in Handling Accidents, Using Equipment, and Disposing of Wastes).
   h. Needles, blades, and other sharp items should be disposed of in rigid, tamper-resistant, puncture-resistant, marked containers.
   i. Materials removed from the laboratory should be free of infectious hazard.
   j. Clinical specimens, cultures, or other potentially infectious materials should be packaged, labeled, and shipped according to federal regulations [80].

Safety Procedure Manual

Every laboratory should have an up-to-date safety manual as an integral part of the laboratory procedure manual. The following information should be included:

1. A designated laboratory safety officer (LSO) and explicit instructions as to how to contact that individual in the event of an accident or exposure. The LSO should lead the educational program for biohazard safety (see Table 18-4).
2. Synopsis of safety components of good laboratory practice and hospital policies for infection control, including universal precautions.
3. Location of necessary emergency equipment and spill cleanup kits.
4. Detailed procedures for cleanup of spills.
5. Instructions for the effective use of biologic safety cabinets.
6. Procedures for safe use of centrifuges and autoclaves.
7. Vaccination policies and tuberculin skin-testing protocols.
8. Procedures for postexposure treatment, prophylaxis, and counseling.

Safety in Handling Accidents, Using Equipment, and Disposing of Wastes
Procedures for Spills and Accidents

Because of the high concentration of microorganisms in patient specimens and cultures in clinical laboratories, special procedures must be used to disinfect spills and other laboratory accidents. The current CDC recommendation is to use "chemical germicides that are approved for use as 'hospital germicides' and are tuberculocidal when used at recommended dilutions" [16, 47] (see Chap. 15). This recommendation applies to all types of spills or other laboratory accidents.

Written procedures should be available in the laboratory safety manual. Employees should be trained to decontaminate and clean up safely spills involving those microorganisms cultured or studied in their laboratory. All necessary disinfectants and cleaning supplies must be readily available in the laboratory. Because spills may occur at any stage of the transport, plating, processing, or storage of microbiologic cultures, specific protocols should be available for spills occurring at each stage and for spills involving routine moderate-risk microorganisms and those of higher risk such as *M. tuberculosis.*

The hazard associated with a spill is dependent on the nature of the spilled agent, the volume of material spilled, the concentration of the agent within the material, and where the spill occurs. Spills involving microorganisms such as *M. tuberculosis, F. tularensis, Brucella* species, *C. immitis,* or *H. capsulatum* may pose a major hazard to laboratory workers. Spills involving large volumes of moderate-risk microorganisms or those occurring in such a manner that aerosols might be generated should also be treated as a major hazard to laboratory workers.

Procedures Used for Routine Spills Involving Low Volumes of Moderate-Risk Microorganisms [22, 80, 82]

1. The affected area should immediately be flooded with a suitable disinfectant and covered with paper towels.
2. Others should be warned to avoid the contaminated area.
3. Personnel should wear gloves and use an autoclavable dustpan and squeegee or forceps to pick up solid materials.
4. Any remaining fluids or other materials should be wiped up with paper towels.
5. Contaminated materials should be disposed of as infectious waste.
6. Unless the laboratory worker is injured or otherwise exposed during the spill or cleanup, no other specific action need be taken.

Procedures for Spills Involving High Volumes of Moderate-Risk Agents or Highly Pathogenic Agents Occurring Outside a Biologic Safety Cabinet [22, 47, 80, 82]

1. Employees should hold their breath, immediately evacuate the room, and close the door.
2. Employees should assist others as needed to protect them from potential exposure.
3. Other personnel should be warned to avoid the contaminated area. Personnel in adjacent areas should be warned of any potential hazard to their safety.

4. Contaminated clothing and protective equipment should be removed and discarded as biohazardous waste.
5. Employees should thoroughly wash exposed skin surfaces.
6. The laboratory safety officer and director should be immediately notified.
7. Biologic safety cabinets should be left running to help decrease the concentration of aerosols in the contaminated room.
8. If the spill occurs in a room under negative pressure, at least 30 minutes should pass before personnel reenter the affected room [82].
9. If the spill occurs in a room not under negative pressure, the cleanup should begin immediately [82].
10. Protective clothing, including a cap, mask, long-sleeved gown, shoe covers, and gloves, should be worn.
11. An appropriate disinfectant should be allowed to run into the spill from the sides. Disinfectant poured directly on the spills may generate aerosols.
12. The area should be covered with paper towels and allowed to stand for 20 minutes.
13. An autoclavable dustpan and squeegee or forceps should be used to clean up pieces of broken glass and other sharp objects.
14. Remaining liquids should be wiped up with paper towels.
15. All materials, including protective clothing, should be discarded as biohazardous waste.

Procedures for Spills Occurring in Biologic Safety Cabinets [22, 80, 82]

1. Biologic safety cabinets (BSCs) should be allowed to operate to minimize further risk to laboratory workers.
2. Cleanup should begin immediately.
3. Gloves, mask, and a gown should be worn during the cleanup.
4. Work surfaces and any catch pans or basins should be flooded with an adequate volume of disinfectant.
5. The flooded area should be allowed to stand for 20 minutes.
6. During this time, the BSC walls, work sur-

faces, and any equipment within the BSC should be cleaned with a germicidal disinfectant (phenolic or iodophor compounds). Flammable organic solvents, such as alcohols, should *not* be used, as these compounds may reach dangerous concentrations within certain BSCs.

7. All contaminated materials and fluids should be disposed of as biohazardous waste.

8. Catch pans and basins should be cleaned per the manufacturer's recommendations.

9. High-efficiency particulate air (HEPA) filters and other components of BSC should *not* be cleaned or disinfected by laboratory personnel. This is not necessary with most spills and should be done only by factory-trained and certified personnel. Major spills or those involving high-risk agents may necessitate formaldehyde decontamination of the BSC. Such decontamination should be performed only by qualified personnel.

Laboratory Equipment

Laboratory safety and diagnostic equipment must be of the proper type and should be tested and maintained according to the manufacturer's recommendations. Equally important is proper use by laboratory personnel. All personnel should be instructed as to the proper use, care, and maintenance of laboratory equipment.

Biologic Safety Cabinets

BSCs are essential for the safe handling of infectious agents. Different BSCs are available; which one to use depends primarily on the infectious agents to be handled.

Class I BSCs (Fig. 18-1) have an open front into which room air flows. All of the exhaust air is discharged through HEPA filters to the outside environment. Although class I BSCs protect the user from exposure to agents within the cabinet, they do not protect materials within the cabinet against contamination. Class I BSCs are unsuitable for use in clinical microbiology laboratories [80].

Class II BSCs (Fig. 18-2) also have an open front into which room air flows. Class II BSCs differ from class I BSCs in that a portion of the exhausted air passing through HEPA filters is recirculated into the cabinet. The filtered air is then used to protect clinical specimens or cultures from contamination. Two basic types of class II BSCs are available. Class

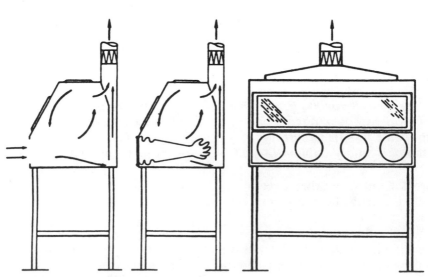

Fig. 18-1. Design of class I biological safety cabinet.

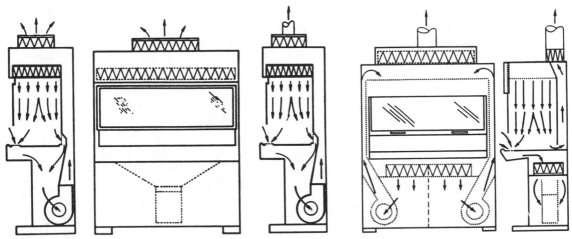

Fig. 18-2. Design of class II biological safety cabinets, types A and B.

II type A BSCs are the most commonly used in clinical laboratories and are sufficient for meeting biosafety level 2 or 3 criteria. Class II type B cabinets may also be used for this purpose but usually are more expensive to purchase and to operate [80].

Class III BSCs (Fig. 18-3) provide the greatest protection to laboratory personnel, but their use is usually restricted to working with highly virulent pathogens in biosafety level 4 laboratories.

Laboratory workers must remember that BSCs are not chemical fume hoods. Toxic, noxious, or flammable chemicals must not be used in these hoods, since the recirculation of exhaust air may allow these chemicals to reach dangerously high levels in the cabinet. BSCs should be installed, tested, and maintained only by qualified personnel. Regular testing and certification of BSCs is crucial for the users' safety. Laboratory personnel should be instructed in the proper use of BSCs and should be aware of their limitations in controlling aerosols. Certain actions by personnel working in a BSC can adversely affect the ability of the cabinet to contain infectious aerosols [56]. Users should consult with the manufacturer as to the potential effect of these and other factors (such as equipment within BSCs) before using a BSC [51]. Finally, personnel should be aware that BSC function

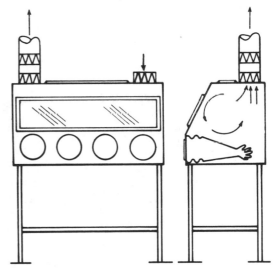

Fig. 18-3. Design of class III biological safety cabinet.

depends on proper airflow patterns and that changes in airflow patterns because of alterations in building air supplies, temporary shutdowns for repairs, and so forth may adversely affect the function of BSCs.

Centrifuges
Centrifuges used to process clinical specimens or cultures should be equipped with sealable, autoclavable, breakage-resistant cups to prevent contamination of the centrifuge

and the release of aerosols should centrifuge tubes break during processing. These cups must be removable from the centrifuge rotor so that they can be cleaned and autoclaved.

Autoclaves

An autoclave should be readily accessible to clinical laboratories. Routine maintenance, testing, and cleaning is essential (see Chap. 15). Autoclaves should be tested for their ability to kill standard bacterial spores [80]. It should be emphasized that autoclave tape indicates that an object has been autoclaved but not necessarily sterilized [32, 71, 82].

Laboratory and Protective Equipment

Other laboratory equipment should be of a type and design that allows for easy cleaning and disinfection. Safety equipment for the cleanup and disinfection of laboratory spills should be readily available. Proper gloves, gowns, masks, and shoe covers should be handy.

Both latex and vinyl disposable gloves have been shown to vary widely in their permeability [23, 50]. It has been shown that washing and reusing gloves is inadvisable and that the proportion of hands contaminated with test microorganisms after gloves are removed varies from 5 to 50 percent [24]. Therefore, health care workers should wash their hands after gloves have been removed. The issue of wearing two pairs of gloves (double gloving) is more contentious. Although it is logical to assume that two barriers offer more protection than one, concerns about loss of tactile sensation and dexterity have led to recommendations against double gloving during routine laboratory procedures [50]. Wearing two pairs of gloves during autopsies and other situations where large amounts of blood are present has been recommended [61].

Disposal of Infectious Materials

Materials contaminated with infectious agents must be disposed of properly to protect the personnel doing the work as well as the general public [80]. Safe disposal of infectious materials begins at the source where these materials are generated. The following are recommended for the safe disposal of infectious materials and waste [71, 80]:

1. Adequate waste bins and sharps containers must be readily available.
2. Waste bins should be lined with two autoclavable bags.
3. All containers should be clearly marked.
4. Laboratory and maintenance personnel should avoid physical contact with these materials; leaking containers should be treated as spills.
5. Infectious materials should be transported in or on carts that can be easily cleaned and disinfected [71].
6. Infectious materials should be autoclaved before disposal; double bagging and overfilling should be avoided, as these practices limit the effectiveness of autoclaving as a means of sterilization [71].
7. Regular monitoring of the adequacy of autoclave sterilization should be part of routine laboratory quality control procedures.

Prevention and Postexposure Treatment
Vaccination

Recommendations for vaccinations for health care workers have recently been reviewed [85], and specific recommendations have been made by the CDC [13, 14] (see Chap. 3). Laboratory workers may or may not have contact with patients but should still follow the recommendations for all health care workers. It should be strongly emphasized that all health care workers should be vaccinated against HBV [13]. Such vaccination should probably be given during the training years, since the risk of occupational exposure to HBV appears to be greatest during that period [14]. Since licensure of HBV vaccine in 1982, approximately 80 percent of the 2.5 million persons vaccinated for HBV have been health care workers [1]. Moreover, the recent 75 percent decline in HBV associated with health care employment is believed to be a direct result of immunization with HBV vaccine and wider use of universal precautions [1]. Nonetheless, it is estimated that only 30 to 40 percent of health care workers have been vaccinated [43]; the goal should be 100 percent.

Before being employed, all hospital workers should provide evidence of immunity to rubella. Persons lacking protective antibody to rubella virus should be vaccinated. Influenza, measles, mumps, and polio vaccines and tetanus-diphtheria toxoid immunization should comply with current guidelines from the Immunization Practices Advisory Committee (ACIP) of the U.S. Public Health Service and should be coordinated with personnel health services (see Chap. 3) in the hospital [12–14, 85].

Postexposure Treatment and Prophylaxis

Specific treatment, prophylaxis, and counseling should be available for all health care workers following exposure to an infectious agent [32]. Such policies and procedures should be made in consultation with the hospital Infection Control Committee. Clinical laboratories should include such policies as part of their laboratory safety and procedure manuals. Specific recommendations have been formulated for exposure to many infectious agents [13, 15]; the reader is referred to Chapter 3 for additional information.

Of special importance to clinical laboratory workers are the recommendations for hepatitis B prophylaxis after percutaneous (needlestick or sharps injury) exposure to blood. Hepatitis B immune globulin (HBIG) should be given immediately, followed by HBV vaccine to individuals who have not been vaccinated against HBV or who lack adequate protective antibodies to HBV (see Chaps. 3, 38).

Laboratory workers with percutaneous exposure to blood samples from patients are also at risk for HIV infection [33] (see Chap. 39). Persons exposed to HIV in the workplace should be informed that there are diverse opinions among physicians about the use of zidovudine (formerly called *azidothymidine* [AZT]) for postexposure prophylaxis and that the U.S. Public Health Service cannot make a recommendation for or against the use of zidovudine for this purpose because of limitations of current knowledge [15]. Workers should be encouraged to have a baseline serum sample obtained for HIV serologic testing and be enrolled in the CDC surveillance system for appropriate long-term follow-up and counseling [10, 15].

Personnel working in mycobacteriology laboratories, and those involved in the processing or disposal of materials likely to be contaminated with mycobacteria, should receive a preemployment Mantoux tuberculin skin test with purified protein derivative (PPD) [48]. The only exceptions are those persons with a previously positive reaction or those who have completed adequate preventive therapy or therapy for active disease that can be documented [9]. Subsequent skin testing of PPD-negative laboratory workers should be done annually and immediately and again 12 weeks after a known hazardous exposure or accident [9, 47]. Exposed persons with skin-test reactions of 5 mm or greater or with symptoms suggestive of tuberculosis should have chest radiographs. Those with skin-test conversions but without active disease should be considered for preventive therapy in accord with published guidelines [9].

Conclusions

Although the incidence of laboratory-acquired infections appears to be decreasing, they still occur at a low rate and are associated with significant morbidity and mortality. Infections caused by HBV and HIV are of particular concern. Laboratory personnel should make every attempt to follow recommended guidelines, policies, and procedures designed to minimize the risk of working with infectious materials. Each laboratory must be designed and constructed in such a way to minimize accidents and facilitate cleanups. It must contain proper and well-maintained safety and diagnostic equipment. Most important, however, is the proper training and supervision of laboratory personnel and adherence to policies and procedures designed to provide a safe working environment. It is the obligation of laboratory directors and administrators to provide such an environment.

References

1. Alter, M.J., et al. The changing epidemiology of hepatitis B in the United States. Need for alternative vaccination strategies. *J.A.M.A.* 263: 1218, 1990.
2. Anderson, R.A., and Woodfield, D.G. Hepatitis B virus infections in laboratory staff. *N. Z. Med. J.* 95:69, 1982.
3. Bachner, P. The epidemiology of fear. Scientific, social, and political responses to the occupational risk of bloodborne infection. *Arch. Pathol. Lab. Med.* 114:319, 1990.
4. Bhatti, A.R., DiNinno, V.L., and Ashton, F.E., and White, L.A. A laboratory-acquired infection with *Neisseria meningitidis. J. Infect.* 4:247, 1982.
5. Blaser, M.J., et al. *Salmonella typhi:* The laboratory as a reservoir of infection. *J. Infect. Dis.* 142:934, 1980.
6. Blaser, M.H., and Lefgren, J.P. Fatal salmonellosis originating in a clinical microbiology laboratory. *J. Clin. Microbiol.* 13:855, 1981.
7. Brown, J.H., Cook, K.M., Ney, F.G., and Hatch, T. Influence of particle size upon the retention of particulate matter in the human lung. *Am. J. Public Health* 40:450, 1950.
8. Centers for Disease Control. Agent summary statement for human immunodeficiency virus and report on laboratory-acquired infection with human immunodeficiency virus. *M.M.W.R.* 37(No. S-4):1, 1988.
9. Centers for Disease Control. Guidelines for preventing the transmission of tuberculosis in health-care settings with special emphasis on HIV-related issues. *M.M.W.R.* 39(No. RR-17):1, 1990.
10. Centers for Disease Control. Guidelines for prevention of transmission of human immunodeficiency virus and hepatitis B virus to health-care and public-safety workers. *M.M.W.R.* 38(No. S-6):3, 1989.
11. Centers for Disease Control. HIV prevalence estimates and AIDS case projections for the United States: Report based upon a workshop. *M.M.W.R.* 39(No. RR-16):1, 1990.
12. Centers for Disease Control. Laboratory-acquired meningococcemia—California and Massachusetts. *M.M.W.R.* 40:46, 1991.
13. Centers for Disease Control. Protection against viral hepatitis. Recommendations of the immunization practices advisory committee (ACIP). *M.M.W.R.* 39(RR-2):1, 1990.
14. Centers for Disease Control. Public health

15. burden of vaccine-preventable diseases among adults: Standards for adult immunization practice. *M.M.W.R.* 39:725, 1990.
15. Centers for Disease Control. Public health service statement on management of occupational exposure to human immunodeficiency virus, including considerations regarding zidovudine postexposure use. *M.M.W.R.* 39(No. RR-1):1, 1990.
16. Centers for Disease Control. Recommendations for prevention of HIV transmission in health-care settings. *M.M.W.R.* 36(Suppl. 25):3S, 1987.
17. Centers for Disease Control. Update: Acquired immunodeficiency syndrome and human immunodeficiency virus infection among health-care workers. *M.M.W.R.* 37:229, 1988.
18. Centers for Disease Control. Update: Universal precautions for prevention of transmission of human immunodeficiency virus, hepatitis B virus, and other bloodborne pathogens in health-care settings. *M.M.W.R.* 37:377, 1988.
19. Centers for Disease Control and National Institutes of Health. *Biosafety in Microbiological and Biomedical Laboratories* (2nd ed.). Atlanta: U.S. Department of Health and Human Services, Public Health Service, Centers for Disease Control, 1988.
20. Collins, C.H. *Laboratory-Acquired Infections* (2nd ed.). London: Butterworths, 1988.
21. Collins, C.H., and Kennedy, D.A. Microbiological hazards of occupational needlestick and 'sharps' injuries. *J. Appl. Bacteriol.* 62:385, 1987.
22. Coyle, M.B., and Schoenknecht, F.D. The Clinical Laboratory. In: J.V. Bennett and P.S. Brachman (Eds.), *Hospital Infections* (2nd ed.). Boston: Little, Brown, 1986. P. 335.
23. DeGroot-Kosolcharoen, J., and Jones, J.M. Permeability of latex and vinyl gloves to water and blood. *Am. J. Infect. Control* 17:196, 1989.
24. Doebbeling, B.N., Pfaller, M.A., Houston, A.K., and Wenzel, R.P. Removal of nosocomial pathogens from the contaminated glove. Implications for glove reuse and handwashing. *Ann. Intern. Med.* 109:394, 1988.
25. Doebbeling, B.N., and Wenzel, R.P. The direct costs of universal precautions in a teaching hospital. *J.A.M.A.* 264:2083, 1990.
26. Evans, M.R., Henderson, D.K., and Bennett, J.E. Potential for laboratory exposures to biohazardous agents found in blood. *Am. J. Public Health* 80:423, 1990.
27. Fahey, B.J., Koziol, D.E., Banks, S.M., and Henderson, D.K. Frequency of nonparenteral occupational exposures to blood and body fluids before and after universal precautions training. *Am. J. Med.* 90:145, 1991.
28. Gardner, L.I., Jr., et al. Evidence for spread of the human immunodeficiency virus epidemic

into low prevalence areas of the United States. *J. Acquir. Immune. Defic. Syndr.* 2:521, 1989.

29. Grist, N.R. Infections in British clinical laboratories 1980–1. *J. Clin. Pathol.* 36:121, 1983.

30. Grist, N.R., and Emslie, J.A.N. Infections in British clinical laboratories, 1982–3. *J. Clin. Pathol.* 38:721, 1985.

31. Grist, N.R., and Emslie, J.A.N. Infections in British clinical laboratories, 1984–5. *J. Clin. Pathol.* 40:826, 1987.

32. Groschel, D.H.M., Dwork, K.G., Wenzel, R.P., and Scheibel, L.W. Laboratory Accidents with Infectious Agents. In: B.M. Miller (Ed.), *Laboratory Safety: Principles and Practices.* Washington: American Society for Microbiology, 1986. Pp. 261–266.

33. Handsfield, H.H., Cummings, J., and Swenson, P.D. Prevalence of antibody to human immunodeficiency virus and hepatitis B surface antigen in blood samples submitted to a hospital laboratory. Implications for handling specimens. *J.A.M.A.* 258:3395, 1987.

34. Harrington, J.M., and Shannon, H.S. Incidence of tuberculosis, hepatitis, brucellosis, and shigellosis in British medical workers. *Br. Med. J.* 1:759, 1976.

35. Harrington, J.M., and Shannon, H.S. Survey of safety and health care in British medical laboratories. *Br. Med. J.* 1:626, 1977.

36. Henderson, D.K., et al. Risk for occupational transmission of human immunodeficiency virus type 1 (HIV-1) associated with clinical exposures. A prospective evaluation. *Ann. Intern. Med.* 113:740, 1990.

37. Hirschowitz, B.I., Dasher, C.A., Whitt, F.J., and Cole, G.W. Hepatitis B antigen and antibody and tests of liver function. A prospective study of 310 laboratory workers. *Am. J. Clin. Pathol.* 73:63, 1980.

38. Hoff, R., et al. Seroprevalence of human immunodeficiency virus among childbearing women: Estimation by testing samples of blood from newborns. *N. Engl. J. Med.* 318:525, 1988.

39. Holmes, M.B., Johnson, D.L., Fiumara, N.J., and McCormack, W.M. Acquisition of typhoid fever from proficiency-testing specimens. *N. Engl. J. Med.* 303:519, 1980.

40. Jacobson, J.T., Orlob, R.B., and Clayton, J.L. Infections acquired in clinical laboratories in Utah. *J. Clin. Microbiol.* 21:486, 1985.

41. Jagger, J., Hunt, E.H., Brand-Elnaggar, J., and Pearson, R.D. Rates of needle-stick injury caused by various devices in a university hospital. *N. Engl. J. Med.* 319:284, 1988.

42. Jagger, J., Hunt, E.H., and Pearson, R.D. Recapping used needles: Is it worse than the alternative? *J. Infect. Dis.* 162:784, 1990.

43. Kane, M.A., Alter, M.J., Hadler, S.C., and Margolis, H. S. Hepatitis B infection in the United States. Recent trends and future strategies for control. *Am. J. Med.* 87(Suppl. 3A):11S, 1989.

44. Kelen, G.D., et al. Human immunodeficiency virus infection in emergency department patients. Epidemiology, clinical presentations, and risk to health care workers: The Johns Hopkins experience. *J.A.M.A.* 262:516, 1989.

45. Kelen, G.D., et al. Unrecognized human immunodeficiency virus infection in emergency department patients. *N. Engl. J. Med.* 318:1645, 1988.

46. Kenny, M.T., and Sabel, F.L. Particle size distribution of *Serratia marcescens* aerosols created during common laboratory procedures and simulated laboratory accidents. *Appl. Microbiol.* 16:1146, 1968.

47. Kent, P.T., and Kubica, G.P. *Public Health Mycobacteriology. A Guide for the Level III Laboratory.* Atlanta: U.S. Department of Health and Human Services, Public Health Service, Centers for Disease Control, 1985.

48. Klein, J.O. Management of infections in hospital employees. *Am. J. Med.* 70:919, 1981.

49. Klein, R.S. Universal precautions for preventing occupational exposures to human immunodeficiency virus type 1. *Am. J. Med.* 90:141, 1991.

50. Kotilainen, J.R., Brinker, J.P., Avato, J.L., and Gantz, N.M. Latex and vinyl examination gloves. Quality control procedures and implications for health care workers. *Arch. Intern. Med.* 149:2749, 1989.

51. Kubica, G.P. Your tuberculosis laboratory: Are you really safe from infection? *Clin. Microbiol. Newslett.* 12:85, 1990.

52. Lauer, J.L., VanDrunen, N.A., Washburn, J.W., and Balfour, H.H., Jr. Transmission of hepatitis B virus in clinical laboratory areas. *J. Infect. Dis.* 140:513, 1979.

53. Leers, W.-D., and Kouroupis, G.M. Prevalence of hepatitis B antibodies in hospital personnel. *Can. Med. Assoc. J.* 113:844, 1975.

54. Levy, B.S., et al. Hepatitis B in ward and clinical laboratory employees of a general hospital. *Am. J. Epidemiol.* 106:330, 1977.

55. Loudon, R.G., Bumgarner, L.R., Lacy, J., and Coffman, G.K. Aerial transmission of mycobacteria. *Am. Rev. Respir. Dis.* 100:165, 1969.

56. Macher, J.M., and First, M.W. Effects of airflow rates and operator activity on containment of bacterial aerosols in a class II safety cabinet. *Appl. Environ. Microbiol.* 48:481, 1984.

57. Mangione, C.M., Gerberding, J.L., and Cummings, S.R. Occupational exposure to HIV: Frequency and rates of underreporting of percutaneous and mucocutaneous exposures by medical housestaff. *Am. J. Med.* 90:85, 1991.

58. Marcus, R., and the CDC Cooperative Needle-

stick Surveillance Group. Surveillance of health care workers exposed to blood from patients infected with the human immunodeficiency virus. *N. Engl. J. Med.* 319:1118, 1988.

59. McCormick, R D., and Maki, D.G. Epidemiology of needle-stick injuries in hospital personnel. *Am. J. Med.* 70:928, 1981.

60. Miller, C.D., Songer, J.R., and Sullivan, J.F. A twenty-five year review of laboratory-acquired human infections at the National Animal Disease Center. *Am. Ind. Hyg. Assoc. J.* 48:271, 1987.

61. National Committee for Clinical Laboratory Standards. *Protection of Laboratory Workers from Infectious Disease Transmitted by Blood and Tissue; Proposed Guideline.* NCCLS Document M29-P. Villanova, PA: National Committee for Clinical Laboratory Standards, 1987.

62. Osterholm, M., and Andrews, J.S. Viral hepatitis in hospital personnel in Minnesota. Report of a statewide survey. *Minn. Med.* 62:683, 1979.

63. Pantelick, E.L., Steere, A.C., Lewis, H.D., and Miller, D.J. Hepatitis B infection in hospital personnel during an eight-year period. Policies for screening and pregnancy in high risk areas. *Am. J. Med.* 70:924, 1981.

64. Pattison, C.P., Boyer, K.M., Maynard, J.E., and Kelly, P.C. Epidemic hepatitis in a clinical laboratory. Possible association with computer card handling. *J.A.M.A.* 230:854, 1974.

65. Pattison, C.P., Maynard, J.E., Berquist, K.R., and Webster, H.M. Epidemiology of hepatitis B in hospital personnel. *Am. J. Epidemiol.* 101:59, 1975.

66. Pike, R.M. Laboratory-associated infections: Incidence, fatalities, causes, and prevention. *Annu. Rev. Microbiol.* 33:41, 1979.

67. Pike, R.M. Laboratory-associated infections: Summary and analysis of 3,921 cases. *Health Lab. Sci.* 13:105, 1976.

68. Pike, R.M. Past and present hazards of working with infectious agents. *Arch. Pathol. Lab. Med.* 102:333, 1978.

69. Pike, R.M., Sulkin, S.E., and Schulze, M.L. Continuing importance of laboratory-acquired infections. *Am. J. Public Health* 55:190, 1965.

70. Reid, D.D. Incidence of tuberculosis among workers in medical laboratories. *Br. Med. J.* 2:10, 1957.

71. Reinhardt, P.A., and Gordon, J.G. Infectious and medical waste management. Chelsea, MI: Lewis Publishers, 1991.

72. Skinhøj, P., and Søeby, M. Viral hepatitis in Danish health care personnel, 1974–8. *J. Clin. Pathol.* 34:408, 1981.

73. St. Louis, M.E., et al. Seroprevalence rates of human immunodeficiency virus infection at sentinel hospitals in the United States. *N. Engl. J. Med.* 323:213, 1990.

74. Standard, P.G., and Kaufman, L. Safety considerations in handling exoantigen extracts from pathogenic fungi. *J. Clin. Microbiol.* 15:663, 1982.

75. Staszkiewicz, J., et al. Outbreak of *Brucella melitensis* among microbiology laboratory workers in a community hospital. *J. Clin. Microbiol.* 29:287, 1991.

76. Steckelberg, J.M., Terrell, C.L., and Edson, R.S. Laboratory-acquired *Salmonella typhimurium* enteritis: Association with erythema nodosum and reactive arthritis. *Am. J. Med.* 85:705, 1988.

77. Stern, E.L., et al. Aerosol production associated with clinical laboratory procedures. *Am. J. Clin. Pathol.* 62:591, 1974.

78. Sulkin, S.E., and Pike, R.M. Laboratory-acquired infections. *J.A.M.A.* 147:1740, 1951.

79. Tomlinson, A.J.H. Infected air-borne particles liberated on opening screwcapped bottles. *Br. Med. J.* 1:15, 1957.

80. U.S. National Research Council, Committee on Hazardous Biological Substances in the Laboratory. *Biosafety in the Laboratory: Prudent Practices for the Handling and Disposal of Infectious Materials.* Washington, DC: National Academy of Sciences, 1989.

81. Vesley, D., and Hartmann, H.M. Laboratory-acquired infections and injuries in clinical laboratories: A 1986 survey. *Am. J. Public Health* 78:1213, 1988.

82. Vesley, D., and Lauer, J. Decontamination, Sterilization, Disinfection, and Antisepsis in the Microbiology Laboratory. In: B.M. Miller (Ed.), *Laboratory Safety: Principles and Practices.* Washington, DC: American Society for Microbiology, 1986. Pp. 182–198.

83. Wedum, A.G. Laboratory safety in research with infectious aerosols. *Public Health Rep.* 79:619, 1964.

84. West, D.J. The risk of hepatitis B infection among health professionals in the United States: A review. *Am. J. Med. Sci.* 287:26, 1984.

85. Williams, W.W., Preblud, S.R., Reichelderfer, P.S., and Hadler, S.C. Vaccines of importance in the hospital setting. Problems and development. *Infect. Dis. Clin. North Am.* 3:701, 1989.

86. Wong, E.S., et al. Are universal precautions effective in reducing the number of occupational exposures among health care workers? A prospective study of physicians on a medical service. *J.A.M.A.* 265:1123, 1991.

87. Wormser, G.P., Rabkin, C.S., and Joline, C. Frequency of nosocomial transmission of HIV infection among health care workers. *N. Engl. J. Med.* 319:307, 1988.

Dialysis-Associated Infections and Their Control

Martin S. Favero
Miriam J. Alter
Lee A. Bland

In the last 25 years, knowledge and application of maintenance dialysis for patients with end-stage renal disease has increased dramatically. In 1967, approximately 1,000 patients were undergoing maintenance dialysis. In 1973, when Medicare included coverage of end-stage renal disease, approximately 11,000 patients were undergoing dialysis in private or hospital-based centers and in homes in the United States. In 1991, there were approximately 120,000 patients undergoing maintenance dialysis, and there were 30,000 staff members in more than 1,900 dialysis centers throughout the United States.

In the early 1960s, hemodialysis was used almost exclusively for the treatment of acute renal failure. Subsequently, the development of the arteriovenous shunt and certain other ancillary technologic advances in dialysis equipment allowed maintenance hemodialysis to become a common procedure. In the 1970s, the primary mode for dialysis treatment was hemodialysis performed with various types of artificial kidney machines. Subsequently, the use of peritoneal dialysis, accomplished by automated machines or by intermittent cycling, increased. In the last 10 years, continuous ambulatory peritoneal dialysis (CAPD) has become popular because patients can perform this procedure at home or while working and do not need lengthy dialysis treatments in a center. Approximately 15 percent of all dialysis patients currently are undergoing some form of peritoneal dialysis.

The purpose of this chapter is to describe the major infectious diseases that can be acquired in the hemodialysis center setting, the important epidemiologic and environmental microbiological considerations, and control procedures. Patients undergoing long-term dialysis have a compromised immune system and other disorders that make them more susceptible to infectious diseases. In addition, several noninfectious complications of dialysis are discussed.

Sources of Bacterial and Chemical Contaminants in Dialysis Systems
High Levels of Gram-Negative Bacteria in Hemodialysis Systems

Technical development and clinical use of hemodialysis delivery systems improved dramatically in the late 1960s and early 1970s. However, a number of microbiologic parameters were not taken into consideration in the design of many hemodialysis machines or their respective water supply systems. As a result, there are many procedural situations in which certain types of gram-negative water bacteria can persist and actively multiply in aqueous environments associated with hemodialysis equipment. This can result in the production of massive levels of gram-negative bacteria, which can directly or indirectly affect patients by septicemia or endotoxemia [20, 45, 46, 51].

In general, a hemodialysis system consists of a water supply, a system for mixing water and concentrated dialysis fluid, and a machine to pump the dialysis fluid through the artificial kidney. This kidney (*dialyzer*) is connected to the patient's circulatory system to remove waste products from the patient's blood. A number of factors can influence microbial contamination of fluids associated with hemodialysis systems (Table 19-1).

The gram-negative water bacteria can be significant contaminants in hemodialysis systems (Table 19-2), and virtually all disinfection strategies for fluid water distribution lines and dialysis machines are targeted to this group of bacteria. Gram-negative water bacteria are capable not only of surviving but also of multiplying rapidly in all types of waters, even those containing relatively small amounts of organic matter such as water treated by distillation, softening, de-ionization, or reverse osmosis. These organisms can attain levels ranging from 10^5 to 10^7 per milliliter of water and, under certain circumstances, can be a

health hazard for patients undergoing dialysis; they constitute a direct threat of septicemia, and they contain bacterial endotoxin (lipopolysaccharide) that can cause pyrogenic reactions [26, 46, 50, 51, 61]. It should be emphasized that virtually any gram-negative water bacterium that can grow in water systems represents a potential problem in a hemodialysis unit. These bacteria are able to adhere to surfaces and form biofilms or glycocalyx and are virtually impossible to eradicate [44, 50].

Gram-negative water bacteria are able to grow even more rapidly in treated water mixed with dialysis concentrate. This mixture results in dialysis fluid that is both a balanced salt solution and a growth medium almost as fertile as conventional nutrient broth [19, 20, 51]. Gram-negative water bacteria growing in distilled, de-ionized, or reverse osmosis–treated water can reach levels of 10^5 to 10^7 organisms per milliliter, but these cell populations are not visibly turbid. On the other hand, these same bacteria growing in dialysis fluids can achieve levels of 10^8 to 10^9 organisms per milliliter and are often associated with a noticeable turbidity.

Nontuberculous mycobacteria (see Table 19-2) also have the capability of multiplying in water. Although they do not contain bacterial endotoxin, they are comparatively resistant to chemical germicides and, as will be discussed later, have been responsible for patient infections as the result of inadequately disinfected dialyzers and peritoneal dialysis machines.

The strategy for controlling the potentially massive accumulation of gram-negative water bacteria and nontuberculous mycobacteria in dialysis systems primarily involves preventing their growth. This can be accomplished by proper disinfection of the water treatment system and the artificial kidney machines. Gram-negative water bacteria and their associated lipopolysaccharides (bacterial endotoxins) and nontuberculous mycobacteria ultimately come from the community water supply, and levels of these bacteria can be amplified depending on the water treatment sys-

Table 19-1.   Factors influencing microbial contamination in hemodialysis systems

Factors	*Comments*
Water supply	
Source of community water	
Groundwater	Contains endotoxin and bacteria
Surface water	Contains high levels of endotoxin and bacteria
Water treatment at dialysis center	
None	Not recommended
Filtration	
Prefilter	Particulate filter to protect equipment; does not remove microorganisms
Absolute filter (depth or membrane)	Removes bacteria but, unless changed frequently or disinfected, bacteria will accumulate and grow through filter; acts as significant reservoir of bacteria and endotoxin
Activated carbon filter	Removes organics and available chlorine or chloramine; significant reservoir of water bacteria and endotoxin
Water treatment devices	
Ion-exchange softener	Both softeners and de-ionizers are significant reservoirs of bacteria
De-ionization	and do not remove endotoxin
Reverse osmosis	Removes bacteria and endotoxin, but must be disinfected; operates at high water pressure
Ultraviolet light	Kills some bacteria, but there is no residual, and ultraviolet-resistant bacteria can develop
Ultrafilter	Removes bacteria and endotoxin; operates on normal line pressure; can be positioned distal to de-ionizer; must be disinfected
Water and dialysate distribution system	
Distribution pipes	
Size	Oversized diameter and length decrease fluid flow and increase bacterial reservoir for both treated water and centrally prepared dialysate
Construction	Rough joints, dead ends, and unused branches can act as bacterial reservoirs
Elevation	Outlet taps should be located at highest elevation to prevent loss of disinfectant
Storage tanks	Undesirable because they act as reservoir of water bacteria; if present, must be routinely scrubbed and disinfected
Dialysis machines	
Single-pass	Disinfectant should have contact with *all* parts of machine
Recirculating single-pass, or recirculating (batch)	Recirculating pumps and machine design allow for massive contamination levels if not properly disinfected. Overnight chemical germicide treatment recommended

Water Supply

tems, dialysate distribution systems, type of dialysis machine, and method of disinfection [24, 25] (see Table 19-1).

Dialysis centers use water from a public supply, which may be derived from either surface or ground waters. The source of the supply may be important in terms of bacterial endotoxin content, since surface sources frequently contain endotoxin from gram-negative water bacteria as well as certain types of blue-green algae. Endotoxin levels are not substantially reduced by conventional municipal water treatment processes and can be high enough to cause pyrogenic reactions in patients undergoing dialysis [60].

Essentially all water supplies are contami-

Table 19-2. Types of water microorganisms that have been found in dialysis systems

Gram-negative water bacteria
  Pseudomonas
  Flavobacterium
  Acinetobacter
  Alcaligenes
  Achromobacter
  Aeromonas
  Serratia
  Xanthomonas
Nontuberculous mycobacteria
  Mycobacterium chelonae
  M. fortuitum
  M. gordonae
  M. scrofulaceum
  M. kansasii
  M. avium
  M. intracellularis

nated with water bacteria, and consequently the water treatment and distribution systems and the dialysis machine are challenged repeatedly with continuous inoculation of these ubiquitous bacteria. Even adequately chlorinated water supplies commonly contain low levels of these microorganisms. Whereas chlorine and other disinfectants added to the city water may prevent high levels of contamination, the presence of these chemicals in dialysis fluids is undesirable because of adverse effects on patients being dialyzed [82]. Further, the dialysis water treatment systems described next effectively remove chlorine, allowing for the unrestricted growth of water microorganisms.

Water Treatment Systems

Water used for the production of dialysis fluid must be treated to remove chemical contaminants. The Association for the Advancement of Medical Instrumentation (AAMI) has published guidelines for the chemical and bacteriologic quality of water used to prepare dialysis fluid [11]. Depending on the area of the United States, a variety of different water treatment systems are used, but most of them are associated with amplification of water bacteria (see Table 19-1). The most common type of treatment is ion exchange using water softeners and de-ionizers. However, neither of these components removes endotoxins or

bacteria, and both provide sites of significant bacterial multiplication [79]. An effective means of treating water for dialysis currently in use is reverse osmosis. Reverse osmosis or de-ionization water treatment systems are used in 99 percent of the U.S. dialysis centers [4]. Reverse osmosis possesses the singular advantage of being able to remove both bacterial endotoxins and bacteria from supply water. However, low numbers of gram-negative and nontuberculous mycobacteria water bacteria can either penetrate this barrier or, by other means, colonize the downstream portion of the reverse osmosis unit. Consequently, reverse osmosis systems must be disinfected routinely.

There are a variety of filters ostensibly used to control bacterial contamination in water and dialysis fluids. Most of these are inadequate, especially if they are not routinely disinfected or changed frequently and disinfected. *Particulate filters,* commonly called *prefilters,* operate by depth filtration and do not remove bacteria or bacterial endotoxins. These filters can become colonized with gram-negative water bacteria, resulting in amplification of the levels of both bacteria and endotoxin in the filter effluent. *Absolute filters,* including the membrane types, temporarily remove bacteria from passing water. However, some of these filters tend to clog, and gram-negative water bacteria can "grow through" the filter matrix and colonize the downstream surface of the filters within a couple of days. Further, absolute filters do not reduce levels of endotoxin present in the effluent water. These types of filters should be changed regularly in accordance with the manufacturer's directions and disinfected in the same manner and at the same time as the dialysis system.

Activated carbon filters are used to remove certain organic chemicals and available chlorine from water, but they too significantly increase the level of water bacteria and do not remove bacterial endotoxins.

Ultraviolet (UV) irradiation is sometimes used to reduce bacterial contamination in water. However, this approach is not recommended [51], because certain populations of gram-negative water bacteria appear to be far more resistant to UV than others, resulting in instances in which significant numbers of bacteria survive theoretically adequate treatment. This problem is accentuated in recirculating dialysis systems where repeated exposures to UV are used to ensure adequate disinfection. Resistance to UV is enhanced because of the multiplication of those microorganisms surviving initial exposure. In addition, bacterial endotoxin is not affected.

As mentioned previously, an effective means of treating water for dialysis is by the correct use of reverse osmosis systems. We recommend using a water treatment system that produces chemically adequate water without massive levels of microbial contamination. Such a system is well suited for hard water and involves the following procedure [41]: Community-supplied water is subjected to prefilters (if necessary), softener, carbon filters, and a particulate filter, and is then passed through first a reverse osmosis unit and then a de-ionization unit. Through these phases, the water becomes progressively chemically pure, but the level of bacterial contamination increases. To compensate, an ultrafilter is included in the final step of the system to remove bacteria and bacterial endotoxins. The ultrafilter consists of similar types of membranes as in a reverse osmosis unit or it may have a polysulfone membrane, but it can be operated at ordinary water line pressure. This entire system can be augmented with other source water treatment devices depending on the chemical quality of the water in question. If this system is adequately disinfected, the microbial content of water should be well within the recommended guidelines discussed under the heading Dialysis Fluids Monitoring.

Distribution Systems

Dialysis centers use one of two general systems for delivering dialysis fluids to individual dialysis machines. In the first type, incoming supply water is treated and distributed to individual freestanding dialysis stations. At each station, the water is mixed with a dialysate concentrate by automatic proportioning. A second type of system, usually found in large dialysis centers, involves the automatic mixing of treated water and dialysate concentrate at a central location, followed by distribution of the warmed dialysis fluid through pipes to individual dialysis stations. In both designs, the distribution system consists of plastic pipes (usually polyvinyl chloride) and appurtenances.

These distribution systems can contribute to microbial contamination in two ways. They frequently use larger-diameter and longer pipes than are necessary to handle the required fluid flow. This slows the fluid velocity and increases both the total fluid volume and the wetted surface area of the system. Gram-negative bacteria in fluids remaining in pipes overnight multiply rapidly and colonize the wetted surfaces of the pipes, producing bacterial populations and endotoxin quantities in proportion to the volume and surface area. Such colonization results in formation of protective biofilm by the bacteria, which is difficult to remove and can protect the bacteria from disinfection [10].

Because pipes can constitute a source of water bacteria in a distribution system, routine disinfection should be performed at least weekly. To ensure that the disinfectant cannot drain from pipes by gravity before adequate contact time is achieved, distribution systems should be designed with the outlet taps at equal elevation and at the highest point of the system. Furthermore, the system should be free of rough joints, dead-end pipes, and unused branches and taps. Fluid trapped in such stagnant areas can serve as reservoirs of bacteria capable of continuously inoculating the entire volume of the system [72].

Incorporation of a storage tank in a distribution system greatly increases the volume of fluid and surface area available to act as reservoirs for the multiplication of water bacteria. Storage tanks should not be used in dialysis systems unless they are frequently drained and adequately disinfected, including scrubbing of the sides of the tank to remove bacterial biofilm. It is also recommended that an ultrafilter be used distal to the storage tank.

Types of Dialysis Systems

Currently in the United States, virtually all centers use single-pass dialysis machines. In the 1970s, most machines were of the recirculating or recirculating single-pass type. It was shown that by the nature of their design, the recirculating dialysis machines contributed to a relatively high level of gram-negative bacterial contamination in dialysis fluid. Single-pass dialysis machines tend to respond to adequate cleaning and disinfection procedures and, in general, have lower levels of bacterial contamination in their dialysis fluid than do recirculating machines. Levels of contamination in single-pass machines are dependent primarily on the bacteriologic quality of the incoming water and on the method of machine disinfection [46, 51].

A frequent error in disinfecting single-pass systems is introducing the disinfectant in the same manner and through the same port as the dialysate concentrate. By so doing, the pipes and tubing of the incoming water are not exposed to a disinfectant, and therefore an environment exists in which bacteria can readily colonize and proliferate, acting as a constant reservoir of contamination. For adequate disinfection of a single-pass system the disinfectant must reach all pertinent parts of the system's fluid pathways.

Types of Dialyzers

In most instances, the dialyzer (artificial kidney) does not contribute significantly to bacterial contamination of the dialysate. Currently, the majority of dialysis centers use hollow-fiber dialyzers rather than plate (parallel-flow) dialyzers, or coil dialyzers [2, 4], which tend not to amplify bacterial contamination in the dialysis systems. The majority of centers (67 percent) also reprocess dialyzers for reuse on the same patient, though improper reprocessing techniques have been the cause of bacteremia and pyrogenic reactions in dialysis patients. This will be discussed in the later section Infections Associated with Hemodialyzer Reuse.

Disinfection Procedures

The objective of a disinfection procedure for a dialysis system is to inactivate bacteria in the fluid pathways associated with the dialysis system and to prevent these organisms from growing to significant levels once the system is in operation. Routine disinfection of isolated components of a dialysis system frequently produces inadequate results in which the hazard to the patient persists. Consequently, the total dialysis system (water treatment system, distribution system, and dialysis machine) needs to be considered when selecting and applying disinfection procedures.

Chlorine-based disinfectants such as sodium hypochlorite solutions are convenient and effective in most parts of the dialysis system when used at the manufacturer's recommended concentration. Also, the test for residual available chlorine to confirm adequate rinsing is simple and sensitive. However, because of the corrosive nature of chlorine, the disinfectant is normally rinsed from the system after a short exposure time—usually 20 to 30 minutes. This practice commonly negates the disinfection procedure because the rinse water invariably contains gram-negative water bacteria that immediately resume multiplication. If permitted to stand overnight, the water will contain significant microbial contamination levels. Therefore, chlorine disinfectants are most effective when applied just before the start-up of the dialysis system rather than at the end of the daily operation. In some large centers where multiple shifts occur, it may be reasonable to use sodium hypochlorite disinfection between shifts (this may not be necessary with single-pass machines if the levels of bacterial contamination are within AAMI limits) and formaldehyde, peroxyacetic acid, or glutaraldehyde disinfection at the end of the day. The latter formulations are commercially available and are designed for use with dialysis machines.

Aqueous formaldehyde, peroxyacetic acid, or glutaraldehyde solutions can produce good disinfection results. They are not as corrosive as hypochlorite solutions and can be allowed to remain in the dialysis system for long periods when the system is not operational, thereby preventing the growth of bacteria in the system. Formaldehyde has good penetrating characteristics but is considered an environmental hazard and potential carcinogen and is also associated with irritating qualities that are objectionable to staff members. Commercial tests (e.g., Formalert, Organon Teknika, Durham, NC) are available that are sensitive for testing for formaldehyde in water at concentrations as low as 1 part per million (ppm). Commercially available glutaraldehyde-based disinfectants and a peroxyacetic acid disinfectant for dialysis systems, when used according to the manufacturer's recommendations, are not corrosive to machines and are good germicides [74, 83]. Furthermore, they are not associated with the irritating qualities and potential health and environmental hazards of formaldehyde.

Some dialysis systems use hot-water disinfection for the control of microbial contamination. In this type of system, water heated to greater than 80°C (176°F) is passed through all proportioning, distribution, and patient-monitoring devices before use. This system is excellent for controlling bacterial contamination.

Surveillance

Pyrogenic reactions and gram-negative sepsis are the most common complications associated with high levels of gram-negative bacterial contamination of dialysis fluid. The former probably results from either the passage of pyrogenic substances of bacterial origin, presumably endotoxins, across the dialysis membrane [54] or stimulation of cytokine production in the patient's blood by endotoxins in the dialysate [59], which most likely is attributable to direct infusion of bacteria into the bloodstream [61, 68].

The higher the level of bacteria and endotoxin in dialysis fluid, the higher the probability that bacteria or endotoxin will pass through the dialysis membrane. It has been shown in an outbreak of febrile reactions among patients undergoing dialysis that the attack rates were directly proportional to the level of bacterial contamination in the dialysis fluid [51].

In 1988, 15 percent of the hemodialysis centers in the United States reported pyrogenic reactions in patients undergoing dialysis [4]. An active surveillance system is essential for early detection and control of these complications. Clinical reactions should be defined as they occur, since this may be the first clue that a problem exists. In addition, the dialysis system should be bacteriologically monitored periodically by methods described later.

Patient Monitoring

Pyrogenic reactions in patients undergoing dialysis are associated with a characteristic set of signs and symptoms. Shaking chills, fever, and hypotension are the most common clinical manifestations. Depending on the type of dialysis system and the level of initial contamination, the onset of an elevated temperature and chills can occur 1 to 5 hours after the initiation of dialysis and usually are associated with a decrease in systolic blood pressure of 30 mm Hg or greater. Other less frequent but characteristic symptoms include headache, myalgia, nausea, and vomiting. We have defined a case of pyrogenic reaction as the onset of objective chills (visible rigors) or fever (oral temperature 37.8°C or higher [100°F]), or both in a patient who was afebrile (oral temperature up to 37.0°C [98.6°F]) and who had no signs or symptoms of infection before the dialysis treatment [58].

Differentiating gram-negative sepsis from a pyrogenic reaction can be difficult, since initially the signs and symptoms of the two are identical. The most reliable means of detecting sepsis is by culturing blood samples taken at the time of the reaction. However, since the results of these cultures take at least 18 to 24 hours to obtain and since therapy for sepsis should not be withheld for this length of time, other less reliable criteria must be used. Most pyrogenic reactions are not associated with bacteremia, and the preceding signs and symptoms generally abate within a few hours after dialysis has been stopped. With gram-negative sepsis, fever and chills may persist, and hypotension is more refractory to therapy [60, 61].

The early detection for pyrogenic reactions or gram-negative sepsis is dependent on the thorough understanding of signs and symptoms of these entities by the dialysis staff and on the careful charting of the patient's symptoms as well as changes in blood pressure and temperature. The following diagnostic procedures are recommended for those patients who meet the criteria of a pyrogenic reaction:

1. A thorough physical examination to rule out other causes of chills and fever (e.g., pneumonia, shunt or fistula infection, urinary tract infection)
2. Cultures of blood samples taken at the time of reactions and cultures of any additional body fluids or secretions indicated by the physical examination as likely sources of infection
3. Collection of dialysis fluid from the dialyzer (downstream side) for quantitative and qualitative bacteriologic assays

Dialysis Fluids Monitoring

In addition to disease surveillance, at least monthly bacteriologic assays of water and dialysis fluids should be performed. It has been recommended that the levels of microbial contamination in water used to prepare dialysis fluid not exceed 200 colony-forming units (cfu) per milliliter and that contamination levels not exceed 2,000 cfu/ml in dialysis fluids [11, 52] (Table 19-3). These particular numbers are based on bacteriologic assays during epidemiologic investigations [52]; they are not considered absolute and should be used as broad guidelines.

The bacteriologic assay is quantitative rather than qualitative, and a standard technique for enumeration should be used. Water samples should be collected at a point as close as possible to where water enters the dialysate-proportioning unit. Samples should be collected at least monthly. Repeat samples should be collected when bacteriologic counts

exceed 200 cfu/ml and after disinfection changes have been instituted. Dialysis fluid samples should be collected during or at the termination of dialysis close to that point where the dialysis fluid either enters or leaves the dialyzer. These types of samples should also be taken at least once monthly.

Samples should be assayed within 30 minutes, or refrigerated and assayed within 24 hours, of collection. Total viable counts (standard plate counts) are the objective of the assays, and conventional laboratory procedures such as the pour plate, spread plate, or membrane filter technique can be used; calibrated loops should not be used—they sample a small volume and are inaccurate. Trypticase soy agar is the culture medium of choice. Colonies should be counted after 48 hours of incubation at 35 to 37°C (95° to 98.6°F) [10a, 10b].

In the event of an outbreak investigation, the assay may need to be qualitative as well as quantitative, and there are some instances in which there might be a concern about NTM in water (see Table 19-2). In such cases, plates should be incubated for 5 to 14 days.

If centers reprocess dialyzers for reuse on the same patient, water used to rinse dialyzers and prepare dialyzer disinfectants also should be assayed at least monthly in the same manner as described previously. It is recommended that microbial or endotoxin contamination not exceed 200 cfu/ml or 1 ng (5 endotoxin units [EU])/ml, respectively (see Table 19-3) [12; 44].

Infections Associated with Peritoneal Dialysis

As mentioned earlier, the number of patients in the United States treated by peritoneal di-

Table 19-3. Microbiologic and endotoxin standards for dialysis fluids

Type of fluid	Bacteria		Endotoxin
Water used to prepare dialysate	<200 cfu/ml		No standard
Dialysate	<2,000 cfu/ml		No standard
Water used to rinse and reprocess dialyzers	<200 cfu/ml	*or*	<1 ng/ml
Water used to prepare dialyzer disinfectant	<200 cfu/ml	*or*	<1 ng/ml

alysis has increased significantly in the past few years, and CAPD especially has gained popularity. In peritoneal dialysis, the patient's peritoneal membrane is used to dialyze waste products from the patient's blood. In the mid-1970s, the development of automated peritoneal dialysis systems made intermittent peritoneal dialysis a viable alternative to hemodialysis for long-term management of patients with end-stage renal disease. Currently, this approach has been replaced by continuous cyclic peritoneal dialysis (CCPD), in which presterilized dialysis fluid is introduced by gravity into a patient's peritoneal cavity continuously and by CAPD. In CAPD, a plastic bag is filled with sterile dialysis fluid which is self-administered by the patient, who has a surgically implanted catheter. The exchanges are done every 4 hours, and the patient can be mobile between exchanges [70].

The most persistent problem in the management of patients treated by peritoneal dialysis is peritonitis [75]. Automated peritoneal dialysis machines must be cleaned and maintained properly to prevent the growth of pathogenic microorganisms that cause this infection. The machines are designed to sterilize and desalinate large quantities of tap water for subsequent mixture with a dialysate concentrate. Theoretically, the incidence of peritonitis should be reduced because the machine functions as a closed system. However, the automated peritoneal dialysis machines may themselves provide a reservoir for pathogens that may cause peritonitis. Several outbreaks of bacterial peritonitis among patients receiving intermittent peritoneal dialysis have been reported, and the etiologic agents have included *Mycobacterium chelonae*–like organisms and *Pseudomonas cepacia* [13, 16]. Both organisms are capable of growing in water, and the investigation of these outbreaks revealed that machines were inadequately cleaned and disinfected, and the product water and dialysis fluid contained the microorganisms responsible for peritonitis [73]. In addition, one group of organisms— the nontuberculous mycobacteria such as *M. chelonae*—are significantly and extraordinarily resistant to the commonly used disinfectants [27]. Berkelman and colleagues [15]

have recommended a set of guidelines that can ensure the production of sterile dialysis fluid and reduce the likelihood of outbreaks of peritonitis for dialysis centers using automated peritoneal dialysis machines. The precise details and protocols differ with each machine type, and the reader is referred to the guidelines for a more complete discussion [15]. Clinical symptoms suggestive of peritoneal infection usually appear 12 to 36 hours after bacterial contamination of the peritoneal cavity. Clinical symptoms include nausea, vomiting, and abdominal pain. Later, vague abdominal tenderness may progress to severe, diffuse, or localized pain associated with fever, abdominal distention, and gastrointestinal dysfunction. The clinical diagnosis should be confirmed by bacteriologic analysis of the peritoneal fluid. Cloudy peritoneal fluid is often the first sign suggestive of infection.

The etiologic agents of peritonitis associated with conventional peritoneal dialysis are usually *Staphylococcus epidermidis* and other gram-positive bacteria, which collectively account for 56 to 78 percent, whereas 12 to 35 percent involve gram-negative organisms such as Enterobacteriaceae, *Pseudomonas aeruginosa*, *P. cepacia*, and *Acinetobacter* species and, in a few cases (less than 10 percent) fungi, yeast, mycobacteria, and anaerobic bacteria. Approximately 15 to 20 percent of cases will be culture-negative [70, 84]. The primary control procedure for peritonitis in this setting is to prevent contamination of the dialysis fluid that enters the peritoneal cavity. This involves (1) aseptic manipulation of the sterile, disposable plastic lines leading into the abdominal catheter, which deliver the dialysis fluid into the peritoneal cavity, and (2) a system for aseptic connection of the sterile dialysis fluid and the patient's catheter.

Infections Associated with Hemodialyzer Reuse

In the early 1960s, the most common dialyzer used in dialysis centers was the Kiil plate dialyzer, which was cleaned and disinfected after each patient use and supplied with a new set of cuprophane membranes. The dialyzer housing, however, was reused each time. With the development of disposable coil and hollow-fiber dialyzers, use of the Kiil dialyzer was discontinued. Disposable dialyzers are medical devices that are supplied in a sterile state and are intended for one-time use. In recent years, as a cost-saving effort, more centers are reusing dialyzers on the same patient after employing an appropriate disinfection procedure. Though it has caused some controversy, this is now standard practice. From 1976 to 1983, the percentage of dialysis centers that reported reuse of disposable dialyzers increased from 18 to 52 percent [5]. This percentage has continued to increase and, in 1988, 67 percent of centers reported that they reused disposable dialyzers; these centers represent 72 percent of dialysis patients. In 1988, the average number of times a dialysis center reused dialyzers was 11 (range, 2 to 50). The mean number of times a disposable dialyzer was *ever* reused was 28 (range, 3 to 131). Dialysis centers most likely to report reuse of dialyzers were those with larger patient populations (more than 40), those located in freestanding facilities, and those operated for profit, compared with centers with smaller patient populations, those located in hospitals, and those not operated for profit [4].

In 1986, the U.S. Public Health Service (PHS) subsumed the AAMI's guidelines for reusing hemodialyzers [12] and recommended these as PHS guidance to the Health Care Financing Administration (HCFA), which in turn made them conditions for participation in Medicare/Medicaid. In effect, the AAMI guidelines, which became PHS guidance, resulted in HCFA regulations. In general, if the procedures involved in reprocessing hemodialyzers are performed according to established and strict protocols, there do not appear to be harmful effects on patients. However, the practice of reusing disposable hemodialyzers should not be considered risk-free. In the last 10 years, outbreaks of patient infections and pyrogenic reactions associated with user error have occurred. Many of these episodes were the result of inadequate reprocessing procedures,

such as the use of incorrect concentrations of chemical germicides and failure to maintain standards for water quality [55]. In addition, in 1986 six dialysis centers reported outbreaks of pyrogenic reactions and septicemia that were associated with the use of a new germicide the active ingredient of which was chlorine dioxide. That germicide, although efficacious for disinfecting dialyzers, appeared to degrade the integrity of cellulosic dialyzer membranes to such an extent that leaks in the membrane developed [32, 68]. Centers that reported using this germicide employed manual reprocessing systems, and most of these centers reused their dialyzers more than 20 times.

In each of 3 successive years (1985–1988), reprocessing dialyzers in a manual reprocessing system was shown consistently to be significantly associated with a higher reported frequency of pyrogenic reactions, even with the use of other germicides, and was not necessarily related to the absolute number of reuses [2–4]. We believe that dialyzer membrane defects may go undetected when manual reprocessing systems are used, because testing for dialyzer membrane integrity, such as by an air-pressure leak test, is generally not performed with this type of system [18]. It is emphasized that adverse reactions associated with reuse of dialyzers are accentuated in dialysis centers that are having problems and that, for the most part, only a small number of centers are experiencing an increased risk with dialyzers that are reused more than 20 times or that include a manual reprocessing system.

The procedures used in dialysis centers for reprocessing hemodialyzers cannot be classified as sterilization procedures but rather constitute high-level disinfection [44]. In 1983, most centers in the United States used 2% aqueous formaldehyde with a contact time of approximately 36 hours for high-level disinfection of disposable dialyzers [4, 5]. Although this procedure may be satisfactory against the presumed microbiologic challenge of gram-negative water bacteria, it is inadequate for the highly germicide-resistant nontuberculous mycobacteria (see Table 19-2).

The CDC investigated an outbreak of infections caused by nontuberculous mycobacteria during which 27 cases of infection occurred among 140 patients [21]. The source of the nontuberculous mycobacteria appeared to be the water used in processing the dialyzers. It was evident that 2% formaldehyde did not effectively inactivate populations of these mycobacteria within 36 hours. It was subsequently shown that 4% formaldehyde with a minimum contact time of 24 hours can inactivate high numbers of nontuberculous mycobacteria and, as a consequence, 4% formaldehyde is recommended as a minimum solution for disinfection of dialyzers [17, 40, 44].

We would point out however, that the use of formaldehyde for reprocessing dialyzers is considered environmentally hazardous to patients and staff members and that this disinfectant is a chemical solution obtained from chemical supply houses rather than a formulation specifically designed for dialyzer disinfection. A number of chemical germicides specifically formulated for this purpose have been shown to be effective and are approved by the Food and Drug Administration (FDA) and the Environmental Protection Agency (EPA) for reprocessing hemodialyzers.

A similar outbreak of systemic mycobacterial infections in 5 dialysis patients, resulting in 2 deaths, occurred when high-flux dialyzers were contaminated with mycobacteria during manual reprocessing and were then disinfected with a commercial dialyzer disinfectant prepared at a concentration that did not ensure complete inactivation of mycobacteria [65]. These two outbreaks of infection in dialysis patients emphasize the need to use dialyzer disinfectants at concentrations that are effective against the more chemically resistant microorganisms such as mycobacteria.

Pyrogenic reactions in dialysis patients, caused by reprocessing dialyzers with water that did not meet AAMI standards (see Table 19-3), have been a factor frequently associated with epidemics investigated by the CDC. In most cases, the water used to rinse dialyzers or to prepare dialyzer disinfectants exceeded AAMI microbial or endotoxin standards because the water distribution system was not disinfected on a frequent basis or the disinfectant was improperly prepared.

Table 19-4 summarizes approximately 20 epidemic investigations of nonviral hemodialysis-associated diseases, giving a brief description, cause of the outbreak, and the primary correction measures recommended.

Acute allergic reactions are a recently recognized problem associated with reused dialyzers; they have occurred in several dialysis centers across the United States [35]. Reactions occurred within 10 minutes of initiating dialysis in patients using reprocessed dialyzers and were characterized by symptoms that included a sensation of warmth, fullness in the mouth and throat, tingling paresthesia, nausea and vomiting, and tightness in the chest. Reactions have not been associated with a specific dialyzer or dialyzer disinfectant.

Infections Associated with High-Flux Dialysis

High-flux dialysis is a very efficient hemodialysis treatment that uses dialyzer membranes with hydraulic permeabilities five to ten times greater than conventional dialyzer membranes. By using highly permeable membranes in dialyzers that have larger membrane surface areas than conventional dialyzers, dialysis treatment times can be dramatically reduced from 4 to 5 hours to 2 to 3 hours. In 1988, 23 percent of the hemodialysis centers in the United States reported using high-flux dialyzer membranes [4]. Because high-flux membranes are so permeable, there is concern that bacteria or endotoxin in the dialysate may penetrate these membranes, causing pyrogenic reactions in the patient. It is also a concern that high-flux dialysis requires the use of bicarbonate dialysate which, unlike the acetate-based dialysate used almost exclusively since the 1970s, is prepared from a concentrate that can support rapid bacterial growth and endotoxin production. Acetate dialysate is prepared from a single concentrate with such a high salt molarity (4.8 M) that most bacteria cannot grow in it. Bicarbo-

Table 19-4. Epidemic investigations by the Centers for Disease Control of nonviral hemodialysis-associated diseases

Description (Reference)	Cause(s) of Outbreak	Corrective Measure(s) Recommended
Microbial and chemical contamination of dialysis fluids		
Pyrogenic reactions in 49 patients [60]	Untreated city water contained high levels of endotoxin	Install reverse osmosis system
Pyrogenic reactions in 45 patients [72]	Inadequate disinfection of dialysis fluid distribution system	Increase frequency of disinfection and disinfectant contact time
Pyrogenic reactions in 14 patients; 2 bacteremias; 1 death [46]	Reverse osmosis water storage tank heavily contaminated with gram-negative bacteria	Remove storage tank from system
Fluoride intoxication of 8 patients; 1 death [29]	Overfluoridated city water treated by dialysis center with de-ionization only	Install reverse osmosis system
Hemolytic anemia in 41 patients [82]	Carbon filter insufficient for fluid flow; chloramines in city water not removed completely	Larger carbon filters connected in series; monitor chloramines after each patient shift
Decreased hemoglobin in 3 pediatric patients [56]	Disinfectant not properly rinsed from fluid distribution system	Thoroughly rinse germicide from system after disinfection; test for residual germicide
Severe hypotension in 9 patients [57]	Dialysate contaminated with sodium azide used as preservative in new ultrafilters	Rinse system after modification or installation of new components
Acute and chronic aluminum intoxication in 27 patients [30]	Exhausted de-ionization tanks unable to remove aluminum from city water	Monitor performance of de-ionization tanks; install reverse osmosis system
Acute formaldehyde intoxication in 5 patients; 1 death [36]	Disinfectant not properly rinsed from fluid distribution system	Modify fluid distribution system to eliminate stagnant flow areas; test for residual germicide after rinse completed
Incorrect concentration of disinfectant		
Mycobacterial infections in 27 patients [21]	Inadequate concentration of dialyzer disinfectant	Increase formaldehyde dialyzer disinfectant concentration to 4%
Gram-negative bacteremia and pyrogenic reactions in 6 patients [31]	Dialyzer disinfectant diluted to improper concentration	Use disinfectant at recommended dilution and verify concentration

Outbreak	Cause	Corrective action
Mycobacterial infection in 5 high-flux dialysis patients; 2 deaths [65]	Inadequate concentration of dialyzer disinfectant	Use greater concentration of disinfectant; more frequent disinfection of water treatment system
Gram-negative bacteremia and pyrogenic reactions in 6 patients [14]	Inadequate mixing of dialyzer disinfectant	Thoroughly mix disinfectant and verify proper concentration
Inappropriate dialyzer disinfectant		
Gram-negative bacteremia in 33 patients at 2 centers [32, 68]	Holes in dialyzer membrane caused by chlorine dioxide–based dialyzer disinfectant	Charge type of disinfectant (disinfectant withdrawn from marketplace by manufacturer)
Errors in dialyzer reprocessing		
Pyrogenic reactions in 3 high-flux dialysis patients [33]	Dialyzer reprocessed with 2 disinfectants; microbial and endotoxin levels of reprocessing water exceeded AAMI standards	Do not disinfect dialyzers with multiple germicides; disinfect water treatment system more frequently
Pyrogenic reactions in 14 high-flux dialysis patients; 1 death [34]	Dialyzers rinsed with city water containing high levels of endotoxin; dialyzers not filled completely with disinfectant; incorrect concentration of dialyzer disinfectant	Do not rinse or clean dialyzers with city water; completely fill dialyzers with disinfectant of proper concentration
Pyrogenic reactions in 18 patients [55]	Dialyzers rinsed with city water containing high levels of endotoxin; microbial and endotoxin levels in reprocessing water exceeded AAMI standards	Do not rinse or clean dialyzers with city water; disinfect water treatment system more frequently
Pyrogenic reactions during high-flux dialysis (CDC: unpublished data)	Dialyzers rinsed with city water; microbial levels in reprocessing water exceeded AAMI standards	Do not rinse or clean dialyzers with city water; disinfect water treatment system more frequently
Allergic reactions of unknown etiology		
Acute allergic reactions in hundreds of patients in at least 31 centers; reactions occur within 10 minutes in patients reusing dialyzers [35]	No cause has been identified; may be related to chemicals used in cleaning dialyzer or inadequate rinsing of germicide prior to dialyzer reuse	No specific recommendation made at this time

AAMI = Association for the Advancement of Medical Instrumentation; CDC = Centers for Disease Control.

nate dialysate, however, must be prepared from two concentrates, an acid concentrate with a pH of 2.8 that is not conducive to bacterial growth and a bicarbonate concentrate with a relatively neutral pH and a salt molarity of 1.2 M. Because the bicarbonate concentration will support rapid bacterial growth and endotoxin production [19], its use can increase bacterial and endotoxin concentrations in the dialysate and, theoretically, may contribute to an increase in pyrogenic reactions, especially when it is used during high-flux dialysis. Some of this concern may be justified. A significant association ($p < .05$) between high-flux dialysis and pyrogenic reactions, compared with conventional dialysis, has been reported [4]. In addition, of those centers that used bicarbonate dialysate, a higher frequency of pyrogenic reactions was reported only in centers that also performed high-flux dialysis. In contrast to these findings, a prospective study of pyrogenic reactions in patients receiving more than 27,000 conventional, high-efficiency, or high-flux dialysis treatments with a bicarbonate dialysate containing high concentrations of bacteria and endotoxin found no association ($p = .12$) between pyrogenic reactions and the type of dialysis treatment [58]. Although there seem to be conflicting data on the relationship between high-flux dialysis and pyrogenic reactions, centers providing high-flux dialysis should be especially mindful of ensuring that dialysate meets AAMI microbial standards (see Table 19-3).

Dialysis Dementia

Dialysis encephalopathy or dialysis dementia is a disorder that affects dialysis patients who, for a variety of reasons, are subjected to water that has a relatively high amount of aluminum, such as community water supplies treated with alum. This complication was first described in 1972 by Alfrey and co-workers [1], and the role of aluminum as a significant contributing factor in this disorder was shown by Schreeder and associates [76] in an epidemiologic study. Case definitions of dialysis encephalopathy include three different groups of objective findings:

1. Speech impairment (stuttering, stammering, dysnomia, hypofluency, mutism)
2. Seizure disorder (generalized tonic-clonic, focal, or multifocal seizures)
3. Motor disturbance (myoclonic jerks, motor apraxia, immobility)

Schreeder's group [76] showed that patients were at increased risk of dialysis dementia when the aluminum content of water used to prepare dialysate was high (greater than 100 ng/L). The number of cases of dialysis dementia reported in 1988 to the Centers for Disease Control (CDC) was 207, an incidence of 0.2 percent. The case fatality rate was 25 percent [4].

The incidence of dialysis dementia reported by hemodialysis centers to the CDC has decreased from 0.4 percent in the years 1980 and 1983–1985 to 0.2 percent in 1988 [4]. Although it is not clear what has been responsible for this decrease, we believe it may be related to increased awareness in the dialysis community of the requirement of good water treatment systems. In 1980, only 26 percent of hemodialysis centers in the United States reported that they employed a reverse osmosis system, either alone or with de-ionization in their water treatment systems. By 1988, 91 percent of the centers were using reverse osmosis alone or in combination with de-ionization as an integral part of their water treatment system [4]. The control of dialysis dementia revolves around adequate water treatment systems and invariably requires the use of reverse osmosis, either alone or with de-ionization [76].

Toxic Reactions

In some instances, chemicals in water or as residual in dialysis systems adversely affect dialyzing patients. Certain chemicals in water may not be toxic when ingested by humans, but the hemodialysis patient may be exposed directly to 150 liters of water per treatment. A few examples will illustrate this problem.

Occasionally, suppliers of community water change water disinfection patterns by increasing chlorine dosages or using chloramines. These changes usually occur without the knowledge of the dialysis staff. Chloramines in water used to prepare dialysis fluid must be removed, or the patient will experience acute hemolysis. If the correct water treatment system (activated carbon) is not present or operating in the dialysis center, patients will be exposed to this chemical. In one instance, a dialysis center changed from acetate to bicarbonate dialysate, adding an additional reverse osmosis unit and tanks for preparation and dilution of the dialysate. No changes were made to increase the capacity of the carbon filter and, within a few weeks, approximately 100 of the center's dialysis patients were exposed to chloramine-contaminated dialysate when the undersized carbon filters failed. A total of 41 patients required transfusion to treat hemolytic anemia caused by the chloramine exposure [82].

Another example of chemical intoxication occurred when a city water treatment plant accidentally fed excessive levels of fluoride into the community water supply, resulting in the death of one dialysis patient and acute illness in several other patients in a hemodialysis center receiving this community water supply. The center's water treatment system was not adequate to remove excessive fluoride from water [29].

In both of the preceding examples, a properly configured water treatment system consisting of adequate carbon filtration for the fluid flow and volume plus the use of reverse osmosis, de-ionization, and ultrafiltration would have prevented toxic reactions.

There have also been instances in which a disinfectant such as formaldehyde was not sufficiently removed from dialysis systems, and patients were exposed to the chemical. This can be prevented by monitoring the system for complete rinsing using a chemical assay sensitive to the chemical. A summary of

toxic reactions in hemodialysis patients that have been investigated by the CDC is given in Table 19-4.

Viral Hepatitis

Hepatitis B virus (HBV) has historically been a risk for dialysis patients as well as hemodialysis staff members. Consequently, in addition to the conventional barrier precautions to prevent infection transmission, several extra precautions are recommended (see Chap. 11). These include routinely testing all patients and staff members for hepatitis B surface antigen (HBsAg), providing patients identified as HBsAg-positive with dialysis in separate areas with the use of separate dedicated dialysis machines, and not including HBsAg-positive patients in dialyzer reuse programs. In contrast, infection control strategies for patients infected with hepatitis C virus (HCV) or human immunodeficiency virus (HIV) include only conventional barrier precautions or what are known as *universal precautions* to prevent transmission (see Chap. 11). Since HBV is the most efficiently transmitted bloodborne virus in the dialysis setting, long-standing precautions developed for its control will be described and used as a model, in part, for the prevention of transmission of other bloodborne infections, such as HCV and HIV.

A concomitant of the large increase in the number of dialysis centers, patients, and staff members in the United States was the realization that viral hepatitis can be a major complication of maintenance hemodialysis. The CDC, which has been conducting surveillance of viral hepatitis in dialysis centers since 1969, reported that in the period between 1972 and 1974, the incidence of HBsAg positivity among patients and staff increased by more than 100 percent to 6.2 and 5.2 percent, respectively [78]. In a separate survey of 15 hemodialysis centers during the same 2-year period, Szmuness and colleagues [80, 81] showed that the point prevalence of HBsAg was 16.8 percent among patients and 2.4 percent among staff. This time period correlated with a significant increase in the number of dialysis centers, patients, and staff members resulting from the federal government's decision to pay for treatment of patients with end-stage renal disease.

In 1977, the CDC issued recommendations for the control of HBV infection in dialysis centers that centered around serologic and disease surveillance of the patients and staff members and separation of HBsAg-positive patients from susceptible patients [28]. Continued nationwide surveillance by the CDC found that by 1983 the incidence of HBV infection had declined to 0.5 percent among both patients and staff (Figs. 19-1, 19-2) [8a]. Over the same time period, the proportion of centers using separation practices increased significantly from 75 percent to 86 percent, and the proportion of centers that screened patients monthly for HBsAg increased from 57 percent to 84 percent. In addition, the risk of acquiring hepatitis B for patients was shown to be highest in those centers that provided dialysis to HBsAg-positive patients but did not separate these patients by room and machine. Other investigators also have shown that segregation of HBsAg-positive patients and their equipment reduces the incidence of HBV infection in hemodialysis units [66, 69]. The success of separation practices in preventing the transmission of HBV can be linked to other control recommendations, including frequent serologic surveillance. Routine serologic surveillance facilitates the rapid identification of patients converting to HBsAg-positive, which allows for the rapid implementation of isolation procedures before cross-infection can occur.

There have also been outbreaks of dialysis-associated non-A, non-B hepatitis [53, 69a]. Primary or reactivated infections with such viruses as herpes virus, Epstein-Barr virus, and cytomegalovirus have been observed in renal transplant recipients and other immunologically suppressed persons (see Chap. 38) [38, 64], but they are not considered as important in dialysis centers as HBV. Viral hepatitis type A, which is spread by the fecal-oral

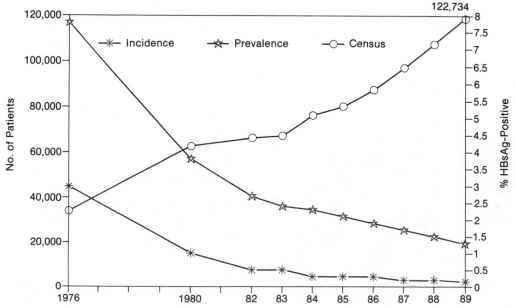

Fig. 19-1   Incidence and prevalence of HBsAg in hemodialysis patients, United States.

route and rarely by blood, has not been reported to occur in hemodialysis units.

Modes of Transmission

A person who is in the acute phase of HBV infection or is a chronic carrier of HBsAg and is also positive for hepatitis B e antigen (HBcAg) has an extraordinary level of HBV circulating in blood—approximately 10^8 per milliliter. With virus titers this high, body fluids containing serum or blood may also contain appreciable levels of HBV [48]. Blood can be diluted until it is no longer visible or chemically detectable and may still contain 10^2 to 10^3 infectious HBV per milliliter. Furthermore, HBV is relatively stable in the environment and has been shown to remain viable for at least 7 days on environmental surfaces at room temperature [22]. Thus, in environments where there is a good deal of blood exposure, a high risk of HBV transmission can exist if proper control measures are not practiced. This is especially true in a hemodialysis center setting.

In the past, HBV infection could be acquired by patients in a dialysis unit by transfusion of infectious blood or blood products. This is very unlikely now since all blood is screened for HBsAg and antibody to hepatitis B core antigen (anti-HBc). Dialysis patients, once infected, frequently become chronic asymptomatic HBsAg carriers who, in turn, become sources of HBV contamination for many environmental surfaces. Indeed, during the early 1970s, HBV infection in dialysis units tended to become endemic because of the presence of chronic carriers who were asymptomatic, the absence of sufficient disease and serologic surveillance systems to detect these carriers, and the lack of infection control measures to prevent transmission.

Given the extraordinarily high level of HBV in blood, one can categorize the various modes of HBV transmission, based on efficiency, as follows [48]:

1. Direct percutaneous inoculation by needle of contaminated serum or plasma

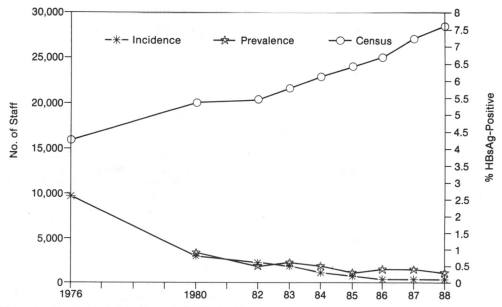

Fig. 19-2 Incidence and prevalence of HBsAg in hemodialysis staff, United States.

2. Percutaneous transfer of infected serum or plasma, such as may occur through cuts, scratches, abrasions, or other breaks in the skin
3. Introduction of infected serum or plasma onto mucosal surfaces such as may occur through inadvertent introduction of these materials into the mouth or eyes
4. Introduction of other known infectious secretions, such as saliva and peritoneal fluid, onto mucosal surfaces
5. Indirect transfer of serum or plasma via inanimate environmental surfaces

No epidemiologic evidence exists to suggest airborne transmission of HBV [71], and no disease transmission occurs by the intestinal route. Splashes of infectious blood that enter the oral cavity may result in HBV infection because the virus enters the vascular system through the buccal cavity but not the intestinal tract.

Various routes of HBV transmission can occur in hemodialysis units (Table 19-5). Staff members may become infected with HBV through accidental needle punctures or breaks in their skin or mucous membranes. These staff members have frequent and continuous contact with blood and blood-contaminated surfaces. Dialysis patients may acquire HBV infection in several ways, including (1) internally contaminated dialysis equipment, such as venous pressure gauges or venous pres-

sure isolators or filters (used to prevent reflux of blood into gauges) that are not routinely changed after each use; (2) injections (if the site of injection is contaminated with HBV); and (3) breaks in the skin or mucous membranes when in contact with blood-contaminated objects.

There is no epidemiologic documentation that HBV has been transmitted from infected hemodialysis staff members to dialysis patients. Hypothetically, this route of transmission is possible but not likely, because infectious blood and body fluids of dialysis personnel are not readily accessible to patients. However, dialysis staff members may physically carry HBV from infected patients to susceptible patients by means of contaminated hands, gloves, and other objects.

Environmental surfaces in the hemodialysis center may play a role in HBV transmission. It has been shown that HBsAg, which can be considered a footprint of HBV, can be detected on environmental surfaces (especially those often touched) in dialysis center settings [49]. For example, HBsAg has been detected on clamps, scissors, dialysis machine control knobs, doorknobs, and other surfaces. If these surfaces or objects are not cleaned or disinfected frequently and are shared among patients using the same or neighboring machines, an almost unnoticeable infection transmission route is created. Although dialysis staff members may rou-

Table 19-5. Routes of hepatitis B transmission in hemodialysis centers

Route	*Comment*
Transfused blood and blood products to patient	Uncommon for hepatitis B due to HBsAg screening; possible for transmission of non-A, non-B hepatitis
Patient to staff member	Transmitted by needle sticks—inapparent percutaneous exposure
Patient to dialysis system to staff member	Transmitted by HBV-contaminated blood on devices, tubes, and environmental surfaces
Patient to dialysis system external surfaces to staff member hands to another patient	Frequently touched dialysis machines or associated environmental surfaces may be reservoirs of HBV; transmitted by staff with contaminated gloves or hands
Staff member to patient	Has never been reported in a dialysis center

HBsAg = hepatitis B surface antigen; HBV = hepatitis B virus.

tinely change gloves after caring for each patient, a new pair of gloves can become contaminated when the staff member touches surfaces previously contaminated with blood from an HBsAg-positive patient. HBV can be transmitted from patient to patient when a staff member, wearing the contaminated gloves, searches for the patient's best site of injection by applying finger pressure or by contaminating that site before injection. The proper procedure here is for a staff member, when donning a pair of new gloves, to refrain from touching any environmental surfaces before performing the injection on the patient.

It is this mode of disease transmission, rather than any phenomenon dealing with internal contamination of dialysis machines, that is the rationale for separating HBsAg-positive patients.

Infection Control Strategies in Dialysis Centers
Surveillance

Routine surveillance of HBsAg and antibody to HBsAg (anti-HBs) should be performed in a dialysis center as part of a comprehensive surveillance and control program to determine whether transmission of HBV is occurring. This surveillance can identify patients and staff as potential sources of infection (i.e., HBsAg-positive), as immune (anti-HBs-positive), or as susceptible (negative for HBsAg and anti-HBs). Patients and staff members should be screened for HBsAg and anti-HBs when they enter the unit to determine their serologic status. HBsAg positivity in staff members does not preclude employment in a dialysis center; disease transmission from dialysis staff members to patients has not been reported, and these individuals may be assigned to care for any patient.

Since 1977, it has been recommended that dialysis patients be tested monthly for HBsAg, alanine aminotransferase, and aspartate aminotransferase, and at least once every 3 months for anti-HBs. At that time, it was also recommended that seronegative staff be tested every 3 months for HBsAg and anti-HBs. With the decline in the incidence of HBV

infection among both dialysis patients and staff, and with the availability of safe and effective hepatitis B vaccines, which are recommended for all susceptible patients and staff [8], these screening strategies have been updated [67], and the following are offered as recommendations:

1. All susceptible patients and staff should receive hepatitis B vaccine (see Table 19-7) (see Chap. 3).
2. Dialysis patients and staff members should continue to be screened for HBsAg and anti-HBs when they enter the center for treatment or employment, respectively. Patients and staff can be identified as either infected (HBsAg-positive), immune (anti-HBs-positive), or susceptible (negative for HBsAg or anti-HBs). Susceptible patients and staff who have not yet received hepatitis B vaccine, are in the process of being vaccinated, or have not adequately responded to vaccination should continue to be tested regularly for HBsAg and anti-HBs (Table 19-6). Susceptible patients should be tested once monthly for HBsAg as previously recommended, but the frequency of anti-HBs testing may be decreased to semiannually. Susceptible staff members should be tested for both HBsAg and anti-HBs on a semiannual basis. The frequency of testing patients and staff who become infected with HBV (positive for HBsAg and IgM anti-HBc) should be based on clinical indications. Only when these persons become HBsAg-negative should they be tested for anti-HBs. Patients and staff who remain HBsAg-positive for 6 months or longer should continue to be tested annually for HBsAg since a small percentage of HBsAg carriers may become HBsAg-negative.
3. Unvaccinated patients found to have anti-HBs on two consecutive tests at a level of at least 10 milli-international units (mIU)/mL need be tested only annually to verify their immune status. If anti-HBs levels decrease to less than 10 mIU/mL, such persons should be considered susceptible and should be vaccinated.

Table 19-6. Recommendations for serologic surveillance in chronic hemodialysis centers

Vaccination and serologic status	Frequency of HBsAg screening		Frequency of anti-HBs screening	
	Patients	Staff	Patients	Staff
Unvaccinated				
Susceptible	Monthly	Semiannually	Semiannually	Semiannually
HBsAg carrier	Annually	Annually	None	None
Anti-HBs-positive*	None	None	Annually	None
Vaccinees				
Anti-HBs-positive	None	None	Annually	None
Low level or no anti-HBs	Monthly	Semiannually	Semiannually	Semiannually

HBsAg = hepatitis B surface antigen; anti-HBs = antibody to HBsAg.
*At least 10 mIU/mL.

4. Staff members who are found to have anti-HBs on two consecutive tests at a level of at least 10 mIU/mL are considered immune and do not need any further routine testing for anti-HBs.
5. Patients and staff who are in the process of receiving hepatitis B vaccine but have not received the complete series should continue to be routinely screened as susceptible.
6. Patients who are initially positive for anti-HBs as a result of vaccination but in whom the level of anti-HBs becomes undetectable should receive a booster dose of the hepatitis B vaccine; staff members who have an adequate response to the vaccine, however, need no further routine testing or booster doses even in the absence of detectable anti-HBs.

Tables 19-6 and 19-7 describe the recommendations for serologic surveillance in hemodialysis centers and the hepatitis B vaccine doses and schedules for adults, respectively. Screening for patients who are infected with HIV, HCV, or delta hepatitis is not necessary for purposes of infection control, but these infections are each discussed in their respective sections later.

Many commercially available tests can be used to assay for various markers of HBV infection. Besides HBsAg and anti-HBs, there are tests for the assay of anti-HBc and for HBcAg and its antibody (anti-HBc). It should be kept in mind that major infection control decisions in dialysis centers are associated almost exclusively with the HBsAg and anti-HBs status of patients. Consequently, other serologic tests are not necessary for infection control purposes.

The infection control staff or the director of the dialysis center should be sure that the most sensitive test methods available for HBsAg and anti-HBs are used. These tests are commercially available and are primarily methods of RIA or EIA.

Record Keeping

As part of the surveillance system, the infection control staff should ensure that the patient's dialysis records are properly kept. These should include the lot number of all blood and blood products used, all mishaps such as blood leaks and blood spills and dialysis machine malfunctions, the location name or number of the dialysis machine used for each dialysis session, and the names of staff members who connect and disconnect the patient to and from a machine. In addition, a log should be maintained to record all hepatitis serologic results. Another log should contain records of all accidental needle punctures and similar accidents sustained by staff members and patients and should include time, place, patient and staff involved, and prophylactic measures if any were taken.

Table 19-7.   Recommended doses and schedules of currently licensed hepatitis B vaccines for adults

	Vaccine	
Group	*Recombivax HB[a]*	*Engerix-B[a,b]*
Dialysis patients	40 μg (1 ml)[c]	40 μg (2 ml)[d]
Healthy adults older than 19 yr	10 μg (1 ml)	20 μg (1 ml)

[a] Usual schedule: three doses at 0, 1, and 6 months.
[b] Alternative schedule: four doses at 0, 1, 2, and 12 months.
[c] Special formulation for dialysis patients.
[d] Two 1.0-ml doses given at one site, in a four-dose schedule at 0, 1, 2, and 6 months.

Specific Infection Control Recommendations

Patients who are HBsAg-positive should be dialyzed in a separate room designated only for HBsAg-positive patients. If this is impossible, they should be separated from hepatitis B seronegative patients in an area removed from the mainstream of activity and should be dialyzed on dedicated machines. Anti-HBs-positive patients may undergo dialysis in the same area as HBsAg-positive patients, or they may serve as a geographic buffer between HBsAg-positive and seronegative patients. Ideally, the same hemodialysis equipment should not be used for both HBsAg-positive and seronegative patients; however, when this is not possible, the machines can be disinfected using conventional protocols and the external surfaces cleaned or disinfected using soap and water or a detergent germicide.

Although there is no evidence that patients or staff in centers that reuse hemodialyzers are at greater risk of acquiring HBV infection [3, 4, 47], we believe that HBsAg-positive patients should not participate in dialyzer reuse programs. HBV can occur in high concentration in blood, and we believe that handling dialyzers during the reprocessing procedures might place staff members at risk for HBV infection.

Outpatients should have specific dialysis stations assigned to them, and chairs and beds should be cleaned after each use. Sharing of ancillary supply equipment such as trays, blood pressure cuffs, clamps, scissors, and other nondisposable items should be avoided.

Nondisposable items should be autoclaved or appropriately disinfected between uses.

Dialysis staff members should not care for both HBsAg-positive and seronegative patients during the same shift but can care for HBsAg-positive and anti-HBs-positive patients during the same shift. Staff members who are HBsAg-positive may be assigned preferentially to care for HBsAg-positive patients. If for some reason staff members must care for both HBsAg-positive and seronegative patients during the same shift, they should ideally change gowns between patients and, more importantly, change gloves and wash hands to prevent cross-contamination. Disposable gloves can be worn by staff personnel for their own protection when handling patients or dialysis equipment and accessories. Gloves should be worn when taking blood pressure, injecting saline or heparin, or touching dialysis machine knobs to adjust flow rates. For the patient's protection, the staff member should use a fresh pair of gloves with each patient to prevent cross-contamination. Gloves also should be used when handling blood specimens. Staff members should wash their hands after each patient contact.

Staff members may wish to wear protective eyeglasses and surgical-type masks for procedures in which spurting or spattering of blood may occur, such as cleaning of dialyzers, centrifugation of blood, and the like. Staff members should wear gowns, scrub suits, or the equivalent while working in the unit and should change out of this clothing at the end of each day.

At the end of each dialysis treatment or dialysis shift, nondisposable equipment should be cleaned and disinfected or sterilized. Special attention should be given to control knobs on the dialysis machines and other surfaces that are frequently touched and potentially contaminated with patients' blood.

In single-pass artificial kidney machines, the internal fluid pathways that supply dialysis fluid to the dialyzer are not subject to contamination with blood. Although the fluid pathways that exhaust dialysis fluid from the dialyzer may become contaminated with blood in the event of a dialyzer leak, it is unlikely that this blood contamination will reach a subsequent patient. In the absence of microbiologic or epidemiologic evidence incriminating these fluid pathways, disinfection and rinsing procedures should be designed to control effectively microbial contamination problems other than those associated with hepatitis.

For dialysis machines that use a dialysate-recirculating system (such as some ultrafiltration control machines), a blood leak in a dialyzer, especially a massive leak, can result in contamination of a number of surfaces that will contact the dialysis fluid of subsequent patients. However, the procedures involving draining, rinsing, and disinfection that are normally practiced after each use will reduce the level of contamination to below infectious levels. Consequently, if a blood leak does occur with either type of dialysis machine, the standard disinfection procedure used for machines in the dialysis center to control bacterial contamination is appropriate. External surfaces of the dialysis machine should also be cleaned or disinfected. Venous pressure isolators or in-line filters should be used to prevent blood contamination of venous pressure monitors. These isolators or filters should not be reused.

Staff members in a hemodialysis unit should not smoke, eat, or drink in the dialysis treatment area or in the laboratory. There should be a separate lounge for this purpose. On the other hand, patients may be served meals even if they are HBsAg-positive and are being treated in a separate area. The glasses, dishes, and other utensils may be cleaned in the usual manner by the hospital staff. No special care of these items is needed.

Crowding of patients and overtaxing of staff may increase the likelihood of HBV transmission in dialysis units. To minimize virus transmission, each patient's station, with its attendant equipment, should occupy sufficient space to permit easy movement of a staff member completely around the patient without interfering with the neighboring station. This will allow for adequate cleaning and proper patient care.

Blood and other specimens such as peritoneal fluid from all patients should be handled with care. Peritoneal fluid can contain high levels of HBsAg and HBV and should be handled in the same manner as the patient's blood. Consequently, if the center performs peritoneal dialysis, the same criteria for separating HBsAg-positive patients who are undergoing hemodialysis apply to those undergoing peritoneal dialysis.

Housekeeping

In general, housekeeping in the dialysis center serves two purposes: (1) to remove soil and waste on a regular basis, thereby preventing the accumulation and concentration of potentially infectious material in the patient-staff environment, and (2) to maintain an environment that is conducive to better patient care. These two purposes are of particular importance in a hemodialysis center because of the critical nature of the procedures performed. The requirement for aseptic access to a patient's blood supply at least twice in each dialysis procedure makes the hemodialysis unit more similar to a surgical suite than to a conventional patient room. Yet, because of crowding and the presence of complex hemodialysis machines with multiple wires, tubes, and hoses, the dialysis unit frequently receives an inferior level of cleaning. If good housekeeping is to be achieved, it is necessary to have adequate space in which to work, as well as special instructions and training for the staff regarding the cleaning of hemodialysis equipment and stations. Although allotted space is often limited and cannot be changed, much can be done to utilize it more efficiently. Elimination of unneeded items, orderly arrangement of required items, and removal of excess lengths of tubes, hoses, and wires from the floor are steps that can provide more accessibility for cleaning.

All disposable items should be placed in bags strong enough to contain the weight of discarded dialyzers and other items. The bags should be thick enough so they do not leak, or double bagging should be practiced. Bags should not be overfilled, requiring the staff to compact the contents by hand to make room for additional waste. Since bags may become contaminated on the outside before they leave the unit, they should be placed in another bag in a "clean" area in the unit before they are picked up. All used needles and syringes should be discarded in puncture-proof containers without being separated. Wastes from a hemodialysis center that are actually or potentially contaminated with blood should be considered infectious and handled accordingly. Eventually, these items of solid wastes should be disposed of properly in an incinerator or sanitary landfill, depending on local ordinances (see Chap. 15).

Nondisposable items such as linen, especially if it is contaminated with blood, also should be considered as potentially infectious and should be handled accordingly (see Chap. 16). These items should be bagged properly, and laundry personnel should wear gloves when handling them and should not work with them in the same area as clean linen. Patients' personal items such as blankets may be taken home by the patient for cleaning.

Cleaning, Disinfection, and Sterilization

Good cleaning and adequate disinfection procedures are an important part of a hemodialysis center's efforts to control and prevent cross-contamination of HBV. Although many of the procedures do not differ from those recommended for medical devices in hospitals and for inanimate surfaces [39, 43] (see Chap. 15), the hemodialysis environment is somewhat unique. In the dialysis procedure, there is an extraordinary amount of blood contamination and concern regarding HBV, which occurs in very high amounts in blood and is relatively stable in dried blood and serum. However, the basic approach is the same as that used in other health care environments: That is, there should be a thorough mechanical cleaning step prior to any sterilization or disinfection process and, depending on the compatibility of materials, especially medical devices, sterilization should be chosen over disinfection.

HBV has not been grown on tissue cultures and, without a simple viral assay system, studies on the precise resistance of this virus to various chemical germicides and heat have not been performed. In the absence of firm data, some investigators have considered HBV to be extremely resistant and have recommended unreasonably long decontamination and sterilization protocols and use of corrosive chemicals. These recommendations are counterproductive because health professionals do not use them. It should be kept in mind that the HBV is a virus, and its resistance to heat and chemical germicides at best may reach the resistance of some other viruses and bacteria but certainly not that of the bacterial endospore. Further, studies have shown that HBV is not resistant to commonly used high-level and intermediate disinfectants [23].

A physical or chemical treatment known to exhibit sporicidal activity should also be virucidal for HBV. Standard autoclave cycles of 121°C (249.8°F) for 15 minutes or ethylene oxide cycles can be used to inactivate HBV. However, in many instances, it is decontamination and not sterilization that is needed. For example, in the hemodialysis unit, blood spills can be adequately decontaminated without using special procedures and corrosive chemical germicides. Immediately after a blood spill, the area should be thoroughly cleaned with a cloth soaked in an appropriate hospital disinfectant. The staff member doing the cleaning should wear gloves, and the towel can be placed in a bucket. After all visible blood is cleaned, a second application of disinfectant using a cloth or towel can be done.

When physically cleaning frequently touched environmental surfaces in a dialysis unit to prevent cross-contamination with HBV, a good detergent or detergent germicide can be employed. Antiseptics such as formulations with povidone-iodine, hexachlorophene, or chlorhexidine should not be used, because these are formulated for use on skin and are not designed for use on hard surfaces.

Hepatitis C

Outbreaks of non-A, non-B hepatitis, a disease primarily transmitted by the bloodborne route, have been reported among hemodialysis patients [62, 69a, 77] (see Chap. 38). A strict case definition for non-A, non-B hepatitis includes serologic exclusion of hepatitis A, hepatitis B, delta hepatitis, cytomegalovirus, and Epstein-Barr virus, as well as the exclusion of other causes of liver inflammation. Recently, a portion of a virus isolated from a chimpanzee experimentally infected with transfusion-associated non-A, non-B hepatitis was cloned and sequenced, and a serologic assay was developed for the diagnosis of what is being called *hepatitis C* [37, 63]. This assay identifies a high proportion (70 to 90 percent) of persons with chronic non-A, non-B hepatitis [6, 7, 9, 63]. For patients with acute non-A, non-B hepatitis, however, a prolonged interval may elapse between exposure (such as blood transfusion) or onset of hepatitis and antibody seroconversion [6, 7, 9]. Persons negative for antibody to hepatitis C virus (anti-HCV) during their acute illness should be retested at least 6 months later to establish a final diagnosis. Patients with a diagnosis of non-A, non-B hepatitis who remain negative for anti-HCV may have hepatitis C but may fail to elicit an immune response detectable by the current assay, they may be infected with a second agent of non-A, non-B hepatitis, or their hepatitis may have another cause (viral or nonviral). Thus, the diagnosis of

acute non-A, non-B hepatitis must continue to rely on the exclusion of other etiologies of liver disease even with the availability of a licensed test for anti-HCV.

Historically, it was recommended that patients be tested monthly for alanine aminotransferase or aspartate aminotransferase to detect possible non-A, non-B hepatitis infections, particularly those occurring in clusters, which might indicate a problem with infection control practices. Isolation of dialysis patients with presumed non-A, non-B hepatitis in separate rooms using dedicated machines was not considered necessary or recommended [42]; instead, the use of basic barrier precautions was emphasized. The availability of a commercial test for anti-HCV does not alter these recommendations for the control of non-A, non-B hepatitis in the dialysis center.

For the control of non-A, non-B hepatitis and hepatitis C in the dialysis center setting, the following recommendations are made:

1. Patients who are positive for anti-HCV or in whom non-A, non-B hepatitis has been diagnosed do not have to be isolated from other patients or dialyzed separately on dedicated machines. In addition, they can participate in dialyzer reuse programs.
2. Infection control strategies should emphasize basic barrier precautions, commonly referred to as *universal precautions* [28, 42].
3. Patients should be monitored for elevations in alanine aminotransferase and aspartate aminotransferase monthly. Elevations in liver enzymes currently are more sensitive indicators of acute HCV infection than is anti-HCV.
4. Routine screening of patients or staff for anti-HCV is not necessary for purposes of infection control. Dialysis centers may wish to conduct serologic surveys of their patient populations to determine the prevalence of the virus in their center and, in the case of patients or staff with a diagnosis of non-A, non-B hepatitis, to determine medical management. In addition, if liver enzyme screening indicates the oc-

currence of an epidemic of non-A, non-B hepatitis in the dialysis setting, anti-HCV screening on serum samples collected during and subsequent to outbreaks may be of value. However, since anti-HCV in an individual cannot distinguish between chronic infection or infection that has resolved, its usefulness for infection control in the dialysis center setting is limited.

Delta Hepatitis

Delta hepatitis is caused by the hepatitis delta virus (HDV), a defective virus that causes infection only in the presence of HDV infection. HDV infection may occur as either coinfection with HBV or superinfection of an HBV carrier. Since HDV is dependent on HBV for replication, prevention of HBV infection by either preexposure or postexposure prophylaxis will prevent HDV infection for a person susceptible to hepatitis B. The prevalence of HDV infection in the United States is relatively low, but a transmission of HDV between hemodialysis patients has been reported [64a]. In addition, HDV exists in extraordinarily high concentrations in circulating blood of persons who are infected; it has been reported that the concentration exceeds that of HBV by one to three orders of magnitude. Consequently, there is a potential for efficient transmission from patient to patient in a dialysis center.

Serologic tests to measure HDV and it antibody are commercially available but, because of the low prevalence of this infection in the United States, we do not believe screening of patients or staff members for HDV infection is warranted.

If a patient is known to be infected with HDV or there appears to be evidence of transmission of HDV in a dialysis center, screening for delta antigen and its antibody would be warranted. Patients who are infected with HDV should be separated from all other dialysis patients, including those who are HBsAg-positive. They should be dialyzed in separate areas and on dedicated machines.

Since the transmission of this virus is very similar to that of HBV, the basic barrier precautions described earlier should be practiced.

Acquired Immunodeficiency Syndrome

When the acquired immunodeficiency syndrome (AIDS) was described in 1982 and it was subsequently determined that its epidemiology was similar to HBV infection (see Chap. 39), concern increased for dialysis patients who were infected with the HIV. However, as the national epidemic progressed and it became evident that the efficiency of transmission of HIV was significantly less than that of HBV, presumably because of the significant difference in the amount of infectious virus circulating in the blood of infected individuals, it was clear that standard infection control strategies utilizing basic barrier precautions could prevent transmission of HIV from patients to staff members, as well as from patient to patient. Routine testing of dialysis patients or staff members for anti-HIV for purposes of infection control is not necessary. Anti-HIV testing for purposes of patient management, medication, and other reasons, however, may be necessary. Testing for anti-HIV among patients who may be considered at risk because of a long history of blood transfusions, especially in those years before donor blood was screened in the United States, is encouraged. The purpose of these tests is not for infection control strategies within the dialysis center setting but rather to prevent HIV transmission between HIV-infected patients and their sexual partners.

Patients with HIV infection can be treated with either hemodialysis or peritoneal dialysis, and they need not be isolated from other patients either in separate rooms or by using dedicated machines. The type of dialysis treatment should be based on the needs of the patient. The standard barrier precautions described earlier (universal precautions) are sufficient to prevent HIV transmission in this setting. Disinfection and sterilization strategies routinely practiced in dialysis centers are adequate to prevent the risk of HIV transmission [42].

In 1985, the CDC added questions pertaining to HIV-infected patients to its dialysis-associated diseases surveillance system. The results have shown that from 1985 to 1988 the percentage of centers that reported providing dialysis for patients with HIV infection increased from 11 to 25 percent [4]. Similarly, the number of patients receiving dialysis who were known to be infected with HIV increased from 0.3 percent in 1985 to 1.2 percent in 1988. Of the 1,253 dialysis patients reported to be infected with HIV in 1988, 670 (53 percent) had clinical symptoms of AIDS, AIDS-related complex, or lymphadenopathy, and 583 (47 percent) were asymptomatic but serologically positive (by both EIA and Western blot) for anti-HIV. In 1988, 19 percent of centers reported routine testing of patients for anti-HIV. Dialysis centers located in hospitals and government and non-profit centers were more likely to test their patients than were freestanding and for-profit centers. Those centers that reported providing dialysis for HIV-infected patients were located in 35 states, the District of Columbia, Puerto Rico, and the Virgin Islands.

To date, transmission of HIV from infected patients to dialysis staff members has not been reported, although such transmission could potentially occur. The absence of such transmission may be attributable to dialysis staff members' use of universal precautions since the early 1970s; in fact, universal precautions are primarily derived from dialysis center infection control strategies.

In summary, HIV-infected patients can be dialyzed in centers without being isolated or separated from other patients and can take part in dialyzer reuse programs. Standard barrier precautions are sufficient to prevent HIV transmission from patient to patient or patient to staff member. Infection control strategies described for the control of HBV infection should be used consistently in all dialysis centers by all personnel.

References

1. Alfrey, A.C., et al. Syndrome of dyscrasia and multifocal seizures associated with chronic hemodialysis. *Trans. Am. Soc. Antif. Intern. Organs* 18:257, 1972.
2. Alter, M.J., et al. National surveillance of dialysis-associated diseases in the United States, 1987. *Trans. Am. Soc. Antif. Intern. Organs* 35:820, 1989.
3. Alter, M.J., et al. Reuse of hemodialyzers. Results of nationwide surveillance for adverse effects. *J.A.M.A.* 260:2073, 1988.
4. Alter, M.J., et al. National surveillance of dialysis-associated diseases in the United States, 1988. *Trans. Am. Soc. Antif. Intern. Organs* 36:107, 1990.
5. Alter, M.J., et al. National surveillance of dialysis-associated hepatitis and other diseases. *Dialysis Transplant.* 12:860, 1983.
6. Alter, M.J., et al. Risk factors for acute non-A, non-B hepatitis in the United States and association with hepatitis C virus antibody. *J.A.M.A.* 264:2231, 1990.
7. Alter, H.J., et al. Detection of antibody to hepatitis C virus in prospectively followed transfusion recipients with acute and chronic non-A, non-B hepatitis. *N. Engl. J. Med.* 321:1494, 1989.
8. Alter, M.J., Favero, M.S., and Francis, D.P. Cost benefit of vaccination for hepatitis B in hemodialysis centers. *J. Infect. Dis.* 148:770, 1983.
8a. Alter, M.J., Favero, M.S., and Maynard, J.E. Impact of infection control strategies on the incidence of dialysis-associated hepatitis in the United States *J. Infect. Dis.* 153:1149, 1986.
9. Alter, M.J., and Sampliner, R.E. Hepatitis C: And miles to go before we sleep. *N. Engl. J. Med.* 321:1538, 1989.
10. Anderson, R.L., et al. Effect of disinfectants on pseudomonads colonized on the interior surface of PVC pipes. *Am. J. Public Health* 80:17, 1990.
10a. Arduino, M.J., et al. Comparison of microbiologic assay methods for hemodialysis fluids. *J. Clin. Microbiol.* 29:592, 1991.
10b. Arduino, M.J., et al. Effect of incubation time and temperature on microbiologic sampling procedures for hemodialysis fluids. *J. Clin. Microbiol.* 24:1462, 1991.
11. Association for the Advancement of Medical Instrumentation. *American National Standard for Hemodialysis Systems.* Arlington, VA: Association for the Advancement of Medical Instrumentation, 1981.
12. Association for the Advancement of Medical Instrumentation. *Recommended Practice for Re-*

use of Hemodialyzers. Arlington, VA: Association for the Advancement of Medical Instrumentation, 1986.

13. Band, J.D., et al. Peritonitis due to a *Mycobacterium chelonei*–like organism associated with intermittent chronic peritoneal dialysis. *J. Infect. Dis.* 145:9, 1982.

14. Beck-Sague, C.M., et al. Outbreak of Gram-negative bacteremia and pyrogenic reactions in a hemodialysis center. *Am. J. Nephrol.* 10:397, 1990.

15. Berkelman, R.L., Band, J.D., and Petersen, N.J. Recommendations for the care of automated peritoneal dialysis machines: Can the risk of peritonitis be reduced? *Infect. Control* 5:85, 1984.

16. Berkelman, R.L., et al. *Pseudomonas cepacia* peritonitis associated with contamination of automatic peritoneal dialysis machines. *Ann. Intern. Med.* 96:456, 1982.

17. Bland, L., et al. Hemodialyzer reuse: Practices in the United States and implications for infection control. *Trans. Am. Soc. Antif. Intern. Organs* 31:556, 1985.

18. Bland, L.A., et al. Effect of chemical germicides on the integrity of hemodialyzer membranes. *Trans. Am. Soc. Antif. Intern. Organs* 34:172, 1988.

19. Bland, L.A., et al. Potential bacteriologic and endotoxin hazards associated with liquid bicarbonate concentration. *Trans. Am. Soc. Antif. Intern. Organs* 33:542, 1987.

20. Bland, L.A., and Favero, M.S. Microbial Contamination Control Strategies for Hemodialysis Systems. In: Joint Commission on Accreditation of Healthcare Organizations, *Plant, Technology and Safety Management Series,* Vol. 3. Oakbrook Terrace, IL: Joint Commission on Accreditation of Healthcare Organizations, 1989. Pp. 30–36.

21. Bolan, G., et al. Infections with *Mycobacterium chelonei* in patients receiving dialysis and using processed hemodialyzers. *J. Infect. Dis.* 152:1013, 1985.

22. Bond, W.W., et al. Survival of hepatitis B virus after drying and storage for one week. *Lancet* 1:550, 1981.

23. Bond, W.W., Favero, M.S., Petersen, N.J., and Ebert, J.W. Inactivation of hepatitis B virus by intermediate-to-high-level disinfection chemicals. *J. Clin. Microbiol.* 18:535, 1983.

24. Carson, L.A., et al. Prevalence of nontuberculous mycobacteria in water supplies of hemodialysis centers. *Appl. Environ. Microbiol.* 54:3122, 1988.

25. Carson, L.A., et al. Factors Affecting Endotoxin Levels in Fluids Associated with Hemodialysis Procedures. In: Novitsky, T.J. and Wastron, S.W. (Eds.), *Detection of Bacterial Endotoxins with the Limulus Amebocyte Lysate Test.* New York: Alan R. Liss, 1987. Pp. 223–234.

26. Carson, L.A., Petersen, N.J., and Favero, M.S. Use of the *Limulus* Amoebocyte Lysate Assay System for Detection of Bacterial Endotoxin in Fluids Associated with Hemodialysis Procedures. In: E. Cohen (Ed.), *Biomedical Applications of the Horseshoe Crab* (Limulidae). New York: Alan R. Liss, 1979. Pp. 453–464.

27. Carson, L.A., Petersen, N.J., Favero, M.S., and Aguero, S.M. Growth characteristics of atypical mycobacteria in water and their comparative resistance to disinfection. *Appl. Environ. Microbiol.* 36:839, 1978.

28. Centers for Disease Control. Control Measures for Hepatitis B in Dialysis Centers. In: *Viral Hepatitis Investigation and Control Series.* Atlanta: Centers for Disease Control, Nov. 1977.

29. Centers for Disease Control. Fluoride intoxication in a dialysis unit—Maryland. *M.M.W.R.* 29:134, 1980.

30. Centers for Disease Control. *Dialysis Dementia from Aluminum.* Epidemic Investigation Report EPI 81-39-2, June 10, 1982. Atlanta: Centers for Disease Control, 1982.

31. Centers for Disease Control. *Clusters of Bacteremia and Pyrogenic Reactions in Hemodialysis Patients—Georgia.* Epidemic Investigation Report EPI 86-65-2, April 22, 1987. Atlanta: Centers for Disease Control, 1987.

32. Centers for Disease Control. Bacteremia associated with reuse of disposable hollow-fiber hemodialyzers. *M.M.W.R.* 35:417, 1986.

33. Centers for Disease Control. *Pyrogenic Reactions in Patients Undergoing High-Flux Hemodialysis—California.* Epidemic Investigation Report EPI 86-80-2, June 1, 1987. Atlanta: Centers for Disease Control, 1987.

34. Centers for Disease Control. *Pyrogenic Reactions in Hemodialysis Patients on High-Flux Hemodialysis—California.* Epidemic Investigation Report EPI 87-12-2, June 1, 1987. Atlanta: Centers for Disease Control, 1987.

35. Centers for Disease Control. Acute allergic reactions associated with reprocessed hemodialyzers—Virginia, 1989. *M.M.W.R.* 38:873, 1989.

36. Centers for Disease Control. *Formaldehyde Intoxication Associated with Hemodialysis—California.* Epidemic Investigation Report EPI 81-73-2, May 7, 1984. Atlanta: Centers for Disease Control, 1984.

37. Choo, Q.L. et al. Isolation of a cDNA clone derived from a blood-borne non-A, non-B hepatitis genome. *Science* 244:359, 1989.

38. Corey, L. et al. HBsAg hepatitis in a hemodialysis unit. Relation to Epstein-Barr virus. *N. Engl. J. Med.* 293:1273, 1975.

39. Favero, M.S., and Bond, W.W. Chemical Disinfection of Medical and Surgical Materials. In: S.S. Block (Ed.), *Disinfection, Sterilization, and Preservation* (4th ed.). Philadelphia: Lea & Febiger, 1991. Pp. 617–641.

40. Favero, M.S. Distinguishing Between High-Level Disinfection, Reprocessing, and Sterilization. In: Association for the Advancement of Medical Instrumentation, *Reuse of Disposables: Implications for Quality Health Care and Cost Containment.* Technical Assessment Report No. 6. Arlington, VA: Association for the Advancement of Medical Instrumentation, 1983. Pp. 19–20.

41. Favero, M.S. Microbiological contaminants. In: *Proceedings of the Association for the Advancement of Medical Instrumentation Technology Assessment Conference: Issues in Hemodialysis,* 1981, Washington, DC: AAMI, 1981. Pp. 30–33.

42. Favero, M.S. Precautions for dialysing Human Immunodeficiency Virus–Infected Patients. In: P.M. Monkhouse (Ed.), *Aspects of Renal Care,* Vol. 3. London: Ballière Tindall, 1989. Pp. 55–61.

43. Favero, M.S., Bond, W.W. Sterilization, Disinfection, and Antisepsis in the Hospital. In: *Manual of Clinical Microbiology.* Washington, DC: American Society for Microbiology, 1991. Pp. 183–200.

44. Favero, M.S., and Bland, L.A. Microbiologic Principles Applied to Reprocessing Hemodialyzers. In: N. Deane, R.J. Wineman, and J.A. Bemis (Eds.), *Guide to Reprocessing of Hemodialyzers.* Boston: Martinus Nijhoff, 1986. Pp. 63–73.

45. Favero, M.S., Carson, L.A., Bond, W.W., and Petersen, N.J. *Pseudomonas aeruginosa:* Growth in distilled water from hospitals. *Science* 173:836, 1971.

46. Favero, M.S., Carson, L.A., Bond, W.W., and Petersen, N.J. Factors that influence microbial contamination of fluids associated with hemodialysis machines. *Appl. Microbiol.* 28:822, 1974.

47. Favero, M.S., Deane, N., Leger, R.T., and Sosin, A.E. Effect of multiple use of dialyzers on hepatitis B incidence in patients and staff. *J.A.M.A.* 245:166, 1981.

48. Favero, M.S., et al. Guidelines for the care of patients hospitalized with viral hepatitis. *Ann. Intern. Med.* 91:872, 1979.

49. Favero, M.S., et al. Hepatitis B antigen on environmental surfaces. *Lancet* 2:1455, 1973.

50. Favero, M.S., et al. Microbial contamination of renal dialysis systems and associated health risks. *Trans. Am. Soc. Antif. Intern. Organs* 20:175, 1974.

51. Favero, M.S., et al. Gram-negative water bacteria in hemodialysis systems. *Health Lab. Sci.* 12:321, 1975.

52. Favero, M.S., and Petersen, N.J. Microbiologic guidelines for hemodialysis systems. *Dialysis Transplant.* 6:34, 1977.

53. Galbraith, R.M., et al. Non-A, non-B hepatitis associated with chronic liver disease in a haemodialysis unit. *Lancet* 1:951, 1979.

54. Gazenfeldt-Gazit, E., and Elaihou, H.E. Endotoxin antibodies in patients on maintenance hemodialysis. *Is. J. Med. Sci.* 5:1032, 1969.

55. Gordon, S., Tipple, M., Bland, L., and Jarvis, W. Pyrogenic reactions associated with the reuse of disposable hollow-fibered hemodialyzers. *J.A.M.A.* 260:2077, 1988.

56. Gordon, S.M., et al. Hemolysis associated with hydrogen peroxide at a pediatric facility. *Am. J. Nephrol.* 10:123, 1990.

57. Gordon, S.M., et al. Epidemic hypotension in a dialysis center caused by sodium azide. *Kidney Int.* 37:110, 1990.

58. Gordon, S.M., et al. A prospective study of pyrogenic reactions in patients receiving conventional, high-efficiency or high-flux hemodialysis with bicarbonate dialysate containing high concentrations of bacteria and endotoxin. *J. Am. Soc. Nephrol.* 5, 1991.

59. Henderson, L.W., Koch, K.M., Dinarello, C.A., and Shaldon, S. Hemodialysis hypotension: The interleukin hypothesis. *Blood Purif.* 1:3, 1983.

60. Hindman, S.H., et al. Pyrogenic reactions during haemodialysis caused by extramural endotoxin. *Lancet* 2:732, 1975.

61. Kantor, R.J., et al. Outbreak of pyrogenic reactions at a dialysis center. *Am. J. Med.* 74:449, 1983.

62. Koretz, R.L., Stone, O., Mousa, M., and Gitnick, G. The pursuit of hepatitis in dialysis units. *Am. J. Nephrol.* 4:222, 1984.

63. Kuo, G., et al. An assay for circulating antibodies to a major etiologic virus of human non-A, non-B hepatitis. *Science* 244:362, 1989.

64. Lang, D.J., and Daniels, C.A. Herpesvirus Hepatitis in Transplant Recipients and Hemodialysis Patients. In: J.L. Touraine et al. (Eds.), *Transplantation and clinical immunology,* Vol. 10. Amsterdam: Excerpta Medica, 1979. Pp. 18–26.

64a. Lettau, L.A., et al. Nosocomial transmission of delta hepatitis. *Ann. Intern. Med.* 104:631, 1986.

65. Lowry, P., et al. *Mycobacterium chelonei* infections among patients receiving high-flux dialysis in a hemodialysis clinic in California. *J. Infect. Dis.* 161:85, 1990.

66. Marmion, B.P., Burrell, C.J., Tonkin, R.W., and Dickson, J. Dialysis-associated hepatitis in

Edinburgh; 1960–1978. *Rev. Infect. Dis.* 4:619, 1982.

67. Moyer, L.A., Alter, M.J., and Favero, M.S. Review of hemodialysis-associated hepatitis B: Revised recommendations for serologic screening. *Semin. Dialysis* 3:201, 1990.

68. Murphy, J., et al. Outbreaks of bacteremia in hemodialysis patients associated with alteration of dialyzer membranes following chemical disinfection (abstr.). *Trans. Am. Soc. Antif. Intern. Organs* 16:51, 1987.

69. Najem, G.R., et al. Control of hepatitis B infection. The role of surveillance and an isolation hemodialysis center. *J.A.M.A.* 245:153, 1981.

69a. Niu, M.T., Alter, M.J., Kristensen, C., and Margolis, H.S. Outbreak of hemodialysis-associated non-A, non-B hepatitis and correlation with antibody to hepatitis C virus. *Am. J. Kidney Dis.* 1992 (in press).

70. Nolph, K.D. (Ed.). *Peritoneal Dialysis* (2nd ed.). Boston: Martinus Nijhoff, 1985.

71. Petersen, N.J. An assessment of the airborne route in hepatitis B transmission. *Ann. N.Y. Acad. Sci.* 353:157, 1980.

72. Petersen, N.J., Boyer, K.M., Carson, L.A., and Favero, M.S. Pyrogenic reactions from inadequate disinfection of a dialysis fluid distribution system. *Dialysis Transplant.* 52:57, 1978.

73. Petersen, N.J., Carson, L.A., and Favero, M.S. Microbiological quality of water in an automatic peritoneal dialysis system. *Dialysis Transplant.* 6:38, 1977.

74. Petersen, N.J., et al. Microbiologic evaluation of a new glutaraldehyde-based disinfectant for hemodialysis systems. *Trans. Am. Soc. Antif. Intern. Organs* 28:287, 1982.

75. Peterson, P., Matzke, G., and Keane, W. Current concepts in the management of peritonitis in patients undergoing continuous ambulatory peritoneal dialysis. *Rev. Infect. Dis.* 9:604, 1987.

76. Schreeder, M.T., et al. Dialysis encephalopathy and aluminum exposure: An epidemiologic analysis. *J. Chronic Dis.* 36:581, 1983.

77. Seaworth, B.J., Garrett, L.E., Stead, W.W., and Hamilton, J.D. Non-A, non-B hepatitis and chronic dialysis—another dilemma. *Am. J. Nephrol.* 4:235, 1984.

78. Snydman, D., Bryan, J., and Hanson, B. Hemodialysis-associated hepatitis in the United States—1972. *J. Infect. Dis.* 132:109, 1975.

79. Stamm, J.M., Engelhard, W.E., and Parsons, J.E. Microbiological study of water softener resins. *Appl. Microbiol.* 18:376, 1969.

80. Szmuness, W., et al. Hepatitis type A and hemodialysis; A seroepidemiologic study in 15 U.S. centers. *Ann. Intern. Med.* 87:8, 1977.

81. Szmuness, W., et al. Hepatitis B infection. A point prevalence study in 15 U.S. dialysis centers. *J.A.M.A.* 227:901, 1974.

82. Tipple, M.A., Bland, L.A., Favero, M.S., and Jarvis, W.R. Investigation of hemolytic anemia after chloramine exposure in a dialysis center. *Trans. Am. Soc. Antif. Intern. Organs* 34:1060, 1988.

83. Townsend, T.R., Siok-Bi, W., and Bartlett, J. Disinfection of hemodialysis machines: An evaluation of three disinfectants. *Dialysis Transplant.* 14:274, 1985.

84. Vas, S. Microbiologic aspects of chronic ambulatory peritoneal dialysis. *Kidney Int.* 23:83, 1983.

The Intensive Care Unit

Didier Pittet
Loreen A. Herwaldt
R. Michael Massanari

The care of critically ill patients in special high-technology units is a primary component of modern medicine. Although the efficacy of critical care has been established for only a few conditions, intensive care units (ICUs) are found in 95 percent of acute-care hospitals in the United States [120]. Invasive diagnostic and therapeutic procedures are essential for the diagnosis and treatment of critically ill patients. However, life support systems disrupt normal host defense mechanisms. Given the severity of the illnesses affecting patients in ICUs, it is not surprising that mortality might exceed 25 percent. In addition, more than one-third of the patients admitted to ICUs experience unexpected complications of medical care. Mortality in the group of patients with complications exceeds 40 percent [1]. Nosocomial infection is one of the most frequent medical complications affecting patients in ICUs. Although ICUs make up only 5 percent of hospital beds and care for less than 10 percent of the hospitalized patients, infections acquired in these units account for more than 20 percent of nosocomial infections [33, 41, 58, 69, 70, 98, 191, 286]. Fortunately, systematic studies of the determinants of nosocomial infections, surveillance for infections, and adherence to protocols for preventing infections have been effective in reducing the risk for patients admitted to ICUs.

Pathogenesis

The dynamics of ICU-acquired infections are complex and depend on the contribution of the host's underlying conditions, the infectious agents, and the unique environment of the ICU. The following discussion will consider the role of each component in the development of infection.

Host Factors
Host Defenses
The ability of patients in ICUs to ward off infections is seriously compromised. Natural host defense mechanisms might be impaired by underlying diseases or as a result of medical and surgical interventions. All patients admitted to an ICU will have at least one, and often multiple, vascular cannulas that break the normal skin barriers and establish direct access between the external environment and the bloodstream. Natural chemical barriers in the stomach are neutralized by administering H_2 blockers or antacids that reduce acidity and allow growth of enteric flora [223]. Physiologic mechanisms for evacuating and cleansing hollow organs are disrupted and circumvented by insertion of endotracheal tubes, nasogastric tubes, and urinary catheters.

Specific host defense mechanisms also might be impaired by the underlying diseases. Patients with malignant disorders might have abnormal immune responses secondary to their disease or to therapies that reduce the number of effective phagocytic cells and blunt the normal immune response. Furthermore, patients admitted to ICUs tend to be at the extremes of age. This population of patients exhibits selected impairments in natural and specific defense mechanisms that increase the risk of nosocomial infection (see Chap. 1).

Because of the precarious condition of the patient in the ICU, normal food intake is often suspended. The prevalence of malnutrition has been estimated to be as high as 10 to 50 percent in some U.S. hospitals [4, 20, 193], and undernutrition in ICUs is an almost universal problem. Moreover, conditions present in ICU patients might increase the level of malnutrition by increasing metabolic demands. Injured tissue, perfusion deficits, and infection cause fever and tachycardia through mechanisms mediated by hormones, cytokines, and bacterial products, such as endotoxin. The physiologic response to these mediators is an increase in the oxygen consumption secondary to an increase in metabolic demand. This results in breakdown of muscle to meet the body's demand for energy. The lean body mass decreases, resulting in deficits in substrates necessary for recovery.

Although its clinical significance in hospitals is not well established, undernutrition has been associated with increased length of stay [7, 216], surgical complications [7, 38, 216], and delayed wound healing [256]. Malnutrition suppresses the cellular immune response and impairs delayed hypersensitivity reactions [186, 245], T-cell formation, lymphocytic response to mitogens, and C3-mediated phagocytosis [77]. Several studies suggest that poor nutritional status is a predisposing factor for nosocomial infections such as pneumonia, urinary tract infection, postoperative wound infections, and bacteremia [7, 74, 91, 101, 175, 219, 245, 256]. Supplemental nutritional support, on the other hand, has been reported to facilitate weaning from mechanical ventilation [14, 153] and to improve prognoses [175, 186, 244, 245].

Host resistance might be decreased in patients who experience major trauma. In a study by Schimpff and colleagues [230], 48 percent of patients with severe trauma developed nosocomial infection, in contrast to only 3 percent of those with minor injuries whose length of stay in the ICU was equal to that of the patients with major injuries. Abnormalities in chemotaxis and neutrophil function secondary to serum inhibitory polypeptide substances have been demonstrated in trauma patients [47, 182]. In addition, abnormalities in T-cell functions have been demonstrated 2 weeks after splenectomy [181]. Moreover, depression of the phagocytic function of the reticuloendothelial system has been demonstrated after traumatic injury or major surgery [3, 54, 134], and enhanced susceptibility to infection has been demonstrated following hemorrhage [10, 247]. Depressed macrophage function [246] and, in particular, decrease in Fc and C3b receptor expression [247], as well as loss of serum opsonizing agents [163, 225], might explain, in part, those impairments in host defense.

Medical Devices
The objectives of intensive care include concurrent monitoring of vital functions and physiologic support of failing organ systems.

The technology necessary to achieve these objectives frequently requires introduction of foreign materials into body orifices or insertion of cannulas percutaneously, often directly into the circulatory system (see Chap. 40). The role of invasive devices in increasing host susceptibility to infections is highlighted in several recent studies [5, 51, 98, 99]. Vascular cannulas traverse the skin barrier and provide a direct portal of entry to the bloodstream. Endotracheal tubes (see Chap. 29) and urinary catheters (see Chap. 28) circumvent local defense mechanisms. Nasotracheal and nasogastric tubes might obstruct the normal flow of secretions from paranasal sinuses and predispose to sinusitis. In addition, enteral nutrition via nasogastric tubes might facilitate retrograde colonization of the upper airways, increasing the risk for subsequent pneumonia [203]. Insertion of cannulas into sterile cavities, such as intracranial "screws" used for monitoring cerebrospinal fluid pressure (see Chap. 32), exposes otherwise sterile, internal environments to exogenous microorganisms. In addition to breaking the normal tissue barriers, the invasive devices tend to enhance colonization with nosocomial pathogens [167, 168, 243, 285].

Medical Therapy

Medical therapy, while administered for its beneficial effects, is often accompanied by adverse effects on host defense. These detrimental effects might be local or systemic. For example, the conventional approach to stress ulcer prophylaxis decreases gastric acidity through antacids or H_2 antagonists. Increasing the gastric pH to greater than 3.5 alters both the qualitative and quantitative flora of the stomach [57, 76, 102, 223]. Alterations in this important chemical barrier lead to colonization of the stomach with nosocomial pathogens, which increases the frequency of retrograde colonization of the oropharynx and trachea with gram-negative organisms. Aspiration of oropharyngeal contents might then lead to gram-negative nosocomial pneumonia [50, 57, 76, 102]. Several studies have compared the rate of nosocomial pneumonias in mechanically ventilated patients who were given conventional antacid therapy to the

rate in those given sucralfate. Although the methodologies have been criticized, at least two studies have shown lower rates of pneumonia in patients treated with sucralfate [73, 261]. Despite the controversy surrounding these studies, they provide important reminders that medical therapy can have unexpected adverse effects on patients.

The adverse effects of cancer chemotherapeutic agents and immunosuppressive therapy are multifarious (see Chap. 41). Some agents are locally toxic to mucosal cells lining the gastrointestinal tract and disrupt mechanical barriers to bacterial invasion. Many agents interfere with synthesis of new phagocytic and immunocompetent cells, significantly impairing the phagocytic and immune systems. Less appreciated are the potential adverse effects of other commonly used agents. Several investigators have reported in vitro evidence for the adverse effects of antimicrobial agents on phagocytic cells [292] and on immune responses [112]. Whether these observations in vitro reflect significant impairment of host defense in vivo is still uncertain. Furthermore, the pharmacokinetics of drugs in ICU patients might be significantly altered by the patients' underlying conditions. Variations in volumes of distribution secondary to fluid retention, sepsis or drug-induced renal tubular damage, decreased drug binding to serum proteins, and age-related diminution in glomerular filtration rates make it difficult to maintain optimal serum concentrations of drugs while avoiding toxicity. Patients in ICUs are usually treated with multiple drugs. Therefore, physicians must be aware of harmful drug interactions that might increase the risk of renal, auditory, hepatic, or central nervous system toxicity or adversely alter the activity of one or more drugs.

Underlying Diseases

ICUs, by design, serve patients with severe illnesses that compromise host defense. Each patient must be assessed individually to determine how the underlying illness might interfere with host defense mechanisms. A simple assessment of the severity of underlying illness was developed by McCabe and Jackson [177], who stratified patients according to whether the underlying disease was fatal, ultimately fatal, or nonfatal. Subsequent studies by Britt and colleagues [31] have demonstrated the utility of this simple assessment for estimating the risk of nosocomial bacteremias. Numerous studies observed increasing rates of infections among patients with more severe illnesses. These observations were confirmed in the Study on the Efficacy of Nosocomial Infection Control (SENIC) Project [110].

Although McCabe's classification has been useful, it was not designed to assess patients admitted to ICUs. More recently, Knaus and colleagues [142] proposed a scoring system for measuring severity of illness in groups of critically ill patients. Their system, the acute physiology and chronic health evaluation (APACHE) classification, is based on a physiology score reflecting the degree of acute illness and the patient's health status before acute illness. Prospective studies have demonstrated that the APACHE score provides reliable estimates of patient outcomes and that it is useful for both patient care and for clinical and epidemiologic studies [143–145, 282]. For the latter, classification of patients according to the severity of illness and the risk of mortality is essential. APACHE scores allow comparison between patients as well as between different hospitals, accurately predicting mortality despite important differences in therapeutic approach [143–145]. APACHE II uses information from fewer clinical measurements but maintains the accuracy of the original scoring system [39, 140]. Physicians involved in critically ill patient care have used APACHE II for a wide variety of research purposes. For instance, it was used to identify patients with a low probability of recovery, to stratify risk in randomized clinical trials, and in decision analysis [24, 64, 141, 146, 179]. In a study of Craven and colleagues [51], an APACHE II score greater than 20 was recorded in 200 of 1,017 patients and in the univariate analysis was associated with a twofold (odds ratio 2.3) increase in the occurrence of nosocomial infection. Although the association of infection with a high APACHE II score did not remain significant in the stepwise logistic regression model, the score accurately predicted mortality.

The sepsis severity score (SSS) is a scoring system that uses subjective as well as objective observations to quantify the pathophysiologic changes in human sepsis [248]. In a study of patients with intraabdominal infections [235], both SSS and APACHE scores were better predictors of outcome than were age, chronic disease, and cause and site of infection. Furthermore, Brannen and colleagues [30] recently compared the physicians' assessment of prognosis with the APACHE II scoring system and found that the latter substantially improved clinical judgment. Thus, scoring systems might be useful for patient care in ICUs. Additional studies are needed to evaluate the association between severity of illness and development of specific nosocomial infections.

To identify ICU patients who are at particularly high risk of nosocomial infection, Gross and colleagues [105] evaluated 148 patients who were admitted to a combined medical ICU–coronary care unit and who stayed in the unit for at least 3 days. They found that 75 patients (51 percent) had three or more active comorbidities at the time of admission. Furthermore, the length of stay, noninfectious complications, and nosocomial infections were all significantly correlated with the number of preexisting comorbidities. Their results highlight the fact that preexisting host conditions are important in the development of nosocomial infections. In addition, they suggest that in clinical trials or for comparisons of infection rates between units or hospitals, patients must be stratified by comorbidities because many of the outcome indicators are significantly affected by the number of preexisting conditions. If these results are confirmed, patients at high risk of infection could be identified prospectively based on the number of active comorbidities present on admission. More intensive surveillance and prevention strategies could be targeted at the patients at highest risk for nosocomial infections.

Infectious Agents

Although ICU patients are susceptible to pathogens causing community-acquired infections, nosocomial infections are usually associated with microbes found in the host's endogenous flora or in the flora of the hospital. The risk of infection depends on multiple factors involving both intrinsic properties of the nosocomial pathogens and the status of the host immune system, as discussed previously. Nosocomial pathogens exhibit various properties that allow them to survive in the hospital environment or within the host.

Adaptability

Pathogens that are common causes of infections in ICUs, such as *Acinetobacter, Pseudomonas aeruginosa,* and *Legionella pneumophila,* are able to adapt to a variety of environmental extremes. For example, *L. pneumophila* can survive in water at temperatures between 5° and 45°C (41° and 113°F) [279]. Pseudomonads have minimal nutritional requirements and can survive in distilled water [122]. The capacity to withstand changes in ambient temperatures enhances the opportunity for transmission from one environmental niche to another. This adaptability allows the organism to establish reservoirs in the ICU environment [52].

Adherence

Adherence to host tissue is the first step in establishing infection. Intrinsic properties of the agent that facilitate adherence enhance the likelihood that an organism will produce disease. Mechanisms promoting the adherence of microorganisms onto cell surfaces, extracellular matrices, or foreign materials differ. *Escherichia coli, Proteus mirabilis,* and other gram-negative bacteria contain fimbriae that enable organisms to attach to selected sites in host tissues (for example, *E. coli* use fimbriae to attach to urinary tract endothelium) (see Chap. 28).

Staphylococci adhere to foreign material, such as intravascular cannulas, prosthetic valves, and joints, through a specific receptor-mediated process [274]. Fibronectin, fibronigen, and laminin possess specific binding sites for staphylococci and serve as ligands mediating bacterial adherence to both inflammatory tissues (e.g., postoperative scars, wounds) and plastic surfaces (e.g., catheters,

prostheses) [116, 148, 274]. The adherence-promoting activity of fibronectin for both *S. aureus* and coagulase-negative staphylococci (see Chap. 40) has been demonstrated on intravenous catheters removed from patients [273]. The high affinity of *Staphylococcus aureus* for traumatized tissues, blood clots, and scars can be explained by the large amount of exposed fibronectin in such conditions.

Oropharyngeal colonization with gram-negative bacilli is associated with both the underlying disease process and the presence of an artificial airway [264]. Abnormal colonization correlates with the alteration in the surface characteristics of the epithelium. Under normal conditions, fibronectin covers the oropharyngeal epithelial cell surface and prevents colonization with gram-negative bacilli [289]. Under the stress of severe illness, excess salivary proteolytic enzymes, particularly elastase, digest cell surface fibronectin, allowing the adherence of gram-negative bacilli [55, 290].

Colonial Protection

After attachment, some bacteria, including *P. aeruginosa* and *Staphylococcus epidermidis,* produce an amorphous substance or biofilm that protects the bacteria from host defenses [46, 200]. Whether pathogenic *P. aeruginosa* organisms utilize this property is still uncertain; however, mucoid-appearing colonies of *Pseudomonas* have been isolated from patients with cystic fibrosis [67]. Some investigators speculate that production of a biofilm might protect the microbe from antibiotics in respiratory secretions. Slime produced by *S. epidermidis* protects the pathogen from normal host defense mechanisms and from the therapeutic effects of antibiotics [46, 232]. In vitro studies demonstrated that slime alters polymorphonuclear cell functions that are important in the inflammatory response and interferes with the normal lymphoproliferative response to mitogens. Epidemiologic studies have shown an association between slime production and strains of *S. epidermidis* causing infection and the failure of medical treatment to eradicate foreign-body infections [59, 117, 208, 291].

Toxin Production

Exotoxins and endotoxins produced by the organisms might be important in the pathogenesis of nosocomial infections. *S. aureus* produces several exotoxins, including leukocidin, which is cytotoxic for neutrophils; enterotoxin F, the toxin responsible for toxic shock syndrome [6]; and exfoliatin, a toxin responsible for the scalded skin syndrome [201]. Exotoxin A is an enzyme released by *P. aeruginosa* that is lethal for mammalian cells and might be important in the pathogenesis of disease in humans [53]. Endotoxin is a virulence factor common to gram-negative bacteria. The active component of endotoxin is lipid A, a structural component of gram-negative bacterial cell walls. Endotoxin plays a pivotal role in gram-negative septicemia and shock by activating several host protein cascade systems, including complement, coagulation, kallikrein-kinin and plasminogen-plasmin pathways [29, 119, 178, 180].

Although some organisms causing nosocomial infections in critically ill patients produce many toxins, pathogens such as *Enterococcus* and *S. epidermidis* produce few toxins but cause clinically significant infections. In fact, these organisms are among the most frequent pathogens causing nosocomial infections, infections that are associated with significant morbidity and mortality [118, 208, 293].

Antimicrobial Resistance

In ICUs, where antibiotics are used more frequently and in greater quantity than in almost any other unit in the hospital, antimicrobial resistance ensures survival of some nosocomial pathogens. Moreover, in ICUs the close proximity of patients facilitates transfer of resistant organisms from patient to patient. Among the most prevalent isolates in ICUs are *S. epidermidis*, *P. aeruginosa*, and *Enterococcus* and *Candida* species (Figs. 20-1 through 20-3), all of which exhibit multiple drug resis-

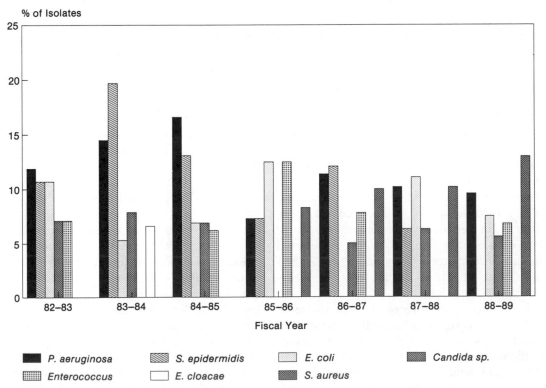

Fig. 20-1. Proportional distribution of the seven most frequently isolated microbes from a medical intensive care unit over 7 years.

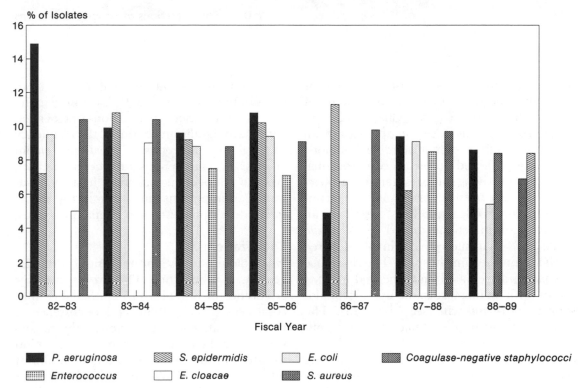

Fig. 20-2. Proportional distribution of the seven most frequently isolated microbes from a surgical intensive care unit over 7 years.

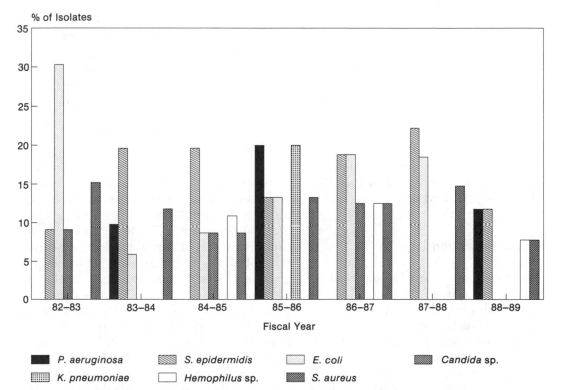

Fig. 20-3. Proportional distribution of the seven most frequently isolated microbes from a pediatric intensive care unit over 7 years.

tance. Antibiotics select resistant organisms and can predispose to the development of nosocomial infections (see Chaps. 12, 13). Organisms such as *Klebsiella* species are an important source of transferable antibiotic resistance [43], and outbreaks of nosocomial infections involving multiresistant Enterobacteriaceae have been reported [34, 35]. Brun-Buisson and colleagues [34] described an outbreak of infections caused by *Klebsiella pneumoniae* that successively involved three ICUs within the same hospital. The resistance was plasmid-mediated and emerged in association with an increase in the use of cephalosporins and amikacin (see Chap. 14). The identical pattern of antimicrobial susceptibility was observed in *E. coli* and *Citrobacter freundii* isolates collected from surrounding symptom-free patients. Numerous other reports have demonstrated spread of antibiotic resistance from ICUs to other hospital units [126, 164, 210, 234].

Axelrod and Talbot [9] studied risk factors associated with the acquisition of gentamicin resistance by enterococci in a general hospital. The most significant factors were length of hospitalization, number and duration of antibiotics received, and admission to ICUs. De Champs and colleagues [61] prospectively studied colonization of ICU patients with Enterobacteriaceae that produced expanded-spectrum β-lactamases. Ten of the 56 patients admitted during the 6-month study period became colonized or infected. Colonization was associated with longer stays in the ICU. The number of colonized patients decreased after the antibiotic policy was changed.

Sources of Colonization
Definitions
The following classification of nosocomial infections as a function of the source of the pathogenic strains is helpful in discussing the dynamics of ICU-acquired infections. *Exogenous infections* are those in which the pathogenic microbe is acquired directly from the external environment. *Primary endogenous infections* are those in which the organism is part of the patient's normal flora. *Secondary endogenous infections* are those that result from modi-

fication of the patient's normal flora or from colonization with hospital flora acquired in the ICU. Whereas modern infection control measures have significantly reduced the frequency of exogenous infections, ICU patients remain at risk for endogenous infections. In both types of endogenous infection, host colonization is an important initial step in the subsequent development of nosocomial infections.

Colonization
Host colonization is a prerequisite for the development of infection. This process involves adherence of organisms to epithelial or mucosal cells, proliferation, and persistence at the site of attachment. Although the factors promoting the progression from colonization to infection are not well understood, almost 50 percent of the ICU-acquired infections are preceded by host colonization with the same microorganism. Factors associated with microbial colonization are similar to those associated with development of infection. These risk factors include the duration of hospitalization and length of stay in an ICU, invasive devices, prolonged antibiotic therapy, and elimination of normal pharyngeal or bowel flora through the use of broad-spectrum antimicrobial agents [51, 168, 218]. Other factors promoting colonization of patients in ICUs include disruption of normal mechanical defense mechanisms (i.e., the bronchial mucociliary "escalator") by drugs and tracheal intubation, changes in protective antibacterial secretions (i.e., lysozyme, lactoferrin, saliva, and gastric acid) in response to stress and therapeutic agents, and disruption of "colonization resistance." The latter refers to the capacity of normal intestinal flora, especially anaerobes, to prevent colonization by new organisms [13, 114, 115, 265–268, 284]. The mechanisms involved are complex and include competition for substrate and mucosal receptors, production of bacteriocins, and physiologic factors such as peristalsis, mucus secretion, and local IgA production. Broad-spectrum antibiotics eliminate many bacterial species in the normal intestinal flora [23, 96, 190], resulting in overgrowth by other organisms, particularly antibiotic-resistant strains

and yeast [13, 96, 131, 132, 187, 190, 229]. Once colonized, mucosal invasion and subsequent bacterial translocation are promoted by postoperative ileus, breaks in the mucosal barriers resulting from surgery, drugs, invasive devices, mesenteric hypoperfusion, and bacterial toxin production.

A vast literature exists regarding the development of colonization and subsequent infection. A few important studies are summarized. Johanson's classic article in 1969 [130] showed that severe illness predisposes to oropharyngeal carriage with gram-negative bacilli. Le Frock [155] reported that illness was associated with intestinal carriage of gram-negative bacilli other than the individual's own *E. coli.* In 1974, Schimpf [230] suggested that, in critically ill patients, the origin of infection is usually the endogenous flora. Several studies have subsequently confirmed that patients are rapidly colonized by gram-negative bacteria after admission to ICUs [8, 76, 191, 271] and later develop infection with the same organisms [137, 149, 252]. Kerver and colleagues [136] showed that the oropharyngeal cavity and lower respiratory tract of 60 percent of patients on mechanical ventilation were colonized by ICU-acquired organisms after 5 days in the ICU. After 10 days, 100 percent of the patients were colonized. In 66 percent of the respiratory tract infections, colonization with the pathogen preceded infection. Flynn and colleagues [82] prospectively studied colonization in patients undergoing cardiac surgery compared with those who underwent coronary angioplasty. Whereas none of the latter became colonized with gram-negative organisms, the majority of surgical patients were colonized with *Enterobacter.* Colonization with *Enterobacter* was correlated with antibiotic prophylaxis, and 14 percent of the patients colonized with *Enterobacter* developed infection. Moreover, phage typing methods confirmed that the patients' newly acquired endogenous flora was the most important source of infection. In a related study, the same authors demonstrated that almost 25 percent of patients colonized with *Enterobacter, Pseudomonas,* and *Serratia* species developed clinical infection [83].

Leonard and colleagues [159] prospectively studied the sequence of colonization and infection in a neonatal ICU. Ninety-eight percent of the patients became colonized with gram-negative bacilli. Colonization was observed in the oropharynx in 19 percent of patients; in the rectum in 58 percent; and simultaneously at both sites in 23 percent. Thirty-eight percent of the infants colonized with *Pseudomonas* subsequently developed infection with the same organism. All infants who developed infection were colonized first in the digestive tract. The average time elapsed between colonization and infection was 7 days. These results suggested that prevention of digestive tract colonization might reduce infection rates in ICU patients. Further prospective studies are needed to determine whether selective decontamination can prevent colonization and infection in critically ill neonates (see Chap. 13). Leonard's results also reinforce the importance of strict infection control measures to prevent transfer of organisms from colonized or infected patients to those recently admitted to the ICU.

Epidemiology
The Agent
Bacteria, fungi, and viruses have been reported as causative agents in nosocomial infections. To illustrate the variety and frequency of organisms responsible for disease in ICUs, 7 years of trended data from the medical (MICU), surgical (SICU), and pediatric (PICU) intensive care units at the University of Iowa Hospitals and Clinics (UIHC) are summarized in Figs. 20-1 through 20-3. The infections were identified through concurrent surveillance by trained epidemiology technicians using modified Centers for Disease Control (CDC) criteria for nosocomial infections. Although these data reflect a small geographic sample of the United States, the trends and distribution of pathogens are representative of ICUs in tertiary care hospitals around the country and the world [32, 51, 58, 285].

On average, 41 different species of bacteria or fungi were isolated each year from SICU-acquired infections, and more than 28 different species were isolated per year from MICU-acquired infections. Figures 20-1 through 20-3 list the five species most commonly causing nosocomial infection in the MICU, SICU, and PICU at the UIHC during 1983–1989. Note that the five most common species accounted for fewer than 50 percent of all infections identified in these units, suggesting that there was no predominant endemic pathogen.

The incidence of infections caused by *Candida albicans* has increased in several ICUs. This trend is in keeping with rates of candidemia across the United States that have been reported to have increased threefold to tenfold. *Candida* species accounted for 10 percent of all nosocomial bloodstream infections at the UIHC between 1983 and 1986 [287].

In the SICU, gram-negative organisms were isolated from a majority of infection sites. *P. aeruginosa* and *E. coli* were the most frequent gram-negative pathogens. The gram-positive bacteria *S. epidermidis* and *S. aureus*

were among the five most common isolated and accounted for 15 to 21 percent of the isolates per annum. Enterococci were among the five most frequent pathogens in 3 of the 7 years, accounting for 7.5 to 8.5 percent of the isolates from the SICU in the same period.

Infection Sites

The frequency with which infections occurred at different sites is illustrated with trended data from the SICU, MICU, and PICU at the UIHC (Figs. 20-4 through 20-6). These data are representative of infections reported from ICUs in other tertiary care hospitals [33, 51, 69, 159, 191]. The rate of nosocomial infections was higher in ICUs than elsewhere in the hospital. Overall rates of nosocomial infections at UIHC ranged between 11 and 16 infections per 1,000 patient-days, compared with 36 to 54 per 1,000 patient-days in the SICU, 23 to 47 per 1,000 patient-days in the MICU, and 14 to 32 per 1,000 patient-days in

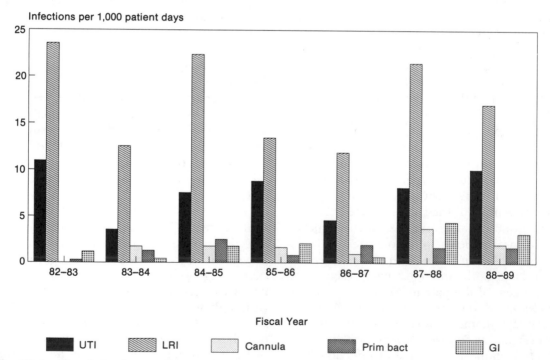

Fig. 20-4. Trends in site-specific nosocomial infection rates (infections per 1,000 patient-days) over 7 years in a medical intensive care unit. UTI = urinary tract infection; LRI = lower respiratory tract infection; Cannula = intravascular cannula entry site infection; Prim bact = primary bacteremia; GI = gastrointestinal tract infection.

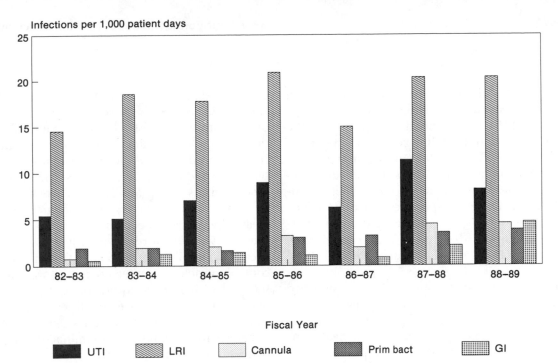

Fig. 20-5. Trends in site-specific nosocomial infection rates (infections per 1,000 patient-days) over 7 years in a surgical intensive care unit. UTI = urinary tract infection; LRI = lower respiratory tract infection; Cannula = intravascular cannula entry site infection; Prim bact = primary bacteremia; GI = gastrointestinal tract infection.

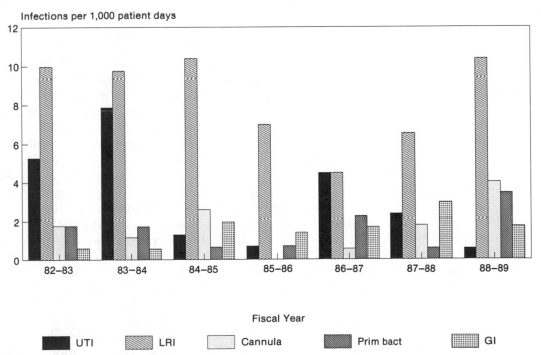

Fig. 20-6. Trends in site-specific nosocomial infection rates (infections per 1,000 patient-days) over 7 years in a pediatric intensive care unit. UTI = urinary tract infection; LRI = lower respiratory tract infection; Cannula = intravascular cannula entry site infection; Prim bact = primary bacteremia; GI = gastrointestinal tract infection.

the PICU. These data (see Figs. 20-4 through 20-6) illustrate several important points. First, rates of infection tended to be higher in the SICU than in the MICU, and rates in both of the adult ICUs were higher than in the PICU. Second, in all three units, the lower respiratory tract was the most common site of infection: Lower respiratory tract infections accounted for approximately 40 percent of infections in the SICU, 37 to 54 percent of those in the MICU, and 20 to 50 percent of those in the PICU. High rates of pulmonary infections relative to other infection sites are unique to critical care units, where patients are frequently admitted because of respiratory distress and require endotracheal intubation. When rates of lower respiratory tract infections have been compared over shorter increments of time (i.e., by month) wide variations were noted. Observations in our units suggested that the level of skilled nursing care relative to patient census may be an important determinant of this variation [254]. Although primary bacteremia and infections secondary to vascular cannulas were less common than lower respiratory tract infections, the mortality associated with these infections was high. The rates of bloodstream infections have increased in all three units over the 7 years reported. Although the PICU has had lower overall rates of infection than the MICU and the SICU, the rates of primary bacteremia and vascular cannula-associated infections have been comparable. Consequently, these infections made up a higher percentage of infections in the PICU than in the MICU and SICU. In fact, in 1988–1989, primary bacteremias and cannula-associated infections accounted for 12.3 and 14.3 percent of nosocomial infections, respectively, in the PICU, compared with 5.7 and 6.0 percent, respectively, in the SICU and 4.8 and 4.3 percent, respectively, in the MICU.

Clusters of Infections in the ICU

Although fewer than 10 percent of hospitalized patients are treated in ICUs, many outbreaks of nosocomial infections occur in this setting [286]. At the University of Vir-

ginia Hospital, 10 of 11 outbreaks identified from 1978 to 1982 occurred in ICUs, and 8 of the outbreaks involved bloodstream infections. Some epidemics were clusters of infections occurring at specific anatomic sites but associated with a variety of nosocomial microorganisms [210]. Similar to the outbreak of polymicrobial bloodstream infections described by Ponce de Leon and colleagues [207], these outbreaks were frequently related to breaks in technique or disregard for infection control guidelines. Other epidemics were associated with specific strains of bacteria and may or may not have been confined to a specific anatomic site [254]. These outbreaks were usually related to a contaminated inanimate or animate reservoir from which the organism was transmitted to the patients.

Although there were unique factors in each epidemic, several generalizations may be made. Epidemics associated with specific pathogens were often associated with bacteria that were (1) relatively resistant to antibiotics [285, 293]; (2) relatively virulent when compared with normal endogenous and environmental flora; (3) capable of withstanding variations in environmental conditions; and (4) transmitted by hand carriage from patient to patient. Pathogens that exemplify these characteristics include *S. aureus* and *Serratia, Klebsiella,* and *Enterobacter* species. Epidemics caused by unusual organisms, such as *Acinetobacter,* were often associated with contaminated equipment or with changes in the environment. It is important to remember that new equipment or a new procedure may simultaneously introduce a new reservoir or mode of transmission into the ICU [52].

A literature search for outbreaks occurring in ICUs from 1983 to the present identified 30 clusters of infections [21, 33, 36, 37, 44, 75, 85, 90, 100, 111, 113, 123, 125, 152, 154, 189, 202, 213, 215, 226, 231, 255, 272, 275, 288]. Five (17 percent) of the outbreaks were associated with *S. aureus,* and five with *Acinetobacter calcoaceticus.* Overall, approximately 40 percent of the outbreaks were caused by gram-negative bacilli and nearly another third by gram-positive bacteria. Three outbreaks were caused by viruses (hepatitis A [75], adenovirus [154], and influenza [255]), and one outbreak was caused by *C. albicans* [37]. Table 20-1 summarizes important features of selected outbreaks.

Clinical Aspects of Infections in the ICU

Critically ill patients are highly susceptible to nosocomial infections. The importance of medical devices in catheter-associated urinary tract infections (see Chap. 28), cannula-derived infections (see Chap. 40), and ventilator-associated pneumonia (see Chap. 29) was discussed earlier. Only selected aspects of infections in patients admitted to an ICU will be discussed in this section.

Pneumonia

Because the respiratory tract is the most common site of infection in patients in ICUs, special aspects of this infection will be discussed here (see Chap. 29). Critically ill patients,

Table 20-1. Summary of recent reports describing outbreaks of nosocomial infections in intensive care units

Type of unit	Organism	Sites of infection or colonization	Study
PICU, SICU	Methicillin-resistant *Staphylococcus aureus*	Multiple sites	Ribner et al. [215]
Burn unit	Methicillin-resistant *S. aureus*	Burn wounds, bacteremia	Ransj et al. [213]
SICU	Methicillin-resistant *S. aureus*	Multiple sites	Bitar et al. [21]
SICU	Methicillin-resistant *S. aureus*	Multiple sites	Gordts [100]
Critical care trauma unit	*Streptococcus pyogenes*	Cellulitis, pneumonia	Lannigan et al. [152]
General ICU	*S. pyogenes*	Bacteremia, pneumonia	Nicolle et al. [189]
SICU burn unit	*S. pyogenes*	Bacteremia, respiratory wounds	Whitby et al. [288]
Burn unit	*S. pyogenes*	Burn wounds	Burnett and Norman [36]
Critical care trauma unit	*Enterococcus faecalis*	Bacteremia, wound	Hussain et al. [123]
General ICU	*Acinetobacter calcoaceticus*	Pneumonia	Cefai et al. [44]
Burn unit	*A. calcoaceticus*	Burn wounds, pneumonia	Sherertz and Sullivan [231]
General ICU	*Ewingella americana*	Bacteremia	Pien and Bruce [202]
Cardiac care unit	*Serratia marcescens*	Bacteremia	Villarino et al. [275]
PICU	*Pseudomonas pickettii*	Pneumonia	Gardner and Shulman [90]
MICU	*Pseudomonas cepacia*	Bacteremia	Henderson et al. [113]

ICU = intensive care unit; PICU = pediatric ICU; SICU = surgical ICU; MICU = medical ICU.

including those who have suffered severe trauma and those who have had major surgery, are at increased risk for subsequent lower respiratory tract infections [50, 91, 160]. ICU-acquired pneumonia is common in patients who die of acute respiratory distress syndrome (ARDS) and multiple organ failure; the overall mortality of these conditions approaches 80 percent [15]. Although common, ICU-acquired pneumonia is difficult to diagnose [258]. Fever, leukocytosis, and lung consolidation, hallmarks of pneumonia in otherwise healthy patients, can result from other pathogenic mechanisms in ICU patients. Infiltrates on chest radiographs may arise from conditions such as pulmonary edema, contusion, atelectasis, pleural effusions, and ARDS [249, 258]. Colonization of the respiratory tract by potential bacterial pathogens, almost universally present in critically ill patients, makes the interpretation of sputum cultures difficult [18, 124, 183, 249, 258]. Prior treatment with antimicrobial agents further confounds the interpretation of sputum cultures.

Multiple factors are probably involved in the pathogenesis of ICU-acquired pneumonia including oropharyngeal colonization with aerobic gram-negative bacilli [128]; increased bacterial adherence to the oropharyngeal mucosa [128, 129, 259]; bypassing of the larynx and other natural defense mechanisms by endotracheal tubes; diminished cough reflex; impairment of ciliary function; decreased macrophage function [149, 217, 248, 258]; hypoxemia; uremia; malnutrition; ventilation-perfusion mismatch; ineffective bronchial toilet; gastric alkalinization; and decreased level of consciousness. In addition, Craven and colleagues [50] found that head trauma and the presence of an intracranial pressure monitor were associated with an increased risk of nosocomial pneumonia in mechanically ventilated patients. The relative contribution of these factors varies with study design and with the population studied. Although mechanical ventilation is not a necessary prerequisite for the development of ICU-acquired pneumonia, it substantially increases the risk of lower respiratory tract in-

fection [49, 50, 160]. Indeed, Langer and colleagues [151] demonstrated that the incidence of pneumonia is directly related to the duration of respiratory support, and the daily rate of acquisition is constant during the first 8 to 10 days of mechanical ventilation. Approximately 5 percent of patients developed pneumonia with each additional day of mechanical ventilation.

Cultures of the lower respiratory tract are important in the diagnosis of ICU-acquired pneumonia. Because the oropharynx of critically ill patients is frequently colonized with potentially pathogenic bacteria, care must be taken to avoid contaminating cultures of the lower airways. Retrieval of culture specimens by bronchoscopy using either a protected brush (PSB) or bronchoalveolar lavage (BAL) has been helpful for this purpose in both non-intubated [133, 257] and intubated patients [45, 107, 127]. In an animal model, both techniques accurately reflected the tissue bacterial content of the lower respiratory tract; however, BAL appeared to be more sensitive [129]. Pugin and colleagues [211] have reported promising results with a new method of nonbronchoscopic BAL sampling. These techniques facilitate quantitative cultures of respiratory secretions that aid in differentiating infection from colonization. Quantification of intracellular organisms, when performed, allows more rapid diagnosis of nosocomial pneumonia [45]. The use of these techniques in the diagnosis of ventilator-associated pneumonia should be strongly encouraged to increase the accuracy of this difficult diagnosis. In fact, some investigators consider PSB, BAL, and transthoracic biopsy to be the only accurate methods for the diagnosis of ventilator-associated pneumonia [127, 133]. Cultures of blood and pleural fluid, although less sensitive, remain important adjuncts in the diagnosis of ICU-acquired pneumonia. In a recent study of 42 patients with SICU-acquired pneumonia, 25 percent had positive blood or pleural cultures [183].

Other assays, including measuring the concentration of elastin fibers or the level of endotoxin in specimens obtained by BAL, have been proposed as adjuncts in the diagnosis of

ICU-acquired pneumonia. Although promising, these assays need extensive evaluation. If PSB, BAL, or biopsy is not available, alternative methods might be used. Mock and colleagues [183] recently described an objective numerical rating system for chest radiographs that provided reasonable discrimination of infection from colonization in patients in an SICU.

Early-Onset Pneumonia

In a prospective survey of 1,107 patients, Mandelli and colleagues [171] reported that more than 50 percent of ICU-acquired pneumonias appeared within the first 4 days following admission to the unit. In a later prospective multicenter study of ICU-acquired pneumonia, these investigators found that 441 of 1,304 admissions were complicated by pneumonia and that 54 percent of the infections were diagnosed within 4 days of admission [150]. Impairment of reflexes that protect the airways was the most important risk factor for early-onset pneumonia. Aspiration of oropharyngeal flora was the presumed mode of inoculation. Mandelli and colleagues [171] suggested that this entity be called *early-onset pneumonia* because the pathogenesis and primary etiologic agents differed from pneumonias arising later in the ICU stay. Because the pathogens causing aspiration pneumonia reflect the oropharyngeal microbial flora at the time of aspiration, the pathogens causing early-onset pneumonia are more likely to reflect normal oral flora or pathogens responsible for community-acquired pneumonia (anaerobes and gram-positive cocci). In one study of patients with multiple traumatic injuries, *S. aureus*, *Streptococcus pneumoniae*, and *Hemophilus influenzae* accounted for 44 percent of pneumonias acquired within the first 48 hours of admission [251].

Currently, it is not clear whether prophylaxis with antimicrobials can prevent early-onset pneumonia. In one small study, 24 hours of systemic antibiotic prophylaxis did not prevent the development of pneumonia [172]. On the other hand, Stoutenbeek [251] has demonstrated the efficacy of 4 days of intravenous antibiotic therapy in preventing early pneumonia in patients with multiple traumatic injures. If early-onset pneumonia indeed reflects a universal subset of nosocomial pneumonias, prospective studies will be necessary to define the etiologic agents, risk factors, and preventive measures for this new clinical entity.

Nosocomial Tracheobronchitis

Nosocomial tracheobronchitis, a recently recognized clinical entity, is defined by the presence of fever, purulent sputum, significant numbers of polymorphonuclear leukocytes on the gram-stain smear, and positive sputum culture in patients who have no radiographic evidence of pneumonia [35, 51, 81, 93, 138, 197, 252, 263]. Although there is no consensus in the literature regarding the need for treatment, most physicians treat tracheobronchitis to prevent subsequent pneumonia. Further studies are needed to define whether tracheobronchitis actually plays a role in the pathogenesis of nosocomial pneumonias.

Sepsis Syndrome

The sepsis syndrome has been defined as the host response to invading organisms [11] and is characterized by hypothermia or hyperthermia, tachycardia, tachypnea, and clinical evidence of infection associated with inadequate perfusion of at least one organ. When the sepsis syndrome is complicated by hypotension unresponsive to fluid therapy, it is classified as *septic shock*. Bone and colleagues [26] recently described this syndrome in a prospective analysis of 191 patients, of whom only 45 percent had documented bacteremia. Seventy percent of the patients developed septic shock within 24 hours of entry into the study, and 25 percent developed acute respiratory distress syndrome. Aside from the development of shock, which occurred more frequently in the group with bacteremia (47 percent versus 30 percent), no differences were demonstrated between bacteremic and nonbacteremic patients. The mortality of normotensive patients was only 13 percent, compared with 43 percent in hypotensive patients. Therefore, early identification and treatment of the sepsis syndrome prior to the onset of shock may reduce mortality in this critically ill population. Additional studies are needed to confirm the validity of this clinical entity and to define the role of endogenous factors, such as tumor necrosis factor or interleukin 1, as possible mediators of this syndrome.

Marshall and Sweeney [173] prospectively studied 210 patients admitted to an SICU to determine the relative contributions of infection and the host response to morbidity and mortality. Using a sepsis score that reflected the host response and was independent of culture results, these authors showed that the intensity of the host response was more highly correlated with morbidity and mortality in the ICU than was documented infection. Thus, the clinical syndrome of sepsis rather than infection per se predicted ICU mortality.

Multiple Organ Failure

With better methods for hemodynamic monitoring and support, the primary cause of death in critically ill patients with infection has shifted from shock to multiple organ failure (MOF). The mortality associated with MOF is 75 percent, even with aggressive management, and correlates with the number of organs involved [141].

The association of organ failure with infection has been noted since the earliest descriptions of the syndrome [165, 236]; whether infection is a necessary prerequisite for the development of MOF remains controversial. Single organ failure, such as ARDS, has been described in patients without significant bacterial infection [15, 79]. Furthermore, susceptibility to other ICU-acquired infections increases as a function of the intensity of the organ failure [174]. The relationship between infection and MOF was clearly demonstrated by Fry and colleagues [88] in a study of 553 consecutive patients who underwent major operative procedures or who sustained severe trauma. Thirty-eight patients developed MOF, 24 (63 percent) of whom had uncontrolled infections. The most common primary sites of infection were pleuropulmonary and intra-abdominal. Other investigators have sug-

gested that organ failure is a sign of occult, usually intraabdominal infection [89, 206]. Marshall and colleagues [174] recently confirmed the importance of the gastrointestinal tract as reservoir of pathogens. In 35 of 54 surgical patients who developed MOF, the site of infection was the peritoneal cavity or the biliary tract. *E. coli, Bacteriodes fragilis,* and enterococci were the predominant pathogens isolated. Whereas intestinal flora was responsible for most of the initial infections, *Candida* species, coagulase-negative staphylococci, and *P. aeruginosa* were the most common ICU-acquired organisms. Moreover, mortality among patients presenting with MOF was more strongly correlated with infections caused by *Candida* species and coagulase-negative staphylococci than with infections caused by other organisms. Finally, some investigators have suggested that exploratory laparotomy is helpful for both diagnosis and treatment of patients with MOF who have no known site of infection [42, 192, 206].

Bacterial translocation and endotoxin release have been proposed as mechanisms for MOF of gastrointestinal origin. Bacterial translocation across the gastrointestinal mucosa has been demonstrated in animals and humans with shock [68, 224, 242]. Positive blood cultures were obtained from patients in shock prior to the restitution of blood pressure, thereby excluding reperfusion injury as the cause. Rush and colleagues [224] showed a relationship between the rates of positive blood cultures and the severity of hypotension in the 50 severely injured patients. In another study, 13 (39 percent) of 33 consecutive patients with cardiac arrest and cardiopulmonary complications had positive blood cultures within 12 hours of the arrest [92]. Twelve of the 13 patients had the same organisms recovered from blood and feces, suggesting that mesenteric ischemia may predispose patients to septicemia. Finally, atrophy of the gastrointestinal mucosal surface because of disuse has been suggested as a possible cause of septic complications in critically ill patients. Endotoxin release by gram-negative bacteria contributes to the clinical and laboratory manifestations of the septic state and organ failure. Serum proteins that bind endotoxin include high-density lipoproteins, alpha$_2$-macroglobulin, Gc-globulin and, possibly, transferrin. Recent studies have reported a correlation between decreasing levels of plasma proteins during the initial postoperative days and the subsequent development of organ failure [17]. Further studies are needed to confirm these interesting observations.

Other ICU-Specific Infectious Problems
The Acquired Immunodeficiency Syndrome and the ICU
Several early studies demonstrated an extremely poor prognosis for patients with the acquired immunodeficiency syndrome (AIDS) and *Pneumocystis carinii* pneumonia who required intubation and mechanical ventilation [228, 277] (see Chap. 39). Despite intensive care, mortality at 3 months was very high, ranging from 85 to 95 percent. However, more recent data documented improved survival for patients with *Pneumocystis* pneumonia and respiratory failure, possibly related to the use of steroid therapy in the later series [86, 184, 220, 278].

Predictors of morbidity and survival need to be better defined in this population, in order to identify subsets of patients who would benefit from intensive support. Smith and colleagues [238] recently reported that the APACHE II scoring system inadequately predicted fatality in this subgroup of patients. The observed mortality of 64 percent was significantly greater than that predicted by the scoring system (46 percent).

Occupational exposure to the human immunodeficiency virus (HIV) is a major concern among health care providers in ICUs (see Chap. 39). A recent study highlighted the frequency of significant exposure to potentially contaminated materials [220]. Over a 6-year period, 56 mucosal splashes and 25 needle-stick injuries occurred in 76 ICU employees. Although none of the health care workers in this study became seropositive for HIV, transmission to health care workers does occur at low rates [94]. Personnel in ICUs must take precautions to avoid contact with blood and body fluids from all patients.

Tuberculosis
Several studies have described unrecognized tuberculosis in hospitalized patients [22, 198, 221] (see Chap. 29). Patients with tuberculosis frequently present with concomitant diseases including AIDS, alcohol abuse, chronic obstructive pulmonary disease, malignancy, and malnutrition. Because many of these patients are acutely ill and require intensive care, tuberculosis may be unrecognized at the time of admission to the ICU [84, 188]. A high index of suspicion is necessary to detect tuberculosis early and prevent secondary transmission.

Sinusitis
Sinusitis frequently complicates nasotracheal or nasogastric intubation (2 to 25 percent) [40, 65, 66]. Mechanical obstruction of the maxillary sinuses usually initiates the process [40], with subsequent spread to the ethmoid and sphenoid sinuses. Fever, leukocytosis, and purulent nasal discharge suggest the diagnosis, but their absence does not exclude this diagnosis [40, 199]. Conventional sinus radiographs and computed tomography scans are useful, but a sinus aspirate allows confirmation of the diagnosis and identification of the etiologic agents. In contrast to community-acquired sinusitis, gram-negative organisms predominated in this setting. *Pseudomonas* and *Klebsiella* species and *Enterobacteriaceae* were the pathogens most commonly recovered [40, 199]. In addition, *S. aureus* and *Candida* were also frequently encountered, and polymicrobial infection was documented in 40 to 100 percent of cases [40, 65, 66]. Complications included unexplained fever [147], pansinusitis [40, 199], orbital cellulitis, brain abscess, osteomyelitis [161], septicemia [65, 194], and nosocomial pneumonia [25]. Treatment required removal of the device and intravenous antibiotic therapy, including coverage for *Pseudomonas* species. Sinus drainage in uncomplicated acute sinusitis remains controversial [25]. Selective decontamination using nasal administration of antibiotics ac-

tive against gram-negative bacteria has been proposed as a prophylactic measure but requires further study [25].

Persistent Peritonitis

The support systems in ICUs facilitate the survival of patients with very severe peritonitis. The course of these patients typically includes prolonged ICU stay, multiple surgical procedures, secondary bloodstream infections, and treatment with broad-spectrum antibiotics [179]. MOF occurs frequently in this setting, and mortality is high, ranging from 60 to 80 percent [87, 179, 241]. Nosocomial pathogens involved in persistent intra-abdominal infections differ from those of patients admitted with acute peritonitis. *S. epidermidis, enterococci,* and *Candida* species are the predominant pathogens in this setting [174, 222, 236]. Management of these severe infections remains controversial; however, a combination of surgical drainage and intravenous antibiotic therapy is certainly indicated.

Acalculous Cholecystitis

Acalculous cholecystitis, also called *postoperative cholecystitis,* commonly complicates both abdominal and nonabdominal surgery in critically ill patients [97, 196]. *P. aeruginosa, E. coli,* and *Enterobacter* are the most commonly isolated pathogens. Severe complications can occur, including gangrene of the gallbladder, perforation, secondary peritonitis, intrahepatic abscesses, and ipsilateral empyema [196]. Treatment requires surgery and appropriate antibiotic therapy.

Toxic Shock Syndrome

Although classically described in young menstruating women using tampons, toxic shock syndrome (TSS) can occur postoperatively and in patients with multiple traumatic injuries [214]. Fever, erythroderma, watery diarrhea, and hypotension occurring 48 hours after surgery (range, 1 to 6 days) suggest this diagnosis (see Chap. 37). In general, the wounds do not appear to be infected, but *S. aureus* can be recovered from cultures of the wound [12]. Staphylococcal toxins are believed to be responsible for this clinical syn-

drome [6]. Antistaphylococcal drugs should be used to eliminate the organisms.

Antibiotic-Associated Colitis

Almost every antibiotic, except vancomycin, has been reported in association with *Clostridium difficile* colitis (see Chap. 30). Critically ill patients are highly susceptible to this entity because they are treated with numerous antibiotics. It is important to note that diarrhea can be absent in patients presenting with postoperative ileus [233]. Health care workers must take precautions to avoid spreading the organism from patient to patient [16, 106].

Noninfectious Fever

The differentiation of the causes of fever in ICU patients is a daily challenge for physicians. Not all fevers are the result of infections. The most common causes of noninfectious fever are listed in Table 20-2.

Control and Prevention of Nosocomial Infections
Surveillance

The recognition of important risk areas and resulting nosocomial infections in ICUs depends on the availability of adequate and accurate data (see Chap. 5). Feedback of information to medical personnel is central to the concept of surveillance and critical to the formation, implementation, and evaluation of control efforts necessary for continued safe care. The multiple risk factors and high cost of intensive care demand continued scru-

Table 20-2. Noninfectious fever in intensive care unit patients

Postoperative fever (during the first 72 hours after surgery)
Central fever in head trauma patients
Atelectasis
Drug-induced fever
Line-associated phlebitis
Phlebothrombosis
Resorption of hematomas
Inflammatory process of the pleura and peritoneum

tiny and documentation of adverse events. Surveillance methods recommended by the CDC have been shown to be successful in determining the causal events responsible for increased nosocomial infection rates. Interventions designed to decrease infection rates should be followed by continued monitoring to ensure their efficacy.

Control

Two types of measures are needed to control nosocomial infections. Engineering controls include controls that are incorporated into the structural design of the unit or equipment and those over which there is limited human control. Administrative controls are guidelines that must be learned and executed by health care workers. The latter are effective only if appropriate changes in behavior are incorporated into the routine activities of health care workers (see Chap. 3).

Engineering Controls

The contribution of the design of critical care units to the control of nosocomial infection is difficult to evaluate. However, it seems prudent to consider several issues when remodeling or designing new units:

1. Adequate space around patients beds is important for placement of support and monitoring equipment, allowing staff access to both the patient and the equipment.
2. Individualized patient cubicles may also be important in reducing transmission of pathogens in the unit [240].
3. Sinks should be located in convenient places to facilitate hand-washing by health care workers and to interrupt the most important mode of microbial transmission in the ICU. Separate, designated sinks should be provided for cleaning equipment.
4. All ICUs should be equipped with one or more class A isolation rooms [209]. Class A isolation rooms include an anteroom for gowning and hand-washing (see Chap. 11). Additional rooms for isolation precautions are necessary in units where patients are located in large open rooms.
5. Consideration should also be given to functional activities in the unit. Attention to traffic patterns, location of clean and dirty utilities, and janitor closets may reduce opportunities for cross-contamination. Clean function and storage should be physically separate from dirty function and waste disposal (see Chap. 15). Housekeeping facilities and equipment should be designated for the specific unit and stored separately from clean and dirty utilities.

Although guidelines for constructing and equipping ICUs seem prudent and might be helpful in controlling infections, several well-designed studies failed to demonstrate improvement in the rates of nosocomial infections after the units were moved into new structures [121, 158, 169]. Studies of postoperative wound infection rates following improvements in the structural design of ICUs have yielded conflicting results. Some investigators have reported reduced infection rates [60, 237, 239], whereas others did not find a significant improvement [158]. Huebner and colleagues [121] conducted a 2-year prospective study after transferring an ICU into a new structure that provided more space and more isolation rooms for infected or colonized patients. They reported that the overall rate of nosocomial infections did not change appreciatively after the move.

Administrative Controls for Medical Equipment

Medical technology is changing rapidly, and new diagnostic and therapeutic devices are constantly being introduced into ICUs. In many instances, the efficacy of the devices has not been adequately evaluated, and the effect of the devices on the incidence of nosocomial infections is unknown. For example, vendors seeking to introduce new catheters claimed to have antimicrobial activity should be challenged to provide data on the efficacy of their product. Cleaning protocols for invasive devices should be provided by the industry and be reviewed by infection control practitioners or hospital epidemiologists to ensure the adequacy of the recommendations. Sufficient numbers of frequently used instruments should be available to allow time for cleaning and disinfection or sterilization. An increase in the initial outlay for equipment may reduce costs and morbidity in the long term.

The routine application of guidelines for the appropriate use of medical devices contributes significantly to the control of nosocomial infections [166, 170]. Guidelines for the use and control of urinary tract catheters (see Chap. 28), intravascular devices (see Chap. 40), respiratory devices (see Chap. 29), and other products have been published by the CDC.

Administrative Controls for Health Care Personnel

Staffing and Training   For the patient to benefit from technologic advances in medical care, health care workers must be well trained in state-of-the-art intensive care. Studies have documented that cooperation among critical care personnel can directly influence outcome from intensive care, suggesting that the use of invasive technologies is important but not sufficient for good patient care [140, 162, 227]. Therefore, health care workers in ICUs should be involved in continuous postgraduate medical education to learn new technologies and the proper use of new medical devices and procedures. They also need periodic updates on new disease entities peculiar to patients in ICUs, including the psychologic problems associated with hospitalization in an ICU. Finally, the level of stress in ICUs exceeds that of most other areas of the hospital. As a result, rates of employee turnover are high in special care units. Loss of highly skilled medical care workers requires extensive training of replacement workers, including in-depth training on infection control procedures. Changes in staff and unrecognized modifications in infection control procedures might contribute to epidemics of nosocomial infections.

The extent and severity of illnesses afflicting patients in ICUs demand a high level of nursing care, and the high rate of nosocomial infections mandates strict application of rigid barrier nursing techniques to control transmission. Breakdown in these techniques during periods of understaffing or overcrowding

has been associated with outbreaks of nosocomial infection [109, 254]. A nurse-to-patient staffing ratio of 1:1 has been recommended to reduce breaks in techniques that lead to person-to-person transmission of pathogens within ICUs [285]. It is important that workers in ICUs understand their responsibility in preventing transmission of infectious diseases. This responsibility includes prevention of spread of pathogens from patient to patient and from the health care worker to the patient. Therefore, it is important that the hospital provide adequate staffing to cover medical absences and personal benefits that will not punish employees who are responsible enough to avoid working when ill (see Chap. 3).

Monitoring Quality of Care   The effectiveness of administrative controls will depend on compliance with established guidelines. Therefore, the performance and behavior of health care providers should be monitored. Failure to comply with guidelines, whether it be by physicians, nurses, or other support personnel, should be addressed promptly to prevent the establishment of bad habits that impose unnecessary risks on patients.

Monitoring the quality of medical care in ICUs is important, albeit controversial, given the complexity of the patients and the procedures performed in these units. Few studies have been published regarding the assessment of the quality of care in ICUs. In one recent study, the clinical and pathologic diagnoses from 100 patients who came to autopsy were compared as measures of quality of care [80]. In 77 percent of the patients, the major clinical diagnoses were confirmed by the autopsy. Of note, myocardial infarction and peritonitis were the most commonly missed diagnoses.

Reviews of autopsy data, although useful, are not sufficient to study the quality of care in ICUs. The APACHE II study will evaluate a nationally representative data file using a measure of the patient's severity of illness to develop an estimate of the number of preventable deaths. This estimate may serve as a monitor of the quality of care in ICUs [72, 280, 281]. The study will collect information using the therapeutic intervention scoring system (TISS). The TISS sensitively measures interpatient as well as interhospital variations in the level of patient care and will facilitate estimates of the costs of ICU care. These data are critical for the assessment of the quality of care in ICUs. A further challenge will be to maintain the quality while reducing the cost of care. In a recent study comparing 13 hospitals, the hospital with the lowest mortality had the highest cost of care [140].

Administrative Controls for Patients

Because of the risk of infection and other complications in ICUs, only patients who will benefit from high-intensity, high-risk care should be admitted to ICUs, and patients should be discharged from the ICU as soon as possible to decrease the risk of nosocomial infection. Unfortunately, there is little published information to assist the physician in those important decisions.

Dragsted and colleagues [71] recently reported results of a 5-year prospective study analyzing outcomes of 1,308 patients from a medical-surgical ICU. When patients were controlled for the level of organ system failure after 48 hours in the unit, sepsis and severity of illness were significant risk factors for mortality during the stay within the ICU. However, no subgroup of patients was identified in which the short-term outcome was so poor as to exclude them from treatment in the ICU.

Surveillance for nosocomial infections, monitoring rates of infection, and reporting results to personnel are important to ensure the quality of medical care in ICUs. Properly conducted surveillance can identify behavioral, environmental, or treatment factors that, when corrected, will decrease endemic rates of infection in the unit. Additional benefits of concurrent surveillance include early identification and intervention in epidemics.

Practical Aspects of Infection Control in the ICU

Methods for preventing nosocomial infections are numerous. Many are discussed elsewhere in the text. Only selected measures will be discussed in this section.

Patient Isolation

More than 50 percent of patients admitted to ICUs are colonized at the time of admission with the organism responsible for subsequent infections. Patients who are readmitted to the hospital may carry and transmit resistant organisms acquired during previous hospitalizations. Not infrequently, unrecognized infection contributes to the decision for entry into the unit. The early diagnosis of potentially transmissible disease requires a high index of suspicion. Patients with suspected infections should be appropriately segregated at the time of admission. The level of isolation should account for each of the following: the site of infection, the mode of transmission, the amount of secretions or excretions, and the virulence and antimicrobial susceptibilities of the etiologic agent. The isolation guidelines published by the CDC are useful in this respect (see Chap. 11).

Specific isolation techniques are beyond the scope of this chapter. It should be recognized that as the duration of stay increases, the frequency of colonization with resistant microflora increases. Patients become animate reservoirs that facilitate transmission to susceptible incoming patients (see Chap. 1). It may be wise, therefore, to separate long-stay patients from the rapid-turnover, short-stay patients who comprise the major portion of the population in the unit. This may be accomplished by moving chronically ill patients to single rooms or relocating groups of patients to a physically separate part of the unit. A dedicated nursing staff for the long-term patients would provide an added barrier to transmission. Frequent transfers of patients through various units and levels of care increase the risk of transmission of resistant organisms throughout the hospital. Moreover, colonized patients are important animate reservoirs of resistant microorganisms during interinstitutional transfers and probably account for the spread of methicillin-resistant *S. aureus* [21, 213] (see Chap. 37). To control the spread of resistant organisms, it is extremely important to document information regarding carriage of antibiotic-resistant microflora in the patient's medical record and to report it to receiving units and facilities.

Hand-Washing

Routine hand-washing before and between patient contact is the most important feature of infection control. Virtually all medical care workers are aware of and agree with this concept [2, 185]. It is dismaying, therefore, to see repeated reports of low levels of compliance with this simple and inexpensive technique. Several reasons have been suggested to account for this low level of compliance, including (1) lack of priority over other required procedures, (2) insufficient time to accomplish hand-washing, (3) inconvenient placement of hand-washing sinks or other hand-washing tools, (4) allergy or intolerance to the hand-washing solutions, (5) lack of leadership by the senior medical staff, and (6) lack of personal commitment to the routine of hand-washing (see Chap. 11).

Barrier Precautions

There is currently little evidence that the addition of gloves in the routine intensive care situation has any benefit over routine hand-washing in controlling infections. However, well-designed studies are extremely difficult to conduct. Whereas a number of studies investigated the role of very sophisticated forms of protective isolation in reducing high rates of nosocomial infections in patients with profound granulocytopenia or full-thickness burns, only a few have evaluated whether simple protective isolation would be beneficial for ICU patients. Klein and co-workers [138] recently conducted a prospective, randomized trial in a pediatric ICU. In this well-designed study, the authors demonstrated the benefit of simple barrier precautions (disposable gown and gloves) on both colonization and subsequent infection. Colonization with ICU bacterial strains occurred an average of 5 days later in isolated patients (n = 32). The daily rate of infection for isolated patients was 2.2 times lower than among patients provided standard care (n = 38, p = .007). Although previous studies reported conflicting results concerning the value of protective isolation in ICU patients, gowns and gloves may be effective in dealing with selected high-risk patients. Further studies are

necessary to determine the cost-effectiveness of this approach in the general ICU population. To draw definitive conclusions regarding the effectiveness of this approach, compliance with isolation precautions should be evaluated also. Only a few studies have analyzed compliance with isolation precautions [2, 103, 138, 156], and most reported less than 50 percent compliance, despite the fact that health care workers were aware that they were under observation [2, 103].

The use of special clothing in ICUs is frequently discussed but has little documentation or support. Carriage of potential pathogens on the gowns and uniforms of health care workers in special care units has been repeatedly studied [191]. Isolation of microorganisms from clothing has been confirmed, and carriage increases with time. However, evidence that clothing is important in the transmission of nosocomial pathogens has been convincingly documented only in a few instances. It appears prudent to avoid contamination of uniforms with organisms. However, there is no evidence that the addition of special surgical scrubs or caps reduces the rates of nosocomial infections.

Prevention of Pneumonia

New approaches in the management of ICU-acquired respiratory infections include prevention of oropharyngeal colonization, maintenance of gastric acidity, and the use of oscillating beds [81, 93, 135, 205]. These procedures, as well as older methods such as postural drainage, tracheal suctioning, and frequent repositioning of the patient, must be studied in a systematic manner to determine whether they actually decrease the rates of ICU-acquired pneumonia (see Chap. 29).

Special Units, Special Problems

Each subspecialty unit uses unique medical and administrative methods in patient care that are, in turn, associated with special risks. Consequently, each unit develops unique endemic and epidemic nosocomial infection problems. The variation in risk of nosocomial infection will be recognized only with active surveillance systems in each unit. In a study evaluating infection reports from 66 hospitals between 1986 and 1990, the rate and distribution of infections by site and pathogen were shown to vary considerably by ICU type [78]. Effective surveillance enables early interception of problems and the development of efficacious, focused interventions.

New Therapeutic Approaches
Selective Digestive Decontamination

Since many nosocomial infections are believed to arise from endogenous flora in the oropharyngeal and gastrointestinal tract, recent innovations in prevention have focused on the control (decontamination) of potential pathogens with oral antimicrobial therapy (see Chap. 13). The aim of selective digestive decontamination (SDD) is to prevent overgrowth of pathogenic gram-negative aerobic bacilli and yeast by using oral nonabsorbable antibiotics that preserve the endogenous anaerobic flora [204].

In 1984, Stoutenbeek and colleagues [252] reported a reduction of ICU-acquired infections from 81 to 16 percent in patients with multiple trauma. Selective decontamination was performed with a mixture of polymyxin E, tobramycin, and amphotericin B (PTA) applied as a paste to the oral cavity and as a suspension via a nasogastric tube. In addition, systemic cefotaxime was administered for several days until decontamination was achieved. The beneficial effects of similar regimens have been demonstrated in a number of studies in ICU patients, including patients in specialized units [48, 137, 250, 263] as well as in combined medical-surgical ICUs [157, 262]. In studies where bacteriologic screening was performed, colonization of the oropharynx, stomach, and lower digestive tract with aerobic gram-negative bacilli increased with the duration of the ICU stay [76, 136, 157, 191, 252, 262]. SDD regimens prevented and eliminated colonization [157, 251–253, 263, 262, 271]. In most studies, a reduction was noted in all categories of ICU-acquired infections. However, results were most marked for respiratory tract infections. In several studies, SDD was also associated with decreased length of stay in the ICU [251] and decreased use of

antibiotics for therapeutic purposes [157]. Although mortality was reduced in specific groups of patients [137, 157, 197, 251], the overall mortality was unaffected except for one randomized trial in which mortality was significantly reduced [262]. The lack of effect on mortality may reflect the small number of patients in the studies and insufficient power to demonstrate a treatment effect.

In addition to its role in preventing ICU-acquired infections, SDD may be of benefit in controlling endotoxemia arising from bowel flora and phenomena associated with endotoxin release, such as MOF, ARDS, and renal failure [212, 270]. However, controversy still exists concerning the use of this approach because the antibiotics may enhance the release of endotoxins by killing bacteria in the bowel.

Another role for SDD may be in the control of nosocomial outbreaks. Brun-Buisson and colleagues [35] reported that intestinal decontamination by oral nonabsorbable antibiotics was important in resolving an outbreak of infection with multiresistant Enterobacteriaceae in an MICU. In units where routine infection control measures fail to control outbreaks [82, 195, 283], careful application of SDD, including the selection of appropriate oral antimicrobial agents and careful monitoring for the efficacy and emergence of new resistant strains, might be an important adjunct to conventional infection control procedures.

The results of clinical trials of SDD are encouraging. However, a few caveats are warranted. First, almost all SDD regimens include concomitant systemic antimicrobial therapy for 4 to 8 days. Although resistance to the third-generation cephalosporins has not been a problem even after several years of use in some units [157, 253, 262], these agents stimulate inducible, chromosomally mediated production of β-lactamases by *Enterobacter* species. Therefore, the enteric flora of patients treated with SDD must be monitored for resistant strains [205]. Second, the role of each component of the SDD regimen must be defined. For example, it is not known whether systemic prophylaxis is necessary. Some investigators have suggested that the oropharyngeal antibiotic paste is the most important facet of SDD [204, 250]. Preliminary results from a randomized controlled trial suggested that the risk of ventilator-associated pneumonia could be reduced by using topical oropharyngeal decontamination alone [211]. On the other hand, preliminary evidence suggests that systemic antibiotics might reduce the rate of early-onset pneumonia [251]. Third, the role of SDD in patients in neonatal ICUs needs to be investigated. Infants rapidly develop colonization with hospital flora and experience high rates of infection arising from the abnormal endogenous flora [159]. Since infants become heavily colonized with gram-positive organisms, it is possible that SDD regimens should include an agent effective against those organisms, particularly coagulase-negative staphylococci. Fourth, the most effective decontamination regimens have not been determined [204], and the cost-effectiveness of SDD has not been established [262]. Fifth and finally, the groups of patients who would benefit most from SDD have not been defined.

Currently, we believe that SDD should be restricted to well-controlled clinical studies or to situations in which efficacy and cost-effectiveness have been well demonstrated. Table 20-3 summarizes situations in which SDD may be beneficial.

New Therapy for Sepsis

Endotoxin release by gram-negative bacteria contributes to the clinical manifestations of

Table 20-3. Possible indications for selective decontamination in patients admitted to intensive care units

Multiple trauma*
Bloodstream infection of gut origin
Sepsis syndrome
Neutropenia*
Outbreak of multiresistant gram-negative bacilli*
Immunocompromised host
Intensive care unit stay > 10 days
Mechanical ventilation > 5 days
Multiple organ failure
Previous radiotherapy

*Efficacy published in the literature.
Adapted with permission from D. Pittet, Decontamination digestive selective aux soins intensifs. *Med. Hyg.* 47:3025, 1989.

sepsis in febrile patients [269]. Consequently, a number of clinical trials have been conducted using either hyperimmune serum or antiendotoxin antibodies for the treatment of septicemia. The initial study by Ziegler and associates [294] was a multicenter, double-blind trial of antiserum prepared by immunizing donors with a "J5" mutant of *E. coli* 0111. Although treatment with the antiserum was associated with reversal of profound shock, little effect on mortality was reported, and no protective antibody titer could be detected. Following this first report, efforts have been made to produce human antiserum by active immunization with other core endotoxin antigens and to produce monoclonal antibodies of murine or human origin. A recent clinical trial of IgG given intravenously was unsuccessful, perhaps due to low levels of antibody to endotoxin [176]. Murine monoclonal antibodies of the IgM isotype have produced encouraging results in both animals and humans.

The results of two large multicenter trials designed to assess the value of monoclonal antiendotoxin antibodies in gram-negative sepsis have been recently reported [104, 295]. In both studies, analysis of the data by intention to treat, which is of critical importance to the practicing physician, failed to demonstrate significant reduction in mortality when the results from the total study populations were analyzed. In each study, a small subgroup of patients appeared to benefit from this therapy; 137 of 468 patients (29 percent) with gram-negative sepsis without shock [104] and 200 of 543 patients (37 percent) with gram-negative bacteremia [295] appeared to benefit from the therapy with monoclonal antiendotoxin antibodies, respectively. Thus, the majority of patients with sepsis syndrome will not benefit from the treatment with either of these antibodies. The results of these studies [104, 295] suggest that the use of this expensive therapy (approximately $3,000 to $4,000 per dose) should be restricted to the subgroups of patients in which it has been shown to be efficacious. Further clinical trials are necessary to determine the role of the use of monoclonal antiendotoxin antibodies in the ICU population.

Tumor necrosis factor (TNF), a cytokine produced by activated macrophage, appears to be a primary mediator of the deleterious effects of endotoxin in animals [19] and in humans [119, 180]. In several studies, a correlation between levels of TNF and mortality has been reported [29, 39, 56]. Plasma TNF levels were increased in patients with meningococcemia [95, 276], gram-negative septicemia [62, 180], septic shock [39, 56], and MOF [29]. Plasma TNF levels have also been reported to be increased in patients with septicemia from gram-positive organisms and yeast [29, 39]. Anti-TNF antibodies might provide a more general therapy for sepsis than antiendotoxin antibodies [260].

The value of corticosteroids in the treatment of gram-negative septicemia has been controversial. In view of the results of recent well-controlled clinical trials [27, 28] that failed to demonstrate a beneficial effect of corticosteroids in the treatment of septic shock and ARDS, this approach cannot be recommended. The use of intravenous immunoglobulins as adjuvant therapy in septic patients needs further investigation [63].

Naloxone, an antagonist of opiates and β-endorphins, has been shown to reverse endotoxic and hypovolemic shock in experimental animals. Despite equivocal clinical data, this agent should be tested in well-controlled clinical trials to determine whether it is of benefit for hemodynamic support [108].

Comments

Considerable progress has been made in providing intensive care and life support to patients who are acutely ill. Unfortunately, each new technologic advance is accompanied by potential risks for the patient, including nosocomial infections. Clinical research is needed to address the benefits and risks associated with these new interventions. To achieve these objectives, collaboration is needed among intensivists, epidemiologists, and infection control practitioners to design appropriate studies, interventions, and policies. Because of problems of small sample size and individual institutions, the generation of useful information will be expedited by the development of multicenter studies evaluating benefits and risks. These objectives may be epitomized in the ancient works of Zenophon of Cyropaedia (circa 400 BC):

> As there are persons who mend torn garments, so there are physicians who heal the sick; but your duty is far nobler and one befitting a great (person)—namely to keep people in health.

The challenge is to avoid undoing the benefits of intensive care by reducing risk of complications to a minimum.

References

1. Abramson, N. S., et al. Adverse occurrences in intensive care units. *J.A.M.A.* 244:1582, 1980.
2. Albert, R. K., and Condie, F. Handwashing patterns in medical intensive care units. *N. Engl. J. Med.* 304:1465, 1981.
3. Altura, B. M., and Hershey, S. G. RES phagocytic function in trauma and adaptation to experimental shock. *Am. J. Physiol.* 215:1414, 1968.
4. Apelgren, K. N., et al. Malnutrition in Veterans Administration surgical patients. *Arch. Surg.* 116:1059, 1981.
5. Armstrong, C. W., et al. Prospective study of catheter replacement and other risk factors for infection of hyperalimentation catheters. *J. Infect. Dis.* 154:808, 1984.
6. Arnow, P. M., et al. Spread of a toxic-shock syndrome associated strain of *Staphylococcus aureus* and management of antibodies to staphylococcal enterotoxin F. *J. Infect. Dis.* 149:103, 1984.
7. Askanazi, J., et al. Effect of immediate postoperative nutritional support on length of hospitalization. *Ann. Surg.* 203:236, 1986.
8. Atherton, S. T., and White, D. J. Stomach as a source of bacteria colonizing the respiratory tract during artificial ventilation. *Lancet* 2:968, 1978.
9. Axelrod, P., and Talbot, G. H. Risk factors for acquisition of gentamicin-resistant enterococci. A multivariate analysis. *Arch. Intern. Med.* 149:1397, 1989.
10. Ayala, A., Perrin, M. M., Wagner, M. A., and Chaudry, I. H. Enhanced susceptibility to sepsis after simple hemorrhage. *Arch. Surg.* 125:70, 1990.
11. Ayres, S. M. SCCM's new horizon's conference on sepsis and septic shock. *Crit. Care Med.* 13:864, 1985.

12. Bartlett, P., et al. Toxic shock syndrome associated with surgical wound infections. *J.A.M.A.* 247:1448, 1982.

13. Barza, M., Giuliano, M., Jacobus, N. V., and Gorbach, S. L. Effect of broad-spectrum parenteral antibiotics on "colonization resistance" of intestinal microflora of humans. *Antimicrob. Agents Chemother.* 31:723, 1987.

14. Bassili, H. R., and Deitel, M. Effect of nutritional support on weaning patients off mechanical ventilators. *J. Parenter. Enter. Nutr.* 5:161, 1981.

15. Bell, R. C., Coalson, J. J., Smith, J. D., and Johanson, W. G. Multiple organ system failure and infection in adult respiratory distress syndrome. *Ann. Intern. Med.* 99:293, 1983.

16. Bender, B. S., et al. Is *Clostridium difficile* endemic in chronic-care facilities? *Lancet* 2:11, 1986.

17. Berer, D., Kitterer, W. R., and Berger, H. G. Are the serum levels of endotoxin-binding proteins reliable predictors of complications in the course of peritonitis? *Eur. J. Clin. Invest.* 20:66, 1990.

18. Berger, R., and Arango, L. Etiologic diagnosis of bacterial nosocomial pneumonia in seriously ill patients. *Crit. Care Med.* 13:833, 1985.

19. Beutler, B., and Cerami, A. Cachectin: More than tumor necrosis factor. *N. Engl. J. Med.* 316:379, 1987.

20. Bistrian, B. R., et al. Prevalence of malnutrition in general medicine patients. *J.A.M.A.* 235:1567, 1976.

21. Bitar, C. M., et al. Outbreak due to methicillin- and rifampin-resistant *Staphylococcus aureus:* Epidemiology and eradication of the resistant strain from the hospital. *Infect. Control* 8:15, 1987.

22. Bobrowitz, I. D. Active tuberculosis undiagnosed until autopsy. *Am. J. Med.* 72:650, 1982.

23. Bodey, G. P., et al. Effect of broad-spectrum cephalosporins on the microbial flora of recipients. *J. Infect. Dis.* 148:892, 1983.

24. Bohnen, J. M. A., Mustard, R. A., Oxholm, S. E., and Schouten, B. D. APACHE II score and abdominal sepsis. A prospective study. *Arch. Surg.* 123:225, 1988.

25. Boles, J-M., Garo, B., and Garre, M. Nosocomial Sinusitis in Intensive Care Patients. In: J. L. Vincent (Ed.), *Update in Intensive Care and Emergency Medicine*, Vol. 8. Berlin: Springer, 1989. P. 133.

26. Bone, R. C., et al. Sepsis syndrome: A valid clinical entity. *Crit. Care Med.* 17:389, 1989.

27. Bone, R. C., et al. A controlled clinical trial of high-dose methylprednisolone in the treatment of severe sepsis and septic shock. *N. Engl. J. Med.* 317:653, 1987.

28. Bone, R. C., et al. Early methylprednisolone treatment for septic syndrome and the adult respiratory distress syndrome. *Chest* 92:1032, 1987.

29. Brandtzaeg, P., et al. Plasma endotoxin as a predictor of multiple organ failure and death in systemic meningococcal disease. *J. Infect. Dis.* 159:195, 1989.

30. Brannen, A. L., II, Godfrey, L. J., and Goetter, W. E. Prediction of outcome from critical illness: A comparison of clinical judgment with a prediction rule. *Arch. Intern. Med.* 149:1083, 1989.

31. Britt, M. R., Schleupner, C. J., and Matsumiya, S. Severity of underlying disease as a predictor of nosocomial infection. *J.A.M.A.* 239:1047, 1978.

32. Brown, R. B., et al. A comparison of infections in different ICUs within the same hospital. *Crit. Care Med.* 13:472, 1985.

33. Brown, R. B., et al. Outbreak of nosocomial *Flavobacterium meningosepticum* respiratory infections associated with use of aerosolized polymyxin B. *Am. J. Infect. Control* 17:121, 1989.

34. Brun-Buisson, C., et al. Transferrable enzymatic resistance to third-generation cephalosporins during nosocomial outbreak of multiresistant *Klebsiella pneumonia. Lancet* 2:302, 1987.

35. Brun-Buisson, C., et al. Intestinal decontamination for control of nosocomial multiresistant gram-negative bacilli. Study of an outbreak in an intensive care unit. *Ann. Intern. Med.* 110:873, 1989.

36. Burnett, I. A., and Norman, P. *Staphylococcus pyogenes:* An outbreak on a burns unit. *J. Hosp. Infect.* 15:173, 1990.

37. Burnie, J. P., et al. Outbreak of systemic *Candida albicans* in intensive care units caused by cross infection. *Br. Med. J. [Clin. Res.]* 290:746, 1985.

38. Buzby, G. P., et al. Prognostic nutritional index in gastrointestinal surgery. *Am. J. Surg.* 139:160, 1980.

39. Calandra, T., et al. Prognostic values of tumor necrosis factor/cachectin, interleukin-1, interferon-gamma, and interferon-alpha in the serum of patients with septic shock. *J. Infect. Dis.* 161:982, 1990.

40. Caplan, E. S., and Hoyt, N. J. Nosocomial sinusitis. *J.A.M.A.* 207:639, 1982.

41. Caplan, E. S., and Hoyt, N. Infection surveillance and control in the severely traumatized patient. *Am. J. Med.* 70:638, 1981.

42. Carrico, C. J., et al. Multiple-organ-failure syndrome. The gastrointestinal tract: The 'motor' of MOF? *Arch. Surg.* 121:197, 1986.

43. Casewell, M. W., and Phillips, I. Aspects of the plasmid-mediated antibiotic resistance and epidemiology of *Klebsiella* species. *Am. J. Med.* 70:459, 1981.

44. Cefai, C., Richards, J., Gould, F. K., and McPeake, P. An outbreak of *Acinetobacter* respiratory tract infections resulting from incomplete disinfection of ventilatory equipment. *J. Hosp. Infect.* 15:177, 1990.
45. Chastre, J., et al. Diagnosis of nosocomial bacterial pneumonia in intubated patients undergoing ventilation: Comparison of the usefulness of bronchoalveolar lavage and the protected specimen brush. *Am. J. Med.* 85:499, 1988.
46. Christensen, G. D., et al. Microbial and Foreign Body Factors in the Pathogenesis of Medical Device Infections. In: A. L. Bisno and F. A. Waldvogel (Eds.), *Infections Associated with Indwelling Medical Devices.* Washington, DC: American Society for Microbiology, 1989. P. 27.
47. Christou, N. V., and Meakins, J. L. Neutrophil function in surgical patients: Two inhibitors of granulocyte chemotaxis associated with sepsis. *J. Surg. Res.* 26:355, 1979.
48. Clasener, H. A. L., Vollaard, E. J., and Van Saene, H. K. F. Long-term prophylaxis of infection by selective decontamination in leucopenia and in mechanical ventilation. *Rev. Infect. Dis.* 9:295, 1987.
49. Craven, D. E., et al. Contamination of mechanical ventilators with tubing changes every 24 or 48 hours. *N. Engl. J. Med.* 306:1505, 1982.
50. Craven, D. E., et al. Risk factors for pneumonia and fatality in patients receiving continuous mechanical ventilation. *Am. Rev. Respir. Dis.* 133:792, 1986.
51. Craven, D. E., et al. Nosocomial infection and fatality in medical surgical intensive care unit patients. *Arch. Intern. Med.* 148:1161, 1988.
52. Craven, D. E., et al. Contaminated medication nebulizers in mechanical ventilator circuits. *Am. J. Med.* 77:834, 1984.
53. Cross, A. S., et al. Evidence for the role of Toxin A in the pathogenesis of infection with *Pseudomonas aeruginosa* in humans. *J. Infect. Dis.* 142:538, 1980.
54. Cuddy, B. G., Loegering, D. J., Blumenstock, F. A., and Shah, D. J. Hepatic macrophage complement receptor clearance function following injury. *J. Surg. Res.* 40:216, 1986.
55. Dal Nogare, A. R., Toews, G. B., and Pierce, A. K. Increased salivary elastase precedes gram-negative bacillary colonization in postoperative patients. *Am. Rev. Respir. Dis.* 135:671, 1987.
56. Damas, P., et al. Tumor necrosis factor and interleukin-1 serum levels during severe sepsis in humans. *Crit. Care Med.* 17:975, 1989.
57. Daschner, F., et al. Stress ulcer prophylaxis and ventilation pneumonia: Prevention by antibacterial cytoprotective agents. *Infect. Control Hosp. Epidemiol.* 9:59, 1988.
58. Daschner, F. D., et al. Nosocomial infections in intensive care wards: A multicenter prospective study. *Intensive Care Med.* 8:5, 1982.
59. Davenport, D. S., et al. Utility of a test for slime production as a market for clinically significant coagulase-negative staphylococcal infections. *J. Infect. Dis.* 153:332, 1986.
60. Davidson, A. I. G., Smylie, H. G., MacDonald, A., and Smith, G. Ward design in relation to postoperative wound infection: Part II. *Br. Med. J.* 1:72, 1971.
61. De Champs, C., et al. Prospective survey of colonization and infection caused by expanded-spectrum-beta-lactamase-producing members of the family Entcrobactcriaccac in an intensive care unit. *J. Clin. Microbiol.* 27:2887, 1989.
62. De Groote, M. A., et al. Plasma tumor necrosis factor levels in patients with presumed sepsis. Results in those treated with antilipid A antibody vs placebo. *J.A.M.A.* 262:249, 1989.
63. De Simone, C., Delogu, G., and Corbetta, G. Intravenous immunoglobulins in association with antibiotics: A therapeutic trial in septic intensive care unit patients. *Crit. Care Med.* 16:23, 1988.
64. Dellinger, E. P., et al. Surgical infection stratification system for intra-abdominal infection. Multicenter trial. *Arch. Surg.* 120:21, 1985.
65. Deutschman, E. C. S., et al. Paranasal sinusitis associated with nasotracheal intubation: A frequent unrecognized and treatable source of sepsis. *Crit. Care Med.* 14:111, 1986.
66. Deutschman, E. C. S., et al. Paranasal sinusitis: A common complication of nasotracheal intubation in neurosurgical patients. *Neurosurgery* 17:296, 1985.
67. Doggett, R. W., Harrison, G. M., and Wallis, E. S. Comparison of some properties of *Pseudomonas aeruginosa* isolated from infections in persons with and without cystic fibrosis. *J. Bacteriol.* 87:427, 1964.
68. Donahoe, M. J., et al. Role of antibiotics in late survival from hemorrhagic shock. *Surg. Forum* 37:62, 1986.
69. Donowitz, L. G. High risk of nosocomial infection in the pediatric critical care patient. *Crit. Care Med.* 14:26, 1986.
70. Donowitz, L. G., Wenzel, R. P., and Hoyt, J. W. High risk of hospital-acquired infection in the ICU patient. *Crit. Care Med.* 10:355, 1982.
71. Dragsted, L., Qvist, J., and Madsen, M. Outcome from intensive care: II. A 5-year study of 1308 patients: Short-term outcome. *Eur. J. Anaesthesiol.* 6:131, 1989.
72. Draper, E., Russo, M., and Wagner, D. Efficiency and nurse staff. *Crit. Care Med.* 17:S217, 1989.

73. Driks, M. R., et al. Nosocomial pneumonia in intubated patients given sucralfate as compared with antacids or histamine type 2 blockers. *N. Engl. J. Med.* 317:1376, 1987.

74. Driver, A. G., McAlevy, M. T., and Smith, J. L. Nutritional assessment of patients with chronic obstructive pulmonary disease and acute respiratory failure. *Chest* 82:568, 1982.

75. Drusin, L. M., et al. Nosocomial hepatitis A infection in a paediatric intensive care unit. *Arch. Dis. Child.* 62:690, 1987.

76. du Moulin, G. C., et al. Aspiration of gastric bacteria in antacid-treated patients: A frequent cause of postoperative colonization of the airway. *Lancet* 1:242, 1982.

77. Edelman, R. Cell Mediated Immune Response in Protein Calorie Malnutrition—A Review. In: R. M. Suskind (Ed.), *Malnutrition and the Immune Response.* New York: Raven Press, 1977.

78. Jarvis, W., Edwards, J. R., and the National Nosocomial Infection Surveillance (NNIS) System. Nosocomial infection rates in adult and pediatric intensive care units in the United States. *Am. J. Med.* 91:3B, 1991.

79. Faist, E., et al. Multiple organ failure in polytrauma patients. *J. Trauma* 23:775, 1983.

80. Fernandez-Segoviano, P., et al. Autopsy as quality assurance in the intensive care unit. *Crit. Care Med.* 16:683, 1988.

81. Fink, M. P., et al. The efficacy of an oscillating bed in the prevention of lower respiratory tract infection in critically ill victims of blunt trauma. A prospective study. *Chest* 97:132, 1990.

82. Flynn, D. M., et al. Patients' endogenous flora as the source of "nosocomial" *Enterobacter* in cardiac surgery. *J. Infect. Dis.* 156:363, 1987.

83. Flynn, D. M., Weinstein, R. A., and Kabins, S. A. Infections with gram-negative bacilli in a cardiac surgery intensive care unit: The relative role of *Enterobacter. J. Hosp. Infect.* 11:367, 1988.

84. Frame, R. N., et al. Active tuberculosis in the medical intensive care unit: A 15-year retrospective analysis. *Crit. Care Med.* 15:1012, 1987.

85. Franks, A., Sacks, J. J., Smith, J. D., and Sikes, R. K. A cluster of unexplained cardiac arrests in a surgical intensive care unit. *Crit. Care Med.* 15:1075, 1987.

86. Friedman, Y., Franklin, C., Rackow, E. C., and Weil, M. H. Improved survival in patients with acquired immunodeficiency syndrome, *Pneumocystis carinii* pneumonia, and severe respiratory failure. *Chest* 96:862, 1989.

87. Fry, D. E., et al. Determinants of death in patients with intraabdominal abscess. *Surgery* 88:517, 1980.

88. Fry, D. E., Pearlstein, L., Fulton, R. L., and Polk, H. C. Multiple system organ failure. The role of uncontrolled infection. *Arch. Surg.* 115:136, 1980.

89. Fulton, R. L., and Jones, C. E. The cause of posttraumatic pulmonary insufficiency in man. *Surg. Gynecol. Obstet.* 140:179, 1975.

90. Gardner, S., and Shulman, S. T. Nosocomial common source outbreak caused by *Pseudomonas pickettii. Pediatr. Infect. Dis.* 3:420, 1984.

91. Garibaldi, R. A., et al. Risk factors for postoperative pneumonia. *J.A.M.A.* 70:677, 1981.

92. Gaussorgues, P., et al. Bacteremia following cardiac arrest and cardiopulmonary resuscitation. *Intensive Care Med.* 14:575, 1988.

93. Gentilello, L., et al. Effect of a rotating bed on the incidence of pulmonary complications in critically ill patients. *Crit. Care Med.* 16:783, 1988.

94. Gerberding, J. L., et al. Risk of transmitting the human immunodeficiency virus, hepatitis B virus, and cytomegalovirus to health care workers exposed to patients with AIDS and AIDS-related conditions. *J. Infect. Dis.* 156:1, 1987.

95. Girardin, E., et al. Tumor necrosis factor and interleukin-1 in the serum of children with severe infectious purpura. *N. Engl. J. Med.* 319:397, 1988.

96. Giuliano, M., Barza, M., Jacobus, N. V., and Gorbach, S. L. Effect of broad-spectrum parenteral antibiotics on composition of intestinal microflora of humans. *Antimicrob. Agents Chemother.* 31:202, 1987.

97. Glenn, F., and Wantz, G. E. Acute cholecystitis following the surgical treatment of unrelated disease. *Surg. Gynecol. Obstet.* 102:145, 1956.

98. Goldmann, D. A., Durbin, W. A., Jr., and Freeman, J. Nosocomial infections in a neonatal intensive care unit. *J. Infect. Dis.* 144:449, 1981.

99. Goldmann, D. A., Freeman, J., and Durbin, W. A., Jr. Nosocomial infection and death in a neonatal intensive care unit. *J. Infect. Dis.* 147:635, 1983.

100. Gordts, B. Epidemic of multiresistant *Staphylococcus aureus* in an intensive care unit. *Acta Anaesthesiol. Belg.* 34:175, 1983.

101. Gorse, G. J., Messner, R. L., and Stephens, N. D. Association of malnutrition with nosocomial infection. *Infect. Control Hosp. Epidemiol.* 10:194, 1989.

102. Goularte, T. A., Lichtenberg, D. A., and Craven, D. E. Gastric colonization in patients receiving antacids and mechanical ventilation: A mechanism of pharyngeal colonization. *Am. J. Infect. Control* 14:88, 1986.

103. Graham, M. Frequency and duration of handwashing in an intensive care unit. *Am. J. Infect. Control* 18:77, 1990.

104. Greenman, R. L., et al. A controlled clinical trial of E5 murine monoclonal IgM antibody

to endotoxin in the treatment of gram-negative sepsis. *J. A. M. A.* 266:1097, 1991.

105. Gross, P. A., et al. Number of comorbidities as a predictor of nosocomial infection acquisition. *Infect. Control Hosp. Epidemiol.* 9:497, 1988.

106. Grube, B. J., Heimbach, D. M., and Marvin, J. A. *Clostridium difficile* diarrhea in critically ill burned patients. *Arch. Surg.* 122:655, 1987.

107. Guerra, L. F., and Baughman, R. P. Use of bronchoalveolar lavage to diagnose bacterial pneumonia in mechanically ventilated patients. *Crit. Care Med.* 18:169, 1990.

108. Hackshaw, K. V., Parker, G. A., and Roberts, J. W. Naloxone in septic shock. *Crit. Care Med.* 18:47, 1990.

109. Haley, R. W., and Bregman, D. A. The role of understaffing and overcrowding in recurrent outbreaks of staphylococcal infection in a neonatal special-care unit. *J. Infect. Dis.* 145:875, 1982.

110. Haley, R. W., et al. Nosocomial infection in U.S. hospitals, 1975–76: Estimated frequency by selected characteristics of patients. *Am. J. Med.* 70:947, 1981.

111. Hartstein, A. I., et al. Multiple intensive care unit outbreak of *Acinetobacter calcoaceticus* subspecies *anitratus* respiratory infections and colonization associated with contaminated, reusable ventilator circuits and resuscitation bags. *Am. J. Med.* 85:624, 1988.

112. Hauser, W. E., and Remington, J. S. Effect of antibiotics on the immune response. *Am. J. Med.* 72:711, 1982.

113. Henderson, D. K., Baptiste, R., Parrillo, J., and Gill, V. J. Indolent epidemic of *Pseudomonas cepacia* bacteremia and pseudobacteremia in an intensive care unit traced to a contaminated bood gas analyzer. *Am. J. Med.* 84:75, 1988.

114. Hentges, D. J. Role of the Intestinal Microflora in Host Defense Against Infection. In: D. J. Hentges (Ed.), *Human Intestinal Microflora in Health and Disease.* New York: Academic, 1983. P. 311.

115. Hentges, D. J., Stein, A. J., Casey, S. W., and Que, J. U. Protective role of intestinal flora against infection with *Pseudomonas aeruginosa* in mice: Influence of antibiotics on colonization resistance. *Infect. Immun.* 47:118, 1985.

116. Herrmann, M., et al. Fibronectin, fibrinogen, and laminin act as mediators of adherence of clinical staphylococcal isolates to foreign material. *J. Infect. Dis.* 158:693, 1988.

117. Herwaldt, L. A., Geiss, M., and Pfaller, M. A. Epidemiologic markers of coagulase-negative staphylococcal true bacteremia. In: *Proceedings of the Third International Conference on Nosocomial Infections* (A29), Atlanta, July 31– August 3, 1990. Washington, DC: American Society for Microbiology, 1990.

118. Herwaldt, L. A., and Kao, C. Coagulase-negative staphylococcal bacteremia: True positive rate. *Clin. Res.* Thorofare, NJ: American Federation for Clinical Research, 38:A159, 1990.

119. Hesse, D. G., et al. Cytokine appearance in human endotoxemia and primate bacteremia. *Surg. Gynecol. Obstet.* 166:147, 1988.

120. *Hospital Statistics.* Chicago: American Hospital Association, 1984.

121. Huebner, J., et al. Influence of architectural design on nosocomial infections in intensive care units—a prospective 2-year analysis. *Intensive Care Med.* 15:179, 1989.

122. Hugh, R., and Gilardi, G. L. *Pseudomonas.* In: E. H. Lennette, A. Balows, W. J. Hausler, Jr., and J. P. Truant, (Eds.), *Manual of Clinical Microbiology* (3rd ed.). Washington, DC: American Society for Microbiology, 1980. P. 288.

123. Hussain, Z., Kuhn, M., Lannigan, R., and Austin, T. W. Microbiological investigation of an outbreak of bacteraemia due to *Staphylococcus faecalis* in an intensive care unit. *J. Hosp. Infect.* 12:263, 1988.

124. Irwin, R. S., and Corrao, W. M. A perspective on sputum analyses in pneumonia. *Respir. Care* 24:503, 1979.

125. Istre, G. R., et al. A mysterious cluster of deaths and cardiopulmonary arrests in a pediatric intensive care unit. *N. Engl. J. Med.* 313:205, 1985.

126. Jarlier, V., et al. Extended broad-spectrum beta-lactamases conferring transferable resistance to newer beta-lactam agents in Enterobacteriaceae: Hospital prevalence and susceptibility patterns. *Rev. Infect. Dis.* 10:867, 1988.

127. Jimenez, P., et al. Incidence and etiology of pneumonia acquired during mechanical ventilation. *Crit. Care Med.* 17:882, 1989.

128. Johanson, W. G., et al. Nosocomial respiratory infections with gram-negative bacilli: The significance of colonization of the respiratory tract. *Ann. Intern. Med.* 77:701, 1972.

129. Johanson, W. G., Jr., et al. Bacteriologic diagnosis of nosocomial pneumonia following prolonged mechanical ventilation. *Am. Rev. Respir. Dis.* 137:259, 1988.

130. Johanson, W. G., Pierce, A. K., and Sanford, J. P. Changing pharyngeal bacterial flora of hospitalized patients. *N. Engl. J. Med.* 281:1137, 1969.

131. Kager, L., et al. Antibiotic prophylaxis with cefoxitin in colorectal surgery. *Ann. Surg.* 193:277, 1981.

132. Kager, L., Malmborg, A. S., Nord, C. E., and Sjostedt, S. The effect of piperacillin prophylaxis on the colonic microflora in patients undergoing colorectal surgery. *Infection* 11:251, 1983.

133. Kahn, F. W., and Jones, J. M. Diagnosing bac-

terial respiratory infection by bronchoalveolar lavage. *J. Infect. Dis.* 155:862, 1987.

134. Kaplan, J. E., and Saba, T. M. Humoral deficiency and reticuloendothelial depression after traumatic shock. *Am. J. Physiol.* 230:7, 1976.

135. Kelley, R. E., Vibulsrest, S., Bell, L., and Duncan, R. C. Evaluation of kinetic therapy in the prevention of complications of prolonged bed rest secondary to stroke. *Stroke* 18:638, 1987.

136. Kerver, A. J. H., et al. Colonization and infection in surgical intensive care patients—a prospective study. *Intensive Care Med.* 13:347, 1987.

137. Kerver, A. J. H., et al. Prevention of colonization and infection in critically ill patients: A prospective randomized study. *Crit. Care Med.* 16:1087, 1988.

138. Klein, B. S., Perloff, W. H., and Maki, D. G. Reduction of nosocomial infection during pediatric intensive care by protective isolation. *N. Engl. J. Med.* 320:1714, 1989.

139. Knaus, W. A., Draper, E. A., Wagner, D. P., and Zimmerman, J. E. APACHE II: A severity of disease classification system. *Crit. Care Med.* 13:818, 1985.

140. Knaus, W. A., Draper, E. A., Wagner, D. P., and Zimmerman, J. E. An evaluation of outcome from intensive care in major medical centers. *Ann. Intern. Med.* 104:410, 1986.

141. Knaus, W. A., Draper, E. A., Wagner, D. P., and Zimmerman, J. E. Prognosis in acute organ system failure. *Ann. Surg.* 202:685, 1985.

142. Knaus, W. A., et al. APACHE—acute physiology and chronic health evaluation: A physiologically based classification system. *Crit. Care Med.* 9:591, 1981.

143. Knaus, W. A., et al. Evaluating outcome from intensive care: A preliminary multihospital comparison. *Crit. Care Med.* 10:491, 1982.

144. Knaus, W. A., et al. A comparison of intensive care in the U.S.A. and France. *Lancet* 2:642, 1982.

145. Knaus, W. A., Wagner, D. P., and Draper, E. A. The value of measuring severity of disease in clinical research on acutely ill patients. *J. Chronic Dis.* 37:455, 1984.

146. Knaus, W., Wagner, D., and Draper, E. Implications. *Crit. Care Med.* 17:S219, 1989.

147. Knoedel, A. R., and Beekman, J. F. Unexplained fevers in patients with nasotracheal intubation. *J.A.M.A.* 248:868, 1982.

148. Kuusela, P. Fibronectin binds to *Staphylococcus aureus*. *Nature* 276:718, 1978.

149. LaForce, F. M. Hospital-acquired gram-negative rod pneumonias: An overview. *Am. J. Med.* 70:664, 1981.

150. Langer, M., et al. Early onset pneumonia: A multicenter study in intensive care units. *Intensive Care Med.* 13:342, 1987.

151. Langer, M., et al. Long-term respiratory support and risk of pneumonia in critically ill patients. *Am. Rev. Respir. Dis.* 140:302, 1989.

152. Lannigan, R., Hussain, Z., and Austin, T. W. *Streptococcus pyogenes* as a cause of nosocomial infection in a critical care unit. *Diagn. Microbiol. Infect. Dis.* 3:337, 1985.

153. Larca, L., and Greenbaum, D. M. Effectiveness of intensive nutritional regimes in patients who fail to wean from mechanical ventilation. *Crit. Care Med.* 10:297, 1982.

154. Larsen, R. A., et al. Hospital-associated epidemic of pharyngitis and conjunctivitis caused by adenovirus (21/H21 + 35). *J. Infect. Dis.* 154:706, 1986.

155. Le Frock, J. L., Ellis, C. A., and Weinstein, L. The impact of hospitalization on the aerobic microflora. *Am. J. Med. Sci.* 277:269, 1979.

156. Leclair, J. M., et al. Prevention of nosocomial respiratory syncytial virus infections through compliance with glove and gown isolation precautions. *N. Engl. J. Med.* 317:329, 1987.

157. Ledingham, I. McA., et al. Triple regimen of selective decontamination of the digestive tract, systemic cefotaxime, and microbiological surveillance for prevention of acquired infection in intensive care. *Lancet* 1:785, 1988.

158. Leissner, K. H. Postoperative wound infection in 32,000 clean operations. *Acta Chir. Scand.* 142:433, 1976.

159. Leonard, E. M., et al. Pathogenesis of colonization and infection in a neonatal surgical unit. *Crit. Care Med.* 18:264, 1990.

160. Leu, H.-S., et al. Hospital-acquired pneumonia. Attributable mortality and morbidity. *Am. J. Epidemiol.* 129:1258, 1989.

161. Lew, D., et al. Sphenoid sinusitis. A review of 30 cases. *N. Engl. J. Med.* 309:1149, 1983.

162. Li, T. C., et al. Staffing in a community hospital intensive care unit. *J.A.M.A.* 252:2023, 1984.

163. Loegering, D. J., and Carr, F. K. Plasma cathepsin activity and reticuloendothelial phagocytic function during hemorrhagic shock. *Circ. Shock* 5:61, 1978.

164. Lowbury, E. J. L., Babb, J. R., and Roe, E. Clearance from a hospital of gram-negative bacilli that transfer carbenicillin resistance to *Pseudomonas aeruginosa*. *Lancet* 2:941, 1972.

165. MacLean, L. D., et al. Patterns of septic shock in a man: A detailed study of 56 patients. *Ann. Surg.* 166:643, 1967.

166. Maki, D. G. Preventing infusion-related infection. *Drug Therapy (Hosp.)* 2:37, 1977.

167. Maki, D. G. Control of colonization and transmission of pathogenic bacteria in the hospital. *Ann. Intern. Med.* 89(Part 2):777, 1978.

168. Maki, D. G. Risk factors for nosocomial infection in intensive care: 'Devices vs nature' and goals for the next decade. *Arch. Intern. Med.* 149:30, 1989.

169. Maki, D. G., Alvarado, C. J., Hassemer, C. A., and Zilz, M. A. Relation of the inanimate hospital environment to endemic nosocomial infection. *N. Engl. J. Med.* 307:1562, 1982.

170. Maki, D. G., Goldmann, D. A., and Rhame, F. S. Infection control in intravenous therapy. *Ann. Intern. Med.* 79:867, 1973.

171. Mandelli, M., Mosconi, P., Langer, M., and Cigada, M. Is pneumonia developing in patients in intensive care always a typical "nosocomial" infection? *Lancet* 2:1094, 1986.

172. Mandelli, M., Mosconi, P., Langer, M., and Cigada, M. Prevention of pneumonia in an intensive care unit: A randomized multicenter clinical trial. *Crit. Care Med.* 17:501, 1989.

173. Marshall, J., and Sweeney, D. Microbial infection and the septic response in critical surgical illness. Sepsis, not infection, determines outcome. *Arch. Surg.* 125:17, 1990.

174. Marshall, J. C., Christou, N. V., Hortn, R., and Meakins, J. L. The microbiology of multiple organ failure. The proximal gastrointestinal tract as an occult reservoir of pathogens. *Arch. Surg.* 123:309, 1988.

175. Martin, T. R. The relationship between malnutrition and lung infections. *Clin. Chest Med.* 8:359, 1987.

176. McCabe, W. R., et al. Immunization with rough mutant of *Salmonella minnesota:* Protective activity of IgM and IgG antibody to the R595 (Re chemotype) mutant. *J. Infect. Dis.* 158:291, 1988.

177. McCabe, W. R., and Jackson, G. G. Gram-negative bacteremia: I. Etiology and ecology. *Arch. Intern. Med.* 110:847, 1962.

178. McCabe, W. R., Treadwell, T. L., and Maria, A. D. Pathophysiology of bacteremia. *Am. J. Med.* 75:1B, 1983.

179. Meakins, J. L., et al. A proposed classification of intra-abdominal infections. Stratification of etiology and risk for future therapeutic trials. *Arch. Surg.* 119:1372, 1984.

180. Michie, H. R., et al. Detection of circulatory tumor necrosis factor after endotoxin administration. *N. Engl. J. Med.* 318:1481, 1988.

181. Miller, C. L., and Baker, C. C. Development of inhibitory macrophages (MO) after splenectomy. *Transplant. Proc.* 11:1460, 1979.

182. Miller, S. E., Miller, C. L., and Trunkey, D. D. The immune consequences of trauma. *Surg. Clin. North Am.* 63:167, 1982.

183. Mock, C. N., Burchard, K. W., Hasan, F., and Reed, M. Surgical intensive care unit pneumonia. *Surgery* 104:494, 1988.

184. Montaner, J. S. G., Russell, J. A., Ruedy, J., and Lawson, L. Acute respiratory failure secondary to *Pneumocystis carinii* pneumonia in the acquired immunodeficiency syndrome: A potential role of systemic corticosteroids. *Chest* 95:881, 1989.

185. Mortimer, E. A., Jr., et al. Transmission of staphylococci between newborns: Importance of the hands of personnel. *Am. J. Dis. Child.* 104:113, 1962.

186. Mullen, J. L., et al. Reduction of operative morbidity and mortality by combined preoperative and postoperative nutritional support. *Ann. Surg.* 192:604, 1980.

187. Mulligan, M. E., et al. Alterations in human fecal flora, including ingrowth of *Clostridium difficile,* related to cefoxitin therapy. *Antimicrob. Agents Chemother.* 26:343, 1982.

188. Neuhaus, A., and Ravikrishnan, K. P. Respiratory failure in pulmonary tuberculosis: A spectrum. *Am. Rev. Respir. Dis.* 115:A404, 1977.

189. Nicolle, L. E., et al. An outbreak of group A streptococcal bacteremia in an intensive care unit. *Infect. Control* 7:177, 1986.

190. Nord, C. E., Kager, L., and Heimdah, I. A. Impact of antimicrobial agents on the gastrointestinal microflora and the risk of infections. *Am. J. Med.* 76:99, 1984.

191. Northey, D., et al. Microbial surveillance in a surgical intensive care unit. *Surg. Gynecol. Obstet.* 139:321, 1974.

192. Norton, L. W. Does drainage of intra-abdominal pus reverse multiple organ failure? *Am. J. Surg.* 149:347, 1985.

193. O'Leary, J. P., et al. Incidence of malnutrition among patients admitted to a VA hospital. *South. Med. J.* 75:1095, 1982.

194. O'Reilly, M. J., et al. Sepsis from sinusitis in nasotracheally intubated patients—a diagnostic dilemma. *Am. J. Surg.* 147:601. 1984.

195. Olson, B., et al. Epidemiology of endemic *Pseudomonas aeruginosa:* Why infection control efforts have failed. *J. Infect. Dis.* 150:808, 1984.

196. Ottinger, L. W. Acute cholecystitis as a postoperative complication. *Ann. Surg.* 184:162, 1976.

197. Peacock, J. E., Jr., et al. Nosocomial respiratory tract colonization and infection with aminoglycoside-resistant *Acinetobacter calcoaceticus* var *anitratus:* Epidemiologic characteristics and clinical significance. *Infect. Control Hosp. Epidemiol.* 9:302, 1988.

198. Pennepalli, R., Franklin, C., and Mizock, B. Severe tuberculosis in the intensive care unit. *Am. Rev. Respir. Dis.* 129:A116, 1979.

199. Perlman, D. M., and Caplan, E. S. Nosocomial sinusitis: A new and complex threat. *J. Crit. Illness* 2:19, 1987.

200. Peters, G., et al. Biology of *S. epidermidis* Extracellular Slime. In: G. Pulverer, P. G. Quie, and G. Peters (Eds.), *Pathogenicity and Clinical Significance of Coagulase-Negative Staphylococci.* Stuttgart: Gustav Fischer Verlag, 1987. P. 15.

201. Piemont, Y., et al. Epidemiological investigation of exfoliative toxin-producing *Staphylo-*

coccus aureus strains in hospitalized patients. *J. Clin. Microbiol.* 19:417, 1984.

202. Pien, F. D., and Bruce, A. E. Nosocomial *Ewingella americana* bacteremia in an intensive care unit. *Arch. Intern. Med.* 146:111, 1986.

203. Pingleton, S. K. Enteral nutrition as a risk factor for nosocomial pneumonia. *Eur. J. Clin. Microbiol. Infect. Dis.* 8:51, 1989.

204. Pittet, D. Decontamination digestive selective aux soins intensifs. *Med. Hyg.* 47:3025, 1989.

205. Pittet, D., and Suter, P. M. Judicious Use of Antibiotics in Critically Ill Patients. In: J. L. Vincent (Ed.), *Update in Intensive Care and Emergency Medicine,* Vol. 8. Berlin: Springer, 1989. P. 154.

206. Polk, H. C., Jr., and Shields, C. L. Remote organ failure: A valid sign of occult intra-abdominal infection. *Surgery* 81:310, 1977.

207. Ponce de Leon, S., Critchley, S., and Wenzel, R. P. Polymicrobial bloodstream infections related to prolonged vascular catheterization. *Crit. Care Med.* 12:856, 1984.

208. Ponce de Leon, S., and Wenzel, R. P. Hospital-acquired bloodstream infections with *Staphylococcal epidermidis. Am. J. Med.* 77:639, 1984.

209. Preston, G. A., Larson, E. L., and Stamm, W. E. The Effect of Private Isolation Rooms on Patient Care Practice—Colonization and Infection in an Intensive Care Unit. In: R. E. Dixon (Ed.), *Nosocomial Infections.* Atlanta: York Medical Books, 1981. P. 285.

210. Price, D. J. E., and Sleigh, J. D. Control of infection due to *Klebsiella* in a neurosurgical unit by withdrawal of antibiotics. *Lancet* 2:1213, 1970.

211. Pugin, J., et al. Accurate diagnosis of ventilator-associated pneumonia using quantitative culture of bronchoalveolar lavage fluid obtained with a nonbronchoscopic catheter. *Am. Rev. Respir. Dis.* 141:A277, 1990.

212. Ramsey, G. Endotoxaemia in Multiple Organ Failure: A Secondary Role for SDD? In: H. K. F. van Saene, C. P. Stoutenbeek, I. McA. Ledingham, and P. Lawin (Eds.), *Update in Intensive Care and Emergency Medicine,* Vol. 7. Berlin: Springer, 1989. P. 135.

213. Ransj, O. U., et al. Methicillin-resistant *Staphylococcus aureus* in two burn units: Clinical significance and epidemiological control. *J. Hosp. Infect.* 13:355, 1989.

214. Reingold, A. L., et al. Toxic-shock syndrome not associated with menstruation. *Lancet* 1:1, 1982.

215. Ribner, B. S., et al. Outbreak of multiply resistant *Staphylococcus aureus* in a pediatric intensive care unit after consolidation with a surgical intensive care unit. *Am. J. Infect. Control* 17:244, 1989.

216. Rich, M. W., et al. Increased complications and prolonged hospital stay in elderly car-

217. Richardson, J. D., DeCamp, M. M., Garrison, R. N., and Fry, D. E. Pulmonary infection complicating intra-abdominal sepsis: Clinical and experimental observations. *Ann. Surg.* 195:732, 1982.

218. Ristuccia, P. A., and Cunha, B. A. Microbiologic Aspects of Infection Control. In: R. P. Wenzel (Ed.), *Prevention and Control of Nosocomial Infections.* Baltimore: Williams & Wilkins, 1987. P. 205.

219. Rochester, D. F., and Esau, S. A. Malnutrition and the respiratory system. *Chest* 83:411, 1984.

220. Rogers, P. L., et al. Admission of AIDS patients to a medical intensive care unit: Causes and outcome. *Crit. Care Med.* 17:113, 1989.

221. Rosenthal, T., Pitlik, S., and Michaeli, D. Fatal undiagnosed tuberculosis in hospitalized patients. *J. Infect. Dis.* 131:S51, 1975.

222. Rotstein, O. D., Pruett, T. L., and Simmons, R. L. Microbiologic features and treatment of persistent peritonitis in patients in the intensive care unit. *Can. J. Surg.* 29:247, 1986.

223. Ruddell, W. S., et al. Effect of cimetidine on the gastric bacterial flora. *Lancet* 1:672, 1980.

224. Rush, B. F., et al. Endotoxemia and bacteremia during hemorrhagic shock: The link between trauma and sepsis? *Ann. Surg.* 207:549, 1988.

225. Saba, T. M., et al. Reversal of opsonic deficiency in surgical, trauma and burn patients by infusion of purified plasma fibronectin: Correlation with experimental observation. *Am. J. Med.* 80:229, 1986.

226. Sacks, J. J., et al. A nurse associated epidemic of cardiac arrests in an intensive care unit. *J.A.M.A.* 259:689, 1988.

227. Safar, P., and Grenvik, A. Organization and physician education in critical care medicine. *Anesthesiology* 47:82, 1977.

228. Schein, R. M. H., et al. ICU survival with the acquired immunodeficiency syndrome. *Crit. Care Med.* 14:1026, 1986.

229. Schimpff, S. C., et al. Origin of infection in acute nonlymphocytic leukemia: Significance of hospital acquisition of potential pathogens. *Ann. Intern. Med.* 77:707, 1972.

230. Schimpff, S. C., Miller, R. M., Polakavetz, S. H., and Hornick, R. B. Infection in the severely traumatized patient. *Ann. Surg.* 179:352, 1974.

231. Sherertz, R. J., and Sullivan, M. L. An outbreak of infections with *Acinetobacter calcoaceticus* in burn patients: Contamination of patients' mattresses. *J. Infect. Dis.* 151:252, 1985.

232. Sheth, N. K., Franson, T. R., and Sohnle, P. C. Influence of bacterial adherence to in-

travascular catheters on *in vitro* antibiotic susceptibility. *Lancet* 2:1266, 1985.

233. Silva, J., Jr., and Fekety, R. Clostridia and antimicrobial enterocolitis. *Annu. Rev. Med.* 32: 327, 1981.

234. Sirot, J., et al. *Klebsiella pneumoniae* and other *Enterobacteriaceae* producing novel plasmid-mediated beta-lactamases markedly active against third-generation cephalosporins: Epidemiologic studies. *Rev. Infect. Dis.* 10: 850, 1988.

235. Skau, T., Nystrom, P.-O., and Carlsson, C. Severity of illness in intra-abdominal infection: A comparison of two indexes. *Arch. Surg.* 120:152, 1985.

236. Skillman, J. J., et al. Respiratory failure, hypotension sepsis, and jaundice: A clinical syndrome associated with lethal hemorrhage from acute stress ulceration of the stomach. *Am. J. Surg.* 117:523, 1969.

237. Smith, G., Logie, J. R. C., MacDonald, A., and Smylie, H. G. Ward design in relation to postoperative wound infection: Part III. *Br. Med. J.* 3:13, 1974.

238. Smith, R. L., Levine, S. M., and Lewis, M. L. Prognosis of patients with AIDS requiring intensive care. *Chest* 96:857, 1989.

239. Smylie, H. G., Davidson, A. I. G., MacDonald, A., and Smith, G. Ward design in relation to postoperative wound infection: Part I. *Br. Med. J.* 1:67, 1971.

240. Snyder, H. G., et al. Ward design in relation to postoperative wound infection: Part II. *Br. Med. J.* 1:72, 1971.

241. Solomkin, J. S., Flohr, A., and Simmons, R. L. *Candida* infections in surgical patients. Dose requirements and toxicity of amphotericin B. *Ann. Surg.* 195:177, 1982.

242. Sori, A. J., et al. The gut as a source of sepsis after hemorrhagic shock. *Am. J. Surg.* 155: 187, 1988.

243. Stamm, W. E. Infections related to medical devices. *Ann. Intern. Med.* 89:764, 1978.

244. Starker, P. M., et al. The response to TPN—a form of nutritional assessment. *Ann. Surg.* 198:720, 1983.

245. Starker, P. M., et al. The influence of preoperative total parenteral nutrition upon morbidity and mortality. *Surg. Gynecol. Obstet.* 162:569, 1986.

246. Stephan, R. N., et al. Mechanism of immunosuppression following hemorrhage: Defective antigen presentation by macrophages. *J. Surg. Res.* 46:553, 1989.

247. Stephan, R. N., et al. Hemorrhage without tissue trauma produces immunosuppression and enhances susceptibility to sepsis. *Arch. Surg.* 122:62, 1987.

248. Stevens, L. E. Gauging the severity of surgical sepsis. *Arch. Surg.* 118:1190, 1983.

249. Stevens, R. M., Teres, D., Skillman, J. J., and Feingold, D. S. Pneumonia in an intensive care unit: A 30-month experience. *Arch. Intern. Med.* 134:106, 1974.

250. Stoutenbeek, C. P., et al. Nosocomial gram-negative pneumonia in critically ill patients. A 3-year experience with a novel therapeutic regimen. *Intensive Care Med.* 12:419, 1986.

251. Stoutenbeek, C. P., et al. The effect of oropharyngeal decontamination using topical nonabsorbable antibiotics on the incidence of nosocomial respiratory tract infections in multiple trauma patients. *J. Trauma* 27:357, 1987.

252. Stoutenbeek, C. P., van Saene, H. K. F., Miranda, D. R., and Zandstra, D. F. The effect of selective decontamination of the digestive tract on colonization and infection rate in multiple trauma patients. *Intensive Care Med.* 10:185, 1984.

253. Stoutenbeek, C. P., van Saene, H. K. F., and Zandstra, D. F. The effect of oral non-absorbable antibiotics on the emergence of resistant bacteria in patients in an intensive care unit. *J. Antimicrob. Chemother.* 19:513, 1987.

254. Streed, S. A., et al. Relationship of nurse staffing patterns to nosocomial infections in a surgical intensive care unit. Presented at the Fourteenth Annual Association for Practitioners in Infection Control Meeting, Miami, May 3–8, 1987.

255. Suspected nosocomial influenza cases in an intensive care unit. *M.M.W.R.* 37:3, 1988.

256. Temple, W. J., Voitk, A. J., Snelling, C. F. T., and Crispin, J. S. Effect of nutrition, diet and suture material on long term wound healing. *Ann. Surg.* 182:93, 1975.

257. Thorpe, J. E., et al. Bronchoalveolar lavage for diagnosing acute bacterial pneumonia. *J. Infect. Dis.* 155:855, 1987.

258. Tobin, M. J., and Grenvik, A. Nosocomial lung infection and its diagnosis. *Crit. Care Med.* 12:191, 1984.

259. Todd, T. R. J., et al. Augmented bacterial adherence to tracheal epithelial cells is associated with gram-negative pneumonia in an intensive care unit population. *Am. Rev. Respir. Dis.* 140:1585, 1989.

260. Tracey, K. J., et al. Anti-cachectin/TNF monoclonal antibodies prevent septic shock during lethal bacteraemia. *Nature* 330:662, 1987.

261. Tryba, M., et al. Prevention of acute stress bleeding with sucralfate, antacids, or cimetidine. *Am. J. Med.* 79(Suppl. 2C):55, 1985.

262. Ulrich, C., et al. Selective decontamination of the digestive tract with norfloxacin in the prevention of ICU-acquired infections: A prospective randomized study. *Intensive Care Med* 15:424, 1989.

263. Unertl, K., et al. Prevention of colonization

and respiratory infections in long-term ventilated patients by local antimicrobial prophylaxis. *Intensive Care Med.* 13:106, 1987.

264. Vallandigham, J. C., and Johanson, W. G., Jr. Infections Associated with Endotracheal Intubation and Tracheostomy. In: A. L. Bisno and F. A. Waldvogel (Eds.), *Infections Associated with Indwelling Medical Devices.* Washington, DC: American Society for Microbiology, 1989. P. 179.

265. Van der Waaij, D. Colonization resistance of the digestive tract: Clinical consequences and implications. *J. Antimicrob. Chemother.* 10:263, 1982.

266. Van der Waaij, D. The Colonization Resistance of the Digestive Tract in Experimental Animals and Its Consequences for Infection Prevention, Acquisition of New Bacteria and the Prevention of Spread of Bacteria Between Cage Mates. In: D. Van der Waaij and J. Verhoef (Eds.), *New Criteria for Antimicrobial Therapy: Maintenance of Digestive Tract Colonization Resistance.* Amsterdam: Excerpta Medica, 1979. P. 43.

267. Van der Waaij, D., Berghuis-de Vries, J. M., and Lekkerkerk-van der Wees, J.E.C. Colonization resistance of the digestive tract in conventional and antibiotic-treated mice. *J. Hyg.* (Camb.) 69:405, 1971.

268. Van der Waaij, D., Vossen, J. M., Korthals Altes, C., and Hartgrink, C. Reconventionalization following antibiotic decontamination in man and animals. *Am. J. Clin. Nutr.* 30:1887, 1977.

269. van Deventer, S. J. H., et al. Endotoxaemia: An early predictor of septicaemia in febrile patients. *Lancet* 1:605, 1988.

270. van Saene, J. J. M., Stoutenbeek, C. P., and van Saene, H. K. F. Prevention of MOF with SDD. In: H. K. F. van Saene, C. P. Stoutenbeek, I. McA. Ledingham, and P. Lawin (Eds.), *Update in Intensive Care and Emergency Medicine,* Vol. 7. Berlin: Springer, 1989. P. 128.

271. Van Uffelen, R., van Saene, H. K. F., Fidle, V., and Lowenberg, A. Oropharyngeal flora as a source of bacteria colonizing the lower airways in patients on artificial ventilation. *Intensive Care Med.* 10:233, 1984.

272. Vandenbroucke-Grauls, C. M., et al. Endemic *Acinetobacter anitratus* in a surgical intensive care unit: Mechanical ventilators as reservoir. *Eur. J. Clin. Microbiol. Infect. Dis.* 7:485, 1988.

273. Vaudaux, P. E., et al. Host factors selectively increase staphylococcal adherence on inserted catheters: A role for fibronectin and fibrinogen or fibrin. *J. Infect. Dis.* 160:865, 1989.

274. Vaudaux, P. E., Lew, D., and Waldvogel, F. A. Host Factors Predisposing to Foreign Body Infections. In: A. L. Bisno and F. A. Waldvo-

gel (Eds.), *Infections Associated with Indwelling Medical Devices.* Washington, DC: American Society for Microbiology, 1989. P. 3.

275. Villarino, M. E., et al. Epidemic of *Serratia marcescens* bacteremia in a cardiac intensive care unit. *J. Clin. Microbiol.* 27:2433, 1989.

276. Waage, A., Halstensen, A., and Espevik, T. Association between tumor necrosis factor in serum and fatal outcome in patients with meningococcal disease. *Lancet* 1:355, 1987.

277. Wachter, R. M., et al. Intensive care of patients with the acquired immunodeficiency syndrome, outcome and changing patterns of utilization. *Am. Rev. Respir. Dis.* 134:891, 1986.

278. Wachter, R. M., Russi, M. G., Hopewell, P. C., and Luce, J. M. The improving survival rate after intensive care for *P. carinii* pneumonia and respiratory failure. In: *Proceedings of the Fifth International Conference on AIDS,* Montreal, Canada, 1989.

279. Wadowsky, R. M., Wolford, R., McNamara, A. M., and Yee, R. B. Effect of temperature, pH, and oxygen level on multiplication of naturally occurring *Legionella pneumophila* in potable water. *Appl. Environ. Microbiol.* 49:1197, 1985.

280. Wagner, D., Draper, E., and Knaus, W. Development of APACHE III. *Crit. Care Med.* 17:S199, 1989.

281. Wagner, D., Draper, E., and Knaus, W. Analysis: Quality of care. *Crit. Care Med.* 17:S210, 1989.

282. Wagner, D. P., Knaus, W. A., and Draper, E. A. Statistical validation of a severity of illness measure. *Am. J. Public Health* 73:878, 1983.

283. Weinstein, R. A. Selective intestinal decontamination—an infection control measure whose time has come (edit.)? *Ann. Intern. Med.* 110:853, 1989.

284. Welling, G. W., et al. Biochemical effects in germ-free mice of association with several strains of anaerobic bacteria. *J. Gen. Microbiol.* 117:57, 1980.

285. Wenzel, R. P., et al. Identification of procedure-related nosocomial infections in high risk patients. *Rev. Infect. Dis.* 3:701, 1981.

286. Wenzel, R. P., et al. Hospital-acquired infections in intensive care unit patients: An overview with emphasis on epidemics. *Infect. Control* 4:371, 1983.

287. Wey, S. B., et al. Risk factors for hospital-acquired candidemia. *Arch. Intern. Med.* 149:2349, 1989.

288. Whitby, M., et al. Streptococcal infection in a regional burns centre and a plastic surgery unit. *J. Hosp. Infect.* 5:63, 1984.

289. Woods, D. E., Straus, D. C., Johanson, W. G., and Bass, J. A. Role of fibronectin in the pre-

vention of adherence of *Pseudomonas aeruginosa* to buccal cells. *J. Infect. Dis.* 143:784, 1981.

290. Woods, D. E., Straus, D. C., Johanson, W. G., and Bass, J. A. Role of salivary protease activity in adherence of gram-negative bacilli to mammalian buccal epithelial cells in vivo. *J. Clin. Invest.* 68:1435, 1981.

291. Younger, J. J., et al. Coagulase-negative staphylococci isolated from cerebrospinal fluid shunts: Importance of slime production, species identification, and shunt removal to clinical outcome. *J. Infect. Dis.* 156:548, 1987.

292. Yourtee, E. L., and Root, R. K. Effect of Antibiotics on Phagocytic-Microbe Interactions.

In: R. K. Root, and M. A. Sande (Eds.), *New Dimensions in Antimicrobial Therapy.* New York: Churchill Livingstone, 1984.

293. Zervos, M. J., et al. Nosocomial infection by gentamicin-resistant *Streptococcus fecalis. Ann. Intern. Med.* 106:687, 1987.

294. Ziegler, E. J., et al. Treatment of gram-negative bacteremia and shock with human antiserum to a mutant *Escherichia coli. N. Engl. J. Med.* 307:1225, 1982.

295. Ziegler, E. J., et al. Treatment of gram-negative bacteremia and septic shock with HA-1A human monoclonal antibody against endotoxin. *N. Engl. J. Med.* 324:429, 1991.

The Newborn Nursery

John D. Nelson

The newborn nursery community is unique from the standpoint of infections. The babies are transients who enter sterile and leave 2 or 3 days later with a full complement of microbial flora without manifesting signs of illness from this initial encounter with microbes, despite their immunologic immaturity. The nursing staff and neonatologists would like to keep the nursery a closed community, but there are necessary intrusions. Technical personnel and medical consultants bring needed skills but also bring potentially dangerous microorganisms from the hospital wards. Parents carry in bacteria and viruses from the outside community.

Natural bacterial interference is a basic concept of infection control in the nursery. The indigenous microbiota of skin and mucous membranes are critical in defense against invasive pathogens. The aims of infection control practices are to permit development of an innocuous microflora while minimizing transmission of potentially dangerous organisms.

The fetus who has not been infected in utero is first exposed to microorganisms during vaginal passage. Subsequently, the normal skin and mucous membrane microflora is established from environmental sources. It is often difficult to ascertain whether an infection has been acquired nosocomially, and the time of onset of disease does not help differentiate among congenital, perinatal, and nosocomial sources as there can be a lag of many days between infection and clinical expression of that infection. Because it is often difficult to ascertain whether a neonatal infection arose from a nosocomial source, the National Nosocomial Infections Surveillance (NNIS) System, conducted by the Centers for Disease Control (CDC), designates as nosocomial all infectious diseases in the first 28 days of life regardless of the actual source of those diseases.

The hospitals participating in the NNIS System reported a mean nosocomial infection rate in newborn nurseries of 1.4 percent, with a range from 0.9 percent in community hospitals to 1.7 percent in large university hospitals [56], but rates as high as 25 percent have been reported in neonatal intensive care units (NICU) [125].

Skin infections, diarrhea, respiratory infections, and septicemia are the most common nosocomial infections encountered in a nursery. Epidemic situations are characteristic of organisms that colonize skin and mucous membranes frequently but cause disease infrequently. In this situation, the organism perpetuates itself in the environment over a prolonged time and, because it causes invasive disease only periodically, it can be difficult to recognize that a nosocomial infection problem exists.

Historically, shifts in major nosocomial etiologic agents have occurred every 10 years or so. In the United States, a severe problem with invasive strains of *Staphylococcus aureus* emerged in nurseries during the 1950s and disappeared in the 1960s, largely unrelated to many attempts that were made to control the problem. Since then, the strains of *S. aureus* causing periodic outbreaks of skin lesions have not been invasive, virulent organisms. In the 1960s, *Pseudomonas aeruginosa* was a serious nosocomial pathogen in many nurseries because of contamination of water in incubators and of respiratory therapy equipment. The 1970s were the decade of group B streptococcal infections and, in the 1980s, methicillin-resistant strains of *S. aureus* and *Staphylococcus epidermidis* emerged as difficult nosocomial problems in NICUs. In the early 1990s, the major nosocomial pathogens in nurseries and NICUs are methicillin-resistant *S. aureus* [98] and coagulase-negative staphylococci [37], enterococci [69] and *Candida* species [124]. Group B streptococci remain important pathogens in vertical transmission from mother to baby, but their role as nosocomial agents, which occurred in some nurseries [14], has diminished.

Occasionally, clusters of cases suggesting nosocomial transmission turn out to be unrelated coincidences when strain markers such as bacteriophage types, restriction endonuclease digestion analysis, or antimicrobial susceptibility patterns are investigated.

Neonatal nosocomial infections are significant determinants of mortality, especially in low-birth-weight infants [63]. Prevention, recognition, and appropriate management of them is an important goal.

Infectious Agents and Methods of Transmission

Babies can acquire infectious agents from fomites, by airborne transmission, from hands or bodies of personnel, or from invasive procedures. The instances of nosocomial infection in newborn nurseries and NICUs are numerous. The foregoing examples are merely representative of the problem.

Intrapartum fetal scalp electrodes have been associated with infections caused by several aerobic gram-positive and gram-negative bacteria, by anaerobes, and by herpes simplex virus (HSV) [34, 92]. The severed umbilical cord stump is at risk of colonization with invasive pathogens [21]. Endotracheal suctioning has resulted in transmission of HSV infection from a physician to a neonate [118].

Outbreaks of infection caused by *P. aeruginosa* and other nonfermenting bacteria have been traced to contaminated eyewash [95], resuscitation equipment [35], and hand carriage by personnel [78]. Contaminated scrub brushes were responsible for an outbreak of *Serratia marcescens* infection [4]. Contaminated hand lotions [79], topical ointments [121], phenolic disinfectants [110], intravenous fluids [64], umbilical cord wash [73], hexachlorophene disinfectants [109], total parenteral nutrition fluids [81], and a blender used to prepare infant formula [86] have also caused outbreaks of infection in nurseries.

Although fomites and contaminated liquids carry a potential risk for spreading infections in nurseries, outbreaks are far more often traced to personnel and poor aseptic techniques. Transmission of pathogens on hands of nursery personnel is the most common cause of outbreaks of infections in neonates [72, 78, 91]. Nasal carriage of staphylococci in personnel can be responsible for outbreaks of skin infections in newborns [12]. Group A streptococcal infections can occur in nurseries [43, 84], as can outbreaks of diarrheal illness caused by toxigenic coliform bacilli [46], rotaviruses [16], *Shigella* [105], *Salmonella* [106], and enteropathogenic *Escherichia coli* [13]. An outbreak of necrotizing enterocolitis was associated with delta toxin–producing, methicillin-resistant *S. aureus* [88]. In most such outbreaks, fecal-oral spread via hands of personnel is the mode of transmission.

Echovirus 11 [58, 77] and respiratory syncytial virus [76] are spread both by droplets and by the hands of personnel touching contaminated objects, since the viruses survive well on hard surfaces in the nursery environment. Coxsackievirus [33, 114] and toxigenic *Clostridium difficile* [128] infections are spread by the fecal-oral route, but the mode of transmission of rotavirus infection is not entirely clear; it may involve fecal-oral, respiratory, and vertical routes of spread [100] (see Chap. 38).

With the concept of aggressive intensive care and with technologic advances came the common use of invasive procedures and devices to manage sick neonates. All carry the risk of nosocomial infection. Intravascular catheters are commonly used to administer fluids and medications and to obtain samples of blood for laboratory tests.

Placement of umbilical vein catheters may introduce bacteria on the umbilical stump into the circulation or dislodge contaminated thrombi [8, 85] (see Chap. 40). Culture of bacteria from the catheter tip following removal has been uncommon in some series and higher than 50 percent in others [8, 97, 119]. The frequency of infection does not appear to correlate with age at time of insertion, local skin care, or duration of catheterization [8, 119]. Infectious complications are less common with umbilical artery catheters [10, 119, 120], very rare with radial artery catheters [1], and virtually never seen with scalp vein needles [93].

Central venous catheters used for administering parenteral nutrition are a serious infection risk from preparation of the fluid, contamination when connections in the line

are violated, and entry wound infections. In several reported series involving more than 2,500 infants receiving parenteral nutrition, bacteremia occurred in none to 23 percent of infants, a broad range. In most series, however, the frequency was from 3 to 8 percent [24, 27, 45, 71]. Candidemia was a serious problem, occurring in approximately 10 percent of cases overall [7, 20]. Nosocomial fungemia has also been associated with intravascular pressure-monitoring devices [111].

Insertion of an umbilical vein catheter to perform exchange blood transfusion induces a transient bacteremia in 10 percent of cases, but this is cleared spontaneously by the infant, and prophylactic antibiotics have no beneficial effect [5, 85].

Banked breast milk that becomes contaminated during collection or storage has caused *Salmonella* [104] and *Klebsiella* [26] infections in preterm infants.

Use of erythromycin ophthalmic ointment for prophylaxis of ophthalmia neonatorum led to an outbreak of erythromycin-resistant staphylococcal conjunctivitis in one nursery [53].

Immunologic Risk Factors

All newborn infants are immunologically deficient. The degree of immunologic deficiency relates principally to immature gestational age, but it is further compromised by intensive care measures. Invasive procedures violate mechanical barriers to infection, and humoral factors and phagocytic cells are depleted by blood drawing.

The skin and mucous membranes are the first lines of defense against microbial invasion. By 37 weeks' gestation, the skin is an effective barrier, but in premature infants with scant stratum corneum, the skin is very permeable [52]. This not only leads to the problem of excessive water loss through the skin; it also allows easy entry of bacteria, especially in the preterm baby of less than 32 weeks' gestation who typically has translucent skin. At approximately 2 weeks after birth, the stratum corneum is fairly well-developed, regardless of the gestational age. The normal microflora of the skin and mucous membrane present in older individuals plays a major role in defense against pathogens. These tissues are sterile at the moment of birth, unless there has been intrauterine infection; hence, this important barrier to pathogens is lacking in most newborns.

Once a pathogen gains entry to blood or other body fluids and tissues, humoral and phagocytic factors are of paramount importance in defense. Polymorphonuclear leukocytes (PMNLs) and monocytes exhibit sluggish migration toward exogenous antigens, with chemotactic activity being only one-half to one-fourth that of adult PMNLs [59, 89]. Neonatal PMNLs have essentially normal phagocytic activity when they are suspended in adult serum, but phagocytosis is decreased in neonatal serum, suggesting the presence of an inhibitory factor [22]. Contrary to the defects in chemotaxis and phagocytosis, intracellular bactericidal activity of neonatal PMNLs is normal [90].

Reticuloendothelial activity is decreased in the term neonate and, in the preterm baby, it is essentially absent [55]. Both the classic and the alternate pathways of the complement system have decreased activity [32], and fibronectin is deficient [42] (see Chaps. 13, 29).

Maternal IgG begins passing transplacentally to the fetus at approximately 15 weeks' gestation, and the fetus begins synthesizing IgM at approximately 30 weeks' gestation. The major portion of maternal antibody is delivered to the fetus during the last trimester by an active mechanism that allows neonatal IgG concentrations in excess of maternal concentrations at term [60]. However, the preterm infant at 32 weeks' gestation has a serum IgG concentration that is less than half that of a term infant. Preterm infants commonly have a large portion of their blood volume withdrawn for diagnostic laboratory tests, thus further depleting humoral factors. The situation is aggravated by the usual practice of replenishing the infant with packed red blood cells rather than with whole blood. As a consequence, many sick preterm babies have severely depleted immunoglobulin stores [122].

Surveillance

Recognition of the existence of a nosocomial infection problem can be difficult in certain situations. Normal term newborns are usually discharged from the nursery at 2 or 3 days of age. Infections acquired in the nursery may not manifest themselves until several days later. Unless the babies' physicians report the information to the nursery director, the existence of a problem may go unrecognized.

Monitoring infectious events that occur in the nursery requires an organized surveillance system and alertness on the part of nursery personnel. There must be collaboration among the microbiology laboratory, the nursery staff, and the infection control practitioner. In addition to monitoring types of illness, antimicrobial resistance patterns should also be monitored. NICUs and special care nurseries demand more intensive monitoring than do term nurseries since prolonged duration of stay and increased antibiotic usage are two strong risk factors for infection [37].

In general, routine surveillance cultures from neonates, personnel, and environmental sources in the nursery are not useful, recommended, or cost-effective. Most nosocomial infections are spread from baby to baby by hands or clothing of personnel. Transmission of infection from baby to personnel or from personnel to baby is an unusual event, and environmental surfaces, solutions, ointments, and the like are not often the source of infection in a modern nursery. In a study of 3,371 infants during a 3-year period, the results of almost 25,000 body surface cultures were compared with the bacteria isolated from babies with illness [30]. The sensitivity was 56 percent, specificity 82 percent, and positive predictive value was only 7.5 percent.

If nosocomial infections continue after a cohorting system has been established and after hand-washing has been reinforced, attention should be paid to the possibility of an environmental or personnel source of the problem. One should be selective in performing cultures of personnel or fomites. The nature of the organism and the anatomic site of the infection often give clues to the possible sources of contamination. For example, if the nosocomial pathogen is an enteric gram-negative bacillus typically transmitted by the fecal-oral route, the overwhelming likelihood is that hands of personnel are responsible for transmission, and environmental cultures are not likely to be worthwhile. However, if the site of infection is the lower respiratory tract of intubated babies, one should look carefully at procedures for suctioning and possible contamination of suctioning equipment. Careful thought about procedures, close scrutiny of their implementation, and good detective work are usually more productive than indiscriminate culturing of the inanimate and animate environment.

Whenever new procedures are introduced in the nursery, the potential for nosocomial infection should be considered. This is particularly important in the case of invasive procedures. Details of the procedure should be discussed with the infection control practitioner. Depending on the nature of the procedure, it may be desirable to do prospective surveillance cultures to monitor for nosocomial infection.

Infection Control for Specific Infections

Recommended infection control practices presented in Table 21-1 are based on guidelines of the CDC [40]. Universal precautions should be practiced in the nursery. Several conditions deserve special comment.

Viral Infections
(See Chapter 38 for additional considerations regarding the following viral infections.)

Herpes Simplex Virus Infection
On rare occasions, intrauterine infection of the fetus with HSV occurs but, in most cases, the infection is acquired during vaginal delivery. The risk of infection is greater when the mother has primary infection than when she has reactivation disease, and prematurity is also a risk factor [83]. Cesarean delivery be-

fore or within 4 hours of rupture of amniotic membranes substantially reduces but does not eliminate the risk of infection when the mother has genital lesions.

Nosocomial transmission of HSV infection is rare, but an outbreak in a nursery has been reported [49] in which the identity of the isolates was confirmed by restriction endonuclease cleavage of viral DNA. HSV type 1 was transmitted to a newborn during endotracheal suctioning by a physician with herpes labialis [118]. It has also been transmitted by fetal scalp electrodes [92] and from oral lesions of nursery personnel [66].

Antenatal maternal cultures are poorly predictive of the infant's risk of exposure to HSV at delivery. Therefore, it is prudent to use contact isolation precautions on babies born vaginally to a mother with a history of genital herpes whether or not lesions are present. Vaginal or cervical cultures should be taken at delivery to guide future management.

Optimal management of an infant at risk for neonatal HSV infection has not been developed by controlled studies, but a consensus of opinion has emerged [87]. The baby with herpetic lesions and the baby at risk for developing HSV infection should be managed with contact isolation precautions in the nursery. Breastfeeding is contraindicated only if the mother has a herpetic lesion on the breast. The mother with genital lesions should be instructed about hand-washing, and the mother with herpes labialis should be instructed not to kiss the baby. On the second day of life, viral cultures of the eye and oral cavity are taken from the baby at risk. If the baby has been born vaginally to a mother with primary genital herpes or, in the case of reactivation disease, if the baby has another risk factor (prematurity, invasive instrumentation, or lacerations), anticipatory antiviral chemotherapy is given until the results of cultures are known. If an infant has been treated for active disease and must remain in the nursery subsequently for other medical reasons, isolation precautions should be maintained because recurrence of skin lesions is common.

Personnel with genital herpes can work in the nursery, provided that strict hand-wash-

Table 21-1. Guidelines for isolation of neonates

Disease or condition	Category of precautions						
	Strict	Contact	Respiratory	Enteric	Drainage/ secretion	Blood and body fluids	Routine
Candidiasis							▲
Chlamydia infection					▲		
Conjunctivitis[a]					▲		
Cytomegalovirus						▲	
Diarrhea				▲			
Gonorrhea		▲					
Hepatitis in mother							
A				▲			
B						▲	
Non-A, non-B						▲	
Herpes simplex		▲					
Human immunodeficiency virus infection						▲	
Meningitis, aseptic				▲			
Meningitis, bacterial							▲
Multiply resistant bacteria (disease or colonization)		▲					
Necrotizing enterocolitis				▲			
Pneumonia		▲					
Respiratory viruses		▲					
Rubella		▲					
Sepsis							▲
Skin infections, funisitis, or omphalitis							
Minor					▲		
Major[b]		▲					
Syphilis							
Mucosal or skin lesions					▲	▲	
Other						▲	
Toxoplasmosis							▲
Tuberculosis							▲
Urinary tract infection							▲
Varicella in mother	▲						

[a]Contact isolation for gonococcal conjunctivitis.
[b]Recommended for any staphylococcal or group A streptococcal infection.
Source: Adapted from J.S. Garner and B.P. Simmons, Guidelines for isolation precautions in hospitals. *Infect. Control* 4:425, 1983.

ing techniques are used. Personnel with herpes labialis should not have direct contact with infants until the lesions are crusted.

Cytomegalovirus Infection

Cytomegalovirus (CMV) infection is the most common congenital infection, and many other babies acquire the virus during delivery or postnatally. The neonate can also acquire infection from breast milk [28] or from blood transfusions [3]. CMV can survive on paper diapers for as long as 48 hours [107], posing a potential hazard to nursery personnel who handle diapers. Transmission of CMV infection among neonates in an intensive care unit has been documented using restriction endonuclease digestion analysis [113]. This technology has also been used to show that suspected nosocomial infections in nurseries were actually caused by different strains [2].

Despite the pervasiveness of CMV in a nursery setting, transmission between babies and personnel is rare [9]. The virus is present in saliva and urine of infected infants, but routine hand-washing appears to be a very effective preventive measure. Although the risk of acquisition of infection by female personnel from an infant is remote, it is prudent to exempt pregnant personnel from attending an infant with known CMV infection, for emotional reasons if not scientific ones.

The diverse opinions about isolation precautions for CMV infection were summarized by Plotkin [94] who recommended that (1) neonates not be routinely screened for CMV infection; (2) "pregnant women precautions" be used for infants with known CMV infection; and (3) female personnel who have the potential for becoming pregnant be screened for their CMV serologic status.

Varicella
The indications for giving varicella-zoster immune globulin (VZIG) to newborns of mothers who have chickenpox in the peripartum period have recently been expanded [75]. The newborn can develop chickenpox when the mother had onset of rash from 28 days before delivery to 28 days following delivery, but the attack rate is highest when the mother's rash begins between 7 days before and 7 days after delivery. Severe neonatal infection occurs most often when the mother's rash began between 4 days before and 2 days after delivery. VZIG to the newborn is recommended when the mother's rash begins 7 days before to 2 days after delivery. VZIG does not always prevent disease in the baby, but it probably modifies the severity of disease.

Hepatitis
Transmission of hepatitis A from mother to newborn is extraordinarily rare. Nevertheless, if the mother had onset of jaundice within a week of delivery, the baby should be considered possibly contaminated by hepatitis virus in her feces, and enteric precautions should be used with the infant. The infant is given human immune serum globulin.

With hepatitis B infection in the mother, the risk of infection of her newborn is very great, particularly if she carries the e antigen. Vertical transmission is effectively prevented by combined use of hepatitis B immune globulin and hepatitis vaccine, or even by vaccine alone [127].

The infant should be considered potentially infected. Gloves should be worn when cleansing the baby's skin after birth. Blood and body fluid precautions are used until the immune status of the infant has been verified at 1 year of age.

Rubella
Congenital rubella has become uncommon in areas where rubella vaccination is widely used. Chronicity of infection is characteristic of intrauterine infection. The virus can be recovered from pharyngeal secretions, urine, conjunctival fluid, and feces for many months and occasionally years. Contact isolation precautions are used in the infant with congenital rubella for at least 1 year.

Bacterial Infections
Syphilis
Skin and mucous membrane lesions of an untreated infant with congenital syphilis are teeming with spirochetes, and such infants have spirochetemia. Therefore, blood precautions are necessary, and gloves should be worn when handling the infant. *Treponema pallidum* in the environment is rapidly killed by drying, heat, and soap [57, 117]. Once treatment with penicillin is started, the organisms are eliminated rapidly [116], and isolation precautions can be discontinued after 24 hours.

Listeriosis
There have been several reports of clusters of cases of neonatal listeriosis and of protracted outbreaks in nurseries [17]. In general, investigations have failed to uncover the source of infection and, specifically, nosocomial sources have rarely been implicated (see Chap. 32). Congenitally infected neonates with listeriosis are managed the same as babies with other types of sepsis or meningitis (see under the heading Sepsis and Meningitis).

Multiply Resistant Bacteria

Antibiotic usage is not common in a nursery for term infants but in NICUs more than half the infants receive antibiotic therapy on one or more occasions [36] (see Chap. 13). Antibiotics alter the normal respiratory and gut flora so that resistant bacteria often replace the antibiotic-susceptible flora. Aminoglycosides are the most commonly used anti-gram-negative antibiotics in nurseries. The common use of one particular aminoglycoside frequently leads to the emergence of coliform bacteria resistant to that aminoglycoside [36]. When kanamycin was the most commonly employed antibiotic, reports of outbreaks caused by kanamycin-resistant strains appeared [54]. Then followed outbreaks of coliform infections resistant to both kanamycin and gentamicin [29] and, finally, with strains resistant to kanamycin, gentamicin, and amikacin [18]. *Klebsiella* and *Serratia* strains are especially likely to develop resistance. The resistance is due to transferable plasmids.

With the advent of new cephalosporin drugs, treatment of disease caused by aminoglycoside-resistant coliform bacteria has been facilitated. However, widespread use of cefotaxime in a nursery because of a problem with gentamicin-resistant *Klebsiella* led to the emergence of cefotaxime-resistant *Enterobacter cloacae* as a problem [15].

Methicillin-resistant *S. aureus* strains resistant to all the penicillins and cephalosporins are common in many tertiary centers. *S. epidermidis* is a common nosocomial pathogen associated with intravascular catheters, and most *S. epidermidis* strains are resistant to β-lactams.

Monitoring antibiotic susceptibilities allows one to detect the emergence of a problem with multiply resistant organisms (see Chap. 9). A search for a source should be undertaken, but generally one will not be found since the infections are usually endogenous from altered flora. All infants in the nursing unit should have cultures of appropriate mucosal surfaces (rectum, throat, trachea) to determine the frequency of colonization with the resistant strain. Identification is facilitated by incorporating an antibiotic to which the organism is resistant into the culture medium. Colonized infants are placed in a cohort, and scrupulous aseptic technique is used in handling them. Ill babies are treated with an appropriate antibiotic, but it is generally futile to try to eliminate asymptomatic colonization with antibiotics. Periodic surveillance cultures are taken, and new cohorts of colonized and uncolonized babies are formed until the epidemic has been controlled. Because some colonized infants require medical care in a low-birth-weight nursery or NICU for a prolonged time, it may take months to clear the unit of all colonized babies.

Fungal Infections

Candidal infection of the oral mucous membranes and diaper area is common in neonates who have received broad-spectrum antibiotics, but nosocomial transmission is not obvious in such cases. *Candida* sepsis is a major problem in infants receiving total parenteral nutrition [7, 20, 53], and nosocomial fungemia has been associated with contaminated transducer domes [111] (also see Chap. 42).

Mixed pulmonary fungal infections occurred in babies in a special care unit secondary to construction activities [61]. The fungi were *Aspergillus*, *Rhizopus*, and *Cryptococcus* species.

Rhizopus contamination of elastic surgical bandages has caused wound infection [23]. Seven nurses working in a newborn nursery developed *Microsporum canis* dermatophytosis of the left forearm. The infection was attributed to their practice of cradling the head of an infant who had *M. canis* infection of the occiput on their unclothed left forearm while feeding the baby [80]. Clusters of cases of *Malassezia furfur* pulmonary infections have been reported [99]. Such episodes are peculiarities and, in general, nosocomial fungal infections other than *Candida* sepsis are rare.

Miscellaneous Infections
Toxoplasmosis

Person-to-person infection with *Toxoplasma gondii* does not occur, so no isolation precautions are necessary for a congenitally infected infant. *Toxoplasma* organisms can be present in the lungs, saliva, sputum, kidneys, and intestine, suggesting a potential risk for nursery personnel. Transmission from such sources, however, has never been proved.

Sepsis and Meningitis

Infants with neonatal sepsis or meningitis are often critically ill and require constant observation and intensive care. Excessive isolation precautions could interfere with their care. The risk of horizontal transmission of sepsis or meningitis in a nursery is virtually nonexistent, so universal precautions are sufficient. A possible exception is the case of *Citrobacter diversus,* an organism with unusual tropism for the central nervous system and a proclivity to cause brain abscesses. Outbreaks related to horizontal transmission of *C. diversus* have occurred [67]. Because the reservoir of that organism is the gastrointestinal tract, enteric precautions are recommended (see Chap. 32).

Aseptic meningitis in the neonate is commonly caused by enteroviruses, and outbreaks are not uncommon [58, 77]. The aseptic meningitis or encephalitis may be accompanied by cardiac and hepatic involvement. Enteric precautions are important in preventing transmission of enteroviruses.

Skin, Soft-Tissue, and Mucous Membrane Infections

S. aureus is the most common cause of nosocomial skin infections in a nursery (see Chap. 37). Prolonged outbreaks are not unusual [12], and control can be difficult.

Daily bathing of infants with hexachlorophene-containing soap decreases skin colonization rates [51] but was not reliable for controlling outbreaks. Rates of skin and mucous membrane colonization do not always correlate with rates of disease [41]. In 1971, the U.S Food and Drug Administration recommended that routine bathing with hexachlorophene be discontinued because of rare but serious toxicity of absorbed hexachlorophene. Outbreaks caused by phage group 2 organisms, which are not invasive and produce bullous impetiginous lesions, are common [12]. Outbreaks of scalded skin syndrome (Ritter's disease) have occurred in nurseries [31].

When multiple cases of staphylococcal disease occur within a limited time frame in a nursery and it is determined by antibiograms and bacteriophage testing that a single strain is involved, the following steps can be undertaken sequentially to control the outbreak:

1. Surveillance cultures (anterior nasal swabs and skin or umbilical cord swabs) of all infants in the nursery define the extent of colonization. Medical care staff should be examined to determine whether any has staphylococcal skin lesions. Strict adherence to hand-washing and other aseptic techniques should be enforced. Colonized babies should be segregated. Surveillance for new cases of disease is carried out. In the majority of instances, these measures suffice to control the outbreak.
2. If, after 1 or 2 weeks of these measures, new cases of disease continue to occur, a cohorting program should be implemented if physical facilities permit. The value of performing nasal cultures of hospital personnel is debatable but, on occasion, a nasal carrier among the staff will be responsible [12]. The carrier should be treated with intranasal bacitracin ointment, gentamicin nose drops, or other agents in an attempt to eliminate carriage (see Chaps. 13, 37). In almost all cases, the cohort system and strict enforcement of aseptic technique terminate the outbreak.
3. Only in the most prolonged and persistent staphylococcal outbreak would one consider implementation of a bacterial interference regimen with *S. aureus* 502A. The methods and results of bacterial interference programs have been reviewed by Shinefield and colleagues [108].

An attempt to control colonization with methicillin-resistant *S. aureus* by applying triple dye to umbilical cords had minimal effect [101].

Group A streptococcal nosomial infection most commonly involves the umbilical cord stump. The funisitis is mild, with little inflammation and minimal secretion, which is characteristically sticky and has a musty odor [84]. Local measures, such as applying triple dye or bacitracin ointment to the umbilical stump, may stop the outbreak, but sometimes it is necessary to give an injection of benzathine penicillin (50,000 units/kg) to all newborns until the epidemic has been stopped [43, 84].

Nosocomial chlamydial infection has not been reported, probably because the disease usually has its onset after babies have been discharged to home. In preantibiotic days, gonococcal infection in a nursery was exceedingly difficult to control [19], but with present-day therapy, gonococcal ophthalmia is not a nosocomial problem. Nevertheless, the CDC recommends that full contact precautions be used instead of drainage/secretion precautions. Contact precautions are also recommended for group A streptococcal and staphylococcal skin or mucous membrane infections.

Respiratory Infections
Pertussis [68] and influenza A [11] are uncommon causes of nosocomial respiratory infections. Most outbreaks are caused by viruses, especially respiratory syncytial virus (RSV) [76]. RSV infection in infants with underlying cardiopulmonary disease is often lethal [70]. Gowning and use of masks is ineffectual in preventing transmission of respiratory infection between infants and personnel because RSV survives on hard surfaces such as the crib or bassinet and is transmitted by hands of personnel [48].

Anterior nasal swab specimens can be used for rapid diagnosis of influenza A or RSV infections by immunoflourescence or enzyme-linked immunosorbent assay (ELISA) methods. This is an exceedingly valuable tool for rapid identification of the cause of an outbreak.

Infants with respiratory symptoms should be housed in nurseries separate from asymptomatic babies. In the NICU, separate isolation facilities should be available. In addition to airborne transmission of virus, to other infants and personnel, transmission of infected secretions by hands or fomites can occur, so it

is recommended that gowns be worn when handling babies. Hand-washing is important. In a controlled trial [82], gowning and masking were not significantly better than hand-washing alone in preventing nosocomial transmission of RSV; nevertheless, these procedures are generally employed during an outbreak for whatever minimal benefit might accrue from their use. Masks should be changed frequently. Wearing eye-nose goggles was the most effective means of preventing nosocomial transmission of RSV in one study [39]. Aerosolized ribavirin therapy shortens the period of shedding of RSV and could help in control.

In pertussis outbreaks, affected infants and personnel are treated with erythromycin to reduce their infectivity. In large and persistent outbreaks, widespread antibiotic prophylaxis and vaccination programs for personnel may be necessary [68].

Respiratory tract colonization with methicillin-resistant *S. aureus* usually persists despite systemic antibiotic therapy. In one case, colonization was eradicated by use of aerosolized vancomycin [123].

Diarrhea and Necrotizing Enterocolitis
Outbreaks of infectious diarrhea in nurseries can be caused by enterotoxigenic [46] or enteropathogenic [13] strains of *E. coli, Shigella* [105], *Salmonella* [106], or viruses [90, 100] (see Chap. 30).

The syndrome of necrotizing enterocolitis (NEC) is probably multifactorial in origin, but clusters of cases associated with intestinal pathogens suggest an important role for infection in pathogenesis. Outbreaks of NEC have been temporally associated with *E. cloacae* [96], rotavirus [102], and enteric coronavirus [103], and with delta toxin–producing *S. aureus* [88]; however, in most outbreaks of NEC, no enteric pathogen is found. The role of toxigenic *C. difficile* in diarrhea or NEC is difficult to assess because many asymptomatic neonates are colonized with these strains [128]. Presumably, the neonate's intestinal mucosa lacks receptors for this toxin.

In isolated cases of diarrhea, or when outbreaks occur, all infants with diarrhea should be housed separately from other infants.

Strict enteric precautions for handling soiled diapers and washing of hands should be stressed. Rectal swab or stool cultures for bacterial pathogens should be performed on sick infants and other infants cared for by the same personnel. Rapid diagnostic tests for rotavirus antigen in stool or electron-microscopic examination for coronavirus can be done. When a bacterial pathogen is responsible for the outbreak, appropriate antibiotic therapy is instituted.

Formerly, it was recommended that nurseries for low-birth-weight infants be closed to admissions and new units open when a substantial outbreak of diarrhea disease occurred. With the measures just outlined, this disruptive, impractical extreme solution should not be necessary.

Prevention
Isolation Precautions for Newborns and Infants

The following recommendations are reprinted verbatim from the CDC *Guidelines for Isolation Precautions in Hospitals* [40]:

> Isolation precautions for newborns and infants may have to be modified from those recommended for adults because (1) usually only a small number of private rooms are available for newborns and infants and, (2) during outbreaks, it is frequently necessary to establish cohorts of newborns and infants. Moreover, a newborn may need to be placed on isolation precautions at delivery because its mother has an infection.
>
> It has often been recommended that infected newborns or those suspected of being infected (regardless of the pathogen and clinical manifestations) should be put in a private room. This recommendation was based on the assumptions that a geographically isolated room was necessary to protect uninfected newborns and that infected newborns would receive closer scrutiny and better care in such a room. Neither of these assumptions is completely correct.
>
> Separate isolation rooms are seldom indicated for newborns with many kinds of infection if the following conditions are met:
>
> 1. An adequate number of nursing and medical personnel are on duty and have sufficient time for appropriate hand-washing.

> 2. Sufficient space is available for a 4- to 6-ft. aisle or area between newborn stations.
> 3. An adequate number of sinks for hand-washing are available in each nursery room or area.
> 4. Continuing instruction is given to personnel about the mode of transmission of infections.

When these criteria are not met, a separate room with hand-washing facilities may be indicated.

Another incorrect assumption regarding isolation precautions for newborns and infants is that forced-air incubators can be substituted for private rooms. These incubators may filter the incoming air but not the air discharged into the nursery. Moreover, the surfaces of incubators housing newborns or infants can easily become contaminated with organisms infecting or colonizing the patient, so personnel working with the patient through portholes may have their hands and forearms colonized. Forced-air incubators, therefore, are satisfactory for limited "protective" isolation of newborns and infants but should not be relied on as a major means of preventing transmission from infected patients to others.

Isolation precautions for an infected or colonized newborn or infant, or for a newborn of a mother suspected of having an infectious disease, can be determined by the specific viral or bacterial pathogen, the clinical manifestations, the source and possible modes of transmission, and the number of colonized or infected newborns or infants. Other factors to be considered include the overall condition of the newborn or infant and the kind of care required, the available space and facilities, the nurse-to-patient ratio, and the size and type of nursery services for newborns and infants.

In addition to applying isolation precautions, cohorts may be established to keep to a minimum the transmission of organisms or infectious diseases among different groups of newborns and infants in large nurseries. A cohort usually consists of all well newborns from the same 24- or 48-hour birth period; these newborns are admitted to and kept in a single nursery room and, ideally, are taken care of by a single group of personnel who do not take care of any other cohort during the same shift. After the newborns in a cohort have been discharged, the room is thoroughly cleaned and prepared to accept the next cohort.

Cohorting is not practical as a routine for

small nurseries or in neonatal intensive care units or graded care nurseries. It is useful in these nurseries, however, as a control measure during outbreaks or for managing a group of infants or newborns colonized or infected with an epidemiologically important pathogen. Under these circumstances, having separate rooms for each cohort is ideal but not mandatory for many kinds of infections if cohorts can be kept separate within a single large room and if personnel are assigned to take care of only those in the cohort.

During outbreaks, newborns or infants with overt infection or colonization and personnel who are carriers, if indicated, should be identified rapidly and placed in cohorts; if rapid identification is not possible, exposed newborns or infants should be placed in a cohort separate from those with disease and from unexposed infants and newborns and new admissions. The success of cohorting depends largely on the willingness and ability of nursing and ancillary personnel to adhere strictly to the cohort system and to meticulously follow patient care practices.

Nursery Design

The preceding CDC statement addresses certain issues about nursery design. It is difficult to generalize about this subject because there is no uniformity in construction or arrangement of newborn nurseries. Some have multiple small rooms and others have one large open area. Some have isolation rooms for individual infants, and others do not. Nevertheless, certain generalizations apply to all nurseries.

Detailed recommendations for design of newborn units are available [6, 38]. The amount of floor space per bassinet for adequate separation of infants is from 20 to 25 sq. ft. in a full-term infant nursery, approximately 50 sq. ft. in an intermediate care nursery, and between 80 and 100 sq. ft. in an intensive care unit. Sinks should be conveniently located throughout the nursery so that it is no more than a few steps from any bassinet to a sink. Foot or knee controls of faucets are preferable to hand controls. Faucet aerators should not be used, and sinks should not be set in countertops.

Floors, walls, counters, bassinets, and other furniture should be made of materials that are easily cleaned and will withstand disinfectant solutions. Disinfectant detergents are recommended for routine cleaning. When a baby is discharged, the bassinet should be disinfected with an iodophor disinfectant.

Routine Procedures

Many restrictive procedures in the past have been shown to be ceremonial rites with little or no impact on nosocomial infection rates. Caps, masks, hairnets, and beard bags have been discarded as routines. Families are no longer barred from nurseries or intensive care units, and medical and surgical consultants are encouraged to enter the newborn unit. Excessive precautionary procedures were not only ineffectual but discouraged personnel from giving optimal hands-on care to babies and decreased the likelihood of adherence to effective procedures.

Hand-Washing

The key to effective infection control in the nursery is strict adherence to hand-washing before and after handling babies. At the time of entering the nursery, personnel should remove rings, watches, and bracelets, and scrub the hands and forearms to the elbows. An antiseptic agent, such as an iodophor, 4% chlorhexidine, or 3% hexachlorophene, should be used for this scrub. Thereafter, hands should be washed for 15 seconds before and after handling an infant or a potentially contaminated object. These washes are preferably done with an antiseptic soap, but plain soap suffices if the individual's skin is sensitive to the antiseptic. Fifteen seconds of washing has no impact on the individual's resident (i.e., permanent) skin flora but effectively removes transient flora acquired by handling a contaminated person or object. Hands should also be washed after touching one's own hair, face, or other parts of the body.

Attire, Gowns, Caps, Masks, and Gloves

(The following recommendations for limited use of gowns are the author's preferences.) Personnel working in the nursery should wear scrub suits. When they leave the nursery temporarily, they should don a long-sleeved gown over the scrub suit. Visitors, consultants, and laboratory and housekeeping personnel should wear a long-sleeved gown over their street clothes. Caps, masks, and hairnets need not be used routinely.

A long-sleeved gown should hang at the side of each bassinet. This is worn whenever the baby's body will come in contact with the body of personnel, such as during feeding. If disposable gowns are not used, the gown should be replaced every 8 hours.

Gowns, caps, masks, and gloves are used when specified for babies on isolation precautions and for performing invasive procedures. Many studies have failed to establish a significant benefit in reducing colonization or disease rates attributable to gowning in term or preterm nurseries. A study in an intensive care unit showed no change in hand-washing rates, infection, or intravascular catheter colonization rates when gowns were used [25]. There is no uniform standard, and each nursery should set policy that is most appropriate for its personnel and the types of problems encountered.

Linens

Traditionally, bassinet linens in the admission observation area and intermediate and intensive care areas have been sterilized by autoclaving. This is recommended by the American Academy of Pediatrics [38]. The need for this practice is debatable since linens after routine laundering are essentially germ-free [74]. Linens and infant clothing are not important sources of infection. Routine laundering is sufficient, provided the hospital's laundry facilities are good. Soiled linens should be placed into plastic bags in receptacles, sealed, and removed from the nursery every 8 hours.

Neonatal Cord and Eye Care and Bathing

Many topical agents and systemic penicillin have been shown to be effective in preventing gonococcal ophthalmia. In most states, the type and method of prophylaxis are precisely defined by law. Credé's prophylaxis with 1% silver nitrate has the disadvantages of causing chemical conjunctivitis frequently and of not preventing chlamydial conjunctivitis. Tetracycline or erythromycin ophthalmic ointments have been proposed to prevent both gonococcal and chlamydial conjunctivitis, but they do not reliably prevent the latter [50]. A single intramuscular dose of 125 mg ceftriaxone has been effective in preventing [62] and treating [47] ophthalmia caused by penicillin-resistant gonococci. Some parents refuse to have anything put in the eyes of their newborns because of theoretic concerns about interference with parent-infant bonding. In such cases, an injection of ceftriaxone should be used.

Immediately after birth, the umbilical cord is tied with sterile tape and cut with sterile instruments. Subsequent care of the umbilical stump is a disputed matter. Application of triple dye, silver sulfadiazine cream, or bacitracin ointment is advocated by some investigators, whereas others prefer keeping the cord dry with periodic swabbing with alcohol. Such disparate results of the various methods of managing the umbilical stump have been reported that it is not possible to identify the most effective method, other than concluding that dyes or antimicrobials more effectively suppress flora than do alcohol or castile soap.

Care of the newborn's skin has also been a debated matter. Current opinion holds that the so-called dry technique decreases trauma, avoids potential toxicity from absorption of chemicals, and interferes least with acquisition of normal flora. Shortly after birth, the skin is cleansed using sterile cotton sponges and sterile water either alone or with mild castile soap. Thereafter, the diaper area is cleansed similarly when necessary.

Equipment

Equipment used on many babies, such as stethoscopes, should be cleaned between uses with alcohol or an iodophor solution. In an NICU, it is common practice to provide a stethoscope at each baby's bed. Nebulization equipment is easily contaminated. It should be autoclaved or gas-sterilized every 8 hours. Water reservoirs are filled only with sterile distilled water and are autoclaved daily. Suction catheters and equipment must be sterilized by autoclaving or gas sterilization. The parts of x-ray equipment that come into contact with an infant should be cleaned with alcohol or an iodophor solution.

Visitors

Parents should follow the same procedure for scrubbing used by personnel before entering the nursery. A long-sleeved gown should be worn over street clothing. They should be instructed not to touch other babies. Parents with respiratory infections or infected lesions on the hands or face should not be permitted in the nursery. Most nurseries permit children who are siblings of critically ill babies to enter the NICU. They are barred from visiting if they have an infectious illness or have been recently exposed to a contagious disease.

Special Procedures
Collection and Storage of Breast Milk

Many mothers like to provide breast milk for their babies who are unable to nurse because of illness or prematurity. Before collecting the specimen, the mother scrubs her hands with an iodophor or other antiseptic. The nipple area does not need special cleansing. The milk is expressed manually or collected by a mechanical device and stored in a sterile bottle under refrigeration until it is used. Milk obtained this way is generally sterile or has small colony counts of nonpathogenic bacteria from normal skin flora [65].

The milk can be safely stored under refrigeration for up to 48 hours [65] and perhaps as long as 5 days [112]. It is not necessary to perform quantitative bacterial cultures of the milk for surveillance.

Formerly, some institutions used banked breast milk collected from multiple donors, but this practice has largely been abandoned and it is not recommended because of outbreaks of infection with *Salmonella* [104], *Klebsiella* [26], and other organisms. If banked milk is used, it is mandatory to perform cultures for bacterial pathogens before it is given to infants.

Blood-Banking Procedures

In addition to routine testing for hepatitis B antigen and human immunodeficiency virus antibody, it is recommended that only blood without CMV antibody be given to neonates. In some hospitals, this restriction is applied only to preterm neonates. An alternative is to use frozen, deglycerolized blood, since that process inactivates CMV [115] or blood from which leukocytes have been filtered [44].

Intravascular Catheters

To insert a radial artery or umbilical vessel catheter, the skin area should be scrubbed with an iodophor and draped with sterile surgical drapes. The operator should wear a cap, mask, and gloves; a gown is optional. The entrance wound should be covered with a sterile dressing that is changed daily. It is common practice to cleanse the entrance wound daily with an iodophor or other antiseptic or to use an antibiotic ointment, but the value of these procedures has not been established.

Insertion of central venous catheters into the jugular or subclavian veins is done in the surgical suite with full surgical sterile technique. Daily dressing changes are done with glove, mask, and cap precautions.

Bacteremia is a small but important complication of intravascular catheters (see Chap. 40). When an infant with an intravascular catheter shows signs of infection, the blood specimen for culture is drawn through the catheter. If the entrance wound becomes infected, the wound itself and the tip of the removed catheter should be cultured in addition to obtaining blood cultures. It is not unusual for catheter tip cultures to be positive in the absence of bacteremia. There are opportunities for contamination of the tip by skin bacteria or in handling the specimen.

Prophylactic systemic antibiotics are not recommended for infants with intravascular catheters.

Fluids for Total Parenteral Nutrition

If fluids are mixed for total parenteral nutrition (TPN) administration, this should be done under a positive-pressure filtered hood.

The connections in the tubing line should not be violated. Because TPN fluids are most commonly given via central venous catheters, the precautions discussed earlier should be followed.

Antibiotic Usage

β-Lactam and aminoglycoside combinations are the mainstay of therapy in newborn nurseries. Because of the widespread use of these antibiotics in low-birth-weight nurseries and NICUs, there is selective drug pressure, encouraging the emergence of resistance to aminoglycosides. A monitoring system to detect emerging resistance of pathogens to the aminoglycoside being administered should be used. Generally, the resistance is specific for one or two of the aminoglycosides, and another aminoglycoside can be selected for routine use.

A broad-spectrum cephalosporin, such as cefotaxime or ceftriaxone, should not be used routinely. These valuable drugs should be held in reserve to be used in the event of nosocomial disease caused by bacteria that are resistant to all aminoglycosides. However, when there is an ongoing nosocomial infection problem with an organism resistant to all aminoglycosides, a cephalosporin should *temporarily* become the drug of choice for empiric therapy of suspected sepsis. Once the problem has disappeared, one should revert to an aminoglycoside for routine use, since, with continued use of the cephalosporin, resistance to that drug is likely to develop [15].

Infants with intravascular catheters are prone to infection with *S. epidermidis*, which is usually resistant to methicillin and other β-lactams. In that situation, or when there is a nosocomial problem with methicillin-resistant *S. aureus*, vancomycin should replace the β-lactam as empiric initial therapy for suspected sepsis.

Immunoprophylaxis

An experimental approach to the prevention of nosocomial infections in low-birth-weight babies is administration of intravenous gamma globulin shortly after birth. There are attractive theoretic considerations to this approach. Antibody production and T cells in the newborn function too slowly to have a significant impact on bacterial disease. The only specific immunity available to the infant is maternally derived immunoglobulin, which is deficient in preterm babies. Another approach is to administer gamma globulin to the mother of a preterm baby during labor; however, the gamma globulin does not cross the placenta until 32 weeks of gestation.

A large body of literature on the use of intravenous gamma globulin in newborns is accumulating, but conflicting results are reported. Therefore, intravenous gamma globulin cannot be recommended for immunoprophylaxis at this time.

Employee Health

General aspects of employee health are discussed in the CDC *Guidelines for Infection Control in Hospital Personnel* [126] (see Chap. 3). Female personnel in the nursery who are of childbearing age should be tested serologically for susceptibility to rubella and, if necessary, given rubella vaccine with appropriate precautions. As discussed earlier, transmission of CMV from infected babies to pregnant personnel is a minimal hazard. Although this appears to be a rare occurrence, prudence dictates that pregnant personnel should not handle infants known to be infected with CMV, and they should pay meticulous attention to hand-washing after diapering any infant.

Personnel with active tuberculosis, pertussis, influenza, and other communicable diseases should be excluded from the nursery. Personnel with bacterial or viral lesions on exposed areas of skin should not handle infants. For other respiratory, gastrointestinal, and cutaneous infections, rigid criteria for exclusion from the nursery are more difficult to establish. Clinical judgment and common sense are weighed against the needs of the nursery. Upper respiratory viral infections are most transmissible during the acute febrile period, but since symptoms often linger for a couple of weeks, employees are often permitted to return before complete resolution of symptoms. Personnel with acute diarrheal illnesses are preferably excluded or permitted to work if it is believed that scrupulous hand-washing will effectively eliminate risk of transmission of the agent. Individuals with acute pharyngitis and fever should be excluded until group A streptococcal infection has been ruled out or treated.

References

1. Adams, J.M., Speer, M.E., and Rudolph, A.J. Bacterial colonization of radial artery catheters. *Pediatrics* 65:94, 1980.
2. Adler, S.P. Nosocomial transmission of cytomegalovirus. *Pediatr. Infect. Dis.* 5:239, 1986.
3. Adler, S.P., Chandrika, T., Lawrence, L., and Baggett, J. Cytomegalovirus infections in neonates acquired by blood transfusions. *Pediatr. Infect. Dis.* 2:114, 1983.
4. Anagostakis, D., et al. A nursery outbreak of *Serratia marcescens* infection. *Am. J. Dis. Child.* 135:413, 1981.
5. Anagnostakis, D., et al. Risk of infection associated with umbilical vein catheterization: A prospective study in 75 newborn infants. *J. Pediatr.* 86:759, 1975.
6. Anonymous. *Planning and Design for Perinatal and Pediatric Facilities.* Columbus, OH: Ross Laboratories, 1977.
7. Ashcraft, K.W., and Leape, L.L. *Candida* sepsis complicating parenteral feeding. *J.A.M.A.* 212:454, 1970.
8. Balagtas, R.C., Bell, C.E., Edwards, L.D., and Levin, S. Risk of local and systemic infections associated with umbilical vein catheterization: A prospective study in 86 newborn patients. *Pediatrics* 48:359, 1971.
9. Balfour, C.L., and Balfour, H.H., Jr. Cytomegalovirus is not an occupational risk for nurses in renal transplant and neonatal units: Results of a prospective surveillance study. *J.A.M.A.* 256:1909, 1986.
10. Bard, H. Prophylactic antibiotics in chronic umbilical artery catheterization in respiratory distress syndrome. *Arch. Dis. Child.* 48:630, 1973.
11. Bauer, C.R., Elie, K., Spence, L., and Stern L. Hong Kong influenza in a neonatal unit. *J.A.M.A.* 223:1233, 1973.
12. Belani, A., et al. Outbreak of staphylococcal infection in two hospital nurseries traced to a single nasal carrier. *Infect. Control* 7:487, 1986.
13. Boyer, K.M., et al. An outbreak of gastroenteritis due to *E. coli* 0142 in a neonatal nursery. *J. Pediatr.* 86:919, 1975.
14. Boyer, K.M., et al. Nosocomial transmission of bacteriophage type 7/11/12 group B streptococci in a special care nursery. *Am. J. Dis. Child.* 134:964, 1980.
15. Bryan, C.S., John, J.F., Jr., Pai, M.S., and Austin, T.L. Gentamicin vs. cefotaxime for therapy of neonatal sepsis. *Am. J. Dis. Child.* 139:1086, 1985.
16. Cameron, D.J.S., Bishop, R.F., Veenstra, A.A., and Barnes, G.L. Noncultivable viruses and neonatal diarrhea: Fifteen-month survey in a newborn special care nursery. *J. Clin. Microbiol.* 8:93, 1978.
17. Canfield, M.A., et al. An epidemic of perinatal listeriosis serotype 1b in Hispanics in a Houston hospital. *Pediatr. Infect. Dis.* 4:106, 1985.
18. Cook, L.N., Davis, R.S., and Stover, B.H. Outbreak of amikacin-resistant Enterobacteriaceae in an intensive care nursery. *Pediatrics* 65:264, 1980.
19. Cooperman, M.B. *Gonococcus* arthritis in infancy. *Am. J. Dis. Child.* 33:932, 1927.
20. Curry, C.R., and Quie, P.G. Fungal septicemia in patients receiving parenteral hyperalimentation. *N. Engl. J. Med.* 285:1121, 1971.
21. Cushing, A.H. Omphalitis: A review. *Pediatr. Infect. Dis.* 4:282, 1985.
22. Dassett, J.H., Williams, R.C., Jr., and Quie, P.G. Studies on interaction of bacteria, serum factors and polymorphonuclear leucocytes in mothers and newborns. *Pediatrics* 44:49, 1969.
23. Dennis, J.E., Rhodes, K.H., Cooney, D.R., and Roberts, G.D. Nosocomial *Rhizopus* infection (zygomycosis) in children. *J. Pediatr.* 96:824, 1980.
24. Dillon, J.D., Jr., Schaffner, W., Van Way, C.W., III, and Meng, H.C. Septicemia and total parenteral nutrition. *J.A.M.A.* 223:1341, 1973.
25. Donowitz, L.G. Failure of the overgown to prevent nosocomial infection in a pediatric intensive care unit. *Pediatrics* 77:35, 1986.
26. Donowitz, L.G., Marsik, F.J., Fisher, K.A., and Wenzel, R.P. Contaminated breast milk: A source of *Klebsiella* bacteremia in a newborn intensive care unit. *Rev. Infect. Dis.* 3:716, 1981.
27. Dudrick, S.J., Groff, D.B., and Wilmore, D.W. Long-term venous catheterization in infants. *Surg. Gynecol. Obstet.* 129:805, 1969.
28. Dworksy, M., Cytomegalovirus infection of breast milk and transmission in infancy. *Pediatrics* 72:295, 1983.
29. Eidelman, A.I., and Reynolds, J. Gentamicin-resistant *Klebsiella* infections in a neonatal intensive care unit. *Am. J. Dis. Child.* 132:421, 1978.

30. Evans, M.E., et al. Sensitivity, specificity, and predictive value of body surface cultures in a neonatal intensive care unit. *J.A.M.A.* 259: 248, 1988.

31. Faden, H.S., Burke, J.P., Glasgow, L.A., and Everett, J.R., III. Nursery outbreak of scalded-skin syndrome: Scarlatiniform rash due to phage group 1 *Staphylococcus aureus. Am. J. Dis. Child.* 130:265, 1976.

32. Farman, M.L., and Stiehm, E.R. Impaired opsonic activity but normal phagocytosis in low birth weight infants. *N. Engl. J. Med.* 281: 926, 1969.

33. Farmer, K., and Patten, P.T. An outbreak of coxsackie B5 infection in a special care unit for newborn infants. *N.Z. Med. J.* 68:86, 1968.

34. Feder, H.M., MacLean, W.C., and Moxon, R. Scalp abscess secondary to fetal scalp electrode. *J. Pediatr.* 89:808, 1976.

35. Fierer, J., Taylor, P.M., and Gezon, H.M. *Pseudomonas aeruginosa* epidemic traced to delivery-room resuscitators. *N. Engl. J. Med.* 276:991, 1967.

36. Franco, J.A., Eitzman, D.V., and Baer, H. Antibiotic usage and microbial resistance in an intensive care nursery. *Am. J. Dis. Child.* 126:318, 1973.

37. Freeman, J., et al. Extra hospital stay and antibiotic usage with nosocomial coagulase-negative staphylococcal bacteremia in two neonatal intensive care unit populations. *Am. J. Dis. Child.* 144:324, 1990.

38. Frigoletto, F.D., and Little, G.A. (Ed.). *American Academy of Pediatrics and American College of Obstetricians and Gynecologists Guidelines for Perinatal Care.* (2nd ed.). Evanston, IL: American Academy of Pediatrics, 1988.

39. Gala, C.L., et al. The use of eye-nose goggles to control nosocomial respiratory syncytial virus infection. *J.A.M.A.* 256:2706, 1986.

40. Garner, J.S., and Simmons, B.P. Guidelines for isolation precautions in hospitals. *Infect. Control* 4:245, 1983.

41. Gehlbach, S.H., et al. Recurrence of skin disease in a nursery: Ineffectuality of hexachlorophene bathing. *Pediatrics* 55:422, 1975.

42. Gerdes, J.S., Yoder, M.C., Douglas, S.D., and Polin, R.A. Decreased plasma fibronectin in neonatal sepsis. *Pediatrics* 72:877, 1983.

43. Gezon, H.M., Schaberg, M.J., and Klein, J.O. Concurrent epidemics of *Staphylococcus aureus* and group A streptococcus disease in a newborn nursery—control with penicillin G and hexachlorophene bathing. *Pediatrics* 51: 383, 1973.

44. Gilbert, G.L., et al. Prevention of transfusion-acquired cytomegalovirus in infants by blood filtration to remove leucocytes. *Lancet* 1: 1228, 1989.

45. Goldmann, D.A., and Maki, D.G. Infection control in total parenteral nutrition. *J.A.M.A.* 223:1360, 1973.

46. Guerrant, R.L., Dickens, M.D., Wenzel, R.P., and Kapikian, A. Z. Toxigenic bacterial diarrhea: Nursery outbreak involving bacterial strains. *J. Pediatr.* 89:885, 1976.

47. Haase, D.A., et al. Single-dose ceftriaxone therapy of gonococcal ophthalmia neonatorum. *Sex. Transm. Dis.* 13:53, 1986.

48. Hall, C.B., and Douglas, R.G., Jr. Modes of transmission of respiratory syncytial virus. *J. Pediatr.* 99:100, 1981.

49. Hammerberg, O., et al. An outbreak of herpes simplex virus type 1 in an intensive care nursery. *Pediatr. Infect. Dis.* 2:290, 1983.

50. Hammerschlag, M.R., et al. Efficacy of neonatal ocular prophylaxis for the prevention of chlamydial and gonococcal conjunctivitis. *N. Engl. J. Med.* 320:769, 1989.

51. Hargiss, C., and Larson, E. The epidemiology of *Staphylococcus aureus* in a newborn nursery from 1970 through 1976. *Pediatrics* 61: 348, 1978.

52. Harpin, V.A., and Eutter, N. Barrier properties of the newborn infant's skin. *J. Pediatr.* 102:419, 1983.

53. Hedberg, K., et al. Outbreak of erythromycin-resistant staphylococcal conjunctivitis in a newborn nursery. *Pediatr. Infect. Dis. J.* 9: 268, 1990.

54. Hill, H.R., Hunt, C.E., and Matsen, J.M. Nosocomial colonization with *Klebsiella*, type 26, in a neonatal intensive care unit associated with an outbreak of sepsis, meningitis, and necrotizing enterocolitis. *J. Pediatr.* 85: 415, 1974.

55. Holroyde, C.P., Oski, F.A., and Gardner, F.H. The "pocked" erythrocyte: Red-cell surface alterations in reticuloendothelial immaturity of the neonate. *N. Engl. J. Med.* 281:516, 1969.

56. Horan, T.C., et al. Nosocomial infection surveillance, 1984. *M.M.W.R.* 35 (No. 1SS): 17SS, 1984.

57. Keller, R., and Morton, H.E. The effect of a hand soap and a hexachlorophene soap on the cultivatable treponemata. *Am. J. Syph.* 36:524, 1952.

58. Kinney, J.S., et al. Risk factors associated with echovirus 11 infection in a hospital nursery. *Pediatr. Infect. Dis.* 5:191, 1986.

59. Klein, R.B., et al. Decreased mononuclear and polymorphonuclear chemotaxis in human newborns, infants, and young children. *Pediatrics* 60:467, 1977.

60. Kohler, P.F., and Farr, R.S. Elevation of cord over maternal IgG immunoglobulin—evidence for an active placental IgG transport. *Nature* 210:1070, 1966.

61. Krasinski, K., et al. Nosocomial fungal infection during hospital renovation. *Infect. Control* 6:278, 1985.

62. Laga, M., et al. Single-dose therapy of gonococcal ophthalmia neonatorum with ceftriaxone. *N. Engl. J. Med.* 315:1382, 1986.

63. LaGamma, E.F., et al. Neonatal infections: An important determinant of late NICU mortality in infants less than 1,000 g at birth. *Am. J. Dis. Child.* 137:838, 1983.

64. Lapage, S.P., Johnson, R., and Hoomes, B. Bacteria from intravenous fluids. *Lancet* 2:284, 1973.

65. Larson, E., Zuill, R., Zier, V., and Berg, B. Storage of human breast milk. *Infect. Control* 5:127, 1984.

66. Light, I.J. Postnatal acquisition of herpes simplex virus by the newborn infant: A review of the literature. *Pediatrics* 63:480, 1979.

67. Lin, F.-Y. Outbreak of neonatal *Citrobacter diversus* meningitis in a suburban hospital. *Pediatr. Infect. Dis.* 6:50, 1987.

68. Linneman, C.C., Jr., et al. Use of pertussis vaccine in an epidemic involving hospital staff. *Lancet* 2:540, 1975.

69. Luginbuhl, L.M., et al. Neonatal enterococcal sepsis: Case-control study and description of an outbreak. *Pediatr. Infect. Dis. J.* 6:1022, 1987.

70. Macdonald, N.E., et al. Respiratory syncytial viral infection in infants with congenital heart disease. *N. Engl. J. Med.* 307:397, 1982.

71. Maki, D.G., Weise, C.E., and Sarafin, H.W. A semiquantitative culture method for identifying intravenous-catheter-related infection. *N. Engl. J. Med.* 296:1305, 1977.

72. Markowitz, S.M., et al. Sequential outbreaks of infection due to *Klebsiella pneumoniae* in a neonatal intensive care unit: Implication of a conjugative R plasmid. *J. Infect. Dis.* 142:106, 1980.

73. McCormack, R.C., and Kunin, C.M. Control of a single source nursery epidemic due to *Serratia marcescens*. *Pediatrics* 37:750, 1966.

74. Meyer, C.L., et al. Should linen in newborn intensive care units be autoclaved? *Pediatrics* 67:362, 1981.

75. Miller, E., Cradock-Watson, J.E., and Ridehalgh, M.K.S. Outcome in newborn babies given anti-varicella-zoster immunoglobulin after perinatal maternal infection with varicella-zoster virus. *Lancet* 2:371, 1989.

76. Mintz, L., et al. Nosocomial respiratory syncytial virus infections in an intensive care nursery: Rapid diagnosis by direct immunoflourescence. *Pediatrics* 64:149, 1979.

77. Modlin, J.F. Perinatal echovirus infection: Insights from a literature review of 61 cases of serious infection and 16 outbreaks in nurseries. *Rev. Infect. Dis.* 8:918, 1986.

78. Morehead, C.D., and Houck, P.W. Epidemiology of *Pseudomonas* infections in a pediatric intensive care unit. *Am. J. Dis. Child.* 124:564, 1972.

79. Morse, L.J., and Schonbeck, L.E. Hand lotions—a potential nosocomial hazard. *N. Engl. J. Med.* 278:376, 1968.

80. Mossovitch, M., Mossovitch, B., and Alkan, M. Nosocomial dermatophytosis caused by *Microsporum canis* in a newborn department. *Infect. Control* 7:593, 1986.

81. Munson, D.P., et al. Coagulase-negative staphylococcal septicemia: Experience in a newborn intensive care unit. *J. Pediatr.* 101:602, 1982.

82. Murphy, D., et al. The use of gowns and masks to control respiratory illness in pediatric hospital personnel. *J. Pediatr.* 99:746, 1981.

83. Nahmias, A.J., et al. Perinatal risk associated with maternal genital herpes simplex infection. *Am. J. Obstet. Gynecol.* 110:825, 1971.

84. Nelson, J.D., Dillon, H.C., Jr., and Howard, J.B. A prolonged nursery epidemic associated with a newly recognized type of group A streptococcus. *J. Pediatr.* 89:792, 1976.

85. Nelson, J.D., Richardson, J., and Shelton, S. The significance of bacteremia with exchange transfusion. *J. Pediatr.* 66:291, 1965.

86. Noriega, F.R., Kotloff, K.L., Martin, M.A., and Schwalbe, R.S. Nosocomial bacteremia caused by *Enterobacter sakazakii* and *Leuconostoc mesenteroides* resulting from extrinsic contamination of infant formula. *Pediatr. Infect. Dis. J.* 9:447, 1990.

87. Overall, J.C., Jr., et al. Prophylactic or anticipatory antiviral therapy for newborns exposed to herpes simplex infection. *Pediatr. Infect. Dis.* 3:193, 1984.

88. Overturf, G.D., Sherman, M.P., Scheifele, D.W., and Wong, L.C. Neonatal necrotizing enterocolitis associated with delta toxin-producing methicillin-resistant *Staphylococcus aureus*. *Pediatr. Infect. Dis. J.* 9:88, 1990.

89. Pahwa, S., Pahwa, R., Grines, E., and Smithwick, E.M. Cellular and humoral components of monocyte and neutrophil chemotaxis in cord blood. *Pediatr. Res.* 5:487, 1977.

90. Park, B.H., Holmes, B., and Good, R.A. Metabolic activities in leucocytes in newborn infants. *J. Pediatr.* 76:237, 1970.

91. Parry, M.F., et al. Gram-negative sepsis in neonates: A nursery outbreak due to hand carriage of *Citrobacter diversus*. *Pediatrics* 65:1105, 1980.

92. Parvey, L.S., and Chien, L.T. Neonatal herpes simplex virus infection introduced by fetal-monitor scalp electrodes. *Pediatrics* 65:1150, 1980.

93. Peter, G., Lloyd-Still, J.D., and Lovejoy, F.H.,

Jr. Local infection and bacteremia from scalp vein needles and polyethylene catheters in children. *J. Pediatr.* 80:78, 1972.

94. Plotkin, S.A. Cytomegalovirus in hospitals. *Pediatr. Infect. Dis.* 5:177, 1986.

95. Plotkin, S.A., and McKitrick, J.C. Nosocomial meningitis of the newborn caused by a flavobacterium. *J.A.M.A.* 198:662, 1966.

96. Powell, J., et al. Necrotizing enterocolitis. *Am. J. Dis. Child.* 134:1152, 1980.

97. Powers, W.F., and Tooley, W.H. Contamination of umbilical vessel catheters. Encouraging information (letter to the editor). *Pediatrics* 49:470, 1972.

98. Reboli, A.C., John, J.F., Jr., and Leukoff, A.H. Epidemic methicillin-gentamicin-resistant *Staphylococcus aureus* in a neonatal intensive care unit. *Am. J. Dis. Child.* 143:34, 1989.

99. Richet, H.M., McNeil, M.M., Edwards, M.C., and Jarvis, W.R. Cluster of *Malassezia furfur* pulmonary infections in infants in a neonatal intensive-care unit. *J. Clin. Microbiol.* 27:1197, 1989.

100. Rodriguez, W.J., et al. Rotavirus: A cause of nosocomial infection in the nursery. *J. Pediatr.* 101:274, 1982.

101. Rosenfeld, C.R., Laptook, A.R., and Jeffrey, J. Limited effectiveness of triple dye in preventing colonization with methicillin-resistant *Staphylococcus aureus* in a special care nursery. *Pediatr. Infect. Dis. J.* 9:290, 1990.

102. Rotbart, H.A., et al. An outbreak of rotavirus-associated neonatal necrotizing enterocolitis. *J. Pediatr.* 103:454, 1983.

103. Rousset, S., et al. Intestinal lesions containing coronavirus-like particles in neonatal necrotizing enterocolitis: An ultrastructural analysis. *Pediatrics* 73:218, 1984.

104. Ryder, R.W., Crosby-Ritchie, A., McDonough, B., and Hall, W.J. Human milk contaminated with *Salmonella kottbus:* A cause of nosocomial illness in infants. *J.A.M.A.* 238:1533, 1977.

105. Salzman, T.C., Scher, C.D., and Moss, R. Shigellae with transferable drug resistance: Outbreak in a nursery for premature infants. *J. Pediatr.* 71:21, 1967.

106. Schroeder, S.A., Aserkoff, B., and Brachman, P.S. Epidemic salmonellosis in hospitals and institutions: A five-year review. *N. Engl. J. Med.* 279:674, 1968.

107. Schupfer, P.C., Murph, J.R., and Bale, J.F., Jr. Survival of cytomegalovirus in paper diaper and saliva. *Pediatr. Infect. Dis.* 5:677, 1986.

108. Shinefield, H.R., Ribble, J.C., and Boris, M. Bacterial interference between strains of *Staphylococcus aureus*, 1960 to 1970. *Am. J. Dis. Child.* 121:148, 1971.

109. Simmons, N.A. Contamination of disinfectants. *Br. Med. J.* 1:842, 1969.

110. Simmons, N.A., and Gardner, D.A. Bacterial contamination of a phenolic disinfectant. *Br. Med. J.* 2:668, 1969.

111. Solomon, S.L., et al. Nosocomial fungemia in neonates associated with intravascular pressure-monitoring devices. *Pediatr. Infect. Dis.* 5:680, 1986.

112. Sosa, R., and Barness, L. Bacterial growth in refrigerated human milk. *Am. J. Dis. Child.* 141:111, 1987.

113. Spector, S.A. Transmission of cytomegalovirus among infants in hospital documented by restriction-endonuclease-digestion analysis. *Lancet* 1:378, 1983.

114. Swender, P.T., Shott, R.J., and Williams, M.L. A community and intensive care nursery outbreak of coxsackievirus B5 meningitis. *Am. J. Dis. Child.* 127:42, 1975.

115. Taylor, B.J., et al. Frozen deglycerolyzed blood prevents transfusion-acquired cytomegalovirus infections in neonates. *Pediatr. Infect. Dis.* 5:188, 1986.

116. Tucker, H.A., and Robinson, R.C.V. Disappearance time of *T. pallidum* from lesions of early syphilis following administration of crystalline penicillin. *Bull. Johns Hopkins Hosp.* 80:169, 1947.

117. Turner, T.B., Bauer, J.A., and Kluth, F.C. The viability of the spirochetes of syphilis and yaws in desiccated blood serum. *Am. J. Med. Sci.* 202:416, 1941.

118. Van Dyke, R.B., and Spector, S.A. Transmission of herpes simplex virus type 1 to a newborn infant during endotracheal suctioning for meconium aspiration. *Pediatr. Infect. Dis.* 3:153, 1984.

119. Van Vliet, P.K.J., and Gupta, J.M. Prophylactic antibiotics in umbilical artery catheterization in the newborn. *Arch. Dis. Child.* 48:296, 1973.

120. Vidyasagar, D., Downes, J.J., and Boggs, T.R., Jr. Respiratory distress syndrome of newborn infants: II. Technic of catheterization of umbilical artery and clinical results of treatment of 124 patients. *Clin. Pediatr.* 9:332, 1970.

121. Wargo, E.J. Microbial contamination of topical ointments. *Am. J. Hosp. Pharm.* 30:332, 1973.

122. Wasserman, R.L. Intravenous gamma globulin prophylaxis for newborn infants. *Pediatr. Infect. Dis.* 5:620, 1986.

123. Weathers, L., Riggs, D., Santeiro, M., and Weibley, R.E. Aerosolized vancomycin for treatment of airway colonization by methicillin-resistant *Staphylococcus aureus*. *Pediatr. Infect. Dis. J.* 9:220, 1990.

124. Weese-Mayer, D.E., Fondriest, D.W., Brouil-

lette, R.T., and Shulman, S.T. Risk factors associated with candidemia in the neonatal intensive care unit: A case-control study. *Pediatr. Infect. Dis. J.* 6:190, 1987.

125. Welliver, R.C., and McLaughlin, S. Unique epidemiology of nosocomial infection in a children's hospital. *Am. J. Dis. Child.* 138:131, 1984.

126. Williams, W.W. Guidelines for infection control in hospital personnel. *Infect. Control* 4: 326, 1983.

127. Xu, Z.-Y., et al. Prevention of perinatal acquisition of hepatitis B virus carriage using vaccine: Preliminary report of a randomized, double-blind placebo-controlled and comparative trial. *Pediatrics* 76:713, 1985.

128. Zedd, A.J., et al. Nosocomial *Clostridium difficile* reservoir in a neonatal intensive care unit. *Pediatr. Infect. Dis.* 3:429, 1984.

The Operating Room

Ronald Lee Nichols

Despite the high standards set for professional performance and equipment, the controlled environment of the operating room remains potentially hostile to both the patient and the surgical team [43]. In the past, authoritative bodies have placed major emphasis on improving the operating room environment in an attempt to reduce the number of infectious complications that followed surgical procedures [20]. The national groups that have spearheaded this challenge over the past three decades include the Committee on Operating Room Environment (CORE) of the American College of Surgeons, the Association of Operating Room Nurses (AORN), the Centers for Disease Control (CDC), the American Hospital Association and the Medical Research Council of Great Britain. Many individuals from different disciplines have contributed valuable insights, but the names of William Altemeier, William Beck, Harvey Bernard, John Burke, Robert Condon, Harold Laufman, Paul Nora, and Carl Walter stand out. The reduction in postoperative wound infections, in two widely quoted national studies, reported in 1964 [1] and in 1985 [24], appears, in part, to be due to these efforts. The more recent study estimates that wound infections accounted for approximately 24 percent of the total number of nosocomial infections, which represented nearly 500,000 wound infections per year or 2.8 per 100 operations performed [24].

Many biologic, physical (electrical, radiation, laser, and new medical devices), and chemical (anesthetics and sterilization techniques) hazards are present in the modern operating room. These hazards need to be monitored, reviewed, and updated continually. Information gained from these reviews needs to be taught to all operating room personnel to provide a safe work environment

[43]. The scope of this chapter will concentrate on the biologic hazards, with consideration given to the patient as host and also as vector. The reader is referred to Chapter 33 for additional considerations of infections in surgical patients.

The Patient as a Risk for Infection

Until the late 1980s, most infection control officers, operating room nurses, and surgeons believed that the type of operative procedure to be accomplished was the most critical factor in predicting the postoperative wound infection rate [55].

Classification of Surgical Wounds

The widely accepted classification of operative procedures is as follows:

Clean wounds are uninfected operative wounds in which no inflammation is encountered and the respiratory, alimentary, genital, and uninfected urinary tracts are not entered.

Clean-contaminated wounds are operative wounds in which the respiratory, alimentary, genital, or urinary tract is entered under controlled conditions and without unusual contamination.

Contaminated wounds include open, fresh, accidental wounds, operations with major breaks in sterile technique or gross spillage from the gastrointestinal tract, and incisions in which acute, nonpurulent inflammation is encountered.

Dirty or infected wounds include old traumatic wounds with retained devitalized tissue and those that involve existing clinical infection or perforated viscera.

The wound infection in clean operations is usually due to exogenous microorganisms such as *Staphylococcus aureus,* whereas the usual etiologic agent or agents in the other categories of surgery generally originate from the polymicrobial aerobic-anaerobic endogenous flora. The often quoted infection rates for the different types of operative procedures are as follows: clean, 1 to 5 percent;

clean-contaminated, 3 to 11 percent; contaminated, 10 to 17 percent; and dirty, more than 27 percent [19].

General Aspects of Risk in the Surgical Patient

Recently, the emphasis concerning the risk factors for development of postoperative infections has shifted somewhat from the type of surgical procedure to the patients themselves. Haley and colleagues [23] were the first to publish a report on the importance of identifying the individual patients who are at high risk of surgical wound infection in each category of operative procedure. To predict the likelihood of surgical wound infection from several risk factors, the authors used information collected on 58,498 patients undergoing operations in 1970 and developed a simple multivariate risk index. Analyzing 10 possible risk factors by stepwise multiple logistic regression techniques, they developed a model containing four risk factors: (1) abdominal operation, (2) operation lasting longer than 2 hours, (3) contaminated or dirty infected operation by traditional wound classification system, and (4) patient having three or more different diagnoses. They utilized the resultant formula to predict an individual patient's probability of developing a postoperative wound infection. This approach was then tested on another group of 59,352 surgical patients admitted in 1975–1976 and was found to be a valid predictor of surgical wound infection. The authors concluded that their simplified index predicts surgical wound infection risk nearly twice as well as the traditional classification of wound contamination. Utilizing this model, low-, medium-, and high-risk levels of developing wound infection were identified in the categories of the traditional wound classification. The overall wound infection rate in this study did progressively increase from clean (2.9 percent), to clean-contaminated (3.9 percent), to contaminated (8.5 percent), to dirty-infected (12.6 percent). The decrease noted in wound infection rates in contaminated and dirty-infected procedures from previous reports may relate to improved surgical techniques and a more common use of proved preventive practices utilized during the last two decades. However, there was noted to be a wide range of infection risk among patients in each category: In clean operations, the level of risk ranged from 1.1 percent in the low-risk category to 15.8 percent in the high-risk group; in clean-contaminated operations, 0.6 percent were low-risk and 17.7 percent were considered high-risk; in contaminated operations, 4.5 percent classified as medium-risk and 23.9 percent were high-risk; and in dirty-infected operations, 6.7 percent were medium-risk and 27.4 percent were high-risk. It should be noted that no low-risk category of patients was identified in contaminated and dirty-infected operations.

Investigators from the CDC have recently reported on a composite risk index [11]. The new risk index uses the traditional wound class but attempts to improve on the previous index in several ways. First, instead of the three discharge diagnoses to identify host factors as a risk for infection, the new risk index uses a dichotomization of the American Society of Anesthesiologists (ASA) score [32]. Its ease for collecting and its objectivity seem advantageous. Second, this risk index uses a procedure-related cutoff point to indicate a long duration of surgery for an individual procedure, rather than a 2-hour cutoff point for all procedures. For some procedures (e.g., cesarean section) the cutoff point is one hour; for other procedures (e.g., coronary artery bypass graft operation), the cutoff point is 5 hours. This procedure-related duration-of-surgery cutoff provides the index with additional discriminating power for specific procedures.

The widespread use of risk indexes such as the ones developed by the CDC investigators will be needed in the future. Hospitals will use the risk indexes to compare wound infection rates by risk category, either for all operations or for a specific procedure. The risk indexes can provide a general guide to potential problem areas for investigation that may need further examination with procedure-specific risk factor information. The risk indexes will also help infection control programs prospectively target their surveillance and control efforts among high-risk surgical patients. (See Chapter 33 for further detail.)

Operating Room Design and Environment

More than 30 years ago, Walter and Kundsin [68] described the bacteriology of various hospital floors, including the operating room, and emphasized the relationship between the bacterial count on the floor and the airborne bacterial count. The authors recommended a standard method to attain a hygienic floor in order to make an impact on the incidence of hospital-acquired infection. Since that time, many reviews have outlined approaches that can reduce the bacterial burden within the operating room environment [19, 36]. It is believed that most surgical wound infections have their origin from the bacteria that enter the operative wound at the time of operation. The causative microorganisms originate from the patient's endogenous microflora, from the operating room environment, or from bacteria shed by the operating room team. Rarely, hematogenous bacterial spread from a site of remote infection occurs during the postoperative course, resulting in wound infection. The previous sections of this chapter have dealt with the individual patient risk factors for infection; the remainder will emphasize the operating room environment and personnel. A postoperative wound infection rate of zero in clean operative procedures appears to be an impossible goal even if rather dramatic techniques are employed. These techniques, primarily studied in orthopedic implant surgery, include excluding the surgeon and team from the operating room environment, sealing the surrounding skin of the patient's operative site, and providing sterile operating room air [72].

Specific Microorganisms Implicated in Operating Room Infections

The microorganisms that are usually isolated from the operating room environment are the so-called ubiquitous nonpathogens or commensals which, in most patients, will not result in postoperative wound infection. This statement does not apply to patients undergoing implant surgery, where these low-virulence microorganisms have been shown to be commonly implicated in postoperative deep and superficial infection [54]. *S. aureus* is a major pathogen related to the skin of the patient or operative team that is frequently implicated in postoperative wound infection.

Staphylococcus epidermidis and other coagulase-negative staphylococci are commonly reported pathogens in implant surgery [33, 54]. These microorganisms can be highly antibiotic-resistant and frequently are associated with mucin production (slime), which acts as a virulence factor allowing for persistence of graft or implant infections [17, 33].

A single outbreak of postoperative infection, including septicemia or mediastinitis and multiorgan failure, has recently been reported, due to multiply β-lactam-resistant *Enterobacter cloacae* in 5 patients undergoing cardiovascular surgery. This same strain was also found in the environmental flora of the cardiovascular operating suite and in a sink reservoir in the surgery department [2]. The authors concluded that the liberal use of cephalosporins, an abundant and constant reservoir of various gram-negative bacteria within the operating room suite, and unsatisfactory infection control procedures had lead to this dilemma. It should be stressed that the usual origin of gram-negative bacterial outbreaks is the intensive care units.

Single-source outbreaks of wound or deep sternal infections due to rarely implicated pathogens have recently been reported following open-heart surgery for coronary revascularization [30, 59]. In one study, *Candida tropicalis* was isolated from sternal wounds in 8 patients during a 2-month period [30]. Environmental surveillance revealed that one scrub nurse harbored the causative microorganism on the fingertips and in the nasopharynx. The removal of the suspect nurse from the cardiac team was noted to be associated with the termination of this cluster outbreak. In another single-source outbreak following open-heart surgery over a 7-month period, 7 patients developed a sternal wound infection due to *Rhodococcus bronchialis* [59]. Environmental surveillance in this outbreak revealed that one circulating nurse was common to all open-heart procedures that resulted in infection and that this individual harbored *R. bronchialis* in her nose, throat, vagina, and fingers. Further investigation resulted in the culturing of this microorganism from the fur of a household pet. The spread to the patients was hypothesized to occur from the nurse's colonized hands by either droplet spread or extrinsically contaminated instruments. Since exclusion of this nurse from open-heart surgery, no further cases of sternal wound infections due to *R. bronchialis* have occurred.

Wound infection outbreaks due to rapidly growing mycobacteria have also been reviewed following cardiac surgery [64] and augmentation mammoplasty [65]. The suggested reservoirs for these outbreaks appear to implicate the surgical environment, including the air and water. These microorganisms are the most common mycobacteria recovered from hospital dust and are known to survive in both soil and water.

Uncommon Vectors for Transmission of Infection

The usual vectors for wound infection that originate within the operating room are the patient followed by the operating room environment and personnel. Wound infection may also be transmitted by some unusual vectors, which will be discussed here. The role that anesthesia technique and equipment play in the development of postoperative respiratory infections is beyond the scope of this chapter [67]. Rarely, septicemia may result from the administration of contaminated intravenous solutions [16]. Central venous catheters placed before surgery in the operating room environment after appropriate skin cleaning and preparation rarely result in bacteremia, although the use of an attachable silver-impregnated catheter cuff may further prevent the development of these infections [45]. Suction devices used to remove blood from the operative field have been shown experimentally to have a higher degree of contamination when aspirated with operating room air [56]. This appears to correlate with a high positive suction tip culture rate when suction is utilized clinically with conventional operating room ventilation [63]. This finding caused the authors to recommend that suction tubes be turned off when not in use and that the tubes be changed during total hip arthroplasty.

Invasive hemodynamic monitoring in a large study of patients undergoing open-heart surgery has shown differing degrees of positive catheter tips following the use of central venous, intravenous, arterial and pulmonary artery catheters [12]. However, the authors observed that no patient developed catheter-related septicemia or endocarditis following the invasive hemodynamic monitoring.

Operating Suite Design

It appears that in most operative procedures the patient and personnel are the chief problem in the control of wound infections. Nevertheless, architectural design concepts have evolved that play a role in the control of surgical infection in modern operating suites. Laufman [36] has previously reviewed the key features of design. These include the isolation of the surgical suite from the mainstream of common corridor traffic and the development of the "clean central core," which serves as the supply center and supposedly offers the cleanest environment. The inner corridors that surround the clean core are designed for use by clean traffic, which includes the preoperative patient, nurses, and surgeons. The peripheral corridors are designated for traffic that includes the postoperative patient as well as surgeons and nurses after operating or between cases. Infected patients should be transferred before and after operation through the peripheral corridors. Floors in the operating room should be nonporous and other surfaces should be as dirt-resistant as possible. The use of tacky or antiseptic mats at the entrance of the operating room is contraindicated [19].

The optimal size for most routine oper-

ating rooms is 20×20 ft with 10 ft ceilings, which allows for easy gowning, draping, circulation of personnel, and the use of equipment without the risk of contact contamination. The door of each operating room should be kept closed except for passage of equipment, personnel, and the patient. The number of personnel allowed to enter each operating room should be kept to an absolute minimum, since the origin of infecting bacteria can sometimes be traced to shedding that occurs during movement of staff within the operating room. Intraoperative surveillance of the number of people in attendance, excessive conversation, number of times the doors are opened, and the pattern of use of antibiotic prophylaxis has led to improvements regarding these factors, which was associated with a decreased postoperative infection rate in implant surgery [8].

Infection Control in the Operating Room Environment

Some of the basic operating room design aspects that appear to help in the control of infection have already been reviewed. Other important considerations are operating room cleansing, ventilation, and the use of ultraviolet light.

Operating Room Cleansing

The operating room environment in the early morning before people have entered is nearly sterile. Wet mopping of the hard-surfaced floors with a phenolic solution between each case and wet vacuuming of the rooms and corridors at night succeeds in keeping the floors clean [36].

The practice of closing for 48 hours a room in which a "dirty" case has been treated is no longer considered necessary [36]. Appropriate cleanup techniques in these cases consist of wet mopping or flooding with a phenolic detergent followed by a wipe-down of all equipment surfaces with 70% alcohol. All rubber and plastic tubing in the room should be replaced, but cleansing of the walls should be done only if direct contamination has occurred. All instruments, linen, and waste should be bagged carefully in these cases, and the gowns, masks, and shoe covers used in the procedure must be left in the room in appropriate containers.

Sterilization of Instruments and Devices

Steam sterilization of manually cleaned instruments remains the technique of choice since the reliable control of this technique was established more than 50 years ago [66]. When performed with the correct temperature and pressure, sterilization is accomplished by the least expensive and time-consuming method. A discussion of the three major types of steam sterilizers—the gravity sterilizer, the high speed (prevacuum) sterilizer, and the table-top sterilizer—is beyond the scope of this chapter (see Chap. 15). Increasing the temperature in a gravity sterilizer allows for faster sterilization, which is done on unwrapped instruments or other equipment (flash sterilization). This technique should be employed only in emergency situations and is not recommended by most national organizations [10].

Ethylene oxide sterilization is a technique that is more complex and expensive and can be hazardous if not handled cautiously [10, 43]. This type of gas sterilization is performed only on clean and dry items and is to be used only as recommended by the manufacturer of heat-sensitive items.

These sterilization processes are reviewed further in Chapter 15 and elsewhere [53].

Operating Room Ventilation Systems

More than 120 years ago, Joseph Lister attempted to prevent "a floating germ" from entering during an operation by using a fine spray of dilute carbolic acid [42]. He believed that this spray would reduce the incidence of postsurgical wound infections by killing the "germs" in the air as well as on the patient's surface drapes and on the surgeon's and assistant's clothing. It appears that Lister at no time considered the use of ventilation for this purpose, and he wrote in 1890, "It seems to follow logically that the floating particles of the air may be disregarded in our surgical

work" [41]. Others earlier in the same century, however, had proposed a method of ventilation to remove from the air of the hospital "pus and matters like pus floating in the air, minute hairs, epidermic scales and also living forms" [39]. Until the 1930s, the only ventilation installed in operating rooms was for the purpose of removing the steam produced by the sterilizers used for instrument cleansing. At this time, spurred by the inability to control the spread of respiratory diseases and childhood fevers, the possible role of airborne transmission of disease became a matter for discussion and evoked scientific interest [70]. Additionally, the persistence of postoperative wound infection, despite the application of aseptic practices, resulted in Meleney's proposal [48] that possibly organisms from the air of the operating room might play a role in their genesis. In England during the 1940s, further insights were gained when sensitive methods for the detection of airborne bacteria were developed. These techniques helped to establish that the activities of the operating room staff were the principal source for these bacteria and that the practice of extract ventilation resulted in the introduction of bacteria from the hospital corridors and wards into the operating room [39]. These advances were largely responsible for the development of the modern practice of a positive-pressure air supply for the operating room. Debate, dispute, and interest concerning the importance of airborne bacteria to postoperative wound infection, discussed first before the time of Lister, continues to the present day.

The modern conventional operating room is virtually free of bacteria or particles larger than 0.5 μm when there are no people in attendance. The source of airborne bacteria within such an operating room is largely the skin of the people present in the room, whereas the quantitative counts depend greatly on the number of people present, their level of activity, and their discipline, knowledge, and application of infection control practices. An excellent review on the subject of aerobiology in the operating room has recently been published by Hambraeus [25]. Despite our present knowledge, the safe level of airborne operating room environmental contamination for different surgical procedures has yet to be determined.

Today, most conventional operating rooms in America are ventilated with 20 to 25 changes per hour of high-efficiency filtered air delivered in a unidirectional vertical flow. High-efficiency particulate air (HEPA) filtration systems are generally utilized, which remove most bacteria that measure 0.5 to 5.0 μm. Therefore, the first air downstream from the HEPA filter is virtually bacteria-free. Bacteria released within the operating room environment remain unaffected by the filter system. At least 20 percent of the air changes per hour should be with fresh air [19]. The air delivered should be at temperatures between 18° and 24°C (65° and 75°F) and with 50 to 55 percent humidity. Inlets should be located as high above the floor as possible and remote from the active exhaust outlets, which are located low on the walls. This arrangement allows for the unidirectionality of the ventilation system. The operating room also should be under positive pressure relative to the surrounding corridors, which minimizes the flow of air into the operating rooms when the doors are opened. Careful maintenance of the ventilation system just described offers an environment that is virtually as clean as more costly special chambers unless personnel abuses occur [36]. The use of this type of air-handling system is clearly indicated for most clean surgical procedures and for all procedures in which the patient's endogenous microflora is released during the surgical procedure. The debate continues as to whether additional highly specialized ventilation systems are advantageous when major implant surgery is to be undertaken (see Chap. 36).

The more costly specialized ventilation systems generally are referred to as *laminar flow* and comprise many types of unidirectional air-blowing systems including those of ceiling or wall diffusers and "curtain-effect" varieties [36]. The laminar flow can be delivered in a horizontal or vertical direction, and each system has its own proponents. The principal characteristic of such a system is the delivery of air at a uniform velocity (0.5 m/sec) over the whole of one wall (horizontal) or, in the case of a vertical system, from the ceiling down, at a sufficient velocity to prevent any retrograde air movements [39]. These systems also utilize HEPA filtration to deliver air free of particles down to 0.3 μm. The first system was devised by Whitfield in 1960 and tested by surgeons soon after [71]. Charnley [9] in 1964 reported on a prototype filtered-air enclosure that was constructed to contain the lower half of the patient's body and 3 surgeons of the operating team. In this system, the filtered air was forced in at the top of the enclosure and the surgeons within the enclosure wore "space suits" with respirators through which their exhaled air was extracted to prevent its mixing with the filtered air of the enclosure. The author reported preliminary results that included a reduction of airborne bacteria within the enclosure, as compared to outside it, and a reduction of wound infections following hip replacement from 9.5 percent to 1.1 percent when the conventional air-handling system was compared to the enclosure system. However, most of the patients did not receive prophylactic systemic antibiotics because of the author's belief that this practice was not effective and may result in increased postoperative infections [39]. In the next decade, many orthopedic surgeons performing thousands of hip replacement operations in conventional operating rooms without laminar flow chambers reported a combined 2-year infection rate of 0.45 percent [35].

In 1982, the results of a multicenter study of infection after total hip or knee replacement in more than 8,000 patients, enrolled from 1974 to 1979, was reported by Lidwell and colleagues [40]. In patients whose implants were inserted in an operating room ventilated by an ultraclean air (laminar flow) system, the incidence of joint infection confirmed at reoperation within a 1- to 4-year period was approximately half (23 infections among 3,922 patients [0.6 percent]) of that observed in those patients whose operation was undertaken in a conventionally ventilated room at the same hospital (63 infections among 4,133 patients [1.5 percent]). In those cases in the ultraclean group for which the surgeons wore whole-body exhaust-ventilated suits, the infection rate was noted to be approximately one-fourth of that found in the cases performed under conventional ventilation. However, the design of the study did not include a strictly controlled test of the effect of prophylactic antibiotics. Their use was associated with a lower incidence of sepsis (34 infections among 5,831 patients [0.6 percent]) when compared to patients undergoing operation without antibiotic prophylaxis (52 infections among 2,221 patients [2.3 percent]).

The results of recent randomized studies of arthroplasty have confirmed that a considerable reduction of sepsis can be obtained by operating in ultraclean air but that similarly low rates of infections can be achieved with normal conventional ventilation when prophylactic antibiotics are routinely given [28, 39]. The question that remains is whether a combination of ultraclean air and prophylactic antibiotics can be shown in a prospective controlled study to offer a significant reduction in infection when compared to the use of either of these preventive measures alone. A recently published review of special clean air, ultraclean air, and partial barrier systems is recommended for those interested in this subject [38].

Use of Ultraviolet Light

The bactericidal effect of ultraviolet (UV) light has long been established [38]. In a large, well-publicized, prospective, randomized study reported in 1964, it was shown that UV irradiation reduced the number of recoverable viable organisms within the operating room by more than 50 percent [1]. Yet, the wound infection rates observed in the same study showed no significant differences between the control operations and those done in the presence of UV irradiation. Another study reported on the value of the use of UF irradiation in preventing infection in refined

clean operations at the Duke University Medical Center [27]. When utilized, the personnel and patients must be protected from the UV irradiation by the wearing of appropriate hoods, masks, and goggles. This approach for the prevention of operating room contamination, although employed by some hospitals, has not recently been the subject of active scientific investigation.

Scheduling of Operations

Practices aimed at scheduling "dirty" operations at the end of the day or in a specific operating room (septic room) should be discouraged [19, 36]. In the modern, well-managed operating suite, the chance of environmentally spread infection remains remote. This is primarily due to the high degree of efficiency in sterilizing instruments and surgical devices, efficient ventilation systems that provide clean air, and the adequacy of the techniques of operating room cleansing between cases.

Maintenance of Surveillance Records

At the present time, it is recommended that all operations be classified and recorded as clean, clean-contaminated, contaminated, or dirty at the time of operation or shortly after [19]. Surgeon-specific, procedure-specific infection rates should be computed periodically and made available to the Infection Control Committee, the department of surgery, and the individual surgeon so that interventions can be designed if apparent increased wound infection rates are reported. All observed increases of the wound infection rates should result in the initiation of appropriate epidemiologic studies to identify possible sources for this occurrence. The hospital committee that is responsible for these functions should be designated by hospital administration.

Operating Room Personnel

The importance of the conduct, personal integrity, and work ethics of operating room personnel to both the level of bacteria within the operating room and to outbreaks of wound infection has already been addressed. To understand the possible significance of the staff's actions, it is necessary to have an ongoing infection control educational and surveillance program that involves all levels of operating room employees (see Chaps. 3, 5). Routine nasopharyngeal cultures of personnel who work in the operating room have been shown not to be necessary [36]. However, the practice of culturing personnel in the presence of an outbreak as part of the epidemiologic investigation should be carried out and is often rewarding. It is important to remember that the presence of a disseminating carrier employee, conventionally masked, gowned, and shod, in any part of the operating room is a hazard to the patient [14, 69].

Surgical Gowns and Related Garb

The primary purpose of wearing a gown around the operating table is to provide a barrier to contamination that may pass from personnel to patient as well as from patient to personnel. Bernard and Beck [5] stressed in 1975 that barrier products could not be properly evaluated unless adequate tests demonstrating consistent efficacy could be established. Laufman and co-workers [37] demonstrated that the bacterial penetration of a given material used in gowns and drapes is relative, depending largely on the degree of stress placed on it, and that the materials used in surgical barriers vary greatly under the same stress. Impermeability to moisture is, of course, a basic necessity of any barrier material because the wicking effect tends to transmit bacteria.

From the late nineteenth century until the 1950s, the standard surgical gown was reusable and constructed of 140-count cotton muslin. Beck and Collette [4] questioned the suitability of this fabric in 1952 when their experiments demonstrated bacterial passage through wet, but not dry, cotton cloth. Bernard and colleagues [6] showed a reduction of bacterial transmission through gowns when a tighter weave of cotton fabric was utilized, whereas Moylan and colleagues [50] later demonstrated that reusable cloth gowns,

even in the dry state, were ineffective bacterial barriers. Still later clinical studies by these investigators showed a significantly reduced postoperative wound infection rate when disposable spun-bonded olefin gowns and drapes were compared to either 140- or 280-thread-count cloth reusables [52]. A similar result was also reported when spun-lace disposable gowns and drapes were compared to 280-thread-count reusables [51]. We have recently tested experimentally the strike-through of blood in 11 types of commonly used disposable and reusable surgical gowns [61]. We have observed that new cloth gowns are more resistant to strike-through than those washed forty times and that spun-bond disposable fabrics are more protective than spun lace. Most reinforced (double-layer) disposables are less vulnerable to the strike-through of blood than a single layer of the same material, and all gowns with a layer of plastic placed between the two layers (impervious) were resistant to blood strike-through. Further clinical and experimental testing, with the establishment of standards, is necessary to better define the efficacy of these barrier products. The emphasis today in regards to barrier efficiency mandates that health care workers be protected from skin contamination with their patient's blood. The materials chosen for these products should be based largely on the level of protection from blood strike-through needed in each operative procedure as well as comfort of the product. Gowns constructed with a complete plastic impervious middle layer would prevent blood strike-through but would be intolerable to wear except in the shortest operative procedures.

Various types of hoods, rather than caps, are being utilized today to cover the hair, which attracts and sheds bacterial particles. The type chosen by each operating room worker should largely be based on the amount and distribution of their scalp and facial hair. As mentioned previously, some authorities recommend the use of ventilated space suits and helmets to isolate the surgeons and assistants completely from their patients' environment during ultraclean implant surgical procedures. Closing of the trouser opening of the surgical scrubs with Velcro tape at ankle level has been shown to reduce the aerial dissemination of skin bacteria [7]. A similar reduction of airborne bacteria did not follow Velcro closure techniques applied to the surgeon's arms or neck. The wearing of disposable shoe covers by operating room personnel, although generally recommended, has not been proved effective as an infection control measure [19, 26].

The Surgical Scrub and Preoperative Skin Preparation

The surgeon and assistants who will touch the sterile surgical field or instruments are required to scrub their hands and forearms in a systematic fashion with an antimicrobial preparation prior to each operative procedure [19]. The duration of this ritual, as late as the 1960s, was 10 minutes, with a stiff brush being used to provide the friction. This technique was abandoned when it was found that bacteria from the deep dermal layers were being isolated at the surface. Today, the usual first daily surgical scrub of at least 5 minutes' duration is accomplished with a sponge impregnated with an antimicrobial-containing preparation [19]. Although the ideal duration of the scrub is not known, times as short as 5 minutes appear safe [13, 18]. Between consecutive operations, the surgical scrub can be as short as 2 to 5 minutes. The cleansing material may be a soap or detergent containing an iodophor, hexachlorophene, or another accepted nonirritating antimicrobial preparation that significantly reduces the number of microorganisms on the intact skin [34]. Appropriate products have been listed in categories, for choice by the hospitals, by the U.S. Food and Drug Administration [73].

Preoperative patient skin preparation is initiated just prior to the time of operative incision by the limited removal of operative site hair by shaving or clipping. This is followed by the systematic washing of the operative site and surrounding areas with similar products as are used in the surgical scrub. The wash is followed by the application of an antimicrobial preparation, working from the center of the planned operative incision to the periphery [19]. Larson [34] has reviewed the agents to be considered for antimicrobial skin preparation. After the patient's skin preparation has been completed, appropriate sterile skin draping is carried out to protect the clean field from the unprepared parts of the patient. The use of plastic impregnated drapes should not be routine, but they can be used in specific cases where isolation of an area from the operative incision is indicated (e.g., ileostomy site).

Surgical Gloves

The surgical team members, after scrubbing, should dry their hands with sterile towels and then don sterile gowns and sterile gloves. If the glove is punctured during operation, it should be promptly changed as dictated by patient safety [29]. Some have recommended double gloving as a routine to lessen the chance of microbial contamination during total joint arthroplasty [46]. Other studies have shown that more than 12 percent of gloves were perforated during surgery and that this occurred in more than 30 percent of operations [15]. Beck [3] has stressed that traditionally gloves have been worn to protect the patient, but today, with the present fear of the transmission of bloodborne disease to the health care worker, there exists an increased level of interest concerning the efficacy of various gloves. He recommends that in the near future industry develop stronger gloves that are resistant to puncture and that, until this occurs, gloves should be changed after each hour of operative time.

Surgical Masks

Everyone who enters the operating room during an operation is required to wear a high-efficiency mask to cover the mouth and nose area fully [19]. If the mask becomes soiled or wet during the procedure, it should be changed. Orr [57] has argued that the efficacy of preventing wound infection with surgical masks has not been established but that their efficiency in reducing bacterial contamination has. He noted no increase in wound infection rate in one operating room where no masks were worn during a 6-month period and concludes "that the wearing of a mask has very little relevance to the well-being of patients undergoing routine general surgery and it is a standard practice that could be abandoned" [57].

Protecting Operating Room Personnel: The Patient as Vector

A great deal of emphasis is currently being placed on protecting the hospital employee from acquiring infectious diseases from an actively infected patient or carrier. The potential for exposure to bloodborne diseases such as human immunodeficiency virus (HIV) and hepatitis B virus (HBV) is high in the operating room. Since operative misadventures such as inadvertent needle stick, sharp injuries, and blood splashes to skin or mucous membranes do occur with regularity to the operative team, it has become popular to predict the probability of occupationally acquiring HIV infection during one's surgical career [29, 44, 47]. This predicted risk of acquiring infection with HIV from operative encounters appears to be primarily related to the amount of time spent in the operating room, type of operations performed, and the local seroprevalence of the patient population. The great differences in seroprevalence of HIV infection in 21 urban populations has been stressed [62]. Thirty-year career risks of HIV seroconversion, due to occupational exposure for surgeons, appear to be as high as 10 percent if the surgeon is actively involved in "bloody" cases in a locality that has a high seroprevalence rate [44, 47].

A recent observational study of more than 1,300 consecutive surgical procedures at San Francisco General Hospital has shown that accidental exposure to the patient's blood occurred in 84 procedures [21]. Parenteral exposure occurred in 1.7 percent of cases, whereas cutaneous exposure was noted in the remainder. The risk of exposure was highest in procedures that lasted more than 3 hours,

when the blood loss exceeded 300 ml, and when major vascular or intraabdominal gynecologic surgery was involved. The authors concluded that surgical personnel are at risk for intraoperative exposure to blood and that preoperative testing for HIV infection did not reduce the frequency of accidental exposure to blood. Universal precautions, which include the limited and careful use of sharps, routine double gloving, use of face shields or glasses with lateral extensions, and the wearing of barrier gowns that prevent blood strikethrough, appear to offer the best protection against accidental exposures to blood that may translate to seroconversion [21, 31, 60, 61].

The role that the HIV-infected surgeon or operating room employee plays in patient seroconversion and whether steps should be taken to curtail the activity of such health care providers remains to be determined [22, 49, 58]. The reader is referred to Chapters 33 and 39 for additional considerations related to HIV infections.

References

1. Ad Hoc Committee of the Committee on Trauma, Division of Medical Sciences, National Academy of Sciences—National Research Council. Factors influencing the incidence of wound infection. *Ann. Surg.* 160 (Suppl): 32, 1964.
2. Andersen, B.M., et al. Multiply beta-lactam resistant *Enterobacter cloacae* infections linked to the environmental flora in a unit for cardiothoracic and vascular surgery. *Scand. J. Infect. Dis.* 21:181, 1989.
3. Beck, W.C. The hole in the surgical glove: A change in attitude. *Bull. Am. Coll. Surg.* 74:15, 1989.
4. Beck, W.C., and Collette, T.S. False faith in the surgeon's gown and surgical drape. *Am. J. Surg.* 83(2):125, 1952.
5. Bernard, H.R., and Beck, W.C. Operating room barriers—idealism, practicality, and the future. *Bull. Am. Coll. Surg.* 60:16, 1975.
6. Bernard, H.R., et al. Reduction of dissemination of skin bacteria by modification of operating-room clothing and by ultraviolet irradiation. *Lancet* 2:458–461, 1965.
7. Blowers, R., and McCluskey, M. Design of

operating-room dress for surgeons. *Lancet* 2: 681, 1965.

8. Borst, M., Collier, C., and Miller, D. Operating room surveillance: A new approach in reducing hip and knee prosthetic wound infections. *Am. J. Infect. Control* 14:161, 1986.

9. Charnley, J. A clean-air operating enclosure. *Br. J. Surg.* 51:202, 1964.

10. Crow, S. *Asepsis, The Right Touch: Something Old Is Now New.* Bossier City, LA: Everett Publishers, 1989.

11. Culver, D.H., et al. Surgical wound infection rates by wound class, operation, and risk index in U.S. hospitals. *Am. J. Med.* 91 (Suppl. 3B): 152, 1991.

12. Damen, J., et al. Microbiologic risk of invasive hemodynamic monitoring in patients undergoing open-heart operations. *Crit. Care Med.* 13:548, 1985.

13. Dineen, P. An evaluation of the duration of the surgical scrub. *Surg. Gynecol. Obstet.* 129: 1181, 1969.

14. Dineen, P., and Drusin, L. Epidemics of postoperative wound infections associated with hair carriers. *Lancet* 2:1157, 1973.

15. Dodds, R.D.A., et al. Surgical glove perforation. *Br. J. Surg.* 75:966, 1988.

16. Duma, R.I., Warner, J.F., and Dalton, H.P. Septicemia from intravenous infusions. *N. Engl. J. Med.* 284:257, 1971.

17. Edmiston, C.E., Jr., Schmitt, D.D., and Seabrook, G.R. Coagulase-negative staphylococcal infections in vascular surgery: Epidemiology and pathogenesis. *Infect. Control Hosp. Epidemiol.* 10:111, 1989.

18. Galle, P.C., Homesley, H.D., and Rhyne, A.L. Reassessment of the surgical scrub. *Surg. Gynecol. Obstet.* 147:215, 1978.

19. Garner, J.S. CDC guidelines for the prevention and control of nosocomial infections: Guideline for prevention of surgical wound infections, 1985. *Am. J. Infect. Control* 14:71, 1986.

20. Garner, J.S., Emori, T.G., and Haley, R.W. Operating room practices for the control of infection in U.S. hospitals, October 1976 to July 1977. *Surg. Gynecol. Obstet.* 155:873, 1982.

21. Gerberding, J.L., et al. Risk of exposure of surgical personnel to patients' blood during surgery at San Francisco General Hospital. *N. Engl. J. Med.* 322:1788, 1990.

22. Gramelspacher, G.P., Miles, S.H., and Cassel, C.K. Aids commentary: When the doctor has AIDS. *J. Infect. Dis.* 162:534, 1990.

23. Haley, R.W., et al. Identifying patients at high risk of surgical wound infection. *Am. J. Epidemiol.* 121:206, 1985.

24. Haley, R.W., et al. The nationwide nosocomial infection rate: A new need for vital statistics. *Am. J. Epidemiol.* 121:159, 1985.

25. Hambraeus, A. Aerobiology in the operating room—a review. *J. Hosp. Infect.* 11:68, 1988.

26. Hambraeus, A., and Malmborg, A.S. The influence of different footwear on floor contamination. *Scand. J. Infect. Dis.* 11:243, 1979.

27. Hart, D., et al. Postoperative wound infections: A further report on ultraviolet irradiation with comments on the recent (1964) National Research Council Cooperative Study report. *Ann. Surg.* 167:728, 1968.

28. Hill, C., et al. Prophylactic cefazolin versus placebo in total hip replacement. *Lancet* 1: 795, 1981.

29. Howard, R.J. Human immunodeficiency virus testing and the risk to the surgeon of acquiring HIV. *Surg. Gynecol. Obstet.* 171:22, 1990.

30. Isenberg, H.D., et al. Single-source outbreak of *Candida tropicalis* complicating coronary bypass surgery. *J. Clin. Microbiol.* 27:2426, 1989.

31. Jagger, J, Hunt, E.H., and Pearson, R.D. Sharp object injuries in the hospital: Causes and strategies for prevention. *Am. J. Infect. Control* 18:227, 1990.

32. Keats, A.S. The ASA classifications of physical status—a recapitulation. *Anesthesiology* 49: 233, 1978.

33. Large, M., et al. A study of coagulase-negative staphylococci isolated from clinically significant infections at an Australian teaching hospital. *Pathology* 21:19, 1989.

34. Larson, E. APIC guidelines for infection control practice. Guideline for use of topical antimicrobial agents. *Am. J. Infect. Control* 16:253, 1988.

35. Laufman, H. Current status of special air handling systems in operating rooms. *Med. Instrum.* 7:7, 1973.

36. Laufman, H. The Operating Rom. In: J.V. Bennett and P.S. Brachman (Eds.), *Hospital Infections* (2nd ed.). Boston: Little, Brown, 1986. Pp.315–324.

37. Laufman, H., et al. Strike-through of moist contamination by woven and nonwoven surgical materials. *Ann. Surg.* 181:857, 1975.

38. Levenson, S.M., Trexler, P.C., and Van der Waaij, D. Nosocomial infection: Prevention by special clean-air, ultraviolet light, and barrier (isolator) techniques (review). *Curr. Prob. Surg.* 23:453, 1986.

39. Lidwell, O.M. Clean air at operation and subsequent sepsis in the joint. *Clin. Orthop.* 211: 91, 1986.

40. Lidwell, O.M., et al. Effect of ultraclean air in operating rooms on deep sepsis in the joint after total hip or knee replacement: A randomised study. *Br. Med. J.* 285:10, 1982.

41. Lister, J. An address on the present position of antiseptic surgery. *Br. Med. J.* 2:377, 1890.

42. Lister, J. On a case illustrating the present as-

pect of the antiseptic treatment in surgery. *Br. Med. J.* 1:30, 1871.

43. LoCicero, J., III, Quebbeman, E.J., and Nichols, R.L. Health hazards in the operating room: An update. *Bull. Am. Coll. Surg.* 72:4–9, 1987.

44. Lowenfels, A.B., Wormser, G.P., and Jain, R. Frequency of puncture injuries in surgeons and estimated risk of HIV infection. *Arch. Surg.* 124:1284, 1989.

45. Maki, D.G., et al. An attachable silver-impregnated cuff for prevention of infection with central venous catheters: A prospective randomized multicenter trial. *Am. J. Med.* 84:307, 1988.

46. McCue, S.F., Berg, E.W., and Saunders, E.A. Efficacy of double-gloving as a barrier to microbial contamination during total joint arthroplasty. *J. Bone Joint Surg.* 63:811, 1981.

47. McKinney, W.P., and Young, M.J. The cumulative probability of occupationally acquired HIV infection: The risks of repeated exposures during a surgical career. *Infect. Control Hosp. Epidemiol.* 11:243, 1990.

48. Meleney, F.L. The control of wound infections. *Ann. Surg.* 98:151, 1933.

49. Mishu, B., et al. A surgeon with AIDS. Lack of evidence of transmission to patients. *J.A.M.A.* 264:467, 1990.

50. Moylan, J.A., Balish, E., and Chan, J. Intraoperative bacterial transmission. *Surg. Gynecol. Obstet.* 141:731, 1975.

51. Moylan, J.A., Fitzpatrick, K.T., and Davenport, K.E. Reducing wound infections. Improved gown and drape barrier performance. *Arch. Surg.* 122:152, 1987.

52. Moylan, J.A., and Kennedy, B.V. The importance of gown and drape barriers in the prevention of wound infection. *Surg. Gynecol. Obstet.* 151:465, 1980.

53. Muhlmann-Weill, M., et al. Preventive Measures in the Care of Infected Patients: Sterilization of Anesthetic Apparatus. In: A. Mathieu, and J.F. Burke (Eds.), *Infection and the Perioperative Period.* New York: Grune and Stratton, 1982. Pp.91–118.

54. Nade, S. Infection after joint replacement—what would Lister think? *Med. J. Aust.* 152:394, 1990.

55. Nichols, R.L. Postoperative wound infection. *N. Engl. J. Med.* 307:1701, 1982.

56. Oeveren, W.V., et al. Airborne contamination during cardiopulmonary bypass: The role of cardiotomy suction. *Ann. Thorac. Surg.* 41:401, 1986.

57. Orr, N.W.M. Is a mask necessary in the operating theatre? *Ann. R. Coll. Surg. Engl.* 63:390, 1981.

58. Rhame, F.S. The HIV-infected surgeon (editorial.) *J.A.M.A.* 264:507, 1990.

59. Richet, H.M., et al. A cluster of *Rhodococcus (Gordana) bronchialis* sternal-wound infections after coronary-artery bypass surgery. *N. Engl. J. Med.* 324:104, 1991.

60. Risi, G.F., Jr., et al. Human immunodeficiency virus: Risk of exposure among health care workers at a southern urban hospital. *South. Med. J.* 82:1079, 1989.

61. Smith, J.W., and Nichols, R.L. Barrier efficacy of surgical gowns: Are we really protected from our patients' pathogens? *Arch. Surg.* 126:756, 1991.

62. St. Louis, M.E. et al. Seroprevalence rates of human immunodeficiency virus infection at Sentinel Hospitals in the United States. *N. Engl. J. Med.* 323:213, 1990.

63. Strange-Vognsen, H.H., and Klareskov, B. Bacteriologic contamination of suction tips during hip arthroplasty. *Acta Orthop. Scand.* 59:410, 1988.

64. Wallace, R.J., Jr., et al. Diversity and sources of rapidly growing mycobacteria associated with infections following cardiac surgery. *J. Infect. Dis.* 159:708, 1989.

65. Wallace, R.J., Jr. et al. Heterogeneity among isolates of rapidly growing mycobacteria responsible for infections following augmentation mammoplasty despite case clustering in Texas and other southern coastal states. *J. Infect. Dis.* 160:281, 1989.

66. Walter, C.W. A reliable control for steam sterilization. *Surg. Gynecol. Obstet.* 67:526, 1938.

67. Walter, C.W. Vectors of Infection in the Operating Room. In: A. Mathieu and J.F. Burke (Eds.), *Infection and the Perioperative Period.* New York: Grune and Stratton, 1982. Pp. 139–166.

68. Walter, C.W., and Kundsin, R.B. The floor as a reservoir of hospital infections. *Surg. Gynecol. Obstet.* 111:1, 1960.

69. Walter, C.W., Kundsin, R.B., and Brubaker, M.M. The incidence of airborne wound infection during operation. *J.A.M.A.* 186:908, 1963.

70. Wells, W.F., and Wells, M.W. Airborne infection. *J.A.M.A.* 107:1698, 1936.

71. Whitcomb, J.C., et al. Ultraclean operating rooms. *The Lovelace Clinic Review* (Albuquerque, NM) 2:65, 1965.

72. Wiley, A.M. Researches in orthopedic wound infections. *Clin. Orthop.* 208:28, 1986.

73. Zanowiak, P., and Jacobs, M.R. Topical Anti-Infective Products. In: *Handbook of Nonprescription Drugs* (7th ed.). Washington, DC: American Pharmaceutical Association, 1982. Pp.525–542.

Ambulatory Care Settings

Marguerite M. Jackson
Patricia Lynch

The vast majority of physician-patient contacts are in ambulatory care facilities. Approximately 75 percent of the population see a physician in a given year, whereas only 10 percent of the population are hospitalized. Annually, there are nearly four times as many visits to physicians on an ambulatory basis as there are hospital days of care [39].

Because of the millions of patient visits in these settings annually, questions frequently arise about the risk for nosocomial infection and about interventions to reduce these risks. Infection risk associated with care in an ambulatory setting is probably very low, although it has not been studied extensively. The majority of patients seen in these settings present with nonurgent problems and are not admitted to hospitals. A substantial proportion of the infections seen in ambulatory care settings are viral respiratory infections and probably carry with them risks of transmission similar to the risks of transmission in the community.

Nosocomial infection risk increases with the number of devices or procedures to which the patient is exposed. Except for emergent and some urgent visits to hospital emergency departments, few ambulatory care patients are exposed to invasive devices or procedures that are known to pose significant infection risk. In addition, the duration of the patient's visit to the facility is usually limited, which is also a factor in reduced risk for nosocomial infection.

This chapter discusses the various types of ambulatory care settings (ACSs), general infection risks associated with these settings, and interventions known or suspected to reduce infection risks for patients seen there.

Ambulatory Care Settings

Ambulatory care may be delivered in various settings, ranging from a single physician's private office to a comprehensive emergency medical services system. The most common types of ACSs are described here.

Emergency Medical Services System

The emergency medical services system (EMSS) was developed partly in response to results from a National Academy of Sciences study of accidental death and disability, conducted in the early 1960s [50]. The Federal EMSS Act, enacted in 1973, outlined 15 separate components, defined 7 patient categories (trauma, burns, spinal cord injuries, poisoning, cardiac, neonatal, behavioral), and provided for a national EMSS framework. At the same time, communities increased emphasis on the timely delivery of care to patients with serious injuries, beginning before arrival at the hospital [60].

Prehospital Care

Prehospital care incorporates all emergency rescue, medical, and transportation services provided to ill or injured patients before they reach the hospital. The functional unit of prehospital care includes the hospital-based emergency department, personnel there who advise the field team, the field team for emergency transport, and the transport vehicle. In addition, some systems incorporate fire department personnel, community-based services, and volunteers.

Emergency Department of a Hospital

The emergency department of a hospital may provide three major services: (1) care of critically ill or injured patients, most of whom are subsequently admitted to the facility; (2) offices where physicians can examine their own patients (e.g., after office hours or when more sophisticated care is necessary than a physician's office can provide); (3) care for persons who are not critically injured or ill but who do not use any other organized ambulatory service or physician's office. Patients

in the latter two categories usually are not admitted to the hospital.

Weinerman and colleagues [75] define three categories used by *providers* to describe requirements for emergency care:

1. *Nonurgent.* Care does not require resources of an emergency service; referral for routine medical care may or may not be needed; disorder is nonacute or minor in severity. Few of these patients require hospital admission.
2. *Urgent.* Condition requires medical attention within the period of a few hours; there is possible danger to the patient if medically unattended; disorder is acute but not necessarily severe. Some of these patients will require hospital admission.
3. *Emergent.* Condition requires immediate medical attention; time delay is harmful to the patient; disorder is acute and possibly threatening to life or function. Many of these patients will require hospital admission and may require intensive care management.

Jonas and colleagues [38] studied 678 patient visits in the summer of 1970 to the emergency department of a 331-bed hospital in New York City. The average distribution by category among patients seen in the emergency department was approximately 53 percent nonurgent, 37 percent urgent, and 5 percent emergent. There are no recent data on this subject, but it is unlikely the situation has changed much [59]. The distribution will vary among hospitals according to the specific nature of the facility; however, this and other studies have consistently reported the majority of visits to be nonurgent in nature.

In two studies of hospital emergency department visits, the two most common responses from patients regarding factors associated with their decision to visit the emergency department were expediency (e.g., available hours or comprehensive care) and immediacy [35, 54]. The patient's perception of these factors may be different from that of the provider. The patient is scheduling care at his or her convenience, often because the emergency department is always open; also, third-party reimbursements may cover emergency department visits but not the same care in a physician's office.

Trauma Units

Trauma units are inpatient facilities that provide immediate and continuing care for patients with severe injuries. Some hospitals admit patients directly into the trauma unit. Infection risks associated with trauma units and the patient care provided there are discussed in Chapter 20.

Emergicenters

Emergicenters are usually freestanding facilities that care for patients with urgent or nonurgent problems. These centers are able to operate at considerably less cost than are emergency departments attached to hospitals because of the limited and exclusive nature of their function. The emergicenter functions like a physician's office with extended hours and may make referrals for more extensive care.

Outpatient Surgery

Surgicenters or ambulatory surgery centers are defined as centers that handle on a same-day basis those surgical procedures that cannot properly be performed in a physician's office or hospital outpatient department but that can be scheduled and performed so that the patient does not need to remain in a hospital overnight. These centers may be freestanding or part of the hospital facility. Administratively, they may be under the jurisdiction of the hospital's operating room or function independently.

According to data collected by the American Hospital Association, outpatient surgery rose 77 percent between 1979 and 1983 at hospitals nationwide, whereas inpatient operations fell 7 percent during the same period [62]. These data, published in 1985, were collected prior to full implementation of the prospective payment system for Medicare patients based on diagnosis-related groups (DRGs). In

an accompanying article [63], reasons given for the growth of ambulatory surgery centers included improvements in technology for laser surgery, improved endoscopic equipment, and development of new anesthetic agents and associated monitoring devices.

Outpatient Diagnostic and Treatment Facilities

Outpatient diagnostic and treatment facilities provide care outside the usual inpatient institutional setting. This may include individual physicians' offices, clinics attached to teaching hospitals, specialty clinics, and clinics or office practices administered by groups of physicians or health maintenance organizations (HMOs). Visits are usually scheduled at the request of the patient and convenience of the care provider and are usually elective in nature.

Data from the National Ambulatory Medical Care Survey were used to determine the most common problems seen in an ambulatory care setting and to identify the medical specialties that provide the greater part of this care [57]. Rosenblatt and co-workers [57] found that 15 diagnosis clusters accounted for 50 percent of all ambulatory care visits, with general medical examination the most frequent diagnosis (approximately 9 percent of all encounters), followed by acute upper respiratory infection (7.3 percent). In addition, they found that general and family physicians, general internists, and general pediatricians accounted for approximately 66 percent of all outpatient visits for the 15 diagnostic clusters.

Hospital Admitting Departments

A visit to the hospital admitting department is the usual first stop for patients with scheduled elective admissions and a prehospitalization step for many patients admitted directly from clinics or emergency departments. Although emergency admissions interact with admitting departments for billing and organizational purposes, many emergency admissions go directly from the emergency department to a nursing unit or intensive care unit and do not visit the admitting department personally.

Nosocomial Infections

A nosocomial infection associated with an ACS can be defined as one that is associated temporally with the visit, with the care provided during the visit (e.g., an inadvertent exposure to a communicable disease while in the waiting room). In other words, it is an infection associated with medical intervention.

Patients seen in an ACS usually leave the facility after the visit and often are not followed up. If an infection develops associated with the visit, it may not be identified to the hospital or facility. The true incidence of these infections is not known, although several reports from ambulatory surgery settings have been published [17, 51].

Risk of Nosocomial Infection in the ACS

Risk of nosocomial infection in the ACS has been demonstrated to be associated with the interaction between host defenses and exposure to potentially infectious agents in a dose sufficient to cause infection (see Chap. 1). Factors of an ACS that are different from the hospital setting include the following:

1. Large numbers of patients are seen in rapid succession.
2. Few procedures are performed in which access to the vascular system (e.g., intravenous therapy) or mucous membranes (e.g., intubation, laryngoscopy) is necessary.
3. A wide variety of ailments may be seen by the same care provider during a single day.
4. Most patients seen in an ACS, including emergency departments, outpatient clinics, or physicians' offices, do not require admission to the hospital.

In summary, most patients in the ACS are seeking care for relatively minor illnesses or injuries that have not compromised their host defenses. The duration of contact with the facility is brief, and contact with potentially infectious agents usually depends on instrumentation. The likelihood of all three factors being sufficient to result in infection is very low.

It is widely accepted that approximately 5 percent of hospitalized patients develop nosocomial infections, primarily of four major types: urinary tract, surgical wound, lower respiratory, and bacteremia (see Chap. 27). Several investigators have estimated that the proportion of these infections that is potentially preventable is approximately 25 to 40 percent [6, 27] and that most of those are related to devices and procedures. The remaining 60 to 75 percent are often judged unavoidable because of the patient's underlying disease combined with other factors such as the duration of hospitalization (see Chap. 27).

The incidence and preventability of nosocomial infections in the ACS have not been investigated adequately. It is reasonable to assume that most nosocomial infections in these settings are largely preventable because the duration of contact with the facility is brief, and those that do occur are usually related to medical devices and procedures.

To answer some of the questions raised about incidence of infection following ACS visits, several investigators have concentrated on patients in ambulatory surgery settings. Complications associated with ambulatory surgery were studied prospectively in 13,433 patients during a 4-year period by Natof [51]. Surgical procedures included tonsillectomy or adenoidectomy (or both), augmentation mammoplasty, submucous resection, and a variety of genitourinary procedures, primarily performed on young, healthy hosts. Only 10 of 13,433 patients developed infections that could be associated with the ambulatory surgery procedure (3 wound infections, 3 gynecologic infections, 2 pneumonias, and 2 upper respiratory infections). The frequency of infectious complications following ambulatory surgery in this series was less than 1 infection per 1,000 patients (less than 0.1 percent).

Craig [17] summarized results of several studies of postoperative infections among ambulatory surgery patients. Despite several differences in study design, when patients and physicians responded to written questionnaires or telephone calls, the infection rate in all studies was no more than 2 percent and usually substantially lower.

Indeed, some procedures likely to pose unacceptably high risks in the acute-care setting can apparently be carried out acceptably in the ACS. A study about aseptic technique in the use and reuse of insulin syringes by diabetic patients was recently conducted at an outpatient clinic of a large teaching hospital [71]. Diabetic outpatients were surveyed at the outset for compliance with recommendations for aseptic handling of syringes. The investigators then studied prospectively the effects of reusing disposable syringes in 56 diabetic patients who reused syringes a mean of 6.6 times (N = 23,664 injections). Although compliance with aseptic precautions was poor, no adverse effects of syringe reuse were identified. The study reviewed other studies and case reports and then raised two important considerations. First, the initial survey established that almost half of the study subjects were reusing disposable syringes, primarily for cost reasons. Second, it found that even with poor aseptic technique associated with reuse of syringes, there were no infections. Although the authors acknowledged that the numbers of patients required to demonstrate safety statistically make it unlikely such a study will ever be done, disposable syringe reuse seems to be a fact of life for large numbers of diabetic patients and should be acknowledged by physicians providing care to diabetic patients.

When the incidence of nosocomial infection is so low, the benefit of an intensive surveillance system is likely to be exceeded by the cost. That is, the time required to follow all patients makes the cost to identify each infection very high; however, the consequences of some nosocomial infections associated with the ACS have been serious [10].

If infections in an ACS are to be monitored by surveillance, it is clear that follow-up with physicians' offices, including telephone calls to those who do not return written requests, will be required. Responsibility for this follow-up rests with various personnel,

depending on the organizational structure of the agency [76].

Personnel Working in the ACS

The key to preventing nosocomial infections is an ACS may lie in the combination of skill in performing procedures and use of aseptic practices. As in any patient care area, personnel in the ACS should not work when they have infectious diseases and should follow the facility's program for personnel health, immunizations, and exposures to communicable diseases (see Chap. 3). Facilities that are not attached to hospitals can also use these guidelines to develop programs.

Training personnel in aseptic practices and ensuring their skills and knowledge of invasive procedures are current is also essential in the ACS. Training patients and home-care givers is increasingly important with the trend toward managing patients with indwelling devices at home. Several reports have described programs for administration of outpatient intravenous antibiotic therapy [2, 21, 23, 44, 55, 64, 68, 69, 70], home parenteral nutrition [24, 37], and ambulatory dialysis [16, 29, 52, 61] (see also Chap. 19). An integral component of all these programs is training for the patient or home-care giver in aseptic practices and recognition of complications. The reported incidence of infectious complications varies with the type of device, reason for and duration of therapy, host susceptibility, and many other factors.

The Inanimate Environment
Cleaning, Disinfection, and Sterilization

The principles of cleaning, disinfection, and sterilization of equipment and devices used in the ACS are the same as in the hospital setting (see Chaps. 15, 16). However, the proportion of patients experiencing device-related procedures in the ACS is much smaller than in the inpatient setting. When a procedure involves contact with the vascular system or with mucous membranes, it is reasonable to expect similar risk in ambulatory patients as in hospitalized patients. There may be differences, however, in the duration of exposure to the device (e.g., intravenous therapy, urinary catheterization), conditions under which the device is inserted (e.g., starting intravenous therapy without adequate preparation of the insertion site), and organisms colonizing skin and mucosal sites (see Chap. 13) involved in device insertion.

Devices that are in contact with the vascular system should be sterile (e.g., instruments used to close lacerations, intravascular devices). Instruments that are in contact with mucous membranes should be sterile or receive high-level disinfection before use (e.g., vaginal specula, sigmoidoscopes, tonometers).

In general, articles and instruments that touch intact skin should be as clean as articles that are readily available in commercial establishments such as restaurants. Proper cleaning includes removal of all soil and body substances and the use of disinfectant agents appropriate to the situation. The more distant and peripheral an article is to any patient, the less infection risk there is associated with it. For example, chairs in the waiting room, cabinets in examining rooms, and curtains present virtually no infection risk.

Because of the possibility of examining tables being soiled by patient secretions, excretions, or blood, there is a common practice in the ACS to provide some barrier between the patient and the table. This is often accomplished by rolls of paper sheets or by linen sheets that are changed between patients. Unless there is soilage of the table surface, disinfection between patients is not necessary. Examination tables, countertops, floors, and other articles in the treatment areas should be cleaned on a regular schedule consistent with need in the facility.

Cleanliness of the physical facility, in general, is most easily accomplished when the number of examination rooms is sufficient and the flow of patients, personnel, and supplies can be accomplished easily.

Ventilation Systems

Airborne transmission of potentially infectious agents via ventilation systems has been studied extensively, and data show that very few agents persist in the air for extended periods of time. The most common organism that persists in the air for extended periods is *Mycobacterium tuberculosis*. To transmit tuberculosis requires that the host be susceptible and in contact with a large enough dose of droplet nuclei for a sufficient time to become infected. Riley and colleagues [56] studied the infectiousness of a series of treated and untreated patients with tuberculosis by experiments in which air from rooms of tuberculosis patients was conducted to an exposure chamber in which guinea pigs in cages were located. Of 61 untreated patients with drug-susceptible organisms, patients were responsible for all of the transmissions to guinea pigs; a patient with tuberculous laryngitis was the most infectious. Riley and colleagues [56] concluded that untreated patients were much more infectious than treated patients and that infectivity was also related to the number of air changes per hour in the room.

Although an ACS may provide the opportunity for the susceptible host to come in contact with a potentially infectious tuberculosis patient, the time interval of contact is usually insufficient to transmit the agent effectively. Whether an examining room in which multiple tuberculosis patients are seen in succession can sustain sufficient droplet nuclei to transmit tuberculosis depends on several factors: the number of infectious patients seen in a short time interval; aerosolization of droplet nuclei by the infectious patients (i.e., the efficiency of dissemination); number of air changes in the examining room per unit of time, whether the air is vented directly to the outside, whether filters or ultraviolet lights are in the ventilation system, and what type of filters they are; and finally, the presence of susceptible patients or personnel in the examination room during or after the same time interval. These factors tend to have an additive effect, and risk is increased accordingly; however, the actual risk is unknown (see Chap. 29).

Many diseases that are spread by droplet contact are seen in the ACS (e.g., measles, rubella, varicella, and other childhood diseases). When a patient presents to an ACS with a fever, skin rash, or other signs characteristic of infection that may be transmitted by droplet contact, expeditious placement in a treatment room alone will reduce the risk to susceptible persons of contact with droplets that may be sneezed or coughed into the patient's immediate environment. In addition, many of these viral agents are transmitted most effectively by direct contact, and handwashing will further reduce the risk of transmission to others [46].

Although droplets that are potentially infectious to the susceptible host do not travel more than 1 m or remain suspended in the air for extended periods of time (see Chap. 1), an outbreak of measles in a pediatric practice in 1981 [8] raised some serious questions about potential airborne transmission of the measles virus by means of droplet nuclei. Bloch and colleagues [8] investigated secondary cases of measles associated with an 11½-month-old child who was in the office for 1 hour on the second day of rash, primarily in a single examining room, and coughing vigorously most of the time. Four of the 7 children had transient contact with the source patient as he entered or exited the waiting room; only 1 of them had face-to-face contact within a meter. In addition, the 3 other children who contracted measles were never in the same room with the source patient; 1 arrived 1 hour after the source patient left. Airflow studies demonstrated that droplet nuclei generated in the examining room used by the source patient were dispersed throughout the entire office suite. The outbreak supports the fact that measles virus, when it becomes airborne, can survive for at least 1 hour. As a result of this outbreak, some physicians may elect not to use an examination room for at least 1 hour after it has been used by a patient diagnosed with measles, especially if the patient is coughing vigorously. This does not address the problem of air circulation throughout an office suite, particularly those in energy-efficient buildings with recirculating air.

Two other studies reported an increase in the proportion of all measles cases that were acquired in medical settings and pointed to the waiting room as a location where a reservoir of susceptible individuals may congregate, allowing for potential exposure to measles and other infectious diseases [19, 31]. They also noted that the primary mode of transmission was face-to-face contact and that airborne transmission appeared to be relatively rare. In Davis's review [19] of measles cases in 30 states from 1980 through 1984, 24 percent of the cases associated with medical facilities were in personnel; 76 percent were in patients or visitors. They concluded that more attention needs to be given to methods to prevent measles in medical facilities, including ensuring that medical personnel are immune to measles (see Chap. 3).

It is becoming increasingly common for emergency physicians to manage hospital employee health services [58] (see Chap. 3) and for the emergency department to care for employees who are exposed to airborne communicable diseases or who have these diseases but are not diagnosed until they report for work. In addition to measles, a common hospital infection control problem is varicella-zoster virus infection (chickenpox). Sayre and colleagues [58] reviewed the literature to determine a rational basis for managing the varicella-zoster virus–exposed employee and pointed out the potential for airborne transmission as an exposure route, especially if ventilation systems are defective. In the absence of a vaccine, attention to prompt patient placement and the use of an examination room with nonrecirculated air (if such is available) will reduce the risks of transmission of varicella-zoster virus, as will assignment of care providers who are known to be immune (see also Chap. 38).

Potentially Infectious Body Substances

Potentially infectious agents may be present in all body substances (e.g., blood, secretions, excretions), and all body substances should be handled as if they are infectious. The implementation of these practices, in reality, is often made difficult because personnel may believe that only patients with diagnosed communicable diseases present a risk of infection. Accordingly, they may not take precautions until a diagnosis is established.

The seriousness of this problem was made clear when Dienstag and Ryan [20] published their report of prevalence of markers for hepatitis B virus (HBV) among various groups of health care workers (HCWs). They found that personnel with the most contact with blood (e.g., emergency room nurses) were most likely to have markers for HBV. The vast majority of such exposures resulted from contacts with patients whose HBV status was not known at the time. Following this report, Jackson, Lynch, and their colleagues [32–34, 47] began to question the efficacy of infection precautions that were initiated at the time a diagnosis was made or suspected and proposed an alternative to traditional isolation techniques. The system was named *body substance isolation* (BSI) and was intended to serve two purposes simultaneously: (1) to reduce the risks of cross-transmission of organisms between patients and (2) to reduce the risks

of transmission of infectious agents from patients to HCWs. At nearly the same time, the Centers for Disease Control (CDC) was also responding to increasing concerns about risks to HCWs for infection with HBV and the human immunodeficiency virus (HIV). The CDC developed a series of recommendations intended primarily to reduce risks to HCWs of infection with HBV, HIV, and other bloodborne pathogens (see Chap. 11). This system was named *universal precautions* or *universal blood and body fluid precautions* [11–14, 30]. Others, including Gerberding [26], have also addressed infection risk reduction strategies for HCWs, and additional information may be found in Chapters 3, 11, 38, and 39 of this text. Table 23-1 presents general precautionary measures, described

Table 23-1. General precautionary measures for handling potentially infectious body substances

Body substance	Examples of infectious agents	Precautions for personnel in direct contact with substance	Precautions for patients or personnel in same room
Blood (e.g., uncontrolled bleeding; lacerations; GI bleed)	Hepatitis B, hepatitis C; HIV	Gloves; cover gowns for large amounts; masks and protective eyewear if splashing is likely	No direct contact, no risk
Saliva, sputum (e.g., purulent sputum, oral secretions)	Viral agents; mixed gram-positive and gram-negative bacteria	Gloves*	No direct contact, no risk*
Feces (e.g., diarrhea, fecal incontinence)	Enteric pathogens; viral agents; other gram-negative bacteria	Gloves; cover gowns for large amounts	No direct contact, no risk
Urine (e.g., incontinence)	Gram-negative bacteria	Gloves	No direct contact, no risk
Wound drainage (e.g., wound infections, abscesses, impetigo)	Gram-positive and gram-negative bacteria	Gloves; cover gowns for large amounts	No direct contact, no risk

GI = gastrointestinal; HIV = human immunodeficiency virus.

*For pediatric or other patients who may have a disease spread by droplet contact (e.g., chickenpox, measles, rubella, mumps), personnel with negative or unknown history of the disease or immunization should not examine the patient. Recent data suggest that some patients with measles and varicella who are coughing vigorously may produce droplet nuclei that can stay suspended in the air for up to 1 hour. Though the predominant mode of transmission of measles is by droplet spread, in facilities where ventilation is poor, consideration should be given to restricting subsequent use of such rooms to patients who are known to be immune to the disease diagnosed in the previous patient for at least an hour after the index case has vacated the room. This practice does not address problems presented by recirculated air in energy-efficient buildings that may result in airborne contamination of the entire medical office; however, transmission in such situations is rare (see text).

Note: Hand-washing is usually sufficient to remove soil and potentially infectious agents from hands; however, regardless of diagnosis, when contact with these substances is anticipated, personnel should glove their hands to reduce the quantity of hand contamination and wash their hands after glove removal. Unless there is direct soilage of articles in the environment, there is no need to perform special cleaning procedures.

according to body substance, that are applicable in the ACS.

Given the concerns of HCWs about potential risks for HIV and HBV infection, several large labor unions approached the Occupational Safety and Health Administration (OSHA) in 1986 to request that a formal rule be made to address the issue. OSHA initiated the rule-making process in 1987, and a final rule was published in December 1991 [73]. In the meantime, enforcement procedures to be used by OSHA inspectors have been developed and revised several times [74]. One of the major concerns of OSHA, the CDC, and others is the lack of compliance by HCWs with obtaining the HBV vaccine, even when it is made available at no cost to the HCW [65, 73] (see Chap. 38). Whether increased emphasis by OSHA about the need for HBV vaccine for HCWs will alter compliance remains to be seen.

Although many of the recommendations by OSHA emphasize the importance of having personal protective equipment (gloves, masks, gowns) readily available for the HCW, it is now well established that the greatest risk for both HIV and HBV infection is puncture injuries. Puncture injuries are often related to the design of the equipment [36], to the situation at the time [48], and to commonly used practices, such as recapping, that have long been acknowledged as risky. In fact, in a recent survey of needle-stick injuries and needle disposal practices in Minnesota physicians' offices [72], recapping of needles was frequent (more than 50 percent of the time) and 44 percent of the offices surveyed reported injuries during the past year.

The Infection Control Practitioner
Hospital-Based Settings
Infection control practitioners (ICPs) who work in hospitals usually have responsibility for infection control in the emergency department, admitting department, and ambulatory care clinics [18] (see Chaps. 4, 5). These responsibilities include education of personnel about measures that reduce infection risks associated with emergency care; cleaning, disinfection, and sterilization; infec-

tion precautions; management of needle-stick injuries and other exposures; and orientation for new personnel. The ICP may also act as a consultant for the development of policies and procedures. Policies and education programs should be specifically tailored for each department.

Freestanding Settings
Most freestanding settings (e.g., surgicenters, emergicenters, physicians' offices) do not have a designated ICP. Consultation about infection control prevention in these settings can frequently be obtained from the local health department and ICPs in hospitals in the community.

Reportable Diseases
State and local health departments require that certain communicable (notifiable) diseases be reported to them. Designation of a person responsible for this task is essential in both the hospital-based and the freestanding ACS. In many hospitals, this is a responsibility of the ICP. In addition, local health departments may provide follow-up for contacts of patients with many infectious diseases (e.g., syphilis, gonorrhea, salmonellosis, viral heptatis, meningococcal disease).

Patient and Personnel Risks for Nosocomial Infections
Emergency Medical Services System
The risks to patients and personnel in the EMSS are increased by the urgency of the patient situation and the need for prompt and efficient patient management. As the urgency for intervention increases (e.g., to provide an airway, control bleeding, stabilize a fracture, provide intravenous fluids), the situation becomes less easily controlled and adherence to aseptic practices by personnel generally decreases.

Prehospital Care
Risks to patients in the prehospital care phase are generally related to aseptic practices. It is important to recognize that the need for careful aseptic practices must be balanced against the patient's need for prompt man-

agement. The duration of contact with the field situation is often brief; however, the devices inserted there and the procedures done to stabilize the patient carry with them certain infection risks. Training programs for personnel working in these situations should include information about and practice in using aseptic techniques. When the urgency of the field situation is such that aseptic practices may be difficult to employ, the decision to compromise them is made *for* the patient and should reflect his or her best interests rather than personnel convenience. When the patient is stabilized, devices inserted under less than optimal conditions should be replaced aseptically and in a timely fashion. Communication among the field team, personnel in the emergency department and, ultimately, the health care providers in the nursing unit where the patient is admitted will help maintain this continuity of care.

Risks to personnel depend on contact with body substances (e.g., blood, feces, saliva) that may be contaminated with an infectious agent. Infection precautions may include the use of barrier techniques (e.g., gloves) to prevent substances from soiling personnel's hands, clothing, and supplies. Personnel reduce the risk of transmitting infectious agents to patients or of acquiring infections themselves by using these barrier techniques along with hand-washing (or antiseptic foams when sinks are not available).

The risks to personnel are rarely known at the onset of a transport situation, and the patient's diagnosis may never be known to the transport personnel. Accordingly, the development of standard procedures—including aseptic practices, when possible—is appropriate in any transport situation.

When communicable diseases are diagnosed, transport personnel should be included in any exposure workups and should receive prophylaxis when indicated. These personnel should follow the same immunization and tuberculin skin-testing routines as do hospital personnel (see Chap. 3).

Fligner and associates [22] recently studied the prevalence of HBV serologic markers in 85 paramedics working in suburban Chicago and compared results to previously reported studies documenting rates ranging from 0.6 to 25 percent. In their study, 7.1 percent of the paramedics were found to be positive. They concluded that prehospital personnel do not constitute a homogeneous occupational category at risk for HBV infection. Using a table comparing six other studies (see [22] for citations), these investigators suggested that prevalence of HBV serologic markers in paramedics is more strongly influenced by the incidence of HBV in the population of the area than by the occupational category of the HCW. They concluded that, when making decisions about the use of prophylactic vaccination versus postexposure prophylaxis and vaccination following documented exposure to blood positive for hepatitis B surface antigen, a cost-effectiveness analysis for HBV vaccine is particularly relevant for EMSSs likely to have low HBV prevalence and attack rates. The logistics of obtaining this information on patients and providing it in a timely manner to EMSS personnel was not discussed.

First responders are also concerned about the potential risk of exposure to HIV-positive blood. In a review of information known to date, Gelb [25] points out many safety issues associated with the prehospital setting when it is the scene of an accident and emphasizes the additional risk introduced by potential HIV transmission. This author concluded by supporting the need for education regarding universal precautions as well as new technologies to allow emergency HCWs to perform procedures rapidly while adequately protecting themselves from exposure. These technologic advances would involve better equipment and clothing as well as affordable disposable equipment or equipment that may be rapidly decontaminated (see also Chap. 39).

The transport vehicle, whether an ambulance, van, or helicopter, should be cleaned on a regular schedule; articles soiled with body substances should be cleaned and disinfected before being used for another patient. Although the patient area of the transport vehicle is a small, closed space, ventilation is easily accomplished, and it is unnecessary to provide extended ventilation times or special decontamination procedures (e.g., fumigation) before the transport of another patient.

Emergency Department of a Hospital

Risks to patients who present to an emergency department of a hospital are related to the patient's underlying condition and the procedures performed for the patient in the emergency department. Few procedures are generally performed for patients in the nonurgent category, and they are at little risk for nosocomial infection; patients in the urgent category undergo more procedures and are at somewhat greater risk; patients in the emergent category may undergo numerous procedures and are at greatest risk. Additionally, it is for these patients that asepsis is most often compromised.

A survey of patient visits to emergency departments has been reported by Moffet [49], who studied 1,145 randomly selected visits to an urban hospital emergency department in 1977. Of these visits, 47 percent were for trauma and 28 percent for infections. The majority of the visits for infections were by patients younger than 18 years; 70 percent of the infections were respiratory infections. Only 1.9 percent of the patients with infections were hospitalized.

Respiratory infections reflect seasonal and community incidence and are usually viral. Risk to emergency department personnel of exposure to many of these infections is probably similar to that in nonhospital settings in which numbers of people are together who may be in the prodromal or acute phase of a viral illness (e.g., schools, offices, stores); however, the concentration of such persons may be greater in an emergency department.

Emergency department personnel are at greater risk for exposure to HBV than are many other hospital workers due to their frequent exposure to blood. In a study by Dienstag and Ryan [20], 624 health workers were surveyed in an urban hospital in Boston. These personnel represented a spectrum of exposure to blood and to patients. Of the 30 emergency department nurses studied, 30 percent were positive for one or more sero-

logic markers for HBV. Among the groups surveyed, this was the group with the highest prevalence for HBV seropositivity. Dienstag and Ryan [20] concluded that emergency department personnel are exposed to the most severely ill patients (including those with uncontrolled bleeding), that emergency department *nurses* are often the first personnel to encounter such patients, and that, at the time of the study, these nurses generally did not wear gloves or protective gowns when providing such care (see Chap. 38).

Recent analysis of the changing epidemiology of HBV in the United States [1] points out that although the overall incidence of HBV remained relatively constant throughout the study period (January 1, 1981, through September 30, 1988), disease transmission patterns changed significantly. Of note was a 75 percent decline in the proportion of HBV patients reporting health care employment, which is primarily attributable to HBV vaccination of HCWs. New recommendations for protection against viral hepatitis, including recommendations for HCWs, were published in 1991 [15].

HBV and HIV infection risk for emergency department personnel has also been hypothesized from studies that have determined the prevalence of HBV and HIV antibody in serum specimens from emergency department patients [3, 40, 43, 45]. The studies have consistently shown that patients who *are not suspected* of being HIV- or HBV-positive, but who *are seropositive*, are regularly seen in emergency departments. These data are used to support the need for consistent use of universal precautions when caring for all patients, although compliance with these recommendations has usually been found to be poor [5]. Similar data about unrecognized seroprevalence for HBV or HIV have also been found for patients admitted to a large teaching hospital when specimens submitted to the hospital laboratory have been tested [28].

In a recent editorial by Kelen [42], the absence of emergency specialists from studies of HCWs was noted, and the comment was made that data were also absent regarding the risk of seroconversion from patients with undiagnosed HIV infection. In an accompanying editorial, Baraff [4] noted concerns about cumulative risk for HCWs using a mathematic model and published data about HIV seroprevalence among emergency department patients. He suggested that if an emergency physician were to suffer one needle stick or similar exposure every year in an emergency department where 5 percent of the patients were HIV-seropositive, and the risk of seroconversion was 0.5 percent per exposure, then the lifetime risk of seroconversion over a 30-year career would be approximately 0.8 percent or 8 per 1,000. To put this in perspective, the risk of death from accidents, suicide, and homicide combined over a 30-year period is approximately 18 per 1,000. Baraff [4] concluded by stating that both of these figures could be modified by behavioral change and noted, "Just as most of us would not consider driving without seatbelts, we should not practice our specialty without employing universal precautions . . ."

With the advent of the HIV and acquired immunodeficiency syndrome (AIDS) epidemic has also come increasing concern about risks associated with mouth-to-mouth resuscitation. In a survey of 5,823 American Heart Association Virginia Affiliate basic cardiac life support (BCLS) instructors, the impact of the HIV and AIDS epidemic on attitudes, beliefs, and behaviors with regard to mouth-to-mouth resuscitation was assessed. They concluded that concern about HIV and AIDS was adversely affecting attitudes, beliefs, and self-reported behaviors of the BCLS instructors regarding mouth-to-mouth ventilation on strangers [53].

Emergicenters

Seriously injured and ill patients are not generally seen in emergicenters; most of the visits are by patients with nonurgent problems. Procedures performed in these facilities are similar to those performed in hospital emergency departments (e.g., laceration repairs, incision and drainage of abscesses, and other minor surgical procedures). The same principles of asepsis apply in this setting as in the hospital emergency department.

Outpatient Surgery

The care of instruments and the quality of aseptic practices should be the same in surgicenters as it is in hospital operating rooms. Written policies and procedures for care of instruments, cleaning of operating rooms, and personnel health practices should be developed following guidelines for hospital operating rooms (see Chap. 22). In addition, Sebben [66, 67] has recently summarized recommendations for sterile technique and prevention of wound infection in office surgery.

Preoperative assessment of the patient should include screening for infection and for presence of communicable disease. Preparation and aftercare management of patients should emphasize prevention of nosocomial infection (e.g., wound care, preoperative and postoperative pulmonary management). Patients should be instructed regarding signs of infection (e.g., fever, redness, pain, swelling, drainage) and whom to contact if questions arise.

It is generally accepted that cleaning after all cases should remove all soil and body substances and that special cleaning after so-called dirty cases is not necessary. Cleaning routines and preparation for subsequent cases should follow the same guidelines that are used for hospital operating rooms (see Chap. 22).

Outpatient Diagnostic and Treatment Facilities

Risk for nosocomial infection in outpatient diagnostic and treatment facilities is generally very low. In some special situations such as oncology or pediatric clinics or physicians' offices, it may be important to identify patients whose compromised immune status may place them at increased risk for infection, especially of the droplet-spread viral respiratory infections. These patients may benefit from reduced contact with other patients in the waiting room. Some pediatric clinics or physicians' offices also have separate waiting rooms for children seeking well care and for those who are ill. Some treatment rooms have doors that open directly to the outside, permitting selected patients to bypass the office waiting room entirely.

Hospital Admitting Department

Generally, infection risk in the admitting department is low. Inadvertent exposures to communicable diseases may occur there because persons with unknown exposure or disease status may be together in the same waiting area for varying lengths of time. This is particularly true in pediatric facilities or hospitals with large pediatric units.

The admitting department can serve a useful role in reducing the risk of transmission of infectious agents between hospitalized patients by being attentive to the room and bed assignments for newly admitted patients and for patients who develop infections while in the hospital. In many hospitals, the ICP conveys information about potentially infectious patients to the admitting department and serves as a consultant for patient placement.

Quality Assurance Issues for the ACS

Berman [7] recently presented the perspective of the Joint Commission on Accreditation of Healthcare Organizations (JCAHO) on the importance of quality assurance monitoring for ACSs. In response to increasing concerns about quality assurance, Kaplowitz [41] described a quality assurance program in a U.S. Coast Guard ambulatory care facility. A method for quality assurance monitoring for ambulatory care centers connected to hospitals was also described by Bradford and Flynn [9], who provided an outline for quality assurance rounds and clinic criteria. Emphasis was on evaluation of the structural and process elements of care. All of these articles stressed the challenges presented by ACSs for developing quality assurance programs that are practical, meaningful, and have a significant positive impact on patient care. None of the authors specifically addressed monitoring for infections associated with care in an ACS, although some of the structural and process

monitoring described by Bradford and Flynn [9] was related to infection risk.

Future Trends

Although ACSs are places where infection risk is generally considered to be low, the increasing use of these settings for surgical procedures, device insertions and management, and outpatient care of increasingly more immunocompromised patients will present interesting challenges for the future. Monitoring for low-frequency events such as nosocomial infections related to care in an ACS is labor-intensive and costly and requires creativity to ensure efficient use of limited resources. The increasing demands presented by the JCAHO [7] to perform these activities and by OSHA [73, 74] to ensure that the ACS environment is a safe one for workers will require agencies to commit resources for personnel to monitor activities and follow protocols that have heretofore been viewed by many agencies as a low priority. This will be one of the challenges of the next decade.

References

1. Alter, M. J., et al. The changing epidemiology of hepatitis B in the United States: Need for alternative vaccination strategies. *J.A.M.A.* 263:1218, 1990.
2. Antoniskis, A., et al. Feasibility of outpatient self-administration of parenteral antibiotics. *West. J. Med.* 128:203, 1978.
3. Baker, J. L., Kelen, G. D., Sivertson, K. T., and Quinn, T. C. Unsuspected human immunodeficiency virus in critically ill emergency patients. *J.A.M.A.* 257:2609, 1987.
4. Baraff, L. J. AIDS: Implications for emergency physicians (edit.). *Ann. Emerg. Med.* 17:1102, 1988.
5. Baraff, L. J., and Talan, D. A. Compliance with universal precautions in a university hospital emergency department. *Ann. Emerg. Med.* 18:654, 1989.
6. Bennett, J. V. Human infections: Economic implications and prevention. *Ann. Intern. Med.* 89(Part 2):761, 1978.
7. Berman, S. Quality assurance in ambulatory health care. *Q.R.B.* 14:18, 1988.

8. Bloch, A. B., et al. Measles outbreak in a pediatric practice: Airborne transmission in an office setting. *Pediatrics* 75:676, 1985.

9. Bradford, M., and Flynn, N. M. Ambulatory care infection control quality assurance monitoring. *Am. J. Infect. Control* 16:21A, 1988.

10. Centers for Disease Control. Amebiasis associated with colonic irrigation: Colorado. *M.M.W.R.* 30:101, 1981.

11. Centers for Disease Control. Recommendations for prevention of HIV transmission in health-care settings. *M.M.W.R.* 36(Suppl. 2S):35, 1987.

12. Centers for Disease Control. Update: Universal precautions for prevention of transmission of HIV, HBV, and other bloodborne pathogens in health-care settings. *M.M.W.R.* 37:277, 1988.

13. Centers for Disease Control. Guidelines for prevention of transmission of HIV and HBV to health-care and public-safety workers. *M.M.W.R.* 38(Suppl. S-6):1, 1989.

14. Centers for Disease Control. Public Health Service statement on management of occupational exposure to HIV, including considerations regarding zidovudine postexposure use. *M.M.W.R.* 39(RR-1):1, 1990.

15. Centers for Disease Control. Hepatitis B virus: Recommendations of the Immunization Practices Advisory Committee (ACIP). *M.M.W.R.* 40(RR-13):1, 1991.

16. Chan, M. K., et al. Three years' experience of continuous ambulatory peritoneal dialysis. *Lancet* 1:1409, 1981.

17. Craig, C. P. Infection surveillance for ambulatory surgery patients: An overview. *Q.R.B.* 9:107, 1983.

18. Crow, S. Infection control in the emergency room. *Nurs. Clin. North Am.* 15:869, 1980.

19. Davis, R. M., et al. Transmission of measles in medical settings: 1980–1984. *J.A.M.A.* 255:1295, 1986.

20. Dienstag, J. L., and Ryan, D. M. Occupational exposure to hepatitis B virus in hospital personnel: Infection or immunization? *Am. J. Epidemiol.* 115:26, 1982.

21. Eisenberg, J. M., and Kitz, D. S. Saving from outpatient antibiotic therapy for osteomyelitis: Economic analysis of a therapeutic strategy. *J.A.M.A.* 255:1584, 1986.

22. Fligner, D. J., et al. The prevalence of hepatitis B serologic markers in suburban paramedics. *J. Emerg. Med.* 7:41, 1989.

23. Frame, P. T. Outpatient intravenous antibiotic therapy (lett.). *J.A.M.A.* 248:356, 1982.

24. Gaffron, R. E., et al. Organization and operation of a home parenteral nutrition program with emphasis on the pharmacist's role. *Mayo Clin. Proc.* 55:94, 1980.

25. Gelb, A. HIV infection control issues concerning first responders and emergency physicians. *Occup. Med.: State Art Rev.* 4 (spec. issue):61, 1989.

26. Gerberding, J. L. Occupational HIV transmission: Risk reduction. *Occup. Med.: State Art Rev.* 4 (spec. issue):21, 1989.

27. Haley, R. W., et al. The efficacy of infection surveillance and control programs in preventing nosocomial infections in U.S. hospitals. *Am. J. Epidemiol.* 121:182, 1985.

28. Handsfield, H. H., Cummings, M. J., and Swenson, P. D. Prevalence of antibody to HIV and hepatitis B surface antigen in blood samples submitted to a hospital laboratory. *J.A.M.A.* 258:3395, 1987.

29. Harrison, J. T. Chronic ambulatory peritoneal dialysis (lett.). *N. Engl. J. Med.* 306:670, 1982.

30. Hughes, J. M. Universal precautions: CDC perspective. *Occup. Med.: State Art Rev.* 4 (spec. issue):13, 1989.

31. Istre, G. R., et al. Measles spread in medical settings: An important focus of disease transmission? *Pediatrics* 79:356, 1987.

32. Jackson, M. M. Implementing universal body substance precautions. *Occup. Med.: State Art Rev.* 4 (spec. issue):311, 1989.

33. Jackson, M. M., et al. Clinical savvy: Why not treat all body substances as infectious? *Am. J. Nurs.* 87:1137, 1987.

34. Jackson, M. M., and Lynch, P. Infection control: Too much or too little? *Am. J. Nurs.* 84:208, 1984.

35. Jacoby, L. E., and Jones, L. S. Factors associated with ED use by "repeater" and "nonrepeater" patients. *J. Emerg. Nurs.* 8:243, 1982.

36. Jagger, J., Hunt, E. H., Brand-Elnaggar, J., and Pearson, R. D. Rates of needle-stick injury caused by various devices in a university hospital. *N. Engl. J. Med.* 319:2114, 1988.

37. Jeejeebhoy, K. N., et al. Total parenteral nutrition at home: Studies in patients surviving 4 months to 5 years. *Gastroenterology* 71:943, 1976.

38. Jonas, S., Flesh, R., Brook, R., and Wassertheil-Smoller, S. Monitoring utilization of a municipal hospital emergency department. *Hosp. Topics* 54(1):43, 1976.

39. Jonas, S., and Rosenberg, S. N. Ambulatory Care. In: S. Jonas (Ed.), *Health Care Delivery in the United States* (3rd ed.). New York: Springer, 1986.

40. Jui, J., et al. Multicenter HIV and hepatitis B seroprevalence survey. *J. Emerg. Med.* 8:243, 1990.

41. Kaplowitz, G. J. Developing and implementing a quality assurance program in a U.S. Coast Guard ambulatory health care facility. *Milit. Med.* 153:625, 1988.

42. Kelen, G. D. Reanalysis of surveillance data regarding health care worker risk of nosocomial

acquisition of HIV (edit.). *Ann. Emerg. Med.* 17:1101, 1988.

43. Kelen, G. D., et al. Unrecognized HIV infection in emergency department patients. *N. Engl. J. Med.* 318:1645, 1988.

44. Kind, A. C., and Williams, D. N., Persons, G., and Gibson, J. A. Intravenous antibiotic therapy at home. *Arch. Intern. Med.* 139:413, 1979.

45. Kunches, L. M., Craven, D. E., Werner, B. G., and Jacobs, L. M. Hepatitis B exposure in emergency medical personnel: Prevalence of serologic markers and need for immunization. *Am. J. Med.* 75:269, 1983.

46. Larson, E. Handwashing: It's essential: Even when you use gloves. *Am. J. Nurs.* 89:934, 1989.

47. Lynch, P., Jackson, M. M., Cummings, M. J., and Stamm, W. E. Rethinking the role of isolation practices in the prevention of nosocomial infections. *Ann. Intern. Med.* 107:243, 1987.

48. Marcus, R. A. Surveillance of health care workers exposed to blood from patients infected with the HIV. *N. Engl. J. Med.* 319:1118, 1988.

49. Moffet, H. L. Common infections in ambulatory patients. *Ann. Intern. Med.* 89(Part 2): 743, 1978.

50. National Academy of Sciences, National Research Council. *Accidental Death and Disability: The Neglected Disease of Modern Society.* Washington, DC: National Academy of Sciences, 1966.

51. Natof, H. E. Complications associated with ambulatory surgery. *J.A.M.A.* 244:1116, 1980.

52. Nolph, K. D., et al. Continuous ambulatory peritoneal dialysis: Three-year experience at one center. *Ann. Intern. Med.* 92:609, 1980.

53. Ornato, J. P., et al. Attitudes of BCLS instructors about mouth-to-mouth resuscitation during the AIDS epidemic. *Ann. Emerg. Med.* 19:151, 1990.

54. Pisarcik, G. Why patients use the emergency department. *J. Emerg. Nurs.* 6(2):16, 1980.

55. Poretz, D. M., et al. Intravenous antibiotic therapy in an outpatient setting. *J.A.M.A.* 248:336, 1982.

56. Riley, R. L., et al. Infectiousness of air from a tuberculosis ward: Ultraviolet irradiation of infected air: Comparative infectiousness of different patients. *Am. Rev. Respir. Dis.* 85:511, 1962.

57. Rosenblatt, R. A., Cherkin, D. C., Schneeweis, R., and Hart, L. G. The content of ambulatory medical care in the United States: An interspecialty comparison. *N. Engl. J. Med.* 309:892, 1983.

58. Sayre, M. R., and Lucid, E. J. Management of varicella-zoster virus–exposed hospital employees. *Ann. Emerg. Med.* 16:421, 1987.

59. Schroeder, S. The increasing use of emergency services. *West. J. Med.* 130:67, 1979.

60. Secord-Pletz, B. Prehospital Emergency Care and Transportation. In: T. C. Kravis, and C. G. Warner (Eds.), *Emergency Medicine: A Comprehensive Review.* Rockville, MD: Aspen Systems Corp, 1983 [2nd ed., 1987].

61. Sewell, C. M., et al. Staphylococcal nasal carriage and subsequent infection in peritoneal dialysis patients. *J.A.M.A.* 248:1493, 1982.

62. Shannon, K. Outpatient surgery up 77 percent: Data. *Hospitals* May 16:54, 1985.

63. Shannon, K. Outpatient surgery owes all to technology. *Hospitals* May 16:56, 1985.

64. Smego, R. A. Home intravenous antibiotic therapy (edit.). *Arch. Intern. Med.* 145:1001, 1985.

65. Spence, M. R., and Dash, G. P. Hepatitis B: Perceptions, knowledge and vaccine acceptance among registered nurses in high-risk occupations in a university hospital. *Infect. Control Hosp. Epidemiol.* 11:129, 1990.

66. Stebben, J. E. Sterile technique and the prevention of wound infection in office surgery: Part I. *J. Dermatol. Surg. Oncol.* 14:1364, 1988.

67. Stebben, J. E. Sterile technique and the prevention of wound infection in office surgery: Part II. *J. Dermatol. Surg. Oncol.* 15:38, 1989.

68. Stiver, H. G., et al. Intravenous antibiotic therapy at home. *Ann. Intern. Med.* 89(Part 1):690, 1978.

69. Swenson, J. P. Training patients to administer intravenous antibiotics at home. *Am. J. Hosp. Pharm.* 38:1480, 1981.

70. Swenson, J. P. Outpatient intravenous antibiotic therapy (lett.). *J.A.M.A.* 249:592, 1983.

71. Thomas, D. R., et al. Disposable insulin syringe reuse and antiseptic practices in diabetic patients. *J. Gen. Intern. Med.* 4:97, 1989.

72. Thurn, J., and Crossley, K. Needlestick injuries and needle disposal in Minnesota physicians' offices. *Am. J. Med.* 86:575, 1989.

73. U.S. Department of Labor and Department of Health and Human Services. Occupational exposure to bloodborne pathogens: Proposed rule and notices of hearings. *Fed. Reg.* 52(219):41818, October 30, 1987; *Fed. Reg.* 52(228):45438, November 27, 1987; *Fed. Reg.* 54(102):23042, May 30, 1989. Final Rule: *Fed. Reg.* 56(235):64004, Dec. 6, 1991.

74. U.S. Department of Labor, Office of Health Compliance Assistance. Enforcement procedures for occupational exposure to hepatitis B virus and human immunodeficiency virus. CPL 2-2.44, January 22, 1988 (rescinded); CPL 2-2.44A, August 15, 1988 (rescinded); CPL 2-2.44B, February 27, 1990. Washington, DC: OSHA, 1990.

75. Weinerman, E. R., et al. Yale studies in ambulatory medical care: V. Determinants of use of hospital emergency services. *Am. J. Public Health* 56:1037, 1966.

76. Yozzo, J. C. Is it feasible to track infections in an ambulatory surgery center? *J. Post Anesth. Nurs.* 4:255, 1989.

Infections in Nursing Homes

Richard A. Garibaldi
Brenda A. Nurse

The U.S. Census Bureau projects that by the year 2050, the segment of the population that is 65 years of age and older will increase by two and one-half times and that the group 85 years of age and older will be six and one-half times larger than in 1982. In numerical terms, this means that the number of persons 85 years of age and older will increase from approximately 2.5 million people to 16 million over the next 60 years. At the present time in the United States, approximately 5 percent of persons 65 years of age and older and 22 percent of persons 85 years of age or older reside in nursing homes. It is estimated that 25 percent of persons who are now older than 65 will spend some time during their life in such facilities [17]. As the population of elderly persons continues to grow, it is anticipated that the need for temporary and permanent nursing-home beds will also grow. In addition, an increasing number of beds will be needed for patients who are not elderly but who have a variety of chronic, debilitating conditions, including the acquired immunodeficiency syndrome (AIDS), that will require long-term, skilled nursing care. Our challenge as health care providers is to ensure that all these patients receive high-quality medical care and are able to maintain active lives without exposing them to the additional risks of diseases associated with institutionalization. This challenge is directed especially toward the infection control practitioner.

Many nursing-home patients are at increased risk for infection because of underlying, debilitating conditions that make them more susceptible to infection. These include diseases that alter immunologic reactivity, cause dysfunction in specific organ systems, limit mobility, impair cognitive skills, decrease ability to maintain personal hygiene, and necessitate the use of therapies that increase the risk of infection. In addition, the nursing-home environment itself provides a unique opportunity for the acquisition and transmission of infectious diseases. In the nursing home, aged patients are clustered together in a relatively confined setting, encouraged to participate in group activities, and cared for by professional and nonprofessional persons who may have limited training in the techniques of infection control. Additionally, due to understaffing, attendants may not follow all the recommended procedures dedicated to preventing the transmission of infection among patients. The combination of a susceptible population and a setting in which infections may be readily spread makes nursing-home patients vulnerable to frequent and serious problems with infections.

Recently, there has been an increased awareness of the magnitude of the problem of infections in the elderly in general and infections in elderly nursing-home patients in particular. Several studies are now available that have attempted to delineate the frequency of endemic and epidemic infections in nursing homes as well as to identify specific risk factors that predispose institutionalized patients to infections. This chapter reviews the epidemiology of infections in nursing homes and outlines aspects of nursing-home residence that promote the acquisition and transmission of these infections. Specific infections that are frequently encountered, including common epidemic infections, are discussed. Strategies to prevent infections and control spread are presented that are based on an understanding of the host factors that predispose nursing-home patients to infection and the unique features of nursing-home life that allow transmission to occur.

Epidemiology
The Nursing-Home Setting
Nursing homes vary in the levels of care that they are able to provide. The different types of nursing homes include day-care centers, domiciliary care homes, chronic-care units, skilled nursing facilities, and rehabilitation centers. Many nursing homes provide a broad range of nursing, psychosocial, and rehabilita-

tive services for patients who require different levels of medical or social supervision. Some nursing homes select patients according to the type of care that they require. Thus an entire nursing home population may be comprised of patients who require close medical supervision and skilled nursing care. Other homes may select patients who are relatively independent and require less assistance with their activities of daily living. Some homes specialize in specific types of rehabilitative or recuperative services, whereas others provide supportive care for the terminally ill. Some homes specialize in providing long-term care for selected subpopulations of patients such as veterans, paraplegics, patients with psychiatric diseases, or the mentally retarded. Some nursing homes have close working agreements with acute-care hospitals that facilitate the exchange of patients between institutions: Hospitalized patients are transferred to the nursing-home unit for less-intensive, lower-cost care or specific rehabilitative services, and nursing-home patients are transferred to the hospital unit for diagnostic evaluations or acute medical management. The demographic characteristics and level of debility of patients in an individual nursing home will vary according to the population for whom care is provided. The types and frequencies of infection will also vary greatly according to the specific referral pattern, patient population, and services provided in the nursing home.

Nursing homes are self-contained environments that provide total daily care for large numbers of needy patients. The nursing-home setting more closely resembles an acute-care hospital than an individual family unit. Bed capacities range from fewer than 50 to more than 300; the majority hold between 100 and 150 beds. Occupancy rates are generally high; in some homes, there is a waiting list for prospective residents. Patients usually occupy semiprivate rooms with 1 or 2 roommates. Private rooms are available for some. Infrequently, a ward with multiple occupants comprises the basic living unit. Patients who are ambulatory usually share a common cleanup area that contains a sink, toilet, and bathing facility. Nonambulatory patients frequently require the assistance of nursing-home employees to help them with personal needs such as washing, bathing, and toileting, which are usually performed in bed or in a chair in the patient's own room. Employees and family members may also assist with meals either in the patient's room or in a common area. Nursing aides or orderlies are often responsible for several patients and move from room to room to perform specified service assignments. These contacts may provide opportunities for the transmission of infectious diseases.

Characteristics of Nursing Homes that Predispose to Infection

Certain activities within the nursing-home setting are particularly conducive to the acquisition and transmission of infections. Nursing-home residents are encouraged to participate in group activities. Ambulatory patients usually eat in a common cafeteria, participate in group physical and occupational therapy sessions, and are gathered together to interact with one another in recreational programs. These activities are designed to encourage social exchanges, but they may also provide opportunities for the transmission of infection. Patients with mild upper respiratory illnesses, diarrhea, or conjunctivitis may not be excluded from group activities and may serve as sources for disease transmission. These risks are much greater for institutionalized patients than for elderly patients cared for at home.

Nursing homes, like hospitals, are reservoirs for potential infectious agents, particularly antibiotic-resistant bacteria [6] (see Chap. 13). Almost 40 percent of nursing-home residents are admitted from acute-care hospitals; more than 20 percent are transferred to the hospital from the nursing home for acute episodes of illness [17]. Patients are likely to become colonized with antibiotic-resistant flora during their hospital stay and to introduce it to the nursing-home environment when they return. The increased prevalence of colonization of nursing-home residents by antibiotic-resistant organisms has been well documented for sites such as the urinary tract, oropharynx, and skin. Asymptomatic colonization of the urinary tract is a

particularly common occurrence in the nursing home; the urine of patients with chronic, indwelling urethral catheters is virtually always colonized with one or more species of bacteria [4, 33]. Patient-to-patient spread of bacteria may occur indirectly by contact with personnel whose unwashed hands may serve as vectors for transmission. The chances for this type of transmission to occur are increased when patients with indwelling catheters are placed in the same room or clustered together in close proximity in group activities. Objects such as urine collection containers, bedpans, and nondisposable equipment may also become contaminated with bacteria and serve as inanimate reservoirs for common-source transmissions. Nursing-home patients with oropharyngeal or skin colonization with antibiotic-resistant organisms are at increased risk for clinical infections with these organisms and may serve as sources for their dissemination to other susceptible patients in the nursing home.

The likelihood for person-to-person transmission in the nursing home is increased because of difficulties in identifying infected patients and diagnosing the site of their infection with accuracy. The clinical presentations of infections in elderly and chronically ill patients are often atypical or nonspecific. Signs or symptoms usually associated with infections may be absent or diminished and may result in delays in diagnosis [5, 31]. For instance, an increased respiratory rate may be the only diagnostic clue for pneumonia; urinary tract infections may present with vague, nonspecific, systemic complaints such as anorexia, nausea, confusion, or memory loss. The detrimental effects of delayed diagnosis are twofold: The initiation of effective treatment may be late in the course of infection, and the spread of infection may occur before the clinical manifestations of the disease are recognized.

Because of the difficulties in clinically identifying infection in nursing home patients, more emphasis needs to be placed on laboratory studies to establish the diagnosis. However, nursing homes are often ill-equipped to do this. The relative lack of availability of adequate clinical microbiology laboratories and other diagnostic facilities may add further delay to the identification of infection. In most nursing homes, cultures are ordered infrequently, communications to and from an outside laboratory are slow, quality of information is unreliable, and interpretation of results may be erroneous. These limitations force physicians to diagnose and treat possible infections on an empiric basis. Thus antibiotics may be prescribed more frequently than is clinically indicated, and broader-spectrum drugs may be chosen to initiate therapy. These actions encourage the selection of antibiotic-resistant bacteria for colonization in treated patients and alter the endemic flora of bacteria in the nursing-home environment.

Certain administrative problems also contribute to the acquisition and spread of infections among patients. These include deficiencies in employee staffing and inadequate training in the basic principles of infection control. In most nursing homes, including skilled care facilities, patients are cared for by orderlies or aides who have little formal training in nursing techniques. Aides are often undertrained, undersupervised, and underpaid, which leads to substantial stress and an annual turnover rate of from 70 to 100 percent [4, 8]. High ratios of nonprofessional to professional staff and high rates of employee turnover in nursing homes make it extremely difficult to establish and maintain efficient programs for infection control.

Most nursing homes have infection control programs and designated infection control practitioners. Infection control programs are usually mandated by state law. In states where surveys have been completed, approximately 90 percent of nursing homes have had written infection control policies and committees that meet at least quarterly [11, 23]. In most nursing homes, however, the designated infection control practitioner has other responsibilities in addition to infection control. Usually, these responsibilities are administrative or supervisory rather than direct nursing care. Most infection control practitioners have had no specific training in infection control techniques or epidemiologic principles. Most nursing homes do not have trained physicians or epidemiologists to oversee their infection control activities. Although surveillance for infections is now routine in most nursing homes, it is usually not considered an adjunct to effective patient care. Programs for employee education in infection control often lack a systematic approach, occur infrequently, and are inadequate to meet the needs of the institution [11]. The combination of ineffective programs and poor compliance with routine infection control practices contributes to the spread of infections in nursing homes.

The difficulties in maintaining effective programs for infection control are compounded by the fact that there are also few standardized guidelines for employee health and infection prevention that focus on the unique problems of the nursing home. Some states have adapted infection control regulations from guidelines intended for patients in acute-care hospitals. Most states mandate that patients and employees be tested for tuberculosis at the time of admission or employment and yearly thereafter. However, there are no national requirements for tuberculin skin testing or for immunizations against influenza, pneumococcal infection, or other infectious agents for either residents or nursing-home staff. Many nursing homes offer immunizations to residents and employees but do not insist on compliance. No regulations exist to establish minimum staffing requirements or minimal levels in health education for nursing-home employees. Most nursing homes have no formal guidelines for monitoring the health status of employees at the time of hiring or during employment. Few nursing homes have formal policies to allow absenteeism for employees with possible communicable diseases. Usually, there is no compensation for sick time; thus, employees with acute infections might choose to go to work rather than remain at home, exposing susceptible nursing home residents to infections from the community.

Nursing-Home Patients

To understand the nature of infectious disease problems in nursing homes and the reasons why they occur, one must be familiar with the types of patients who receive care in this setting. The majority of patients are elderly and functionally disabled. The average age of nursing-home patients ranges between 80 and 85 years. In most institutions, as many as 20 percent of patients are 90 years of age or older. Approximately 75 percent of the residents of nursing homes are women; 96 percent are white. Patients are usually admitted to nursing homes for functional disabilities, such as dementia, incontinence, falls, or diminished levels of self-sufficiency, and because their family or community is unable to provide adequate support [14]. More than 90 percent of nursing-home patients require assistance in providing for their activities of daily living, such as bathing, dressing, toileting, maintaining continence, and transferring from bed or chair. In general, today's nursing-home residents are more functionally disabled and dependent than their counterparts in the 1970s [17]. In skilled nursing facilities, 35 to 50 percent of the population are nonambulatory and confined to bed and chair status; up to 5 percent are totally bedridden. As many as 50 percent of nursing-home residents are incontinent of urine and 30 to 40 percent are incontinent of feces. Many incontinent patients have substantial cognitive impairment and limited mobility. Between 5 and 10 percent of patients require chronic urinary drainage despite the known hazards of long-term catheterization and attempts by many nursing homes to avoid this invasive procedure if possible.

In addition to being old and functionally disabled, the typical nursing-home patient also has a variety of concurrent chronic conditions that may involve multiple organ systems. The average nursing-home patient has more than three diagnosed conditions recorded in the medical chart. Organic brain syndrome or dementia is the most common diagnosis, affecting up to 50 percent of nursing-home residents [17]. Other common problems include organic heart disease, cerebrovascular accidents, hypertension, arthritis, and previous fractures, each affecting more than 20 percent of patients [4]. Because of their long list of underlying medical problems, most nursing-home patients receive a large number of medications. Drugs are prescribed to treat underlying diseases, regulate body functions, control behavior, induce sleep, and prevent infections. Studies have shown that the average nursing-home patient receives between three and seven medications per day, many of which may be unneeded or ineffective. Cathartics, analgesics, and tranquillizers are the most commonly prescribed drugs. Antibiotics account for a relatively small percentage of all prescriptions and are often used in an attempt to suppress urinary tract infections. Presently, relatively few patients in nursing homes have intravenous lines, tracheostomies, gastrostomies, or nasogastric tubes; however, this may change as acute-care hospitals come under increasing economic pressure to discharge patients early.

Host Factors that Predispose Nursing-Home Patients to Infection

Many of the functional defects and underlying diseases that characterize nursing-home patients are also risk factors that predispose them to infection. These factors can be classified as either normal physiologic consequences of aging or pathologic processes related to disease conditions that accelerate the aging process. Physiologic changes that occur with normal aging include alterations in the composition of body water and fat, decreased efficiency of tissue repair and regeneration, depression of homeostatic mechanisms and responses to stress, and declines in the functional reserves of organs such as the kidneys, lungs, and brain [W. A. Tisdale; personal communication, 1989]. Some of these changes are associated with an increased risk of infection. Thus elderly nursing-home patients are often less tolerant to lipid-soluble drugs such as the benzodiazepines that can predispose to aspiration. Poor wound healing increases the risk for infected decubitus ulcers. Decreased gastric acidity permits infections with gastrointestinal pathogens that cause diarrheal diseases. Diminished vital capacity, impaired gag and cough reflexes, decreased ability to clear secretions, loss of lung elastic recoil, and weakened respiratory muscles are risk factors for lower respiratory tract infections [12]. Incomplete bladder emptying, impaired generation of acid urine, poor perineal hygiene, and postmenopausal estrogen deficiency predispose to urinary tract infections in the elderly. On the other hand, aging alone does not have a major impact on senescence or deterioration of immunologic functions. With increasing age, subtle changes have been noted in the humoral response to immunizing agents and skin test reactivity. However, diminished reactivity is usually associated with the presence of other underlying diseases that are known to depress immunologic response. Old age, per se, is not associated with significant physiologic deterioration or immunologic dysfunction that increases susceptibility to infection.

A variety of clinical conditions frequently found in nursing-home patients can predispose to infections. Examples of these include underlying diseases, severe levels of debility, impaired mentation, and receipt of medications that alter mental status or affect normal flora. These factors reflect pathologic changes that are consequences of the process of growing old. Patients with certain chronic diseases are predisposed to infectious complications that are directly or indirectly related to their primary disease process. For instance, patients with neurologic disorders or dementia may be unable to feed themselves, communicate effectively, recognize danger, protect themselves with reflex actions, or move in bed; they are at increased risk for aspiration pneumonia and pressure sores that may become subsequently infected. In addition, they are likely to be incontinent of urine or feces and to be treated with long-term, indwelling urinary catheterization. Often, they are agitated and require sedative or tranquillizing medications that additionally diminish their physiologic responsiveness and increase their risk for infection. Similarly, patients with other underlying diseases also have increased susceptibility for other infections. For instance, patients who are smokers or who have chronic pulmonary disease are at risk for respiratory infections because they are likely to have oropharyngeal colonization with gram-negative bacteria, dysfunctional mucociliary clearance, and depressed immunocyto-

logic responsiveness (see Chap. 29). Likewise, patients with congestive heart failure and chronic hypoxemia also have diminished pulmonary defenses and increased risks for pneumonia. Patients with hiatal hernias, esophageal motility disorders, autonomic neuropathy involving the esophagus or stomach, or unsuspected tumors are also at increased risk for aspiration. Patients with obstructive urinary flow secondary to prostatic hypertrophy, calculi, or uterine prolapse are at risk for urethral catheterization and urinary tract infection (see Chap. 28).

In addition to their underlying diseases, chronically ill nursing-home patients are plagued by a number of other limitations or frailties that increase their susceptibility to infections. Systemic conditions such as glucose intolerance, osteoporosis, and degenerative arthritis are common among all elderly. Gait disturbances, difficulty with balance, impaired coordination, easy fatigue, and subtle muscle weakness increase the likelihood for falls, fractures, and subsequent immobility. Nonambulatory patients are more likely than ambulatory patients to be incontinent, require urinary catheterization, develop pressure sores, and aspirate. Depression is a common problem in the elderly that may manifest itself by a loss of appetite, loss of energy, loss of involvement, or loss of a will to live. The presence of ill health and diminished levels of activity in chronically debilitated elderly nursing-home patients enhances their susceptibility to infection.

Surveys have shown that between 30 and 40 percent of chronically ill, debilitated nursing-home patients suffer from some degree of protein-calorie malnutrition. Malnourished patients frequently are unable to respond to skin test antigens, suggesting that they have significant impairments in cell-mediated immunity. Elderly patients with depressed skin test reactivity have a higher mortality (48 percent) during the 6-month period following testing than patients who are able to react (13 percent) [26]. Animal studies have shown associations between protein-calorie malnutrition and increased adherence of *Pseudomonas aeruginosa* to tracheal cells, decreased respiratory tract secretory IgA levels, and defective recruitment of macrophages into infected lungs. Deficiencies in vitamins, particularly vitamin B_6 and folate, and zinc ion may impair antibody responsiveness to antigens. Thus malnutrition in nursing-home patients may be another important factor in increasing their susceptibilities to infections.

Medications and other therapies prescribed for nursing-home patients may also predispose to infection. Use of sedatives and tranquillizers encourage aspiration; narcotic and atropine derivatives decrease mucociliary clearance function. Drugs that decrease lower esophageal sphincter pressure such as beta$_2$-agonists, caffeine, benzodiazepines, and calcium channel blockers increase the likelihood of gastric reflux and aspiration. Antibiotics alter the indigenous flora of the gastrointestinal tract, oropharynx, vagina, and perineum. Patients being treated with antibiotics are frequently colonized with antibiotic-resistant bacteria and are at increased risk for infection with these organisms (see Chap. 12). Antacids, H_2 blockers, and drugs that interfere with gastrointestinal motility predispose to enteric infection. Fortunately, invasive procedures are used infrequently in nursing homes with the exception of indwelling urinary catheters. At this time, there are no data to show that alternatives to chronic indwelling urethral catheterization, such as condom drainage, intermittent catheterization, or suprapubic drainage, are less likely to induce infection.

Endemic Infections

As yet, there are no comprehensive studies that use standard methodology to establish generalizable rates of endemic infections among nursing-home residents. Published data give inconsistent results from survey to survey. Overall prevalence rates vary from 2.7 to 17 percent [2, 4, 15, 21, 25]. The differences in rates reflect differences in patient populations, definitions of infection, case identification methodologies, and surveillance techniques. Lower rates are reported in surveys that include nursing homes that agreed to participate, use chart reviews as the sole methods for case finding, define infections stringently, and limit surveillance to specific sites. Higher rates are observed when chart reviews are augmented by patient examinations, definitions are less strict, infections at all sites are included, and asymptomatic as well as symptomatic patients are counted.

Urinary Tract Infections

Urinary tract infections are the most common type of institutionally acquired infection (see Chap. 28). In prevalence surveys, the rates of urinary tract infection among nursing-home residents range between 1.2 and 3.1 percent. Rates are higher in nursing homes where a large segment of the resident population is being treated with long-term, indwelling urinary catheters and in studies in which asymptomatic colonized patients are included. In most nursing homes, between 5 and 10 percent of the patients are catheterized. In some nursing homes that care for more debilitated patients or patients with spinal cord injuries, as many as 50 percent of the population may be catheterized. The longer the patients are catheterized, the more likely it is that bacteria will be found in their urine. Urinary colonization is in a constant state of influx, is usually polymicrobial, and involves organisms that are often resistant to commonly prescribed antibiotic agents [33]. Alternatives to indwelling, long-term urinary catheters (i.e., suprapubic catheters, intermittent catheters, condom catheters, and diapers) have not been well studied.

There is still some controversy concerning the significance of asymptomatic bacteriuria in noncatheterized elderly and how to manage it when it is found. The prevalence of bacteriuria in young and middle-aged women is approximately 5 percent and in men is less than 0.1 percent. In patients older than 65 years, rates of bacteriuria are higher in both sexes, with 20 to 30 percent of women and 10 to 15 percent of men being affected [1]. Rates are even higher in elderly residents in nursing homes than in elderly men and women living at home. As the functional status of the patient decreases, the rate of bacteriuria increases. The higher rates seen in nursing-home and hospitalized patients correlate well with a more debilitated clinical status, which is often complicated by fecal incontinence, bladder dysfunction, and an increased incidence of catheterization. Boscia and co-workers [1] identified positive urine cultures in 36 percent of nursing-home residents from whom three urine samples were collected at 6-week intervals. Often there was spontaneous resolution of asymptomatic bacteriuria without specific intervention, although some patients did go on to develop symptomatic infection. Nicolle and colleagues [19, 20] reported no improvement in rates of morbidity or mortality when asymptomatic bacteriuria was treated with antibiotic therapy.

In a prevalence survey, Garibaldi and associates [4] identified 14 symptomatic urinary tract infections among 532 residents of seven Salt Lake City nursing homes, for a rate of 2.6 percent. In these homes, 63 of the 532 patients were chronically catheterized. Eighty-five percent of the urine specimens taken from chronically catheterized patients revealed bacteriuria with at least 10^5 colony-forming units (cfu) per milliliter of urine. The rates of bacteriuria were similar in patients receiving chronic suppressive therapy and in those who did not. An average of two bacterial species was recovered from each positive urine specimen. The most common isolates were enterococci, *Proteus vulgaris, Escherichia coli, Proteus mirabilis,* and *Providencia stuartii.* Two-thirds of the bacterial isolates were resistant to ampicillin, two-thirds to cephalothin, one-third to trimethoprim-sulfamethoxazole, and one-fifth to gentamicin.

Other studies of chronically catheterized nursing-home patients have revealed results similar to these. In one study in which weekly cultures were collected, the prevalence of bacteriuria approached 100 percent with a mean of 2.6 organisms identified in each specimen [33]. In these patients, changes in bacterial strains were detected every 2 weeks. Episodes of bacteriuria with *P. stuartii, P. mirabilis, E. coli,* and *P. aeruginosa* were frequently identified. The persistence of colonization

varied with different organisms. For example, when *P. stuartii* gained access to the urinary tract, it persisted for an average of 10 weeks; some episodes of bacteriuria with this organism lasted as long as 36 weeks. In contrast, most gram-positive organisms, with the exception of enterococci, were recovered in only a single weekly culture. Other gram-negative organisms persisted for 2 to 5 weeks. Thus it appears that bacterial colonization of the chronically catheterized urinary tract is in a constant state of flux. The changing pattern of urinary colonization undermines the rationale for collecting routine urine surveillance cultures. It is imperative for physicians to obtain a fresh urine culture before treating symptomatic urinary tract infections in catheterized patients.

Skin Infections

Rates of skin and subcutaneous infection vary from 1.1 to 6 percent in prevalence surveys. Two studies in which the prevalence of superficial skin infections was 5 percent and 6 percent used clinical criteria to define an infection [4, 13]. Studies that have reported lower rates have used stricter definitions. Skin and wound infections often occur in sites of decubitus ulcers.

It is estimated that up to 3 percent of patients in acute-care facilities develop decubitus ulcers during their hospital stay, whereas 45 percent in chronic-care facilities are at risk [22]. The prevalence of pressure ulcers among patients on admission to skilled nursing facilities ranges from 15 to 25 percent [18]. There are a number of factors that, either alone or in conjunction with others, can cause decubitus ulcers. They include extrinsic factors such as unrelieved pressure (by far the most important); shearing, which occurs when a person's body changes position without a compensatory change in skin position; friction, which removes the stratum corneum and increases risk for early superficial ulceration; and moisture secondary to perspiration and urinary or fecal soilage. The intrinsic factors that can play a role include obesity, anemia, joint contractures and spasticity, diabetes mellitus, edema, and malnutrition [22]. Often, it is difficult to distinguish uninfected pressure sores from superficial skin infections. Wound cultures should not be obtained from decubitus ulcer sites that have no clinical evidence of infection. Positive cultures in such a situation may only reflect colonization of the site and do not support the use of antibiotic therapy (see Chap. 37).

Respiratory Tract Infections

Respiratory tract infections are reported to be present in between 0.3 and 3.6 percent of nursing-home residents; approximately 50 percent involve the lower respiratory tract. Pneumonia and influenza constitute the leading cause of death secondary to infection in the elderly and are the fourth most common cause of death overall (see Chap. 29). Many of the patients who develop pneumonia have underlying disease processes that have predisposed them to the infection. Examples of conditions that increase risk include emphysema, chronic obstructive pulmonary disease (COPD), bronchitis, and alcohol use and abuse. Indirect factors include cancer, malnutrition, cerebrovascular disease, and medications that increase risk of aspiration.

The prevalence of respiratory tract infections varies according to the time of year and occurrence of infections in the community. In the nursing home, the diagnosis of respiratory tract infection is often ambiguous. Objective verification is uncommon. Roentgenograms are not usually available and physical examination findings are often not included in the medical record. Gram stain and cultures of sputum are not always obtained because of difficulty in getting adequate specimens; when this information is available, it can be difficult to interpret. Patients with pneumonia in nursing homes are infected with organisms more like those seen in hospitalized patients with nosocomial pneumonias than those found in patients with community-acquired pneumonia [2]. In the nursing home, bacteria such as *Klebsiella pneumonia, E. coli, Proteus species,* and *Staphylococcus aureus* are more commonly seen. Organisms identified in nursing-home pneumonias are likely to be resistant to commonly prescribed

antibiotics. It is prudent for clinicians to know the prevalence of antibiotic-resistant bacteria in the nursing home where they practice and to obtain appropriate cultures before initiating therapy. When empiric therapy is prescribed, broad-spectrum antibiotics should be used; the spectrum of coverage should be narrowed once sensitivities are known.

Other Infections

There is a growing concern about *methicillin-resistant S. aureus* (MRSA) in chronic-care facilities that parallels its increasing incidence in acute-care hospitals [29] (see Chaps. 12, 37). Once introduced into the nursing home, MRSA can be extremely difficult to eradicate. The common mechanism of spread is person-to-person, frequently being carried on the hands of a health care worker and transmitted in the course of patient care. It is often difficult to determine whether the patient is actively infected with the organism or only colonized. The most frequent sites of colonization are wounds, decubitus ulcers, indwelling bladder catheters, and the anterior nares. Risk factors for colonization include serious or chronic underlying disease, prior hospitalization, exposure to a colonized health care worker or patient, presence of invasive devices and, most importantly, prior receipt of broad-spectrum antibiotics [30].

Given the nursing-home environment, it is extremely difficult to isolate patients colonized with MRSA. Unless a respiratory source is found, patients should be routinely cared for under the umbrella of universal precautions. Staff having significant touch contact with a colonized patient should wear gloves or gowns. When possible, the patient should be placed in a private room. If more than one patient is infected or colonized, it is reasonable to cohort them until they are cleared of the organism. Combination therapy with trimethoprim-sulfamethoxazole (if the organism is sensitive) and rifampicin may be prescribed in an effort to eliminate asymptomatic colonization with MRSA; also, a topical agent such as mupirocin may be applied to the anterior nares. The addition of an antimicrobial cleanser to the patient's bath once daily may further decrease significant bacterial counts from the skin. Even with aggressive therapy, success in eradicating the organism is not guaranteed, and relapses after treatment are frequent (see Chap. 37).

Epidemic Infections

A number of reports have been published concerning outbreaks of infections in nursing homes. However, most clusters of nosocomial infection go unrecognized because they are either not identified or not thoroughly investigated.

Respiratory Infections
The respiratory tract is, by far, the most frequent site of epidemic infection in the nursing home (see Chap. 29). This is a consequence of the community atmosphere that is encouraged in many nursing homes and the close contacts that patients have with one another. There have been several reports of tuberculosis clusters in susceptible nursing-home residents as well as outbreaks of such viral infections as influenza A and B, respiratory syncytial virus (RSV), and parainfluenza.

Infections with influenza viruses can be severe in debilitated nursing-home patients. The reported case fatality ratio for influenza A is as high as 30 percent [7]. Epidemic influenza infections usually occur concurrently with community outbreaks. Influenza is introduced into the institution by employees or visitors who interact with patients. In nursing homes, the attack rate for clinical infection among unvaccinated patients usually ranges between 25 and 40 percent. Although influenza A and B rarely cause primary pneumonia, they can increase susceptibility to secondary bacterial pneumonias with *Streptococcus pneumoniae, S. aureus,* or *Hemophilus influenzae.* This underscores the importance of an aggressive annual influenza immunization program in nursing homes that encompasses both patients and employees. Although there is conflicting information on the efficacy of vaccine in preventing influenza infections among older patients, immunization appears

to reduce substantially the risk of dying from influenza.

RSV usually causes infection in young children but can be seen in any age group. There have been outbreaks of RSV reported in nursing homes. Morales and colleagues [16] have suggested that RSV infections in the elderly may be reinfections in individuals who are no longer immune. Parainfluenza virus has also been implicated in nursing-home outbreaks. Infection with parainfluenza virus may cause either upper respiratory infection or pneumonia; the diagnosis is made by serology.

The tuberculosis case rate in nursing-home residents older than 65 years is four times higher than that in community residents of the same age [1]. Epidemics of tuberculosis in nursing homes have been documented as well. In one outbreak, 47 of 102 previously uninfected residents (46 percent) became infected from a single index case [27]. Stead and co-workers [28] have observed a low prevalence of tuberculosis skin test reactivity at the time of nursing-home admission in Arkansas. In follow-up, however, there was an annual increase in infection rate of between 3.5 and 5.0 percent, suggesting exogenous infection [28]. At this time, it is recommended to treat elderly skin test convertors since many elderly patients in nursing homes are not immune and are susceptible to progressive primary infection. Although there is a reported incidence of hepatotoxicity with the use of isoniazid (INH) that increases with increasing age, this should not prohibit the use of INH in the elderly. In one report, only 3 of 39 (7.7 percent) elderly nursing-home patients receiving preventive therapy with INH were unable to complete therapy because of hepatitis. In the 36 treated patients, there were no documented cases of subsequent disease; however, 2 of 5 convertors who were not treated developed disease [27]. Today, most nursing homes have policies for initial and annual purified protein derivative of tuberculin (PPD) skin testing of patients and employees, but the effectiveness of such programs is hampered by lack of compliance with policies, anergic reactions to skin tests, and inaccurate interpretation of results.

Gastroenteritis

Occurrences of other types of epidemic infections among nursing-home patients are reported less commonly [9]. Outbreaks of diarrheal disease secondary to Salmonella infection have been reported in the nursing-home setting (see Chap. 30). Often, there is significant morbidity and mortality with these infections, given the already debilitated status of many nursing-home patients. Case clusters of salmonellosis have been associated with both person-to-person transmission and common-source spread, from tube feedings or other food items contaminated with this organism.

Outbreaks of virus-mediated diarrhea have been seen as well. Rotavirus has been described as the causative agent in at least three outbreaks involving long-term care facilities in Norway, London, and Nova Scotia. The Norwalk-like agents have also been implicated in an outbreak of gastroenteritis in a nursing home in Maryland, with an attack rate of 46 percent; the spread of illness suggested person-to-person transmission [10]. There have been instances of diarrhea outbreaks in nursing homes with *E. coli* 0157:H7 causing hemorrhagic colitis. In the elderly, this agent can be associated with a hemolytic uremia syndrome with a high rate of mortality [24]. Lastly, clusters of cases of diarrhea and pseudomembranous colitis secondary to *Clostridium difficile* infection have now been reported from several long-term care facilities. The occurrence of this problem is very likely related to increased antibiotic use in these patients, with transmission by person-to-person contacts and contaminated objects. It is important to recognize that many of these infections can involve staff as well as patients.

Urinary Tract Infection

Scattered outbreaks of epidemic catheter-associated urinary tract infections have been described, particularly from chronic-care facilities that manage large numbers of patients with long-term indwelling urinary catheters.

Infection is believed to be transmitted from patient to patient by passive carriage of bacteria on the hands of personnel. These outbreaks are characterized by high rates of infection or asymptomatic colonization with bacterial species such as *P. stuartii, Proteus rettgeri,* or *Serratia marcescens* that are resistant to multiple antibiotics. Often, an individual nursing home will have its own pattern of endemic flora colonizing the urinary tracts of both catheterized and noncatheterized patients [4]. Among chronically catheterized patients, colonization by *Providencia* or *Proteus* species occurs frequently; these organisms appear to have unique abilities to persist in the catheterized urinary tract, perhaps because of their adherence to the surface of the catheter itself [32].

The Infection Control Program

An effective infection program should provide timely recognition of nosocomial infection problems and prevent disease transmission in the nursing home. Standards outlined by the Joint Commission for Accreditation of Healthcare Organizations (JCAHO) and other regulatory bodies have influenced many of the basic components found in infection control programs in both acute-care hospitals and nursing homes. The key to successful infection control is a commitment to the purpose and an understanding of the necessity for such a program. This includes the active participation of personnel interested in infection control, a regular system of surveillance to identify problems, and the implementation of procedures to prevent the acquisition of infections and control their transmission. The primary goal of any program is disease prevention. The major objectives of infection control programs in nursing homes are very similar to those in the acute-care setting; however, some of the specific problems and solutions may be very different (see Chap. 4).

The Infection Control Committee

The core element for an effective infection control program is the Infection Control Committee and the cooperative efforts of its members (see Chap. 4). In many nursing homes, the position of chairperson is delegated to the medical director or to an attending physician who has an interest in infectious diseases or infection control. A physician as chairperson or co-chairperson lends both credibility and authority to the committee and enables it to deal more effectively with other physicians and administrators. Critical members of the committee include an infection control practitioner, the nursing-home administrator, and director of nursing.

The role of the infection control practitioner is pivotal for program operations in any setting; this is even more true in the nursing home or chronic-care facility. Not every facility has a full-time infection control practitioner. In some nursing homes, the infection control practitioner is also the director of nursing. In others, the job may span two departments, incorporating employee health responsibilities with infection control. To be able to function effectively, the infection control practitioner should have a basic understanding of infectious diseases, microbiology, epidemiology, and public health, as well as an in-depth knowledge of nursing technique and aseptic practice. It is also important to have excellent communication skills, have the respect of the staff, and have a desire to become educated in the discipline of infection control. With widespread concerns today involving work-related exposures and life-threatening infectious agents, including the human immunodeficiency virus, the role of the infection control practitioner has expanded to include that of advisor and confidante as well as teacher.

The facility's administrator plays an important role on the Infection Control Committee. At committee meetings, he or she will participate in discussions with appropriate staff about infection control issues and become informed about state or national standards that require compliance. The administrator needs to be informed about infectious diseases that are prevalent in the nursing home and plans for infection control. In return, the administrator can provide the committee with realistic expectations of the institution's ability to comply with the committee's recommendations. Ultimately, he or she will be critical in the communication, implementation, and enforcement of facilitywide decisions.

The other members of the Infection Control Committee should represent the interdisciplinary nature of infection control activities throughout the facility. Representatives from nursing, dietary services, pharmacy, housekeeping and building services, maintenance, and other specialty departments, if present within the facility, should be included as well. Often a member from the local health department is invited to attend, although his or her presence is not mandatory at meetings.

Surveillance

Rates of infection should be determined by periodic surveys of disease incidence or prevalence. The procedures used to perform surveillance will vary from institution to institution. In conducting surveillance, it is important to use the same methodologic techniques of data collection in each survey, utilizing standard definitions of infection, reproducible methods for case identification, and consistent data sources for the calculation of rates (see Chap. 5). By using standard techniques, individual nursing homes will be able to generate data that will establish relative norms to characterize the pattern and identify trends in endemic infections for their institution. With this information, they will be able to evaluate changes in nosocomial infections and identify clusters or outbreaks. Documentation of clinical infections with bacteriologic cultures is essential for an effective surveillance program.

The surveillance program should describe institutionally acquired infections by site, etiology, room location, date of onset, and relationship to iatrogenic manipulations. A number of approaches may be needed to identify new infections in the nursing-home setting; routine chart reviews will not identify the onset or even the presence of most infections. Daily temperature elevations may not be recorded on a regular basis, making review of the vital signs sheet an incomplete source of information to screen for infections. Even when daily temperature recordings are available, the information may be misleading; elderly patients frequently do not respond to infection with a febrile reaction. There is no effective substitution for regular rounds of the nursing units, where the infection control practitioner can talk to the nurses and nursing assistants who provide daily, direct patient care. Review of the staff nurses' notes in the medical record or bedside chart may provide helpful clues to identifying infections. Personnel working on the nursing unit should be encouraged to report newly diagnosed nosocomial infections. Specially designated liaison nurses can be trained to become infection control extenders and encouraged to participate in surveillance activities on their nursing units. Surveillance of new prescriptions for antibiotics can also identify newly infected patients. Routine collection of surveillance cultures from environmental sources or patients, even urine from chronically catheterized patients, is not recommended. It is the responsibility of the infection control practitioner to compile the results of surveillance activities on a regular basis for presentation to the Infection Control Committee.

When an unusual clustering of cases is noted, the infection control practitioner should perform an epidemiologic investigation (see Chap. 6). The investigation should include the identification of the problem, a case count that documents the number of patients involved, and an analysis of cases by time, place, and person. In most instances, this type of investigation will reveal the extent of the epidemic and the pattern of disease transmission. With this information, the infection control practitioner can recommend appropriate control measures to the Infection Control Committee. On rare occasions, the extent of the problem may be great, or seemingly appropriate control measures may be ineffective. In these situations, the nursing-home administrator or medical director should be alerted and outside help obtained. Sources of outside help include infection control practitioners in other institutions, the local health department, infectious disease practitioners from the community, epidemi-

ologists at a local acute-care hospital, the state health department, or the Centers for Disease Control, Atlanta.

Infection Control Procedures

When an infection control problem is identified, it is the infection control practitioner's responsibility to implement effective intervention. The problem may be an increased frequency of a specific type of infection, a breakdown in aseptic technique, failure to understand or initiate specific isolation precautions, or a possible epidemic occurrence of infection. In each of these situations, the infection control practitioner needs to intervene with an action plan to correct the problem and educate the involved staff. The practitioner should maintain contact with the staff on a regular basis to make sure that the problem is resolved.

An appropriate time to introduce the concepts and application of infection control to new employees is during their initial orientation to the institution. At this time, the infection control practitioner can review the risks of infections in the nursing home and the techniques of infection control. This is also a time to evaluate the new employees' knowledge and performance of infection control practices. For all employees, ongoing educational programs should be scheduled to review new techniques in infection control. These sessions may also serve as problem-solving exercises in which issues raised by employees are discussed. There are many issues on which the infection control practitioner can focus during employee updates. She or he may want to devote some of this time to the review of proper techniques of indwelling urinary catheter care or decubitus ulcer prevention. Educational programs should discuss the value of hand-washing and emphasize the concept of universal precautions (see Chap. 11). Universal precautions stress the potential infectivity of all blood and body fluids. The switch from disease-specific precautions to universal precautions incorporates appropriate isolation techniques with the use of gloves, gowns, and goggles when contact with blood or secretions is likely. Most diseases, except for those that are spread by the respiratory route, such as tuberculosis and varicella, are adequately managed by universal precautions. Universal precautions also provide protection for employees who care for patients infected with the human immunodeficiency virus (see Chap. 39).

Both patients and employees with communicable diseases should be identified early, and proper precautions should be taken to prevent the spread of infection within the institution. Patients with infectious diseases should have their activities restricted. The type and severity of isolation precautions must be individualized according to the type of infection and the patient's total needs. Ill employees should remain at home. Visitors with symptoms of acute infection should not be allowed to see patients in the facility.

Employee Health

The surveillance and control of infections in employees is as important as the prevention of infection in patients (see Chap. 3). Nursing homes should have a system for monitoring the health of their personnel. At the time of employment, all personnel should be evaluated to rule out the presence of acute or chronic infectious disease (e.g., PPD skin testing to rule out tuberculosis). An employee's immunization status should be questioned, checked, and updated. This information can be collected by the employee's private physician, with results sent to the nursing home, or by the infection control practitioner, who in many institutions also serves as the employee health nurse. Even though the size of the facility may preclude the feasibility of a formal employee health program, all nursing homes should maintain a file of health-related problems for each of their employees and provide a means to evaluate acutely ill staff members who might be infected. Employees who develop acute infections should be encouraged to seek early medical evaluation to determine their infectivity. Infected personnel should be given time off from work without being penalized. Lastly, appropriate vaccinations should be offered to all employees in a timely manner. For instance, an annual influenza vaccination for employees will protect not only the medical staff but also the patients with whom they work.

Administrative Considerations

An effective infection control program requires more than surveillance and control activities by an infection control practitioner. Nursing homes must provide a professional staff of adequate size during each shift to care for patients and maintain sound infection control practices. Staff members should have a basic understanding of techniques to prevent disease transmission. Appropriate financial or fringe-benefit incentives must be offered to attract professionally trained personnel to nursing homes and reverse the trend of high employee job turnover. A stable, conscientious, well-educated team of patient care providers is likely to exercise good infection control practices and respond to educational efforts. Such a team, together with a competent infection control practitioner, will have a great impact on diminishing the spread of infections within the nursing home.

References

1. Boscia, J.A., et al. Epidemiology of bacteriuria in an elderly ambulatory population. *Am. J. Med.* 80:208, 1986.
2. Cohen, E.D., Hierholzer, W.J., Schilling, C.R., and Snydman, D.R. Nosocomial infections in skilled nursing facilities: A preliminary survey. *Public Health Rep.* 94:162, 1979.
3. Garb, J.L., Brown, R.B., Garb, J.R., and Tuthill, R.W. Differences in etiology of pneumonias in nursing home and community patients. *J.A.M.A.* 240:2169, 1978.
4. Garibaldi, R.A., Brodine, S., and Matsumiya, S. Infections among patients in nursing homes: Policies, prevalence and problems. *N. Engl. J. Med.* 305:731, 1981.
5. Garibaldi, R.A., and Nurse, B.A. Infections in the elderly. *Am. J. Med.* 81 (Suppl. 1a):53, 1986.
6. Gaynes, R.P., Weinstein, R.A., Chamberlin, W., and Kabins, S.A. Antibiotic-resistant flora in nursing home patients admitted to the hospital. *Arch. Intern. Med.* 145:1804, 1985.
7. Goodman, R.A. et al. Impact of influenza A in a nursing home. *J.A.M.A.* 247:1451, 1982.
8. Institute of Medicine, Committee on Nursing

Home Regulations. *Improving the Quality of Care in Nursing Homes.* Washington, DC: National Academy Press, 1986.

9. Jackson, M.M., and Fierer, J. Infections and infection risk in residents of long-term care facilities: A review of the literature, 1970–1984. *Am. J. Infect. Control* 13:63, 1985.

10. Kaplan, J.E., et al. Epidemiology of Norwalk gastroenteritis and the role of Norwalk virus in outbreaks of acute nonbacterial gastroenteritis. *Ann. Intern. Med.* 96:756, 1982.

11. Khabbaz, R.F., and Tenney, J.H. Infection control in Maryland nursing homes. *Infect. Control Hosp. Epidemiol.* 9:159, 1988.

12. Krumpe, P.E., Kundson, R.J., Parsons, G., and Reiser, K. The aging respiratory system. *Clin. Geriatr. Med. North Am.* 1:143, 1985.

13. Lester, M.R. Looking inside 101 nursing homes. *Am. J. Nurs.* 64:111, 1964.

14. Libow, L.S., and Starer, P. Care of the nursing home patient. *N. Engl. J. Med.* 321:93, 1989.

15. Magnussen, M.H., and Robb, S.S. Nosocomial infections in a long-term care facility. *Am. J. Insect. Control* 8:12, 1980.

16. Morales, F., et al. A study of respiratory infections in the elderly to assess the role of RSV. *J. Infect.* 7:236, 1983.

17. National Center for Health Statistics and Hing, E. *Use of Nursing Homes by the Elderly: Preliminary Data from the 1985 National Nursing Home Survey.* Advance Data from Vital and Health Statistics, no. 135. D.II.II.S. Pub. No. (P.H.S.) 87-1250. Hyattsville, MD: Public Health Service, May 14, 1987.

18. National Pressure Ulcer Advisory Panel. Pressure ulcers: Prevalence, costs and risk assessment: Consensus development conference statement. *Decubitus* 2(2):24, 1989.

19. Nicolle, L.E., et al. The association of bacteriuria with resident characteristics and survival in elderly institutionalized men. *Ann. Intern. Med.* 106:682, 1987.

20. Nicolle, L.E., Mayhew, W.J., and Bryan, L. Prospective randomized comparison of therapy and no therapy for asymptomatic bacteriuria in institutionalized elderly women. *Am. J. Med.* 83:27, 1987.

21. Nicolle, L.E., McIntyre, M., Zacharias, H., and MacDonnell, J.A. Twelve-month surveillance of infections in institutionalized elderly men. *J. Am. Geriatr. Soc.* 32:513, 1984.

22. Nurse, B.A., and Collins, M.R. Skin Care and Decubitus Ulcer Management in the Elderly Stroke Patient. In: R. V. Erickson (Ed.), *Physical Medicine and Rehabilitation. Medical Management of the Elderly Stroke Patient,* Vol. 3. Philadelphia: Hanley & Belfus, 1989. P. 549.

23. Price, L.E., Sarabbi, F.A., and Rutala, W.A. Infection control programs in twelve North Carolina extended care facilities. *Infect. Control* 6:437, 1985.

24. Ryan, C.A., et al. *E. coli* 0157:H7 diarrhea in a nursing home: Clinical epidemiological and pathological findings. *J. Infect. Dis.* 154:631, 1986.

25. Scheckler, W.E., and Peterson, P.J. Infections and infection control among residents of eight rural Wisconsin nursing homes. *Arch. Intern. Med.* 146:1981, 1986.

26. Shaver, H.J., Loper, J.A., and Lutes, R.A. Nutritional status of nursing home patients. *J.P.E.N.* 4:367, 1980.

27. Stead, W.W. Tuberculosis among elderly persons: An outbreak in a nursing home. *Ann. Intern. Med.* 94:606, 1981.

28. Stead, W.W., Lofgren, J.P., Warren, E., and Thomas, C. Tuberculosis as an endemic and nosocomial infection among the elderly in nursing homes. *N. Engl. J. Med.* 312:1483, 1985.

29. Storch, G.A., Radcliff, J.L., Meyer, P.L., and Hinrichs, J.H. Methicillin-resistant *Staphylococcus aureus* in a nursing home. *Infect. Control* 8(1):24, 1987.

30. Thompson, R.L., Cabezudo, I., and Wenzel, R.P. Epidemiology of nosocomial infections caused by methicillin-resistant *Staphylococcus aureus. Ann. Intern. Med.* 97:309, 1982.

31. Verghese, A., and Berk, S.L. Bacterial pneumonia in the elderly. *Medicine* 62:271, 1983.

32. Warren, J.W. *Providencia stuartii:* A common cause of antibiotic-resistant bacteriuria in patients with long-term indwelling catheters. *Rev. Infect. Dis.* 8:61, 1986.

33. Warren, J.W., et al. A prospective microbiologic study of bacteriuria in patients with chronic indwelling urethral catheters. *J. Infect. Dis.* 146:719, 1982.

25

Cost-Benefit Analysis of Infection Control Programs

Robert W. Haley

Economic Analysis in Infection Control

Economic concerns have taken on increasing importance in infection control since the mid-1970s. The increase in published scientific articles on economic aspects of infection control have followed closely both the proliferation of organized infection control programs and the nationwide expenditures on health care in the United States [86] (Fig. 25-1). During these years, the growing recognition of the preventive value of organized infection control programs was stimulating pressure on hospital administrators to allocate more resources to such programs, while they were simultaneously being pressured to reduce overhead costs to keep their hospitals financially viable. Both their patients and their medical staffs were pressing for more patient care programs but, while the advocates for prevention were relatively few, their voices were sustained largely by the force of the accreditation process. Faced with having to decide whether to put available financial resources into new patient care programs that generate direct revenue and profit or into infection prevention programs that do not, tough-minded administrators have been understandably reluctant to invest in prevention programs without some reasonable assurances that the programs would be effective in reducing nosocomial infection risks and thereby would contribute to the hospital's financial solvency. To compete successfully for resources, the advocates of infection control programs have responded with an increasingly sophisticated array of economic analyses substantiating the economic benefits of their programs. Since the decisions on hospital expenditures are influenced by authorities both in hospitals and in advisory and

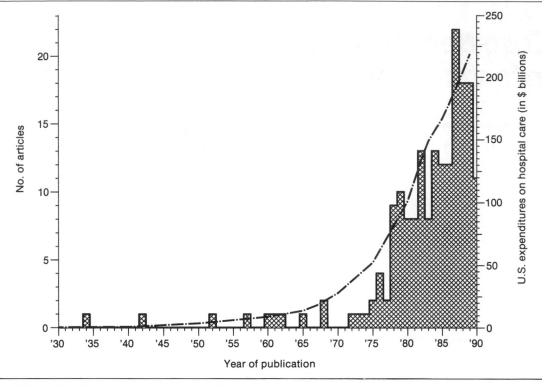

Fig. 25-1. The increase in the number of articles on the economics of nosocomial infections and infection control in scientific journals (histogram) in relation to the increases in expenditures for hospital care in the United States (broken line). (Hospital care expenditures data from S.W. Letsch, K.R. Levitt, and D.R. Waldo. National health expenditures, 1987. *Health Care Financ. Rev.* 10:1019, 1988.)

regulatory agencies outside of hospitals, the economic arguments have been targeted at both the hospital level and at the national or international levels.

Current estimates of the economic impact of nosocomial infections can be found in Chapter 27 under the heading Adverse Effects of Nosocomial Infections. This chapter will focus on the issues involved in conducting and interpreting studies on the economics of nosocomial infections and infection control.

Types of Economic Analyses
Studies on the economics of nosocomial infections and infection control have been mainly of the following four types: (1) estimates of the costs, and thus the potential benefits through prevention, of nosocomial infections (cost estimates); (2) comparisons of

the costs of providing an infection control program and its potential economic benefits (cost-benefit analyses); (3) estimates of the financial savings to be obtained by an infection control program's eliminating unnecessary, often ritualistic, practices in patient care or in their own programs (cost-containment studies); and (4) comparisons of the relative efficiency of alternative strategies for bringing about given improvements in particular patient outcomes (cost-effectiveness analyses). Whereas the distinctions among these different types of analyses have often been blurred, from the frequency with which they have been used and reported, each appears to have been used persuasively in convincing hospital administrators to invest resources in infection control.

This chapter will deal primarily with cost

estimates and cost-benefit analyses (recognizing, of course, that the first is a necessary component of the second), because they should ultimately prove the most convincing to administrators. This is not to discourage cost-containment studies [7, 22, 24, 40, 44, 52, 97, 99, 117, 148] and cost-effectiveness studies [36, 96, 116, 134, 141] related to infection control, for they also can be useful. Nonetheless it must be recognized that, while the latter two techniques deal with more immediate and tangible financial savings, their ultimate financial impact is substantially less than the potential savings from reductions in nosocomial infections brought about by effective infection surveillance and control programs, which is measured by cost-benefit analysis.

Cost-Benefit Analysis

Cost-benefit analysis is the exercise of estimating, in comparable economic units (usually a particular monetary currency, such as U.S. dollars), all of the costs and benefits of a proposed program regardless of to whom they accrue, over as long a period as is pertinent and practicable [78]. The balance, or ratio, of the costs and benefits provides a measure of the value of the program, which can be compared with similar measures for competing programs, even though the programs and health outcomes of the programs are entirely disparate. For example, it would be reasonable to compare the cost-benefit ratio of an infection control program with that of a proposed renal dialysis center or radiologic imaging device. (Note that cost-effectiveness analysis, which compares the costs of alternative strategies for achieving a given outcome, cannot be used to compare programs that affect different outcomes.)

Although the basic concept of cost-benefit analysis seems straightforward, serious methodologic problems surface as soon as one begins to design an analysis of a particular program to influence a specific decision maker. For instance, one must decide whether *all* the costs and benefits are to be included or only those of interest to the particular decision maker to whom the study is directed. A complete cost-benefit analysis would estimate all the costs of nosocomial infections that are to be saved by effective infection control, including the physicians' fees and costs to the patient from time off work, but few published studies have included these because they may be of little strategic interest to hospital administrators. Similarly, one must decide whether to measure hospital charges attributable to nosocomial infection, which are easily obtained from the patient's hospital bill, or actual costs incurred by the hospital as a result of the patient's nosocomial infection, which is far more difficult to obtain, requiring a type of cost-accounting system that exists in few hospitals. Since patient charges are different from hospital costs, can they be compared with the costs incurred by the hospital for supporting its infection control program? These and the other equally troublesome methodologic decisions listed in Tables 25-1 and 25-2 explain the wide variation in designs and methods used in the published cost-benefit studies of infection control.

It is of interest that cost-benefit analysis is of rather recent origin, its first serious applications appearing in the late 1950s [78]. Consequently, its quantitative methods are still developing. The major advances in its application to infection control have occurred since the early 1980s. It is no wonder, then, that many methodologic questions remain to be answered.

With the financial pressures on hospitals likely to become increasingly intense, it can be expected that there will be an increasing demand for cost-benefit studies that are more and more convincing to decision makers. It is not unlikely that more sophisticated cost-benefit analyses will compare the cost-benefit ratio of infection control with those of newly proposed patient care services or alternative preventive programs and that the results will be used to direct resources to the programs with the most favorable cost-benefit ratios. This expectation justifies greater attention to the methodologic issues in performing cost-benefit studies of infection control.

Table 25-1. Methodologic issues in performing cost-benefit studies of infection control: estimating the costs of nosocomial infections

Basic design	Patient selection	Setting	Scope	Design for attributing extra days and costs	Currency	Summary measure	Unit of analysis
Cross-sectional	Incidence series	In-hospital	Hospital	Crude weighting	Hospital costs	Mean	Patient
Longitudinal	Prevalence series	Postdischarge follow-up	Nation	Direct attribution	Hospital charges	Median	Infection
Demonstration of a change in the infection rate	Epidemics	Readmissions	Developing countries	Comparative attribution	Components of cost or charges	Geometric mean	
	High-cost patients	Outpatient clinics	Site	Randomized trial	Hospital days	Percentage	
			Service		Lost wages	Total	
			Pathogen		Intangibles		
			Surgical procedure		Cost to third parties		
					Adjustments for DRG payments		
					Deaths		
					Antimicrobial use		
					Antimicrobial resistance		
					Environmental damage		

Table 25-2. Methodologic issues in performing cost-benefit studies of infection control (IC): estimating the costs of infection control programs

Components assessed	Effect on patient care practices	Indirect effects	Revenue from IC services	Issues affecting the estimation of both nosocomial infections and IC programs
IC practitioners	Burden on nursing time	Malpractice losses	Charging for services	Adjusting for inflation in costs to compare estimates obtained in different years
Hospital epidemiologist	Expense of supplies used	Hospital marketing		Discounting future costs
IC Committee	Quantity of supplies used			Providing convenient methods for cost estimates to be used for making economic projections in individual hospitals
Clerical	Number of tests (cultures) done			
Equipment	Isolation and private rooms			
Maintenance/operations				
Space				
Utilities				
Administrative overhead				

Methodologic Issues in Estimating the Costs of Nosocomial Infections

The many methodologic issues that are inherent in the published cost and cost-benefit studies of infection control are listed in Tables 25-1 and 25-2. That there are far more issues in estimating the costs of nosocomial infections than in estimating the costs of the infection control programs may reflect only the fact that the former has been studied more extensively.

The eight main issues in the design of studies to estimate the costs of nosocomial infections are listed in Table 25-1. Within each column of the table, the methodologic choices are not necessarily mutually exclusive and, in many studies several of them are used simultaneously. The large number of possible combinations of choices across the columns explains the enormous diversity of study designs as well as the considerable difficulty in trying to understand and compare studies. Such a classification of issues is helpful in comparing the results of many studies, because it allows the identification of subtle methodologic differences that can produce large disparities in the final estimates. Besides these eight issues, one must also consider the many methodologic issues common to all epidemiologic studies, including the use of valid definitions for nosocomial infections as well as the complete and accurate ascertainment of infections (see Chap. 5).

Basic Design

The most fundamental issue is whether the study is of cross-sectional or longitudinal design (see Table 25-1). Either can produce valid estimates of the costs of nosocomial infections, but longitudinal studies including an infection control intervention can be more insightful by providing a more convincing estimate of a reduction in the infection rate. Depending on how well the intervention study is designed, an empiric demonstration of a reduction may constitute a more convincing estimate of the economic impact that an infection control program can have than may a hypothetical estimate or one taken from

other published studies [59, 62]. Most studies on the costs of nosocomial infections, however, are cross-sectional.

Patient Selection

There are four ways in which patients have been selected for estimating the costs of nosocomial infections. These include incidence studies covering either endemic periods or epidemics, prevalence studies, and special cohorts of "high-cost patients."

Incidence Series

In the vast majority of cost-benefit studies of infection control, the patients constitute an incidence series—that is, all patients admitted or operated on during a defined, usually prolonged, time period. Most of these studies have been based on endemic incidence series, although there is an increasing literature on the costs of epidemics [5, 14, 39, 50, 72, 74, 84, 95, 121, 149].

Prevalence Series

At least two studies have used data collected in prevalence studies to estimate the costs of nosocomial infections [42, 145]. Although prevalence studies, usually involving surveying every bed in a hospital on a single day, can be done with relatively little effort and expense, the results are difficult to interpret. The difficulty arises from the fact that prevalence is a function of incidence times duration of the illness. Thus patients found to be in the hospital and to have an active nosocomial infection on the day of a prevalence survey will predictably be the longer-staying patients, those with a higher risk of nosocomial infection, and those with the more long-lasting (more severe) infections. Consequently, in the same patient population the prevalence rate can be expected to be one and a half to two times higher than the incidence rate, and the average prolongation of stay and extra costs attributable to infection will be similarly longer in the prevalence series than in the corresponding incidence series.

In the first economic study from a prevalence study, Freeman and colleagues [42] estimated that the average length of stay of patients identified as having nosocomial infections in a prevalence study was 13.0 days longer than uninfected patients selected from a concurrent incidence series, matched on age, diagnosis, and operative procedure. In a follow-up report, these investigators found that the prolongation of stay due to nosocomial infection, similarly estimated, was 13.3 days for infections identified in the same prevalence series but only 7.3 days for infections identified in a concurrent incidence series assembled from the same population of patients [41]. They concluded, "Results from prevalence and incidence series must be clearly distinguished because the same events will be perceived differently in the two types of series" [41]. In a later study, Thomann [145] attempted to correct this bias by estimating the incidence rate from their prevalence study and multiplying the prevalence rate by two-thirds before projecting the costs. While this might correct the estimated number and rate of infections, it would not correct for the selection bias in the higher average severity and costliness of the patients selected in the prevalence series.

In general, prevalence studies should not be used for making economic projections because of the uncertainty in trying to correct for the large selection bias inherent in the prevalence survey method. If they are used, conversion models, similar to those for estimating the incidence rate from a prevalence series [123], should be developed.

High-Cost Patients
A particularly insightful group of patients to study is comprised of those who suffer the most costly nosocomial infections. Successfully identifying risk factors unique to these more serious infections might lead to the development of intervention strategies that prevent them selectively. Such strategies would be likely to have a particularly high level of cost-effectiveness relative to other infection control measures.

In 1979, Schroeder and co-workers [135]

studied the characteristics of high-cost patients in a general hospital population without regard to nosocomial infection to estimate the implications for a national catastrophic health insurance. The fact that a relatively small percentage of patients with nosocomial infection (25 percent) account for a disproportionately large share (64 to 86 percent) of the total extra days and costs of nosocomial infection was demonstrated in three hospitals by Haley and colleagues [64] and corroborated by Green [54] and Wakefield [152] and their associates using different methods. A follow-up analysis of high-cost infections by Pinner and co-workers [114] found that surgical patients with wound infections after injuries and medical patients with lower respiratory nosocomial infections were likely to have the most costly infections. Numerous studies have shown that multiple nosocomial infections and secondary bacteremia are also associated with more costly infections [35, 41, 54, 64].

Setting
Most of the studies have concentrated on patients whose nosocomial infections were detected while they were in a hospital. Recognizing that many surgical patients are now being discharged from the hospital soon after their operations, some investigators have excluded from surveillance, or from the analysis, all patients who remained in the hospital less than 48 hours or, in studies of surgical patients, less than 48 hours after the operation [1, 28]. As the duration of hospitalization continues to decrease in hospitals in the United States and in some other countries, it will become increasingly important to continue surveillance after discharge to measure some infection rates accurately, particularly surgical wound infections. For economic studies, however, as long as the objective of the cost-benefit study is to demonstrate the impact of nosocomial infections on the hospital's financial balance, studies can concentrate on detecting patients whose infections begin before discharge, those readmitted to the hospital for treatment of a nosocomial infection, or those seen in an outpatient clinic, if run by

the hospital. This would not be adequate, however, for true cost-benefit studies in which *all* the costs are to be enumerated [78].

Scope

The scope of the study—that is, the nature and extent of the target universe to which the investigator wishes to project the cost or cost-benefit projection—varies widely in the published studies. Most commonly, studies have attempted to estimate the costs of nosocomial infections in an individual hospital, but they often make imprecise extrapolations of their findings to nationwide estimates for the United States [6, 9, 13, 30, 58, 59, 77, 136] and for other countries [4, 22, 28, 29, 35, 48, 52, 75, 77, 88, 89, 92, 107, 111, 113, 119, 143, 146, 150, 156].

Some studies have estimated costs for each site of infection, particularly surgical wound infections [3, 10, 12, 15, 16, 20, 27, 32, 34, 35, 37, 42, 46, 53, 59, 64, 76, 87, 90, 105, 109, 110, 126, 129, 131, 133, 138, 140, 142, 144, 157], nosocomial urinary tract infections [19, 42, 49, 59, 64, 81, 108, 116, 126–128, 131, 133], bacteremia [42, 59, 64, 93, 125, 131, 133, 139], and pneumonia [36, 42, 64, 91, 131, 133, 137]. Others have reported their estimates stratified by service [8, 28, 64] or for a particular service, usually the neonatology service [48, 67], intensive care units [28], orthopedics [27, 87], or other surgical services. Estimates for particular pathogens have most commonly focused on infections involving *Staphylococcus aureus* [15, 121, 147, 151].

Design for Attributing Extra Days and Costs

The methodologic issue that has received the most critical attention is the series of design strategies used to estimate how many extra hospital days and how much extra cost are *attributable* to nosocomial infections. A classification of these design strategies is shown in Table 25-3. Four basic strategies have been used to estimate attributable days and costs. The strategies are not mutually exclusive; that is, often investigators have used more than one of them in a particular study, although each usually requires its own separate

Table 25-3. Classification of types of study designs used to estimate the number of days and costs that are attributable to nosocomial infections

I. Crude weighting
II. Direct attribution
A. Clinician's subjective judgment
B. Variation from a predicted value
C. Standardized case review protocol
III. Comparative attribution
A. Unmatched group comparison
B. Matching on multiple characteristics
C. Matching on summary measures of confounding
D. Stratification with indirect standardization
IV. Randomized trial

statistical analysis and possibly even its own separate database [28, 41, 65, 152]. In view of the fact that the imprecise terms used to describe these methods have led to considerable confusion among them, the following discussion will explain each method in detail, following the terminology given in Table 25-3.

Crude Weighting

The simplest method is to select some constant that estimates the average extra costs or the average number of extra days to be expected for each nosocomial infection and use it to weight (multiplying by the constant) the number of nosocomial infections detected in the study to estimate an overall cost of infections in the setting of the study. The constant is usually obtained from a previous study using one of the other attribution methods. A table of constants can be used for more precise weighting of stratified analyses: For example, site-specific cost constants can be used to weight infections stratified by site. Additional constants can be used to project the estimates to wider target universes, such as a nation or the world.

While this strategy, often referred to as the "back-of-the-envelope" method, is quick, its accuracy is limited by a number of factors, particularly the intrinsic accuracy of the constants and their appropriateness to the set of data being weighted. This method was frequently used in most of the initial cost-benefit studies, particularly those intended to create political urgency for directing resources to preventive services in the United States [6, 13, 30, 58, 136] and abroad [77, 88, 113, 119, 143, 145]. It is still used to provide an "economic punch" at the conclusion of epidemiologic descriptions of emerging nosocomial infection problems [18–20, 81, 98, 110] and in editorials and reviews on the subject [43, 52, 96, 118, 130].

Direct Attribution

The second main approach is to attempt to measure directly for each infected patient how many hospital days or costs are attributable to the infection. Three important variations have been used for making attributions by the direct approach.

Clinician's Subjective Judgment Most often it has been done by having a physician, infection control practitioner, or trained technician visit each infected patient daily to study the medical and nursing record and to speak with the physicians or nurses or examine the patient as needed to decide which days, services, and costs are attributable to the infection [7, 34, 51, 64, 65, 75, 76, 84, 131, 133, 142, 144, 157]. This method has the advantage of an expert's being at the bedside each day to ferret out whatever evidence is needed to attribute days and costs accurately [60, 65]. It has two basic disadvantages. First, it is, to one extent or another, subjective and not amenable to exact replication from study to study [41]. Second, since the physician surveyors have generally been conservative in their judgments, attributing extra days only in the face of definite evidence that the patient would have been discharged absent the infection, they are prone to overlooking attributable services and extra days. Consequently, this method has an inherent tendency to underestimate the attributable days and costs [41, 65].

Variation from a Predicted Value In several studies investigators have obtained an *a priori* estimate of the patient's expected length of stay in the absence of nosocomial infection based on the diagnoses, operations, and other

factors, and they have subtracted this reference value from each patient's actual length of stay to estimate the extra hospital days attributable to nosocomial infection [15, 50, 64, 65, 109, 133]. In two studies, the investigators used as the reference durations the average length of stay of all patients, or of all uninfected patients, in the hospital's population at risk [15, 50]. In others, the investigators used the published figures for the fiftieth or seventy-fifth percentiles of the distribution of length of stay of all patients in the same region of the country, stratified by age, diagnosis, and operation [17], as the reference value for *otherwise uncomplicated patients* who developed nosocomial infection, but they relied on subjective clinical judgments for complicated cases, thus combining design types IIA and IIB [64, 65, 133]. In a study of surgical wound abscesses, Olson and Allen [109] used the length of postoperative stay up until the onset of the signs and symptoms of the abscess as the expected length of stay in the absence of infection. The advantages of using predicted values of length of stay is that they can be applied easily, particularly to the large number of otherwise uncomplicated patients who develop nosocomial infections and, as the precision of criteria used widely in routine utilization review increases in the future, the *a priori* estimates may become increasingly precise. There are several disadvantages. First, in many circumstances the *a priori* reference values may not be accurate. Second, the rationale behind choosing the fiftieth or seventh-fifth percentiles is not well established. Choosing the fiftieth percentile is perhaps too liberal, leading to an overestimate of attributable stay, because it assumes that the distribution of the length of stay of patients who get nosocomial infections is the same as those who do not; whereas, the seventy-fifth percentile, which may be as much as twice as long as the fiftieth [41], may be too conservative, leading to an underestimate of the attributable length of stay.

Standardized Case Review Protocol Clearly, the greatest innovation to the methods of attributing extra days and costs has been the introduction of a standardized case review protocol. Known as the *appropriateness evaluation protocol*, this method was developed as a standardized technique for patient care reviewers to detect unnecessary days of hospitalization [47, 124]. In the late 1980s, Wakefield and colleagues [151, 152] adapted the method for use in estimating the number of extra days that are attributable to nosocomial infection. The method involves having trained record reviewers review the medical records of discharged patients who had nosocomial infections and apply standardized criteria for classifying each hospital day into one of three categories: those attributable to the patient's reason for admission (or to noninfectious complications), those attributable to both the reason for admission and nosocomial infection, and those attributable only to nosocomial infection [152]. The days in the last category are the ones that are counted in estimating the costs of nosocomial infection. The method has been subjected to validation and found to produce very high levels of interreviewer agreement [47, 124].

The advantages of this method are that it is simple enough to be applied in scientific studies or in routine infection control work; being standardized, it is replicable from setting to setting; it has been validated; and, by incorporating it into routine utilization review screening, it could potentially be applied to large numbers of patients or over long time periods. Its disadvantage is that it relies on the clinical information available in medical records, which are less complete in some hospitals than in others [61, 94].

Comparative Attribution   The third main approach is to compare the lengths of stay and costs of patients with nosocomial infection (infected patients) with patients who did not suffer a nosocomial infection (uninfected patients). Investigators who favor this method have referred to it as the *case-control method* or the *epidemiologic approach*. In actuality, the design of these studies is not strictly a case-control design, as the term is currently used in epidemiology [79]. In a true case-control study, the subjects are initially selected and

classified on the outcome variable and are then studied to determine their exposure to the risk factor. In comparative attribution studies on the costs of nosocomial infections, the patients are selected and classified on the basis of the risk factor (presence or absence of nosocomial infection), and then their lengths of stay or costs (the outcome variable) are compared. This constitutes a cohort, or follow-up, study design rather than a case-control design. Four types of comparative attribution studies have been used to estimate the extra days and costs attributable to nosocomial infections (see Table 25-3).

Unmatched Group Comparison   The earliest, and still the least sophisticated, of the comparative attribution studies involves comparing the lengths of stay or costs of a group of infected patients with those of a group of uninfected patients, the difference between the means or totals of the two groups being accepted as the amount that is attributable to nosocomial infection [3, 12, 15, 16, 28, 32, 41, 46, 65, 67, 87, 122, 129, 140, 155]. From the beginning, most investigators who used this method acknowledged that it overestimates the amount that is actually attributable to infection, because patients who develop nosocomial infections are generally more severely ill and thus are destined for longer hospitalization even if the infection had not occurred [28, 37, 41, 48, 54, 65, 67, 93, 125, 139, 140, 143]. This phenomenon, which pervades all discussion of the comparative attribution methods, will be referred to as the *severity bias*. One indication of its possible presence is the fact that in several studies the preoperative stay of patients who later got wound infections is longer than that of patients who did not get a wound infection [119]. The severity bias causes all unmatched group comparison studies to overestimate substantially the extra days and costs attributable to nosocomial infection. Consequently, this method should never be reported.

Matching on Multiple Characteristics   In an effort to overcome the severity bias, numerous investigators have tried various schemes for matching uninfected patients (controls) to the infected patients (cases) to set up a comparison between groups that have the same predicted length of stay and cost before the infections supervened [8, 27, 28, 35, 37, 41, 42, 48, 49, 53, 54, 60, 65, 90, 93, 105, 125, 126, 133, 138, 139]. These studies have been known by the misnomer *matched case-control studies,* when in fact they are cohort studies with matched exposure groups, or matched infected and uninfected patient groups.

In most of these studies, the investigators have matched the infected and uninfected patients on several parameters. Most commonly, they have chosen one uninfected match for each infected patient, but two or three matched "controls" have been used to advantage in some studies [37, 41]. The number of matching parameters used has varied from one to eight, with four or five being the number most often used. The parameters most commonly used in matching are patients' age (with ± 5 years), sex, service, main discharge diagnosis, first-listed surgical procedure, and month or year of discharge. Other interesting parameters that have been used uncommonly are the Quetelet index of obesity, smoking, and social class [27]; subjective estimate of severity of underlying illness from medical record review [1]; the presence or absence of unspecified "major confounding factors" [54]; and the number of valves replaced or the number of coronary vessels bypassed in cardiac surgery [132].

Recognizing that matching on these parameters may not entirely control for the severity bias, some investigators have required the length of stay, or the postoperative stay, of the uninfected patient(s) to be at least as long as that of the infected patient before the onset of the infection [41, 54, 93, 139], or for all infected and uninfected patients included in the analysis to have stayed at least 7 days [126]. Freeman and McGowan [41] demonstrated that, after matching for several of the usual characteristics, this further restriction had a very small, though measurable, impact on the estimated prolongation of stay due to nosocomial infection (only 0.8 days of the average of 13 extra days).

The more matching parameters that are required to accept a match and the more categories contained in each matching variable, the larger the pool of potential uninfected patients that is needed to find matches for all the infected patients. Consequently, in many of these studies a substantial number of the infected patients have had to be excluded from the analysis for lack of a match, and these excluded patients tend to have longer lengths of stay and more severe infections than those who remain in the analysis [48, 54, 65, 93, 125, 131]. This introduces a bias that tends to underestimate the extra days and costs attributable to nosocomial infection.

A related pitfall, referred to previously, is the bias that results from selecting matched controls from an *incidence* series, matched to infected patients who were identified in a *prevalence* study [42]. Since the prevalence study design selectively identifies longer-staying patients with longer-lasting infections, this selection bias will cause the comparison of infected patients from a prevalence series with uninfected patients from an incidence series to overestimate the attributable extra stay and costs [41].

In the analysis of matched comparison studies, opinions differ over whether to maintain the matching in the analysis. Examples of statistical techniques used for analyzing matched data include McNemar's test, the paired *t*-test, and the Mantel-Haenszel technique [80]. While several studies have employed the correct statistical methods for matched data [41, 48, 65, 90, 131], the majority have analyzed the matched series as if they were unmatched groups of infected and uninfected patients [8, 27, 28, 37, 48, 49, 53, 93, 105, 125, 126, 138]. Failure to maintain the matching may lead to underestimating the true magnitude of the difference and to overestimating its variance. These errors, however, are usually far less important in matched cohort studies, such as matched comparison studies of cost, than for true case-control studies [80].

There are several advantages to the method of matching on multiple characteristics. First, it is relatively easily done on computerized databases collected by routine surveillance or in outbreak investigations, and the patients' lengths of stay, or postoperative stay, and total hospital bill are easily obtained and merged into the database. Second, the matching on these convenient parameters clearly does reduce the effects of the severity bias that are more evident in the unmatched comparison studies [65]. Its main disadvantages are the need for rather large pools of uninfected patients from which to select the matches and the selection bias resulting from excluding unmatched infected patients. Another drawback is the difficulty of knowing how much of the severity bias was eliminated by the matching and, conversely, how much overestimation remains uncontrolled in the estimates of the attributable extra stay and costs.

Matching on Summary Measures of Confounding Despite the widespread use of matching on multiple characteristics, it has been suggested that the usual matching characteristics may not be the ones that best control for the severity bias [60]. It is conceivable that infected and uninfected patients may be perfectly matched on age, sex, diagnosis, operation, and length of stay until onset of infection, and yet the infected patients still have a longer expected stay apart from the additional stay conferred by the infection. This is because, even within the strata defined by the intersection of these usual matching characteristics, it is intuitively apparent that the severity of illness, infection risk, and expected length of stay and cost may differ substantially among patients. If true, these matching parameters will not completely eliminate the effects of the severity bias. In addition, matching on multiple characteristics, with some (such as diagnosis and operation) having thousands of diagnosis or procedure categories, often makes it difficult to obtain enough matches.

These problems have led to a search for more aggregate measures that control more efficiently for the severity bias. The ideal aggregate measures should meet the following three conditions: First, they should be truly

confounding variables in the analysis of the association of nosocomial infection with length of stay or cost [60]; second, they must have face validity for controlling much of the variance in length of stay due to diagnoses, operations, and severity of illness, but not that attributable to nosocomial infection; and third, they must contain as few categories as possible to maximize the number of infected patients for whom a match can be found. Statistical methods for reducing many confounding variables to summary measures have been described [70, 100].

Presently, the available measure considered the most powerful predictor of length of stay and resource utilization is the system of diagnosis-related groups (DRGs), used in the United States as the basis for the federal government's paying hospitals to care for its elderly citizens under the Medicare system [66, 154]. For the DRG variable to qualify as a useful matching parameter, two conditions would have to be met. First, it would have to be augmented by another simple indicator of patient severity of illness, since DRGs are known to leave some amount of severity uncontrolled [60]. Several measures of severity of illness have been proposed, including complex measures such as the Medical Illness Severity Grouping System (MEDISGRPS) and the Acute Physiology and Chronic Health Evaluation (APACHE) system and simple ones such as a count of the number of discharge diagnoses [55, 60, 73, 102, 103]. Second, to qualify as a confounding variable, a parameter must have been shown to be reasonably strongly associated with both the risk factor and the outcome variable in the analysis [85]. Satisfactory resolution of this issue has been frustrated by the lack of large enough databases containing all of the required variables along with accurately ascertained nosocomial infections.

A reanalysis of the large database from the Study on the Efficacy of Nosocomial Infection Control (SENIC Project) addressed this problem [60]. The 169,526 patients were divided into two arbitrary groups, and multivariate linear models were fit to each half separately to determine the multivariate association of DRG, number of diagnoses, and their interaction with length of stay and with nosocomial infection. The results, summarized in Table 25-4, support the following conclusions. First, DRG is strongly associated with both length of stay and nosocomial infection, making it a true confounding variable. Second, the number of diagnoses increased the explanatory power of DRGs by approximately 10 percent (e.g., an increase in R^2 from 0.31 to 0.34) for both length of stay and nosocomial infection, suggesting that it provides additional control of severity of illness within DRG categories. Third, all these findings were corroborated by the finding of virtually identical results in both halves of the database and by the additional validation analyses (see Table 25-4). These findings suggest that matching on DRG and the number

of diagnoses might be a better way of estimating the extra stay and costs attributable to nosocomial infection in comparative attribution studies using matching or stratification with indirect standardization. Additional studies are needed to compare results obtained by matching on the traditional characteristics with those obtained by matching on DRG and the number of diagnoses.

Recently, Boyce and colleagues [8] reported a study in which they used DRGs along with age (± 7 years), sex, urgency of surgery and type of surgery, and number of vessels, bypasses, or valves replaced as matching parameters in estimating the extra stay and costs attributable to postoperative infections in open-heart surgery. Even though there were only a small number of DRG categories represented in those patients, the study ap-

Table 25-4. Values of explained variance from general linear models and contingency tables of the SENIC database of 169,526 patients from 1975–1976 [66],[a] demonstrating that DRGs and the number of diagnoses (coded 1, 2, or 3+) and their interaction constitute true confounding variables in the analysis of nosocomial infection and length of hospital stay.

Dependent variable	Predictors in the models	First half[b]	Second half[b]	Validation analysis[c]	Both halves combined[d] Linear model R^2	Both halves combined[d] Contingency table U
Log(LOS)[e]	DRG only	0.32	0.31	0.30	0.31	
Log(LOS)	Number of diagnoses only	0.07	0.07	0.07	0.07	
Log(LOS)	DRG, number of diagnoses, and their interaction	0.35	0.34	0.32	0.34	
Nosocomial infection[f]	DRG only	0.18	0.16	0.15	0.16	0.27
Nosocomial infection	Number of diagnoses only	0.01	0.01	0.01	0.01	0.02
Nosocomial infection	DRG, number of diagnoses, and their interaction	0.19	0.18	0.16	0.18	0.29

DRGs = diagnosis-related groups.

[a] The 147 DRGs (31%) that contained fewer than 100 patients each were excluded, eliminating 6,979 patients (4%) from the analyses. All linear models were generated with the general linear models (GLM) procedure of the Statistical Analysis System (SAS), and were statistically significant at $p <.0001$.

[b] The database was arbitrarily divided into two halves containing 80,805 and 81,742 patients, respectively. The numbers in the table are R^2 values unless otherwise stated.

[c] To validate the models, the coefficients from the first-half model were used to generate predicted values of the dependent variable in the second-half data, and these were regressed on the dependent variable in the second-half data; model R^2 values are reported.

[d] Since the R^2 values obtained in the first and second halves of the database were similar, final estimates of R^2 from linear models were generated from the complete database and, for the analyses of nosocomial infection, were compared with the asymmetric uncertainty coefficient (U) from contingency table analyses [2].

[e] Logarithmic transformation of length of stay (LOS).

[f] Coded 1 if the patient had any nosocomial infection and 0 otherwise.

Source: R.W. Haley, Measuring the costs of nosocomial infections: Methods for estimating economic burden on the hospital. *Am. J. Med.* 19 (Suppl. 3B): 325, 1991. With permission from the *American Journal of Medicine*.

pears to be the most thoroughly controlled of the comparative attribution studies using matching on multiple characteristics.

Stratification with Indirect Standardization In 1982, Fabry and associates [35] reported a study on the costs of nosocomial infections in abdominal surgery in which they used stratification and indirect standardization instead of matching to reduce the severity bias. A similar method was used several years later in a report by Le Coutour and colleagues [84]. This method attempts to include as many of the uninfected patients as possible in the analysis by stratifying on the confounding parameters instead of matching.

The infected patients and the uninfected patients were separately stratified on the intersection of several confounding variables. Fabry's group [35] used age, surgical procedure, and level of *medical risk,* defined by "infection at entry, heavier surgery and associated chronic condition." Uninfected patients in strata containing no infected patients were excluded from the analysis. Within each of the resulting strata, the mean length of stay (or costs) of the uninfected patients was weighted by the proportional distribution of the infected patients in the strata and summed across strata to derive the *expected* mean length of stay. The difference between this expected mean length of stay and the mean length of stay of the infected patients was considered to be the average extra days attributable to infection.

Le Coutour's group [84] stratified according to whether the patient had an infection on admission, four classes of admitting illness, and a severity-of-illness measure (described by Le Gall and colleagues [85]) used for only two classes of admitting illness. Although the stratification table was set up similarly to Fabry's, Le Coutour and co-workers calculated the attributable mean length of stay in each stratum by subtracting the means of the infected and uninfected patients, and then calculated a weighted average of the stratum-specific attributable means to obtain an overall estimate of the attributable length of stay per infected patient. This constitutes

the calculation of a weighted mean rather than the method of indirect standardization used by Fabry and associates.

These two approaches offer the advantage over the matching methods of using all, or almost all, of the information available in the population of uninfected patients for estimating the expected length of stay or costs, while matching uses only 1 or 2 uninfected patients per infected patient. The effectiveness of both methods, however, ultimately depends on how well the stratifying parameters, like the matching parameters, control for the severity bias while minimizing the number of strata.

To clarify the place of this method in the classification of study design (see Table 25-3), indirect standardization resembles, though it improves on, the comparison of infected patients' length of stay with an *a priori* predicted expected length of stay (design type IIB). The reason it is classified separately is that comparison with a predicted value (design type IIB) is usually applied prospectively in the data collection stage, whereas stratification with indirect standardization (design type IIID) has been applied in the analytic stage.

Randomized Trial

The fourth main approach to estimating the attributable extra stay and costs is to conduct a prospective, randomized clinical trial. How a randomized trial would be designed to address this question most effectively has not yet been addressed in the literature on the economics of nosocomial infection, but a clever clinical trial on prophylactic antibiotic therapy conducted by Stone and colleagues [142] in the late 1970s deserves serious study. In that trial, the investigators randomized 463 patients undergoing elective stomach, biliary tract, or colon operations into two groups, one receiving cefazolin and the other a placebo intramuscularly 8 to 12 hours and 1 hour preoperatively, in the recovery room after the operation, on the morning following the day of surgery, and on that same afternoon. Infections of the wound or peritoneal cavity developed in 11 (4.7 percent) of the 232 patients in the cefazolin group and in 36 (15.6 percent) of the 231 patients in the placebo group. Since the patients were randomly assigned, the lengths of stay and hospital costs of the two groups should have been equal except for those resulting from the difference in the number of infections due to the use of the effective prophylactic antibiotic in the experimental group.

Although the investigators then sacrificed the advantage of the randomized trial methodology by resorting to direct attribution by subjective judgment (design type IIA) to estimate the attributable days and costs, they supplied the basic data with which the true difference in length of stay between the two groups could be calculated. From the calculations shown in Table 25-5, the patients in the placebo group had 25 more wound and peritoneal infections and spent a total of 428 more postoperative days in the hospital than those in the experimental group, amounting to an average of 17.1 extra postoperative days per infection. Still, however, this figure may be an overestimate because the 11 infections in the experimental group appear to have been less serious on average than the 36 in the placebo group (average excess postoperative days by the clinician's subjective assessment, 13.3 versus 17.0), possibly due to an ameliorating effect of the prophylactic antibiotic in addition to the demonstrated preventive effect. Against this interpretation, however, is the finding that the average ex-

cess postoperative stay estimated by the clinician's subjective judgment was 17.0 days for all 36 infections in the placebo group, agreeing with the figure of 17.1 days for the overall trial, calculated in Table 25-5.

The estimate of 17 extra days per postoperative wound infection is among the highest of all in the literature. Its derivation from a randomized trial may shed doubt on the much smaller estimates from the many direct and comparative attribution studies, although the higher figure may reflect the mix of more serious surgery studied in this randomized trial. Because of the promise of this method, future designers of randomized antibiotic trials should consider including measurements and analyses to estimate the extra days and costs of wound infections.

Currency

A central concept of cost-benefit analysis is to express both the costs and benefits of a program in a common currency so that they can be meaningfully compared. Although financial currencies are most often used, the costs of nosocomial infections are often expressed in a wide variety of currencies, including true economic costs, hospital charges, components of costs or charges, hospital days, lost wages, intangible costs, costs to third parties, deaths, excessive antimicrobial use and resistance and, possibly, environmental damage (see Table 25-1). Even though these diverse currencies do not conform to the conventions of

Table 25-5. Estimation of the extra hospital days attributable to postoperative wound and peritoneal infections in a randomized clinical trial of cefazolin in intraabdominal operations

	Preoperative antibiotics		*Preoperative placebo*
Total patients[a]	232		231
Average postoperative hospital days[a]	10.9		12.8
Total postoperative hospital days	2,529		2,957
Difference in postoperative hospital days		428	
Postoperative infections[a]	11		36
Difference in postoperative infections		25	
Average extra days per infection		17.1	
Average excess postoperative days per infection[a,b]	13.3		17.0

[a] Data from H.H. Stone et al., Prophylactic and preventive antibiotic therapy: Timing, duration and economics. *Ann. Surg.* 189:691, 1979.
[b] Derived by clinician's subjective judgment (design type IIA).

cost-benefit analysis, many do seem to have been useful in conveying the seriousness of the problem of nosocomial infections and in focusing attention on the need to reduce infection risks.

Extra Days and Charges
By far the most commonly used currencies in studies estimating the costs of nosocomial infections have been hospital days and hospital charges attributable to nosocomial infections [42, 53, 59, 64, 151]. These recur repeatedly in studies because they are the most readily measured variables that get relatively close to what concerns hospital administrators, namely hospital costs. Patients' length of stay (Julian discharge date minus admission date) can be obtained quickly from diverse sources, such as the hospital's medical records system and patient accounting system, and patients' charges can be obtained from their itemized hospital bills or from the billing system. Extra days has the advantage of appearing to be a "harder" measure that varies less from year to year, whereas extra charges is more inclusive but also more variable due to inflationary pressures. Most often both are reported.

Components
A number of investigators have attempted to disaggregate the total charges due to nosocomial infection [7, 27, 28, 35, 48, 64, 84, 122, 129, 139, 142, 151]. The components of the costs can best be viewed in two major categories: routine and ancillary costs [64]. *Routine costs* are those due to the extra days of hospitalization and are often referred to as the *per diem*, or *hotel*, costs. They include nursing care and other recurring expenses and vary widely among different locations in the hospital (e.g., routine costs are higher in intensive care units than in general ward areas). *Ancillary costs* are those resulting from definable services performed in the treatment of the infection, such as antibiotics, respiratory therapy, microbiologic cultures, other laboratory services, and radiologic examinations. While the proportional distribution of these components varies among different type of nosocomial infections, overall the routine and ancillary components each account for ap-

proximately half of the costs of nosocomial infections [64].

Extra Hospital Costs
An issue of increasing concern to investigators in this area is how to estimate the actual costs to the hospital of nosocomial infection [60]. The review by Finkler [38] pointed out the potential biases inherent in using hospital charges to estimate hospital costs. Briefly, third-party payers tend to underpay, or refuse to pay, for some hospital patients or services and will pay more for others. To maintain financial balance, hospitals tend to shift their charges for underreimbursed costs to those with which they can recover more than their costs. This means that the charges for a given service may be far higher or lower than the hospital's actual cost for delivering it. As a result, depending on the mix of services that are attributable to nosocomial infections, the charges may or may not reflect the hospital's costs accurately.

Realization of this pitfall has led a few investigators to use new methods to generate estimates that are closer to actual hospital costs [8, 60, 83, 151]. These generally involve itemizing the actual services provided for treatment of the nosocomial infection and weighting each service by a cost weight that reflects the costs to the hospital of the goods and personnel services used to deliver the service. For example, the cost of administering a dose of an antibiotic would include the price paid by the hospital for the dose and the salary and benefits costs of the personnel time required to order, store, dispense, and administer the dose. To date, methods for estimating true hospital costs are still crude, and the resulting estimates appear little different from those derived from charges, but the advent of more detailed cost-accounting systems in hospitals is likely to provide more accurate estimates of the true costs in the future. The alternative approaches were recently reviewed in detail [64].

Adjustments for Insurance Reimbursements
In attempting to estimate the impact of nosocomial infections on hospitals' costs, it is

potentially important to adjust for reimbursement payments that the hospital might receive specifically for complications such as nosocomial infections. Under fee-for-service reimbursement, hospitals passed their costs for nosocomial infections directly through to the payers who reimbursed them entirely [1, 22, 122, 131]. Under that system, hospitals bore little or none of the costs; instead, they were borne by the third-party payers who passed them on to the public through higher health policy premiums. When the prospective payment system (PPS) using DRGs was introduced into the U.S. hospital system, several investigators predicted that by reimbursing hospitals a set fee based on the admitting diagnosis, the DRG system would provide little reimbursement for the occurrence of a nosocomial infection [1, 6, 21, 30, 31, 118, 131]. The added provisions that the costs of complications were built into the adjusted standard amount on which DRG payments are based and that patients in some DRGs are moved to higher-paying DRGs when they suffer a complication made it impossible to estimate how much of the costs of nosocomial infections are actually recovered by hospitals through reimbursements. Later studies, however, confirmed empirically that only 5 percent or so of hospitals' costs for caring for nosocomial infections are returned in added reimbursement under the PPS in all U.S. hospitals [66], and similar findings were obtained in special settings [8, 105, 121, 152]. These findings indicate that there appears to be a strong financial incentive for hospitals to prevent nosocomial infections under the PPS form of hospital reimbursement.

Indirect Costs

Though almost all of the research has dealt with estimating the direct costs of nosocomial infections, Fabry and colleagues [35, 83] in France and Schäfer [129] in Germany have estimated some of the important indirect costs to patients attributable to nosocomial infections. Among their findings were that after surgical patients returned home, surgical wound infection prolonged their absence from work an average of 13.8 and 20 days [35, 129]. These rather larges estimates suggest the need for additional research to document the extent of morbidity and indirect costs due to nosocomial infections.

Deaths

An important cost of nosocomial infection is the occurrence of death. Most of the studies on the mortality related to nosocomial infection have studied matched infected and uninfected patients (design type IIIB) but, just as for attributing extra days and economic costs, it is not clear that the matching has completely controlled for the severity bias in attributing deaths to nosocomial infection [28, 56, 93, 115, 125, 139]. The best estimates of the frequency of deaths due to nosocomial infections came from a combined analysis of data from the National Nosocomial Infections Surveillance (NNIS) System and the SENIC Project [59]. In the NNIS System, the collaborating infection control practitioners followed a protocol to examine every death in a patient with nosocomial infection and make a clinical determination of the extent to which the death was caused by the infection (design type IIA). The findings indicate that 10 percent of patients with nosocomial infection die in the hospital, which breaks down as follows: In 6 percent, the death is unrelated to the nosocomial infection; in 3 percent, the nosocomial infection contributes to, but is not the main cause, of death; and in 1 percent, nosocomial infection is the main cause of death. By applying these figures to the nationally representative SENIC data, it is estimated that nosocomial infections directly cost more than 20,000 lives per year in U.S. hospitals and contribute to an additional 60,000 deaths per year [59]. To date, no estimates of the economic costs of premature death from nosocomial infections have been made.

In studies to estimate the economic costs of nosocomial infection, it has been suggested that patients who die in the hospital should be excluded from analysis to avoid underestimating the extra days and costs attributable to the nosocomial infections when length of stay is cut short by death. Whereas some patients' length of stay is clearly shortened by death, other patients linger for long periods with nosocomial infection before dying. As a result, further empiric study of this question is needed to determine the impact of death on estimates of the costs of nosocomial infection.

Antimicrobial Use for Treating and Preventing Nosocomial Infection

A substantial body of literature has been generated to analyze the costs of antibiotics used either to prevent or to treat nosocomial infections [7, 11, 33, 46, 57, 68, 71, 91, 106, 120, 134, 141, 153]. Although this might be viewed as only a component of the overall costs of nosocomial infections, this component has arisen as a subject of interest in its own right (see Chap. 12).

Antimicrobial Resistance

Another unique currency in which the costs of nosocomial infections can be expressed is the emergence of antimicrobial resistance [69, 112, 151]. Under the pressure of broad-spectrum antimicrobial treatment, highly resistant strains of microorganisms emerge in the hospital and become preferentially involved in nosocomial infections (see Chaps. 12, 14). As cross-infection spreads these resistant strains among patients, causing more nosocomial infections, resistance becomes increasingly widespread. Through this mechanism, nosocomial infections have greatly increased the costs of hospital care, not only by incurring costs to care for the patients during more prolonged illnesses, but also by requiring the development and increasing use of new, more powerful antimicrobial drugs.

Environmental Damage

A final currency is the impact on the environment of measures taken to prevent nosocomial infections. Daschner [23] has pointed out the enormous amount of waste and environmental pollution that is introduced into the environment as a direct result of efforts to prevent nosocomial infections in hospitals. The major offending elements include disposable equipment and supplies, detergents, washing agents, disinfectants, chlorides, and phosphates. To date, no estimates of the cost

to society of environmental damage has been made, but clinical efforts to control infection clearly contribute to this problem. An important role that organized infection control programs can play is in limiting the environmentally damaging products to at least those that actually lead to the reduction in infection risks.

Summary Measures

In describing the quantitative impact of nosocomial infections, it is necessary to calculate summary measures that express the central or overall magnitude of the problem. Although the various articles on the subject use standard statistical measures, the choice of summary measures is controversial and requires careful consideration by future investigators.

The most commonly used summary measures are the arithmetic mean, the percentage, and the total of the estimated attributable extra days or costs. The total extra days (or costs) is used to express the overall impact of the problem in a hospital or country. It is simply the sum of the extra days, or cost, of all of the patients with nosocomial infection in a study or the total from a study projected, or extrapolated, to a larger population.

The percentage is used to indicate the relative magnitude of the extra days and costs to the total hospital days and costs of hospitalization. The most carefully derived percentages were reported by Wakefield and co-workers [151, 152] from their study using direct attribution by standardized case review protocol (design type IIC). As found by other investigators, they reported that fewer than half (38 percent) of patients with nosocomial infection have their hospital stay prolonged by the infection but that, in those patients whose stay was prolonged, the extra stay constituted half (52 percent) of their total length of stay, and the magnitude of the prolongation (average of 20 extra days per infection) was more severe than appreciated by calculations of the overall average prolongation of stay.

Whereas the total and percentage are straightforward measures, the mean has almost always been used incorrectly. The problem arises because the distribution of extra days, or costs, is almost always skewed positively by a relatively few, very-high-cost nosocomial infections [54, 64, 114, 152]. This skewness causes the arithmetic mean to overestimate the central tendency of the distribution, as discussed thoroughly by Green and colleagues [54]. For matched comparison studies (design types IIB and IIC), they recommended using either the geometric mean of the *difference* in length of stay, or cost, between infected and uninfected patients in the matched pairs or the geometric mean of the *ratio* of the values in the matched pairs. The former retains the advantage that its interpretation is closer to that of the familiar arithmetic mean, whereas the latter conveys the length of stay of the infected patients as a percentage of that of their uninfected matches. The median could also be used.

Unit of Analysis

A methodologic issue that has been little noticed is the distinction between analyzing nosocomial infections or patients with nosocomial infection. In the former, the extra days, or costs, attributable to each infection are counted separately, whereas in the latter, the extra days, or costs, of all infections in a given patient are summed for that patient. These will be different to the extent that individual patients have more than one nosocomial infection. On a nationwide basis, 18 percent of patients with nosocomial infection have more than one episode or site affected [63] and, in another study of 3 hospitals, 15 percent had more than one infection [64]. Whereas the average extra days and costs are higher in patients with more than one infection than in those with only one [35, 41, 42, 54, 64], the amount that can be separately attributed to a second infection is usually far less than that attributed to the first infection, except when the second infection is nosocomial pneumonia [64]. The importance of knowing the unit of analysis is that estimates of the average extra days and costs are approximately 15 percent higher for studies for patients with nosocomial infection than for studies of nosocomial infections [64, 84].

Estimating the Costs and the Cost-Benefit Ratio of Infection Control Programs

Despite a great deal of research on measuring the costs of nosocomial infections, less work has been done toward estimating the costs to the hospital for conducting an organized infection control program and the ratio of its costs and benefits. The first study on the costs of infection control was published in 1959 by Gee [45]. Since the study predated recommendations for surveillance and full-time infection control staff, it is no surprise that Gee enumerated the costs of changes in hospital practice that were brought about by starting a new infection control program. These included one-time costs such as construction and physical changes, adding sterilizers, and increasing the numbers of thermometers, masks, gowns, and shoe covers, amounting to approximately $43,000 (in 1958 dollars), and recurring costs such as additional personnel in the laboratory, housekeeping, and laundry, and more disposable supplies and equipment and soaps and disinfectants, amounting to approximately $44,000 per year.

Ten years later, using Gee's method, Sperry and Craddock [140] estimated the start-up cost of their program at $90,000 and annual recurring costs at $60,000, and compared these to the estimated economic benefits of preventing nosocomial infections, under varying assumptions of the percentage (20, 50, and 80 percent) of nosocomial infections prevented by the program. Dividing the costs attributable to their infection control program by the anticipated benefits from preventing infections, they derived the first cost-benefit ratio for an infection control program (incorrectly referred to as a *cost-effectiveness ratio*). They estimated that at 20 percent preventive efficacy, the costs would outweigh the benefits by 30 percent; at 50 percent efficacy, the costs would constitute only 51 percent of the benefits; and at 80 percent efficacy, they would constitute only 32 percent of the benefits. Their estimates of the potential benefits (i.e., the costs of nosocomial infections) were derived by the comparative attribution method (design type IIIA).

As part of the planning of the SENIC Project, Haley [58] derived a cost-benefit analysis that was later used for generating policy support for infection control programs in the United States [136] and internationally [58]. Since that analysis was generated after the beginning of the infection control movement in the 1970s, the cost of the infection control program focused on the salary costs of one infection control nurse, a part-time infection control physician, clerical assistance, and miscellaneous expenses, amounting to $20,000 per 250 hospital beds in 1975 dollars. These infection control program costs were then projected to the universe of U.S. hospitals, amounting to $71,840,000 nationwide. To estimate the potential benefits from prevention nationwide, the costs of nosocomial infection were estimated with the crude weighting method (design type I), arriving at a nationwide estimate of approximately $1 billion. From these assumptions, the costs of having an infection control program in every U.S. hospital amounted to approximately 6 percent of the costs of all nosocomial infections. Thus, at 6 percent preventive efficacy, the costs of the program would be exactly balanced by the benefits from infection costs averted; at 20 percent efficacy, there would be a $155 million nationwide savings; and at 50 percent efficacy, there would be a half billion dollar savings, all in 1975 dollars.

In 1986, Haley [59] updated the estimates of the costs and benefits of infection control to 1985 dollars and reformatted the analysis to allow infection control staff in individual hospitals to make estimates for their own institutions. On the basis of nationwide figures from the SENIC Project and the NNIS System and infection costs derived by the direct attribution method (design type IIA) updated for inflation, estimates were provided for the ratio of extra days, dollars, and deaths to total hospital beds for use in projecting these numbers to hospitals of varying sizes. Models were given for making cost-benefit calculations for hospitals of any size. Examples were given for assumed levels of preventive efficacy of 6, 32,

and 50 percent, and a detailed form was included for estimating a program's level of preventive efficacy from a profile of its surveillance and control program activities and personnel, based on SENIC findings [59].

Subsequently, several investigators have compared the estimated costs and the benefits of their infection control programs with varying degrees of sophistication [16, 18, 52, 58, 82, 83, 101, 110, 121, 122]. The most interesting of these recent contributions is the analysis by Miller and colleagues [101]. Using the Haley methods [59] on data from the University of Virginia Hospitals, they estimated the costs of running their infection control program and the actual savings from nosocomial infections prevented, and they used these estimates to derive a fee that should be charged to patients and third-party payers to reimburse hospitals for these preventive services. Although the suggestion does not appear to have been adopted in practice, probably due to the inability to render charges under the PPS, the concept is an interesting one that might someday prove useful as hospital reimbursement systems evolve further.

Since relatively little research has been done in the area of estimating the costs and cost-benefit ratios of infection control programs, many methodologic issues remain to be addressed. Some of the more obvious ones are listed in Table 25-2. In estimating the costs of infection control programs, it is important to decide what components of the programs are to be counted. Certainly, all would agree on the salary of the infection control practitioner, the time of the infection control physician and committee, any direct costs for clerical assistance, maintenance and operations costs, and a portion of the hospital's overhead costs (utilities, space, administrative costs, etc.), but there has been little discussion of whether to include the myriad patient care practices that are done wholly or in part to prevent cross-infection (e.g., closed-system urinary drainage, isolation and handwashing costs, prophylactic antibiotic costs). The prevailing view appears to be that these costs now constitute a minimal standard of care, irrespective of whether there is an organized infection control program, and that the enumeration of the costs of the infection control program should be limited to those costs incurred directly by the infection control practitioners and the infection control committee. Opposing this view, however, is the growing body of articles pointing to the savings produced for the hospital by reductions in wasteful patient care practices initiated to control infection but eliminated at the suggestion of infection control staff [7, 22–26, 40, 44, 52, 97, 99, 117, 148]. If savings from phasing out ineffective practices should be credited to infection control, should not the costs of continuing useful practices be counted on the other side?

A potentially useful study would be a complete enumeration of all of the economic costs borne by hospitals to control and prevent nosocomial infections and all of the economic costs to society for nosocomial infections, distinguishing those that are preventable from those that are not. Whereas such a complete cost-benefit study has not been attempted, the progress in the methods for studying the economics of this problem provides a rich base for attempting it [25, 28, 36, 41, 43, 65, 104, 116, 141, 152]. In view of the rapidly changing economic forces in health care, further research of this problem is likely to continue to interest decision makers.

Summary Recommendations for Hospitals

Infection control personnel wishing to estimate how much nosocomial infections are costing to elevate interest in the problem might consider three alternative study designs. The best crude estimates for the least time expenditure can be obtained by simply multiplying the estimated numbers of nosocomial infections at various sites by the site-specific cost weights (cost per infection) derived from the SENIC study and published by Haley [59] (design type I). Probably the most precise measurements within a hospital for the least time commitment involve using the Appropriateness Evaluation Protocol (design

type IIC), described for this purpose by Wakefield and colleagues [151, 152], possibly with the hospital's actual cost weights obtained from a detailed cost-accounting system. Although approaches for refining the matched comparison methods (design type IIIC) are improving [60], definitive estimates of the costs of nosocomial infections might best be obtained from prospective, randomized, clinical trials (design type IV), possibly as a byproduct of studies of antimicrobial agents or other interventions, after the model of Stone and colleagues [142].

References

1. Aber, R.C. Nosocomial infections—1979. *Delaware Med. J.* 51:635, 1979.
2. Agresti, A. *Categorical Data Analysis.* New York: Wiley, 1990. Pp. 24–35.
3. American College of Surgeons, Committee on Control of Surgical Infections, Committee on Pre- and Post-operative Care. *Manual on Control of Infection in Surgical Patients.* Philadelphia: Lippincott, 1976. Pp. 11–15.
4. Apostolopoulou, E. Nosocomial infections [Gre]. *Noseleutike* 29:23, 1990.
5. Barnass, S., et al. The tangible cost implications of a hospital outbreak of multiply-resistant *Salmonella. Epidemiol. Infect.* 103:227, 1989.
6. Bennett, J.V. Human infections: Economic implications and prevention. *Ann. Intern. Med.* 89:761, 1978.
7. Beyt, B.E., Jr., Troxler, S., and Cavaness, J. Prospective payment and infection control. *Infect. Control* 6:161, 1985.
8. Boyce, J.M., Potter-Bynoe, G., and Dziobek, L. Hospital reimbursement patterns among patients with surgical wound infections following open heart surgery. *Infect. Control Hosp. Epidemiol.* 11:89, 1990.
9. Brachman, P.S. Nosocomial infection control: An overview. *Rev. Infect. Dis.* 3:640, 1981.
10. Brachman, P.S., et al. Nosocomial surgical infections: Incidence and cost. *Surg. Clin. North Am.* 60:15, 1980.
11. Briceland, L.L., et al. Antibiotic streamlining from combination therapy to monotherapy utilizing an interdisciplinary approach. *Arch. Intern. Med.* 148:2019, 1988.
12. Brote, L. Gillquist, J., and Tarnvik, W. Wound infections in general surgery. *Acta Chir. Scand.* 142:99, 1976.
13. Brown, A., and Magnussen, M. H. Infection

control problems. A survey of the Veterans Administration medical centers in the northeastern United States. *Milit. Med.* 146:348, 1981.

14. Choi, M., et al. *Salmonella* outbreak in a nursing home. *J. Am. Geriatr. Soc.* 38:531, 1990.

15. Clarke, S.K.R. Sepsis in surgical wounds, with particular reference to *Staphylococcus aureus. Br. J. Surg.* 44:592, 1957.

16. Collier, C., Miller, D. P., and Borst, M. Community hospital surgeon-specific infection rates. *Infect. Control* 8:249, 1987.

17. Commission on Professional and Hospital Activities. *Length of Stay in PAS Hospitals, United States, Regional Reports.* Ann Arbor: Commission on Professional and Hospital Activities, 1980.

18. Condon, R.E., Schulte, W.J., Malangoni, R.A., and Anderson-Teschendorf, M.J. Effectiveness of a surgical wound surveillance program. *Arch. Surg.* 118:303, 1983.

19. Cox, C.E. Nosocomial urinary tract infections. *Urology* 32:210, 1988.

20. Cruse, P.J.E., and Foord, R. The epidemiology of wound infection: A 10-year prospective study of 62,939 wounds. *Surg. Clin. North Am.* 60:27, 1980.

21. Daschner, F. Patient-oriented prevention and control of hospital-acquired infections (author's transl.) [Ger]. *Klinische Wochenschrift* 1203, 1979.

22. Daschner, F. Economic aspects of hospital infections. *J. Hosp. Infect.* 3:1, 1982.

23. Daschner, F. Cost-effectiveness in hospital infection control—lessons for the 1900s. *J. Hosp. Infect.* 13:325, 1989.

24. Daschner, F.D. Practical aspects for cost reduction in hospital infection control. *Infect. Control* 5:32, 1984.

25. Daschner, F.D. The cost of hospital-acquired infection. *J. Hosp. Infect.* 5 (Suppl. A):27, 1984.

26. Daschner, F.D., and Frank, U. Controversies in hospital infection control. *Europ. J. Clin. Microbiol.* 6:335, 1987.

27. Davies, T.W., and Cottingham, J. The cost of hospital infection in orthopaedic patients. *J. Infect.* 1:329, 1979.

28. de Clercq, H., De Decker, G., Alexander, J.P., and Huyghens, L. Cost evaluation of infections in intensive care. *Acta Anaesthesiol. Belg.* 34:179, 1983.

29. de Martín, M.C., de Cajar, S., Abrego, G., and Díz, O. Economic impact of nosocomial infections on the Metropolitan Hospital Complex of the Social Security Fund (from January through December 1987) [Spa]. *Rev. Med. Panama* 15:112, 1990.

30. Dixon, R.E. Effect of infections on hospital care. *Ann. Intern. Med.* 89:749, 1978.

31. Dunk-Richards, G. Cost factors associated with hospital acquired infection. *Aust. Nurs. J.* 8:36, 1961.

32. Edwards, L.D. The epidemiology of 2056 remote site infections and 1966 surgical wound infections occurring in 1865 patients: A four year study of 4,923 operations at Rush-Presbyterian-St. Luke's Hospital, Chicago. *Ann. Surg.* 184:758, 1976.

33. Ehrenkranz, N.J. Containing costs of antimicrobials in the hospital: A critical evaluation. *Am. J. Infect. Control* 17:300, 1989.

34. Eliason, E.L., and McLaughlin, C. Postoperative wound complications. *Ann. Surg.* 100:1159, 1934.

35. Fabry, J., et al. Cost of nosocomial infections: Analysis of 512 digestive surgery patients. *World J. Surg.* 6:362, 1982.

36. Fedson, D.S. Prevention and control of influenza in institutional settings. *Hosp. Pract.* 24:87, 1989.

37. Fekety, F.R. The Epidemiology of Infections in Surgical Patients. In: B. S. Berlin and M. Hilbert (Eds.), *Control of Infections in Hospitals: Proceedings of an Institute Held at the University of Michigan, March 1–3, 1965.* Ann Arbor: University of Michigan School of Public Health, 1965. Pp. 24–38.

38. Finkler, S.A. The distinction between cost and charges. *Ann. Intern. Med.* 96:102, 1982.

39. Finn, A., Anday, E., and Talbot, G.H. An epidemic of adenovirus 7a infection in a neonatal nursery: Course, morbidity, and management. *Infect. Control Hosp. Epidemiol.* 9:398, 1988.

40. Franck, J.N. Literature search reveals focus of cost savings. *J. Hosp. Infect.* 5 (Suppl. A):115, 1984.

41. Freeman, J., and McGowan, J.E., Jr. Methodologic issues in hospital epidemiology: III. Investigating the modifying effects of time and severity of underlying illness on estimates of cost of nosocomial infection. *Rev. Infect. Dis.* 6:285, 1984.

42. Freeman, J., Rosner, B.A., and McGowan, J.E. Adverse effects of nosocomial infection, *J. Infect. Dis.* 140:732, 1979.

43. Fuchs, P.C. Hospital infection in orthopaedic patients [lett.] *J. Infect.* 2:185, 1980.

44. Garner, J.S., Emori, T.G., and Haley, R.W. Operating room practices for the control of infection in U.S. hospitals, October 1976 to July 1977. *Surg. Gynecol. Obstet.* 155:873, 1982.

45. Gee, D.A. How infection control affects the hospital. *Mod. Hosp.* 93 (Sept.):63, 1959.

46. Germiniani, R. Prevention of infections in surgery. Costs and benefits of infections of surgical wounds and of their prevention with antibiotics [Ita.] *Minerva Chirurgica* 44:789, 1989.

47. Gertman, P.M., and Restuccia, J.D. The ap-

propriateness evaluation protocol: A technique for assessing unnecessary days of hospital care. *Med. Care* 19:855, 1981.

48. Girard, R., et al. Costs of nosocomial infection in a neonatal unit. *J. Hosp. Infect.* 4:361, 1983.

49. Givens, C.D., and Wenzel, R.P. Catheter-associated urinary tract infections in surgical patients: A controlled study on the excess morbidity and costs. *J. Urol.* 124:646, 1980.

50. Goetz, A., Yu, V.L., and O'Donnell, W.F. Surgical complications related to insertion of penile prostheses with emphasis on infection and cost. *Infect. Control Hosp. Epidemiol.* 9(6):250, 1988.

51. Goodall, J.W.D. Cross-infection in hospital wards: Its incidence and prevention. *Lancet* 1:807, 1952.

52. Grazebrook, J. Hospital-acquired infection. Counting the cost of infection. *Nursing Times,* 82:24, 1986.

53. Green, J.W., and Wenzel, R.P. Postoperative wound infection: A controlled study of the increased duration of hospital stay and direct cost of hospitalization. *Ann. Surg.* 185:264, 1977.

54. Green, M.S., Rubinstein, E., and Amit, P. Estimating the effects of nosocomial infections on the length of hospitalization. *J. Infect. Dis.* 145:667, 1982.

55. Gross, P.A., et al. Description of case-mix adjusters by the Severity of Illness Working Group of the Society of Hospital Epidemiologists of America (SHEA). *Infect. Control Hosp. Epidemiol.* 9:309, 1988.

56. Gross, P.A., and Van Antwerpen, C. Nosocomial infections and hospital deaths: A case-control study. *Am. J. Med.* 75:658, 1983.

57. Guimaraes, R.X., et al. Hospital infection: Reduction of antibiotics consumption due to the action of the Hospital Infection Control Committee of the Hospital do Servidor Publico Municipal de Sao Paulo [Por]. *Rev. Paulista Med.* 104:274, 1986.

58. Haley, R.W. Preliminary Cost-Benefit Analysis of Hospital Infection Control Programs (The SENIC Project). In F. Daschner (Ed.), *Proven and Unproven Methods in Hospital Infection Control: Proceedings of an International Workshop at Baiersbronn, September 24–25, 1977.* New York: Gustav Fischer Verlag, 1978. Pp. 93–95.

59. Haley, R.W. *Managing Hospital Infection Control for Cost-Effectiveness.* Chicago: American Hospital Association, 1986.

60. Haley, R.W. Measuring the costs of nosocomial infections: Methods for estimating economic burden on the hospital. *Am. J. Med.* 19 (Suppl. 3B):325, 1991.

61. Haley, R.W., et al. Increased recognition of infectious diseases in US hospitals through increased use of diagnostic tests, 1970–1976. *Am. J. Epidemiol.* 121:168, 1985.

62. Haley, R.W., et al. The efficacy of infection surveillance and control programs in preventing nosocomial infections in US hospitals. *Am. J. Epidemiol.* 121:182, 1985.

63. Haley, R.W., et al. Nosocomial infections in U.S. hospitals, 1975–1976: Estimated frequency by selected characteristics of patients. *Am. J. Med.* 70:947, 1981.

64. Haley, R.W., et al. Extra charges and prolongation of stay attributable to nosocomial infections: A prospective interhospital comparison. *Am. J. Med.* 70:51, 1981.

65. Haley, R.W., et al. Estimating the extra charges and prolongation of hospitalization due to nosocomial infections: A comparison of methods. *J. Infect. Dis.* 141:248, 1980.

66. Haley, R.W., White, J.W., Culver, D.H., and Hughes, J.M. The financial incentive for hospitals to prevent nosocomial infections under the prospective payment system. An empirical determination from a nationally representative sample. *J.A.M.A.* 257:1611, 1987.

67. Hemming, V.G., Overall, J.C., and Britt, M.R. Nosocomial infections in a newborn intensive-care unit: Results of forty-one months of surveillance. *N. Engl. J. Med.* 294:1310, 1976.

68. Hemsell, D.L., Hemsell, P.G., Heard, M.C., and Nobles, B.J. Piperacillin and a combination of clindamycin and gentamicin for the treatment of hospital and community acquired acute pelvic infections including pelvic abscess. *Surg. Gynecol. Obstet.* 165:223, 1987.

69. Holmberg, S.D., Solomon, S.L., and Blake, P.A. Health and economic impacts of antimicrobial resistance. *Rev. Infect. Dis.* 9:1065, 1987.

70. Hooton, T.M., et al. The joint associations of multiple risk factors with the occurrence of nosocomial infection. *Am. J. Med.* 70:960, 1981.

71. Huckleberry, S.D. Antibiotic cost-containment. *Drug Intelli. Clin. Pharm.* 20:589, 1986.

72. Hyams, P.J., Stuewe, M.C., and Heitzer, V. Herpes zoster causing varicella (chickenpox) in hospital employees: Cost of a casual attitude. *Am. J. Infect. Control* 12:2, 1984.

73. Jencks, S.F., Dobson, A., Willis, P., and Feinstein, P. Evaluating and improving the measurement of hospital case mix. *Health Care Financ. Rev.* Nov. (Annu. Suppl.):1, 1984.

74. Johnston, J.M., and Burke, J.P. Nosocomial outbreak of hand-foot-and-mouth disease among operating suite personnel. *Infect. Control* 7:172, 1986.

75. Jorup-Rönström, C., and Britton, S. The nosocomial component of medical care. A

prospective study on the amount, spectrum and costs of medical disturbances in a department of infectious diseases. *Scand. J. Infect. Dis.* 36:150, 1982.

76. Kaiser, A. B., et al. Efficacy of cefazolin, cefamandole, and gentamicin as prophylactic agents in cardiac surgery. *Ann. Surg.* 206:791, 1987.

77. Kereselidze, T., and Maglacas, A.M. Nosocomial infections—what WHO is doing. *J. Hosp. Infect.* 5(Suppl. A):7, 1984.

78. Klarman, H.E. Application of cost-benefit analysis to the health services and the special case of technologic innovation. *Int. J. Health Serv.* 4:325, 1974.

79. Kleinbaum, D.G., Kupper, L.L., and Morgenstern, H. Typology of Observational Study Designs. In: *Epidemiologic Research: Principles and Quantitative Methods.* Belmont, CA: Lifetime Learning Publications, 1982. Pp. 62–95.

80. Kleinbaum, D.G., Kupper, L.L., and Morgenstern, H. Matching in Epidemiologic Studies. In: *Epidemiologic Research: Principles and Quantitative Methods.* Belmont, CA: Lifetime Learning Publications, 1982. Pp. 377–402.

81. Krieger, J.N., Kaiser, D.L., and Wenzel, R.P. Nosocomial urinary tract infections: Secular trends, treatment and economics in a university hospital. *J. Urol.* 130:102, 1983.

82. Lambert, D.C. The cost of nosocomial infection and its prevention. Projection and limitations of an economic analysis [Fre.]. *Agressologie* 28:1123, 1987.

83. Lambert, D.C., and Fabry, J. Cost-benefit and cost-effectiveness methods and evaluation of additional costs due to hospital infection [Fre]. *Agressologie* 26:173, 1985.

84. Le Coutour, X., et al. The cost of hospital acquired infections [Fre]. *Agressologie* 30:275, 1989.

85. Le Gall, J.R., Loirat, P., and Alperovitch, A. Simplified acute physiologic score for intensive care patients. *Lancet* 2:741, 1983.

86. Letsch, S.W., Levitt, K.R., and Waldo, D.R. National health expenditures, 1987. *Health Care Financ. Rev.* 10:109, 1988.

87. Lidgren, L., and Lindberg, L. Duration and costs of hospitalization because of orthopaedic infections and proposed cooperation between orthopaedic departments and departments of infectious diseases. *Acta Orthop. Scandinav.* 43:355, 1972.

88. Losos, J., and Trotman, M. Estimated economic burden of nosocomial infection. *Can. J. Public Health* 75:248, 1984.

89. Lossa, G.R., and Valzacchi, B. Estimation of the cost of hospital infections [Spa]. *Bol. Ofic. Sanitar. Panamericana* 101:134, 1986.

90. Lowenthal, J. Sources and sequelae of surgical sepsis. *Br. Med. J.* 1:1437, 1962.

91. Mangi, R.J., et al. Cefoperazone versus ceftazidime monotherapy of nosocomial pneumonia. *Am. J. Med.* 85:44, 1988.

92. Martïn, D.A. Repercussions at the individual and social level of hospital infections [Spa]. *Rev. Enferm.* 8:81, 1985.

93. Martin, M.A., Pfaller, M.A., and Wenzel, R.P. Coagulase-negative staphylococcal bacteremia: Mortality and hospital stay. *Ann. Intern. Med.* 110:9, 1989.

94. Massanari, R.M., Wilkerson, K., Streed, S.A., and Hierholzer, W.J., Jr. Reliability of reporting nosocomial infections in the discharge abstract and implications for receipt of revenues under prospective reimbursement. *Am. J. Public Health* 77:561, 1987.

95. Matson, D.O., and Estes, M.K. Impact of rotavirus infection at a large pediatric hospital. *J. Infect. Dis.* 162:598, 1990.

96. McGowan, J.E., Jr. Cost and benefit in control of nosocomial infection: Methods for analysis. *Rev. Infect. Dis.* 3:790, 1981.

97. McGowan, J.E., Jr. Cost and benefit—a critical issue for hospital infection control. Fifth Annual National Foundation for Infectious Diseases Lecture. *Am. J. Infect. Control* 10:100, 1982.

98. Mead, P.B., et al. Decreasing the incidence of surgical wound infections: Validation of a surveillance-notification program. *Arch. Surg.* 121:458, 1986.

99. Meers, P.D. Facts and fancies in hospital infection. *Ann. Acad. Med. Singapore* 16:671, 1966.

100. Miettinen, O.S. Stratification by a multivariate confounder score. *Am. J. Epidemiol.* 104:609, 1976.

101. Miller, P.J., Farr, B.M., and Gwaltney, J.M., Jr. Economic benefits of an effective infection control program: Case study and proposal. *Rev. Infect. Dis.* 11:284, 1989.

102. Munoz, E., et al. Financial risk, hospital cost, and complications and comorbidities in medical non-complication and comorbidity-stratified diagnosis related groups. *Am. J. Med.* 84:933, 1988.

103. Munoz, E., et al. Financial risk, hospital cost, complications, and comorbidities in surgical noncomplication- and noncomorbidity-stratified diagnostic related groups. *Ann. Surg.* 305, 1988.

104. Munoz, E., et al. Financial risk, hospital cost, and complications and comorbidities (CCs) in the non-CC-stratified pulmonary medicine diagnostic-related group Medicare hospital payment system. *Am. Rev. Respir. Dis.* 137:998, 1988.

105. Nelson, R.M., and Dries, D.J. The economic implications of infection in cardiac surgery. *Ann. Thorac. Surg.* 42:240, 1987.

106. Neu, H.C. Antimicrobial activity, bacterial re-

sistance, and antimicrobial pharmacology. Is it possible to use new agents cost-effectively? *Am. J. Med.* 78:17, 1985.

107. Norberg, B. Hospital infections cost money and suffering [Swe]. *Vardfacket* 10:24, 1986.

108. O'Leary, M.P. Economic considerations in management of complicated urinary tract infections. *Urology* 35:22, 1990.

109. Olson, M.M., and Allen, M.O. Nosocomial abscess. Results of an eight-year prospective study of 32,284 operations. *Arch. Surg.* 124:356, 1989.

110. Olson, M.M., and Lee, J.T., Jr. Continuous, 10-year wound infection surveillance: Results, advantages, and unanswered questions. *Arch. Surg.* 125:794, 1990.

111. Pastorová, J., et al. Results of a prospective study of the economic importance of nosocomial infections in the surgical department in a type I polyclinic hospital [Cze]. *Rozhledy V Chirugii* 60:433, 1981.

112. Phelps, C.E. Bug/drug resistance. Sometimes less is more. *Med. Care* 27:194, 1989.

113. Piffaut, V. Nosocomial infections. Position of the Council of Europe. Impact legal, economic and at the social security level [Fre]. *Agressologie* 28:1133, 1987.

114. Pinner, R.W., et al. High cost nosocomial infections. *Infect. Control* 3:143, 1982.

115. Platt, R., et al., Mortality associated with nosocomial urinary-tract infection. *N. Engl. J. Med.* 307:637, 1982.

116. Platt, R., Polk, B.F., Murdock, B., and Rosner, B. Prevention of catheter-associated urinary tract infection: A cost-benefit analysis. *Infect. Control Hosp. Epidemiol.* 10:60, 1989.

117. Pobanz, R.B. The economic impact of universal precautions on a surgical unit. *Nurs. Management* 20:38, 1942.

118. Polakavetz, S.H., Dunne, M.E., and Cook, J.S. Nosocomial infection: The hidden cost in health care. *Hospitals* 52:101, 1978.

119. Prabhakar, P., et al. Nosocomial surgical infections: Incidence and cost in a developing country. *Am. J. Infect. Control* 11:51, 1983.

120. Quintiliani, R., Cooper, B.W., Briceland, L.L., and Nightingale, C.H. Economic impact of streamlining antibiotic administration. *Am. J. Med.* 82:391, 1987.

121. Rao, N., Jacobs, S., and Joyce, L. Cost-effective eradication of an outbreak of methicillin-resistant *Staphylococcus aureus* in a community teaching hospital. *Infect. Control Hosp. Epidemiol.* 9:255, 1988.

122. Reinarz, J.A., Megna, M.J., and Brown, G.T. Nosocomial infection: Time for accountability. In: D.N. Gilbert and J.P. Sanford (Eds.), *Infectious Diseases: Current Topics*, Vol. 1. New York: Grune & Stratton, 1979. Pp. 219–240.

123. Rhame, F.S., and Sudderth, W.D. Incidence and prevalence as used in the analysis of the occurrence of nosocomial infections. *Am. J. Epidemiol.* 113:1, 1981.

124. Rishpon, S., Lubacsh, S., and Epstein, L.M. Reliability of a method of determining the necessity of hospitalization days in Israel. *Med. Care* 24:279, 1986.

125. Rose, R., Hunting, K.J., Townsend, T.R., and Wenzel, R. P. Morbidity/mortality and economics of hospital-acquired blood stream infections: A controlled study. *South. Med. J.* 70:1267, 1977.

126. Rubinstein, E., et al. The effects of nosocomial infections on the length and costs of hospital stay. *J. Antimicrob. Chemother.* 9 (Suppl. A):93, 1982.

127. Rutledge, K.A., and McDonald, H.P., Jr. Costs of treating simple nosocomial urinary tract infection. *Urology* 26:24, 1985.

128. Rutledge, K.A., and McDonald, H.P., Jr. Costs and strategies for managing nosocomial urinary tract infections. *Drug Intellig. Clin. Pharm.* 20:587, 1986.

129. Schäfer, U. Cost analysis in nosocomial infections. A 1-year study in the Surgical Department of Riesa District Hospital [Ger]. *Zentralblatt Fur Chirugie* 112:1552, 1987.

130. Schaffner, W. Infection control: Time to justify the costs. *Hospitals* 53:125, 1979.

131. Scheckler, W.E. Septicemia and nosocomial infections in a community hospital. *Ann. Intern. Med.* 89:754, 1978.

132. Scheckler, W.E. Nosocomial infections in a community hospital: 1972 through 1976. *Arch. Intern. Med.* 138:1792, 1978.

133. Scheckler, W.E. Hospital costs of nosocomial infections: A prospective three-month study in a community hospital. *Infect. Control* 1:150, 1980.

134. Scheife, R.T., Cox, C.E., McCabe, R.E., and Grad, C. Norfloxacin vs best parenteral therapy in treatment of moderate to serious, multiply-resistant, nosocomial urinary tract infections: A pharmacoeconomic analysis. *Urology* 32:24, 1988.

135. Schroeder, S.A., Showstack, J.A., and Roberts, H.E. Frequency and clinical description of high-cost patients in 17 acute-care hospitals. *N. Engl. J. Med.* 300:1306, 1979.

136. Sencer, D.J., and Axnick, N.W. Utilization of cost/benefit analysis in planning prevention programs. *Acta Med. Scand.* 576 (Suppl.):123, 1975.

137. Septimus, E.J. Nosocomial bacterial pneumonias. *Semin. Resp. Infect.* 4:245, 1989.

138. Simchen, E., and Sacks, T. Infection in war wounds—experience during the 1973 October war in Israel. *Ann. Surg.* 182:754, 1975.

139. Spengler, R.F., and Greenough, W.B. Hospital costs and mortality attributed to nosocomial bacteremias. *J.A.M.A.* 240:2455, 1978.

140. Sperry, H.E., and Craddock, J. It pays to

spend money for infection control. *Mod. Hosp.* 111:124, 1968.

141. Stevenson, R.C., Blackman, S.C., Williams, C.L., and Bartzokas, C.A. Measuring the saving attributable to an antibiotic prescribing policy. *J. Hosp. Infect.* 11:16, 1988.

142. Stone, H.H., et al. Prophylactic and preventive antibiotic therapy: Timing, duration and economics. *Ann. Surg.* 189:691, 1979.

143. Suwanakoon, P., et al. Symposium: Impact of nosocomial infections on Thailand. *J. Med. Assoc. Thailand* 71(Suppl. 3):52, 1988.

144. Thoburn, R., Fekety, F.R., Cluff, L.E., and Melvin, V.B. Infections acquired by hospitalized patients. *Arch. Intern. Med.* 121:1, 1968.

145. Thomann, J. An attempt at evaluating the costs of nosocomial infections [Fre]. *Agressologie* 28:1221, 1987.

146. Trilla, A., and Mirö, J.M. Control of nosocomial infections: Who? how? and how much does it cost? (edit.) [Spa]. *Medicina Clinica* 92:217, 1989.

147. Turnidge, J. MRSA—is control worthwhile and feasible? *Med. J. Aust.* 152:225, 1990.

148. Valenti, W.M., Sovie, M.D., Reifler, C.B., and Douglas, R.G., Jr. Cut costs by revising policies and procedures. *Hospitals* 54:84, 1980.

149. Van Voris, L.P., Belshe, R.B., and Shaffer, J.L. Nosocomial influenza B virus infection in the elderly. *Ann. Intern. Med.* 96:153, 1982.

150. Verbrugh, H.A., Mintjes-de Groot, A.J., and Verkooyen, R.P. Registration and prevention of hospital infections in a general hospital [Dut]. *Nederlands Tijdschrift Voor Geneeskunde* 134:490, 1990.

151. Wakefield, D.S., et al. Cost of nosocomial infection: Relative contributions of laboratory, antibiotic, and per diem costs in serious *Staphylococcus aureus* infections. *Am. J. Infect. Control* 16:185, 1988.

152. Wakefield, D.S., Pfaller, M.A., Hammons, G.T., and Massanari, R.M. Use of the appropriateness evaluation protocol for estimating the incremental costs associated with nosocomial infections. *Med. Care* 25:481, 1987.

153. Weinstein, M.C., et al. Cost-effective choice of antimicrobial therapy for serious infections. *J. Gen. Intern. Med.* 1:351, 1986.

154. Wenzel, R.P. Nosocomial infections, diagnosis-related groups, and study on the efficacy of nosocomial infection control. Economic implications for hospitals under the prospective payment system. *Am. J. Med.* 78(Suppl. 6B):3, 1985.

155. Westwood, J.C.N., Legrace S., and Mitchell, M.A. Hospital-acquired infection: Present and future impact and need for positive action. *Can. Med. Assoc. J.* 110:769, 1974.

156. Williams, R.E.O. Infection and the injured patient: Lessons and opportunities. *Injury* 9:227, 1978.

157. Williams, R.E.O., McDonald, J.C., and Blowers, R. Incidence of surgical wound infection in England and Wales. *Lancet* 2:659, 1960.

26

Legal Aspects of Hospital Infections

Karen Rose Koppel Kaunitz
Andrew M. Kaunitz

As the sophistication of medical practice along with patient expectations continue to grow, our society's appetite for litigation continues to increase. These synergistic trends have expanded legal liability related to nosocomial infections.

Today's human immunodeficiency virus (HIV) epidemic has certainly intensified such liability. By reviewing how liability related to hospital infection may occur, this chapter seeks to help hospitals and clinicians minimize their exposure to legal consequences of these infections.

Introduction to Law and the Legal System

Sources of the law include federal and state constitutions, statutes, administrative law, and judicial decisions (common law). A legal *cause of action* may be created by a constitutional right, a statute, or by common law. A cause of action is composed of several elements, each of which must be proved before the plaintiff can establish legal liability on the part of the defendant. Each cause of action consists of its own distinct elements but, in general, the following must exist before legal liability occurs:

1. The plaintiff must have an interest that is protected by law.
2. There must be a legal duty.
3. A breach of duty by the defendant must be proved.
4. An injury must be shown—damage to the protected interest.
5. It must be proved that the breach caused the injury.

Initially, the burden of proof rests with the plaintiff. The plaintiff must establish each element at least by a preponderance of the evidence. If the plaintiff succeeds in this, the burden shifts to the defendant to offer a legal defense. If liability is established, the plaintiff must then prove damages [101].

In some cases, the court decides that there are no material fact issues and that the required elements of the cause of action do or do not exist (or that a legal defense does exist). In these cases, the court grants summary judgment in favor of the prevailing party, and there is no trial.

Negligence

Malpractice refers to a tort, or civil wrong, committed by a professional acting in his or her professional capacity. Negligence is the most common cause of action in medical malpractice cases. *Negligence* is legally defined as "a violation of the duty to use care" [28]. It arises where injury results from the failure of the wrongdoer (the tort-feasor) to exercise due care. To establish liability, the four elements of the tort of negligence must be satisfied [87].

1. The existence of a standard or duty owed to the plaintiff
2. The defendant's failure to perform that duty or satisfy the standard of care owed
3. The plaintiff's demonstration that his or her injury resulted directly or proximately from the defendant's failure to perform the duty or to meet the standard of care
4. The occurrence of damages attributable to the injury

To prevail in litigation when alleging damages due to a hospital infection, a plaintiff must therefore establish that an infection was contracted in the hospital, that the hospital breached its duty to the plaintiff through an act of negligence, and that this negligence directly caused both the infection and any damages sustained [63]. The test for negligence in an infection control case might be framed in the following way: "Was the hospital care or lack of care in some way responsible for the infection; and did the hospital act in a reason-

able and prudent manner in recognizing, reporting and trying to control the infection?" [10]. Negligence in the treatment of infection can also result in liability [27, 29, 52].

Standard of Care and Breach of the Standard

A fundamental component of establishing liability involves delineating which particular duties hospitals and physicians have toward patients. The *duty of due care* requires all persons to conduct themselves as any average reasonable person would do in similar circumstances. In the health care context, these duties translate to the *standard of care*. To prevail in negligence actions, therefore, plaintiffs must establish that a provider has failed to meet such a standard of care. The standard of care required relates, in turn, to the circumstances of the particular case. Local, state, or national practices may determine a standard of care. The traditional rule, which was favorable to providers, held that practices should conform to the standards of other providers in the same locality. Under this *customary practice standard* of the local community, or *locality rule,* a provider's performance was measured against the level of care delivered by reasonably competent persons or institutions of equivalent skill in the same geographic community. The court's sole function, therefore, was to determine whether the providers did something that was not customary or failed to do something that was [61]. This standard was subsequently expanded to include those practices common in similar communities; hence, the standard was same or similar communities.

The same or similar locality custom standard has been replaced by a *national standard*. This nationwide approach is based on the assumption that there should be one prevailing level of care. The standard of care in the provider's locality, or in a similar locality, therefore, has become simply one factor in determining whether the standard of care has been met [7, 31, 52]. National accreditation standards promulgated by the Joint Commission on Accreditation of Healthcare Organizations (JCAHO) and state licensure requirements and guidelines such as those published by the Centers for Disease Control

(CDC) and the American Hospital Association (AHA) have encouraged courts to hold providers to a national standard of care. Application of a national standard of care has also allowed the use of experts from outside the defendant's locality.

Standard of Care in Nosocomial Infection Cases

Although hospitals have a duty to protect patients from injury due to infections, courts have never maintained that hospitals guarantee their patients will not acquire nosocomial infections. A hospital, however, may be liable for a patient's infection if it can be shown that the infection was caused by the negligence of the hospital or any of its agents. Hospitals' duties to monitor medical care include conducting infection control reviews. If a plaintiff establishes that an excessive number of infections has occurred at a defendant hospital, the hospital may have to prove that it could not have discovered the pattern any sooner and that, on discovery, measures were immediately undertaken to correct the problem. To minimize the risk of failing to meet the standard of care, hospitals should vigorously educate personnel in aseptic technique and infection control procedures and should institute monitoring mechanisms to establish that proper procedures are indeed being followed.

A spectrum of standards rather than a single standard of infection control applies to hospitals. In determining the standards of care within a hospital, courts have looked to various sources. One source is based on the hospital's own internal rules; these include protocols, procedures manuals, and bylaws. In *Robinson* v. *St. John's Medical Center,* 508 S.W.2d 7 (Mo. 1974), for example, the hospital's operating procedure manual was used to establish nurses' duties in the operating room. This established the standard of care for which the hospital was subsequently liable. In *Helman* v. *Sacred Heart Hosp.,* 381 P.2d 605 (Wash. 1963), there was evidence that hospital personnel moved from one patient to another without washing their hands, failing to follow hospital policy designed to prevent the spread of infection. The court,

therefore, ruled that the hospital breached its duty to the patient. In *Kapuschinsky* v. *United States,* 248 F. Supp. 732, 259 F. Supp. 1 (D.S.C. 1966), the court cited the hospital's failure to follow the standard of care it voluntarily assumed in its own procedure manual. This case involved nurses' aides working with preterm infants, a practice explicitly prohibited by the hospital's procedure manual. (See under the heading Exposure to Contagious Personnel for details of this case [p. 544].)

A hospital's failure to follow its own rules and procedures may lead to a liability claim against which it may be particularly difficult to defend:

> . . . [T]he hospital should be very careful to make sure that its own hospital regulations and procedures are followed assiduously. Because these items may be taken as the duties or standards of care incumbent upon a hospital, the failure to perform such duties or to meet such standards of care may allow the plaintiff to show the first two elements of negligence; then he [she] would only have to show that such failure to perform the duty or failure to meet a standard of care was the direct cause of his [her] injury and to show the amount of his [her] damages [78].

In addition to promoting staff compliance with internal regulations, hospitals should establish in their internal manuals procedures that are as practicable as possible.

Accreditation requirements, federal and state laws, and regulations governing hospitals may also establish standards of care. In some instances, they may serve as a substitute for expert testimony. In most states, hospitals are subject to government rules regulating the practice of hospital infection control. These requirements vary considerably from state to state; hence, hospital administrators and counsel should consult their own state's regulations. Some states allow considerable latitude in procedures, providing little guidance. Other states, such as Illinois, set forth explicit requirements for infection control procedures, including requirements for the sterilization of equipment, instruments, utensils, water, and supplies. In some circumstances, regulations even specify the particular methods of sterilization to be used. Courts have sometimes ruled that these regulations establish guidelines for minimum standards of hospital care.

Plaintiffs alleging damages resulting from violations of state regulations may be able to establish negligence. For example, in *Suburban Hosp Ass'n* v. *Hadary*, 22 Md. App. 186, 322 A.2d 258 (Md. 1974), the hospital's failure to comply with a licensing regulation requiring the segregation of sterile and nonsterile needles established the hospital's negligence. In the case of *Derrick* v. *Ontario Community Hosp.*, 120 Cal. Rptr. 566, 47 Cal. App.3d 145 (1975), a state law requiring hospitals to report communicable diseases to the local health officer was cited by the plaintiff in establishing a cause of action against the hospital, which failed to report a particular communicable disease. Even though the court stated that it might be difficult to prove that the defendant hospital's failure to report a communicable disease to the local health officer resulted in the plaintiff's injury, it found that the statute imposed a duty on the hospital to report such a case. The appellate court reversed the trial court and concluded that, at trial, the plaintiffs would have to prove not only that the hospital violated its duty under the statute but also that this violation was the proximate cause of the plaintiff's injuries.

Mere compliance with minimum statutory or regulatory standards and licensure provisions, however, may not preclude liability for negligence. Hospitals may be held to a higher degree of care due to local practices and requirements of good medical practice or because the court rejects an existing standard as inadequate to protect the public.

Government agencies such as the Health Care Financing Administration [71] and the CDC [18] issue regulations and guidelines for health care. Private organizations such as the JCAHO, AHA, and professional associations also issue standards and recommendations. All these may play a role in establishing a particular standard of care.

The *Darling* decision, described later under the heading Corporate Negligence Theory, held that the standards of the JCAHO along with the hospital's medical staff bylaws were admissible as evidence in determining negligence. Finding that the defendant hospital failed to abide by its own rules and failed to maintain JCAHO standards, the court determined the hospital to be liable [17].

Whereas accreditation standards have ordinarily applied only to accredited hospitals, these standards may receive such acceptance in a given community that courts will employ accreditation standards in determining negligence in nonaccredited hospitals as well. In its chapter on infection control, the JCAHO [58] lists the following standards:

Standard 1.   There is an effective hospitalwide program for the surveillance, prevention, and control of infection.

Standard 2.   A multidisciplinary committee oversees the program for surveillance, prevention, and control of infection.

Standard 3.   Responsibility for the management of infection surveillance, prevention, and control is assigned to a qualified person(s).

Standard 4.   There are written policies and procedures for infection surveillance, prevention, and control for all patient care departments/services.

Standard 5.   Patient care support departments/services, such as central services, housekeeping services, and linen and laundry services, are available to assist in the prevention and control of infections and are provided with adequate direction, staffing, and facilities to perform all required infection surveillance, prevention, and control functions.

Each standard is accompanied by an interpretive section to assist hospital personnel in understanding the standards and their application.

The CDC *Guidelines for the Prevention and Control of Nosocomial Infections* [18] were developed to update and consolidate recommendations for infection surveillance and control. The guideline topics include prevention of catheter-associated urinary tract infections, environmental control of nosocomial infections, prevention of intravascular infections, prevention of surgical wound infections, prevention of respiratory tract infections, isolation techniques, role of the microbiology laboratory in infection surveillance and control programs, employee health services and objectives, and methods of surveillance. To help infection control staff critically assess the value of the recommendations, a three-category ranking scheme was developed: Category I, strongly recommended for adoption; category II, moderately recommended for adoption; and category III, weakly recommended for adoption. Category I recommendations "are judged to be applicable to the majority of hospitals regardless of size, patient population, or endemic nosocomial infection rate, and are considered practical to implement" [18]. Category II recommendations "are not to be considered a standard of practice for every hospital" [18]. Although the CDC recommendations are likely to influence standards of care on a national basis, the standard of care is ultimately established on a case-by-case evaluation [65].

To summarize, courts look to a variety of sources, including national practices, local or national rules, and guidelines, when determining the standard by which a defendant is judged.

Establishing the Standard of Care

When a plaintiff alleges a defendant has failed to meet a standard of care, the plaintiff must first establish the standard and then prove that it was breached. This proof is normally accomplished by the use of expert testimony. When negligence has been admitted, however, or when the neglect is obvious to a layperson, expert testimony may not be required. Other alternatives to expert testimony include the use of medical texts, journals, state and federal laws, regulations, and guidelines to establish the standard; direct cross-examination of the provider; and the use of the doctrine of *res ipsa loquitur.*

The Doctrine of *Res Ipsa Loquitur*

The doctrine of *res ipsa loquitur, (res ipsa:* "the thing speaks for itself") is related to the expert testimony requirement [34, 49]. The precedent-setting case of *Ybarra* v. *Spangard,*

25 Cal.2d 486, 489, 154 P.2d 687 (1944), established that the use of the *res ipsa* doctrine requires three elements:

1. The accident must be of a kind that ordinarily does not occur in the absence of someone's negligence.
2. It must be caused by an agency or instrumentality within the exclusive control of the defendant.
3. It must not have been due to any voluntary action or contribution on the part of the plaintiff.

Because the main rationale for use of *res ipsa* is the plaintiff's inability to discover the cause of injury, some states have applied a fourth requirement that the defendant must have superior knowledge of the cause of the accident. When circumstantial evidence indicates that the defendant's negligence is the most plausible explanation for the injury, the doctrine of *res ipsa* may apply despite the absence of direct evidence.

Res Ipsa *and Infection Cases*

Because infections indeed occur in the absence of negligence, courts have infrequently applied *res ipsa* when plaintiffs attempt to establish liability for infections. Two recent cases reflect this principal: In *Roark* v. *St. Paul Fire and Marine Insurance Co., et al.,* 415 So.2d 295 (La. 1982), the court stated that a certain number of hospital patients will contract a staphylococcal infection regardless of the hospital's conduct. An essential element of *res ipsa* was absent, therefore, in that the plaintiff's infection could indeed have occurred without negligence. In *Wilson* v. *Stilwill,* 411 Mich. 587, 284 N.W.2d 773 (1981), the defendant hospital's postoperative infection rate was well below the national average. The plaintiff sought to apply *res ipsa* by establishing that the low incidence of infection at the hospital implied that infection did not ordinarily occur. The court, however, was not persuaded: "Although it is true that statistically infections did not ordinarily occur at the defendant hospital, this fact does not suggest that when an infection does occur, it is the result of negligence."

The doctrine of *res ipsa* has been held applicable, however, in other hospital infection cases. In *Southern Florida Sanitarium and Hosp.* v. *Hodge,* 215 S.2d 753 (Fla. 1986), *res ipsa* was allowed because testimony established that thrombophlebitis would not have occurred if proper sterile technique had been maintained by the defendant hospital throughout an injection procedure. This testimony fulfilled the three required elements for *res ipsa:* (1) Thrombophlebitis ordinarily should not occur in the absence of neglect; (2) the injection was performed by an agent or instrumentality under the control of the hospital; and (3) the thrombophlebitis was not caused by any voluntary action or contribution by the plaintiff.

The case of *Sommers* v. *Sisters of Charity of Providence in Oregon,* 277 Or. 549, 561 P.2d 603 (1977), demonstrates that use of the *res ipsa* doctrine may involve certain pitfalls. In this case, a patient sued the hospital for negligence after a *Staphylococcus aureus* infection developed at the site of an intravenous cannula. The patient alleged that hospital nurses did not properly disinfect her skin before inserting the cannula. Medical experts testified that it was impossible to sterilize skin completely. They also stated that the patient had a poison oak rash associated with large numbers of bacteria; hence, the patient was probably the source of her own infection. Had the plaintiff not relied on the doctrine of *res ipsa,* she might have been able to establish that a reasonably prudent nurse should not cannulate an area where a rash is present [25].

Causation, Damages, and Infection Liability

To prevail in a negligence action, a plaintiff must prove that a provider's failure to exercise the required standard of care resulted in the plaintiff's injury [100]. If a patient can establish that he or she suffered injury due to an infection resulting from hospital or staff negligence, the hospital or its staff may be liable. A hospital's responsibility for the prevention and control of infections extends to patients, personnel, and visitors. As was discussed earlier, however, hospitals neither ensure nor guarantee patients' safety; hence,

liability is not established on mere proof that a plaintiff developed an infection, nor would *res ipsa* apply. In *Rohdy* v. *James Decker Munson Hosp.,* 170 N.W.2d 67 (Mich. 1969), for instance, a plaintiff alleged that the hospital was responsible for a staphylococcal infection occurring on the same arm as an injection received 1 month earlier. The court held, however, that *res ipsa* could not be applied because there was no certainty that the infection resulted from the injection.

Because nosocomial infections are common, unpredictable, and may be difficult to prevent, courts have recognized that such infections may occur despite reasonable care. In addition, it is often difficult or impossible to establish that a particular negligent act or omission specifically resulted in infection (the element of proximate causation) [36]. In *Kaster* v. *Woodson,* 123 S.W.2d 981 (Tex. Civ. App. 1938), the court noted that infections may arise from a variety of sources; hence, there must be affirmative proof of such negligence or lack of care and proof that the injuries complained of must have resulted from this negligence. In *Wilson* v. *Stilwill,* 411 Mich. 587, 284 N.W.2d 773 (1981), the plaintiff alleged that the occurrence of an arm infection following hospital treatment indicated negligence. Because there was no testimony establishing that the treatment was negligent or contrary to any professional standard of conduct, however, the jury decided against the plaintiff. The court stated: "The mere occurrence of a postoperative infection is not a situation which gives rise to an inference of negligence when no more has been shown than the fact that an infection has occurred and that an infection is rare" [16, 24, 70, 97].

A hospital was held liable in *St. Paul Fire and Marine Insurance Co.* v. *Prothro,* 590 S.W.2d 35 (Ark. 1979), when a patient developed an infection after a metal basket lowering him into a whirlpool bath broke, struck him, and reopened his surgical wound. The appeals court supported the plaintiff's assertion that the infection was caused by the fall into the bath.

Only rarely are patients awarded damages for hospital-acquired infections. As methods of typing microorganisms improve, however, the ability to trace the specific sources of infections, thereby proving proximate causation, may also improve. Moreover, knowledge in the field of nosocomial infections is growing rapidly, and conditions long believed to be unavoidable may soon be considered preventable. Likewise, currently accepted procedures may become substandard practices. As discussed earlier, plaintiffs may also attempt to use the doctrine of *res ipsa* to establish negligence without proving proximate cause.

Defenses to Negligence

Legal defenses can avoid or reduce liability even if the plaintiff can establish all the necessary elements of a cause of action. Examples of defenses are failure to initiate suit within the statute of limitations (required time period), contributory negligence (an absolute defense to the plaintiff's cause of action whereby the defendant proves the plaintiff's conduct breached the duty of self-protection and contributed as a legal cause of the injury), and comparative negligence. This latter type of defense compares the fault of the plaintiff with that of the defendant to determine an appropriate recovery, thereby affirming a percentage of respective negligence to each party. Other defenses include the assumption of risk (if the patient failed to act as would a reasonable, prudent person and if this negligence contributed in any way to the injury), a release executed by a patient subsequent to treatment, good samaritan statutes, worker's compensation, and government immunity [101].

Theories of Liability

Liability for nosocomial infections may be imposed on any health care provider, including hospitals, physicians, and nurses [26, 56, 59]. Nosocomial infections occur in an estimated 5.7 percent of hospitalized patients. They are believed to add more than 7.5 million extra hospital days and well in excess of $1 billion annually in hospital charges [45]. The number of substantial awards from health care providers as a result of nosocomial infections has grown in recent years as patients have be-

come sensitive to treatment complications, including infections [92].

A variety of legal theories may be used to impose liability, including negligence, warranty, and strict tort liability, as well as government statutes and regulations. Hospital liability for negligence arises under two different theories. The first theory is based on the doctrine of *respondeat superior* ("let the master answer"), arising from the negligence of one or more employees or agents. The second theory holds that a hospital corporation itself may be negligent if it fails to perform a legally recognized corporate duty—the corporate negligence theory. If a staff physician, resident, nurse, or other hospital employee is negligent with respect to a patient, negligence may be imputed to the hospital, and the patient may have a cause of action against both the employee and the hospital-employer [42].

Doctrine of Respondeat Superior *(Agency)*

Under the classic principal of agency (*respondeat superior*), a master is liable for the actions of his servants. Accordingly, an employer may be held liable for the wrongful acts of an employee, even though the employer is itself without fault (vicarious liability) [94]. Hospitals in general are not liable for the wrongful conduct of private physicians working in the hospital as independent contractors. Recent case law using the corporate theory, however, has expanded the responsibilities of hospitals to monitor the activities of independent medical personnel within their facilities. Hospitals have been held liable for the torts of independent physicians under a theory of *apparent or ostensible agency,* which holds that a hospital is responsible when a patient is led to believe he or she is being treated by an agent of the hospital, typically when specialists under contract with the hospital are furnished by the hospital rather than personally selected by the patient [81].

Even if an employer is found to be liable under the principle of agency, the employee who actually committed the tort can also be held personally liable for his or her wrongful act or omission [100]. The plaintiff may sue any such parties separately or all of them together. The plaintiff is not, however, permitted to collect judgment in full from two or more defendants. If the plaintiff collects the judgment from the employer, the employer may have a right of indemnification from the negligent employee. This right is most likely to be asserted when employer and employee are insured by different carriers.

Corporate Negligence Theory

The second theory of liability, the corporate negligence theory, recognizes that hospitals owe certain duties and responsibilities imposed by courts or legislatures directly to patients, visitors, and employees. If, by failing to meet these duties, the hospital causes harm, the hospital itself may be held liable.

Under the traditional rule, enunciated in *Scoendorff* v. *Society of New York Hosp.*, 105 N.E. 92 (N.Y. 1914), hospitals were not liable for torts committed by physicians because physicians, not hospitals, practice medicine. The landmark case of *Darling* v. *Charleston Community Memorial Hosp.*, 211 N.E.2d 253 (Ill. 1965), *cert. denied* 383 U.S. 946, 86 S. Ct. 1204 (1966), departed from this rule and expanded the obligations of hospitals to monitor the quality of patient care services in the following three ways [83].

1. The hospital must not allow an independent staff physician to violate a specific hospital requirement for patient safety.
2. The hospital must ensure that its employees will detect apparent dangers to the patient and bring such dangers to the attention of the hospital medical staff and the administration so that the administration can act to alleviate the danger.
3. The hospital must supervise the actions of independent staff physicians.

In *Darling*, an emergency department patient with a fractured leg was assigned to a general practitioner on call who applied a cast. Despite easily recognizable signs that the leg had become ischemic, the physician failed to recognize or react to this complication. Although the nurses were aware that the patient was developing complications, the hospital administration failed to take steps to obtain consultation as required by hospital bylaws. The plaintiff's leg became infected and was ultimately amputated. The court held the hospital liable for failing to ensure the provision of quality medical care. Mere reliance on self-regulation, according to the court, was inadequate. Cases after *Darling*, particularly those in the area of medical staff selection and review, have expanded malpractice liability by recognizing the independent duty of hospitals to ensure the provision of quality medical care [32, 57, 72, 74, 88, 96].

Case law, however, stops short of providing that hospitals are guarantors of the adequacy of medical care. The isolated acts of otherwise competent physicians, therefore, remain the sole responsibility of that physician [64]. Some cases have gone even further than requiring careful selection and review and suggest that a hospital has a duty to supervise the competency and quality of its physicians. In these cases, however, the defendant hospitals were aware physicians were providing substandard care but failed to intervene [81, 108]. This theory, however, was rejected in *Scheneck* v. *Gov't of Guam*, 609 F.2d 387 (9th Cir. 1979).

Corporate Obligations

Hospitals have been found to owe a variety of obligations directly to patients and the public. These obligations include [50]:

1. The duty to furnish and maintain proper equipment, supplies, and services and to exercise reasonable care in the selection and use of such equipment, supplies, and services
2. The duty to exercise reasonable care in the selection and retention of appropriate personnel
3. The duty to exercise reasonable care with respect to the maintenance of buildings and grounds, including keeping the environment clean and sanitary with the aim of preventing infection
4. The duty to comply with policies and procedures which, whether established by the hospital or by outside agencies, have as

their objective the safety and well-being of patients and the public

Because such duties include the obligation to promulgate and enforce rules to protect patients from infections, hospitals that fail to establish proper procedures, organizations, and techniques of infection control may be liable. In addition, hospitals may have a duty to monitor infection rates by specific physicians and to intervene if excessively high rates are noted [41, 53]. Given current availability of computers as a resource for infection control information management, hospitals are well advised to utilize this technology [107].

The JCAHO [58] mandates the presence of ". . . an, effective, hospital wide program for the surveillance, prevention, and control of infection." A required characteristic is that there are written policies and procedures for infection surveillance, prevention, and control for all patient care department services. Medicare Conditions of Participation for Hospitals constitute federal regulation of hospital infection control programs (42 C.F.R. Sec.482.42) and state that "the hospital must provide a sanitary environment to avoid sources and transmission of infections and communicable diseases. There must be an active program for the prevention, control, and investigation of infections and communicable diseases" [71]. Specifically, the following is required [46, 69, 84]:

1. *Standard: Organization and policies.* A person or persons must be designated as infection control officer or officers to develop and implement policies governing control of infections and communicable diseases.
   a. The infection control officer or officers must develop a system for identifying, reporting, investigating, and controlling infections and communicable diseases of patients and personnel.
   b. The infection control officer or officers must maintain a log of incidents related to infections and communicable diseases.
2. *Standard: Responsibilities of chief executive officer, medical staff, and director of nursing*

services. The chief executive officer, the medical staff, and the director of nursing services must:
   a. Ensure that the hospitalwide quality assurance program and training programs address problems identified by the infection control officer or officers.
   b. Be responsible for the implementation of successful corrective action plans in affected problem areas.

Claims Data

According to data published in 1990 by the St. Paul Fire and Marine Insurance Co., infection, contamination, and exposure ranks thirteenth of 16 categories in claims reported by St. Paul–insured hospitals during 1988 and 1989, with the average cost of each claim being $76,458 [92].

Medical Staff Obligations

The medical staff as well as the hospital has an obligation to prevent and control infections. Physician responsibilities include appropriate clinical care; in certain cases, serving as a member of the Infection Control Committee or as a hospital epidemiologist or infection control officer; and, in general, setting a proper example in practicing medical asepsis. Physicians may incur liability for failure to adhere to appropriate standards of care. In addition, as the availability of physicians specializing in infectious disease grows, liability may even be imposed for failure to consult with a specialist [82, 103].

Examples of Liability Risk Exposure for Nosocomial Infections

The failure to diagnose the presence of infection is a common allegation against hospitals and physicians. According to claim data from St. Paul Fire and Marine Insurance Co. for 1986–1987, it is the eighth most common allegation by frequency in negligence cases brought against physicians, numbering 350 claims and costing on average $81,523. Alleged improper treatment of infection resulted in 332 claims [102]. Physicians and hospitals have a duty to evaluate and monitor patients in a timely manner so as to prevent or reasonably control an infection. Examples of representative cases follow:

Failure to respond to a high fever in a case of a plaintiff who allegedly suffered organic brain damage led to an $800,000 jury verdict. In this case, between the hours of 8 AM and 1 PM, the hospital personnel knew of the plaintiff's extremely high temperature and critical medical condition, yet failed to provide medical treatment necessary to alleviate the crisis. See *Robert* v. *Chodoff*, 259 Pa. Super. 332, 393 A.2d 853 (1979).

In *Harris* v. *State through Huey P. Long Memorial Hosp.*, 378 So. 2d 383 (La. 1979), a court held that despite a distinct odor in the patient's room and a rise in the patient's temperature associated with incipient gás gangrene infection, there was no indication of failure to perform medical services or observation adequately.

In *Celeste Pierre* v. *Booker,* Alameda County (CA) No. 536866-0, a defense verdict resulted in a suit alleging that negligent treatment of a postsurgical infection prolonged the plaintiff's hospital stay by 1 month. The defendants argued that infection is a recognized and inherent risk of the procedure.

In the case of *Dora Lewis* v. *Dr. Badr Ghumranis,* Cugohoga County (OH) Court of Common Pleas, Case No. 1346034, the plaintiff's decedent, a 74-year-old man, was allegedly infected during a bronchoscopy. When he returned to the defendant 10 to 12 days later with clear signs of infection in his lung, it is alleged the defendant failed to perform tests that would have diagnosed the infection, resulting in a delay in the administration of proper antibiotics. The plaintiff died after a 7-week hospitalization due to the infection. The jury returned a verdict for $607,921.81.

In *Doan* v. *Tucson Surgical Specialist, M.D.,* Puma City (AZ) Superior Court, Case No. 220239, the plaintiff, a 21-year-old woman, injured her knee while hiking. Postopera-

tively, she developed an infection in the joint, and the plaintiff alleged the defendants failed to recognize there was an infection and failed to treat it in a timely manner. Allegedly, the infection was not diagnosed until the seventh postoperative day. A jury award of $175,000 compensatory damages was the result.

Patient Notification of the Presence of Infection or Disease

Some lawsuits have involved plaintiffs' allegations that they were not informed of the presence of hospital infections. In *Jones* v. *Sisters of Charity,* 173 S.W.639 (Tex. 1915), the plaintiff alleged that his wife died from smallpox because the hospital failed to notify his wife that there was a case of this disease in the hospital. Because strict quarantine was maintained and there was no concealment, the court found for the defendant hospital. In *Robey* v. *Jewish Hosp. of Brooklyn,* 20 N.E.2d 6 (N.Y. 1939), the court took a similar stand when damages for the infection of a newborn infant were alleged. In this case, an expectant mother was not warned of infection currently affecting infants in the hospital; the court ruled, however, that the record failed to show any actionable negligence on the part of the hospital. In *Aetna Casualty and Surety Co.* v. *Pilcher,* 244 Ark. 11, 424 S.W.2d 181 (1968), the hospital's failure to warn the plaintiff before surgery that pathogens existed in the hospital was not found to be the proximate cause of infection.

Hospitals have an obligation to patients sharing a room with another patient with a contagious disease. It is recommended that physicians treating such patients be informed; the physicians can then determine appropriate care. The patients likewise should be informed of exposure in such situations [86].

Negligent Handling of Patients

Infections resulting from negligent handling of patients have resulted in liability. For example, in *Inderbitzen* v. *Lane Hosp.,* 124 Cal.

App. 462, 12 P.2d 744, 13 P.2d 905 (1932), the plaintiff, a woman in active labor, received vaginal examinations by 2 medical students with unsterilized hands; the plaintiff developed postpartum endometritis. Noting the risk of infection for receiving vaginal examinations with unsterilized hands while in labor, the court found the hospital liable.

In *Kirchoff* v. *St. Joseph's Hosp.*, 260 N.W. 509 (Minn. 1935), a hospital was found liable after a nurse gave a mother the wrong baby, which was infected with impetigo. The mother was infected by this infant and subsequently transmitted the disease to her own child.

A hospital was found negligent in *Helman v. Sacred Heart Hosp.*, 62 Wn. 2d 136, 381 P.2d 605 (1963), for failing to prevent cross-infection of the plaintiff. The plaintiff contracted a staphylococcal infection after being placed in a room with a patient who had a staphylococcal infection; testimony indicated that the 2 patients were infected with the same strain of coagulase-positive *S. aureus*. The court noted that the hospital attendants did not observe the sterile techniques prescribed by the hospital for infected cases, and they did not wash their hands between administering to the patients. In addition, the court indicated that when the presence of an infected patient presented a serious risk to the well-being of another patient, the hospital may have a corporate duty to isolate the infected patient [79]. Other cases on point include the following:

In the case of *Anonymous* v. *American Medical International, Inc.*, Haines County (TX), A technician's sneezing on the plaintiff's back and instrument tray allegedly caused infection resulting in a $170,000 settlement. An infectious disease specialist determined that the infectious agent was α-streptococcus, which is known to live in nasal passages, and a physician also testified that the technician's sneezing on the plaintiff's back or on the instruments led to the introduction of the organism into the plaintiff's spinal column during the myelogram and resulted in the plaintiff's meningitis.

In *Yvonne Vogt* v. *Dr. Katz*, St. Louis County (MO) Circuit Co. CV 184-2889 CCJ2-Div. 2, the 40-year-old plaintiff alleged that the defendant physician injected his elbow joint with cortisone to treat a tennis elbow condition without sterilizing the needle and staphylococcal infection developed. The defendant alleged he used alcohol to sterilize the needle. A defense verdict resulted.

Exposure to Contagious Patients

Liability may be imposed for failure to isolate patients with communicable diseases or for failure to guard against cross-infection. Hospital licensure regulations in most states require isolation facilities for patients with communicable disease.

Courts have held that defendants are liable should a patient contract an infection after being negligently exposed to a contagious patient. An early case involving patient-to-patient contact was *Gadsen General Hosp.* v. *Bishop*, 96 So. 145 (Ala. 1923); in this suit, a patient's administrator alleged that the deceased patient died from smallpox acquired in the hospital. The court assumed that proper care and attention would include preventing a patient from being exposed to a contagious disease from another patient in the hospital. To recover damages, the court ruled the following five elements would need to be established: (1) The patient died of smallpox; (2) he acquired the disease while a patient in the hospital; (3) the infection was transmitted to him from another patient in the hospital during the patient's stay; (4) hospital staff knew that the other patient had smallpox; and (5) hospital staff negligently exposed the deceased to the infected patient. The court ruled that the plaintiff did not meet all these requirements.

In *Bush* v. *Board of Managers of Binghamton City Hosp.*, 251 App. Div. 601, 297 N.Y.S. 991 (1937), the plaintiff alleged that his wife contracted fatal diphtheria because she was placed too close to patients with diphtheria at the defendant hospital. Although the lower court held for the plaintiff, the appellate division reversed the judgment; it found neither evidence of the defendant's failure to employ safe and suitable methods and equipment nor adequate proof that the decedent had in fact contracted diphtheria.

The following cases also exemplify liability related to exposure to contagious patients: In the case of *Ryan* v. *Frankford Hosp.*, Court of Common Pleas, Philadelphia County (PA), Sept. Term 1983, Case No. 1754, the minor plaintiff, Sean Ryan, was hospitalized and, during his hospitalization, was placed in a room with another minor, Donald Cummings. A sign above the bed of the Cummings child read "Enteric Conditions and/or Precautions." In their complaint, the plaintiffs alleged that at no time throughout Sean Ryan's hospitalization at the defendant hospital were they advised that their child's roommate had a contagious infection, shigellosis. Interaction between the minor plaintiff and infected roommate was encouraged, and meals were served to the two minor patients at the same table. The minor plaintiff was discharged from the hospital on March 29, 1982. On March 22, his pregnant mother, as a result of her contact with Donald Cummings or the minor plaintiff, was admitted to Jeanes Hospital with the diagnosis of shigellosis. Shortly thereafter, she underwent a therapeutic abortion. Court documents show that the case was settled before Common Pleas Court Judge Abraham J. Gafni on October 31, 1988, but the amount of the settlement was not disclosed.

In yet another case, 5 patients in Sequoia Hospital in Redwood City, California, were infected with hepatitis B virus, and a lawsuit alleges that an anesthesiologist gave a local anesthetic to patients from a contaminated multidose vial. The anesthesiologist routinely administered lidocaine anesthetic from a 50-ml vial. During this procedure, blood from a hepatitis-infected patient was aspirated into the container. When lidocaine was given to subsequent patients, the hepatitis virus was transmitted. Although many patients were believed to be exposed to the virus, only 5 agreed to be tested (reported in *Hospital Risk Management*, September 1989).

A hospital may avoid liability when it is not aware of a contagious patient. In *Gill* v. *Hart-*

ford Accident and Indemnity Co., et al., 337 So.2d 420 (Fla. Dist. Ct. App. 1976), for instance, a physician neglected to notify hospital personnel that a patient was contagious.

Restrictions on Infected Patients

The acquired immunodeficiency syndrome (AIDS) epidemic has raised issues regarding the proper scope of infection control measures. Suit was filed against a psychiatric hospital under the Federal Rehabilitation Act alleging the patient was the subject of discrimination due to unnecessarily restrictive infection control procedures by the hospital. The plaintiff alleged he was restricted to his room and not allowed to shower or eat with other patients and that hospital personnel who came in contact with him were fully masked, gowned, and gloved. The case was dismissed on the grounds that damages for mental anguish were unavailable and any action for injunctive relief would be moot (*Rhodes* v. *Charter Hospital*, CA J89-0062 [S.D. Miss. 1989]) (see also p. 563).

Exposure to Contagious Personnel

Hospitals in most states are required to screen personnel for infectious disease by testing new employees and periodically screening existing personnel. For example, in Illinois, periodic physical examinations of hospital staff are recommended, and personnel absent from work because of any communicable disease may not return to work until examined by a physician [55, 64]. Medicare and Medicaid Conditions of Participation require that "a continuing process is enforced for inspection and reporting of any hospital employee with an infection who may be in contact with patients, their food, or laundry" [21]. The failure to recognize obvious symptoms of an employee's poor health and to remove such an employee from duty may also generate liability. Hospitals must minimize patient contact with staff who are carriers of infection. Detecting, reassigning, and even removing contagious staff from duty, therefore, are all parts of a hospital's duties. Liability related to hospital employee health is discussed in greater detail later in this chapter.

Many suits have been brought alleging that patients contracted diseases resulting from negligent exposure to hospital staff. For example, in *Taaje* v. *St. Olaf Hospital,* 199 Minn. 113, 271 N.W.109 (1937), the court held the hospital was negligent because a nurse with a severe cough, of which other nurses were aware, attended a newborn. The nurse was later found to have tuberculosis. The court found that the death of the infant from acute military tuberculosis was caused by contact with the nurse and the hospital breached its duty by failing to take the infected nurse off duty. In *Hurley* v. *Nashua Hospital Association,* 191 A. 649, 650 (N.H. 1937), however, the plaintiff's evidence was insufficient to establish that the plaintiff's nosocomial pneumonia was caused by a nurse suffering from a severe cold.

Cases in which injury resulted because hospital policies or standards of care were blatantly violated often result in hospital liability. In *Kapuschinsky* v. *United States,* 248 F. Supp. 732, 259 F. Supp. 1 (D.S.C. 1966), hospital policy was violated when a nurses' aide was allowed to care for a sick premature infant. The infant developed a severe staphylococcal infection; subsequently, the aide's nose and throat were found to be colonized with *S. aureus.* The court found the government, which operated the hospital, remiss in its duty in two respects, either one of which was sufficient to prevail [75]:

1. It permitted an inexperienced aide to come in "critical contact" with the plaintiff, whose susceptibility to infection was well known, in violation of proper medical standards.
2. It permitted this "critical contact" without a complete physical examination of the aide, including appropriate laboratory tests, before she began to work in the premature nursery.

In the case of *Thompson* v. *Methodist Hospital,* 367 S.W.2d 134 (Tenn. 1962), an action was brought against a hospital based on injuries allegedly sustained by a newborn and his parents from a staphylococcal infection contracted by the baby. The baby allegedly transmitted the infection to his parents. The plaintiffs attempted to show that an intern who examined the baby's mother when she was at the hospital was a carrier of the infection, that a practical nurse with a boil appeared in the hospital from time to time, and that there had been other failures to follow aseptic technique. The court dismissed the case, finding that there was no evidence that either the intern or the nurse in question had ever come in contact with the infant or that the alleged events had, in fact, occurred while the infant and his mother were patients in the hospital. The court stated that the infant's infection could be attributed to other causes and that the degree of care exercised by the hospital at the time met, in every detail, the local standard of care. The court concluded that if, given the circumstances in this case, the hospital were held liable for the infection, then few hospitals could afford the financial risks of having a child born within their walls.

The case of *Peck* v. *Charles B. Towns Hospital,* 275 App. Div. 302, 898 N.Y.S.2d 190 (1949), is another example of the need to provide a higher standard of care in special situations. The plaintiff, a drug abuser, established that the skin of drug addicts is highly susceptible to infection. The court held that the hospital should have been aware of his unusual susceptibility to infection and therefore his skin should have been disinfected more carefully before placement of an intravenous catheter.

Contagious Patients Seeking Premature Hospital Discharge

When a patient who is actively infected with a communicable disease seeks discharge from the hospital against medical advice, the general rule that a patient of sound mind may leave the hospital at any time he or she chooses does not apply. In such cases, hospitals generally have the lawful authority to detain the patient. In fact, many states' public health laws provide the authority to restrain a contagious patient from leaving. Hospital legal counsel and public health authorities should be consulted immediately in such situations.

Informed Consent

Regarding consent, "every human being of adult years and sound mind has a right to determine what should be done with his own body" (*Schoendorff* v. *Society of New York Hospitals,* 105 N.E.92 N.Y. 1914). Failure to obtain informed consent may subject the doctor to criminal and civil liability for assault and battery or negligence.

Patients should be fully informed of the risk of medical procedures, including the risk of contracting infection. However, a dissertation on the intricacies of nosocomial infections is not required. The doctrine of informed consent requires reasonable disclosure of the available choices with respect to proposed therapy and the dangers inherently and potentially involved in each. Generally, this is sufficient compliance with the disclosure rule when the patient has been informed of the possibility of infection and given some idea of the probability of its occurrence under the circumstances. Decisions in some cases have suggested that, because infection is an inevitable risk over which the physician and hospital have no control, there is no legal obligation to warn of its dangers, which are widely known to the public. For example, in *Butler* v. *Berkeley,* 25 N.C. App. 325, 213 S.E.2d 571, 582 (1975), the court ruled that risk of infection is known to any person of ordinary sophistication and that "the probability of infection was not so great as to warrant advising plaintiff of the possibility." Failure to inform the plaintiff that an infection could have resulted from surgery did not result in liability in *Tripp* v. *Pate,* N.C. App. 271 S.E.2d 407 (1980), because the failure to inform the patient of the risk was not a proximate cause of the injury.

In another case involving a postoperative infection, *Contreras* v. *St. Luke's Hospital,* 78 Cal. App. 3d 919, 144 Cal. Rptr. 647, 653

(1978), the court found that the defendant physician, who informed the plaintiff before surgery that infections occurred in 1 of 100 operations, had complied with the disclosure rule. The court concluded, "It is a matter of common knowledge that infections may have serious consequences and at times are stubbornly resistant to treatment, and . . ." the doctor was not required to calculate and give information as to how long the plaintiff might have to be hospitalized or as to what specific treatment might be required in the unlikely event that an infection occurred. In *Cobbs* v. *Grant,* 8 Cal. 3d 229, 502 P.2d 1 (1972), the defendants were found to have adequately informed the patient of the risks of surgery when he was told that infection occurred in 1 of 100 operations.

The current trend in decisions, however, indicates that patients are entitled to all relevant information to assess risks associated with their medical care. In *Harwell* v. *Pittman,* No. 82 CA 0397, Court of Appeal of Louisiana, First Cir., Slop Opinion, Feb. 22, 1983, the court concluded that the patient was not adequately informed of the material risks of postoperative infection. The plaintiff underwent an elective cholecystectomy without being informed that the risks of infection were greater in his case due to his obesity. The plaintiff alleged that had he been so advised, he would not have consented to the proposed surgery.

In general, the responsibility to obtain informed consent rests with the physician. In *Baltzell* v. *Baptist Medical Center,* 718 S.W.2d 140 (Mo. 1986), a woman brought suit against her physician and the hospital, charging that she was subjected to surgical assault when she was not warned of the dangers of infection prior to undergoing surgery for the removal of a breast lump. The court held that the trial court properly directed a verdict in favor of the hospital in the absence of evidence that the hospital, as opposed to the attending physician, had any duty to inform the patient of risks. The verdict should not have been directed in favor of the physician, however, since jury issues were raised by the testimony of the plaintiff's expert that the applicable standard of care required that the patient be warned that the surgery in question carried a 5 to 10 percent risk of staphylococcal infection.

To establish patients' awareness of hospital infections, some attorneys have suggested that hospital admission consent forms should state that infections are a risk associated with any hospitalization and that there is no assurance that the patient will not contract an infection. Operative consent forms in many hospitals state that infections are a possible complication of surgical procedures [77].

As discussed in the section Posttransfusion Infection and Litigation, the patient's risk of contracting from blood products viruses that cause hepatitis or AIDS should be discussed, if appropriate, when obtaining informed consent. In the case of *Moore* v. *Underwood Memorial Hospital,* 371 A.2d 105 (N.J. Super. Ct. APP. Div. 1977), a physician was sued for failing to warn the patient of the risks of posttransfusion hepatitis. The physician avoided liability because the patient had taken a course in hematology, was the son of a physician, and was presumed to be familiar with such risks. A federal appeals court, interpreting Tennessee law, found that the physician need not have warned the patient of the risk of contracting hepatitis because the likelihood at the defendant hospital of contracting this infection was remote (*Sawyer* v. *Methodist Hospital,* 522 F.2d 1102 [6th Cir. 1975]). Despite the finding in this case, advising patients of the risk of infection associated with transfusions is appropriate for both the patient's information and the provider's protection.

HIV testing has focused attention on informed consent issues. Some argue that hospital general consent forms signed at admission will allow physicians to order diagnostic tests necessary to treat their illness. This is based on the argument that specific consent is not customarily obtained prior to performing blood tests in that consent is implied due to the routine nature of the procedure. Others contend that informed consent prior to testing is required, since a positive test result has significant personal and social consequences and may create psychologic distress, form a basis for discrimination, and affect the availability of health and life insurance. Many

states, by law or regulation, require informed consent prior to testing. A number of states have enacted legislation to allow exceptions to the informed consent requirement in the case of occupational exposures of health care workers to individuals who are potentially infected with HIV.

In the absence of law or regulations, common law and ethical principals of informed consent suggest it is advisable to obtain consent before HIV testing. Industry guidelines are uniform in recognizing that consent should be obtained prior to testing. Hence, liability for failure to obtain consent may be established because a standard of practice has evolved through policy statements of several leading health care organizations including the AHA, CDC, and the American Medical Association (AMA).

Unless dictated by state law, consent to testing does not need to be in writing. However, it is strongly advisable to document the consent process. Regarding the scope of disclosure for an informed consent, industry guidelines should be consulted. The April 1987 CDC Guidelines for HIV Antibody Counseling and Testing in *Prevention of HIV Infection and AIDS* (April 30, 1987) states, "Ideally, a person who requests testing or for whom testing is recommended should have a reasonable understanding of the medical and social aspects of HIV infection and the process of post-test counseling before consent." Patients should be told that the test is being done; that it is intended to indicate whether they have been exposed to HIV, the virus that causes AIDS; that the test can result in false negatives or positives; and that they have the right to refuse testing. In addition to disclosures regarding the nature, scope, and effects of the testing, some suggest that physicians discuss potential adverse personal social consequences before testing.

Following the test, the patient should be counseled by trained personnel regarding interpretation. The American Medical Record Association has issued a pamphlet titled "Guidelines for Handling Health Data on Individuals Tested for HIV Virus," which includes forms for request and consent for testing and a recommended procedure for conducting a confidential screening program. (For further information contact the American Medical Record Association, 875 N. Michigan Avenue, Suite 1850, Chicago, IL 60611.) Sample forms are also included in a publication prepared in November 1989 by the AIDS Task Group of the American Academy of Hospital Attorneys of the American Hospital Association. It is available from the AHA, 840 North Lake Shore Drive, Chicago, IL 60611.

Postoperative Infections

Many malpractice claims filed against surgeons involve infections. As in all categories of potential liability, one key element in such suits is whether the provider met the standard of care. In *Fluhrer* v. *Ritter,* Sup. Ct. Nassau Co., 845-1956, N.Y.L.J. p. 12, col. 2, (April 1962), the plaintiff successfully sued the hospital because its employees negligently allowed him to contract a postoperative infection in the operating room. The testimony of a pathologist and an orthopedic surgeon established that the plaintiff's "clean" operation had been performed in the same operating room that had previously been used for a "dirty" (contaminated) operation and that this was at variance with good hospital practice. In *Bartlett* v. *Argonaut Insurance Companies,* 258 Ark. 221, 523 S.W.2d 385 (1975), a malpractice action against a hospital was brought by a patient who developed a postoperative staphylococcal infection. The court ruled that although hospital floors were not swept daily and some nurses wore their uniforms from home, there was no proof that these hospital activities, inappropriate as they were, caused the patient's infection. The court held that "one of the known hazards to hospitalization and to conducting surgical procedures is postoperative infection" and that the germ causing the infection "could have entered her body in many ways and from many sources." The court, refusing to apply *res ipsa,* stated, "It is impossible for a hospital to be in complete control of a staph germ which may be brought in by the patient."

In *Denneny v. Siegel,* 407 F.2d 433 (3rd Cir. 1969), the plaintiff alleged her infection occurred because she was wheeled into an operating room for emergency surgery by a person wearing street clothes rather than operating room attire. This plaintiff lost the case because there was no evidence to prove a connection between the alleged negligence and the subsequent infection.

Organisms causing postoperative infection are those frequently present in many normal people. This observation had been used to counter plaintiffs' allegations of negligence in cases involving postoperative infections. For example, in *Roark* v. *St. Paul Fire and Marine Insurance Company,* 415 So.2d 295, 297 (La. 1982), a staphylococcal infection occurred at the plaintiff's surgical site. Evidence established that standard procedures were followed by the hospital to establish the sterility of the supplies and instruments and that the environment met or exceeded national standards. An expert testified that:

> Most individuals who contract a staph infection after surgery had the bacteria on their skin prior to surgery. Since the bacteria is found within the subcutaneous sweat glands and hair follicles of some patients, the organism may survive the cleansing of the skin with antiseptics.

The physician also testified that susceptibility to staphylococcal infection varies from individual to individual. "With the present state of medicine, there is no practical way to determine prior to surgery who may be more susceptible to staph infection or who may be a 'carrier' of the staph bacteria." The expert concluded that staphylococcal infections are an unavoidable risk of surgery.

Obligation to Inform Patients of Nosocomial Infection

Providers should inform patients when a nosocomial infection has occurred [22]. Courts have become increasingly insistent that physicians have a duty to disclose fully all pertinent facts concerning their patient's condition, even if the physician is convinced that he or she is acting in the patient's best interest by remaining silent. This obligation exists regardless of whether the condition is the result of negligence of the physician, a colleague, or the hospital. Failure to inform patients in such situations may result in liability for fraud (constructive fraud or fraudulent concealment), by conspiracy, as well as negligence. Punitive as well as compensatory damages may be awarded in such situations. In addition, courts have held that allegation of fraud stops the running of the statute of limitations [66, 110].

Infections due to Medical Equipment and Devices

As many as 45 percent of all nosocomial infections (or more than 850,000 per year) may be related to the patient's exposure to a medical device; the most common of these is the urinary catheter [104]. Hospitals have an obligation to ensure proper cleaning, handling, storage, and sterilization of equipment and supplies. Infections caused by contaminated instruments, equipment, or appliances may result in liability. Such cases often have involved the use of improperly sterilized needles or unclean catheters [60, 73, 85, 95, 99]. In *Kalmus* v. *Cedars of Lebanon Hosp.*, 281 P.2d 872 (Cal. 1955), a nurse failed to sterilize a needle used for an injection.

When purchased presterilized supplies become contaminated, however, and the contamination is not the result of hospital negligence, hospital liability should not result unless it can be established that the hospital should have been aware of the contamination. In *Shepard* v. *McGinnis*, 131 N.W.2d 475 (Iowa 1964), for example, the court held the hospital and physician liable for an infection because they should have been aware that certain sutures were contaminated. Other cases involving infections due to devices and equipment include the following:

In *St. Paul Fire and Marine Insurance Co.* v. *Protho*, 266 Ark. 1020, 590 S.W.2d 35 (1979), a hospital was held liable when a patient with a surgical wound developed a staphylococcal infection several days after the wound reopened as he was lowered into a whirlpool bath. The wound came into contact with unsterile bath water and towel; it was not cleaned after the incident but merely closed with surgical tape. The subsequent infection caused permanent damage to the patient, who was awarded $75,000.

The plaintiff in *Gordon* v. *St. Mary's Hosp. of Kansas City,* Jackson County (MO) Superior Court, Case No. CV82-11383, alleged an unsterile needle was used to give a tetanus shot, which resulted in an infection that caused loss of use of the arm and an inability to be gainfully employed. The verdict was for the defendant.

In *Ernest Chester* v. *Mercy Catholic Medical Center of South-eastern Pennsylvania,* Philadelphia County (PA) Court of Common Pleas, May 1984, Case No. 2555, the plaintiff developed a staphylococcal infection that caused an enlarged heart and mitral valve prolapse. He claimed the infection was caused by improper placement and monitoring of equipment, which allowed the intravenous site to become contaminated. The plaintiff also claimed the infection was not properly diagnosed. An undisclosed settlement was reached in February 1989.

The reuse of disposable, single-use medical devices can be problematic. Some providers have reused devices such as hemodialyzers, transducer domes, balloon-tipped catheters, cardiac catheters, catheter guide wires, biopsy needles, endotracheal tubes, anesthesia face masks, irrigating syringes, and manual resuscitators. At least 44 medical devices have been identified as reusable disposables [68]. Although it is not illegal to reuse such devices, manufacturers often recommend against it. The Health Industry Manufacturers Association (HIMA) has assembled a number of clinical case reports and reports of court verdicts suggesting dire consequences for those who reuse disposables. They describe a $970,000 verdict against a physician and hospital who reprocessed an intravenous catheter that subsequently broke during use inside the patient; 27 bacteremia cases among patients treated with reused dialyzers; 18 cases of hepatitis B in a physician's office where a nurse reused single-use blood lancets for hemoglobin testing; and four bacteremia deaths caused by contaminated pressure-monitoring domes originally sold presterilized for single-use only [38]. In addition, professional organizations, associations, and government agencies have policies against such reuse. An indepth report of a U.S. Senate Special Committee on Aging investigation questioned the safety of hemodialyzer reuse, a cost-savings practice performed at more than 60 percent of dialysis centers nationwide. Although the JCAHO [59] has stated in the past that "disposable items should not be reused," the current manual requires that "there are written policies and procedures addressing the reuse of disposable items and these policies and procedures address the reprocessing of disposable items to be reused" [58]. When the devices are explicitly labeled "for single use only," hospitals and physicians bear the burden of proving that reuse poses no threat to the quality of care they provide. Guidelines and protocols regarding reuse procedures should be established, and careful detailed records should be kept to substantiate that reuse does not jeopardize patient care.

The American Society for Hospital Central Service Personnel issued guidelines for the reuse of disposable medical devices in February 1986. They recommend that decisions about the reuse of single-use-only (disposable) medical devices should not be made "on the spot" and that the consistency of practice in all areas of the institution is of utmost concern. Unless an institution can demonstrate and document that patient safety and device effectiveness are not compromised by reprocessing a disposable medical device, reprocessing is not recommended [6].

If disposable devices are being reused, patients should be informed regarding the rationale and risks associated with the reuse of disposable products [98]. Administering special consent forms may also be appropriate in this situation [9]. The California Department of Health Services' licensing and certification division recently devised dialyzer reuse regulations that include a section on informed consent. One other precaution for providers reusing disposable devices is to obtain documentation that physicians are aware of and approve of such reuse. When reuse of certain disposable devices is acceptable to a substantial segment of the medical community, this practice may indeed become acceptable to courts.

Antibiotics

When antibiotics are used inappropriately, litigation may result [33]. Suits alleging negligence have focused on the injudicious use of antibiotics for surgical prophylaxis, failure to perform indicated cultures before administering antibiotics, and prescription of antibiotics that are either not clinically indicated or actually contraindicated for a particular patient [82]. In addition, the emergence of organisms resistant to multiple antibiotics may increase litigation in this area.

In principal, it should be possible for a patient who develops a nosocomial infection caused by a resistant organism to recover damages resulting from the organism's resistance, if he or she can prove that the resistance was caused by the physician's or hospital's indiscriminate use of antibiotics. In hospitals where antibiotic usage is not left entirely to the discretion of individual physicians, and the hospital can take affirmative steps to control the use of antibiotics, legal exposure may extend to the hospital.

In *Lewis* v. *Golden State Memorial Hospital et al.*, Los Angeles County Superior Court No. NWC 40143, a jury awarded a patient $1,225,000 in damages after gentamicin prescribed for a surgical infection resulted in renal failure. This jury found that the presence of preoperative albuminuria should have alerted the physicians to the increased risk of nephrotoxicity in the patient. *Haynes* v. *Baton Rouge General Hospital*, 298 S.2d 149 (1974), involved the use of an antibiotic (cephalexin [Keflex]) for the treatment of the organism

Enterobacter. The product information indicated the antibiotic was not effective against most strains of that organism. Fortunately for the defendant, there had been a culture and sensitivity testing that showed the organism involved was sensitive to the antibiotic prescribed. The plaintiff in *Sims* v. *United States,* 645 F. Supp. 47 (D.C. Mo., 1986), alleged negligence by Veterans Administration physicians following surgery to repair a hip fracture. Specifically, the plaintiff alleged that a postoperative infection might have been controlled had the defendants administered an adequate dose of ampicillin. The plaintiff was awarded more than $600,000.

JCAHO standards require that hospitals monitor their antibiotic use in their quality assurance audit programs. The 1992 JCAHO *Accreditation Manual for Hospitals* [58], in the chapter entitled "Medical Staff," states, "Drug usage evaluation is performed by the medical staff as a criteria-based, ongoing, planned and systematic process designed to continuously improve the appropriate and effective use of drugs." The JCAHO [58] goes on to state that "the process for monitoring and evaluating the use of drugs may include the use of screening mechanisms to identify, for more intensive evaluation, problems in or opportunities to improve the use of a specific drug or category of drugs . . . When an individual has performance problems that he/she is unable or unwilling to improve, modifications are made in clinical privileges or job assignments as indicated or some other appropriate action(s) is taken." Medicare and Medicaid Conditions of Participation require that "there are measures which control the indiscriminate use of preventive antibiotics in the absence of infection, and the use of antibiotics in the presence of infection is based on necessary cultures and sensitivity tests" [20].

Clinical review of hospital antibiotic use may be performed by the medical staff as a whole, by a medical staff committee, or by a hospital clinical department. Such review should access clinical aspects of infections occurring in hospitalized patients, pharmacy data on antibiotic use, and trends in pathogen resistance reported by the hospital microbi-ology laboratory. Institutional observations, actions, and recommendations regarding hospital antibiotic use should be documented in writing. Should it be appropriate to restrict the use of a particular antibiotic, this decision should be implemented through the medical staff or departmental chairpersons.

Duties to Nonpatients

Providers' obligations extend to persons other than their patients. A duty of reasonable care extends to all employees, volunteers, and visitors on the premises. An individual who visits during regular visiting hours and remains in those parts of the premises open to visitors is an invitee to whom the hospital owes the duty of exercising ordinary care [52]. If a third party develops an infection from a patient because of the provider's negligence, case law has established that damages may be awarded to the third party [7, 53].

Visitors of isolation patients, for example, should be warned of the risk of contracting the disease, and documentation should be made indicating the visitor was so advised [39]. The AHA recommends that suitable regulations pertaining to visitors are imperative in the control of nosocomial infection, and states [5]:

> To visit a patient is basically a privilege. Visits often have therapeutic value—or the converse— and hence should be subject to the control of the attending physician. The rules and regulations regarding visiting should take into consideration such aspects as the areas of special risks of infection, the particular needs of individual patients, and the peak work periods of staff.

The case of *Livingston* v. *Gribetz,* 549 F. Supp. 238, (S.D.N.Y. 1982), provides an example of litigation arising from alleged exposure to a contagious patient. In this case, a nurse alleged that she contracted herpetic encephalitis from an infant suffering from herpes virus infection. The nurse sued the infant's pediatrician on the grounds that the pediatrician failed to institute or monitor proper isolation procedures for the child and the nurse. The pediatrician prevailed, however, because the court held that there was no evidence of a duty owed to the nurse or breach of duty. Furthermore, proximate cause was not established since there was no proof that room placement, use of gloves, or donning of masks and gowns would have prevented the nurse from becoming infected.

The court in *Kniere* v. *Albany Medical Center Hospital,* 500 NYS 2d 490 NY Supp. 1986, held that a hospital has no duty to warn the public, assuming it would be possible, that one of its employees had contracted a communicable disease from a patient. The plaintiff was a nurse who contracted scabies and transmitted the disease to her family. The court "declined to impose a duty upon a hospital to warn the general public that one of its staff members had been exposed to an infectious disease."

In *DiMarco* v. *Lynch Homes-Chester County, Inc.,* Pennsylvania Superior Court, April 14, 1989, 559 A.2d 530 (PA Super 1989), a phlebotomist suffered a puncture wound when a nursing home patient from whom she was drawing blood kicked her. The phlebotomist sought consultation and treatment from her physician, who advised her that if she had contracted hepatitis, it would appear within 6 weeks, and that she should refrain from sexual relations during that time. When no symptoms appeared after 8 weeks, she resumed her relationship with her boyfriend. In September 1985, hepatitis was diagnosed in the phlebotomist; in December, it was also diagnosed in her boyfriend. He sued the physicians and nursing home, but the trial court dismissed the case. The court reasoned that the defendants might have a duty to prevent a patient's spouse from contracting an infectious disease, but there was no duty to a third party who was sexually involved with an individual to whom he was not married. The boyfriend appealed, and the Pennsylvania Superior Court concluded that he had stated a cause of action in that the public policy which favored preventing the spread of infectious disease outweighed the policy supporting marriage and family. The court concluded that one who renders services to another that

he or she should recognize as necessary to protect a third party may be liable to a third party who is injured in reliance.

Strict Liability or Breach of Implied Warranty

Liability is usually based on finding fault, or negligence. Attorneys, however, have sought to assert that providers are liable on a theory of strict liability in tort or breach of implied warranty [15, 46, 84]. Under those theories, a plaintiff need not allege or prove a negligent act or omission to establish liability. These theories originate in the Uniform Commercial Code's section on implied warranty of fitness for a particular purpose. This section provides that when a merchant knows that a product is purchased for a particular use and is relied on to provide the correct product, an implied-in-law warranty arises that the product provided should be suitable for the particular use. Attorneys who wish to apply this theory to health care litigation argue that the implied warranty applies to a hospital room and warrants that the room is infection-free. This argument has not prevailed to date. Plaintiffs may be more successful by establishing that an implied contract, under which the hospital had infection control obligations, arose between a patient and the hospital at the time of admission. In *Hall* v. *City of Huntsville,* 278 S.2d 708, 710 (Ala. 1973), for example, the court found an implied contract, but only to ensure a reasonable degree of infection control. The plaintiff developed a hip infection after numerous injections. There was no proof, however, that the infection resulted from the defendant's failure to give proper care and attention to the plaintiff. The plaintiff was still obligated to establish negligence or nonperformance because "to charge an implied contract to keep the plaintiff safe from infection and then to prove merely that an infection did occur would amount to equating the hospital's duty to that of an insurer." Although efforts to establish liability without negligence have failed in most cases involving infections, courts have applied strict liability in tort and warranty liability in cases in which a patient contracted viral hepatitis following a blood transfusion [100].

Posttransfusion Infection and Litigation

Liability for negligence may be imposed when a patient contracts an infection from a blood transfusion [13, 52, 89, 93, 111]. Infections acquired through blood transfusions include viral hepatitis, syphilis, malaria, toxoplasmosis, brucellosis, cytomegalovirus, and HIV [64]. In general, liability can be established only when a reliable test to detect the particular infection in the donor blood is available. Since tests are available to detect the presence of syphilis, failure to identify this infection in donor blood has resulted in liability, as in *Giambozi* v. *Peters,* 127 Conn. 380, 16 A.2d 833 (1940). Because posttransfusion viral hepatitis is not universally preventable by donor screening, however, contraction of this disease per se does not imply negligence.

Early cases, such as *Perlmutter* v. *Beth David Hospital,* 308 N.Y. 100, 123 N.E.2d 792 (1954), rehearing denied, 308 N.Y. 812, 125 N.E.2d 869 (1955), held that a hospital was performing a serivce rather than a sale in furnishing blood to its patients; therefore, no warranty of fitness was implied. Under this interpretation, hospitals could not incur liability related to administering blood without proof of negligence. As a reaction to difficulty in establishing negligence in posttransfusion cases, some courts have categorized the administration of blood components as the sale of a product, using product liability or implied warranty of fitness theories to impose liability. As the following case attests, it is crucial whether blood is classified as a service or as a product.

Cunningham v. *MacNeal Memorial Hospital,* 266 N.E.2d 897 (Ill. 1970), held that because a transfused patient acquired hepatitis, the hospital was liable even though not negligent. This decision was made despite the lack of a reliable test for the presence of hepatitis virus in donor blood. The court apparently preferred to compensate the innocent patient rather than find for those who provided the blood for a fee [11]. In *Hoffman* v. *Misericordia Hosp. of Philadelphia,* 439 Pa. 501, 267 A.2d 867 (1970), a plaintiff successfully used a breach of implied warranty theory in a case regarding the transfusion of "impure" blood. Most decisions, however, have denied liability under the warranty theory. Since the Cunningham decision, virtually every state has enacted remedial legislation (blood-shield statutes), which classifies blood transfusion as services (adopting the *Perlmutter* rule and precluding strict liability). Such legislation limits liability for adverse effects to those unusual cases in which negligence can be demonstrated [12, 69]. In many states, however, these statutes fail to state explicitly that blood banks and hospitals that administer blood components are immune from liability in the absence of negligence [100].

Efforts to apply *res ipsa* generally fail in posttransfusion cases because the first criterion (the injury does not ordinarily happen without negligence) is not met. In *Morse* v. *Riverside Hospital,* 44 Ohio App.2d 422, 339 N.E.2d 846, 848 (1974), for instance, the court stated that "no presumption that the hospital is negligent can be drawn solely from the fact that the patient contracted hepatitis following a blood transfusion, and the patient cannot recover damages on the theory of *res ipsa.*"

Established blood bank practices, accreditation standards, and state and federal statutes, regulations, and guidelines may all play a role in establishing standards of care for transfusion services. Public Health Service (PHS) recommendations for the prevention of HIV infection, for example, might be utilized by a court seeking to establish the appropriate standard of care [19].

Although hospitals normally are not held responsible for contaminated blood obtained from community blood banks, hospitals should scrutinize the source from which they obtain blood, ascertaining that the supplier is in fact screening donors in accordance with professional standards. Federal requirements promulgated by the Food and Drug Administration provide that blood must be labeled "paid donor" or "volunteer donor" [23]. Many states also require such labeling. The Illinois statute requires that blood obtained from paid donors may be administered only after the attending physician documents the reason for the transfusion in the patient's medical records [54]. An Oklahoma Supreme Court decision relates to the practice of using blood from paid donors. In *Gilmore* v. *St. Anthony Hospital et al.*, 598 P.2d 1200 (Okl. 1979), the court ruled that a woman who contracted posttransfusion hepatitis could sue the blood bank for negligence because the bank may have failed to ensure safe sources. The observation that hepatitis occurs more frequently in a paid donor system determined the outcome of this case.

Considerable posttransfusion infection litigation involves HIV. A recent survey found that 14 such cases have been settled and 15 are pending [37]. Many of these cases concern the failure of blood collection centers to assess HIV risk factors among donors during the early years of the epidemic, prior to the availability in 1985 of antibody tests for HIV. Some courts have awarded substantial damages (*Carroll* v. *Blood Center of S.E. Wisconsin*, Wisc. Cir. Ct. Milwaukee Cty), and one federal circuit court ruled that a blood supplier could be held liable for the transfusion of HIV-contaminated blood (*Doe* v. *Miles Lab and Cutter Lab*, 675 F. Supp. 1966 [D.Md 1987]). Even when a blood supplier has exercised due care, transfusion of HIV-contaminated blood may occur. Unable to recover damages for failure to screen or to defer high-risk donors, infected patients have turned to other claims for relief. These include failure to warn a patient about the risk of transfusion-associated HIV infection before obtaining consent and failure to inform the patient about alternatives to transfusions from the general blood supply, such as directed or autologous donations [35]. Clearly, liability may be imposed on physicians and hospitals for transfusions that result in HIV infections if the transfusions are deemed medically inappropriate or if informed consent is not obtained. In *Valdiviez* v. *United States*, 884 F.2d

196 (5th Cir. 1989) [1], the Fifth Circuit Court of Appeals held that a jury could find that a patient could have refused a blood transfusion if informed of the risk. (Also see *Doe* v. *Werner*, Cir. Ct. Milwaukee Cty, WI [2]; *Doe* v. *Johnson, Iowa Methodist*, Ctr. Dist. Ct., Polk Cty, CA [3]; and *Quintana* v. *United Blood Serv.*, Dist. Ct., Denver, CO [4].)

In the spring of 1986, the American Red Cross, the American Association of Blood Banks, and the Council of Community Blood Centers instituted the Look-Back Program to identify and notify all recipients of blood that were known to be or suspected of being HIV-positive [30]. One state, Texas, has legislated a duty to fully implement the Look-Back Program [106]. Since the implementation of the Look-Back Program, providers may be found liable for the failure to trace recipients. Liability exposure may extend from the patient to any third party, such as the patient's spouse, who might be at risk. Once physicians and hospitals are notified of the potential exposure of one of their former patients, they have a duty to notify the patient and advise further testing. It is prudent to document all efforts to locate the patient, especially if tracing efforts are unsuccessful.

Another issue raised by the AIDS epidemic concerns protecting the confidentiality of blood donors' identities. To prove the plaintiff contracted HIV from a blood transfusion, litigants have sought to discover the identity of the donor. Blood banks and hospitals have uniformly opposed the disclosure of the donor's identity, arguing that if suppliers are forced to reveal the identity of donors, it could undermine the voluntary and confidential nature of the blood supply system. If disclosure were allowed, people might decline to donate blood to avoid being personally involved in subsequent litigation. Theories invoked by hospitals and blood banks to protect blood donors include [14]:

1. The identities of blood donors fall within the scope of the physician-patient privilege and are thus not discoverable.
2. An order compelling disclosure of donors'

names and addresses is an unconstitutional infringement of the donor's fundamental right to privacy.
3. State abuse-of-discovery rules may be applied to protect the identities of blood donors.

Courts of Florida, New York, Pennsylvania, Tennessee, Ohio, and Michigan have ruled that privacy and public health interest are more important than the plaintiff's need for the information. In contrast, those who argue on behalf of disclosure have said it is necessary for the administration of justice. The Texas Supreme Court ruled that litigants have the right to confidential donor information because the donor's identity does not fall within the protected physician-patient privilege, the donor's right to privacy is not compelling, and the volunteer blood supply is not unreasonably harmed. The U.S. Supreme Court refused to hear an appeal of this issue. Disclosure of donor information was allowed by courts in Kentucky, Colorado, and Nevada. A Pennsylvania judge ruled that a blood transfusion recipient who acquired AIDS was entitled to learn about, but not to identify, the donor or other recipients.

Role of Medical Records in Hospital Infection Liability

Statutes and regulations concerning medical records vary from state to state. Some states require that the record contain minimum categories of information. Other statutes stipulate that records should be "adequate," "accurate," or "complete." Other jurisdictions set out requirements for medical records in greater detail, addressing such concerns as timeliness, retention procedures, and requirements for maintenance, signature, and filing. Medicare and Medicaid regulations and the standards of the JCAHO should be followed.

Medical records often play a critical role in defending against a charge of negligence. Failure to maintain accurate, complete, and

current records has frequently enhanced plaintiffs' assertions of negligence. Speculative comments should not be included in the chart, nor should blame be assigned for an outbreak. The notation of "nosocomial infection," for instance, should be written in a chart only after such an infection is confirmed.

If a patient has been determined to pose a risk of spreading infection to other patients, recommendations of the infection control practitioners should be recorded in the medical record and filed with the hospital administration [40]. Although some have suggested that infection control reports in cases of nosocomial infection should not be included in the progress notes of the patient's chart, others believe that such reports should indeed appear in the physician's progress notes to establish that the managing physician knows of the report [51].

Infection Control Committee Reports

According to the JCAHO [58], hospital infection control programs are to include a multidisciplinary committee that "oversees the program for surveillance, prevention, and control of infection." Plaintiffs' attorneys, not surprisingly, may become interested in the proceedings, records, and reports of these committees. Accordingly, protection of the patient's confidentiality, names of personnel involved in hospital infection surveillance, and the infection control reports themselves have become controversial issues. Whether these records may be disclosed remains unresolved. Courts have sought to balance the desire of infection control personnel to maintain confidentiality with plaintiffs' need for information to support their allegations. In response to court decisions that have found infection control program records discoverable, the majority of states have enacted statutes to protect such records. The protection such statutes offer varies considerably among states, however. In *Davidson* v. *Light*, 79 F.R.D. 137, 25 F.R. Serv.2d 173 (Colo. 1978), the defendant hospital was ordered to produce the infection control report of the hospital's Infection Control Committee. The court concluded that free discussion among hospital employees during committee meetings should be relatively unaffected by the discovery of factual data used in producing the committee's report.

In *Spears* v. *Mason,* 303 So.2d 260 (La. 1974), which concerned an alleged postoperative infection, the court ordered the defendant hospital to disclose hospital Infection Control Committee reports related only to the plaintiff's case and the period of his hospitalization. *Young* v. *King,* 136 N.J. Super. 127, 344 A.2d 792 (1975), involved a fatal staphylococcal infection. The plaintiff's subpoena for the records was allowed because the court held that the statutory privilege protecting the records of the Utilization Review Committee applied only to that committee. Records of other committees, even if they were also involved in quality review functions, were not held to be protected.

In a contrasting decision, an Oklahoma court, in *City of Edmond* v. *Parr,* 587 P.2d 56, 57 (Okl. 1978), agreed that the records of the Hospital Infectious Disease Control Committee were protected by the statute that prevented disclosure of "all information, interviews, reports, statements, memoranda, or other data relating to the condition and treatment of any person . . . for the purpose of reducing morbidity or mortality . . . (by) . . . any in-hospital staff committee." In a broader opinion, *Texarkana Memorial Hospital, Inc.* v. *Jones,* 551 S.W.2d 33 (Tex. 1977), the Texas Supreme Court held that the Texas statute protected the records and proceedings of any hospital committee. A petition to require a hospital to produce records of the Infectious Disease Control Committee was denied based on statutory immunity by a Florida Court (*Palm Beach Gardens Community Hospital* v. *Shaw,* 446 So.2d 1090 [Fl. 1984]).

In *Lang* v. *Abbott Laboratories,* 59 A.D.2d 734, 398 N.Y.S.2d 577 (1977), the plaintiff alleged she contracted septicemia from contaminated intravenous fluids manufactured by the defendant. The plaintiff's attempt to obtain records documenting the incidence of septicemia during the years before and following her admission was denied by the lower court. Because the hospital and staff were not parties to the suit, however, the appellate court allowed release of the records.

In an action against a hospital by an infant plaintiff who contracted a staphylococcal infection following her birth, the plaintiffs sought not only a statement from the defendant as to the nature and extent of staphylococcal infection at the hospital during the relevant period but also to ascertain the nature and extent of such infections by examination of records of the hospital review committee. Because these latter records were protected by statute, the court denied the plaintiffs' motion for discovery. A 1988 Illinois court decision reaffirmed protection of similar hospital committee records (*Farley* v. *County of Nassau* [1983, 2d Dept] 92 App. Div. 583, 459 N.Y.S.2d 470; and *Sakoski* v. *Memorial Hospital,* 522 N.E.2d 273 [Ill. 1988]).

The New Hampshire Supreme Court ruled that the defendant hospital's Infection Control Committee minutes and epidemiologist's report were privileged and not subject to disclosure in an action brought by a plaintiff diagnosed with herpes after giving birth at the hospital. The concerns of the plaintiff's husband led the hospital's nurse epidemiologist to conduct an investigation to determine whether the plaintiff could have contracted the infection while in the hospital. The findings were reported to the Infection Control Committee. The state statute provided that records created to evaluate patient care or treatment for quality assurance are privileged. The trial court found that the privilege only applied to committee records related to quality assurance and since the hospital had separate quality assurance and Infection Control committees the records were not privileged. The Supreme Court, however, found the Infection Control Committee was indeed a quality assurance committee and that the reports were privileged, since the Infection Control Committee was serving its quality assurance function when it investigated the source of the plaintiff's infection (*In re K.*, 132 N.H.4, 561 A.2d 1063 [1989]).

By avoiding written speculation when recording observations, members of hospital Infection Control Committees can minimize potential medicolegal problems [76]. An infection control nurse's written observations on an *S. aureus* outbreak in a newborn nursery exemplifies this type of written speculation: The nurse's report stated that the use of float personnel and inadequate facilities "contributed to" the outbreak. In the absence of data documenting the source of the outbreak, using the phrase "may have contributed" would be more accurate and less damaging to the hospital should litigation occur [51].

Employee Health

Health care providers have a duty to protect the health of personnel as well as patients (see Chap. 3). Health care workers are exposed to a wide array of health and safety hazards including exposure to biologic agents, physical agents, stress, injury, and chemical agents [91]. Under the common law, employers had a duty to provide reasonably safe working conditions for their employees or to warn of unsafe conditions they might not discover on their own. Courts have held that health care workers must be warned of contagious patients where necessary to protect them, as in the case of *Thigpen* v. *Executive Committee of the Baptist Convention*, 114 Ga. App. 839, 152 S.E. 2d 920 [1966], in which a nurses' aide was not warned how to avoid staphylococcal infection.

The Occupational Safety and Health Administration (OSHA) has codified such requirements and obligates private employers, including health care providers, to take all feasible measures necessary to recognize and eliminate significant occupational hazards. In the absence of specific federal and state occupational safety and health laws and regulations, an employer has the "general duty" to provide a safe workplace. The Occupational Safety and Health Act's general duty clause provides that:

(E)ach employer . . . shall furnish to each of his [her] employees employment and a place of employment which are free of recognized hazards that are causing or are likely to cause death or serious physical harm to his [her] employees (29 U.S.C. Section 645 (a) (1) (1982).

OSHA has the authority to levy fines. Violations directly related to job safety and health but unlikely to result in death or serious physical harm can lead to discretionary penalties of up to $1,000 per violation. Violations creating a substantial probability that death or serious physical harm could result will result in higher mandatory penalties. Violations committed intentionally and knowingly by the employer (the employer knows there are hazardous conditions that violate a standard or other statutory obligation and makes no reasonable effort to abate them) may result in penalties of up to $10,000 per violation. Citations may also be issued and penalties proposed for repeated violations (fines up to $109,000 per violation), failure to correct prior violations (penalty up to $1,000 per day beyond the abatement date shown on the citation), failure to observe citation-posting requirements (up to $1,000), and for other activities related to the compliance process. State laws also should be examined for employee safety requirements. In addition, under 43 C.F.R. Part 85A, OSHA has broad powers to investigate workplaces and employer records and to conduct medical examinations to ensure that employees have a safe workplace.

Transmission of infection both to and from employees has been described in hospital outbreaks of rubella, pertussis, hepatitis B, measles, and Legionnaires' disease. The following publications address responsibilities of hospitals in the area of employee health and are likely sources of the applicable standard of care: the JCAHO's *Accreditation Manual* [58], the CDC's *Guidelines for the Prevention and Control of Nosocomial Infections* [18], and the AHA's *Infection Control in the Hospital* [5] (recommendations of the AHA's Committee on Infections Within Hospitals).

Medical Examination of Prospective Employees

A health inventory on all new employees is critical. It has been recommended that the inventory should include immunization status, past health conditions that might predispose the employee to certain communicable diseases, and any history of certain communicable diseases. The health inventory should be used as a guide to determine on an individual basis whether an examination or laboratory studies are needed. CDC guidelines, published in 1983, delineate the elements of a personnel health service for infection control as follows [18]:

1. A health inventory should be obtained from personnel who will have patient contact.
2. For infection control, complete physical and laboratory examinations should not be routinely required for all personnel but should be done when indicated; for example, the need for an examination or laboratory test may be determined from results of the health inventory.
3. Health assessments of personnel other than placement evaluations should be done depending only on need; for example, as required to evaluate work-related illness or exposures to infectious disease.
4. Routine culturing of personnel, such as taking cultures of the nose, throat, or stool, should not be done as part of the placement evaluation or thereafter.

(See also CDC *Guidelines for the Prevention and Control of Nosocomial Infections,* personnel health, and Chap. 3.)

Surveillance of Personnel and Medical Staff

Hospitals should monitor infectious disease and carrier states in personnel. Special effort should be made to monitor staff in high-risk areas such as nurseries and hemodialysis units [43].

The Study on the Efficacy of Nosocomial Infection Control (the SENIC Project) included interviews with selected hospital personnel involved in infection surveillance and control in a sample of 433 hospitals. The authors made the following observations regarding hospital employees [44]:

> The majority of U.S. hospitals are routinely performing the recommended tests to detect potentially contagious infections among their employees, and hospitals with employees at presumably higher risk of acquiring such infections (e.g., those with hemodialysis units) are more likely to be performing the appropriate screening tests. There appears to be, however, a sizable minority of hospitals in which the appropriate screening tests are not being offered and many in which unnecessary but expensive screening procedures (for example, routine culturing of employees) are continuing despite recommendations to the contrary.

Whether or not a provider knows of any medical staff member infected with HIV, it should take steps to protect its patient population and other health care personnel from infection. Providers should rigorously monitor and enforce continued compliance with CDC guidelines to reduce the risk of patients' exposure to HIV and other pathogens from health care workers, including physicians. A provider or its medical staff may also choose to adopt a policy under which physicians have responsibility for disclosing to patients any physical impairment that might adversely affect patient care. Such a policy would theoretically compel a physician to disclose to patients that he or she has AIDS or HIV infection. In addition to patient disclosure policy, the hospital or medical staff may consider a policy requiring disclosure of physician HIV or AIDS infection to the hospital itself. For example, some hospitals' medical staff bylaws require that physicians disclose their health status on application for privileges and also require routine disclosure of any changes in their health status while on the medical staff.

OSHA announced in August 1987 that it would enforce CDC bloodborne guidelines to protect health care workers from exposure to disease (CDC guidelines issued August 31, 1987, which call for universal precautions) and will develop its own bloodborne disease control regulations over the next 2 years. A Joint Advisory Notice was issued by the Department of Labor and Department of Health and Human Services on October 30, 1987, (*Federal Register* 52FR 41818), entitled "Protection Against Occupational Exposure to Hepatitis B Virus (BHV) and Human Immunodeficiency Virus (HIV)." The notice announced that OSHA was beginning a program of enforcement, including inspections, to ensure that existing general regulations were being followed.

The first Advance Notice of Proposed Rule-Making was issued November 27, 1987, which notice outlined interim enforcement measures and invited public comment from the health care community and public. On January 9, 1989, a draft proposed rule was made public. According to the Department of Labor, only 25 AIDS cases have been traced to on-the-job exposures. In contrast, approximately 12,000 health care workers are infected with hepatitis B annually, resulting in 200 deaths (see OSHA instructions CPL 2-2.44A).

A revised version of the proposed standard, entitled "Proposed Standard for Occupational Exposure to Bloodborne Pathogens," was issued May 30, 1989 (*Federal Register* 54FR 23042). The proposed rule will cover nearly 4.7 million health care workers in facilities such as hospitals and physician and dentist offices and another 600,000 who work in law enforcement, fire and rescue, correctional facilities, research laboratories, blood banks, and the funeral industry.

The OSHA standard covers all occupational exposures to blood or other potentially infectious body fluids as defined by the CDC. Under the proposal, employers would be required to evaluate routine tasks and procedures in the workplace that involve exposure to blood or potentially infectious materials, identify the workers performing such tasks, and use a number of methods, including personal protective equipment and engineering controls, to reduce the risks of exposure. The proposal would also incorporate the CDC's universal precautions, which recommend that workers consider all blood and body fluids as potentially infectious (see Chap. 11). Under this proposal, employers would be required

to offer hepatitis B virus vaccine free to workers who have occupational exposures on an average of one or more times monthly. OSHA estimated that the average annual cost of complying with the proposed rule will be $1,373 per facility, ranging from an average of $32,875 per year for a hospital to $141 per year for a funeral parlor. OSHA will continue to use its existing bloodborne infectious disease compliance guidelines as the basis for enforcement until a final standard is published. If employees do not follow policies and procedures, OSHA expects employers to take punitive or disciplinary action against the employee to correct the situation.

OSHA requires the recording of needlestick injuries on the OSHA 200 Form whenever such injuries result in medical treatment. The revised manual permits the use of needle resheathing instruments and other mechanical means of needle recapping. According to the manual, standard violations involving physicians who are members of a professional corporation working in a hospital may result in citation for both the corporation and the hospital. The hospital will not be cited when the physician is a sole practitioner or partner in a practice and exposes only himself or herself (OSHA Instruction CPL 2-22.44B).

Regarding OSHA authority to cite hospitals for physician failure to observe universal precautions, the Occupational Safety and Health Act of 1970 specifically governs health- and safety-related rights and responsibilities between employers and employees; it does not address hospital responsibilities related to physicians and other health care professionals who are independent contractors. As a caveat, regardless of OSHA requirements, hospitals have strong incentives to ensure that independent contractors follow CDC guidelines. To the extent barrier precautions provide protection for employees, physicians, and patients, liability considerations mandate their use by all persons potentially exposed to blood or body fluids.

Immunization of Personnel

Immunization of personnel is an important component of hospital infection control programs (see Chap. 3). Records of the immunization status of employees should be maintained. The PHS's Immunization Practices Advisory Committee (ACIP), the AHA's Committee on Infections within Hospitals, and some medical specialty organizations routinely issue immunization recommendations. A number of states also require specific immunizations.

In light of OSHA's directive that employers must undertake all feasible measures necessary to eradicate substantial and recognized occupational hazards, health care providers should carefully design policies to implement abatement procedures, including offering the hepatitis B vaccine to at-risk employees. Failure to offer, and pay for, the vaccine may subject the provider to sanctions under the Act and may expose providers to liability.

Some states have issued immunization recommendations. The Massachusetts Department of Public Health recommends an immunizations program for hospital employees younger than 30 years of age who provide patient care [62]. The New York State Hospital Code mandates immunity to rubella for health care workers regardless of age or sex. The CDC *Guidelines for Infection Control in Hospital Personnel* recommends vaccinating personnel who are likely to have contact with patients with rubella or pregnant patients, regardless of age or sex [109]. In the absence of state or local requirements, immunization recommendations issued by such groups as the AHA Advisory Committee on Infections, ACIP, and medical specialty organizations are likely to establish a nationwide standard of care. Hospitals are thus well advised to monitor such recommendations. If a hospital decides not to follow such recommendations, the reasons for the decision should be fully documented. Recommendations in this controversial area, however, may be conflicting. Whether hospitals indeed should have special obligations in the area of employee immunizations remains unresolved. For example, even though the CDC, the AHA Advisory Committee, and the American College of Obstetricians and Gynecologists currently recommend rubella immunizations of hospi-

tal employees, a published report did not find an increased risk of rubella transmission to pregnant patients in the healthcare setting compared to the community. This study concluded that "rubella screening and immunization of health care personnel will escalate health care costs without substantially decreasing the incidence of congenital rubella except in young female health care workers who voluntarily consent to immunization" [47]. A debate among members of the Vanderbilt University Hospital Infection Control Committee on the issue of mandatory immunization of hospital staff articulates the spectrum of opinions in this area [90]:

Counterpoint. In the absence of state and local laws or regulations, one can anticipate legal difficulties in requiring immunization of current and new employees, especially those who are not actual employees of the hospital (e.g., community physicians, volunteers, private duty nurses). Many believe immunization should remain a personal, not an institutional, decision.

Point. The question of whether hospitals may require serologic evidence of rubella immunity or immunization as a condition of employment or practice in the hospital should not be a major legal issue. Our society often has supported compliance with health requirements for certain groups. For example, food handlers must pass health examinations and children in most states must have certain immunizations before they may attend school. If the Infection Control Committee recommended evidence of rubella immunity for employment or practice in the hospital and the policy were adopted by the hospital's governing board, the decision very likely would be supported by the courts.

In the absence of relevant case law, administrators and attorneys advising hospitals formulating a staff immunization policy should consider the following areas:

1. Applicable state and local statutes and regulations

2. Consent forms that specifically address potential vaccine side effects
3. Potential liability arising from either hospital administration of the vaccine or the hospital requirement of immunization as a condition of employment
4. Current hospital liability insurance coverage vis-à-vis the program
5. Applicability of the state workers' compensation law to claims that may arise
6. Potential religious objections that might be raised by requiring vaccination

It is likely that a court would decide that the health and safety of the public outweighs any individual interests asserted by employees challenging hospital immunization policy. If an employee in a critical patient contact area (e.g., an obstetric clinic) refuses rubella immunization, the employee should, if possible, be offered transfer to a noncritical area; if this is not a viable option, ultimately termination may be appropriate. Publicizing requirements and maintaining open communications with employees, medical staff, and volunteers should be an important component of any hospital staff immunization program.

When an Employer Discovers an Employee Has an Infection

Questions arise as to how to deal with problems raised when an employer discovers that an employee is infected with HIV. Public relations concerns are often a problem for employers in the health care field. Employers often face a difficult dilemma and are forced to make a business decision between facing charges of employee discrimination or facing the repercussions stemming from public hysteria.

Once a provider learns an employee is infected with HIV, it should approach the employee and verify this status with sensitivity in a private and confidential manner. If HIV infection is confirmed, the provider should take appropriate action to protect the employee, other health care workers, and the patient population, with the assistance of the pro-

vider's infection control staff. The provider and employee should attempt to agree on appropriate and reasonable protection measures, following CDC guidelines, which in some circumstances could include limiting tasks to noninvasive procedures, double gloving, and other safety procedures. When an employee does not agree with the procedures that the provider deems necessary, the provider's actions should be fully documented, and disciplinary measures may be considered if the employee will not comply.

When Providers Refuse to Care for Contagious Patients

Patients suffering from incurable infections such as Jacob-Creutzfeld disease and HIV have at times encountered difficulty in obtaining care. Historically, private hospitals had no legal obligation to accept nonemergency patients they did not desire. Traditional rules governing a hospital's responsibility in this area, however, have undergone many changes in reaction to legal theories, statutes, and licensing agency regulations. Aside from discrimination, providers must consider other restrictions on their ability to refuse care. As mandated by law in most states and to avoid sanctions and civil liability under the anti-dumping provisions of the Social Security Act, emergency care must be rendered by hospitals whenever requested.

Denials based on such factors as race or handicap are illegal. Any hospital that receives federal financial assistance bears an obligation under Section 504 of the Federal Rehabilitation Act of 1973 to provide nondiscriminatory treatment. Discrimination against AIDS patients clearly is unethical and may be illegal under federal and state laws prohibiting discrimination against handicapped persons. These laws provide that hospitalization or treatment cannot be denied to a person merely because that person is handicapped.

Once a hospital admits a patient, it is obligated to provide appropriate care or risk potential liabilty for abandonment; hence, if the hospital staff refuse to care for a patient with a contagious disease, the hospital has a responsibility to see to it that care is rendered, even if this means a transfer of the patient to another facility where appropriate care will be provided.

Although there is generally no duty for a hospital to provide nonemergency services, failure to follow established hospital policy, such as failure to follow hospital admission policies for reasons related to race, sex, age, religion, or national origin, may result in liability under state discrimination statutes. An AIDS patient might allege sexual orientation discrimination if, for example, a hospital treated transfusion-associated AIDS but refused to treat sexually transmitted AIDS. Discrimination against individuals who are HIV-infected because of employee fear of infection may violate federal and state anti-discrimination laws.

Health care personnel should not be excused from providing care to patients with infectious diseases. The provider's personnel policies and procedures (or handbook) should specifically address employee insubordination or unreasonable refusals to treat patients. Employee educational programs have been very effective in assuaging the fears of personnel. Employees should be reminded that the hospital provides gowns, gloves, masks, goggles, and the like to protect against transmission of infectious diseases. If an employee, after individual education and counseling, still refuses to perform his or her duties in caring for infected patients, the hospital may either attempt to accommodate the employee by job reassignment or institute disciplinary action for insubordination [105]. In doing this, the hospital will have to act within any relevant limitations imposed by the National Labor Relations Act or collective bargaining agreement.

The American Nurses Association issued a statement from their Committee on Ethics entitled "Risk v. Responsibility in Providing Nursing Care." The committee delineated four fundamental criteria regarding providing nursing care:

1. The patient is at significant risk of harm, loss or damage if the nurse does not assist.

2. The nurse's intervention or care is directly relevant to preventing harm.
3. The nurse's care will probably prevent harm, loss, or damage to the patient.
4. The benefit the patient will gain outweighs any harm the nurse might incur and does not present more than minimal risk to the health care provider.

The statement concludes that, in most instances, it would be considered morally obligatory for a nurse to give care to an AIDS patient.

As was discussed earlier, OSHA provides that each employer must furnish employees an environment free from recognized hazards likely to cause serious physical harm. The Joint Advisory Notice provides detailed guidelines for employer precautions. This act also prohibits an employer from taking any adverse action against an employee who, after first seeking correction of the health hazard from his or her employer, refuses to expose himself or herself to a health hazard that he or she reasonably believes to pose a real danger of death or serious injuries. However, if the hospital educates employees about HIV transmission risks and enforces all recommended precautions, an employee's refusal to work with a co-worker or patient who has AIDS probably will not be protected by OSHA because the fear, while real, will not be considered reasonable.

The following cases recognize the duty to provide care to contagious persons:

A $15,000 settlement resulted in the case of *Willimae Williams* v. *United States*, U.S.D.C. PA No. 86-348, for the premature discharge of an AIDS patient without proper arrangements for care. According to court records, throughout the plaintiff's hospitalization the hospital staff and employees "conducted a campaign to attempt to have him discharged from the hospital even though they knew he was never well enough to leave."

A federal judge ruled on June 30, 1988, that an asymptomatic HIV carrier who was excluded by Centinela Hospital from a federally funded program for alcohol and drug treatment because of fear of contagion was found to be handicapped within the meaning of Section 504 of the Vocational Rehabilitation Act of 1973 (*Doe* v. *Centinela Hospital*, DC, Calif., No. CV 87-2514 PAR [PX]). On January 10, 1989, Centinela agreed to drop the requirement, and the lawsuit was settled on the day the trial was to begin.

A discrimination suit filed in federal court February 10, 1989, against a Jackson, MS, psychiatric hospital was dismissed. The plaintiff charged he was restricted to his room, not allowed to participate in group therapy, not allowed to shower or eat with patients, and restricted in his activities without cause. Charter personnel who came in contact with him were fully masked, gowned, and gloved while in his room. The court granted Charter's motion to dismiss, holding that damages for emotional distress are not recoverable under Section 504 and that Charter's treatment of the plaintiff did not involve state action (*Rhodes* v. *Charter Hospital*, 730 F.Supp. 1383 [S.D. Miss. 1989]).

Medical Staff Issues and AIDS

Physicians' obligation to treat HIV-infected patients should be addressed by hospital and medical staff policies. Some surgeons have publicly announced their refusal to operate on HIV-infected patients. Others argue that patients should be treated based on their clinical condition: If such a patient is judged to be a candidate for cardiac surgery, for example, neither AIDS nor HIV infection should, in and of itself, be considered a contraindication.

Though hospitals cannot require physicians to accept AIDS patients in their private practices, the legal and ethical principles that require employees to provide care to AIDS patients also apply to physicians. In view of hospitals' duty to treat emergency patients and to render appropriate care to admitted patients, they should have policies establishing physicians' obligation to treat. Although such policies should rely on education and counseling, they need to include provisions for withdrawal of staff privileges (after a hearing and appeal) in the case of persistent physician noncompliance. Courts should uphold disciplinary actions based on bylaw provisions where it can be demonstrated that a physician's conduct endangered patient welfare.

The AMA's Council on Ethical and Judicial Affairs on November 13, 1987, stated that physicians have an obligation to treat HIV-infected patients. Previous AMA policy held that physicians should have the freedom, except in emergencies, to choose whom to serve. This same policy indicated, however, that during an epidemic, ". . . a physician must continue his [her] labors without regard to the risk of his [her] own health."

Individual state medical organizations have not felt bound by the AMA's recommendations. The Arizona State Board of Medical Examiners, for example, issued a statement that endorses the right of a physician to refuse to treat patients who have AIDS. The Texas Medical Association, in 1987, also determined that physicians could ethically refuse treatment to patients with AIDS.

The Deans of New York medical schools, in December 1987, announced that refusal of faculty, residents, or medical students to treat AIDS or HIV patients would be grounds for dismissal or other sanctions. The American College of Physicians and the Infectious Disease Society of America, in a March 1988 statement, indicated that "physicians, other health professionals, and hospitals are obligated to provide competent and humane care to all patients, including patients with AIDS and AIDS-related conditions as well as HIV-infected patients with unrelated medical problems. The denial of appropriate care to patients for any reason is unethical" [48].

Employee Insistence Regarding Precautions

An employee may lawfully refuse to work in proved unsafe conditions and may also insist on wearing safety equipment while working. OSHA does not permit employees to leave the job because of potential unsafe work conditions. Rather, the employees are to inform their employer of the conditions or request an OSHA inspection of the workplace under OSHA guidelines if no action is taken by the employer (29 C.F.R., Section 1977.12[b] [1]). If an employee is confronted with a condition presenting a real danger of serious injury or death, he or she may refuse in "good faith" to work (29 C.F.R., Section 1977.12 [b] [2]). (See also *Whirlpool Corp.* v. *Marshall,* 445 U.S. 1 [1980].) For the employee to be protected, the perceived hazard must be such that a reasonable person would believe it to present a real danger of death or serious injury and that the danger was of such an urgent nature that the use of normal channels of solving the problem would be ineffective.

When an employee insists on wearing more protective gear than the employer health care provider believes is necessary to prevent disease transmission, the employer is advised to investigate the employee's rationale and then to educate employees regarding appropriate infection control techniques. If, after this process, the employee still insists on following procedures contrary to the recommended approach based on the most recent medical information, legal advice should be sought regarding state law on the subject. Predisciplinary legal consultation is appropriate because some states forbid discrimination against employees for complaining about health hazards, even if there is no actual danger, as long as the employee has a reasonable belief that a danger exists (California Labor Code Sections 6310-11). A California court held that disciplining an employee for complaining about a health hazard, even if one did not actually exist, may constitute "wrongful termination," subjecting an employer to compensatory and punitive damages (*Hunter* v. *Singer,* 138 Cal. App. 3d).

Restrictions of Duties of Health Care Workers

A complaint was filed in 1987 by a nurse at New York Hospital who sought relief from the New York City Commission on Human Rights due to a transfer in job assignments. The complaint alleged that the nurse decided she wanted to become pregnant and sought to take advantage of the confidential HIV-testing program made available through the hospital's employee health service. After a positive result occurred, the nurse was informed by her employer that she would be transferred out of the surgical intensive care unit to another position in emergency critical care with the same salary and benefits. The nurse declined the transfer and filed the discrimination action. In 1988, an administrative law judge denied prehearing motions challenging the commission's jurisdiction on grounds that the decision to reassign the nurse was made in good faith based on medical judgment (*Doe* v. *New York Hospital,* Complaint No. GA-000350 41487 DN [N.Y. Comm. Human Rights, Oct. 3, 1988]).

When Employees Contract Diseases

Disease acquired on the job by employees is ordinarily covered under state workers' compensation laws [67]. Specified amounts of compensation are provided if an employee is killed or disabled from an accidental injury that arises out of, and is within the scope of, employment. Workers' compensation is normally the claimant's sole remedy, precluding the claimant from filing a negligence action against the employer. Generally, because workers' compensation is the exclusive remedy for employees who contract occupational disease, employees are entitled to recover without proof of fault or negligence on the part of the employer. The employee must generally establish that his or her illness is an occupational disease that was contracted on the job (arose from and occurred in the course of employment).

In certain circumstances, hospital employees acquiring work-related infections may be eligible for remuneration beyond that provided by the workers' compensation system. If it can be established that an employer was aware of and intentionally disregarded an infection risk in the workplace, an infected employee may prevail in bringing suit against the employer. In certain states, accidental infectious disease statutes provide compensation for employees becoming infected at the workplace. Finally, criminal actions have been brought against employers who knowingly exposed employees to life-threatening conditions in the workplace. The authors, however, are not aware of any such actions involving infected hospital workers. In an unusual case, an extern at Kings County Hospital pricked her finger on a needle used to draw blood from a patient dying of AIDS in January 1983. The plaintiff tested positive for AIDS in March 1985. The plaintiff alleged that the defendants failed to dispose of used needles properly, claiming that needle boxes should have been provided in each room. The parties ultimately settled for $1,350,000 in cash in March 1990 (*Veronica Prego* v. *The City of New York,* Kings County Hospital, New York City Health and Hospital Corporation, Kings County [NY] Supreme Court, Index No. 14974/88, as reported in *Medical Malpractice Verdicts, Settlements and Experts,* March 1989 and April 1990).

When seeking coverage under workers' compensation laws, a hospital employee alleging he or she contracted an infection on the job must establish that the infection was not acquired outside the working environment. Such an employee may also have to prove that the risk of acquiring the infection as a hospital employee was greater than the general public's risk.

If an employee becomes infected with HIV in the course of employment, workers' compensation benefits are a proper remedy. The worker would have to demonstrate a "causal connection" between his or her HIV infection and his or her employment. Specifically, the employee would need to establish that an incident occurred on the job involving a documented needle-stick injury, puncture wound, or other exposure to HIV-contaminated blood or body fluids. In this situation, the worker's personal lifestyle will probably come into play. A negative serologic workup for HIV at the employee's time of exposure and a positive test 8 weeks later can establish

the likely initial absence of infection in the employee.

Preemployment health evaluations may prove useful later should an employee allege contraction of infection on the job. Detailed histories regarding previous infections and immunizations, preemployment tuberculin tests, chest radiographs, and serologic studies may be helpful in this context. In addition, it may be useful to keep records of the room location of patients (for this purpose, there is no need to use patient names) infected with contagious disease to help determine possible exposure to a specific infection.

If a worker becomes psychiatrically disabled due to the perception that he or she has developed, or is at high risk of developing, AIDS, some states might award compensation, even if the perception is unfounded (Michigan and California have upheld such claims). In such cases, the worker must demonstrate that the work environment played an "active role" in the development of the psychiatric condition and was not a mere "passive element." If a worker quits because of contracting AIDS, unemployment benefits may be available if the worker can show that he or she believed in good faith that continued employment would jeopardize his or her health. The burden, however, is on the worker to show the decision to quit was of a compelling nature.

Cases involving claims for emotional distress include the following:

A San Francisco General Hospital nurse was granted $5,000 workers' compensation based on the development of ulcers from the stress of treating AIDS patients (*Vernales* v. *City and County of San Francisco,* Case Nos. 11-17001-1, 11-17001-2, 11-17001-3, and 11-17001-4 [Cal. Dept. of Industrial Relations, Division of Labor Standards Enforcement, Sept. 9, 1985]).

No unemployment compensation for fear of AIDS was the ruling in *Vinokurov* v. *Mt. Sinai Hospital, Unemployment Compensation Appeals Bureau,* Docket No. 88-31586, March 29, 1988. The claimant was employed in a research laboratory and knew part of her duties included maintaining HIV cultures. One of her co-employees caused a spill of the virus August 1987 by placing a flask containing the virus upside down. The claimant stated that she was afraid and was quitting. The Appeals referee held that in cases of voluntary quitting it is incumbent on the claimant to show by a preponderance of the evidence that the quitting was for good cause and attributable to the employer.

A New York Court of Claims judge rejected a claim by a health care worker for damages for emotional distress stemming from the "AIDS-phobia" he suffered after being bitten by a patient, a prison inmate who was rumored to have AIDS. The worker consistently tested negative for HIV antibodies. The judge said the evidence "is simply too speculative and remote" to award damages on the basis of unsubstantiated risk (*Hare* v. *State of New York*, NY CTOS [55, 80].

Workers' compensation cases involving nosocomial infections include the following:

In *Russell* v. *Camden Community Hospital*, 359 A.2d 607 (Me. 1976), a nurses' aide was awarded compensation after applying hospital prescribed ointment to a tuberculous ulcer and subsequently developing pulmonary tuberculosis.

An electroencephalography (EEG) technician in *Melamed* v. *Montefiore Hospital*, 182 Pa. Super. 482, 128 A.2d 129 (1956), alleging she developed tuberculosis from exposure to infected patients at work, was awarded compensation after it was established that several hundred people with tuberculosis had been inpatients during this woman's period of employment. That the technician had not performed EEG on any of these patients did not influence the award.

In *Evans* v. *Indiana University Medical Center*, 121 Ind. App. 679, 100 N.E.2d 828 (1951), a plumber who occasionally worked in an isolation ward and was once in a room occupied by a patient with tuberculosis was denied compensation, because his exposure to the disease was considered too uncertain.

In *Furchtsam* v. *Binghamton General Hospital*, 24 App. Div.2d 786, 263 N.Y.S.2d 746, 747 (1965), a general duty nurse who developed a staphylococcal middle ear infection was awarded compensation. The court held that ". . . the close contacts of a hospital nurse inherent in caring for infected patients enhances the risk of contracting the disease."

Compensation was awarded to the wife of a laboratory technician who died after being exposed to viral hepatitis. The court in *Booker* v. *Duke Medical Center*, 256 S.E.2d 189 (N.C. 1979), ruled that even though viral hepatitis may be contracted by people outside the laboratory environment, the technician's job "exposed him to a greater risk of contracting the disease than members of the public or employees in general." In addition, there was no evidence that he was exposed to viral hepatitis outside of the laboratory or that he had received any previous injections or transfusions.

In *Sacred Heart Medical Center* v. *Department of Labor & Industries*, 600 P.2d 1015 (Wash. 1979), workers' compensation was awarded to a nurse who contracted hepatitis. There was no evidence to establish that she had contracted the disease at work. After examining her lifestyle, however, the court concluded it was most likely that she acquired hepatitis in the course of her employment.

An emergency medical technician applied for Special Disability Retirement, contending he contracted hepatitis B during the course of his employment. The hearing examiner awarded the benefits, finding the plaintiff was free of the disease when he began employment and that there was no suggestion that he had been exposed to hepatitis outside the course of his work. On appeal, the circuit court reversed this decision, concluding that the plaintiff had failed to meet his burden of proof that the injury arose of and in the course of the actual performance of duty. The Court found that the plaintiff's evidence amounted to "mere possibility or speculation" that he contracted the disease during the course of his work (*Board of Trustees of the Fire and Police*

Employees Retirement Systems v. *Powell,* No. 955, Maryland Court of Special Appeals, March 8, 1989).

A plaintiff developed chronic persistent hepatitis associated with hepatitis B virus during her first year of employment at her employer-hospital. In her claim to the Industrial Commission, an arbitrator found that the plaintiff had not established the requisite causal connection prescribed by statute. Although the plaintiff testified she often pricked herself with sharp operating room instruments that had been exposed to patients' blood, she failed to identify a single occurrence wherein transmission was likely to have occurred or evidence that she treated any infected patient. On review, the Industrial Commission affirmed the arbitrator's decision. The circuit court upheld the commission's action, which was reversed by the appellate court on the grounds that proof of a causal connection for a health care worker's exposure to an occupational disease could be inferred indirectly by showing that the employee worked in an environment where exposure was likely. The Supreme Court, however, rejected the appellate court's statutory interpretation, holding that a disease is deemed to arise out of employment only if the connection was apparent to the rational mind on consideration of all the circumstances (*Sperling* v. *Industrial Commission,* No. 67533 [Sup. Ct. Ill. May 17, 1989]).

In *Gatlin* v. *Truman Medical Center,* 770 S.W.2d 510 (MD App. 1989), a malpractice claim based on the assertion of contracting an occupational disease was denied. While employed at the defendant medical center, the plaintiff nurse came in contact with the blood and body fluids of a patient carrying the hepatitis B virus and contracted hepatitis. The nurse sought workers' compensation and damages for medical negligence. The Missouri Court of Appeals upheld the trial court's dismissal of the plaintiff's cause of action for malpractice, finding a claim under Missouri's workers' compensation law was the exclusive remedy.

The New York Supreme Court in Kings County ruled in 1990 that the exclusive remedy for a nurses' aide who allegedly suffered injuries as a result of an accidental needle stick inflicted by a co-worker was workers' compensation (*Peters* v. *New York City Health and Hospitals Corp.,* Sup. Ct. Kings Cty, Index No. 22907-89, 3/29/90).

A resident physician acquired HIV from a patient while working at a well-known teaching hospital. In a letter to the *New England Journal of Medicine,* he stated [8]:

> [W]orkers' compensation works well to cover medical expenses and income lost because of occupational injuries that result in temporary or minor disabilities such as muscle tears or bone fractures. But these are not the accidents that a physician is likely to suffer at work. The main threats today are catastrophic, and workers' compensation is grossly inadequate for catastrophic illness.

Employee Exposure to Blood and Body Fluids

The stigma associated with AIDS has added to the dilemma hospitals face when deciding how to treat workers accidentally exposed to patient's blood and body fluids. Hospitals have faced a similar dilemma for years with workers filing false workers' compensation claims for hepatitis B and back injuries. Workers' compensation laws usually cover infections employees acquire on the job. Employees may try filing claims outside the workers' compensation system for negligent failure to disclose harmful conditions at the workplace, malicious intent to conceal, or failure to use due care in keeping the workplace safe. Should it be determined there is no entitlement to workers' compensation benefits, the provider's hospitalization and medical care benefits program may cover needed care, absent any exclusions from coverage on account of preexisting conditions or on other grounds.

The CDC recommends that after a health care worker has a parenteral or mucous membrane exposure to blood or other body fluids or has a cutaneous exposure involving large amounts of blood, the source patient should be informed of the incident and should be tested for serologic evidence of HIV infection after informed consent is obtained. If the source patient is positive for HIV or refused HIV antibody testing, the health care worker should be counseled and evaluated clinically and serologically for evidence of HIV infection as soon as possible after the exposure. If the source patient is seronegative, it is advisable that the health care worker still be provided a baseline HIV antibody test. The CDC recommends that no further follow-up of the exposed worker is necessary unless the patient is at high risk of HIV infection. Because of heightened employee concern, many hospitals have chosen to make serologic testing available to all workers who are fearful they may have been infected.

If the source patient, after being informed of the incident, refuses HIV testing, the hospital's options depend on state law.

In some states, state law forbids testing without written informed consent. In a few states (such as Colorado and Florida), state law expressly allows testing regardless of consent. In at least one state (Maine), one may apply for a court order requiring testing of the source patient.

Releasing Information Regarding Communicable Disease

Engrained in American society is the deeply held belief that individuals have a right to privacy. This right is tempered, however, by the obligation to disclose information needed by others to protect themselves from injury. In most states, an obligation exists to report communicable diseases to health officials. Individuals or organizations such as hospitals who hold privileged information are expected to protect it from disclosure to those without a legitimate need to know. Confidentiality rights flow from constitutional and statutory rights and from physician-patient privilege. This is expressed in statutes and regulations at federal and state levels that restrict access to information contained in medical records,

as well as such certain common-law theories as defamation. Statutes mandating the reporting of communicable diseases contain strict confidentiality requirements and are evidence of public policy to protect this information. Illinois, Florida, and Maine have statutes that, with limited exceptions, provide for the confidentiality of all HIV test results.

The duty to maintain confidentiality should not be viewed as absolute. Under appropriate circumstances, it may be outweighed by competing responsibilities to others. In *Tarasoff* v. *The Regents of the University of California*, (551 P.2d 334, 1976), a psychiatrist was found to have a duty to warn a young woman that one of his patients had repeatedly threatened to kill her. The court found the psychiatrist's duty to the victim overruled his duty to keep his patient's confidences. Based on the Tarasoff precedent, some courts have limited the duty to warn others to cases of explicit threat (harm to specific identified individuals), whereas other courts have accepted a broader duty simply to act prudently to prevent reasonably foreseeable harm.

The legal risks for divulging a patient's HIV status, whether publically or to a single person, differ greatly from state to state. If a hospital, physician, blood bank, laboratory, school, employer, or insurance company releases information concerning diagnosis of AIDS or a positive HIV test in an individual, it may be subject to liability under various traditional legal theories. A breach of confidentiality can result in civil liabilities for injury under the causes of action of defamation and invasion of privacy. Recognizing the sensitive nature of HIV-related information, many states have enacted statutes establishing the confidentiality of such information as test results, the identity of persons seeking testing, or reports to health departments. These statutes provide for civil or criminal damages for breach of confidentiality. For example, California has a law specifying a $10,000 penalty for divulging a patient's serostatus without his or her permission.

A hospital can be liable for disclosing to a third party that a patient has AIDS or is infected with HIV unless the patient consents to the disclosure or a situation exists that overrides the patient's right of privacy. Health care providers have been found liable for posting names of HIV-positive patients on a laboratory bulletin board to allay the fears of technicians, for permitting news media in waiting rooms, and for disclosing a patient's HIV status to family, friends, or employers [37]. Damages that may be alleged include loss of employment, loss of housing, loss of or inability to obtain insurance, school expulsion, social stigma, harassment, and mental anguish. The disclosure of inaccurate information implying that a person is infected with HIV will be "actionable per se" in most states, implying there is no requirement to prove specific damages.

Unfortunately, health care providers can also be sued by an infected third party for *failing* to disclose an individual's HIV status. In such bedeviling situations, providers may find themselves forced to choose between potential liability for breach of confidentiality and potential liability for wrongful death. Before ordering an HIV test in such a setting, it is advisable to inform the patient that positive results may be reported to third parties.

As an example of the type of litigation that may arise, a former patient sued a hospital, a church, and its minister for compensatory and punitive damages, claiming that hospital employees falsely told the minister that the patient was suffering from AIDS and the minister conveyed the erroneous information to the patient and others. Although the plaintiff ultimately determined he did not have AIDS, he alleged suffering "severe emotional distress and great anguish" and sought damages in excess of $20,000 (*Burton* v. *Yaeger, Quakertown Community Hosp., et al.*, Ct. Com Pleas, Bucks County, Pa. No. 87-287-03-2).

In another case, a jury in Lawrence County Common Pleas Court found for a Florida man who claimed that while he was a patient in Lawrence County Medical Center, rumors circulated among employees that he had AIDS. The jury awarded $50,000 and also recommended the hospital issue a public apology. The hospital has appealed (AP, Thurs. July 28, 1988).

A patient's AIDS diagnosis or HIV infection may be disclosed to hospital personnel who require such information to care for the patient. In addition, the patient's diagnosis may be recorded in the medical record, where only authorized personnel are allowed access to it. Disclosure to enable hospital personnel who are at risk to protect themselves from exposure to HIV is also permissible and may be required by OSHA. However, it is recommended that personnel should observe infection control precautions whenever exposed to any blood or other body fluids (universal precautions) rather than relying on information as to the patient's HIV status (see Chap. 11).

A growing number of doctors and legislators have begun to argue that the sanctity of the doctor-patient relationship and the patient's right to privacy must give way to society's need to protect itself. Clearly, HIV-infected patients have an obligation to warn potential victims. However, because HIV sometimes attacks the brain, patients may lack the capacity to warn, or fear of repercussions from disclosure may interfere with one's duty to warn contacts. A move away from absolute privacy is reflected in the large number of states considering laws to identify and trace victims of the disease and carriers of the virus. The American College of Physicians, the CDC, and the AMA all urge physicians to notify third parties of a patient's HIV status when necessary to protect the third party's health. A breach of confidentiality should be considered only when it is medically necessary to protect someone and is not appropriate when responding to requests from an employer or insurer.

In a major policy change, the AMA, at its December 1989 annual meeting, decided to recommend name reporting of HIV-positive patients to state health departments for tracing and notification of sexual contacts. The development of such treatments as zidovudine and aerosolized pentamidine occasioned this shift, which represents a change from the AMA's previous policy of balancing the infected individual's right to privacy with the exposed individual's right to know. Left unchanged was the AMA's recommendation that states give serious consideration to protecting individuals' confidentiality and privacy.

Federal regulations that decrease the requirement that laboratories performing HIV tests maintain names and identifications of patients went into effect January 3, 1989. A laboratory seeking payment for tests through Medicare or Medicaid must still maintain such records, but the facility may use identifiers other than the patient's name. These final rules (*Federal Register* 53FR 48645) further protect confidentiality of HIV test results and encourage voluntary testing.

Testing and Screening Issues

HIV antibody testing raises a number of legal issues. Health care providers have been drawn into the debate about testing all hospitalized patients for HIV. The balancing of the rights of the infected and the rights of the uninfected to exercise self-protection is at the core of this issue. State laws differ on the treatment of this information, and many legislative proposals have been introduced at the state and federal level regarding confidentiality; hence, providers should remain current regarding evolving law in this area. The CDC initially specified that hospitals should not screen patients or health care workers. The August 21, 1987, recommendations for prevention of HIV transmission in health care settings stated that "decisions regarding the need to establish testing programs for patients should be made by physicians or individual institutions." The following types of abuses in HIV testing were cited by the CDC:

1. Ordering tests for hospitalized patients under false names
2. Failing to inform patients they are being tested or failing to inform patients of the result
3. Failing to report test results to the state health department

Since there are circumstances in which an HIV test may be indicated to care for a patient, a provider may request the test for di-

agnosis and treatment. If a patient refuses to consent to the test, diagnosis and treatment should continue without the test. The patient's refusal, together with the discussion of risks and consequences of the decision, should be fully documented in the medical record. A national policy of mandatory testing of all hospitalized patients for HIV has been opposed by the AMA, AHA, and public health officials. The fear is that mandatory testing will drive those infected underground, further exacerbating difficulties in controlling the spread of the virus. They point to the observance of universal precautions as a more appropriate course of action. Technical limitations of currently available tests are also relevant here. A negative test does not necessarily prove an absence of HIV infection, and therefore a broad testing program would create a false sense of security in some. In addition, testing is expensive and carries with it obligations for counseling, confidentiality, and reporting that may be challenged as unlawful discrimination. In the absence of state law authorizing testing without a patient's consent, testing is not advisable unless as part of a formal research project or surveillance that provides for the removal of patient-identifying information. The following cases involve testing issues:

The U.S. District Court for the Eastern District of Louisiana ruled in March, 1989, that a nurse who was fired for refusing to communicate his HIV test results to his hospital employer did not show he was handicapped or perceived to be handicapped and therefore was not protected under the Vocational Rehabilitation Act of 1973. The plaintiff claimed the hospital requested the test because his roommate of 8 years had recently died of AIDS. He was fired for insubordination after continuing to refuse to be tested. The judge stated the hospital had a "legitimate and nondiscriminatory reason for firing Lockett: the need of a health care institution to monitor the health status of employees who have been exposed to infectious diseases, particularly diseases such as AIDS . . . in order to protect patients and co-workers and to accommodate any current or future handicap of the employee." The decision was affirmed by a three-judge panel of the U.S. Court of Appeals for the Fifth Circuit (*Lockett* v. *Hospital District No. 1,* CA 5, No. 89-3256). In 1988, the U.S. District Court for the District of Nebraska ruled that the mandatory employee testing at a Nebraska facility for the mentally retarded violated the Fourth Amendment's ban on unreasonable searches and seizures. The court issued a permanent injunction in the class action filed by some 400 staff members at the Eastern Nebraska Community Office of Retardation. The court stated the medical evidence "is overwhelming that the risk of transmission in the (facility) is trivial to the point of non-existence. Such a theoretical risk does not justify a policy which interferes with the constitutional rights of the staff members." A testing program might be upheld under the Constitution when a risk of transmission "is real and tangible." The appellate court affirmed this decision (*Glover* v. *Encor,* CA 8, CA 88-1678, U.S. Court of Appeals [8th Cir.] Feb. 6, 1989).

References

1. *AIDS Lit. Reptr.* (3/24/89).
2. *AIDS Lit. Reptr.* (5/27/88).
3. *AIDS Lit. Reptr.* (9/9/88).
4. *AIDS Lit. Reptr.* (6/10/88). Westtown, PA: Andrews Publications, 1988.
5. American Hospital Association. *Infection Control in the Hospital* (4th ed.). Chicago: American Hospital Association, 1979. Pp. 39–40.
6. The American Society for Hospital Central Service Personnel. Guidelines for the reuse of disposable medical devices. *Infect. Control* 11:562, 1987.
7. Annas, G.J., Glantz, L.H., and Katz, B.F. Malpractice Litigation. In: *The Rights of Doctors, Nurses, and Allied Health Professionals: A Health Law Primer.* New York: Avon, 1981. P. 246.
8. Aoun, H. When a house officer gets AIDS. *N. Engl. J. Med.* 321(10): 695, 1989.
9. Attorneys explain liability of hemodialyzer reuse. *Hosp. Infect. Control* 9:129, 1982.
10. Attorneys outline basics of IC malpractice cases. *Hosp. Infect. Control* 7:32, 1980.
11. Bernstein, A.H. *A Trustee's Guide to Hospital Law* Chicago: Teach 'Em, Inc., 1981, P. 59.
12. Bernstein, A.H. Legal implications of administering blood. *Hospitals* 55:43, 1981.
13. Bock, J.A. Liability for Injury or Death from Blood Transfusion, 59 A.L.R.2d 768.
14. Bollow, R.C., and Capp, D.J. Protecting the confidentiality of blood donors' identities in AIDS litigation through state abuse of discovery rules. *J. Health Hosp. Law* 22(2): 37, 1989.
15. Carmichael, M.C. Liability of Hospital or Medical Practitioner under Doctrine of Strict Liability in Tort, or Breach of Warranty, for Harm Caused by Drug, Medical Instrument, or Similar Device Used in Treating Patient, 54 ALR3d 258.
16. *Carpenter* v. *Campbell,* 149 Ind. App. 189, 271 N.E.2d 163 (1971).
17. Castle, M. *Hospital Infection Control.* New York: Wiley, 1980. P. 233.
18. Centers for Disease Control. *Guidelines for the Prevention and Control of Nosocomial Infections. Introduction.* Springfield, VA: National Technical Information Service, U.S. Department of Commerce, 1981.
19. Centers for Disease Control. Prevention of acquired immune deficiency syndrome (AIDS): Report of the inter-agency recommendations. *M.M.W.R.* 32:101, 1983.
20. 42 C.F.R. §405.1022(c)(6).
21. 42 C.F.R. §405.1022(c)(8).
22. Chavigny, K.H., and Helm, A. Ethical dilemmas and the practice of infection control. *Law Med. Health Care* 10:169, 1982.
23. Classification Labeling Requirements, 21 C.F.R. 606. 120 and 640.2, *et seq.*
24. *Contreras* v. *St. Luke's Hospital,* 78 Cal. App.3d 919; 144 Cal. Rptr. 647 (1978).
25. Cram, S. The hospital's obligation to protect patients from carriers of infectious diseases. *Medicolegal News* 7:11, 1979.
26. Creighton, H. Legal aspects of nosocomial infection. *Nurs. Clin. North Am.* 15:789, 1980.
27. *Criss* v. *Angelus Hospital Association of Los Angeles et al.,* 13 Cal. App.2d 4 12, 56 P.2d 1274 (1936), 37 ALR2d 1290, Section 5.
28. Crook, G.B. Negligence. In: 57 Am. Jur. 2d, Municipal, School, and State Tort Liability, Section 1.
29. Davis, R.P. Hospital's Liability for Injury or Death in Obstetrical Cases, 37 ALR2d 1284.
30. Dornette, W. *AIDS and the Law* New York: Wiley, 1987. P. 235.
31. Drechsler, C.T. Physicians, Surgeons, and Other Healers. In: 61 Am. Jur. 2d, Perpetuities and Restraints on Alienation, Section 219.
32. *Elam* v. *College Park Hospital,* 132 Cal. App.3d 332 (1982), opinion modified 122 Cal. App.3d 94a (1982).

33. Fifer, W.R. Infection control is quality control. *Am. J. Infect. Control* 9:121, 1981.

34. Frechette, A.L., and Swarthout, A.M. *Res Ipsa Loquitur* in Action Against Hospital for Injury to Patient, 9 ALR3d 1315.

35. *Fridena* v. *Evans,* 622 P.2d 463 (Ariz. 1980).

36. Frumer, L.R. (Ed.). *Personal Injury: Actions, Defenses, Damages, Hospitals and Asylums* 1.06{5}. New York: Matthew Bender, 1982.

37. Gostin, L. The AIDS Litigation Project. *J.A.M.A.* 263:14, 1961, 1962, 1965, 1990.

38. Greene, V.W. Reuse of disposable medical devices: Historical and current aspects. *Infect. Control* 75(10): 512, 1986.

39. Griffith, J.L. Advise visitors of risks from isolated patients. *Hosp. Infect. Control* 7:53, 1980.

40. Griffith, J.L. Document recommendations in chart, with administration. *Hosp. Infect. Control* 8:111, 1981.

41. Griffith, J.L. Hospitals have legal duty. *Hosp. Infect. Control* 9:52, 1982.

42. Griffith, J.L. Legal commentary. *Hosp. Infect. Control* 5:11, 1978.

43. Haley, R.W., and Emori, T.G. The employee health service and infection control in U.S. hospitals, 1976–1977: II. Managing employee illness. *J.A.M.A.* 256:962, 1981.

44. Haley, R.W., and Emori, T.G. The employee health service and infection control in U.S. hospitals, 1976–1977: I. Screening procedures. *J.A.M.A.* 246:847, 1981.

45. Haley, R.W., et al. The nationwide nosocomial infection rate: A new need for vital statistics. *Am. J. Epidemiol.* 121:159, 1985.

46. Harrison, D.B. Application of Rule of Strict Liability in Tort to Person or Entity Rendering Medical Services, 100 ALR3d 1205.

47. Hartstein, A.I., et al. Rubella screening and immunization of health care personnel: Critical appraisal of a voluntary program. *Am. J. Infect. Control* 11:8, 1983.

48. Health and Public Policy Committee of the American College of Physicians and Infectious Diseases Society of America. *The Acquired Immunodeficiency Syndrome (AIDS) and Infection with the Human Immunodeficiency Virus (HIV).*

49. Henry, H.H. Physicians and Surgeons: *Res Ipsa Loquitur,* or Presumption or Inference of Negligence in Malpractice Cases, 82 ALR2d 1262.

50. Horty, J. Negligence, Liability, Hospital Corporate Negligence. In: *Hospital Law.* Pittsburgh: Action-Kit for Hospital Law 1978, 1981. Pp. 2, 6.

51. Hospital records: Friends or foes in the courtroom? *Hosp. Infect. Control* 7:25, 1980.

52. Hospitals and Asylums, 40 Am. Jur. 2d, Highways, Streets, and Bridges, Sections 14.5, 26, 29, 33, 35.

53. Iffy, L., and Wecht, C.H. Medical-Legal Aspects of Perinatal and Surgical Infections. In: *Legal Medicine 1980.* Philadelphia: Saunders, 1980. P. 177.

54. Ill Rev. Stat. Ch. 111 '12, Section 620-6.

55. Illinois: Hospital Licensing Requirements 1977, Sections 4-1.4 and 4-1.5.

56. Infection control in nursing care: Legalities. *Regan Report on Nursing Law* 22:1, 1982.

57. *Johnson* v. *Misericordia Community Hospital,* 301 N.W.2d 156 (Wisc. 1981).

58. Joint Commission on Accreditation of Healthcare Organizations. *Accreditation Manual for Hospitals* Chicago: Joint Commission on Accreditation of Healthcare Organizations, 1992. Pp. 39–42, 66–67.

59. Joint Commission on Accreditation of Hospitals. *Accreditation Manual for Hospitals* Chicago: Joint Commission on Accreditation of Hospitals, 1983. Pp. 70–75.

60. *Kalmus* v. *Cedars of Lebanon Hospital,* 132 Cal. App.2d 243, 281 P.2D 872 (1955).

61. Keeton, P. Medical negligence: The standard of care. *Tex. Tech. L.R.* 10:351, 1979.

62. Klein, J.O. Management of infections in hospital employees. *Am. J. Med.* 70:920, 1981.

63. Kraut, J. Hospital's Liability for Exposing Patient to Extraneous Infection or Contagion, 96 ALR2d 1205.

64. Lasky, P.C. Principles of Liability. In: P.C. Lasky (Ed.), *Hospital Law Manual.* Rockville, MD: Health Law Center, Aspen Systems Corporation, 1983. Pp. 4, 21, 37–38, 75.

65. Lawyers predict new CDC guidelines will become standard of care. *Hosp. Infect. Control* 8:73, 1981.

66. LeBlang, T.R. Disclosure of injury and illness: Responsibilities in the physician-patient relationship. *Law Med. Health Care* 9:4, 1981.

67. Malone, W.S., and Plant M.L. *Cases and Materials on Workmen's Compensation.* St. Paul, MN: West, 1963.

68. Mayhall, G. Commentary: Types of disposable medical devices reused in hospitals. *Infect. Control* 7(10): 491, 1986.

69. *McAllister* v. *American National Red Cross,* 240 S.E.2d 247 (Ga. 1977).

70. *McCall* v. *St. Joseph's Hospital,* 184 Neb. 1, 165 N.W.2d 85 (1969).

71. Medicare and Medicaid Conditions of Participation, 42 C.F.R. 405.1011 *et seq.,* Section 505.1022(c)(1)–(8).

72. *Mitchell County Hospital Authority* v. *Joiner,* 189 S.E.2d 412 (Ga. 1972).

73. *Moses* v. *St. Barnabas Hospital,* 130 Minn 1, 153 N.W. 128, (1915).

74. Nadel, A.G. Hospital's Liability for Negligence in Failing to Review or Supervise Treatment Given by Doctor, or to Require Consultation, 12 ALR4th 57.

75. Nottebart, H.C., Jr. Hospital-acquired staphylococcal infection transmitted by hospital personnel. *Infect. Control* 1(3): 190, 1980.

76. Nottebart, H.C., Jr. Infection Control Committee reports. *Infect. Control* 1(1): 47, 1980.

77. Nottebart, H.C., Jr. The law and infection control: The myth of negligence. *Infect. Control* 2(2): 158, 1981.

78. Nottebart, H.C., Jr. Legal Aspects of Infection Control. In: K.R. Cundy and W. Ball (Eds.), *Infection Control in Health Care Facilities: Microbiological Surveillance*. Baltimore, MD: University Park Press, 1977. P. 199.

79. Nottebart, H.C., Jr. Staphylococcal infection in hospital roommates. *Infect. Control* 1(2): 105, 1980.

80. N.Y.L.J., 4, Col. 3, p. 23.

81. O'Brien, J.P. Emerging malpractice trends. *Hospitals* 57:60, 1983.

82. Olson, M. Nosocomial infections next target for malpractice suits. *Hosp. Med. Staff* 10:19, 1981.

83. Orlikoff, J.E., Fifer, W.R., and Greeley, H. *Malpractice Prevention and Liability Control for Hospitals*. Chicago: American Hospital Association, 1981. P. 9.

84. Peters, B.M. The application of reasonable prudence to medical malpractice litigation: The precursor to strict liability? *Law Med. Health Care* 9:21, 1981.

85. *Posthuma* v. *Northwestern Hospital*, 197 Minn 304, 267 N.W. 221 (1936).

86. Practitioner outlines isolation problems. *Hosp. Infect. Control* 7:70, 1980.

87. Prosser, W.L. *Handbook of The Law of Torts* (3rd ed.). St. Paul, MN: West, 1964. P. 146.

88. *Purcell* v. *Zimbelman*, 500 P.2d 335 (Ariz. App. 1972).

89. Purver, J.M. Liability for Injury or Death from Blood Transfusion, 45 ALR3d 1364.

90. Recommendations from AHA Office of the General Counsel. Hospital rubella control alert: Immunization recommendations, May 1981. *Infect. Control* 2(5): 410, App. A, 1981.

91. Rutala, D.M., and Hamory, B. Infection control. *Hosp. Epidemiol.* 10(6): 261, 1989.

92. Salman, S.L., and Click, N. Risk manager must interact with infection control expert. *Hospitals* 54:52, 1980.

93. Shafer, N., Wilkenfeld, M., and Shafer, R. Blood Transfusion Reactions. In: C. Wecht

(Ed.), *Legal Medicine 1980*. Philadelphia: Saunders, 1980. P. 207.

94. Shaw, J.W., Jr. Hospital's Liability for Negligence in Selection or Appointment of Staff Physicians or Surgeons, 51 ALR3d 981.

95. *Sheehan* v. *Strong*, 257 Mass 525, 154 N.E. 253 (1926).

96. Shipley, W.E. Hospital's Liability for Negligence in Failing to Review or Supervise Treatment Given By Individual Doctor, or to Require Consultation, 14 ALR3d 873.

97. *Shurpit* v. *Brah*, 30 Wis.2d 388; 141 N.W.2d 266 (1966).

98. Single-use devices should not be reused. *Hospitals* 54:157, 1980.

99. *Sommers* v. *Sisters of Charity of Providence in Oregon*. 561 P.2d 603 (Ore. 1977).

100. Southwick, A. *The Law of Hospital and Health Care Administration*. Ann Arbor, MI: Health Administration Press, 1978. Pp. 128, 351–352, 355, 358.

101. Southwick, A. *The Law of Hospital and Health Care Administration*. Ann Arbor, MI: Health Administration Press, 1988. Pp. 71–77.

102. The St. Paul's 1989 Annual Report to Policyholders. St. Paul, MN: St. Paul Fire and Marine Insurance Co., 1990. Pp. 4–5.

103. The St. Paul's 1990 Annual Report to Policyholders. St. Paul, MN: St. Paul Fire and Marine Insurance Co., 1991. Pp. 4–5.

104. Stamm, W.E. Nosocomial infections due to medical devices. *Q.R.B.* 5:23, 1979.

105. Stickler, B.K. *Labor Law and Liability Considerations of Acquired Immune Deficiency Syndrome* (handout). Chicago: Wood, Lucksinger, & Epstein.

106. Tex Rev. Civ. Stat. Ann. Art. 4419-1.5, Sec 3(g) effective Aug. 31, 1987.

107. Troxler, S. Infection control software for microcomputers. *Infect. Control* 7(9): 470; 1986.

108. *Tucson Medical Center* v. *Misevch*, 545 P.2d 958 (Ariz. 1976).

109. Valenti, W. Rubella Prevention Programs. *Infect. Control* 6(8): 329, 1985.

110. Vogel, J., and Delgado, R. To tell the truth: Physicians' duty to disclose medical mistakes. 28 U.C.L.A. L. Rev. 52-94 (1980).

111. Zitter, J.M. Liability of Hospital, Physician, or Other Individual Medical Practitioner for Injury or Death Resulting from Blood Transfusion, 20 ALR4th 136.

Endemic and Epidemic Hospital Infections

Incidence and Nature of Endemic and Epidemic Nosocomial Infections

William J. Martone
William R. Jarvis
David H. Culver
Robert W. Haley

One of the central concepts of modern infection control is that one must have a thorough knowledge of the occurrence of infection problems to control them most effectively. Although there is no substitute for timely information from ongoing surveillance of the current infection situation in one's own hospital, a valuable perspective can be gained from studying the incidence and nature of nosocomial infections in the nation as a whole and in hospitals similar to one's own. Such information not only points out national infection problems and trends that are likely to be mirrored in local situations but also alerts infection control personnel to potentially useful concepts and techniques that can be adopted and to potential pitfalls that can be avoided.

The problem of nosocomial infections is usually discussed in two different contexts: epidemics of infections and endemic occurrences. Epidemics have been very important in the development of the modern approach to hospital infection control by presenting emergency situations that have focused concern and effort on the problem; consequently, epidemics of infections have received much attention from infection control personnel and have been the focus of much of the scientific literature on the subject. When epidemics occur, they often provoke crises that call for intensive investigation and decisive control measures. Since, however, only approximately 2 to 4 percent of nosocomial infections occur as part of epidemics [29, 74], descriptions of nosocomial infections reflect almost entirely the nature of endemic infections and give little insight into epidemic problems.

The purpose of this chapter is, first, to describe the nationwide incidence and distribution of endemic nosocomial infections in U.S. hospitals from several studies recently completed; second, to characterize the nature of epidemics and trends in their occurrence, including the troublesome problem of pseudoepidemics; and third, to discuss methods of estimating the adverse consequences of these problems in terms of prolongation of hospital stay, extra costs, and death.

Endemic Nosocomial Infections
Overall Infection Rates

The effort to estimate rates of nosocomial infections began with surveillance studies of the prevalence [39] and incidence [17, 65] of infections in individual hospitals. The first effort to estimate the magnitude of the problem on a wider scale was made by the Centers for Disease Control (CDC) in a collaborative study of eight community hospitals known as the Comprehensive Hospital Infections Project (CHIP) [17]. Performed in the late 1960s and early 1970s, this contract-supported study involved very intensive surveillance efforts to detect both nosocomial and community-acquired infections. Validation studies were performed by CDC epidemiologists who visited the hospitals on a regular basis to estimate the percentage of infections detected by the hospitals' surveillance personnel. Based on an overall rate of 3.2 infected patients per 100 discharges and an adjustment for the percentage of true infections detected, it was estimated that in 1970 approximately 5 percent of patients in community hospitals developed one or more nosocomial infections (the *infection percentage;* see Chap. 5) [8], an estimate that was subsequently widely held to be the national rate of nosocomial infection.

In 1970, the CDC studies were extended to a group of approximately 80 volunteer hospitals of diverse sizes and types and called the National Nosocomial Infections Surveillance (NNIS) System. Although the same general surveillance methods were used, the quality control techniques used in CHIP were not feasible in the NNIS Study; however, the advantages of the NNIS System were that the group contained a substantial number of hospitals representing the major types of hospitals in the United States, and the system could continue reporting data over a number of

years. The overall infection rates reported from the NNIS hospitals, unadjusted for completeness of ascertainment, have remained relatively stable at approximately 3.2 infections per 100 discharges (the *infection ratio;* see Chap. 5) from 1970 through 1982, although some interesting secular trends have been observed and are described in this section and under the heading Secular Trends. Assuming that the completeness of ascertainment of infections in the NNIS System was similar to that in CHIP, we could derive an estimate of the nationwide infection rate in the same range as the 5 percent figure estimated from CHIP. Although the design of these two surveillance studies limited the precision of the estimates, they gave the first consistent estimates of the order of magnitude of the problem.

One of the objectives of the Study on the Efficacy of Nosocomial Infection Control (SENIC) (see Chap. 4) was to derive a more precise estimate of the nationwide nosocomial infection rate from a statistical sample of U.S. hospitals [31]. On the basis of direct estimates made in 338 randomly selected general medical and surgical hospitals with 50 beds or more and statistically derived extrapolations to groups of small and specialty hospitals, the report from the SENIC Project estimated that at least 2.1 million nosocomial infections occurred among the 37.7 million admissions to the 6,449 acute-care U.S. hospitals in a 12-month period in 1975–1976 [24]. Thus nationwide there were approximately 5.7 nosocomial infections per 100 admissions (the infection ratio), and approximately 4.5 percent of hospitalized patients experienced at least 1 nosocomial infection (the infection percentage). Given that patients stayed a total of almost 299 million days in U.S. hospitals in 1976, the incidence-density of infections was approximately 7 infections per 1,000 patient-days (see Chap. 5).

The SENIC Project applied specifically to the 6,449 acute-care U.S. hospitals and did not account for a substantial number of additional institutional infections that occur each year in chronic-care hospitals, nursing homes (see Chap. 24), children's hospitals, and federal hospitals. On the basis of the one study from which incidence rates in nursing homes can be estimated, as many as 3.3 infections per 1,000 resident-days may be occurring, an incidence-density approaching half that in acute-care hospitals [24, 43]. Since there are somewhat more total institutional days spent by residents in nursing homes than by patients in hospitals (approximately 451 million versus 299 million), nursing homes may be accounting for as many as 1.5 million institutional infections per year. If these figures and the secular trends are reasonably accurate, the total number of nosocomial and other institutional infections in the 1980s may exceed 4 million per year, a number substantially larger than the total number of yearly hospital admissions for all cancers, accidents, and acute myocardial infarctions combined [69].

Rates by Site of Infection

Nosocomial infections involve diverse anatomic sites, but the risks of these various types of infections, and consequently their relative frequency, appear to be very similar in most hospitals. Table 27-1 lists the estimated nationwide infection rates and the relative

Table 27-1. Rates and relative frequencies of the major types of nosocomial infections, SENIC Project 1975–1976

	Nationwide infection rates[a]	Percentage distribution
Urinary tract infection	2.39	42
Surgical wound infection	1.39[b]	24
Lower respiratory infection	0.60	11
Bacteremia[c]	0.27	5
Other sites	1.07	18
All sites	5.72	100

[a] Ratio of number of infections to number of admissions multiplied by 100 (i.e., number of nosocomial infections per 100 admissions). From R.W. Haley et al., The efficacy of infection surveillance and control programs in preventing nosocomial infections in U.S. hospitals. *Am. J. Epidemiol.* 121:159, 1985.
[b] The ratio of surgical wound infections to total operations was 2.79 per 100 operations.
[c] Includes primary and secondary bacteremias.

frequency of the most common sites found in the SENIC Project [24]. These estimates, as well as those from past studies, support the following conclusions: Nosocomial urinary tract infections make up approximately two-fifths of all nosocomial infections; surgical wound infections, nearly one-fourth; respiratory tract infections, approximately one-eighth; bacteremia, about one-sixteenth; and all other types of nosocomial infections collectively account for the remainder. Although these data are expected to vary from hospital to hospital, they have been remarkably consistent in most reported studies.

Rates by Pathogen

Currently, the best source of information for gaining insight into the nationwide patterns of microorganisms involved in nosocomial infections is the NNIS System. Data from the hospitalwide component of the NNIS System in the period 1986–1990 indicate that cultures were obtained in 89 percent of reported nosocomial infections and, in 85 percent, at least one causative pathogen was isolated. Among these infections of known cause, 85 percent involved aerobic bacteria; 4 percent, anaerobic bacteria; 9 percent, fungi; and the remaining 2 percent, a miscellaneous group of viruses, protozoa, and parasites. On the basis of other studies [33, 70], it appears that viral nosocomial infections are substantially underreported in the NNIS System, a fact that mirrors the underrecognition of viral infections in hospitals generally.

The relative frequency of the 10 most commonly isolated pathogens for each of the four major sites of infection is shown in Figure 27-1. In nosocomial urinary tract infections, *Escherichia coli* was by far the most commonly isolated pathogen, and this held true for all services except urology, where *Enterococcus faecalis* was isolated with nearly equal frequency. The second most common urinary pathogen was *E. faecalis,* although it was slightly exceeded by *Pseudomonas* in cardiac, orthopedic, and plastic surgery patients and by *Klebsiella* in pediatric patients. Urinary tract infections were uncommon in newborns.

In surgical wound infections, *Staphylococcus*

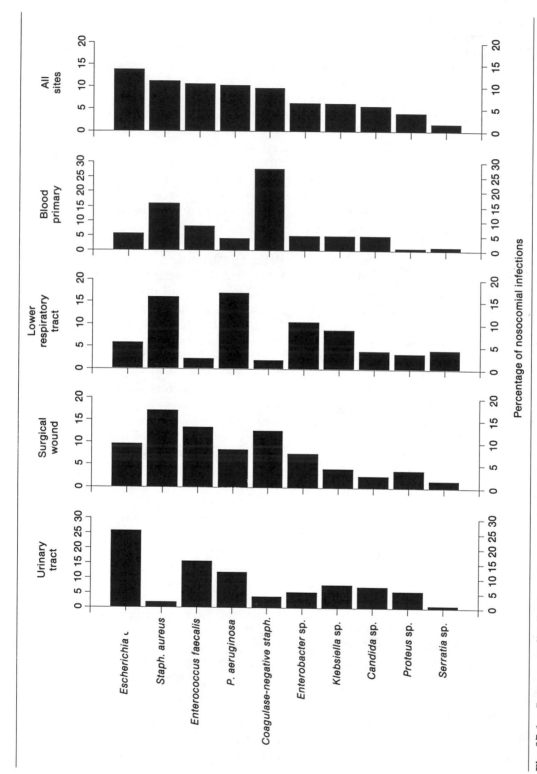

Fig. 27-1. Percentage distribution of nosocomial infections by primary pathogen at the major sites of infection, National Nosocomial Infections Surveillance System, 1986–1990.

aureus was the most common pathogen, followed by *E. faecalis*. *E. faecalis* was the most common pathogen in burn or trauma, general surgery, and urology patients, whereas coagulase-negative staphylococci played a predominant role in cardiac surgery and high-risk nursery patients.

In lower respiratory infections, *S. aureus* and *Pseudomonas aeruginosa* were encountered with almost equal frequency overall. *S. aureus* was the most common pathogen in burn or trauma, neurosurgery, orthopedic, pediatric, and high-risk nursery patients. *P. aeruginosa* was the most common pathogen in cardiac surgery, general surgery, plastic surgery, urology, and medical patients. Viruses were the second most common pathogen reported in pediatric and well-baby nursery patients.

Primary bacteremias are culture-documented bloodstream infections in which no other site of infection was found to be seeding the bloodstream. The microbiologic features of primary bacteremia have changed over the past 10 years, with coagulase-negative staphylococci emerging as the most significant nosocomial pathogen [4]. Coagulase-negative staphylococci made up approximately 29 percent of infections overall and were the most frequently reported isolate on all services except in obstetrics and well-baby nursery patients, where group B streptococci predominated. The predominance of group B streptococci in obstetrics and well-baby nursery patients may be an indication that some primary bacteremias are, in fact, secondary bacteremias in which the primary site of infection was never ascertained. *S. aureus* was the second most common cause of primary bacteremia.

On the basis of its microbiologic features, secondary bacteremia (not included in Fig. 27-1) appears to be a different disease from primary bacteremia. The risk of secondary bacteremia is highest following lower respiratory infections (6.7 percent), surgical wound infections (5.6 percent), and urinary tract infections (4.1 percent). Complications of infection by secondary bacteremia were most common on the oncology service (10.6 per-

cent), followed by the cardiac surgery service (9.1 percent), the high-risk nursery (8.7 percent), the burn or trauma service (7.2 percent), and the urology service (6.9 percent). Secondary bacteremia was least likely on the otolaryngology service (2.7 percent), the orthopedic service (2.6 percent), and the gynecology service (1.8 percent). Secondary bacteremia was also more likely in large teaching hospitals. The organisms most commonly involved were *S. aureus* (22 percent), *E. coli* (13.6 percent), *P. aeruginosa* (10.8 percent), *E. faecalis* (6.1 percent), and *Enterobacter* species (6.0 percent).

E. coli is the most commonly isolated pathogen from all nosocomial infections, regardless of site, because of its predominance in urinary tract infections and its substantial role in infections at all other sites. *S. aureus* is the second most commonly isolated pathogen overall, because of its frequent involvement in all types of infections except those of the urinary tract, where it is uncommonly found. The high frequency of enterococci, the third leading pathogen, has perhaps not been well enough appreciated in the past. The important role of *Pseudomonas* as the fourth most common pathogen is not surprising because of its well-known involvement in all types of nosocomial infections. Recently, coagulase-negative staphylococci have emerged as the fifth most common pathogen, largely because of their increasing importance in bloodstream infections. Improvements in surveillance and laboratory techniques are needed to clarify the roles of coagulase-negative staphylococci, anaerobic bacteria, and viruses, whose true frequencies have probably been misjudged, and perhaps more attention should be given to the endogenous mechanisms and nosocomial transmission of group B streptococci in the obstetric and newborn areas.

Patient Risk Factors

The strongest determinants of the risk of nosocomial infection are the characteristics and exposures of patients that predispose them to infection. Like the so-called chronic diseases, such as coronary heart disease and cancer, nosocomial infections arise from the complex interactions of multiple causal factors, and these factors interact differently in predisposing to the different types of infection (see Chap. 1). Much epidemiologic and clinical research has been devoted to studying the characteristics associated with the occurrence of nosocomial infection [13, 15, 16, 19, 20, 23, 27, 34, 35, 40, 47, 63]. It has not always been clear whether the associations are truly causal, however, and these characteristics are often referred to as *risk factors*—that is, factors associated with, but not necessarily causing, infection. Undoubtedly, some of these risk factors are true causes of infection; others are only coincidentally associated with infection because they frequently follow infection or occur along with the truly causal factors. Complicating matters further is the fact that two or more risk factors often occur simultaneously in the same patient, sometimes exerting additive, or even synergistic, effects. In this respect, it is said that these risk factors are strongly intercorrelated.

To design strategies for preventing infections, it is important to try to differentiate among coincidental indicators of risk, independent causal factors, and synergistic interactions of causal factors. There have been several attempts to study multiple risk factors using modern techniques of multivariate statistical analysis. Much of this work can be illustrated by the results of analyses of risk factors performed on a group of 169,526 patients who made up a representative sample of patients admitted to acute-care U.S. hospitals in 1975–1976 as part of the SENIC Project [23, 27, 34]. In an initial descriptive analysis, population estimates of infection rates for each of the four major types of infection were calculated within each category of exposure to between 10 and 20 separate risk factors [27]. A striking finding was that all of the risk factors were associated with infection at all four sites. At first this seems surprising, since one would not expect a direct causal association between being treated on a respirator, for example, and acquiring a urinary tract infection. The explanation, of course, is that some of the associations are indicative of direct causal relationships; others

are indicative of partial causal relationships, potentiated or diminished by other concurrent influences; and others (such as that between respirators and urinary tract infection) represent largely coincidental associations (most patients on respirators also have indwelling urinary catheters that predispose them to urinary tract infection).

The two factors that appeared to exert the strongest causal influences in all four sites of infection were indicators of the degree of the patient's underlying illness: (1) in surgical patients, the duration of the patient's operation, and (2) an index of the number and type of distinct diagnoses and surgical procedures recorded (intrinsic risk index). After these, several factors were strongly associated with infections at one or two sites but not with all four. Having a combined thoracic-abdominal operation was strongly associated with pneumonia and surgical wound infection; undergoing a "dirty" (or contaminated) operation was associated with surgical wound infection; having an indwelling urinary catheter was linked to urinary tract infection; being on a respirator, with pneumonia and bacteremia; previous nosocomial infection, with bacteremia; and receiving immunosuppressive therapy, with bacteremia. Examples of risk factors that had weaker associations with all four sites were age, sex, previous community-acquired infection, and length of preoperative hospitalization.

Another way of viewing these complex multivariate associations is to hypothesize that there are two general categories of causes: those that allow microorganisms access to vulnerable areas of the patient (e.g., operations, catheters, and endotracheal tubes) and those that reduce the patient's capacity for resisting the multiplication and injurious effects of the microorganisms (e.g., immunosuppressive therapy and metabolic sequelae of lengthy operations). In a later multivariate analysis of the SENIC data, this concept was tested using surgical wound infection as an example [23]. The resulting multivariate model indicated that two factors—the familiar surgical wound classification [2] and undergoing an abdominal operation—both represent the likely degree of contamination of the operative wound. These measured a portion of the risk of surgical wound infection largely separate from that measured by the other two factors—the duration of the operation and the number of diagnoses recorded. These later two factors represent the patient's degree of susceptibility to infection. Moreover, one might infer that the degree of contamination of the wound and the patient's susceptibility were of nearly equal importance in the genesis of surgical wound infections because each of these four factors was about equally important in the multivariate model (see Chap. 7).

Although multivariate modeling of risk factors for nosocomial infection is still in an early stage, several conclusions appear reasonable, pending additional research. The risk of infection is primarily determined by definable causal factors reflecting the patient's underlying susceptibility to infection or the degree to which microorganisms have access to vulnerable body sites. Modification of one or more of these factors can alter a patient's risk. Multivariate statistical models can be developed to predict accurately a patient's risk of nosocomial infection from measurable risk factors. The aggregate infection risk of a hospital, or of a subgroup of patients in a hospital—measured by its overall nosocomial infection rate—is primarily determined by the mix of patients, that is, by the causal factors present when patients are admitted and to which they are exposed in diagnosis and treatment. These conclusions form the basis for understanding much of the variation in nosocomial infection rates described in the following sections.

Rates by Service
Differences in the average risk of infection among groups have been most readily noticed in relation to the well-known differences in infection rates of different services or specialty areas. Analyses of the SENIC data showed that surgical patients were not only at highest risk of surgical wound infections but also had rates of infection for the other main sites almost three times higher than medical patients (approximately four times higher for

pneumonia and approximately one and one-half times higher for urinary tract infection and bacteremia). Moreover, even though surgical patients constituted only 42 percent of general medical and surgical patients, they accounted for 71 percent of nosocomial infections of the four major types (virtually all surgical wound infections, 74 percent of pneumonias, 56 percent of urinary tract infections, and 54 percent of bacteremias) [27]. Analysis of data collected in the NNIS System from 1986 through 1990 showed a stepwise decrease in nosocomial infection rates (calculated as the number of infections per 1,000 patient-days) by service as follows: burn or trauma service (11.5), cardiac surgery service (11.2), neurosurgery service (10.2), general surgery service (9.5), high-risk nursery (9.5), and oncology service (8.2). Lowest rates were found on the plastic surgery service (excluding the burn service) (3.0), the well-baby nursery (2.0), and the ophthalmology service (0.5). Other investigators have quantitated the inordinately high risks of patients in special care units (see Chap. 20).

Rates by Type of Hospital
It has long been apparent that overall nosocomial infection rates differ substantially from one hospital to another. In the mid-nineteenth century, Sir James Y. Simpson [62] found that the rate of death from infection of amputated extremities varied directly with the size of the hospital in which the operation was performed (with larger hospitals having higher rates), a phenomenon he called "hospitalism." The rates of surgical wound infection in the five hospitals participating in the National Research Council's prospective evaluation of ultraviolet light were found to vary from 3.2 to 11.0 percent [35]. The average infection rates of hospitals participating in the NNIS System were reported to vary from 1.7 percent in small community hospitals to more than 11 percent in chronic disease hospitals [8].

A multivariate analysis of the SENIC data was performed to determine what institutional characteristics of the hospitals best predicted their nosocomial infection rates. Of the many characteristics studied, those found to differentiate best were affiliation with a medical school (teaching versus nonteaching), size of the hospital (indicated by the number of beds), type of control or ownership of the hospital (municipal, nonprofit, investor-owned), and region of the country [30]. The overall nosocomial infection rates averaged 3.7 percent in small (fewer than 200 beds) nonteaching hospitals, 5.1 percent in large (200 beds or more) nonteaching ones, 7.6 percent in nonprofit teaching hospitals, and 8.5 percent in the municipal teaching hospitals. These relationships tended to be consistent for each of the four major sites of infection. Since nonprofit teaching hospitals tend to have fewer than 500 beds, and municipal teaching hospitals tend to have more than 500, teaching hospitals could be subclassified almost as well by size as by ownership-control. In addition, within these four hospital groups, rates of urinary tract infection, surgical wound infection, and bacteremia were generally higher in the northeast and north central regions, whereas rates of pneumonia were higher in the West. A similar analysis of NNIS data from 1980–1982 found the lowest rates in nonteaching hospitals, intermediate levels in teaching hospitals with fewer than 500 beds, and highest rates in teaching hospitals with 500 beds or more [31]. This relationship held consistently for infection rates at each site, on every service, and for all pathogens.

To test the hypothesis that these differences were largely due to differences in the mix of patients typically treated in the various types of hospitals, the SENIC data were additionally analyzed to try to explain the differences. Indeed, indexes of the patients' risk factors explained the greatest part of the interhospital differences and, after controlling for indexes of patients' risk factors, average length of stay, and measures of the completeness of diagnostic workups for infection (e.g., culturing rates), the differences in the average infection rates of the various hospital groups virtually disappeared. These findings indicate that much of the difference in observable infection rates of various types of hospitals is

due to differences in the intrinsic degree of illness of their patients and related factors and, because of this, the overall infection rate per se usually gives little insight into whether the hospital's infection control efforts are effective.

Trends Over Time

The occurrence of nosocomial infections is a dynamic process. Changes are constantly occurring in the types of patients admitted to hospitals, risk factors to which they are exposed, character of the pathogens predominating in the hospital milieu, quality of patient care, thrust of infection control efforts, and other important factors. Two indicators of the dynamic nature of the problem are the seasonality of certain types of nosocomial infections and the long-term secular trends that may occur.

Seasonality

Analysis of the data from the NNIS System has repeatedly shown seasonal variations in the occurrence of nosocomial infections involving certain gram-negative rods [1, 36, 52]. The report of the 1980–1982 results shows clear seasonal peaks of infections in the summer and early fall with certain gram-negative bacteria, specifically *Klebsiella, Enterobacter, Serratia,* and *Acinetobacter* species as well as *P. aeruginosa.* In contrast to the seasonal occurrence of pyogenic infections in the community [7], staphylococcal and streptococcal infections show no significant seasonal variation in the hospital. There also seems to be no seasonality of infections with other common bacteria, such as *E. coli,* enterococcus, *Enterobacter,* and anaerobes. Nosocomial viral respiratory infections occur mostly during the seasons in which they occur in the community (e.g., influenza and respiratory syncytial virus infections in the winter and early spring) [33].

Secular Trends

Changes in nosocomial infection rates over time are difficult to study. In prevalence studies performed over several decades, the relatively small sample sizes have hampered the detection of secular changes. An analysis of secular trends in the NNIS System from 1970–1979 suggested that surgical wound infections may have decreased slightly over the decade, bacteremias may have increased, and other types of infections remained unchanged [1]. More recent analysis of hospital-wide NNIS data demonstrates a remarkable increase in nosocomial bloodstream infection rates, largely attributable to coagulase-negative staphylococci and *Candida albicans* [4]. The inability to control these analyses for other factors that could have accounted for the changes, however, rendered these findings difficult to interpret.

To address this issue, the rates from the two time periods of the SENIC Project, 1970 and 1975–1976, were compared after controlling for the most likely biasing factors [25]. After controlling for changes in levels of patient risk, length of stay, and completeness of ascertainment of infections, overall nosocomial infection rates in acute-care hospitals were found to have increased by a statistically significant 10 percent over the 5-year period. Additional analysis, however, revealed three contrasting trends in different groups of hospitals. In the group that established no substantial infection surveillance and control programs, the overall infection rate increased by 18 percent; in the group in which moderately intensive programs were established, the rates tended to show no significant change; and in the group that established very intensive programs for preventing infections at all four of the major sites, the overall rate decreased by 36 percent. These findings suggest strongly that the overall nationwide trend of a 10 percent increase was really the result of two forces that were affecting the nationwide rate in opposite directions: (1) the continuing introduction of more invasive and immuno-compromising techniques into the care of hospitalized patients, which tended to increase the infection rates, and (2) the efficacy of newly established infection surveillance and control programs, which tended to decrease them. This indicates that future secular trends in the rates of endemic nosocomial infections could be in either direction, depending strongly on the balance that hospitals achieve between technologic innovations in patient care and investments in infection surveillance and control programs.

Epidemic Nosocomial Infections
Incidence, Recognition, and Control

Although many scientific articles have been written to describe individual outbreaks of nosocomial infections, very little work has been done to estimate the frequency of these epidemics. The earliest study on this subject was performed in the CDC's CHIP study in the early 1970s [29]. Among seven community hospitals participating in CHIP during 12 months in 1972–1973, a computerized threshold program screened the regularly reported cases of nosocomial infection for clusters of infection that might indicate an outbreak, and a CDC epidemiologist additionally analyzed the data to eliminate purely coincidental clusters. Then CDC staff members visited the hospitals that had potential outbreaks to confirm the nature of the problem and suggest control measures if needed. From these data it was estimated that one true outbreak occurred for every 10,000 hospital admissions and that outbreaks accounted for somewhere in the range of 2 percent of patients with nosocomial infections. More recently, Wenzel and colleagues [74] estimated that 3.7 percent of nosocomial infections in a large university-affiliated referral hospital occurred in outbreaks. Although confined to a relatively small number of hospitals, these estimates appear to confirm the prevailing view that outbreaks account for a fairly small proportion of nosocomial infections.

One of the main reasons that infection control personnel are concerned about outbreaks, aside from the attention they often provoke, is that control measures can often stop outbreaks if they are recognized and investigated, thus bringing about demonstrable reductions in morbidity and mortality. In the CHIP investigations, despite the fact that the seven hospitals had very active surveillance systems, one-third of the clusters had not been recognized before the CDC visit. This fact points out the difficulty of recognizing outbreaks even in the best of circumstances and suggests the usefulness of inventive computerized systems to screen surveillance data for potential epidemics (see Chaps. 5, 8). It also suggests that hospitals which appear never to have outbreaks may simply be failing to recognize them.

The CHIP investigations also demonstrated that 40 percent of the outbreaks appeared to have resolved spontaneously, whereas the remaining 60 percent continued until control measures were instituted [29]. Half of the outbreaks that continued were controlled by measures taken by the hospitals' infection control staff and the other half were completely resolved only after measures suggested by the outside investigators. The rate of spontaneous resolution explains the origin of opinions against surveillance expressed by some persons, but if these figures are representative of community hospitals in general— and it must be recalled that these were hospitals with very active infection surveillance systems—then a large number of outbreaks may currently be going unrecognized and uncontrolled, despite the advanced state of infection surveillance and control programs.

Characteristics of Epidemics

The recognition, investigation, and control of epidemics requires an understanding of the epidemiology of nosocomial outbreaks, including the most common sources, modes of transmission, and effective control measures. Each year, numerous publications describe outbreaks at individual institutions and the results of their investigation and control. From 1956 to 1990, more than 381 hospital outbreak investigations were conducted by the CDC. Many factors influence the types of investigations conducted by the CDC, including which outbreaks are recognized and brought to the CDC's attention, which outbreaks are of sufficient potential public health importance (by causing significant morbidity or mortality) to warrant CDC investigation, investigator availability, and whether a CDC investigation may add to the infection control knowledge to help prevent or control similar outbreaks

in the future. Thus, these outbreaks reflect problems that are unique, urgent, perplexing, or difficult to control.

The 252 hospital outbreak investigations conducted by the CDC from 1956 to 1979 have been summarized by Stamm and co-workers [64]. In the early years (1956–1962), the two most common problems investigated included epidemics of gastrointestinal disease, primarily due to *Salmonella* species and enteropathogenic *E. coli,* or staphylococcal infections; both types of epidemics were most frequently encountered in newborn nurseries. In the early 1960s, the investigation of staphylococcal infections abruptly decreased, which was followed in the 1970s by a decrease in the number of gastrointestinal outbreaks investigated. This probably reflects a decrease in the incidence of such outbreaks because of improved understanding of the epidemiology and control of such infections and the improved ability of hospital infection control personnel to recognize and control these outbreaks without CDC assistance. From the late 1960s until the 1980s, there was an increase in investigations of outbreaks caused by gram-negative pathogens, bacteremias, surgical wound infections, and problems related to intensive care units, newly introduced medical devices, and invasive procedures. During the 1970s, outbreaks of bacteremia were the most common problem investigated. Other problems emerging during the 1970s were outbreaks of hepatitis A and B; necrotizing enterocolitis in nurseries; sternal wound infections following open-heart surgery, particularly those caused by rapidly growing mycobacteria; and nosocomial Legionnaires' disease. Also during this period, there was the emergence of the continuing problem of outbreaks due to microorganisms resistant to multiple antimicrobials, particularly, aminoglycoside-resistant gram-negative bacilli and methicillin-resistant *S. aureus.*

Outbreak investigations conducted by the CDC from 1980 to 1990 have recently been reviewed by Jarvis [38]. A total of 129 outbreaks were investigated; the most common sites of infection were the bloodstream or surgical wounds. Many of the bloodstream infections resulted from inadequately disinfected transducers in intensive care unit patients [6]. During this period, there have been no investigations of epidemics of urinary tract infections, and fewer than 10 percent of the outbreaks have involved nosocomial pneumonia. This probably reflects the recognition of bloodstream and surgical wound infections as serious causes of morbidity and mortality and the difficulties involved in identifying the pathogen causing nosocomial pneumonia. Furthermore, this may reflect the fact that nosocomial pneumonia most commonly results from the patient's endogenous flora or from organisms transmitted by the hands of medical personnel, whereas bloodstream or surgical wound infection clusters frequently can be traced to an invasive device, procedure, or personnel carrier (see Chaps. 29, 40).

From 1980 to 1990, the majority of investigated outbreaks were caused by bacteria. Although gram-negative organisms accounted for more than half of the outbreaks, from 1985 to 1990 outbreak investigations increasingly involved gram-positive organisms. Also during this decade, fungi, viruses, or mycobacterial outbreaks were responsible for a larger proportion of the investigations. Rapidly growing mycobacteria were recognized as causes of surgical wound infections, chronic otitis media, and infections following hemodialysis [41, 42, 55], Outbreak investigations also implicated noninfectious causes, such as E-Ferol toxicity in neonates in intensive care units and pyrogenic reactions and chemical toxin exposures in hemodialysis centers (e.g., chloramine, hydrogen peroxide) [21, 45, 66].

In the 1980s, investigations probably reflected the increasing use of invasive procedures and devices and the introduction of an ever-increasing number of products. Approximately 33 percent of the outbreaks investigated occurred in intensive care settings, and nearly 25 percent of the outbreaks involved surgical patients. More than 50 percent of the outbreaks investigated were associated with products, procedures, or devices. For example, 9 cases of *Yersinia enterocolitica* sepsis were associated with transfusion of contaminated packed red blood cells [67]. Each

of these independent events was traced to mildly symptomatic or asymptomatic infection in the blood donor. Prolonged storage of the blood cells allowed proliferation of the *Y. enterocolitica,* which resulted in sepsis or endotoxin shock when the blood was transfused [3]. In another outbreak, five separate episodes of bloodstream infection or surgical wound infection were traced to extrinsic contamination of a newly introduced anesthetic agent [11]. The manufacturer of this soybean oil–based product, which does not contain a preservative, did not recommend refrigeration. Laboratory studies demonstrated that when contaminated with low numbers of microorganisms, rapid microbial proliferation ensued [11].

Interestingly, the sites of infection involved in epidemics investigated by the CDC differ markedly from those involved in endemic infections (Table 27-2). Of the epidemics investigated, bloodstream infections predominated, followed by surgical wounds, pneumonia, gastrointestinal infections, and meningitis. Among endemic infections, however, urinary tract infections predominate, followed by surgical wounds, pneumonia, and bloodstream infections, in that order. Similarly, the distribution of pathogens varies markedly between epidemic and endemic infections. *Pseudomonas* and *Serratia* species, *S. aureus,* and *Candida* species were the most common organisms causing epidemics, whereas *E. coli,* coagulase-negative staphylococci, and *S. aureus* predominated among endemic infections. Epidemic infections also commonly involved more unusual organisms, such as *Ewingella americana, Tsukamurella* species, *Rhodococcus bronchialis,* mycobacteria, viruses, and fungi [38, 49, 53, 54, 68]. This probably reflects that nosocomial infections vary by service or location (i.e., intensive care unit versus nonintensive care unit) and that clusters of infections caused by unusual organisms or usual organisms with unusual antimicrobial susceptibility patterns are more easily recognized, whereas clusters of infections caused by common organisms with unremarkable antimicrobial susceptibility patterns are probably not recognized. Also, these differences reflect the fact that unusual outbreaks are more likely to be investigated, as are outbreaks in which a common-source or personnel carrier is involved, rather than the more common problem with endemic infections whereby usual organisms are frequently transferred from patient to patient on the hands of medical personnel.

A number of selection biases influence which outbreaks are investigated by the CDC. First, a problem must be recognized at the hospital level. Once recognized, whether local expertise exists influences whether CDC assistance is requested. Second, if a problem at the hospital level is recognized and brought to the attention of the state health department, interest or expertise at the state level determines whether the state concurs with the hospital's request for CDC assistance. Since the CDC is a nonregulatory agency, any request for CDC assistance must include both an invitation by the hospital's administration and the state health department. Last, if the CDC is asked to conduct an on-site epidemiologic investigation, several factors determine the CDC's response. The likely public health

Table 27-2. Comparison of types of infections and pathogens involved in endemic and epidemic infections

	Endemic infections[a] (%)	Epidemic investigations[b] (%)
Type of infection		
Urinary tract infection	37	5
Surgical wound infection	17	10
Pneumonia	16	12
Cutaneous infection	2	13
Bacteremia	11	20
Meningitis	<1	5
Gastroenteritis	3	18
Hepatitis	<1	7
Other	12	10
Total	100	100
Pathogen		
Escherichia coli	13.8	<1
Enterococcus	10.7	<1
Staphylococcus aureus	11.2	5
Pseudomonas	11.2	16
Proteus	3.9	<1
Klebsiella	6.2	2
Enterobacter	6.3	4
Group A streptococcus	0.2	3
Serratia	1.7	5
Salmonella	<1	2
Hepatitis	<1	<1
Coagulase-negative staphylococci	9.7	<1
Candida species	7.1	5
Mycobacteria	<1	5
Other	15	48
Total	100	100

[a] National Nosocomial Infections Surveillance System, 1986–1990.
[b] Source of data for 1971–1979 adapted from W.E. Stamm et al., Comparison of endemic and epidemic nosocomial infections. *Am. J. Med.* 70:393, 1981; and for 1980–1990 adapted from W.R. Jarvis, Nosocomial outbreaks: The Centers for Disease Control's Hospital Infections Program experience, 1980–1990. *Am. J. Med.* 91 (Suppl. 3B): 101S, 1991.

importance of the problem is the most important: If an outbreak is potentially product-related or is causing significant morbidity or mortality, all efforts will be made to respond. In addition, if the outbreak appears to be caused by an unusual pathogen or a common pathogen with unusual characteristics or it involves an unusual or uncommon reservoir or mode of transmission, and if personnel are available, an on-site epidemiologic investigation by the CDC will be conducted. All investigations are conducted as collaborative efforts, and close working relationships with local, state, and federal personnel are desirable. These and other selection biases undoubtedly contribute to this profile of nosocomial epidemic problems. Of greatest value to infection control is the knowledge gained by investigation about the most common sources and modes of transmission of various pathogens in outbreaks. These data help infection control practitioners focus their preventive interventions on the areas most likely to result in containment of ongoing outbreaks. In general, outbreaks can be classified into five groups according to their most likely mode of transmission: (1) common source, (2) human transmitter (carrier), (3) cross-infection (person to person), (4) airborne (microorganism traveling more than a few feet), and (5) uncertain modes of transmission. When outbreaks are classified this way, certain site-pathogen combinations, often specific to certain patient groups, become apparent (Table 27-3).

Knowledge of these site-pathogen com-

Table 27-3. Likely modes of transmission of common nosocomial outbreak pathogens

Mode of transmission	Site or type of infection	Pathogen	Service or group
Common source	Blood	*Pseudomonas cepacia*	All
		Pseudomonas fluorescens	All
	GI	*Salmonella* species	All
	Peritonitis	*P. cepacia*	All
	Blood	*Candida parapsilosis*	All
	Blood, SWI	*Serratia marcescens*	ICU, surgical
	Blood, SWI	Mycobacteria	Hemodialysis, surgical
Human disseminator	SWI	*Staphylococcus aureus*	Surgical, obstetric
	Cutaneous	*S. aureus*	Nursery
	Hepatitis	Hepatitis A or B	All
Cross-infection	SWI	*S. marcescens*	Surgical
	Pulmonary	*Xanthomonas maltophilia*	ICU
	Meningitis	*Citrobacter diversus*	Neonates
		GBS	
	Gastroenteritis	*Salmonella* species	
		Clostridium difficile	All
	Urinary tract	Gram-negative bacilli	All
	Pneumonia	Respiratory syncytial virus	Nursery
	Meningitis	Enteroviruses	Nursery
	Cutaneous	*S. aureus*	Nursery
	Hepatitis	Hepatitis A	Nursery
	SWI, pulmonary, cutaneous	MRSA	All
Airborne	Pulmonary	*Aspergillus* species	Oncology
	Pulmonary	*Mycobacterium tuberculosis*	All
	Varicella	Varicella-zoster virus	All
	Pulmonary	*Legionella*	All

GI = gastrointestinal; SWI = surgical wound infection; ICU = intensive care unit; GBS = Guillain-Barré syndrome; MRSA = methicillin-resistant *S. aureus*.

binations can facilitate initial investigative efforts by focusing on the most likely source or modes of transmission. For example, although nosocomial *Salmonella* infections can be transmitted from person to person, most outbreaks are traced to a common-source food (see Chap. 17). Clusters of *Pseudomonas cepacia* infections or pseudoinfections should alert infection control personnel to the possibility of contaminated solutions, including antiseptics such as povidone-iodine solution [10]. Group A streptococcal surgical wound infections are almost always traced to a personnel carrier; carriage can involve the rectum, vagina, scalp, or other sites [46]. Intensive care unit outbreaks of gram-negative bacteremia frequently are traced to inadequately disinfected intraarterial pressure-monitoring transducers [5, 6] (see Chap. 20). Clusters of *Legionella* or *Aspergillus* species pulmonary infections, particularly in the immunocompromised patient, should stimulate a search for an environmental source for airborne transmission [71] (see Chap. 29).

The most common cause of both endemic and epidemic infections is cross-infection, whereby organisms are transferred from patient to patient by medical personnel. Although almost any organism can be transmitted by cross-infection, gram-negative organisms and *S. aureus* are the most commonly recognized. Nosocomial viral infections, which frequently occur in pediatric patients, also are often transmitted by cross-infection.

Multihospital Epidemics

As hospitals become more and more specialized, the possibility of multiple hospital outbreaks becomes a greater concern. This occurs most commonly by interhospital spread and less commonly through the national distribution of products that cause or predispose to infection. First, a pathogen involved in an epidemic in one hospital may be introduced into a patient population at another hospital, generally by one of three modes of transmission: (1) transfer of colonized or infected patients, particularly those with burns or decubitus ulcers [51, 56, 57, 60, 73, 75], (2) transfer of colonized or infected medical

house staff [61, 70], and (3) transient colonization of hands of nurses or technicians who rotate among different hospitals [58]. Since the transfer of house staff and seriously ill patients occurs primarily among large, university-affiliated, tertiary referral hospitals, interhospital spread appears to occur most frequently in these and, less commonly, among smaller community hospitals [26]; however, the increasing trend of nurses and technicians toward working in cooperatives serving several hospitals may encourage more interhospital spread. Interhospital transmission of outbreaks has been observed primarily in epidemics involving pathogens with important antimicrobial resistance patterns, such as multiply resistant *Serratia* species [58], aminoglycoside-resistant gram-negative bacilli [73], and methicillin-resistant *S. aureus* [26, 75] (see Chaps. 12–14, 37). This association could be due to the genetic colinkage of antimicrobial resistance with factors that facilitate spread. For example, strains of diverse genera that are prevalent in nosocomial infections have been shown to share the genetic information that confers resistance to important antimicrobial agents [59]. Similarly, the diversity of phage types involved in epidemiologically clear outbreaks of methicillin-resistant *S. aureus* infections suggests the spread of genetic information among different strains that have strong predispositions to infect hospital patients. Alternatively, the association could be due merely to the fact that resistance provides a dramatic marker that increases the likelihood that an epidemic will be recognized. If so, as infection control personnel in hospitals develop more sensitive means for recognizing outbreaks and more effectively share surveillance data with their counterparts in other local hospitals (e.g., through areawide surveillance systems supported by local health departments), interhospital transmission of infection will probably be recognized more commonly.

In the second type of multiple-hospital involvement, a widely distributed product used in patient care may cause infections in many hospitals simultaneously, due to either intrinsic contamination of the product in the factory

[44] or design flaws or common usage errors that encourage in-use contamination in the hospitals [9, 14] (see Chaps. 40, 42). After a series of nationwide epidemics due to intrinsically contaminated products in the early 1970s, it appeared that intrinsic product contamination would become a common problem (44). Subsequent experience has shown, however, that in-use contamination is a far more common explanation for infections related to newly introduced products and devices. Although intrinsic contamination is still recognized [10, 67, 68], extrinsic contamination of products during manipulation is much more common [11].

In recent years, the widespread use of an unlicensed intravenous vitamin E preparation in neonates led to a nationwide problem of unusual illness with high fatality in neonates [45]. The recognition of this new syndrome in several neonatal intensive care units in some states led to the identification of the source and U.S. Food and Drug Administration (FDA) recall of the product. Similarly, the recent outbreak of bloodstream infections or surgical wound infections in five states led to the identification of a newly introduced intravenous anesthetic as the source [11]. Although only one species of organism was involved in each outbreak, different institutions had different pathogens, including *S. aureus*, *Moraxella* species, and *C. albicans*. On-site epidemiologic investigations at each hospital identified contamination of the product during preparation by anesthesia personnel. These experiences highlight the fact that infection control personnel should remain alert to the possibility of infections or toxic reactions associated with newly introduced products or procedures. Suspicion of such problems should immediately be reported through the state health department to the CDC and the FDA.

Pseudoepidemics

Not all clusters of reported nosocomial infections constitute true epidemics of disease. In the prospective study of outbreaks in the CDC CHIP project, approximately 80 percent of the clusters of infection identified statistically by a computerized threshold program were judged to be coincidental, illustrating the need for epidemiologic evaluation of surveillance data to detect outbreaks [29]. More importantly, of those clusters that appeared to represent real outbreaks epidemiologically, approximately one-third (37 percent) were found not to be true outbreaks after thorough investigations. Most of these pseudoepidemics were traced to systematic errors or changes in the definition of infection used, the clinical diagnosis of infection, or in reporting of infection by the infection surveillance staff. These results show the importance of using the same definitions over time, using the same surveillance methodology, and realizing that changes in the frequency of performance of various diagnostic tests will influence the detection of infections. Systematic errors in the microbiology laboratory accounted for fewer than one-fourth of the pseudoepidemics. From 1959 to 1979, 11 percent of the CDC's hospital outbreak investigations were, in fact, pseudoepidemics. Approximately one-half of these were attributed to processing errors in the microbiology laboratories [64, 72]. From 1980 to 1990, 6 percent of outbreaks investigated were pseudoepidemics. Of these, 75 percent were traced to contaminated products, 12.5 percent were traced to environmental contamination, and 12.5 percent were traced to contamination of the culture during laboratory processing.

The difference in results between the CHIP study and the CDC outbreak investigation experience is probably due to the more extensive investigation usually done by hospital personnel to rule out artifactual problems before the CDC epidemiologists undertake a formal investigation. Consequently, in the routine practice of infection control in most hospitals, the majority of pseudoepidemics may be due to diagnostic and reporting errors as reflected by the CHIP investigation, although truly perplexing pseudoepidemics may more often be traced to contaminated equipment or errors in the microbiology laboratory, as reflected in the CDC investigations (see Chap. 6).

Adverse Consequences of Nosocomial Infections

In reading the scientific literature on the subject of nosocomial infections, one is struck by the disproportionately large number of articles on the adverse consequences—prolongation of hospital stay, extra hospital costs or charges, and deaths—of these infections. The importance of these studies stems from two factors: First, in contrast to most other hospital services, hospitals have not traditionally been able to charge patients or their insurance carriers directly for the costs of their infection surveillance and control programs; and second, it has been difficult to demonstrate how many nosocomial infections these programs prevent. Consequently, it has been necessary, or at least very helpful, in many hospitals to estimate the magnitude of adverse effects of nosocomial infections on the patients to justify the expenditures of mounting and sustaining a preventive program. The adverse outcomes most often studied are deaths and costs attributable to infection. Despite their usefulness, such estimates must be interpreted with caution because of controversies over the methods used [12, 18, 32].

Nationwide estimates of the number of deaths attributable to nosocomial infections have varied even more widely. By combining data from the SENIC Project [24] and from a concurrent assessment of mortality performed in the NNIS System [37], 19,000 deaths nationwide per year were estimated to be directly attributable to nosocomial infections and, in 58,000 more deaths, nosocomial infections contributed but were not the only cause (Table 27-4). At the other extreme, a recent study using multivariate logistic regression techniques, with the same drawbacks as the matched comparison approach, estimated 300,000 deaths per year nationwide attributable to nosocomial urinary tract infections alone [50]. Regardless of which estimates are used, however, the large number of deaths from nosocomial infections is a cause for concern. Counting only the 19,000 deaths directly caused by nosocomial infections—the lowest estimate derived from the NNIS System and SENIC—would place nosocomial infection just below the tenth leading cause of death in the U.S. population. These figures indicate the need for an accurate counting of nosocomial infections in our national systems for vital and health statistics [24].

Until the serious methodologic problems are solved, it seems prudent to use the more conservative estimates derived from concurrent assessments, even though they may underestimate the magnitude of the problem. Table 27-4 lists the estimates of extra days and costs derived from concurrent assessments in the SENIC pilot studies [30] and estimates of deaths derived from the NNIS System [37] and SENIC [24]. In view of the new strategies of prospective reimbursement for hospital care and the evidence for the efficacy of infection surveillance and control programs, it is likely that the direct cost reductions produced by infection control will be sufficiently obvious even if derived from the most conservative estimates (see Chap. 25).

Preventability of Nosocomial Infections

That large numbers of endemic as well as epidemic nosocomial infections are preventable has periodically been reaffirmed by milestone reports such as that of Semmelweis, studies on the effects of proper care of urinary catheters and respirators, and the virtual elimination of epidemic bacteremia caused by intrinsic contamination of commercial intravenous solutions. Yet when a representative sample of infection control program heads were asked to estimate the percentage of nosocomial infections presently occurring in U.S. hospitals that are preventable, the responses varied from 1 percent to 100 percent, with a mean of approximately 50 percent; the program heads who had served in their positions longer and who were more knowledgeable about infection control tended to give lower estimates [22]. There are at least two reasons for this lack of agreement among those working most closely with the problem. First, it is

Table 27-4. Estimated extra days, extra charges, and deaths attributable to nosocomial infections annually in U.S. hospitals

	Extra days		Extra charges			Deaths directly caused by infections		Deaths to which infections contributed	
	Avg. per infection[a]	Est. U.S. total[b]	Avg. extra charges per infection in 1975 dollars[a]	Avg. extra charges per infection in 1992 dollars[c]	Est. U.S. total in 1992 dollars[b]	Percent[d]	Est. U.S. total[b]	Percent[d]	Est. U.S. total[b]
Surgical wound infection	7.3	3,726,000	$838	$3,152	$1,609,000,000	0.64	3,251	1.91	9,726
Pneumonia	5.9	1,339,000	$1,511	$5,683	$1,290,000,000	3.12	7,087	10.13	22,983
Bacteremia	7.4	762,000	$935	$3,517	$362,000,000	4.37	4,496	8.59	8,844
Urinary tract infection	1.0	903,000	$181	$680	$615,000,000	0.10	947	0.72	6,503
Other site	4.8	1,946,000	$430	$1,617	$656,000,000	0.80	3,246	2.48	10,036
All sites	4.0[e]	8,676,000	$560[e]	$2,100	$4,532,000,000	0.90[e]	19,027	2.70[e]	58,092

[a] Adapted from R.W. Haley et al., Extra days and prolongation of stay attributable to nosocomial infections: A prospective interhospital comparison. *Am. J. Med.* 70:51, 1981, by pooling data from the three SENIC pilot study hospitals.

[b] Estimated by multiplying the total number of nosocomial infections estimated in the SENIC Project (R.W. Haley et al., The nation-wide nosocomial infection rate: A new need for vital statistics. *Am. J. Epidemiol.* 121:159, 1985) by the average extra days, average extra charges, or percentage of infections causing or contributing to death, respectively.

[c] 1992 dollars estimated from R.W. Haley et al., *Am. J. Med.* 70:51, 1981, by pooling data from the three hospitals and adjusting for the annual rate of inflation of hospital expenses from 1976 to 1992 (range 5.0 to 12.3 percent) obtained from the American Hospital Association's National Panel Survey. Estimates for inflation rates in 1991 and 1992 were projected 1987-tc-1990 trend.

[d] Unpublished analyses of data reported to the National Nosocomial Infections Surveillance (NNIS) System in 1980–1982 (J.M. Hughes et al., *Abstracts of the Twenty-Second Interscience Conference on Antimicrobial Agents and Chemotherapy,* Miami Beach, FL, October 4–6, 1982.

[e] Nationwide estimate obtained by summing the products of the site-specific estimate of the average extra days, average extra charges, or the percentage of infections causing or contributing to death, respectively, from the SENIC pilot studies (R.W. Haley et al., *Am. J. Med.* 70:51, 1981), and the nation-wide estimate of the proportion of nosocomial infections affecting the site from the main SENIC analysis (R.W. Haley et al., *Am. J. Epidemiol.* 121:159, 1985).

difficult to demonstrate that infections have been prevented or to infer whether active infections were preventable [48]. Second, because new risk factors for infection are constantly appearing, necessary control measures are continually evolving, and ability to manage the patient care behavior of hospital personnel is changing, the true percentage of infections that are preventable probably changes from time to time.

Consequently, the only meaningful way of framing the preventability question is to ask what percentage of nosocomial infections can be prevented by maintaining an intensive infection surveillance and control program that continually adjusts to the new risks and attempts to manage patient care behavior. Since this was precisely the question framed in the SENIC Project, there is an approximate answer. Among U.S. hospitals in the 1970s, approximately one-third of all nosocomial infections were preventable by maintaining infection surveillance and control programs with particular characteristics [25] (see Chap. 4). The fact that the approaches found to be effective were general preventive strategies aimed at managing infection control (i.e., surveillance and control programs), rather than individual preventive practices (e.g., catheter care), suggests that the SENIC estimate of preventability will remain reasonably accurate for the foreseeable future.

References

1. Allen, J.R., Hightower, A.W., Martin, S.M., and Dixon, R.E. Secular trends in nosocomial infections: 1970–79. *Am. J. Med.* 70:389, 1981.
2. Altemeir, W.A., et al. (Eds.). *Manual on the Control of Infection in Surgical Patients.* Philadelphia: Lippincott, 1976. Pp. 29–30.
3. Arduino, M.J., et al. Growth and endotoxin production of *Yersinia enterocolitica* and *Enterobacter agglomerans* in packed erythrocytes. *J. Clin. Microbiol.* 27:1483, 1989.
4. Banerjee, S.N., et al. Secular trends in nosocomial primary bloodstream infections in the United States, 1980–89. *Am. J. Med.* 91(Suppl. 3B): 86S, 1991.
5. Beck-Sague, C.M., et al. Epidemic bacteremia

due to *Acinetobacter baumanni* in five intensive care units. *Am. J. Epidemiol.* 132:723, 1990.
6. Beck-Sague, C.M., and Jarvis, W.R. Epidemic bloodstream infection associated with pressure transducers: A persistent problem. *Infect. Control Hosp. Epidemiol.* 10:54, 1989.
7. Benenson, A.S. Staphylococcal Disease. In: A.S. Benenson (Ed.), *Control of Communicable Diseases in Man* (15th ed.). Washington, DC: American Public Health Association, 1990. Pp. 358–366.
8. Bennett, J.V., Scheckler, W.E., Maki, D.G., and Brachman, P.S. Current National Patterns: United States. In: *Proceedings of the International Conference on Nosocomial Infections, August 3–6, 1970.* Chicago: American Hospital Association, 1971. Pp. 42–49.
9. Centers for Disease Control. Nosocomial Bacteremia from Intravascular Pressure Monitoring Systems. In: *National Nosocomial Infections Study Report.* Atlanta: Centers for Disease Control, 1977 (issued 1979). Pp. 31–36.
10. Centers for Disease Control. Contaminated povidone-iodine solution—Texas. *M.M.W.R.* 38:133, 1989.
11. Centers for Disease Control. Postsurgical infections associated with an extrinsically contaminated intravenous anesthetic agent. *M.M.W.R.* 39:426, 1990.
12. Clark, S. Sepsis in surgical wounds with particular reference to *Staphylococcus aureus. Br. J. Surg.* 44:592, 1957.
13. Cruse, P.J.E., and Foord, R. The epidemiology of wound infection: A 10-year prospective study of 62,939 wounds. *Surg. Clin. North Am.* 60:27, 1980.
14. Donowitz, L.G., Marsick, F.J., Hoyt, J.W., and Wenzel, R.P. *Serratia marcescens* bacteremia from contaminated pressure transducers. *J.A.M.A.* 242:1749, 1979.
15. Dukes, C. Urinary infections after excision of the rectum: Their cause and prevention. *Proc. R. Soc. Med.* 22:259, 1928.
16. Ehrenkrantz, N.J. Surgical wound infection occurrence in clean operations: Risk stratification for interhospital comparisons. *Am. J. Med.* 70:909, 1981.
17. Eickhoff, T.C., Brachman, P.S., Bennett, J.V., and Brown, J.F. Surveillance of nosocomial infections in community hospitals: I. Surveillance methods, effectiveness, and initial results. *J. Infect. Dis.* 120:305, 1969.
18. Finkler, S.A. The distinction between costs and charges. *Ann. Intern. Med.* 96:102, 1982.
19. Freeman, J., and McGowan, J.E., Jr. Risk factors for nosocomial infection. *J. Infect. Dis.* 138:811, 1978.
20. Garibaldi, R.A., et al. Risk factors for predicting postoperative pneumonia. *Am. J. Med.* 70:677, 1981.
21. Gordon, S.M., Tipple, M., Bland, L.A., and

Jarvis, W.R. Pyrogenic reactions associated with the use of processed disposable hollow fiber hemodialyzers. *J.A.M.A.* 260:2077, 1988.

22. Haley, R.W. The "hospital epidemiologist" in U.S. hospitals, 1976–1977: A description of the head of the infection surveillance and control program. *Infect. Control* 1:21, 1980.

23. Haley, R.W., et al. Identifying patients at high risk of surgical wound infection: A simple multivariate index of patient susceptibility and wound contamination. *Am. J. Epidemiol.* 121:206, 1985.

24. Haley, R.W., et al. The nation-wide nosocomial infection rate: A new need for vital statistics. *Am. J. Epidemiol.* 121:159, 1985.

25. Haley, R.W., et al. The efficacy of infection surveillance and control programs in preventing nosocomial infections in U.S. hospitals. *Am. J. Epidemiol.* 121:182, 1985.

26. Haley, R.W., et al. The emergence of methicillin-resistant *Staphylococcus aureus* infections in United States hospitals: Possible role of the house staff–patient transfer circuit. *Ann. Intern. Med.* 97:297, 1982.

27. Haley, R.W., et al. Nosocomial infections in U.S. hospitals, 1975–1976. Estimated frequency by selected characteristics of patients. *Am. J. Med.* 70:947, 1981.

28. Haley, R.W., et al. Extra days and prolongation of stay attributable to nosocomial infections: A prospective interhospital comparison. *Am. J. Med.* 70:51, 1981.

29. Haley, R.W., et al. How frequent are outbreaks of nosocomial infection in community hospitals? *Infect. Control* 6:233, 1985.

30. Haley, R.W., Morgan, W.M., Culver, D.H., and Schaberg, D.R. Differences in nosocomial infection rates by type of hospital: The influence of patient mix and diagnostic medical practices. Presented at the Interscience Conference on Antimicrobial Agents and Chemotherapy, Miami, FL, October 4, 1982.

31. Haley, R.W., Quade, D.H., Freeman, H.E., and the CDC SENIC Planning Committee. Study on the efficacy of nosocomial infection control (SENIC Project): Summary of study design. *Am. J. Epidemiol.* 111:472, 1980.

32. Haley, R.W., Schaberg, D.R., Von Allmen, S.D., and McGowan, J.E., Jr. Estimating the extra charges and prolongation of hospitalization due to nosocomial infections: A comparison of methods. *J. Infect. Dis.* 141:248, 1980.

33. Hall, C.B. Nosocomial viral respiratory infections: Perennial weeds on pediatric wards. *Am. J. Med.* 70:670, 1981.

34. Hooton, T.M., et al. The joint associations of multiple risk factors with the occurrence of nosocomial infection. *Am. J. Med.* 70:960, 1981.

35. Howard, J.M., et al. Postoperative wound infections: The influence of ultraviolet irradiation of the operating room and of various other factors. *Ann. Surg.* 160(Suppl.):1, 1964.

36. Hughes, J.M., et al. Nosocomial infection surveillance, 1980–1982. *M.M.W.R.* 32:1SS, 1983.

37. Hughes, J.M., et al. Mortality Associated with Nosocomial Infections in the United States, 1975–1981. In: *Abstracts of the Twenty-Second Interscience Conference on Antimicrobial Agents and Chemotherapy.* Miami Beach, FL, October 4–6, 1982. Washington, DC: American Society for Microbiology, 1982. P. 189.

38. Jarvis, W.R. Nosocomial outbreaks: The Centers for Disease Control's Hospital Infections Program experience, 1980–1990. *Am. J. Med.* 91(Suppl. 3B): 101S, 1991.

39. Kislak, J.W., Eickhoff, T.C., and Finland, M. Hospital-acquired infections and antibiotic usage in the Boston City Hospital. *N. Engl. J.Med.* 271:834, 1964.

40. Lidwell, O.M. Sepsis in surgical wounds: Multiple regression analysis applied to records of post-operative hospital sepsis. *J. Hyg.* (Camb.) 59:259, 1961.

41. Lowry, P.W., et al. *Mycobacterium chelonae* infection among patients receiving high-flux dialysis in a hemodialysis clinic, California. *J. Infect. Dis.* 161:85, 1990.

42. Lowry, P.W., et al. *Mycobacterium chelonae* causing otitis media in the ear-nose-and-throat practice. *N. Engl. J. Med.* 319:978, 1988.

43. Magnussen, M.H., and Robb, S.S. Nosocomial infections in a long-term care facility. *Am. J. Infect. Control* 2:12, 1980.

44. Maki, D.G., Rhame, F.S., Mackel, D.C., and Bennett, J.V. Nationwide epidemic of septicemia caused by contaminated intravenous products. I. Epidemiologic and clinical features. *Am. J. Med.* 60:471, 1976.

45. Martone, W.J., et al. Illness with fatalities in premature infants: Association with an intravenous vitamin E preparation. *Pediatrics* 78:591, 1986.

46. Mastro, T.D., et al. An outbreak of surgical-wound infections due to group A *streptococcus* carried on the scalp. *N. Engl. J. Med.* 323:968, 1990.

47. McCabe, W.R., and Jackson, G.C. Gram-negative bacteremia. I. Etiology and ecology. *Arch. Intern. Med.* 110:847, 1962.

48. McGowan, J.E., Jr., Parrott, P.L., and Duty, V.P. Nosocomial bacteremia: Potential for prevention of procedure-related cases. *J.A.M.A.* 237:2737, 1977.

49. McNeil, M.M., et al. *Ewingella americana:* Recurrent pseudobacteremia from a persistent environmental reservoir. *J. Clin. Microbiol.* 25:498, 1987.

50. Platt, R., et al. Mortality associated with noso-

comial urinary tract infection. *N. Engl. J. Med.* 307:637, 1982.

51. Price, E.H., Brain, A., and Dickson, J.A.S. An outbreak of infection with a gentamicin- and methicillin-resistant *Staphylococcus aureus* in a neonatal unit. *J. Hosp. Infect.* 1:221, 1980.

52. Retailliau, H.F., et al. *Acinetobacter calcoaceticus:* A nosocomial pathogen with an unusual seasonal pattern. *J. Infect. Dis.* 139:371, 1979.

53. Richet, H.M., et al. A cluster of *Rhodococcus (Gordona) bronchialis* sternal wound infections after coronary-artery bypass surgery. *N. Engl. J. Med.* 324:104, 1991.

54. Richet, H.M., McNeil, M.M., Edwards, M.C., and Jarvis, W.R. Cluster of *Malassezia furfur* pulmonary infections in infants in a neonatal intensive care unit. *J. Clin. Microbiol.* 27:1197, 1989.

55. Safranek, T.J., et al. *Mycobacteria chelonae* wound infections after plastic surgery employing contaminated gentian violet skin marking solution. *N. Engl. J. Med.* 317:197, 1987.

56. Sapico, F.L., Mongomerie, J.Z., Canawati, H.N., and Aeilts, G. Methicillin-resistant *Staphylococcus aureus* bacteriuria. *Am. J. Med. Sci.* 281:101, 1980.

57. Saraglou, G., Cromer, M., and Bisno, A.L. Methicillin-resistant *Staphylococcus aureus:* Interstate spread of nosocomial infections with emergence of gentamicin-methicillin-resistant strains. *Infect. Control* 1:81, 1980.

58. Schaberg, D.R., et al. An outbreak of nosocomial infection due to multiply resistant *Serratia marcescens:* Evidence of interhospital spread. *J. Infect. Dis.* 134:181, 1976.

59. Schaberg, D.R., et al. Evolution of antimicrobial resistance and nosocomial infection: Lessons from the Vanderbilt experience. *Am. J. Med.* 70:445, 1981.

60. Shanson, D.C. Antibiotic-resistant *Staphylococcus aureus. J. Hosp. Infect.* 2:11, 1981.

61. Shanson, D.C., and McSwiggan, D.A. Operating theatre-acquired infection with a gentamicin-resistant strain of *Staphylococcus aureus:* Outbreaks in two hospitals attributable to one surgeon. *J. Hosp. Infect.* 1:171, 1980.

62. Simpson, J.Y. Our existing system of hospitalism and its effect. Part I. *Edinburgh Med. J.* 14:816, 1869.

63. Stamm, W.E., Martin, S.M., and Bennett, J.V. Epidemiology of nosocomial infections due to gram-negative bacilli: Aspects relevant to development and use of vaccines. *J. Infect. Dis.* 163(Suppl.):S151, 1977.

64. Stamm, W.E., Weinstein, R.A., and Dixon, R.E. Comparison of endemic and epidemic nosocomial infections. *Am. J. Med.* 70:393, 1981.

65. Thoburn, R., Fekety, F.R., Cluff, L.E., and Melvin, V.B. Infections acquired by hospitalized patients. *Arch. Intern. Med.* 121:1, 1968.

66. Tipple, M.A., Bland, L.A., Favero, M.S., and Jarvis, W.R. Investigation of hemolytic anemia after chloramine exposure in a dialysis center. *Trans. Am. Soc. Artif. Intern. Organs* 34:1060, 1988.

67. Tipple, M.A., et al. Sepsis associated with transfusion of red blood cells contaminated with *Yersinia enterocolitica. Transfusion* 30:207, 1990.

68. Tokars, J.I., et al. *Mycobacterium gordonae* pseudoinfection associated with a contaminated antimicrobial solution. *J. Clin. Microbiol.* 28:2765, 1990.

69. United States National Center for Health Statistics. *Utilization Patterns and Financial Characteristics of Nursing Homes in the United States: 1977 National Nursing Home Survey.* (Data from the National Health Survey, Series 13, No. 53. DHHS publication no [PHS]81,1714) Hyattsville, MD: National Center for Health Statistics, 1981.

70. Valenti, W.M., et al. Nosocomial viral infections: Epidemiology and significance. *Infect. Control* 1:33, 1980.

71. Weems, J.J., et al. *Candida parapsilosis fungemia* associated with parenteral nutrition and contaminated blood pressure transducers. *J. Clin. Microbiol.* 25:1029, 1987.

72. Weinstein, R.A. Pseudoepidemics in hospital. *Lancet* 2:862, 1977.

73. Weinstein, R.A., and Kabins, S.A. Strategies for prevention and control of multiple drug–resistant nosocomial infection. *Am. J. Med.* 70:449, 1981.

74. Wenzel, R.P., et al. Hospital acquired infections in intensive care unit patients: An overview with emphasis on epidemics. *Infect. Control* 4:371, 1983.

75. Winn, R.E., et al. Epidemiological, bacteriological, and clinical observations on an interhospital outbreak of nafcillin-resistant *Staphylococcus aureus. Curr. Chemother.* 2:1096, 1979.

Nosocomial Urinary Tract Infections

Walter E. Stamm

Incidence

According to data from numerous hospitals [39, 53, 60] and from multihospital collaborative studies (see Chap. 5), nosocomial urinary tract infections have consistently been responsible for 35 to 45 percent of all hospital-acquired infections. Thus approximately 2 per 100 patients admitted to acute-care hospitals in the United States, or more than 0.8 million patients per annum, acquire nosocomial bacteriuria. In the National Nosocomial Infections Surveillance (NNIS) System, urinary tract infections have consistently accounted for 40 percent of all hospital-acquired infections, with little change evident over the period 1970–1990. In this survey, the proportion of nosocomial bacteriuria cases associated with or contributing to mortality was less than 3 percent (see Chap. 5).

Endemic Versus Epidemic Infections

Endemic acquisition accounts for the majority of nosocomial urinary tract infections, but numerous examples of epidemic transmission have been reported [71, 81]. Epidemics of nosocomial bacteriuria have resulted from inadequately disinfected cystoscopes, nonsterile irrigating solutions used on multiple patients, contaminated disinfectants in catheter insertion trays and, most commonly, person-to-person transmission on crowded hospital wards where aseptic catheter care practices were not being used [71, 81]. Frequent catheter irrigation appeared to be an important causal factor in several epidemics. Multiply drug-resistant strains of *Serratia, Proteus, Klebsiella,* and *Pseudomonas* possessing unique antimicrobial susceptibility patterns have afforded opportunities to trace the epidemiology of nosocomial urinary tract infections in the epidemic setting. Most often, epidemic investigations have demonstrated transmission of organisms from one catheterized patient to another via the hands of hospital personnel. In several epidemics, patients with unrecognized asymptomatic bacteriuria lasting for weeks or even months served as an important reservoir, with temporal and spatial clustering of subsequent cases in proximity to these source patients.

Most likely, a proportion of infections classified as endemic actually result from clusters or microepidemics of cross-infection on hospital wards. Using tertiary marker systems (e.g., pyocin typing, serotyping, and phage typing) to trace cross-infection attributable to common organisms such as *Escherichia coli*, Schaberg and co-workers [70] demonstrated that approximately 15 percent of endemic nosocomial infections occur in clusters suggestive of cross-infection. *Pseudomonas* and *Serratia* infections were most often clustered, and *E. coli* infections least often. Thus attention to the same factors that prevent or terminate epidemics of nosocomial bacteriuria (see under the heading Prevention) presumably would prevent some endemic infections as well.

Risk Factors

Nearly all nosocomial urinary tract infections occur in patients with indwelling urinary catheters (approximately 80 percent) or after other types of transient urologic instrumentation (nearly 20 percent). Specific host factors associated with an increased risk of infection during or after instrumentation include female gender, older age, and an increasing degree of underlying illness (Table 28-1). The risk of developing nosocomial bacteriuria in women exceeds the risk in men by approximately twofold in each decade of life [31, 80], but men more often manifest secondary bacteremia. For both men and women, the risk of catheter-associated bacteriuria increases with age [31, 80]. In addition, 95 percent of deaths and 83 percent of bacteremic episodes occur in patients older than 50 years [80].

In addition to host factors (which, for the most part, cannot be altered), the risk of urinary infection relates directly to the type and duration of urologic instrumentation. After a single in-and-out catheterization, between 1 and 20 percent of patients acquire bacteriuria [76, 89]; lower rates occur in healthy outpatients and higher rates in older hospitalized patients. Indwelling urethral catheters draining into an open collecting vessel result in bacteriuria in 100 percent of patients within 4 days [36]. With the sterile closed collecting systems used in most hospitals today, bacteriuria occurs on the average in 10 to 25 percent of catheterized patients [17, 43, 88]. In hospitals with active prevention programs, rates of less than 10 percent have been reported (see Chap. 5). In prospective studies carried out in general hospital populations between 1966 and 1990 [17, 19, 34, 44, 66, 86, 96], there has been an apparent trend toward a reduced prevalence of catheter-associated bacteriuria (Table 28-2). Many factors may account for this decrease, including increased antimicrobial use in catheterized patients, decreasing lengths of catheterization and

Table 28-1. Risk factors associated with infection during catheterization

Alterable factors	Unalterable factors
Indications for catheterization	Female gender
	Older age
Length of catheterization	Severe underlying illness
Catheter care techniques	Meatal colonization
Type of drainage system	
Receipt of antimicrobials	

Table 28-2. Prevalence of catheter-associated urinary tract infections in prospective studies, 1966–1990

Study	Prevalence (%)
Kunin 1966 [44]	23
Finkelberg 1969 [17]	21
Garibaldi 1974 [19]	23
Warren 1978 [96]	17
Platt 1983 [66]	9
Thompson 1984 [86]	10
Johnson 1990 [34]	10

hospitalization, and more effective infection control efforts. The per-day risk of developing bacteriuria appears comparable throughout catheterization (3 to 6 percent), but the cumulative risk increases with duration of catheterization [18, 20]. Thus approximately 50 percent of hospitalized patients catheterized longer than 7 to 10 days develop bacteriuria [18, 43] (Fig. 28-1).

Bacteriuria develops more frequently in patients not receiving systemic antimicrobials and in patients in whom catheter cure violations have occurred [34, 68].

Etiology

Aerobic gram-negative rods account for the vast majority of catheter-associated urinary tract infections. In recent data collected by the NNIS System (Table 28-3) [26], Enterobacteriaceae and pseudomonads accounted for more than 80 percent of all culture-positive infections. Of the gram-positive organisms, group D streptococci accounted for approximately 14 percent, whereas staphylococci collectively caused about 5 percent. Increasingly, the aerobic gram-negative rods causing nosocomial bacteriuria have been characterized by multiple antimicrobial resistance, often mediated by transmissible plasmids (see Chap. 14) [46]. Candidal infections of the catheterized urinary tract appear to have increased over the last decade (see Chap. 5).

The relative proportion of infections accounted for by an individual species, as well as their antimicrobial susceptibility patterns, vary widely from hospital to hospital and fluctuate with time in each hospital. In two studies, *E. coli* and *Proteus* accounted for a progressively smaller percentage of nosocomial urinary tract infections as the period of hospitalization and catheterization lengthened [41, 80]. Conversely, *Serratia* and *Pseudomonas aeruginosa* accounted for a progressively greater proportion of infection as hospitalization increased. These observations suggest that a proportion of catheter-associated infections are, in fact, not newly acquired but may represent recognition of previous covert bacteriuria after insertion of a urinary catheter.

Pathogenesis

Occasionally, nosocomial urinary tract infections result from direct introduction of urethral microorganisms at the time of catheterization, other instrumentation (usually cystoscopy), or surgery. Based on time of onset,

Table 28-3. Pathogens causing nosocomial urinary tract infections (n = 54,940)

Pathogen	Percent
Escherichia coli	31.9
Group D streptococci	14.4
Pseudomonas aeruginosa	11.5
Klebsiella	8.8
Proteus mirabilis	6.7
Candida species	4.4
Enterobacter	4.1
Staphylococcus epidermidis	3.4
Staphylococcus aureus	1.9
Serratia	1.6
Group B streptococci	1.2
Pseudomonas species	1.1
Morganella	0.9
Others	8.1
Total	100.0

Source: From R.W. Haley et al., The nationwide nosocomial infection rate: A new need for vital statistics. *Am. J. Epidemiol.* 121:159, 1985.

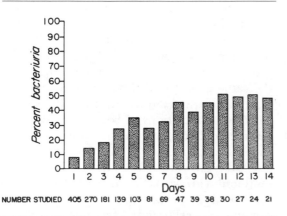

NUMBER STUDIED 405 270 181 139 103 81 69 47 39 38 30 27 24 21

Fig. 28-1. Percent of catheterized patients with bacteriuria by day of catheterization. (From R.A. Garibaldi et al., Factors predisposing to bacteriuria during indwelling urethral catheterization. *N. Engl. J. Med.* 291:216, 1974. Reprinted by permission of *The New England Journal of Medicine.*)

however, most catheter-associated infections arise later in the period of catheterization. Microorganisms causing these infections enter the catheterized urinary tract either through the lumen of the catheter (intraluminal route) or along its external surface in the mucous sheath between the catheter and urethral mucosa (transurethral route) (Fig. 28-2). Women appear to be at greater risk than men of transurethral infection. In one study, approximately two-thirds of women who developed catheter-associated bacteriuria were shown to have previous urethral and rectal colonization with their infecting strain, compared with only one-third of men [11]. Thus the pathogenesis of catheter-associated infections in many women resembles the pathogenesis of noncatheter-associated infections. Studies of community-acquired bacteriuria in women suggest that fecal organisms establish introital, vaginal, and urethral colonization before urinary tract infection with these strains occurs [49, 75]. Since only one-third of men who develop catheter-associated bacteriuria can be demonstrated to have antecedent urethral and rectal colonization, the urethral route of entry may be less important in men. In either sex, however, establishment of urethral colonization with a gram-negative rod apparently confers an increased risk of subsequent infection. Garibaldi and co-workers [19] showed that the increased risk of sub-

sequent nosocomial bacteriuria associated with a positive meatal culture was approximately fourfold in women and twofold in men. However, periurethral colonization is not invariably followed by bacteriuria and, when bacteriuria does occur, it is often more than 72 hours after the establishment of periurethral colonization [72].

Bacteriuria may also result from microorganisms that enter the collecting system and ascend through the lumen of the urinary catheter into the bladder (intraluminal route). In studies assessing this mode of entry, approximately 15 to 20 percent of infected patients can be demonstrated to have their infecting organism in the collecting bag before entry into the bladder [19, 72, 94]. Retrograde spread of the organism from the collecting bag to the bladder occurs within 24 to 48 hours in nearly all such patients [19]. Once in the bladder, small numbers of microorganisms (e.g., 100 colony-forming units [cfu] per milliliter) increase to large numbers (more than 100,000 cfu/ml) in less than 24 hours [82]. Thus contamination of the collecting bag or introduction of organisms by disconnection of the distal catheter and proximal collection tube can allow entry of organisms that produce nosocomial bacteriuria. Rarely, nosocomial bacteriuria arises secondary to hematogenous seeding of the genitourinary tract or as a complication of surgical procedures involving the urinary tract or adjacent structures.

Studies in the last decade have demonstrated an important role for attachment and growth of bacteria on the inner surface of the catheter in the pathogenesis of catheter-associated urinary tract infection [9, 10, 63, 64]. Two populations of bacteria exist in the catheterized urinary tract, those growing within the urine itself (planktonic growth) and those growing on the surface of the catheter (biofilm growth). The growth of a bacterial biofilm on the urinary catheter progresses according to a well-defined sequence of events: Bacteria attach to the urinary catheter, initiate a biofilm form of growth in which sheets of organisms coat the catheter, and secrete an extracellular matrix of bacterial glycocalyces

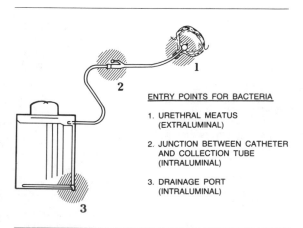

ENTRY POINTS FOR BACTERIA

1. URETHRAL MEATUS
   (EXTRALUMINAL)

2. JUNCTION BETWEEN CATHETER
   AND COLLECTION TUBE
   (INTRALUMINAL)

3. DRAINAGE PORT
   (INTRALUMINAL)

Fig. 28-2. Entry points for bacteria causing catheter-associated urinary tract infection.

in which they become embedded. In addition, host urinary proteins such as Tamm-Horsfall protein and urinary salts are incorporated into this biofilm. Subsequently, this material leads to encrustation of the inner catheter surface. Examination of catheters by electron microscopy has demonstrated this biofilm growth on the inner surface of catheters removed from both patients and animals [9, 10, 63, 64]. Certain genera of bacteria, particularly *Proteus* and *Pseudomonas,* are frequently associated with a propensity for biofilm growth and catheter obstruction [59].

In patients without urinary catheters who develop urinary tract infections, it has been demonstrated that a small number of "urovirulent clones" of *E. coli* produce most serious infections [78, 79]. These clones are defined on the basis of a limited number of O, K, and H serotypes and by the presence in these clones of specific virulence genes for P fimbriae, hemolysin, and siderophores. Studies to determine whether similar strains frequently infect the catheterized urinary tract have shown that the urovirulent strains seen in community-acquired urinary tract infections rarely cause bacteremic catheter-associated urinary tract infections [34, 35]. The diversity of species causing catheter-associated urinary tract infections implies that compromised host defenses are probably more important than specific bacterial virulence factors in the genesis of these infections [37, 74, 80, 100]. However, specific bacterial properties may be of importance in some settings. It has been demonstrated, for example, that specific strains of bacteria adhere more avidly to either catheter materials themselves or to uroepithelial cells from patient's bladders [12]. Better understanding of the interaction of bacteria and host epithelial cells could lead to novel approaches for preventing catheter-associated urinary tract infection.

Though catheter-associated bacteriuria has been clearly linked to subsequent bacteremia, the mechanism through which such bacteremia occurs has not been elucidated. Bacteremia could occur secondary to mucosal ulcerations resulting from bladder wall damage during catheterization. Cystoscopic examination of catheterized patients and animals suggests such ulcerations are common after 7 days of catheterization [32, 60]. Alternatively, the well-known association of bacteremia with either insertion or withdrawal of urinary catheters or other urologic instruments suggests that bacteremia may result from the mucosal trauma associated with these events [84]. Finally, as in non-catheter-associated urinary tract infections, bacteremia may result when infection ascends beyond the bladder to involve the kidney, prostate, or other portions of the upper urinary tract.

At present, the various mechanisms through which bacteremia may develop have not been distinguished in studies of catheter-associated bacteriuria. To address this issue, localization of the site of infection in patients with catheter-associated bacteriuria and bacteremia requires additional study. Certainly, few patients with an unobstructed urinary tract develop characteristic clinical evidence of renal infection. The antibody-coated bacteria (ACB) test has been used in patients with catheter-associated bacteriuria to assess the frequency of asymptomatic renal involvement and, in some studies, has suggested the presence of clinically inapparent upper tract infection in 15 to 20 percent of those with bacteriuria [22, 87]. However, comparison of the ACB test with other localization tests in catheterized patients has not been carried out, and thus the actual significance of a positive result has not been established.

Sequelae

From the short-term clinical perspective, most catheter-associated urinary tract infections appear benign. Because only 20 to 30 percent cause symptoms, most episodes can be classified as asymptomatic bacteriuria [27, 61]. Pyuria accompanies most episodes of catheter-associated bacteriuria, however, suggesting host invasion rather than simple bladder colonization [62, 77]. Not many patients with catheter-associated bacteriuria have undergone localization studies, and thus the proportion of patients with bladder, prostate, or kidney infections has not been determined. In studies using the ACB test, as many as one-fourth of episodes of catheter-associated bacteriuria were positive, suggesting upper tract infection [22, 87]. Clinically recognized ascending infection, including prostatitis, epididymitis, seminal vesiculitis, and renal infection, may arise from bacteriuria originating during catheterization, but the frequency of such infections remains ill-defined. In general, these complications arise primarily in patients with long-term indwelling catheters and are rare in patients whose catheterization lasts less than 10 days.

The major systemic complication of catheter-associated bacteriuria has been secondary bacteremia [14]. Although the risk of secondary bacteremia is small in any given patient, taken collectively bacteremia arising from catheter-associated bacteriuria accounts for a large proportion of all nosocomial bacteremias. Most series of hospitalized patients with gram-negative bacteremia demonstrate that 30 to 40 percent of all gram-negative bacteremias acquired in the hospital originate in the urinary tract [16, 40, 83, 99], making this the most commonly recognized source of gram-negative sepsis. Estimates of the frequency of secondary bacteremia associated with catheterization range from 1 per 50 to 1 per 150 catheterized bacteriuric patients. In one prospective study, however, 8 percent of patients had bacteremia after urinary catheterization [84]. Bacteremia thus may occur more often than is recognized clinically, especially on insertion, withdrawal, manipulation, or obstruction of the catheter.

Epidemiologic studies have related nosocomial bacteriuria with an increased mortality [66]. After adjustment for other factors, such as type of underlying disease, severity of illness, age, and sex, an approximately threefold relative increase in risk of death was observed by Platt and colleagues [66]. The mechanism through which bacteriuria might produce increased mortality has not been elucidated but may relate to unrecognized septicemia [66, 92]. To date, catheter-associated bacteriuria has not been associated with long-term renal damage, but the natural history of this condition has not been studied prospectively.

Several authors have attempted to estimate whether increased hospital stay results from nosocomial urinary tract infection [21, 23, 65]. In a case-control study, Givens and Wenzel [21] found that urinary infections occurring in surgical patients resulted in 2.4 days of increased hospitalization and a cost of $558 per patient. Other estimates of increased hospitalization attributable to catheter-associated infection have ranged from 1 to 4 days, and estimates of increased costs have ranged from none to $1,100 [23, 65] (see Chap. 25).

Clinical Manifestations

Only 20 to 30 percent of patients with catheter-associated bacteriuria experience symptoms attributable to infection, and thus most cases can be classified as asymptomatic bacteriuria [61]. When present, symptoms include dysuria, urgency, frequency, and hematuria. Fever, flank pain, or other clinical manifestations of pyelonephritis develop in fewer than 1 percent of patients with catheter-associated bacteriuria [62, 77]. Despite the absence of symptoms in most patients with catheter-associated bacteriuria, the presence of pyuria suggests host invasion and actual infection rather than simple bladder colonization. Clinical findings characteristic of gram-negative bacteremia accompany bacteremia secondary to bacteriuria. Interestingly, the onset of bacteremia usually occurs within 24 hours of the onset of bacteriuria except for *Serratia marcescens* infections, in which bacteremia most commonly originates days after the onset of bacteriuria [41].

Diagnosis

Most physicians diagnose catheter-associated bacteriuria by obtaining a urine specimen for culture via aspiration through a sampling port on the catheter itself. Since specimens so collected presumably represent actual bladder urine, contamination is infrequent. In recent studies, catheter aspiration corresponded with cultures obtained by suprapubic aspiration in at least 90 percent of cases

[3]. Urine cultures obtained from the catheter sampling port may not always reflect true bacteriuria in patients who have organisms growing on a biofilm on the inner surface of the catheter. Rather, bladder urine may be sterile but organisms from the catheter biofilm may contaminate the aspirated urine culture. Such contamination would be more likely to occur in patients with catheters in place for a week or more.

Quantitative culture results may demonstrate organisms ranging in quantity from 10 to more than 10^5 cfu/ml. Various authors have used quantitative bacterial counts ranging from at least 10^2 to at least 10^5 cfu/ml to define infection in catheterized patients. However, prospective studies to establish a specific quantitative level as more or less indicative of infection have not been carried out. For clinical purposes, bacteriuria of 10^2 cfu/ml or more, especially when associated with pyuria, can probably be taken as evidence of bladder infection. Catheter-tip cultures should not be used to diagnose urinary infection [24].

Treatment

Since most patients with catheter-associated bacteriuria lack associated symptoms, treatment need not be undertaken unless the patient is at high risk for complications such as bacteremia or renal infection. Thus treatment of asymptomatic bacteriuria may be useful in patients with neutropenia, obstructed urinary tracts, renal transplants, pregnancy, or other specific situations in which bacteriuria in and of itself may be of significant risk. In most patients without such complicating clinical features, however, treatment of bacteriuria should not be undertaken. In such patients, bacteriuria often resolves spontaneously with removal of the catheter; if one anticipates removal of the catheter, treatment should be postponed until that time. After catheter removal, the patient can either be observed for a period of time and subsequently treated if the bacteriuria does not resolve spontaneously, or treated empirically after the catheter has been removed. The latter may be particularly useful in elderly women. Treatment with the catheter in place often results in emergence of resistant strains, and eradication of bacteriuria in the presence of an indwelling catheter has been largely unsuccessful [7]. Since the antimicrobial susceptibility patterns of strains causing catheter-associated bacteriuria vary widely, choice of a specific antimicrobial agent should be guided by the in vitro antimicrobial sensitivities of the infecting organisms (see Chap. 12).

Prevention

Guidelines for prevention of catheter-associated bacteriuria have been published by the Centers for Disease Control [101]. Until more has been learned about the pathogenesis of nosocomial bacteriuria, preventive efforts must be focused largely on aseptic care of the urinary catheter (Table 28-4). These measures are directed primarily at preventing entry of bacteria into the sterile closed drainage system and have been most effective when the period of catheterization is less than 7 days. Probably the single most effective preventive measure is to avoid use of the indwelling catheter whenever possible. Indications for continued catheterization should be reviewed on a daily basis, since the risk of bacteriuria associated with catheterization can be markedly reduced by removing catheters as soon as possible. Catheters should be inserted aseptically under sterile conditions. In addition, the closed drainage system should be considered a sterile site, and aseptic precautions should be observed when manipulating any portion of the system. Inadvertent or pur-

Table 28-4. Methods for prevention of catheter-associated infections

Avoid catheterization.
Decrease duration of catheterization.
Use intermittent catheterization.
Insert catheters aseptically.
Use a closed sterile drainage system.
Use a condom catheter in cooperative patients.
Maintain gravity drain.
Apply topical meatal antimicrobials in women.
Separate infected and uninfected patients.

poseful disconnection of the catheter and collecting system predisposes to bacteriuria, as does use of nonsterile technique when emptying urine from the collecting vessel. Continuous downhill gravity flow drainage should be maintained at all times. Both hospital personnel and catheterized patients should be taught the importance of these principles.

Many technologic improvements in catheters and drainage systems have been proposed as means of preventing bacteriuria. These include polymeric silicone (Silastic) rather than rubber catheters; baffles, vents, or other devices for preventing reflux or retrograde infection; instillation of antimicrobial or antiseptic agents into the catheter bag; culture vents on the side of the urinary catheter; permanent junctions between the distal catheter and collecting system; and antimicrobial substances impregnated into the catheter itself. Most of these technologic improvements make sense from the standpoint of the pathogenesis of these infections, but it has been difficult in controlled trials to prove the effectiveness of most such innovations. Since opening the closed collecting system has been clearly shown to predispose to infection, sampling ports that permit cultures to be obtained without opening the system are preferred. Although sometimes inconvenient, drainage systems marketed as a single unit extending from the bladder catheter to the collecting bag prevent inadvertent disconnection of the catheter and collecting system. In a randomized, controlled trial, Platt and colleagues [67] found that sealed-junction catheters significantly reduced the risk of urinary tract infection and also reduced the risk of death in individuals not receiving systemic antimicrobials.

More controversial has been the value of using antimicrobial substances such as hydrogen peroxide or chlorhexidine in the collecting bag. In one study, Maizels and Schaeffer [48] demonstrated that hydrogen peroxide in the collecting bag successfully eradicated microorganisms introduced into the collecting system and prevented retrograde infection. In another study, use of hydrogen peroxide in the drainage spigot prevented retrograde

infection [13]. On the other hand, some studies have failed to find benefit attributable to either system [69, 86]. In part, the potential benefit of such a system relates to the proportion of infections acquired via the intraluminal route. In previous studies, an estimated 15 to 20 percent of infections occurred in this manner [56], and thus the majority of infections may not be preventable through control measures aimed at interrupting this route of bacterial ingress. Such measures may, however, reduce reservoirs of organisms available for transfer from one catheterized patient to another on the hands of personnel. In hospitals in which technique is not optimal and intraluminal infection occurs more often, these preventive approaches may have greater benefit.

Since many infections acquired during catheterization arise following urethral meatal colonization with the infecting strain, topical application of antiseptic agents to these areas has been advocated as a preventive measure. In a large and careful study addressing this topic, Burke and co-workers [5] were unable to ascribe benefits to twice-daily application of povidone-iodine solution followed by povidine-iodine ointment. In a subsequent study, Burke and colleagues [6] demonstrated reduced infection rates using a twice-daily polyantimicrobial ointment applied at the meatal-catheter junction; however, the benefit was seen only in a specific high-risk group: women with previous meatal colonization. Thus although the overall efficacy of this approach remains in doubt, it is apparently effective in some patients.

Alternative means of blocking urethral colonization and ascension of organisms from the urethral meatus surface are now being investigated. Many years ago, antimicrobial impregnation of catheters was assessed [8]. Although the technique was not successful in those studies, newer approaches using silver-impregnated catheters have recently been undertaken. This approach has an appealing logical basis in that silver ions are bactericidal, can be applied to catheters, are nontoxic and, when used topically, have been effective in other settings such as controlling burn wound infections. Shaeffer and colleagues [73] demonstrated that silver-coated catheters (in conjunction with a silver catheter tubing–junction connector and an antiseptic-filled drainage bag) reduced the incidence of catheter-associated urinary tract infections and delayed their onset in chronically catheterized patients. In a recently published trial by Liedberg and Lundeberg [47], excellent results were also obtained in short-term catheterized patients utilizing a silver-coated catheter. They demonstrated that 10 percent of the patients catheterized with the silver-coated latex catheter had urinary tract infections versus 37 percent of those receiving a Teflon control catheter [47]. However, other studies of the silver-coated catheter in general hospital populations have demonstrated less benefit [34]. Further study of these catheters appears warranted.

Irrigation of the bladder with antimicrobial solutions is another technique that has been used to prevent catheter-associated bacteriuria [2]. Martin and Bookrajian [50] first reported prevention of infections using acetic acid or a neomycin–polymyxin B irrigant in an open collecting system. Instillation of chlorhexidine into the bladder has also been reported as efficacious [38]. However, Warren and colleagues [96], in a carefully controlled trial, were unable to ascribe any benefits to continuous irrigation with polymyxin-neosporin and found that patients on irrigation developed infections with more resistant organisms.

Systemic antibiotic agents have been demonstrated to decrease the likelihood of bacteriuria during the first 5 to 7 days of catheterization [5, 6, 43, 61, 96]. In addition, in one controlled trial, systemic antimicrobials were associated with a decreased rate of catheter-associated bacteriuria [4]. Thus systemic antimicrobial agents probably reduce the likelihood of bacteriuria developing during short-term catheterization. However, whether the risks, side effects, and costs of such antimicrobials warrant their use for this purpose requires additional study. It may be reasonable to consider systemic antimicrobials as a preventive measure in high-risk patients who have an antici-

pated short duration of catheterization. In patients with long-term urinary catheterization, continued antimicrobial use results in the emergence of resistant strains and probably should be avoided [95]. Antimicrobial prophylaxis has been of clear benefit in preventing postoperative urinary infection among men with sterile urine undergoing urologic surgery [16, 29].

A recent study has demonstrated the value of selective decontamination of the gut (see Chap. 13) in preventing catheter-associated urinary tract infections [93]. According to Vollaard and colleagues [93], oral norfloxacin plus oral amphotericin B administered to patients with urinary catheters decreased the occurrence of catheter-associated urinary tract infections and delayed their onset.

Daily culture monitoring of catheterized patients to detect bacteriuria before onset of symptoms or bacteremia has been advocated [43]. However, Garibaldi and colleagues [20] found monitoring to be of little benefit since most symptomatic infections and bacteremias occurred within 24 hours of the onset of bacteriuria. Alternative methods of urinary drainage such as condom drainage, suprapubic catheterization, or intermittent catheterization (see next section) may be preferable in selected patients. Condom catheters have been most successfully used in alert, cooperative patients receiving meticulous skin care to prevent meatal ulceration [28, 33]. In this setting, condom catheters used for 2 to 4 weeks appear to have an infection risk lower than that of indwelling catheters. In uncooperative patients who manipulate the condom catheter, however, infections occur at least as frequently as in comparable patients with indwelling catheters [87]. Suprapubic catheterization has been largely used by gynecologists and urologists for short-term catheterization after surgical procedures. Reported experience suggests that this technique may be less often associated with bacteriuria than is indwelling urethral catheterization, but a direct prospective comparison of the two techniques has not been published [30, 51]. Suprapubic catheterization eliminates the urethral route of infection and thus might be expected to cause less bacteriuria than urethral catheterization.

Chronic Catheterization

Bacteriuria occurs in essentially all patients who require chronic catheter drainage because of spinal cord injury or other causes of neurogenic bladder [90]. Prospective evaluation of such patients has shown that they experience multiple sequential episodes of bacteriuria, usually with a different species each episode (reinfection), but occasionally with a single persisting species [55, 97]. Polymicrobial infections commonly occur. Some strains, specifically Proteeae, pseudomonads, and enterococci, appear to be persistent within the urinary tract once present, whereas other strains frequently cycle in and out of the urinary tract [94, 97]. This may be because the persisters are able to adhere more avidly to the catheter. For *Providencia stuartii*, specific fimbriae (the MR/K fimbriae) have been shown to promote adherence to the catheter and persistence in the urinary tract [57]. On the other hand, *E. coli* type 1 fimbriae have been shown to promote persistence in the urinary tract by increasing avidity of adherence to uroepithelial cells [57]. Thus there may be two populations of organisms in such patients—namely, those that attach to the catheter and those that attach to bladder uroepithelial cells. Alternatively, *Proteeae* have been found as persistent colonizers of the groin in nursing-home patients, and such colonization may provide a reservoir from which infection originates [15].

The vast majority of bacteriuric episodes are asymptomatic, but bacteremia, pyelonephritis, epididymitis, and renal calculi occur with sufficient frequency to be of major concern [55, 97, 98]. These conditions probably contribute in part to deterioration in renal function, a major cause of death in this population [96].

A recurrent problem in these patients is that of catheter encrustation and eventual obstruction. The pathogenesis of catheter encrustation is similar in many ways to that of an infection stone [97]. Bacteria adhere to the catheter and produce encrustation as described previously. The encrustation consists of bacteria, their glycocalyces, host proteins such as Tamm-Horsfall protein and, eventually, urinary crystals such as struvite and apatite. This process is accelerated by urease-producing bacteria, especially *Proteus mirabilis*, which has a very potent urease [52, 58]. The urease results in products that alkalinize the urine, promote crystallization of struvite and apatite, and promote the encrustation and obstruction process. Patient-related factors may play a role here as well in that some patients' urine leads to catheter obstruction more rapidly than others. Further study of the process of encrustation and catheter blockage would be of great interest in these patients.

Prevention of infection has been difficult in patients with chronic indwelling catheters. Aseptic techniques applied to patients with short-term catheterization have not been successful in those with longer-term catheterization. Antimicrobial treatment of asymptomatic bacteriuric episodes had no apparent impact on the frequency or natural history of infection according to one study and instead selected for antibiotic-resistant strains [97]. Similarly, antimicrobial prophylaxis or the use of urinary antiseptics has not been successful in these patients [54, 85, 91]. Most bacteriuria in these patients is accompanied by pyuria, suggesting that more than simple bladder colonization has occurred, but studies to localize such infections to the lower or upper urinary tract have been largely unsuccessful [42, 55]. Patients with chronic catheterization should probably receive antibiotic treatment only for clinically apparent pyelonephritis, epididymitis, or bacteremia—not for asymptomatic bacteriuria. Treatment should be guided by in vitro sensitivities, since these patients develop infections with multiply resistant hospital-acquired strains.

Recent experience suggests that intermittent catheterization, even if done in a nonsterile fashion, may be a significant advance over chronic indwelling catheterization. Infection reportedly can be avoided altogether in some patients and occurs periodically in others on intermittent catheterization [25, 45]. In addition, low-dose continuous antimicrobial prophylaxis may be effective in patients with intermittent catheterization [96], but it is generally not effective in patients with indwelling catheters.

References

1. Barrett, F.F., Casey, J.I., and Finland, M. Infections and antibiotic use among patients at Boston City Hospital. *N. Engl. J. Med.* 278:5, 1968.
2. Bastable, J.R.G., Peel, R.N., Birch, D.M., and Richards, B. Continuous irrigation of the bladder after prostatectomy: Its effect on postprostatectomy infections. *Br. J. Urol.* 49: 689, 1977.
3. Bergquist, D., Bronnestam, R., Hedelin, H., and Stahl, A. The relevance of urinary sampling methods in patients with indwelling Foley catheters. *Br. J. Urol.* 52:92, 1980.
4. Britt, M.R., et al. Antimicrobial prophylaxis for catheter-associated bacteriuria. *Antimicrob. Agents Chemother.* 11:240, 1977.
5. Burke, J.P., et al. Prevention of catheter-associated urinary tract infections: Efficacy of daily meatal care regimens. *Am. J. Med.* 70: 655, 1981.
6. Burke, J.P., et al. Evaluation of daily meatal care with poly-antibiotic ointment in prevention of catheter-associated bacteriuria. *J. Urol.* 129:331, 1983.
7. Butler, H.K., et al. Evaluation of specific systemic antimicrobial therapy in patients on closed catheter drainage. *J. Urol.* 100:567, 1968.
8. Butler, H.K., and Kunin, C.M. Evaluation of polymyxin catheter lubricant and impregnated catheters. *J. Urol.* 100:560, 1968.
9. Cox, A.J., et al. An automated technique for in vitro assessment of the susceptibility of urinary catheter materials to encrustation. *Eng. Med.* 6:37, 1987.
10. Cox, A.J., Hukins, D.W.L., and Sutton, T.M. Infection of catheterized patients: Bacterial colonization of encrusted Foley catheters shown by scanning electron microscopy. *Urol. Res.* 17:349, 1989.
11. Daifuku, R., and Stamm, W.E. Association of rectal and urethral colonization with urinary tract infection in patients with indwelling catheters. *J.A.M.A.* 252:2028, 1984.
12. Daifuku, R., and Stamm, W.E. Bacterial adherence to bladder uroepithelial cells in catheter-associated urinary tract infection. *N. Engl. J. Med.* 314:1208, 1986.
13. Desautels, R.E., Chibaro, E.A., and Lang, R.J. Maintenance of sterility in urinary drainage bags. *Surg. Gynecol. Obstet.* 154:838, 1982.
14. Dupont, H.L., and Spink, W.W. Infections due to gram-negative organisms: An analysis of 860 patients with bacteriuria at the University of Minnesota Medical Center 1958–1966. *Medicine* 48:307, 1969.
15. Ehrenkranz, N.J., Alfonso, B.C., Eckert, D.G., and Moskowitz, L.B. Proteeae species bacteriuria accompanying Proteeae sp. groin skin carriage in geriatric outpatients. *J. Clin. Microbiol.* 27:1988, 1989.
16. Falkiner, F.R., et al. Antimicrobial agents for the prevention of urinary tract infections in transurethral surgery. *J. Urol.* 129:766, 1983.
17. Finkelberg, Z., and Kunin, C.M. Clinical evaluation of closed urinary drainage systems. *J.A.M.A.* 207:1657, 1969.
18. Garibaldi, R.A., et al. Meatal colonization and catheter-associated bacteriuria. *N. Engl. J. Med.* 303:316, 1980.
19. Garibaldi, R.A., et al. Factors predisposing to bacteriuria during indwelling urethral catheterization. *N. Engl. J. Med.* 291:215, 1974.
20. Garibaldi, R.A., Mooney, B.R., Epstein, B.J., and Britt, M.R. An evaluation of daily bacteriologic monitoring to identify preventable episodes of catheter-associated urinary tract infections. *Infect. Control* 3:466, 1982.
21. Givens, C.D., and Wenzel, R.P. Catheter-associated urinary tract infections in surgical patients: A controlled study on the excess morbidity and costs. *J. Urol.* 124: 646, 1980.
22. Gonick, P., Falkner, B., Schwartz, A., and Pariser, R. Bacteriuria in the catheterized patient: Cystitis or pyelonephritis? *J.A.M.A.* 233:253, 1975.
23. Green, M.S., Rubinstein, E., and Amit, P. Estimating the effects of nosocomial infections on the length of hospitalization. *J. Infect. Dis.* 145:667, 1982.
24. Gross, P.A., Harlzavy, L.M., Barden, G.E., and Kerstein, M. Positive Foley catheter tip cultures: Fact or fancy. *J.A.M.A.* 228:72, 1979.
25. Guttman, L., and Frankel, H. The value of intermittent catheterization in the early management of traumatic paraplegia and tetraplegia. *Paraplegia* 4:63, 1966.
26. Haley, R.W., et al. The nationwide nosocomial infection rate: A new need for vital statistics. *Am. J. Epidemiol.* 121:159, 1985.
27. Hartstein, A.I., et al. Nosocomial urinary tract infection: A prospective evaluation of 108 catheterized patients. *Infect. Control* 2: 380, 1981.
28. Hirch, D.D., Fainstein, V., and Musher, D.M.

Do condom catheter collecting systems cause urinary tract infections? *J.A.M.A.* 242:340, 1979.

29. Hirschmann, J.V., and Inui, T.S. Antimicrobial prophylaxis: A critique of recent trials. *Rev. Infect. Dis.* 2:1, 1980.

30. Hodgkinson, C.P., and Hodrari, A.A. Trocar suprapubic cystostomy for postoperative bladder drainage in the female. *J. Obstet. Gynecol.* 96:773, 1966.

31. Hooton, T.M., et al. The joint association of multiple risk factors with the occurrence of nosocomial infections. *Am. J. Med.* 70:960, 1981.

32. Isaacs, J.H., and McWhorter, D.M. Foley catheter drainage systems and bladder damage. *Surg. Gynecol. Obstet.* 132:889, 1971.

33. Johnson, E.T. The condom catheter: Urinary tract infection and other complications. *South. Med. J.* 76:579, 1983.

34. Johnson, J.R., et al. Prevention of catheter-associated urinary tract infections with a silver oxide–coated urinary catheter: Clinical and microbiological correlates. *J. Infect. Dis.* 162:1145, 1990.

35. Johnson, J.R., Moseley, S.L., Roberts, P.L., and Stamm, W.E. Aerobactin and other virulence factor genes among strains of *E. coli* causing urosepsis—association with patients' characteristics. *Infect. Immun.* 56:405, 1988.

36. Kass, E.H. Asymptomatic infections of the urinary tract. *Trans. Assoc. Am. Physicians* 69:56, 1956.

37. Kennedy, R.P., Plorde, J.J., and Petersdorf, R.G. Studies on the epidemiology of *E. coli* infections: IV. Evidence for a nosocomial flora. *J. Clin. Invest.* 44:193, 1965.

38. Kirk, D., Bullock, D.W., Mitchell, J.P., and Hobbs, S.J.F. Hibitane bladder irrigation in the prevention of catheter-associated urinary infections. *Br. J. Urol.* 51:528, 1979.

39. Kislak, J.W., Eickhoff, T.C., and Finland, M. Hospital-acquired infection and antibiotic usage in the Boston City Hospital. *N. Engl. J. Med.* 271:834, 1964.

40. Kreger, B.E., Craven, D.E., Carling, P.C., and McCabe, W.R. Gram-negative bacteremia: III. Reassessment of etiology, epidemiology, and ecology in 612 patients. *Am. J. Med.* 68:332, 1980.

41. Krieger, J.N., Kaiser, D.L., and Wenzel, R.P. Urinary tract etiology of bloodstream infections in hospitalized patients. *J. Infect. Dis.* 148:57, 1983.

42. Kuhlemeier, K.V., Lloyd, L.K., and Stover, S.L. Localization of upper and lower urinary tract infections in patients with neurogenic bladders. *Sci. Digest* 4:29, 1982.

43. Kunin, C.M. *Detection, Prevention, and Management of Urinary Tract Infections* (4th ed.). Philadelphia: Lea & Febiger, 1985.

44. Kunin, C.M., and McCormack, R.-C. Prevention of catheter-induced urinary tract infections by sterile closed drainage. *N. Engl. J. Med.* 274:1155, 1966.

45. Lapides, J., Diokno, A.C., Lowe, B.S., and Kalish, M.D. Followup on unsterile, intermittent self-catheterization. *J. Urol.* 3:184, 1974.

46. Levy, S.B. Antibiotic resistance. *Infect. Control* 4:195, 1983.

47. Liedberg, H., and Lundeberg, T. Silver alloy coated catheters reduce catheter-associated bacteriuria. *Br. J. Urol.* 65:379, 1990.

48. Maizels, M., and Schaeffer, A.J. Decreased incidence of bacteriuria associated with periodic instillations of hydrogen peroxide into the urethral catheter drainage bag. *J. Urol.* 123:841, 1980.

49. Marsh, F.P., Murray, M., and Panchamia, P. The relationship between bacterial cultures of the vaginal introitus and urinary infection. *Br. J. Urol.* 44:368, 1972.

50. Martin, C.M., and Bookrajian, E.N. Bacteriuria prevention after indwelling urinary catheterization. *Arch. Intern. Med.* 110:703, 1962.

51. Mattingly, R.F., Moore, D.E., and Clark, D.O. Bacteriologic study of suprapubic bladder drainage. *Am. J. Obstet. Gynecol.* 114:732, 1972.

52. McLean, R., Nickel, J.C., Noakes, V.C., and Costerton, J.W. An in vitro ultrastructural study of infectious kidney stone genesis. *Infect. Immun.* 49:805, 1985.

53. McNamara, M.J., et al. A study of bacteriologic patterns of hospital infections. *Ann. Intern. Med.* 66:486, 1967.

54. Merritt, J.L., Erickson, R.P., and Opitz, J.L. Bacteriuria during followup in patients with spinal cord injury: II. Efficacy of antimicrobial suppressants. *Arch. Phys. Med. Rehabil.* 63:413, 1982.

55. Merritt, J.L., and Keys, T.F. Limitations of the antibody-coated bacteria test in patients with neurogenic bladders. *J.A.M.A.* 247:1723, 1982.

56. Milles, G. Catheter-induced hemorrhagic pseudopolyps of the urinary bladder. *J.A.M.A.* 193:196, 1965.

57. Mobley, H.L.T., et al. MR/K hemagglutination of *Providencia stuartii* correlates with catheter adherence and with persistence in catheter-associated bacteriuria. *J. Infect. Dis.* 157:264, 1988.

58. Mobley, H.L.T., and Warren, J.W. Urease-positive bacteriuria and obstruction of long-term urinary catheters. *J. Clin. Microbiol.* 25:2216, 1987.

59. Mobley, H.L.T., and Warren, J.W. Urease-positive bacteriuria and obstruction of long-term urinary catheters. *J. Clin. Microbiol.* 25: 2216, 1987.

60. Moody, M.L., and Burke, J.P. Infections and antibiotic use in a large private hospital. *Arch. Intern. Med.* 130:261, 1972.

61. Mooney, B.R., Garibaldi, R.A., and Britt, M.R. Natural History of Catheter-Associated Bacteriuria (Colonization, Infection, Bacteremia): Implication for Prevention. In: J.D. Nelson and C. Grassi (Eds.), *Current Chemotherapy and Infectious Diseases,* Vol. 2. Washington, DC: American Society of Microbiology, 1980. Pp. 1083–1084.

62. Musher, D.M., Thorsteinsson, S.B., and Airola, V.M. Quantitative urinalysis. Diagnosing urinary tract infection in men. *J.A.M.A.* 236:2069, 1976.

63. Nickel, J.C., Grant, S.K., and Costerton, J.W. Catheter-associated bacteriuria, an experimental study. *Urology* 26:369, 1985.

64. Nickel, J.C., Gristina, P., Costerton, J.W. Electron miscoscopic study of an infected Foley catheter. *Can. J. Surg.* 28:50, 1985.

65. Pinner, R.W., et al. High cost nosocomial infections. *Infect. Control* 3:143, 1982.

66. Platt, R., Polk, B.F., Murdock, B., and Rosner, B. Mortality associated with nosocomial urinary tract infection. *N. Engl. J. Med.* 307:637, 1982.

67. Platt, R., Murdock, B., Polk, B.F., and Rosner, B. Reduction of mortality associated with nosocomial urinary tract infection. *Lancet* 1:1893, 1983.

68. Platt, R., Polk, B.F., Murdock, B., and Rosner, B. Risk factors for nosocomial urinary tract infection. *Am. J. Epidemiol.* 124:977, 1986.

69. Sarubbi, F.A., Rutala, W.A., and Samsa, G. Hydrogen peroxide instillations into the urinary drainage bag: Should we or shouldn't we? *Am. J. Infect. Control* 10:72, 1982.

70. Schaberg, D.R., et al. Nosocomial bacteriuria: A prospective study of case clustering and antimicrobial resistance. *Ann. Intern. Med.* 93:420, 1980.

71. Schaberg, D.R., Weinstein, R.A., and Stamm, W.E. Epidemics of nosocomial urinary tract infection caused by multiply resistant gram-negative bacilli: Epidemiology and control. *J. Infect. Dis.* 133:363, 1976.

72. Schaeffer, A.J. Catheter-associated bacteriuria. *Urol. Clin. North Am.* 4:735, 1986.

73. Schaeffer, A.J., Stony, K.O., and Johnson, S.M. Effect of silver oxide/trichloroisocyanuric acid antimicrobial urinary drainage system on catheter-associated bacteriuria. *J. Urol.* 139:69, 1988.

74. Sobel, J.D., and Kaye, D. Host factors in the pathogenesis of urinary tract infection. *Am. J. Med.* 76 (Suppl.): 122, 1984.

75. Stamey, T.A., et al. Recurrent urinary infection in adult women: The role of introital enterobacteria. *Calif. Med.* 155:1, 1971.

76. Stamm, W.E. Guidelines for prevention of catheter-associated urinary tract infections. *Ann. Intern. Med.* 82:386, 1975.

77. Stamm, W.E. Measurement of pyuria and its relationship to bacteriuria. *Am. J. Med.* 75 (Suppl.): 53, 1983.

78. Stamm, W.E. Recent developments in the diagnosis and treatment of urinary tract infections. *West. J. Med.* 137:213, 1982.

79. Stamm, W.E., et al. Urinary tract infections: From pathogenesis to treatment. *J. Infect. Dis.* 159:400, 1989.

80. Stamm, W.E., Martin, S.M., and Bennett, J.V. Epidemiology of nosocomial infections due to gram-negative bacilli: Aspects relevant to development and use of vaccines. *J. Infect. Dis.* 136S(Suppl.): S151, 1977.

81. Stamm, W.E., Weinstein, R.A., and Dixon, R.E. Comparison of endemic and epidemic nosocomial infections. *Am. J. Med.* 70:393, 1981.

82. Stark, R.P., and Maki, D.G. Bacteriuria in the catheterized patient. What quantitative level of bacteriuria is relevant? *N. Engl. J. Med.* 311:560, 1984.

83. Steere, A.C., Stamm, W.E., Martin, S.M., and Bennett, J.V. Gram-negative Rod Bacteremia. In: J.V. Bennett and P.S. Brachman (Eds.), *Hospital Infections.* Boston: Little, Brown, 1979. Pp. 507–518.

84. Sullivan, N.M., et al. Clinical aspects of bacteremia after manipulation of the genitourinary tract. *J. Infect. Dis.* 127:49, 1973.

85. Sweet, D.E., et al. Evaluation of H_2O_2 prophylaxis of bacteriuria in patients with long-term indwelling Foley catheters: A randomized controlled study. *Infect. Control* 6:263, 1985.

86. Thompson, R.L., et al. *Effect of Periodic Instillation of Hydrogen Peroxide (H_2O_2) into Urinary Drainage Systems in the Prevention of Catheter-Associated Bacteriuria.* Program and Abstracts of the Twenty-Second Interscience Conference on Antimicrobial Agents and Chemotherapy, October 4–6, 1982, No. 769. Washington, DC: American Society of Microbiology, 1982.

87. Thorley, J.D., Barbin, G.K., and Reinarz, J.A. The prevalence of antibody-coated bacteria in urine. *Am. J. Med. Sci.* 275:75, 1978.

88. Thornton, G.F., and Andriole, V.T. Bacteriuria during indwelling catheter drainage: II. Effect of a closed sterile drainage system. *J.A.M.A.* 214:339, 1970.

89. Turck, M., Goffee, B., and Petersdorf, R.G. The urethral catheter and urinary tract infection. *J. Urol.* 88:834, 1962.

90. Turck, M., and Stamm, W.E. Nosocomial infection of the urinary tract. *Am. J. Med.* 70: 651, 1981.

91. Vainrub, B., and Musher, D.M. Lack of effect of methanimine in suppression of or prophylaxis against chronic urinary infections. *Antimicrob. Agents Chemother.* 12:625, 1977.

92. van Dventer, S.J.H., et al. Endotoxemia, Bacteria, and Urosepsis. In: *Bacterial Endotoxins: Pathophysiological Effects, Clinical Significance, and Pharmacological Control.* London: Alan R. Liss, 1988. Pp. 213–224.

93. Vollaard, E.J., et al. Prevention of catheter associated Gram-negative bacilluria with norfloxacin by selective decontamination of the bowel and high urinary concentration. *J. Antimicrob. Chemother.* 23:915, 1989.

94. Warren, J.W. Catheter-associated urinary tract infections. *Infect. Dis. Clin. North Am.* 1:823, 1987.

95. Warren, J.W., Anthony, W.C., Hoopes, J.M., and Muncie, H.L. Cephalexin or susceptible bacteriuria in afebrile, long-term catheterized patients. *J.A.M.A.* 248:454, 1982.

96. Warren, J.W., et al. Antibiotic irrigation and catheter-associated urinary tract infections. *N. Engl. J. Med.* 299:570, 1978.

97. Warren, J.W., et al. A prospective microbiologic study of bacteriuria in patients with chronic indwelling urethral catheters. *J. Infect. Dis.* 146:719, 1982.

98. Warren, J.W., Muncie, H.L., Bergquist, E.J., and Hoopes, J.M. Sequelae and management of urinary tract infection in the patient requiring chronic catheterization. *J. Urol.* 125: 1, 1981.

99. Wenzel, R.P., Osterman, C.A., and Hunting, K.J. Hospital-acquired infections: I. Infection rates by site, service, and common procedures in a university hospital. *Am. J. Epidemiol.* 104:645, 1976.

100. Winterbauer, R.H. Turck, M., and Petersdorf, R.G. Studies on the epidemiology of *E. coli* infections: V. Factors influencing acquisition of specific serologic groups. *J. Clin. Invest.* 46:21, 1967.

101. Wong, E.S., and Hooton, T.M. Guidelines for prevention of catheter-associated urinary tract infections. *Infect. Control* 2:125, 1982.

Lower Respiratory Tract Infections

F. Marc LaForce

Hospital-acquired pneumonia is defined as a lower respiratory tract infection which was neither present nor incubating on admission. These serious infections are largely confined to patients recovering from thoracic or abdominal surgery, to patients requiring ventilatory support for respiratory insufficiency, and to patients recovering from a community-acquired pneumonia [13, 21, 37, 49]. The clinical criteria used to establish the diagnosis vary with different studies, but most investigators have used four measures to establish the diagnosis as definite or probable: (1) radiographic appearance of a new or progressive infiltrate, (2) fever, (3) leukocytosis, and (4) presence of purulent tracheobronchial secretions. Presence of all four criteria allows for a definite diagnosis, whereas presence of three criteria allows for the diagnosis of a probable infection [45]. A good working rule is to consider the diagnosis in a patient who has been hospitalized for more than 72 hours, although most nosocomial pneumonias occur after 7 days of hospitalization.

Nosocomial pneumonia is particularly important because of the formidable mortality reported with these infections and the general refractoriness of these infections to further reductions in attack rates [49]. One important, although not well studied, issue is an assessment of the proportion of fatal nosocomial pneumonias that are truly preventable and what fraction represent an inexorable progression of irreversible disease. Gross and his associates [35] studied the impact of nosocomial infections on deaths at a university and a community hospital. In a series of 200 consecutive deaths, there were 88 nosocomial infections in 63 patients. Deaths in 52 of 63 of these patients were believed to be directly attributable to nosocomial infections. Lower respiratory infections made up 31 of these fatal infections or 15.5 percent of all the deaths in this series. These authors also noted that two-thirds of the patients who died during hospitalization had been classified on admission as having a disease likely to end fatally in 6 months. Gross and Van Antwerpen [36] then matched each of 100 fatal cases from the community hospital to a survivor, using age, type, and severity of disease as matching criteria. They examined the impact of nosocomial diseases on both groups. Nosocomial infections were found in one-third of the cases and in 11 percent of the controls. Not surprisingly, the case group consisted of a much higher fraction of patients whose condition was believed likely to end fatally within 6 months (76 percent versus 11 percent). Nonetheless, 11 of 24 patients who died but were not believed to have a terminal condition on admission had a nosocomial infection, and 7 of the 11 infections were pneumonias [36].

Bryan and Reynolds [11] evaluated 172 bacteremic episodes due to nosocomial pneumonia in Columbia, South Carolina, from 1977 to 1981. The overall mortality was 58 percent. In 59 patients, death was directly attributed to pneumonia, and nearly all of these patients had severe underlying disease. Only 4 of the 59 patients, 2 infants and 2 adults, lacked severe and irreversible disease. Most of these deaths were considered to be nonpreventable with currently available preventive and treatment modalities.

These data show that fatal nosocomial pneumonia occurs predominantly in the very ill and in patients noted to be suffering from a terminal condition at the time of admission. However, nosocomial pneumonia seems to play an important role in patients who are expected to survive their hospitalization but who die. Better prospective studies are needed to answer the question of preventability and how many lives might be realistically saved. It is likely that most of the nosocomial pneumonias that are preventable are those occurring in surgical intensive care units and that control activities in these units ought to be emphasized in the hope that more focused interventions may be more productive.

Incidence

Nosocomial pneumonias account for nearly 20 percent of all nosocomial infections [13, 37]. Surveillance data from the National Nosocomial Infections Surveillance (NNIS) System (discussed in Chap. 27) are particularly helpful because they are based on a standard data collection system begun in 1970. It is important to note that 61 percent of the hospitals in the NNIS network are teaching hospitals. Patients who are at higher risk of developing nosocomial pneumonia are concentrated in these hospitals, and their nosocomial infection rates tend to be higher. Thoracic and upper abdominal surgery are important risk factors, and the explosion in coronary bypass surgery has significantly increased the pool of patients at risk. In 1986, 250,000 coronary bypass operations were done, as compared to 114,000 in 1978.

From 1970 to 1984, the incidence of nosocomial lower respiratory tract infections has increased by almost 40 percent: In 1970, there were 4.3 such infections per 1,000 hospital discharges, 5.1 in 1980–1982, and 6.0 in 1984 [13]. For the first time, in 1984, nosocomial pneumonias in the NNIS network hospitals were more common than postoperative wound infections [13]. Table 29-1 summarizes the 1984 NNIS data for lower respiratory tract infections by teaching status for medical and surgical services. Incidence rates in large teaching hospitals are more than twice the rates in community hospitals [13].

These infections are not evenly distributed

Table 29-1. Nosocomial lower respiratory tract infection rates, 1984 (cases/1,000 discharges)

Hospital category	Infection rate		
	Medicine	Surgery	Total
Nonteaching	5.2	5.4	3.6
Small teaching	7.5	7.8	5.4
Large teaching	10.2	11.2	7.7

Source: Data from the National Nosocomial Infections Surveillance System, as reported by the Centers for Disease Control, *CDC Surveillance Summaries*, Vol. 35, 1986. Pp. 17SS–29SS.

among clinical services, with approximately 80 percent of nosocomial pneumonias occurring on medical and surgical services. Because of the importance of respiratory tract instrumentation as a risk factor for nosocomial pneumonia, cases tend to cluster in intensive care units [18]. Hence, smaller hospitals with moderately active surgical services will not consider nosocomial pneumonia a major problem, whereas the reverse is often true in many tertiary care institutions with active cardiothoracic and transplantation units.

Microbiologic Features

Table 29-2 lists the most frequently isolated pathogens in patients with nosocomial pneumonia. These data are taken from the NNIS 1984 information base and have been fairly consistent for several years [13]. The most important pathogens are aerobic gram-negative rods, which make up 55 percent of all isolates. Gram-positive organisms are less important, and only *Staphylococcus aureus* and *Streptococcus pneumoniae* occur with enough frequency to be considered major pathogens.

Nosocomial pneumococcal pneumonia is reported from hospitals with high-risk patients. Most of the published series of nosocomial pneumococcal bacteremia have originated from veterans' hospitals or large

Table 29-2. Most frequently isolated pathogens in nosocomial lower respiratory tract infections, 1984

Pathogen	Percent isolated
Staphylococcus aureus	12.9
Pseudomonas aeruginosa	16.9
Escherichia coli	6.4
Klebsiella species	11.6
Enterobacter species	9.4
Proteus species	4.2
Serratia species	5.8
Candida species	4.0
All others	28.8

Source: Data from the National Nosocomial Infections Surveillance System, as reported by the Centers for Disease Control, *CDC Surveillance Summaries,* Vol. 35, 1986. Pp. 17SS–29SS.

municipal medical centers, where nosocomial cases have comprised from 22 to 59 percent of these bacteremic pneumococcal infections [2, 61, 73]. These patients were, for the most part, on medical or long-term care services, and many suffered from chronic obstructive lung disease, alcoholism, and cancer. Such high-risk patients may also develop pneumonia due to *Hemophilus influenzae* and *Moraxella catarrhalis.* Among gram-positive organisms, the most important pathogen is *S. aureus,* which is most often isolated postoperatively or after viral infection.

Aerobic gram-negative rods make up the bulk of infecting pathogens in cases of nosocomial pneumonia. These organisms are generally of low virulence and, under appropriate circumstances, can proliferate extensively as colonizing organisms in the oropharynx and trachea. These organisms are robust and can be spread by direct contact or indirect contact by fomites. Lastly, they often show antibiotic resistance patterns commensurate with their isolation from a high-antibiotic-use environment.

Viruses tend to be underrepresented because they are not cultured frequently. In one teaching hospital, viruses accounted for at least 5 percent of nosocomial infections and one-third of hospital-acquired pediatric infections [93]. Respiratory viruses, including respiratory syncytial virus (RSV), influenza, parainfluenza, adenovirus, and rhinovirus, account for 70 percent of the nosocomial viral pathogens [33]. Viral infections in the hospital tend to mirror the activity of these agents in the community, and circulating viruses are regularly brought into the hospital environment where they can spread. Viral agents are more infectious than the usual bacterial pathogens, and illnesses may occur in any susceptible individual rather than preferentially infecting high-risk patients.

Pathophysiology

The pathophysiology of most nosocomial lower respiratory tract infections can be described as occurring in two phases. The first phase is that of colonization with aerobic gram-negative rods of either or both the oropharynx and the stomach; each of these bacterial reservoirs regularly spill some of their contents into the trachea. The second phase is the struggle between aspirated bacteria and intrapulmonary antibacterial defenses. Nosocomial pneumonia occurs when these defenses are incapable of neutralizing the challenges, and bacterial proliferation ensues. A schematic diagram of the interplay between these components is shown in Figure 29-1. Each of the components will be discussed separately, but it is important to remember that they are interconnected and that the development of colonization in one area of the body has an effect on the other.

The clinical significance of colonization is most clear when the incidence of nosocomial pneumonia is compared in colonized and uncolonized patients. Johanson and colleagues [45] showed that 85 percent of the patients who developed nosocomial pneumonia were colonized with gram-negative rods, whereas only 3 percent of the uncolonized patients developed hospital-acquired pneumonia.

Oropharyngeal Colonization

The oropharynx is a complicated bacterial ecosystem that, under normal circumstances, is very stable. Aerobic gram-negative rods are not often isolated from pharyngeal swabs taken from normal volunteers and, if present, occur in small numbers [43, 72]. Normal volunteers rapidly clear huge inoculums of Enterobacteriaceae from the pharynx after gargle challenge [51]. Salivary flow is an important defense mechanism, since an atropine-induced decrease in salivary flow is associated with decreased clearance of a technetium radiolabeled sulfur colloid with the same size characteristics as bacteria [52].

Bacterial interference is an important guarantor of stability in oropharyngeal flora. Viridans streptococci are known to be inhibitory to gram-negative rods. Sprunt and Redman [80] evaluated the role of inhibitory flora in persons receiving large doses of antibiotics. All 10 patients given penicillin and streptomycin prior to cardiac surgery became colonized with gram-negative rods, and there was a reciprocal relationship between α-streptococci and enteric bacilli. Within 10 days after the cessation of antibiotic therapy, oral flora of most patients had returned to normal, with disappearance of gram-negative rods. More recent studies have reconfirmed the validity of these observations [74]. Some oral anaerobes such as *Bacteroides melaninogenicus* are also known to inferfere with coliforms, but the overall role of oral anaerobes requires better definition [60]. Suffice it to say that high doses of antibiotics perturb normal mouth flora and are associated with increased colonization rates.

Despite these potent oral defense mechanisms, there are a variety of clinical conditions that appear to be associated with the phenomenon of oral colonization (Table 29-3). Alcoholics, diabetics, and persons with viral pharyngitis have higher colonization rates [30, 54, 68]. Colonization varies widely in the elderly, depending on their health at the time the culture is taken; colonization was noted in only 9 percent of elderly persons living independently, as compared to 60 percent in patients who were bedded on hospital wards. Multivariate analysis suggested that respiratory disease and a bedridden existence

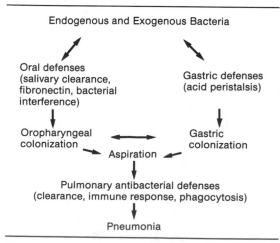

Endogenous and Exogenous Bacteria

Oral defenses
(salivary clearance, fibronectin, bacterial interference)

Gastric defenses
(acid peristalsis)

Oropharyngeal colonization ⟷ Gastric colonization

Aspiration

Pulmonary antibacterial defenses
(clearance, immune response, phagocytosis)

Pneumonia

Fig. 29-1. Pathogenesis of nosocomial pneumonia.

Table 29-3. Oropharyngeal colonization rates with aerobic gram-negative rods

Population	Number cultured	Number positive	Positive rate (%)	Reference
Normal subjects	82	2	2	[43]
Clinic patients	100	18	18	[72]
Alcoholics	25	12	48	[30]
Diabetics	33	13	39	[54]
Viral pharyngitis	82	38	46	[68]
Hospitalized				
Moderately ill	81	26	32	[43]
Moribund	23	16	70	[43]
Medical intensive care unit	213	95	45	[45]
Elderly				
Independent	48	3	6	[95]
Skilled nursing facility	223	50	22	[95]
Hospital ward	25	10	40	[95]

were the two most important variables in predicting colonization [95].

Adherence Studies

As summarized earlier, many descriptive studies have demonstrated that local conditions in the oropharynx can change such that gram-negative rods that are unable to establish themselves as successful colonizers under normal conditions may become highly successful. A great deal of effort has been expended in trying to understand the mechanisms whereby this change can occur. Fortunately, this research question was posed at a time when the general phenomenon of bacterial colonization of mucosal surfaces was receiving much attention. Using in vitro models of adherence, several investigators have found that bacteria adhere to oral epithelial cells and that, in general, resident species adhere in greater numbers [7, 32].

Adherence of bacteria to mammalian epithelial cells was shown to be dependent on specific characteristics of the host cell and the bacterium. Bacterial cells are endowed with specific adhesions, principally located on surface appendages such as pili or fimbriae, which interact with epithelial cell surface receptors [7].

Johanson and his associates [44] first tested the hypothesis that a change in adherence characteristics of buccal epithelial cells would favor colonization with gram-negative rods. Of 32 patients undergoing surgery and followed prospectively, 11 became colonized postoperatively. Their buccal epithelial cells, when tested in vitro, were shown to accept more gram-negative rods than buccal cells from uncolonized patients. Intensive care unit patients were similarly studied and, in general, buccal cells from colonized patients showed greater in vitro adherence for *Pseudomonas aeruginosa* when compared to adherence characteristics of cells from uncolonized patients [46].

Fibronectin, a high-molecular-weight glycoprotein normally present on oral epithelial cells, has been shown to play an important role in the inhibition of adherence of gram-negative rods [96]. Immunofluorescence studies have shown that buccal epithelial cells that resist colonization with *P. aeruginosa* are positive for fibronectin. This glycoprotein is highly susceptible to proteases, and brief trypsin treatment of normal buccal epithelial cells in vitro decreased cell surface fibronectin at the same time it increased the ability of these treated cells to bind *Pseudomonas* organisms [101]. Fibronectin facilitates interaction with gram-positive bacteria, and loss of cell surface fibronectin has been correlated with increased gram-negative colonization in vivo [102]. Sixteen patients undergoing coronary bypass surgery were prospectively studied; 6

of them became colonized, and salivary samples from these patients were shown to have high elastase activity and the ability to degrade fibronectin [23]. Inhibition studies showed that the elastase activity likely originated from polymorphonuclear leukocytes. These data are consistent with the hypothesis that increased salivary elastase levels digest fibronectin and allow for the expression of gram-negative bacterial receptors, which facilitates the colonization of these cells with gram-negative rods. These results also allow for the intriguing possibility that colonization could be blocked by locally enhancing anti-elastase activity to preserve fibronectin coating of epithelial cells.

Gastric Colonization

A major development over the last decade has been the recognition of the role of the stomach as an important site for aerobic gram-negative rod colonization [16]. Gastric acidity is a built-in and highly effective antibacterial system which insures that stomach contents have low to absent bacterial counts. However, most patients who are in intensive care units now receive antacid or H_2 blocker therapy to prevent bleeding from superficial stress ulcers. Rates of gastric hemorrhage have been reduced but at the microbiologic price of regular colonization of the stomach with aerobic gram-negative rods. As gastric pH rises, the level of microbial contamination increases concomitantly. The stomach can then serve as an internal bacterial reservoir that is anatomically connected to the oropharynx and, by aspiration, to the lung itself.

Several studies have described concordance between bacteria found in stomach contents and those recovered from the trachea. Atherton and White [5] found the same organism in tracheal aspirate and stomach in 6 of 10 patients, with the organism having been noted first in gastric cultures one-half of the time. In a larger study, duMoulin and colleagues [27] cultured the same organism from the trachea and the stomach in 52 of 60 consecutive patients and, in 17 of these 52 patients, the organism appeared first in the gastric contents. In a study of 142 patients, Daschner and co-workers [24] showed that retrograde colonization from the stomach to the trachea occurred in one-third of the patients.

Enteral therapy has also been shown to be an important risk factor for oropharyngeal colonization. Enteral feeding solutions have a pH of between 6.4 and 7.0. Pingleton and associates [67] serially cultured the oropharynx, trachea, and stomach in patients admitted to a respiratory intensive care unit who were simultaneously being enterally fed. Gastric cultures were positive throughout the study. Tracheal colonization occurred in 16 of the 18 study patients; primary colonization occurred in 6 patients, whereas secondary tracheal colonization occurred in 10 patients. Definite or probable nosocomial pneumonia occurred in 11 of the 18 patients. This was an important study because tracheal, oropharyngeal, and gastric cultures were taken simultaneously and the colonization sequences could be accurately determined. The results unequivocally showed that tracheal colonization could occur as a primary event or, as was seen more frequently, could follow oropharyngeal or gastric colonization.

Role of Tracheal Intubation

Patients bedded in intensive care units are at the highest risk of developing nosocomial pneumonia. One important reason for this association is the extent of respiratory instrumentation in these patients [22, 37]. All studies of nosocomial pneumonia in intensive care units have noted a positive relationship between the length of tracheal intubation and the risk of infection. Constant movement of the low pressure cuff allows secretions between the cuff and the wall of the trachea to be massaged toward the lungs [74]. This accounts for the concordance between oropharyngeal and tracheal flora in intubated patients. Additionally, intubation of the patient largely eliminates aerodynamic filtration as a pulmonary defense against aerosolized particles measuring greater than 10 μm in diameter. Almost all such patients have nasogastric tubes for nutritional support. Nasogastric tubes provide a conduit by which bacteria may migrate to and from the oropharynx [67].

Aspiration

Colonization of the stomach or oropharynx with aerobic gram-negative rods creates a precarious clinical situation in which the lungs are at constant risk of being soiled by these organisms. Aspiration occurs frequently and is universal in intubated patients because of the continuity of oropharyngeal and tracheal secretions. The sequential colonization studies that were previously cited offer indirect yet strong evidence consistent with the universality of aspiration in such patients [5, 27, 45, 67]. Direct evidence for the frequency of aspiration has come from the use of dye or radiolabel markers to monitor aspiration events: At least 70 percent of patients with impaired consciousness aspirate oropharyngeal contents during sleep, as do 50 percent of control patients [41].

Clinical Manifestations
Risk Factors

Common risk factors associated with nosocomial pneumonia are as follows:

Intubation
Presence in intensive care unit
Treatment for pneumonia
Thoracic or abdominal surgery
Advanced age
Chronic cardiopulmonary disease
Immunosuppression

One-half of all nosocomial pneumonias occur after surgery. Garibaldi and colleagues [31] prospectively followed 520 patients after thoracic or abdominal surgery, and 91 patients (17.5 percent) developed pneumonia. Preoperative markers of the severity of underlying disease, such as a low serum albumin or classification of high risk by the anesthesiologist, were strongly associated with pneumonia. Length of preoperative stay, duration

of surgery, and thoracic or upper abdominal sites of surgery were also significantly associated. Just as importantly, this study identified individuals who were at low risk for nosocomial pulmonary infection; factors associated with low risk were short duration of surgery, lower abdominal operation, normal preoperative serum albumin, and no history of smoking. Pulmonary infiltrates in these patients would then suggest diseases other than pneumonia.

Treatment of a community-acquired pneumonia is also an important risk factor, because antibiotic treatment facilitates colonization and because many of these patients have severely compromised pulmonary antibacterial defenses. In one report, 59 percent of 149 hospitalized patients treated for pneumonia with narrow-spectrum antibiotics (e.g., penicillin or erythromycin) eventually became colonized with either staphylococci or gram-negative enteric bacilli in the respiratory tract [88]. Of this group, 16 percent developed actual superinfection with these potential pathogens.

Clinical Evaluation

From the clinician's standpoint, the diagnosis of nosocomial pneumonia is first considered when a high-risk patient develops fever and a new or worsening infiltrate on the chest roentgenogram. However, many other conditions, such as congestive heart failure, pulmonary emboli, cancer, and atelectasis, can also present in this fashion and should be considered as diagnostic possibilities. An orderly clinical and laboratory evaluation is necessary, realizing that the rather ominous prognosis associated with nosocomial pneumonia will necessitate prompt treatment with broad-spectrum agents.

The diagnosis of nosocomial pneumonia can be made with confidence in a febrile postoperative patient with a new pulmonary infiltrate, an increase in leukocyte count, and a sputum smear showing abundant gram-negative rods and polymorphonuclear leukocytes. Frequently, patients fall into less certain categories. Congestive heart failure, atelectasis, and pulmonary embolism may all confuse the clinical picture. Elderly and immunosuppressed patients often do not manifest the classic signs of infection seen in younger patients. Further, the isolation of potential bacterial pathogens from sputum or endotracheal aspirate cultures in the absence of positive blood cultures often cannot differentiate between colonization and infection. Not infrequently, the diagnosis remains unclear, and patients are treated empirically. This is particularly true in granulocytopenic patients, for whom a delay in therapy may be fatal.

The physical examination should concentrate on evaluating the overall status of cardiopulmonary function (vital signs, cardiac and pulmonary examination), assessing oxygenation (skin color, mentation), and examining for other major organ dysfunction and evidence of metastatic infection.

A chest roentgenogram, with particular attention paid to the presence of pleural effusions, complete blood cell count, and blood gases should be obtained as soon as possible. Examination and culture of sputum and pleural effusions, if present, should be done. Blood cultures should always be taken. Many of these patients are intubated and so access to respiratory secretions is simple. However, confusion between colonization and infection often clouds the results of sputum or bronchial aspirate cultures. The need to use more invasive diagnostic procedures such as bronchoscopy and bronchoalveolar lavage is greatest in immunosuppressed patients or in patients with chronic pneumonia that may be of infectious or noninfectious etiology. The tendency to delay such procedures should be avoided; in general, once proposed, they ought to be done. Vigorous efforts should be expended in identifying an etiologic agent so that sensitivity studies on these recovered organisms can help direct antimicrobial therapy.

Therapy

Empiric therapy for pneumonia in the hospitalized patient must consider the level and type of imunosuppression of the patient to be

treated, resistance patterns of hospital flora, and severity of illness. Initial empiric therapy in the absence of a specific bacterial isolate should be broad enough to encompass *Klebsiella, E. coli, S. aureus, P. aeruginosa,* and *Enterobacter, Proteus,* and *Serratia* species, which account for approximately 70 percent of nosocomial lower respiratory tract infections [13]. If cultures of sputum, endotracheal aspirate, blood, or invasively obtained materials reveal pure or predominant growth of a pathogen, specific therapy can be instituted. More often, however, sputum Gram stains are nondiagnostic, and cultures are pending, nondiagnostic, or yield mixed flora. Local antimicrobial resistance patterns are important, and what may be appropriate antibacterial therapy in a community hospital may be ineffective in the setting of a large referral center.

For the most part, empiric therapy is straightforward. The most likely organisms (Table 29-2) must be covered, with particular attention paid to local resistance patterns. Gram-positive infections are treated with semisynthetic penicillins or cephalosporins. If chronic lung disease is present, antibiotic coverage for *H. influenzae* should also be included.

Aminoglycosides plus a cephalosporin or a broad-spectrum penicillin have been a cornerstone of therapy for nosocomial pneumonia. There are data suggesting that synergistic antimicrobial combinations give a better therapeutic result when treating gram-negative infections. Sculier and Klastersky [76] reviewed records of 79 bacteremic patients (30 with granulocytopenia) in whom serum bactericidal studies had been performed. Among patients with normal granulocyte counts, a peak serum bactericidal titer below 1:8 was associated with clinical failure in all patients, but serum bactericidal titers of 1:8 or more were associated with clinical success in 98 percent. In granulocytopenic patients, a peak serum bactericidal titer of 1:8 or less was associated with failure in 83 percent, and a peak serum bactericidal titer of 1:16 or more was associated with clinical success in 87 percent. There were 9 patients with bacteremic pneumonia in this study. One was granulocytopenic and responded (mean serum bactericidal titer, $1:32$). Eight were not granulocytopenic; there were 5 responders, with a mean serum bactericidal titer of $1:32$, and 3 nonresponders, all with serum bactericidal titers of $1:4$. The 3 clinical failures involved single isolates of *Klebsiella, Proteus,* and *Pseudomonas* species that were resistant to the β-lactam antibiotics being used in the study.

These data are consistent with an increasingly persuasive body of literature that correlates serum bactericidal levels to clinical cures, particularly in more difficult infections such as bacterial endocarditis [98]. Further studies should be done to confirm the relationship between successful clinical outcome and a given serum bactericidal activity. If these studies are consistent with the data of Sculier and Klastersky [76], measurement of serum bactericidal activity might constitute a useful clinical marker for the treatment of nosocomial pneumonia.

It seems intuitive that successful treatment of a lower respiratory tract infection would depend on the ability of an antibiotic given systemically to penetrate to alveolar and bronchial sites [9]. There are major differences in the ability of antibiotics to penetrate into pulmonary secretions. For example, pulmonary secretions are 10 to 45 percent of simultaneously measured serum aminoglycoside levels. Because of the relatively narrow therapeutic to toxic ratio of aminoglycosides, the fractional penetration may result in respiratory tract levels that are low in relation to the minimal inhibitory concentration (MIC) of most Enterobacteriaceae [65]. This explanation has been proposed as a reason for the rather poor results in treating gram-negative pneumonias. Respiratory tract levels of third-generation cephalosporins are approximately 30 percent of serum levels. A prospective study that compares antibiotic concentrations or bactericidal activity in blood and respiratory secretions to clinical outcome still remains to be done. Until these data are available, it is difficult to make specific comments as to the importance of intrabronchial penetration of antibiotics and the success of systemic treatment of nosocomial pneumonia.

Moore and co-workers [55] have made an important observation regarding blood levels of aminoglycosides and successful treatment of pneumonia. Reviewing their data from several randomized controlled studies, these investigators compared clinical outcome with 1-hour postinfusion levels of gentamicin, tobramycin, and amikacin. Patients with mean peak levels of 7 μg/ml or greater for gentamicin or tobramycin or 28 μg/ml for amikacin more often had successful outcomes (78 percent) than those with lower levels (32 percent). Similar results were noted by Cipolle and co-workers [15], who documented an 88 percent success rate with tobramycin in the treatment of lower respiratory tract *Pseudomonas* infections. The mean peak tobramycin level in the study was 7.9 μg/ml. These data are in contrast to several studies that describe combination therapy to treat nosocomial pneumonia but have aimed at aminoglycoside levels approximately 20 percent lower than the levels reported in the previously cited studies.

In recent years, several broad-spectrum antibiotics have been introduced that have excellent activity against many of the organisms capable of causing nosocomial pneumonia. These agents have introduced the real possibility of monotherapy for treating such infections [50]. For example, the aminothiazoxyl penicillins are very active against a wide variety of aerobic gram-negative rods and have the major advantage of being less toxic than aminoglycosides. Agents such as ceftazidime and cefoperazone, when used as monotherapy, have shown serum bactericidal levels exceeding those obtained with standard synergistic combinations against bacteria isolated from patients with nosocomial pneumonias. Results from controlled clinical trials show that monotherapy is at least as good as combination therapy in nongranulocytopenic patients. Table 29-4 summarizes treatment

Table 29-4.   Treatment of nosocomial pneumonia in nongranulocytopenic patients by bacterial isolate

Organism	Drugs of choice
No organism (cultures pending)	Ceftazidime, cefoperazone, or aztreonam
Escherichia coli	Ceftazidime, cefoperazone, or aztreonam
Klebsiella species	Ceftazidime, cefoperazone, or aztreonam
Enterobacter species	Ceftazidime, cefoperazone, or aztreonam *plus* aminoglycoside
Serratia species	Ceftazidime, cefoperazone, or aztreonam *plus* aminoglycoside
Pseudomonas aeruginosa	Antipseudomonas penicillin, ceftazidime, cefoperazone, or aztreonam *plus* tobramycin

Source: From F.M. LaForce, Systemic antimicrobial therapy of nosocomial pneumonia: Monotherapy versus combination therapy. *Eur. J. Clin. Microbiol.* 8:61, 1989.

regimens according to bacterial species. Until better studies are available, granulocytopenic patients with hospital-acquired pneumonia should receive combination therapy.

Control Measures
Centers for Disease Control Recommendations

In 1982, the Centers for Disease Control (CDC) developed guidelines for the prevention of nosocomial pneumonia [79]. These recommendations have proved to be a useful template for Infection Control Committees and intensive care unit personnel. The procedure followed to arrive at the recommendations was a modified Delphi technique, whereby a draft of recommendations was prepared and widely circulated to experts who categorized each recommendation or statement according to a ranking scheme presented in Table 29-5. A smaller group then met to discuss the specific recommendations, which were then published and are reproduced here as Table 29-6.

Table 29-5.   Ranking scheme for recommendations

Category I: Strongly recommended for adoption* Measures in category I are strongly supported by well-designed and controlled clinical studies that show effectiveness in reducing the risk of nosocomial infections or are viewed as useful by the majority of experts in the field. Measures in this category are judged to be applicable to the majority of hospitals regardless of size, patient population, or endemic nosocomial infection rate, and are considered practical to implement.

Category II: Moderately recommended for adoption Measures in category II are supported by highly suggestive clinical studies or by definitive studies in institutions that might not be representative of other hospitals. Measures that have not been adequately studied but have a strong theoretical rationale indicating that they might be very effective are included in this category. Category II measures are judged to be practical to implement. They are not to be considered a standard of practice for every hospital.

Category III: Weakly recommended for adoption Measures in category III have been proposed by some investigators, authorities, or organizations but, to date, lack both supporting data and a strong theoretical rationale. Thus they might be considered important issues that require additional evaluation; they might be considered by some hospitals for implementation, expecially if such hospitals have specific nosocomial infection problems or sufficient resources.

*Recommendations that advise against the adoption of certain measures can be found in the guidelines in Table 29-6. These negative recommendations are also ranked into one of the three categories depending on the strength of the scientific backing or opinions of the members of the working group. A negative recommendation in category I means that scientific data or prevailing opinion strongly indicates that the measure not be adopted. A negative recommendation in category III means that, given the available information, the measure under consideration should probably not be adopted; such a measure, however, requires additional evaluation. Source: B.P. Simmons and E.S. Wong, CDC guidelines for the prevention and control of nosocomial pneumonia. *Am. J. Infect. Control* 11:230, 1983.

Respiratory Equipment
Gases used in respiratory devices are free of water vapor, and their continuous use would result in dessication of the airways. Therefore, increasing the water vapor in inspired

Table 29-6. CDC guidelines for prevention of nosocomial pneumonia: recommendations

1. Perioperative measures for prevention of postoperative pneumonia
   a. Patients who will receive anesthesia and will have an abdominal or thoracic operation or who have substantial pulmonary dysfunction, such as patients with chronic obstructive lung disease, a musculoskeletal abnormality of the chest, or abnormal pulmonary function tests, should receive preoperative and postoperative therapy and instruction designed to prevent postoperative pulmonary complications such as pneumonia. The therapy and instruction, which are recommended below in *b* through *g*, should be given by a person trained to administer them. *Category I*[a]
   b. Whenever appropriate, preoperative therapy should include treatment and resolution of pulmonary infections, efforts to facilitate removal of respiratory secretions (e.g., by use of bronchodilators and postural drainage and percussion), and discontinuance of smoking by the patient. *Category I*
   c. Preoperative instruction should include discussions of the importance in the postoperative period of frequent coughing, taking deep breaths, and ambulating (as soon as medically indicated). During the discussions, the patient should demonstrate and practice adequate coughing and deep breathing. *Category I*
   d. An incentive spirometer should be used for preoperative instruction in deep breathing and for postoperative care. *Category III*
   e. Postoperative therapy and instructions should be designed to encourage frequent coughing, deep breathing and, unless medically contraindicated, moving about in the bed and ambulating. *Category I*
   f. If conservative measures (mentioned in *e* above) do not remove retained pulmonary secretions, postural drainage and percussion should be done to assist the patient in expectorating sputum. *Category II*
   g. Pain that interferes with coughing and deep breathing should be controlled, for example, by use of analgesics, appropriate wound support for abdominal wounds (such as placing a pillow tightly across the abdomen), and regional nerve blocks. *Category I* (Caution: Narcotics may reduce the urge to cough and breathe deeply.)
   h. Systemic antibiotics should not be routinely used to prevent postoperative pneumonia. *Category I* (Caution: This recommendation may be reevaluated in light of recent publications on the strategy of selective decontamination to prevent nosocomial pneumonias.)
2. Hand-washing
   Hands should be washed after contact with respiratory secretions, whether or not gloves are worn. Hands should be washed before and after contact with a patient who is intubated or has had a recent tracheostomy. (See CDC Guidelines on Infection Control. *Guidelines for Hospital Environmental Control: Antiseptics, Handwashing, and Handwashing Facilities, 1985.* Hospital Infections Program, Center for Infectious Diseases, CDC, Atlanta, GA.) *Category I*
3. Fluids and medications
   a. (1) Only sterile fluids should be nebulized or used in a humidifier. These fluids should be dispensed aseptically; that is, contaminated equipment should not be allowed to enter or touch the fluid while it is being dispensed. *Category I*
      (2) After a large container (bottle) of fluid intended for use in a nebulizer or humidifier has been opened, unused fluid should be discarded within 24 hours. *Category II*
   b. Either single-dose or multidose vials can be used for respiratory therapy. If multidose vials are used, they should be stored (refrigerated or at room temperature) according to directions on the vial label or package insert. Vials should be used no longer than the expiration date given on the label. *Category II*
4. Maintenance of in-use respiratory therapy equipment
   a. (1) Fluid reservoirs should be filled immediately before—but not far in advance of—use. Fluid should not be added to replenish partially filled reservoirs; that is, if fluid is to be added, the residual fluid should first be discarded. *Category II*
      (2) Water that has condensed in tubing should be discarded and not allowed to drain back into the reservoir. *Category I*
   b. (1) Venturi wall nebulizers and their reservoirs should be routinely changed and replaced with sterilized or disinfected ones every 24 hours. *Category I*
      (2) Other nebulizers (including medication nebulizers) and their reservoirs and cascade (high-volume) humidifiers and their reservoirs should be changed and replaced with sterilized or disinfected ones every 24 hours. *Category II*

Table 29-6.   (*continued*)

(3) Room air humidifiers that create droplets to humidify (and thus are really nebulizers) should not be used. *Category I*

c.   Reusable humidifier reservoirs for use with wall oxygen outlets should be cleaned, rinsed out, and then dried daily. *Category II* (Disposable reservoirs for use with wall oxygen outlets may be safe for long periods, and it is not known whether these need to be routinely changed before they are empty.)

d.   The tubing (including any nasal prongs) and any mask used to deliver oxygen from a wall outlet should be changed between patients. *Category I*

e.   Breathing circuits (including tubing and exhalation valve) should be routinely changed and replaced with sterilized or disinfected ones every 24 hours. *Category II* (Caution: New data [17] suggest that tubing need only be replaced every 48 hours.)

f.   When a respiratory therapy machine is used to treat multiple patients, the breathing circuit should be changed between patients and replaced with a sterilized or disinfected one. *Category II*

5. Disposable equipment
   No pieces of respiratory therapy equipment that are designed for single use (disposable) should be reused. *Category I*

6. Processing reusable equipment (See also CDC Guidelines on Infection Control. *Guideline for Hospital Environmental Control: Cleaning, Disinfection, and Sterilization of Hospital Equipment, 1985*. Hospital Infections Program, Center for Infectious Diseases, CDC, Atlanta, GA.)

a.   All equipment to be sterilized or disinfected should be thoroughly cleaned to remove all blood, tissue, food, or other residue. It should be decontaminated before or during cleaning if it is marked *contaminated* and received from patients in certain types of isolation. *Category I*

b.   Respiratory therapy equipment that touches mucous membranes should be sterilized before use on other patients; if this is not feasible, it should receive high-level disinfection. *Category I*

c.   Breathing circuits (including tubing and exhalation valves), medication nebulizers and their reservoirs, venturi wall nebulizers and their reservoirs, and cascade humidifiers and their reservoirs should be sterilized or receive high-level disinfection. *Category I*

d.   Since coolant chambers for ultrasonic nebulizers are difficult to disinfect adequately, these chambers should be gas-sterilized (ethylene oxide) or have at least 30 minutes of contact time with a high-level disinfectant. *Category I*

e.   The internal machinery of ventilators and breathing machines should not be routinely sterilized or disinfected between patients. *Category I* (Disinfection or sterilization may be necessary only after a machine is potentially contaminated by extremely dangerous agents, such as Lassa fever virus.)

f.   Respirometers and other equipment used to monitor several patients in succession should not directly touch parts of the breathing circuit. Rather, extension pieces should be used between the equipment and breathing circuit and should be changed between patients. If no extension piece is used and such monitoring equipment is directly connected to contaminated equipment, the monitoring equipment should be sterilized or receive high-level disinfection before use on other patients. *Category II*

g.   Once they have been used for one patient, hand-powered resuscitation bags (e.g., Ambu[b] bags) should be sterilized or receive high-level disinfection before use on other patients. *Category I* (There are no data to suggest that these bags need to be changed routinely during use on one patient.)

7. Microbiologic monitoring

a.   In the absence of an epidemic or high endemic rate of nosocomial pulmonary infections, the disinfection process for respiratory therapy equipment should not be monitored by cultures; that is, routine sampling of such equipment should not be done. *Category I* (This recommendation differs slightly from a previous CDC recommendation. See text of this guideline for a discussion of this recommendation).

b.   Because of the difficulty in interpreting results, routine microbiologic sampling of respiratory therapy equipment while it is being used by a patient is not recommended. *Category I*

8. Patients with tracheostomy

a.   Tracheostomy should be performed under aseptic conditions in an operating room, except when strong clinical indications for emergency or bedside operation intervene. *Category I*

b.   Until a recent tracheostomy wound has had time to heal or form granulation tissue around the tube, "no-touch" technique should be used or sterile gloves should be worn on both hands for all manipulations at the tracheostomy site. *Category II*

Table 29-6. *(continued)*

---

   c. (1) When a tracheostomy tube requires changing, a sterile tube or one that has received high-level disinfection should be used. *Category I*

     (2) Aseptic technique, including the use of sterile gloves and drapes, should be employed when a tube is changed. *Category II*

9. Suctioning of respiratory tract

   a. Risk of cross-contamination and excessive trauma increases with frequent suctioning. Thus suctioning should not be done routinely but only when needed to reduce substantial secretions, which may be indicated by increased respiratory difficulties or easily audible "gurgling" breathing sounds. *Category I*

   b. Suctioning should be performed using "no-touch" technique or gloves on both hands. *Category I* (Although fresh gloves should be used for each suctioning, sterile gloves are not needed.)

   c. A sterile catheter should be used for each series of suctioning (defined as a single suctioning or repeated suctioning done with only brief periods intervening to clear or flush the catheter). *Category I*

   d. If tenacious mucus is a problem and flushing of the catheter is required, sterile fluid should be used to remove secretions from it; fluid that becomes contaminated during use for one series of suctioning should then be discarded. *Category I*

   e. (1) Suction collection tubing (up to the canister) should always be changed between patients. *Category I*

     (2) Suction collection canisters when used on one patient need not be routinely changed or emptied. *Category III*

     (3) Unless used in short-term care units (recovery or emergency rooms), suction collection canisters should be changed between use on different patients. *Category II*

     (4) If used in short-term care units, suction collection canisters need not be changed between patients but should be changed daily. *Category III*

     (5) Once they are changed, reusable suction collection canisters should be sterilized or receive high-level disinfection. *Category II*

   f. With portable suction devices, which may discharge contaminated aerosols, high-efficiency bacterial filters should be used between the collection bottle and vacuum source. *Category III* (When used with wall suction units, such filters have not been shown to be useful for infection control.)

10. Protection of patients from other infected patients or staff

   a. Patients with potentially transmissible respiratory infections should be isolated according to the current edition of *Isolation Techniques for Use in Hospitals* [11a].[c] (This recommendation is not categorized.)

   b. Personnel with respiratory infections should not be assigned to the direct care of high-risk patients, for example, neonates, young infants, patients with chronic obstructive lung disease, or immunocompromised patients. *Category II*

   c. If an influenza epidemic is anticipated, a prevention program should be started for all patient care personnel and high-risk patients. This program could include use of influenza vaccine and antiviral chemoprophylaxis. *Category I*

---

[a] The reader is referred to Table 29-5 for an explanation of the ranking scheme of the various recommendations.
[b] Use of trade names is for identification only and does not constitute endorsement by the Public Health Service, U.S. Department of Health and Human Services.
[c] See also Chapter 11.
Source: From B.P. Simmons and E.S. Wong, CDC guidelines for the prevention of nosocomial pneumonia. *Am. J. Infect Control* 11:230, 1983.

gases is necessary. Humidification and nebulization are the two methods used to increase water vapor (Fig. 29-2). Nebulizers, when they become contaminated, have been unequivocally shown to increase the risk of nosocomial infection due to gram-negative rods [69]. Humidifiers are devices that saturate gas with water vapor, usually by bubbling gas through water; such devices are used in virtu-

ally all currently manufactured respiratory support equipment. They do not aerosolize bacteria and have not been implicated in the occurrence of nosocomial pneumonia.

Reservoir nebulizers easily become contaminated by endogenous secretions, residual fluid in respirator tubing, or personnel. Bacteria multiply within the reservoir fluid, which results in the generation of contami-

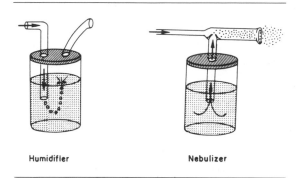

Humidifier   Nebulizer

Fig. 29-2. Differences in principles of operation of humidifiers and nebulizers. (Reprinted with permission from J.P. Sanford and A.K. Pierce. In P.S. Brachman and T.C. Eickhoff (Eds.), *Proceedings of the International Conference on Nosocomial Infections.* Chicago: American Hospital Association, 1971.)

nated aerosols. These aerosolized bacteria are capable of penetrating into the distal recesses of the lung where they can multiply. In the mid-1960s, clinical investigators in Dallas demonstrated the importance of contaminated reservoir nebulizers in the epidemiology of nosocomial lower respiratory tract infections [66, 69]. These researchers documented a significant increase in the incidence of necrotizing pneumonia in ventilator patients at a time when better than 80 percent of the nebulization equipment was contaminated with gram-negative rods. Routine acetic acid decontamination of respiratory equipment was begun in 1965, and by 1967 the incidence of necrotizing pneumonia had decreased to levels seen before the widespread use of inhalation equipment [66].

Small medication nebulizers can become contaminated and may produce small-particle bacterial aerosols capable of penetrating to the distal lung. Craven and colleagues [19] prospectively studied the microbiology of in-line medication nebulizers and found that 15 of 19 nebulizers were culture-positive, with 13 having bacterial colony counts greater than 10^4 organisms per milliliter. Quantitative studies of the aerosols that were generated by these nebulizers showed that some particles measuring less than 3.3 μm were generated and capable of penetrating to the distal lung. These nebulizers should be cleaned after every use, or a switch to dis-

posable medication nebulizers should be made.

The fluid in the respirator tubing frequently becomes contaminated, and it is important that this fluid not be allowed to drain into the patient as this could result in sudden soilage of the bronchopulmonary tree [20]. In general, these fluids ought to be drained out as they accumulate. Respirator tubing should be replaced regularly. Initial recommendations from the CDC suggested this should be done every 24 hours (Table 29-6, 4e), but a prospective study done at the Boston City Hospital showed that respirator tubing need not be changed more frequently than every 48 hours [17].

Preventing Gastric Colonization with Sucralfate

Sucralfate is an agent shown to be effective in preventing stress ulcer bleeding while not significantly altering gastric pH. In a controlled study, Driks and colleagues [26] found that 7 of 61 patients (12 percent) treated with sucralfate developed nosocomial pneumonia, as compared with 16 of 69 patients (23 percent) in the antacid-treated or cimetidine-treated group. Colonization with gram-negative rods was higher in the stomach, pharynx, and trachea of patients randomized to antacids or H_2 blockers compared to patients treated with sucralfate. Similar results were also noted in a randomized study of ventilator patients by Tryba [89], who documented nosocomial pneumonia in 3 of 29 patients (10 percent) treated with sucralfate, as compared to 11 of 34 patients (32 percent) treated with antacids.

These data are consistent with the hypothesis that low stomach pH plays an important role in helping to minimize the gastric bacterial burden and, in so doing, decreases tracheal soilage with aerobic gram-negative rods. Daschner and co-workers [24] have extended these observations by clearly showing in a prospective study of ventilated patients that the incidence of nosocomial pneumonia largely depended on the pH of gastric fluid; furthermore, these authors were able to show that sucralfate has direct antibacterial activity against the common colonizing organisms so that the pH-dependent protective effect of sucralfate was also enhanced by the agent itself. The direct antibacterial activity of sucralfate may prove to be an important factor, since gastric secretory failure has been reported in critically ill patients, and a recent study of gastric pH and colonization in sucralfate-treated intensive care unit patients showed that approximately 50 percent were colonized and that their mean gastric pH was 4.7 [99].

Blocking Colonization with Locally Applied Oropharyngeal Antibiotics

The most detailed studies of local oropharyngeal antibiotics for the control of nosocomial lower respiratory tract infections were those done by the Beth Israel group in Boston [34, 48]. In a series of well-planned and well-executed studies, the group was able to show that daily aerosolization of the oropharynx with polymyxin in intensive care unit patients significantly reduced oral colonization and pneumonia due to *P. aeruginosa*, a pathogen that had been a particular problem on this unit [34, 48]. Polymyxin was chosen because it is poorly absorbed through an intact mucosa, absorbs to epithelial cells, and is bactericidal for a wide variety of gram-negative rods. However, continuous use of aerosolized polymyxin as a preventive maneuver was followed by an outbreak of fatal lower respiratory tract infections caused by polymyxin-resistant organisms [29]. The use of local polymyxin as a means of decreasing nosocomial pneumonia was abandoned. These were important studies because, first, they unequivocally showed the relationship between oropharyngeal colonization and pneumonia and, second, they demonstrated that rates of nosocomial pneumonia would fall if colonization could be prevented. However, the overall poor results of these studies had another important negative effect in that American clinical investigators were directed away from further study of chemotherapeutic approaches to preventing colonization as a method of decreasing nosocomial pneumonia.

Selective Decontamination

In the 1970s and early 1980s, the data showing the interrelationship between gastic,

oropharyngeal, and tracheal colonization became clearer. This led to the consideration that the stomach and gastrointestinal tract were key elements in the colonization–to–respiratory infection cascade (see Fig. 29-1). At the same time, studies evaluating antimicrobial prophylaxis in granulocytopenic patients proposed that nonabsorbed antibiotics could eliminate or greatly reduce the population of aerobic gram-negative rods and yeasts in the gastrointestinal tract while retaining the anaerobic flora so as to prevent colonization and overgrowth with resistant strains, a phenomenon called *colonization resistance*.

With these concepts, Stoutenbeek and co-workers [84–87] in the early 1980s developed a new, more comprehensive prophylactic approach, called *selective decontamination of the digestive tract* (SDD), to prevent nosocomial lower respiratory tract infections (see also Chap. 13). They reasoned, as did the original Boston researchers, that if colonization could be avoided, rates of pneumonia should decrease. They conceived and subsequently studied a prophylactic regimen that was far broader than the single-drug polymyxin treatment and one that specifically addressed the upper gastrointestinal tract. Working with seriously ill trauma patients, decontamination was achieved with a mixture of tobramycin, polymyxin E, and amphotericin B, which was applied as a paste to the mouth and was administered by nasogastric tube to the stomach. In addition, parenteral cefotaxime was used in all patients early in the regimen as a broad-spectrum antibacterial agent. Antibiotics that would affect anaerobic gut flora as little as possible were deliberately chosen. This regimen resulted in marked reduction in the colonization of the oropharynx, and the incidence of nosocomial lower respiratory tract infections rates fell from 81 percent in historical controls to 16 percent in patients receiving selective decontamination. An added benefit was a generalized reduction in all nosocomial infection rates in patients given selective decontamination. A summary of the published series testing selective decontamination is presented in Table 29-7.

Stoutenbeek's original observations [84–

Table 29-7. Selective decontamination as a means of decreasing rates of nosocomial pneumonia in intensive care units

Study site	Prophylactic regimen	Patient population	Types of controls	Oropharyngeal colonization rate (%)		Pneumonia rate (no./total [%])		Total infection rate (no./total [%])		Reference
				Study	Control	Study	Control	Study	Control	
Holland 1979–1983	Colistin, tobramycin, amphotericin PO and by oral ointment *plus* IV cefotaxime	Severely traumatized ventilator patients	None, open study	2	65	5/63 (8)	35/59 (59)	NA	NA	[86]
Germany 1984–1985	Polymyxin B, gentamicin PO and local and amphotericin orally	Severely traumatized ventilator patients	Prospective and randomized	0	85	1/19 (5)	9/20 (45)	NA	NA	[91]
Scotland 1985–1986	Colistin, tobramycin, amphotericin PO and by oral ointment *plus* IV cefotaxime	General ICU; >60% on ventilators	Historical, non-concurrent	0	30	3/98 (3)	18/94 (19)	10/98 (10)	23/94 (24)	[53]

Holland 1986–1987	Colistin, tobramycin, amphotericin PO and by oral ointment *plus* IV cefotaxime	Surgical ICU; all on ventilators	Prospective, randomized	0	55	6/49 (12)	40/47 (85)	19/49 (39)	38/47 (81)	[47]
Holland 1986–1987	Colistin, norfloxacin, amphotericin PO and by oral ointment *plus* trimethoprim	General ICU; >75% on ventilators	Prospective, randomized	0	85	3/48 (6)	23/52 (44)	25/48 (52)	40/52 (77)	[90]
France 1987	Colistin, neomycin, nalidixic acid PO and povidone-iodine locally to all patients	Medical ICU	Historical and concurrent	ND	ND	6/50 (12)	3/35 (9)	32/50 (64)	23/35 (66)	[10]

ICU = intensive care unit; ND = no data; NA = not available.

87] were made with a highly select group of patients, trauma victims who were likely to have extended stays in an intensive care unit. His technique has been carried into other specialized [90] and unspecialized intensive care units with the same results. Ledingham and colleagues [53] applied Stoutenbeek's approach to consecutive patients admitted to a general intensive care unit. They noted a sharp drop in nosocomial infection rates in patients undergoing prophylaxis.

Two randomized controlled trials have studied intestinal decontamination in intensive care unit patients. Using Stoutenbeek's protocol, Kerver and co-workers [47] randomized consecutive patients to selective decontamination or standard therapy. Gram-negative rod colonization of the respiratory tract fell from 60 percent in control patients to 10 percent in the treated patients. Forty of 47 patients (85 percent) in the control group developed gram-negative pneumonias as compared to 6 of 49 (15 percent) in the treated group. In a second study, Ulrich and co-workers [90] randomly assigned intensive care unit patients to a control group or to a group receiving an intestinal decontamination protocol that included colistin, norfloxacin, and amphotericin given orally and applied as an oral ointment. The incidence of nosocomial pneumonias due to aerobic gram-negative rods was 27 percent in the control group and only 4 percent in the treatment group. The overall mortality was significantly reduced from 54 percent in the control group to 31 percent in the group receiving prophylaxis [90].

A recent study of intestinal decontamination has been reported from Paris [10]. The medical intensive care unit at the Henri Mondor Hospital was having a problem with multiresistant *Klebsiella* infections, intestinal colonization being an important reservoir for these organisms. A protocol for intestinal decontamination using oral colistin, nalidixic acid, and neomycin lowered intestinal colonization of multiresistant *Klebsiella* from 10 percent in controls to 1 percent in patients receiving prophylaxis. The study was not specifically designed to evaluate respiratory tract

infections, and all tracheally intubated patients (60 percent of both groups) received oral disinfection with povidone-iodine on a regular basis. The rates of nosocomial pneumonia in this group were half the rate noted in 122 historical controls studied 3 months earlier, but the report is unclear as to whether the intubated historical controls also received oropharyngeal povidone treatments.

An important concern in all these studies has been the possibility that a strategy of intestinal decontamination could lead to the proliferation of resistant bacteria. To date, despite a thorough search for resistant organisms, this has not been seen. As a group, these papers are persuasive even though some are methodologically flawed. The positive findings are consistent within studies and congruous with a great deal of prior pathophysiologic research. One disturbing issue is the inability of most studies to show that lowering rates of nosocomial pneumonia has led to improved survival. Nonetheless, it is very likely that use of this approach will increase, particularly in intensive care units with high endemic nosocomial infection rates [1, 42].

Special Problems
Legionnaires' Disease
Legionella pneumophila is an important cause of nosocomial pneumonia. The organism is ubiquitous in water and hence is regularly present in the hospital environment [8, 28]. The key to preventing nosocomial legionellosis is recognizing this organism as a cause of disease. The development of charcoal yeast agar has markedly facilitated the isolation of *Legionella* species, which is well within the capabilities of most hospital microbiology laboratories. Nonetheless, many hospitals do not culture for *Legionella* and nosocomial cases are often not recognized. Tracheal aspirates and pleural fluids should be cultured for *Legionella* in cases of hospital-acquired lower respiratory tract infections in which the microbiologic diagnosis is unclear. This is especially true of infections in immunosuppressed patients, who have been shown to be

particularly at risk for *Legionella* infections. Because *L. pneumophila* is not spread person to person, identification of cases in a hospital setting usually means that an environmental source is present which, if not identified and corrected, may lead to more cases.

The early studies of epidemic legionellosis focused on the importance of airborne spread and contaminated cooling systems as disseminators of *Legionella* organisms. The report by Dondero and co-workers [25] of a hospital-centered outbreak in Memphis is one such example. In the summer of 1978, there was a sudden outbreak of 44 cases of *Legionella* pneumonia that were all epidemiologically related to a single hospital. The epidemic coincided with the use of an auxiliary cooling unit that had not been used for the previous 2 years. Differential attack rates showed that patients in the east wing of the hospital were more at risk. The cooling tower in question was on the eastern side of the hospital. There were two air intakes 3½ stories up the eastern side of the hospital and approximately 15 m from the cooling tower. Tracer smoke studies showed that smoke rose from the cooling tower to the eastern face of the building.

Microbiologic studies of the cooling tower showed the presence of *L. pneumophila,* and the cause of the epidemic became clear: *Legionella,* probably from potable water, was introduced into the cooling tower and multiplied. The aerosol that was produced as part of normal tower operation was drawn into the ventilation system of the hospital where it was distributed. New cases stopped when the auxiliary cooling unit ceased to be used. This and other outbreaks have focused attention on the importance of cooling towers and evaporative condensers as reservoirs for nosocomial legionellosis.

Legionella can be eliminated from these units with disinfectants. However, the optimal disinfectant for contaminated systems has not yet been determined. Periodic cleaning and hyperchlorination are prudent measures until more specific recommendations can be offered. Irrespective of the maintenance schedules of these units, it is important that the location of all building air vents in relation to cooling towers and evaporative condensers be reviewed and changed, if necessary.

A more vexing problem has been that of *Legionella* in potable water and what role this aqueous contamination plays in the epidemiology of nosocomial legionellosis. Over the last decade, an impressive body of epidemiologic and microbiologic data has led to the inescapable conclusion that potable water can be an important reservoir for nosocomial infections. Data for this assertion come from a variety of sources. One of the first indications that potable water may play an important role in the epidemiology of nosocomial legionellosis came from the well-publicized epidemic at the Wadsworth Veterans Administration Medical Center [77]. Cases occurred over a 3-year period despite chlorination of the main cooling tower. Epidemiologic and microbiologic studies showed that cases were related to the degree of contamination in potable water. The outbreak did not stop until hyperchlorination of the potable water supply was accomplished.

In 1981, a French hospital reported 4 cases of nosocomial legionellosis due to serogroup 1 [62]. There was a direct association between development of disease and exposure to hot potable water. Monoclonal antibody testing showed that the cases and potable water isolates were the same subgroup but different from the serogroup 1 *L. pneumophila* isolate from a cooling tower. Three of the cases were tightly clustered in time and, although on different floors, were all in rooms supplied by one of 18 possible hot-water pipes that cultured positive for the epidemic strain.

A major epidemic of legionellosis occurred at the University of Iowa Hospital in 1981 [38]. Twenty-four cases of nosocomial disease were documented; most of the patients were immunosuppressed. A thorough investigation of the ventilation system showed no evidence of faulty function. The epidemic ceased after water use by patients bedded in the hematology-oncology unit was stopped. Detailed microbiologic studies of the isolates using restriction endonuclease plasmid analysis identified a unique strain of *L. pneumophila* from both patients and potable water samples. Continuous hyperchlorination of the water system was begun in January 1982 and has been continued to the present. Potable water samples have been negative for *Legionella* species, and 4 sporadic cases of Legionnaires' disease have been reported in the hematology-oncology unit from 1982 to 1987 [39]. The isolates from these cases were different from the original epidemic strain.

Stout, Yu, and their associates [82, 83, 103] have clearly shown that widespread contamination of potable water is common and associated with nosocomial legionellosis. Shower heads were early in-hospital sites for the isolation of *Legionella* and have always been an attractive explanation for nosocomial cases (i.e., that aerosolization of *Legionella* occurred during the shower and disease resulted from inhalation of these·contaminated aerosols). Woo [100] was unable to demonstrate aerosolization of *Legionella* during use of contaminated showers, but he and Arnow [4, 100] have clearly shown that use of *Legionella*-positive potable water in humidifiers can result in airborne transmission of *Legionella* in the hospital. *L. pneumophila* could be directly instilled into the respiratory tree if contaminated tap water is used to rinse an instrument or a catheter that is then used orally or intratracheally. *Legionella* need not be aerosolized to cause disease, since a well-characterized guinea pig infection model relies on an aspiration challenge [28a].

The final and perhaps most persuasive data implicating potable water and nosocomial legionellosis were generated by a three-hospital prospective study by Yu and colleagues [104]. The three hospitals were chosen because they were believed not to have problems with nosocomial legionellosis. Hospital 1 was colonized with *L. pneumophila* type 1; hospital 2 was colonized by serogroup 5 *L. pneumophila*, a strain not associated with disease; and hospital 3 was free of environmental *Legionella*. Respiratory specimens from all patients with respiratory infections were cultured for *Legionella* species for 6 months. Results of the study are summarized in Table 29-8. Nosocomial Legionnaires' disease occurred only in the hospital with the most contaminated water supply. Laboratories in hospitals 2 and 3 were capable of growing *Legionella* since they diagnosed cases of community-acquired disease during the same time period. In a follow-up study, 4 more cases of serogroup 1 *L. pneumophila* pneumonia occurred in hospital 1.

In a thoughtful and provocative analysis of modes of spread of *L. pneumophila*, Muder and associates [58] have made the following observations: Simple environmental contamination with *Legionella* rarely causes disease; the infection rate is proportional to the degree of exposure to contaminated aerosols; and contact with aspirated *Legionella* occurs frequently, but disease may be more a function of compromised host defenses.

Given these data, there exists little doubt

Table 29-8. Prospective study of nosocomial legionellosis

| Hospital | Positive environmental cultures (%) | | Legionella serogroup | Nosocomial pneumonias, Legionella pneumophila isolated | | |
	Water tanks	Distal sites		Total	No.	%
1	11	48	1	32	3[b]	9
2	67	22	5	26	0	0
3	0	2[a]	—	38	0	0

[a] Single isolate of *L. pneumophila* (serogroup 1).
[b] Subtype same as environmental isolates.
Source: From V.L. Yu et al., Routine culturing for *Legionella* in the hospital environment may be a good idea: A three-hospital prospective study. *Am. J. Med. Sci.* 294:97, 1987.

that nosocomial legionellosis can occur as a result of environmental contamination with *Legionella* species. When to obtain environmental cultures for *Legionella* and when to decontaminate the hospital water system are not as clear-cut and can present a major headache for hospital epidemiologists.

Specific guidelines for environmental culturing have not been developed. In general, culturing potable water for the presence of *Legionella* species is discouraged unless nosocomial cases are observed. This recommendation has little meaning unless the hospital microbiology laboratory is capable of culturing *Legionella* or referring to an appropriate laboratory clinical specimens from patients with nosocomial pneumonia in whom the microbiologic diagnosis is unclear.

If cases of nosocomial legionellosis occur, a thorough epidemiologic investigation, including environmental samples, is indicated. If geographic clustering of cases has occurred, it is appropriate to substitute a new source of potable water until the preliminary environmental sampling studies are finished. If water samples are positive for *Legionella* in the setting of nosocomial cases, a representative sample of the isolates should be subtyped to determine, as precisely as possible, the relationship between the clinical and environmental isolates. Factors that promote colonization with *Legionella* include water heaters set to temperatures lower than 50°C (122°F), scale and sediment accumulation, stagnation, holding tanks, and commensal microflora, particularly free-living protozoa [59].

There are no specific rules as to when water systems ought to be treated to eliminate or reduce contamination with *Legionella*, but the following indications for decontamination are presented as general guides: (1) when the site has been implicated in an outbreak of Legionnaires' disease; (2) when environmental *Legionella* cultures are positive in conjunction with high-risk patients such as bone marrow transplant recipients; and (3) when *Legionella* organisms are found in the water supply of a building not used for a long time, since colony counts, in such settings, may be very high.

Muraca and associates [59] have written a particularly useful summary of the methodologies that can be used to disinfect water distribution systems contaminated with *Legionella*. A comparative assessment of the disinfection strategies is presented in Table 29-9. Several hospitals have successfully used hyperchlorination to control environmental contamination with *Legionella*. Suppression requires residual levels of chlorine greater than 3 parts per million. One major disadvantage is system corrosion; in one study, the average number of pipe leaks increased from 0.17 per month prechlorination to 5.2 per month 3 years after hyperchlorination had begun [39].

L. pneumophila are killed at temperatures greater than 60°C (140°F). Hospital epidemiologists and engineers have used this temperature sensitivity in developing a "heat and flush" method to eradicate *Legionella*. The basic technique requires that hot-water tank temperature be elevated to greater than 70°C (158°F), followed by the running of all shower heads and faucets to kill *Legionella*. The method provides effective short-term control, and colonization can be minimized by keeping hot-water tank temperatures at 60°C (140°F). The simplest approach for new construction is the installation of an instantaneous steam heating system that flash heats incoming water to 88°C (190.4°F) and blends this hot water with cold water to achieve the desired temperature.

L. pneumophila is susceptible to ultraviolet light, and continuous ultraviolet treatment of incoming water has been used to render water *Legionella*-free. Such an approach has been particularly useful to disinfect water in special units where high-risk patients are bedded. Because this technique ensures only that incoming water is clean, the entire system must be disinfected beforehand.

Disinfecting a hospital's water and entire hot-water system is no easy task. A coordinated approach that employs the specialized skills of the hospital engineer, microbiologist, hospital administrator, and epidemiologist is essential. Consultation with state and local health officials and with personnel from hos-

Table 29-9.   Comparative assessment of disinfection modalities

Method	Ease of application or installation	Expense	Maintenance	Short-term efficacy	Long-term efficacy	Disadvantages
Hyperchlorination	Difficult	High	Fair to difficult	Good	Fair to good	System corrosion, carcinogenic by-products
Thermal eradication	Easy	Low	Easy	Good	Poor*	Recolonization at lower temperatures, labor-intensive
Instantaneous heaters	Difficult	Moderate	Difficult	NA	NA	Maximal efficiency requires installation as original system in new building
Ozonation	Difficult	High	Difficult	NA	NA	Ozone rapidly decomposes system, corrosion
Ultraviolet irradiation	Fair	Moderate	Difficult	Good	Fair	Quartz sleeve subject to scale, servicing requires electrical personnel
Metal ionization	Fair	Moderate	Fair	NA	NA	Metallic ions added to drinking water

NA = not available.
*Long-term efficacy is fair to good if hot water temperature is maintained at 60°C (140°F)
Source: From P.W. Muraca, V.L. Yu, and A. Goetz. Disinfection of water distribution systems for *Legionella:* A review of application procedures and methodologies. *Infect. Control Hosp. Epidemiol.* 11:79, 1990.

pitals who have successful environmental control programs for *Legionella* is strongly encouraged.

Aspergillosis

Aspergillus spores are found universally in unfiltered air [71]. Because of their size, *Aspergillus* spores remain suspended in air for long periods of time. When inhaled, they penetrate to the distal lung where they are inactivated by normal cellular defenses. *Aspergillus* is very hardy and, once introduced into an environment, persists for long periods of time. High concentrations in the hospital have been found in false ceiling dust, polystyrene linings of fireproofed doors, and fireproofing material.

The most important nosocomial infection due to *Aspergillus* is pneumonia in immuno-

suppressed patients [78]. Since the treatment of pulmonary aspergillosis in the immunosuppressed patient is very unsatisfactory, primary prevention is of great importance, particularly in hospitals with high-risk patients. Ambient air *Aspergillus* counts are the most important predictor of the incidence of these infections. Most hospital outbreaks of pulmonary aspergillosis have occurred in transplant or granulocytopenic patients and have been traced to an increase in airborne contamination with *Aspergillus* spores. Nosocomial outbreaks of *Aspergillus* infection have been correlated with building construction and external contamination of intake air.

During a 6-month period, a sixfold increase in *Aspergillus* isolates was noted in a North Carolina hospital [75]. Most of these new isolates came from patients in an older wing of the hospital that was adjacent to a construction site where a new hospital was being built. A study of the ventilation system in the wing with high isolation rates of *Aspergillus* showed that the major intake vent was directly above the construction site. Cultures of the louvers yielded *Aspergillus flavus,* and it was noted that the filters were defective. Outside sampling in the vicinity of the construction showed massive amounts of fungi. The filtering system was rebuilt and high-efficiency filters were installed, the result being that *Aspergillus* isolation rates fell to preconstruction levels.

Several outbreaks of aspergillosis have been associated with hospital construction. From 1981 to 1983, 11 patients at a military hospital in Colorado became infected [63]. All of the patients were immunocompromised, and the cases were associated with a major renovation project within the hospital. Air sampling showed airborne spore counts of 4.2 per cubic meter. Control strategies included sealing the construction areas from the patient areas and placing the construction area in negative pressure with vents to the outside air. Copper-8-quinolinolate was used as a surface decontaminant in the special-care areas, and portable high-efficiency particulate air (HEPA) filters were placed in rooms where high-risk patients were bedded. Airborne spore counts fell dramatically with copper-8-quinolinolate treatment and were at very low levels in rooms with HEPA filters. There were no new cases that occurred after the implementation of these control measures, despite continuation of the hospital renovation.

Hopkins and co-workers [40] described an interesting epidemic of aspergillosis that underscored the point that patients may become exposed to *Aspergillus* outside their rooms. The epidemic consisted of 6 cases of nosocomial aspergillosis that occurred in a single month, as compared to 4 cases over the prior 12 months. The only common geographic area to these cases was the radiology suite, which had been undergoing extensive renovation. Obviously, the highest-efficiency room filters cannot protect susceptible pa-

tients from exposures in other areas. Whenever possible, diagnostic studies should be done within the protective environment of the patient's room, and, if a patient must be moved, this should be done in the most expeditious manner possible.

The prevention of nosocomial aspergillosis, like legionellosis, requires the cooperation of engineering and housekeeping services. The key point is that prevention is dependent on reducing the spore content of the patient's ambient air. Outside air has 1 to 10 *Aspergillus* colonies per cubic meter [70]. Ambient spore concentrations in the range of 0.01 per cubic millimeter can be achieved with HEPA filtration, air exchange rates of 10 per hour, efforts at decreasing contamination from outside air, and attention to corridor air [70]. Walsh and Dixon [97] have proposed preventive and corrective measures for the control of nosocomial aspergillosis (Table 29-10).

Tuberculosis

Nosocomial tuberculosis does not result in an acute pulmonary infection, but rather the hospital serves as a locus where susceptible patients with active tuberculosis are hospitalized because of a chronic febrile respiratory illness that has a characteristic chest roentgenogram. Unfortunately, this pattern has become blurred with the increase of atypical clinical cases in the elderly and in patients with the human immunodeficiency virus infection [3].

Infection control personnel usually become involved with tuberculosis under two circumstances: (1) as consultants to employee health personnel who are responsible for the annual tuberculin testing program at the hospital, and (2) as consultants to floor nurses, physicians, and other employees when tuberculosis is suspected or diagnosed. Valenti [92] has published useful guidelines for a hospital-based tuberculin testing program for employees. A two-step initial tuberculin test is recommended to avoid the confusion associated with the booster effect.

Hospitalized patients in whom tuberculosis is undiagnosed present the greatest hazard to

Table 29-10. Preventive and corrective measures for nosocomial aspergillosis

Construction

1. Avoid building materials with high concentrations of *Aspergillus conidia*.
2. Relocate patients before starting construction.
3. Construct barriers (plastic or drywall) impermeable to *A. conidia* from floor to ceiling between patient care areas and construction areas.
4. Clean work areas of construction and new wards before patients enter the area.
5. Vacuum areas above false ceilings located under or adjacent to construction areas.
6. Direct pedestrian traffic through construction areas to prevent dust from being tracked into patient areas.
7. Ventilate construction areas with negative pressure relative to patient areas.
8. Eliminate any damp paper, pulp, or wood-base material that can harbor *Aspergillus*.
9. Use copper-8-quinolinolate (efficacy in sustained environmental control remains to be clarified).

Ventilation systems

1. Routinely inspect air supply ducts to high-risk patient care areas.
2. Install quality high-efficiency particulate air filters in rooms supporting patients with profound, protracted granulocytopenia.
3. Prevent access by roosting birds to hospital intake ducts.
4. Coordinate repairs on air supply and exhaust fans and ducts with hospital engineering.
5. Vacuum contaminated air-conditioning equipment, air supply ducts, and rooms.

Source: From T.J. Walsh and D.M. Dixon. Nosocomial aspergillosis: Environmental microbiology, hospital epidemiology, diagnosis and treatment. *Eur. J. Epidemiol.* 5:131, 1989.

other patients and staff. *Mycobacterium tuberculosis* is spread by the airborne route, and patients who are expectorating viable tubercle bacilli contaminate the surrounding airspace. Aerosolized tubercle bacilli tend to form droplet nuclei and can remain suspended in air for long periods of time. These organisms can be inhaled by susceptible patients and staff and lead to primary tuberculosis infection. Patients with tuberculosis who are being ventilated may be more infectious. Currently, nosocomial spread of multidrug-resistant strains is becoming a significant problem [105].

Catanzaro [12] described an outbreak of tuberculosis in an intensive care unit setting that resulted in 14 of 45 susceptible staff becoming infected. The patient was admitted to the unit with respiratory insufficiency, presumably because of seizure-induced aspiration. The patient underwent bronchoscopy and placement of an endotracheal tube and was ventilated for 3 days. Sputum samples were smear-negative, but two of the sputum cultures later grew *M. tuberculosis*. The outbreak was not recognized until one of the physicians caring for the patient developed fatigue, cough, and a markedly positive skin test. His only patient contact for the last 6 months had been in the intensive care unit, which prompted a retrospective review of smear and culture data. Further investigation showed that of the 13 susceptible staff who were present at the time of bronchoscopy, 10 converted (77 percent).

Patients and staff who are exposed to an active case of tuberculosis should first have their tuberculin status carefully reviewed. Known tuberculin-positives are not a problem since their positivity conveys protection [81]. Persons who do not know their tuberculin status should have an intermediate tuberculin test done and, if negative, a second test within 2 weeks to identify those persons in whom a booster response is needed to define their positivity. Persons who are negative to both tuberculin tests are considered true negatives unless they have a medical reason (such as immunosuppression or intercurrent viral illness) that might blunt a delayed hypersensitivity response. Tuberculin-negative patients and staff should be retested in 6 weeks; those who test positive at this point are classified as converters and should be offered isoniazid prophylaxis.

Influenza

The majority of the reported outbreaks of nosocomial influenza have originated from nursing homes and other chronic-care settings [14]. General hospital wards are at risk for influenza epidemics but are less easily noticed and reported, probably because of the rapid turnover of patients. Nonetheless, when these outbreaks occur, they are explosive and cause major disruption.

Influenza virus may be introduced into the hospital setting by patients as well as by hospital staff who are either incubating or suffering from influenza [64]. Nosocomial influenza presents with fever, myalgia, headache, coryza, and cough. The elderly and patients with chronic cardiac, pulmonary, or metabolic disease suffer increased morbidity and mortality after influenza infection. Since these high-risk patients make up the bulk of patients on general medical wards, it is important for infection control personnel to be alert to the possibility of nosocomial influenza infection on those units.

The capacity for airborne transmission of influenza is remarkable. In a rather unfortunate set of circumstances, 54 persons were grounded for 3 hours prior to a transoceanic flight in an airliner without ventilation. A single person with influenza was on the plane, and 72 percent of the passengers acquired clinical influenza within 72 hours [56].

The control of influenza is based predominantly on prevention by immunization or through chemoprophylaxis. Annual immunization is recommended for all high-risk individuals, such as the elderly and patients of all ages with chronic cardiac, pulmonary, renal, or metabolic disease. Unfortunately, only 20 percent or so of high-risk persons in the United States are immunized on an annual basis. Because influenza can be introduced by hospital personnel, it is prudent to emphasize their immunization as a means of decreasing risk to hospitalized patients. Unfortunately, influenza vaccine has not been well received by hospital employees even when provided conveniently and at low cost.

Current influenza vaccines are preparations of formalin-inactivated virus growth in the allantoic fluid of chick embryos. The vaccines are trivalent, containing equal amounts of the hemagglutinin (15 μg) of each of the three types of influenza that have been prevalent for the last 10 years. These are two subtypes of influenza (A/H3N2 and A/H1N1)

and influenza B. The vaccines are highly purified, and most of the pyrogenic components that plagued the earlier influenza vaccines have been removed. The antigens contained in the vaccines are changed frequently to accommodate to the continuing antigenic drift, particularly of the influenza A/H3N2 type.

In most years, vaccination should be done in the early fall. However, individuals who have not been vaccinated should receive vaccine along with amantadine in the event that influenza A appears at any time during the winter [57]. This is particularly important in closed populations such as nursing homes or for individuals who are at particularly high risk and who have close contact with persons with influenza.

Reactions to the vaccine in the elderly are infrequent and minor, consisting mainly of low-grade fever and a few hours of malaise, which can usually be controlled with analgesic preparations. Vaccine should not be given to individuals who have a definite history of allergy to eggs. Several properly designed controlled studies have shown that amantadine is an effective chemoprophylactic agent to prevent influenza A. Amantadine does not interfere with the antibody response to influenza vaccine, and a recommended approach for dealing with a high-risk unprotected population, such as hospitalized patients, during an epidemic is to vaccinate and treat with amantadine for 2 weeks, by which time protective antibody titers would be present. Rimantadine has also been shown to be an effective chemoprophylactic agent against influenza A with fewer side effects, but it is not yet licensed. Amantadine and rimantadine ought not to be considered substitutes for routine influenza B, are more expensive than influenza vaccine, and have important side effects. Confusion occurs in approximately 15 percent of elderly patients given 200 mg daily of amantadine. In one study of amantadine prophylaxis in the acute-care hospital setting, a significant reduction in the attack rate of nosocomial influenza was noted in patients given amantadine (4 percent) when compared to controls (20 percent) [6].

For adults, comprehensive influenza prophylaxis would include yearly immunization of high-risk patients and hospital personnel and chemoprophylaxis plus immunization for those not immunized earlier in the season. Additional disease control measures would include warning visitors and hospital personnel not to visit the hospital or come to work while they are ill. Infected patients who are hospitalized should be grouped together, with special attention to personnel caring for these patients, who should have been vaccinated or using amantadine chemoprophylaxis [94]. General guidelines for the use of cohort isolation are presented in Table 29-11.

Table 29-11. General guidelines for use of cohort isolation

1. Patients should be separated into cohorts of infected and noninfected patients.
2. Only persons with proved or suspected infection should be admitted to the infected cohort.
3. All exposed (potentially infected) individuals should be included with the cohort of infected patients. In some instances, the potentially infected cohort may be separated into a third cohort.
4. The infected cohort should be closed to new, uninfected admissions, and all new, uninfected admissions should be placed in the uninfected cohort.
5. Personnel working with the infected cohort should be immune to the illness in question by either previous history of illness or vaccination whenever possible.
6. Personnel should be assigned so that separate groups work with the infected and uninfected cohorts whenever possible. Crossover between cohorts should be discouraged, especially during a single shift, to minimize the risk of cross-infection of the uninfected cohort.
7. When members of the staff must work in both areas, they should work in the uninfected area first, then work in the infected area.
8. The infected cohort area will be closed as patients are discharged from the hospital and may be used for new, uninfected admissions after thorough cleaning of the area and its equipment.

Source: From W.M. Valenti and M.A. Menegus. Nosocomial viral infections: IV. Guidelines for cohort isolation, the communicable disease survey, collection and transport of specimens for virus isolation, and considerations for the future. *Infect. Control* 2:236, 1981.

References

1. Alcock, S.R., and Cole. D.S. Selective decontamination of the digestive tract (SDDP), ICU-acquired pneumonia and selection of antibiotic-resistant bacteria. *J. Hosp. Infect.* 15(2):195, 1990.
2. Alvarez, S., et al. Nosocomial pneumococcal pneumonia. *Arch. Intern. Med.* 146:1509, 1986.
3. Alvarez, S., Shell, C., and Berk, S.L. Pulmonary tuberculosis in elderly men. *Am. J. Med.* 82:602, 1987.
4. Arnow, P.M., et al. Nosocomial Legionnaires' disease caused by aerosolized tap water from respiratory devices. *J. Infect. Dis.* 146:460, 1982.
5. Atherton, S.T., and White, D.J. Stomach as source of bacteria colonizing respiratory tract during artificial ventilation. *Lancet* 2:968, 1978.
6. Atkinson, W.L., et al. Amantadine prophylaxis during an institutional outbreak of type A (H1N1) influenza. *Arch. Intern. Med.* 146:1751, 1986.
7. Baddour, L.M., Christensen, G.D., Simpson, W.A., and Beachey, E.H. Microbial Adherence. In: G.L. Mandell, R.G. Douglas, Jr., and J.E. Bennett (Eds.), *Principles and Practice of Infectious Diseases* (3rd ed.). New York: Churchill Livingstone, 1990. Pp. 9–25.
8. Bartlett, C.L.R., et al. *Legionella* in hospital and hotel water supplies. *Lancet* 2:1315, 1983.
9. Bergogne-Berezin, E. Pharmacokinetics of Antibiotics in Respiratory Secretions. In: J.E. Penninton (Ed.), *Respiratory Infections: Diagnosis and Management.* New York: Raven Press, 1983. Pp. 461–479.
10. Brun-Buisson, C., et al. Intestinal decontamination for control of nosocomial multiresistant Gram-negative bacilli. Study of an outbreak in an intensive care unit. *Ann. Intern. Med.* 110:873, 1989.
11. Bryan, C.S., and Reynolds, K.L. Bacteremic nosocomial pneumonia. Analysis of 172 episodes from a single metropolitan area. *Am. Rev. Respir. Dis.* 129:668, 1984.
11a. CDC Guidelines on Infection Control. Isolation techniques for use in hospitals. *Infect. Control* 4:249, 1983.
12. Catanzaro, A. Nosocomial tuberculosis. *Am. Rev. Respir. Dis.* 125:559, 1982.
13. Centers for Disease Control. Nosocomial Infection Surveillance, 1984. In: *CDC Surveillance Summaries,* Vol. 35 (No. 1SS), 1986. P. 1755.
14. Centers for Disease Control. Prevention and control of influenza. Recommendations of

the Immunization Practices Advisory Committee (ACIP). M.M.W.R. 39 (No. RR-7):1, 1990.

15. Cipolle, R.J., Seifert, R.D., Zaske, D.E., and Strate, R.G. Hospital-acquired Gram-negative pneumonias: Response rate and dosage requirements with individualized tobramycin therapy. *Ther. Drug Monit.* 2:359, 1980.

16. Craven, D.E. Nosocomial pneumonia: New concepts on an old disease. *Infect. Control Hosp. Epidemiol.* 9:57, 1988.

17. Craven, D.E., et al. Contamination of mechanical ventilators with tubing changes every 24 or 48 hours. *N. Engl. J. Med.* 306:1505, 1982.

18. Craven, D.E., et al. Nosocomial infection and fatality in medical and surgical intensive care unit patients. *Arch. Intern. Med.* 148:1161, 1988.

19. Craven, D.E., et al. Contaminated medication nebulizers in mechanical ventilator circuits. *Am. J. Med.* 77:834, 1984.

20. Craven, D.E., Goularte, T.A., and Make, B.J. Contaminated condensate in mechanical ventilator circuits. *Am. Rev. Respir. Dis.* 129:625, 1984.

21. Craven, D.E., and Steger, K.A. Nosocomial pneumonia in the intubated patient. *Infect. Dis. Clin. North Am.* 3:843, 1989.

22. Cross, A.S., and Roup, B. Role of respiratory assistance devices in endemic nosocomial pneumonia. *Am. J. Med.* 70:681, 1981.

23. Dal Nogare, A.R., Toews, G.B., and Pierce. A.K. Increased salivary elastase precedes Gram-negative bacillary colonization in postoperative patients. *Am. Rev. Respir. Dis.* 135:671, 1987.

24. Daschner, F., et al. Stress ulcer prophylaxis and ventilation pneumonia: Prevention by antibacterial cyptoprotective agents? *Infect. Control Hosp. Epidemiol.* 9:59, 1988.

25. Dondero, T.J., et al. An outbreak of Legionnaires' disease associated with a contaminated air-conditioning cooling tower. *N. Engl. J. Med.* 302:365, 1980.

26. Driks, M.R., et al. Nosocomial pneumonia in intubated patients given sucralfate as compared with antacids or histamine type 2 blockers. *N. Engl. J. Med.* 317:1376, 1987.

27. du Moulin, G.C., et al. Aspiration of gastric bacteria in antacid-treated patients: A frequent cause of postoperative colonization of the airway. *Lancet* 1:242, 1982.

28. Edelstein, P.H. Environmental aspects of *Legionella*. *A.S.M. News* 51:460, 1985.

28a. Edelstein, P.H., Calarco, K., and Yasui, V.K. Antimicrobial therapy of experimentally induced Legionnaires' disease in guinea pigs. *Am. Rev. Respir. Dis.* 130:849, 1984.

29. Feeley, T.W., et al. Aerosol polymixin and pneumonia in seriously ill patients. *N. Engl. J. Med.* 293:471, 1975.

30. Fuxench-Lopez, Z., and Ramirez-Ronda, C.H. Pharyngeal flora in ambulatory alcoholic patients. Prevalence of Gram-negative bacilli. *Arch. Intern. Med.* 138:1815, 1978.

31. Garibaldi, R.A., et al. Risk factors for postoperative pneumonia. *Am. J. Med.* 70: 677, 1981.

32. Gibbons, R.J., and van Houte, J. Bacterial adherence in oral microbial ecology. *Ann. Rev. Microbiol.* 29:19, 1975.

33. Graman, P.S., and Hall, C.B. Epidemiology and control of nosocomial viral infections. *Infect. Dis. Clin. North Am.* 3:815, 1989.

34. Greenfield, S., et al. Prevention of gram-negative bacillary pneumonia using aerosol polymixin as prophylaxis: I. Effect on the colonization pattern of the upper respiratory tract of seriously ill patients. *J. Clin. Invest.* 52:2935, 1973.

35. Gross, P.A., et al. Deaths from nosocomial infections: Experience in a university hospital and a community hospital. *Am. J. Med.* 68:219, 1980.

36. Gross, P.A., and Van Antwerpen, C.V. Nosocomial infections and hospital deaths. *Am. J. Med.* 75:658, 1983.

37. Haley, R.W., et al. Nosocomial infections in U.S. hospitals, 1975–1976. *Am. J. Med.* 70:947, 1981.

38. Helms, C.M., et al. Legionnaires' disease associated with a hospital water system. *J.A.M.A.* 259–2423, 1988.

39. Helms, C.M., et al. Legionnaires' disease associated with a hospital water system: A cluster of 24 nosocomial cases. *Ann. Intern. Med.* 99:172, 1983.

40. Hopkins, C.C., Weber, D.J., and Rubin, R.H. Invasive *Aspergillus* infection: Possible nonward common source within the hospital environment. *J. Hosp. Infect.* 13:19, 1989.

41. Huxley, E.J., et al. Pharyngeal aspiration in normal adults and patients with depressed consciousness. *Am. J. Med.* 64:564, 1978.

42. Johanson, W.G. Infection prevention by selective decontamination in intensive care. *Intensive Care Med.* 15417, 1989.

43. Johanson, W.G., Pierce, A.K., and Sanford, J.P. Changing pharyngeal bacterial flora of hospitalized patients. Emergence of Gram-negative bacilli. *N. Engl. J. Med.* 281:1137, 1969.

44. Johanson, W.G., Higuchi, J.H., Chaudhuri, T.R., and Woods, D.E. Bacterial adherence to epithelial cells in bacillary colonization of the respiratory tract. *Am. Rev. Respir. Dis.* 121:55, 1980.

45. Johanson, W.G., Jr., Pierce, A.K., Sanford, J.P., and Thomas, G.D. Nosocomial respira-

tory infections with Gram-negative bacilli. The significance of colonization of the respiratory tract. *Ann. Intern. Med.* 77:701, 1972.

46. Johanson, W.G., Jr., Woods, D.E., and Chaudhuri, T. Association of respiratory tract colonization with adherence of Gram-negative bacilli to epithelial cells. *J. Infect. Dis.* 139:667, 1979.

47. Kerver, A.J.H., et al. Prevention of colonization and infection in critically ill patients: A prospective randomized study. *Crit. Care Med.* 16:1087, 1988.

48. Klick, J.M., et al. Prevention of gram-negative bacillary pneumonia using aerosol polymixin as prophylaxis: II. Effect on the incidence of pneumonia in seriously ill patients. *J. Clin. Invest.* 55:514, 1975.

49. LaForce, F.M. Hospital-acquired Gram-negative rod pneumonias: An overview. *Am. J. Med.* 70:664, 1981.

50. LaForce, F.M. Systemic antimicrobial therapy of nosocomial pneumonia: Monotherapy versus combination therapy. *Eur. J. Clin. Microbiol.* 8:61, 1989.

51. LaForce, F.M., Hopkins, J., Trow, R., and Wang, W.L.L. Human oral defenses against gram-negative rods. *Am. Rev. Respir. Dis.* 114:929, 1976.

52. LaForce, F.M., Thompson, B., and Trow, R. Effect of atropine on oral clearance of a radiolabeled sulfur colloid. *J. Lab. Clin. Med.* 104:693, 1984.

53. Ledingham, IMcA., et al. Triple regimen of selective decontamination of the digestive tract, systemic cefotaxime, and microbiological surveillance for prevention of acquired infection in intensive care. *Lancet* 1:785, 1988.

54. Mackowiak, P.A., Martin, R.M., and Smith, J.W. The role of bacterial interference in the increased prevalence of oropharyngeal Gram-negative bacilli among alcoholics and diabetics. *Am. Rev. Respir. Dis.* 120:589, 1979.

55. Moore, R., Smith, C.R., and Lietman, P.S. Association of aminoglycoside plasma levels with therapeutic outcome in gram-negative pneumonia. *Am. J. Med.* 77:657, 1984.

56. Moser, M.R., et al. An outbreak of influenza A aboard a commercial airliner. *Am. J. Epidemiol.* 110:1, 1979.

57. Mostow, S.R. Prevention, management, and control of influenza: Role of amantadine. *Am. J. Med.* 82(Suppl. 6A):35, 1987.

58. Muder, R.R., Yu, V.L., and Woo, A.H. Mode of transmission of *Legionella pneumophila*. *Arch. Intern. Med.* 146:1607, 1986.

59. Muraca, P.W., Yu, V.L., and Goetz, A. Disinfection of water distribution systems for *Legionella:* A review of application procedures and methodologies. *Infect. Control. Hosp. Epidemiol.* 11:79, 1990.

60. Murray, P.R., and Rosenblatt, J.E. Bacterial interference by oropharyngeal and clinical isolates of anaerobic bacteria. *J. Infect. Dis.* 134:281, 1976.

61. Mylotte, J.M., and Beam, T.R. Comparison of community-acquired and nosocomial pneumococcal bacteremia. *Am. Rev. Respir. Dis.* 123:265, 1981.

62. Neill, M.A., et al. Nosocomial legionellosis, Paris, France. Evidence for transmission by potable water. *Am. J. Med.* 78:581, 1985.

63. Opal, S.M., et al. Efficacy of infection control measures during a nosocomial outbreak of disseminated aspergillosis associated with hospital construction. *J. Infect. Dis.* 153:634, 1986.

64. Pachucki, C.T., et al. Influenza A among hospital personnel and patients. Implications for recognition, prevention, and control. *Arch. Intern. Med.* 149:77, 1989.

65. Pennington, J.E. Penetration of antibiotics into respiratory secretions. *Rev. Infect. Dis.* 3:67, 1981.

66. Pierce, A.K., Sanford, J.P., Thomas, G.D., and Leonard, J.S. Long-term evaluation of decontamination of inhalation therapy equipment in nosocomial pulmonary infections. *N. Engl. J. Med.* 282:528, 1970.

67. Pingleton, S.K., Hinthorn, D.R., and Chien, L. Enteral nutrition in patients receiving mechanical ventilation. *Am. J. Med.* 80:827, 1986.

68. Ramirez-Ronda, C.H., Fuxench-Lopez, Z., and Nevarez, M. Increased pharyngeal colonization during viral illness. *Arch. Intern. Med.* 141:1599, 1981.

69. Reinarz, J.A., Pierce, A.K., Mays, B.B., and Sanford, J.P. The potential role of inhalation therapy equipment in nosocomial pulmonary infections. *J. Clin. Invest.* 44:831, 1965.

70. Rhame, F.S. Nosocomial aspergillosis: How much protection for which patients? *Infect. Control Hosp. Epidemiol.* 10:296, 1989.

71. Rhame, F.S., Streifel, A.J., Kersey, J.H., Jr., and McGlave, P.B. Extrinsic risk factors for pneumonia in the patient at high risk of infection. *Am. J. Med.* 76(5A):42, 1984.

72. Rosenthal, S.R., and Tager, I.B. Prevalence of Gram-negative rods in the normal pharyngeal flora. *Ann. Intern. Med.* 83:355, 1975.

73. Ruben, F.L., Norden, C.W., and Korica, Y. Pneumococcal bacteremia at a medical/surgical hospital for adults between 1975 and 1980. *Am. J. Med.* 77:1091, 1984.

74. Sanderson, P.J. The sources of pneumonia in ITU patients. *Infect. Control* 7(2):104, 1986.

75. Sarubbi, F.A., Jr., et al. Increased recovery of *Aspergillus flavus* from respiratory specimens during hospital construction. *Am. Rev. Respir. Dis.* 125:33, 1982.

76. Sculier, J.P., and Klastersky, J. Significance of

serum bactericidal activity in Gram-negative bacillary bacteremia in patients with and without granulocytopenia. In: A.E. Brown and D. Armstrong (Eds.), *Infectious Complications of Neoplastic Disease.* New York: Yorke, 1985: Pp. 35–48.

77. Shands, K.N., et al. Potable water as a source of Legionnaires' disease. *J.A.M.A.* 253:1412, 1985.

78. Sherertz, R.J., et al. Impact of air filtration on nosocomial *Aspergillus* infections. Unique risk of bone marrow transplant recipients. *Am. J. Med.* 83:709, 1987.

79. Simmons, B.P., and Wong, E.P. Guidelines for prevention of nosocomial pneumonia. *Infect. Control* 3:327, 1982.

80. Sprunt, K., and Redman, W. Evidence suggesting importance of role of interbacterial inhibition in maintaining balance of normal flora. *Ann. Intern. Med.* 68:579, 1968.

81. Stead, W.W. Tuberculosis among elderly persons: An outbreak in a nursing home. *Ann. Intern. Med.* 94:606, 1981.

82. Stout, J., et al. Potable water supply as the hospital reservoir for Pittsburgh pneumonia agent. *Lancet* 1:471, 1982.

83. Stout, J., et al. Ubiquitousness of *Legionella pneumophila* in the water supply of a hospital with endemic Legionnaires' disease. *N. Engl. J. Med.* 306:466, 1982.

84. Stoutenbeek, C.P., et al. The prevention of superinfection in multiple trauma patients. *J. Antimicrob. Chemother.* 14(B):203, 1984.

85. Stoutenbeek, C.P., et al. Nosocomial gram-negative pneumonia in critically ill patients. *Intensive Care Med.* 12:419, 1986.

86. Stoutenbeek, C.P., et al. The effect of oropharyngeal decontamination using topical nonabsorbable antibiotics on the incidence of nosocomial respiratory tract infections in multiple trauma patients. *J. Trauma* 27:357, 1987.

87. Stoutenbeek, C.P., van Saene, H.K.F., Miranda, D.R., and Zandstra, D.F. The effect of selective decontamination of the digestive tract on colonisation and infection rate in multiple trauma patients. *Intensive Care Med.* 10:185, 1984.

88. Tillotson, J.R., and Finland M. Bacterial colonization and clinical superinfection of the respiratory tract complicating antibiotic treatment of pneumonia. *J. Infect. Dis.* 119:597, 1969.

89. Tryba, M. Risk of acute stress bleeding and nosocomial pneumonia in ventilated intensive care unit patients: Sucralfate versus antacids. *Am. J. Med.* 83:117, 1987.

90. Ulrich, C., et al. Selective decontamination of the digestive tract with norfloxacin in the prevention of ICU-acquired infections: A prospective randomized study. *Intensive Care Med.* 15:424, 1989.

91. Unertl, K., et al. Prevention of colonization and respiratory infections in long-term ventilated patients by local antimicrobial prophylaxis. *Intensive Care Med.* 13:106, 1987.

92. Valenti, W.M. Infection control and employee health. *Infect. Control* 6:169, 1985.

93. Valenti, W.M., et al. Nosocomial viral infections: I. Epidemiology and significance. *Infect. Control* 1:33, 1980.

94. Valenti, W.M., and Menegus, M.A. Nosocomial viral infections: IV. Guidelines for cohort isolation, the communicable disease survey, collection and transport of specimens for virus isolation, and considerations for the future. *Infect. Control* 2:236, 1981.

95. Valenti, W.M., Trudell, R.G., and Bentley, D.W. Factors predisposing to oropharyngeal colonization with gram-negative bacilli in the aged. *N. Engl. J. Med.* 298:1108, 1978.

96. Vercellotti, G.M., et al. Bacterial adherence to fibronectin and endothelial cells: A possible mechanism for bacterial tissue tropism. *J. Lab. Clin. Med.* 103:34, 1984.

97. Walsh, T.J., and Dixon, D.M. Nosocomial aspergillosis: Environmental microbiology, hospital epidemiology, diagnosis and treatment. *Eur. J. Epidemiol.* 5:131, 1989.

98. Weinstein, M.P., Stratton, C.W., and Ackley, A. Multicenter collaborative evaluation of a standardized bactericidal test as a prognostic indicator in infective endocarditis. *Am. J. Med.* 78:262, 1985.

99. Winter, R., et al. Gastric pH and colonization in sucralfate treated patients. *Intensive Care Med.* 15:479, 1989.

100. Woo, A.H., Yu, V.L., and Goetz, A. Potential in-hospital modes of transmission of *Legionella pneumophila. Am. J. Med.* 80:567, 1986.

101. Woods, D.E., et al. Role of fibronectin in the prevention of adherence of *Pseudomonas aeruginosa* to buccal cells. *J. Infect. Dis.* 143:784, 1981.

102. Woods, D.E., et al. Role of salivary protease activity in adherence of gram-negative bacilli to mammalian buccal epithelial cells in vivo. *J. Clin. Invest.* 68:1435, 1981.

103. Yu, V.L., et al. Legionnaires' disease: A new clinical perspective from a prospective pneumonia study. *Am. J. Med.* 73:357, 1982.

104. Yu, V.L., et al. Routine culturing for *Legionella* in the hospital environment may be a good idea: A three-hospital prospective study. *Am. J. Med. Sci.* 294:97, 1987.

105. Centers for Disease Control. Nosocomial transmission of multidrug-resistant tuberculosis among HIV-infected persons—Florida and New York. *M.M.W.R.* 40:585, 1991.

Infectious Gastroenteritis

Herbert L. DuPont
Bruce S. Ribner

Microorganisms that cause outbreaks of food-borne illness in the community also have the potential for causing similar events in hospitalized patients. However, certain forms of gastroenteritis—such as that caused by food-borne toxins of *Clostridium perfringens, Clostridium botulinum, Staphylococcus aureus,* and *Bacillus cereus,* as well as that produced by the ingestion of food contaminated with group A streptococci and *Vibrio parahaemolyticus*—have not been recognized to be transmissible from person to person within the hospital. The control of these diseases in the hospital depends on safe food-handling practices as discussed in Chapter 17, and such forms of gastroenteritis are not considered additionally in this chapter.

Infectious or communicable gastroenteritis caused by *Salmonella* other than *S. typhi, Escherichia coli, Shigella,* and rotavirus receive primary attention in this chapter. In addition, the chapter separately addresses *Clostridium difficile* (an agent with a high degree of communicability that causes antibiotic-associated colitis), *Yersinia enterocolitica* (an agent that has produced communicable nosocomial infections involving the gastrointestinal tract), staphylococcal enterocolitis (a noncommunicable form of nosocomial gastroenteritis), and necrotizing enterocolitis (a disease of uncertain, possibly infectious cause). Nosocomial transmission of *Vibrio cholerae* has produced nosocomial infectious gastroenteritis in areas endemic for this disease, but the agent will not be discussed here because of the rarity of endemic cases in the United States.

Infectious gastroenteritis differs from most other hospital-associated infections, which characteristically result from endogenous organisms in persons with markedly altered resistance. Enteric infections caused by the agents just mentioned are nearly always exogenously acquired, often occur in clusters or epidemics, and are usually due to the introduction of a virulent organism through the ingestion of contaminated foods or medications, through short-term carriers among patients and hospital staff, or through patient-to-patient transmission on the hands of personnel. Although host factors such as age and debility are important, healthy patients and hospital personnel also are frequently involved in outbreaks of these infections.

Incidence

Although the true incidence of nosocomial infectious gastroenteritis is not known, it is evident that its occurrence is greatly underestimated. The common occurrence of non-infectious diarrhea among patients and personnel, the lack of standard criteria for the diagnosis of nosocomial infectious gastroenteritis, and the limited ability of many hospital laboratories to identify the most common agents responsible for infectious gastroenteritis have all contributed to the underreporting of this condition. These factors have also contributed to the great differences in rates of nosocomial infectious gastroenteritis reported by investigators in the literature.

It is important to distinguish between nosocomial diarrhea and nosocomial infectious gastroenteritis. Nosocomial diarrhea has been reported to occur in 7.7 to 41 percent of the patients admitted to adult intensive care units [20, 23], 1.2 to 2.1 percent of all patients admitted to pediatric teaching hospitals [2], and 1.5 percent of children admitted to two pediatric wards [23]. When compared to nosocomial infections occurring at other body sites in the same populations, nosocomial diarrhea represented either the first or second most common nosocomial illness. However, most studies do not require the isolation of a pathogen for the diagnosis of nosocomial diarrhea. Where sought, pathogens are found in slightly more than half of the affected patients in unselected populations [36] and in as few as 17 percent of the patients who develop

nosocomial diarrhea while receiving tube feedings [9]. Thus, nosocomial infectious gastroenteritis accounts for only a portion of those patients who experience nosocomial diarrhea.

The National Nosocomial Infections Surveillance (NNIS) System (see Chap. 27) for the period January 1986 through December 1989 found that, for hospitals reporting all nosocomial infections, 1.55 patients per 1,000 patients discharged experienced a nosocomial gastrointestinal infection. There were marked differences among services. The highest rates were found in high-risk nurseries (9.30 per 1,000), reflecting the underlying susceptibility of the hosts and the ease of transmission of the pathogens responsible for infectious gastroenteritis in this age group. Surgical services had the next highest rate (3.55 per 1,000), followed by medicine and pediatrics (1.88 and 1.36 per 1,000, respectively). Obstetric services had the lowest rates of enteric nosocomial infection (0.16 per 1,000 discharges).

Causative pathogens also tended to differ substantially by service. On pediatric services and in high-risk nurseries, rotaviruses were responsible for 75 percent and 51 percent, respectively, of all instances of nosocomial infectious gastroenteritis. In contrast, *C. difficile* accounted for 95 percent of such disease on general surgery services and 97 percent on medical services.

Diagnostic Criteria
Clinical and Microbiologic Criteria
There is wide variation in the clinical symptoms experienced by patients with these enteric infections. Some patients become asymptomatic excreters of a potential pathogen, whereas others show varying forms of diarrheal disease. Organisms that invade the intestinal epithelial lining often elicit a febrile response in addition to causing diarrhea. In infections with pathogens that invade the colonic mucosa primarily, symptoms of colitis occur, including urgency, tenesmus, and passage of bloody, mucoid stools (dysentery). Diarrhea or loose stools in a patient with un-

explained fever should be diagnosed as infectious gastroenteritis, regardless of culture results for bacterial pathogens. When diarrhea or loose stools occur in an afebrile patient or in a febrile patient whose fever has other likely causes, the identification of a recognized pathogen in stools or by serologic testing is necessary for this diagnosis.

Diarrhea of noninfectious origin—such as that caused by cathartics, inflammatory diseases of the gastrointestinal tract, and surgical resections and anastomoses—should be carefully differentiated from the diarrhea of infectious gastroenteritis. Alterations in the gastrointestinal flora because of antibiotic administration are commonly associated with diarrhea; such cases of diarrhea should not be reported as gastroenteritis unless enterocolitis occurs, in which event they should be reported as noninfectious gastroenteritis.

Classification of Infections

Diarrhea with onset after admission that is associated with a positive culture for organisms recognized as causative of infectious gastroenteritis should be regarded as a nosocomial infection. The interval between the time of admission and the onset of clinical symptoms must be greater than the known incubation period for that agent (see subsequent sections) unless there are associated cases among other hospital patients or personnel. Alternatively, nosocomial infections may be diagnosed if a stool culture obtained shortly before or just after admission is negative for the pathogen in question and the pathogen is subsequently cultured from the patient.

Predisposing Host Factors
Defective Gastric Defenses

There is evidence to indicate that gastric acid plays an important role in the defense against ingested organisms. The bactericidal action of stomach acid greatly reduces or eradicates ingested organisms and thus reduces the inoculum of organisms that subsequently reaches the intestine. Physiologic or pathologic achlorhydria, which is most common in premature infants and elderly patients, may

underlie the increased risks of certain enteric infections seen in these groups. Although unstudied, variations in gastric acidity may also partly determine which person becomes ill following the ingestion of a contaminated common vehicle. Antacid use has been shown to facilitate greatly colonization of the intestine with vaccine strains of *Shigella* and to increase the frequency of gastrointestinal acquisition of nosocomial strains of aerobic gram-negative rods. Similar effects are produced by agents such as cimetidine. It is probable that anticholinergic medications act similarly. Persons with histories of gastric resection and vagotomy are known to be at higher risk of acquiring cholera than normal persons.

The time during which ingested substances are in contact with gastric acid may be important. Water without food tends to traverse the stomach more rapidly than solid food, reaching the neutralizing secretions of the duodenum more rapidly. The inoculum of organisms required to produce infection is probably reduced when transmitted by water. Waterborne outbreaks of salmonellosis have occurred when low concentrations of the organism are present, whereas large numbers are usually required for foodborne transmission of these organisms.

Antibiotic Therapy

The oral or systemic administration of antibiotics to which an epidemic strain is resistant greatly facilitates cross-colonization and infection (see Chap. 12). These effects presumably occur because of a reduction in the competitive interference of normal, sensitive flora against the ingested strains, which in effect reduces the inoculum required for establishment of the pathogen. The continued administration of the drug following acquisition of the pathogen may permit the selective outgrowth of the pathogen and result in much greater concentrations of the organism in the feces than might otherwise occur. The chances of transmission and risk of disease are thereby increased.

Antibiotic administration may also predispose certain patients to diarrhea by enteric pathogens sensitive to the antibiotic. This may occur during therapy or shortly after termination of the antibiotic. In such cases, the pathogen is able to replicate more rapidly than the suppressed normal flora, reaching concentrations not normally achievable when the normal flora is at pretherapy levels. These elevated concentrations may lead to enteritis and increase the risk of cross-infection in a manner similar to that of resistant pathogens.

Crowding and Staffing Factors
A ratio of staff to patients that is insufficient encourages infractions in hand-washing and isolation techniques, especially in critical care areas. Even careful hand-washing, however, is sometimes ineffective in removing gram-negative rods from the hands, and a slight but definite risk of transmitting organisms by direct contact with successive patients exists even after hand-washing. Thus inordinately low staff-to-patient ratios may lead to increased risk of cross-colonization and infection. Crowding of patients also increases the risk of cross-infection. While crowding of patient is often accompanied by insufficiencies in staff, it may be independently important in that it increases the risk of indirect contact spread through environmental sources, especially in nurseries.

General Control Measures

In controlling the spread of enteric infections within the hospital environment, a number of general measures can be taken regardless of the specific pathogen responsible. The most important mode of cross-infection for enteric bacterial pathogens in the hospital is usually the fecal-oral route, where indirect contact spread of organisms occurs from patient to patient on the hands of personnel. Outbreaks may also result from the ingestion of contaminated food, medication, or test materials.

Hand-Washing
Since the most important means of spread of enteric bacterial pathogens is via hand transfer, effective hand-washing is among the most important measures to prevent disease trans-

mission. Although it is unlikely that all potentially pathogenic microorganisms can be removed by hand-washing, the level of contamination can be reduced, in most cases, below that necessary for disease transmission among healthy children and adults. Among debilitated patients or newborn infants, the dose of enteropathogens needed to produce disease probably is substantially lower. In areas housing such patients, additional measures for the prevention of cross-infection may be required.

Surveillance
It is necessary to have an alert hospital surveillance program that continually reviews clinical patterns of infection in the hospital and evaluates bacteriologic reports from the diagnostic microbiology laboratory. Such a program is often instrumental in defining the extent of an outbreak before it has reached serious proportions and represents the foundation of an effective infection control program (see Chap. 5).

Surveillance must include hospital personnel, particularly food handlers, as well as patients. One important means of minimizing nosocomial diarrheal disease is to establish an effective personnel health service. Food handlers, nurses, and ancillary staff having direct contact with patients should be encouraged to communicate with the personnel health service when an episode of acute gastroenteritis occurs among themselves. Stool cultures should be performed and the ill person removed from work until culture results and the clinical course of the disease can be evaluated (see Chap. 3).

All personnel with an acute diarrheal illness should be removed from food handling and direct patient contact until the diarrhea has resolved. If stool cultures reveal the presence of an infectious pathogen, the employees should not return to food handling and should not care for patients in high-risk areas (e.g., intensive care units, newborn nurseries, transplant services) until two stool specimens obtained a minimum of 24 hours apart are negative for the pathogen. Employees from whom an enteric pathogen is isolated may care for patients in low-risk areas on resolution of diarrhea and before elimination of the infectious pathogen from the stool. However, such employees must be instructed to pay careful attention to thorough hand-washing after use of toilet facilities.

No infant born of a mother with diarrhea or with stool cultures positive for an enteric pathogen should be admitted to the nursery ward. Any infant with loose, watery, or bloody diarrhea should be handled with enteric precautions until a noninfectious cause for the diarrhea has been identified.

Similarly, patients of all ages admitted to the hospital with unexplained diarrhea, or developing diarrhea while in the hospital, should be placed in enteric isolation until an infectious etiology has been ruled out. Historically, such patients have led to well-documented outbreaks of nosocomial gastroenteritis by both bacterial and viral agents.

Use of Antispasmodic Drugs

Treatment of acute gastroenteritis with drugs to decrease the motility of the gut and produce symptomatic relief of diarrhea may have undesirable side effects in select patients. In persons with severe illness due to invasive pathogens (*Shigella, Salmonella,* and *Campylobacter*), worsening of clinical illness may result. Drugs such as diphenoxylate hydrochloride and atropine (Lomotil) or loperamide (Imodium) should be avoided in the treatment of nosocomial gastroenteritis when patients have significant fever or are passing bloody mucoid stools.

Prompt Investigation of Cases

The occurrence of 2 or more cases of nosocomial infectious gastroenteritis caused by the same organism within a few weeks should prompt a review of the exposures common to these cases (see Chap. 6). Case-control investigations are less likely to establish the source of infections conclusively when the number of cases is small, and microbiologic sampling of foods, medications, or equipment common to cases may be of special value in this circumstance. Culture surveys of other patients hospitalized in the same patient care areas as those with cases of disease and of employees working in these areas may identify asympto-

matically infected persons, and such persons should be included with symptomatic patients for purposes of epidemiologically establishing possible sources.

Hospital outbreaks of enteric disease may be caused by patients or hospital personnel who are short-term carriers of a specific pathogen. Comparison of the exposures of cases and controls to specific personnel (see Chap. 6) and culture surveys of hospital personnel and asymptomatic patients may help to identify the carriers responsible for such outbreaks. Occasionally, environmental factors such as air, dust, bedside tables, thermometers, and mattresses are important in contact spread. If a common vehicle such as food, contaminated equipment, or contaminated oral medication or test solution can be identified, its removal or disinfection may assist in terminating the outbreak.

Secondary cases often occur following disease outbreaks caused by contaminated vehicles, and the chance of epidemiologically identifying responsible sources may be improved in such situations by focusing attention on early cases and on patients whose illnesses seem unlikely to have derived from person-to-person spread.

On occasion, epidemiologic studies may indicate that the central kitchen is responsible for the dissemination of a bacterial pathogen. Removal of food handlers with recent diarrheal disease or kitchen personnel with positive cultures on culture surveys may result in termination of the epidemic. In the vast majority of instances, however, foodborne outbreaks of nosocomial gastroenteritis derive from inadequate handling of products from food-producing animals rather than from contamination of the food by food handlers.

Outbreak Management

During an epidemic, it is usually helpful to isolate patients with asymptomatic as well as symptomatic infections in separate rooms with separate lavatory facilities. Enteric precautions are necessary, of which glove-gown-stool precautions should be a part.

In nurseries in which enteric isolation of individual cases is not possible, cohort systems (see Chap. 21) should be employed during an epidemic to minimize the risk of cross-infection. Successful control of outbreaks sometimes requires repeated culture surveys coupled with a special type of cohorting. Infants who are ill or colonized with the epidemic organism can sometimes be grouped together into a cohort that is physically separated from noninfected infants. Personnel caring for these infants must not care for non-infected infants, and no equipment should be shared between the two groups. Only milk packaged in sterile containers should be used, common equipment shared among babies should be removed, and infants should be confined to their own bassinets or Isolettes. To prevent additional spread of infection, infants born outside the hospital should not enter the nursery during an epidemic of diarrhea. Unnecessary contact with babies by hospital personnel or contact between infants should be eliminated during epidemics. An adequate-sized nursing and hospital staff is especially important in the management of nursery epidemics.

Not only is it important to isolate patients with active disease as long as indicated (see Chap. 11), but infected patients should be discharged from the hospital as soon as their condition allows them to be managed at home. Uninfected patients should also be discharged as soon as possible from hospital areas experiencing an outbreak of nosocomial gastroenteritis.

Salmonella Infections
General Aspects
Clinical and Microbiologic Features

In salmonellosis, fever, nausea, and vomiting develop and are followed shortly thereafter by abdominal pain and watery diarrhea. Frequently, mucous strands can be found in stool specimens, whereas gross blood is found in slightly fewer than 10 percent of cases. In shigellosis and *Campylobacter* enteritis, stools are bloody in approximately 50 percent of cases.

Newborns have a predisposition to disease. Approximately 50 percent of exposed infants

develop illness once a case is introduced into a nursery. *Salmonella* infections in infants may result in septicemia or disseminated focal disease such as meningitis, abscesses or osteomyelitis. They may also result in asymptomatic intestinal colonization. Some neonates become persistent intestinal carriers of salmonellae, and their cultures may remain positive for more than a year.

Others who are at high risk are the aged and the debilitated. Patients with malignant disease have an unexplained predisposition to the development of salmonellosis, and the frequency of bloodstream invasion in such patients is quite high. Persons housed in nursing homes represent another segment of hospitalized patients in whom explosive outbreaks may occur with high fatality rates.

In a patient with acute gastroenteritis, the isolation of *Salmonella* from a stool culture is generally sufficient to establish the cause of the disease. This is true because of the relatively high degree of pathogenicity of these enteric bacteria, plus the fact that long-term carriers are unusual.

Therapy

Antimicrobial therapy has been shown in numerous studies to prolong the intestinal excretion of salmonellae. Mild, uncomplicated *Salmonella* gastroenteritis should not be treated. However, in patients in whom bloodstream invasion occurs—most commonly newborn or extremely debilitated patients, particularly those with malignant disease—antimicrobials often are instrumental in recovery from infection and may be lifesaving. In general trimethoprim-sulfamethoxazole, ciprofloxacin (adults), and possibly aztreonam provide the most effective therapy.

In addition to prolonging the period of excretion of the infecting strains, the administration of antimicrobial agents may, on occasion, make the clinical infection more severe or cause clinical relapse of infection when the drug administered is one to which the infecting strain is resistant. Antimicrobial therapy also increases the chance of the infecting organism acquiring additional resistances (see Chap. 12).

Epidemiologic Considerations
Classification of Infections
Incubation periods for salmonellosis vary from 6 to 72 hours. The incubation period varies inversely with the size of the infecting dose. Patients with positive cultures and an onset of gastroenteritis 72 hours or more after admission should be considered to have nosocomial infections. Persons with onsets within 6 to 72 hours of admission should be considered to have nosocomial infections only when epidemiologic evidence makes nosocomial acquisition likely. Isolation of salmonellae from a patient's stool in the absence of clinical symptoms of gastroenteritis should be reported as a nosocomial infection only if previous stool cultures during hospitalization were negative.

Transmissibility
Whereas person-to-person transmission of *Salmonella* strains is unusual among healthy persons outside of the hospital environment, these organisms can be transmitted on the hands of health care workers or by person-to-person spread among the aged, debilitated, or newborn patients in the hospital setting. Communicability of this organism from patients to hospital personnel or to community contacts is uncommon because larger doses are necessary to infect healthy persons and the precautions routinely used by hospitals in managing patients with gastroenteritis are generally effective.

Incidence
Approximately 50 percent of infections occur on the newborn service or pediatric floor. The remaining cases occur mainly among patients on the surgical or medical services.

Since 1963, the Centers for Disease Control has maintained nationwide surveillance of salmonellosis. Between 1963 and 1972, 112 (or 28 percent) of the total reported outbreaks occurred in institutions (hospitals, nursing homes, and custodial institutions) [1]. Approximately 3,500 cases were reported in these outbreaks among institutionalized populations, which represented 13 percent of the total reported cases. In 1979, 13 percent of reported outbreaks in the United States occurred in institutions. These outbreaks accounted for only 1.4 percent of all the cases occurring in outbreaks that year. The average institutional outbreak involved 6 patients, contrasting with the average noninstitutional outbreak, which involved 69 patients.

Sources and Modes of Acquisition
The nosocomial salmonellosis that occurs in the pediatric population, especially in newborns, is characteristically spread from person to person. The organism is typically introduced into the nursery by an infant who acquired the infection from its mother at delivery, but it can also be introduced by a carrier among the personnel or, more rarely, through foods and medications. Spread from infant to infant within the nursery then occurs on the hands of personnel. Fomites may be important in cross-infections, and persistence of the organism in dust and other environmental sites is sometimes responsible for perpetuating an outbreak. Epidemics have been traced to contaminated delivery-room resuscitation equipment and the water baths used for heating infant formula [31]. A commercially distributed, special nutritional formula that contains contaminated egg albumin has caused *Salmonella infantis* outbreaks when administered orally or by tube feeding. Outbreaks of *S. kottbus*, a serotype that has a tendency to be excreted from infected bovine mammary glands, have been traced to contamination of human breast milk collected to feed premature infants. Although it is unclear whether the breast milk was primarily or secondarily contaminated, inadequate storage and handling of the milk following collection allowed the organisms to proliferate to significant levels.

Outbreaks in nurseries are generally smaller than those commonly seen in nosocomial *Salmonella* infections in adults [1]. In adult infections, a common source can usually be incriminated. The common source may be previously contaminated, raw or undercooked meats or other products of food-producing animals (e.g., eggs or milk products), or food that has become contaminated after cooking because of organisms on equipment or surfaces in the kitchen [19, 24]. Food contaminated by a short-term *Salmonella* carrier working in the kitchen is much less commonly responsible. On occasion, a medication contaminated by *Salmonella* serves as a vehicle, especially medications containing enzymes and hormones of animal origin (e.g., pepsin, bile salts, vitamins, and endocrine gland extracts). Sporadic cases caused by intermittent exposure to infrequently used medications can produce a puzzling epidemiologic problem that requires a careful case-control approach for its solution (see Chap. 6).

In homes for the aged, epidemics often are initiated by the ingestion of contaminated food, and the epidemic may be perpetuated by cross-infection among debilitated patients by means of health care workers (see Chap. 24).

Less frequent sources of *Salmonella* infections include yeast, dried coconut, carmine dye, and inadequately disinfected equipment used on successive patients (e.g., Gomco suction and endoscopy equipment).

The specific serotype of *Salmonella* may provide a clue to the source. Some serotypes commonly infecting humans, such as *S. typhimurium*, derive from a variety of sources, but some have strong associations with particular sources that may be likely in human infection: *S. choleraesuis* is associated with porcine sources; *S. cubana*, with cochineal insects used to prepare carmine dye; *S. dublin*, with bovines; *S. pullorum*, with poultry sources; and so on. Many additional correlations exist between serotypes and sources among the more than 2,000 serotypes of *Salmonella*. Establishing that several different cases were caused by the same serotype may also be of value in suggesting a common source of infection. This is especially true when cases have occurred sporadically in different hospital areas. For this reason, all *Salmonella* isolated from nosocomial infections should be serotyped.

Control

Safe food-handling practices, as outlined in Chapter 17, are especially important in the prevention of nosocomial salmonellosis. In addition to the prompt epidemiologic identification and removal of common sources and implementation of the measures mentioned earlier in this chapter concerning outbreak management, thorough cleaning and disinfection of fomites and environmental surfaces in a nursery after discharge of infected infants is also important (see Chap. 21). Prophylactic antibiotics are contraindicated as a control measure.

Escherichia coli Infections
General Aspects
Clinical and Microbiologic Features

E. coli can produce gastroenteritis in children and adults by several different mechanisms. Strains that produce keratoconjunctivitis in the guinea pig eye (the Sereny test) tend to produce an invasive *Shigella*-like illness. Disease caused by such strains appears rare in the United States, although large common-source outbreaks have been documented. Loose, watery diarrhea, usually mild but sometimes severe and resembling that of cholera, is associated with certain strains of *E. coli* that produce enterotoxin. Both heat-labile and heat-stable toxins have been identified. Disease can be produced by either type of enterotoxin, although both are frequently produced by the same strain. Enterotoxin-producing strains appear to be major causes of travelers' diarrhea and are frequent causes of gastroenteritis in developing countries. Enterotoxigenic *E. coli* occasionally causes outbreaks of diarrhea in the United States, characteristically traced to contaminated food or water. One large hospital nursery outbreak has been reported [28].

E. coli belonging to the classic enteropathogenic serotypes (EPEC) appears to produce disease by mechanisms not yet fully understood, since disease caused by such strains cannot be explained on the basis of the previously described mechanisms [14]. In more recent studies, a high percentage of EPEC strains have been enteroadherent, as seen in HEp-2 tissue culture cells [4]. EPEC has previously been considered a common cause of nursery outbreaks, which sometimes were explosive with high attack rates and fulminating clinical courses [33]. Reports of such outbreaks are not common in the United States in recent years. Undoubtedly, this relates at least in part to the decreasing availability of serotyping procedures in hospital diagnostic laboratories over the past 10 years. During any hospital outbreak of diarrhea, particularly when it has occurred in the newborn nursery, EPEC should be considered in the differential diagnosis.

The clinical expression of EPEC infections varies considerably—probably as a result of differences in pathogenic mechanisms—from minimal, watery diarrhea to fulminating disease with septicemia. There appears to be a great deal of unexplained variability even among strains with the same serotype, and occasional outbreaks occur in newborn nurseries in which attack rates exceed 50 percent and mortality is high. EPEC outbreaks are almost totally confined to newborn nurseries, and infants and young children, especially those younger than 2 years, appear to be primarily at risk. The association of EPEC disease with the very young may not be totally correct, because such strains are generally considered to occur only in children younger than 4 with diarrhea, and appropriate laboratory tests are performed only in this age group.

Clinicians should be aware that the laboratory procedures used to determine the serogroup of isolates have certain deficiencies. Non-EPEC serotypes that cross-react with EPEC serotypes can agglutinate in pooled test sera to give a false-positive test result that can be identified only by complete serotyping. Also, *E. coli* implicated in cases of diarrhea not belonging to EPEC serotypes and not producing the conventional heat-labile or heat-stable toxins of enterotoxigenic *E. coli* may be enteroadherent in HEp-2 cells.

Therapy

Disease caused by enterotoxin-producing strains of *E. coli* was shown to respond favorably to antibiotics to which the organisms are sensitive in studies conducted in Mexico, an area where such disease has a high endemic frequency [25a]. The duration and severity of diarrhea are reduced by such therapy. Although controlled trials have not been conducted, antibiotic therapy would appear to be indicated on clinical grounds for *Shigella*-like disease caused by invasive strains, and responses comparable to those seen in treatment of shigellosis (see under the heading *Shigella* Infections) might be anticipated.

The value of antimicrobial therapy for EPEC disease is presently controversial, part of this controversy doubtlessly deriving from the difficulty in ensuring that EPEC was the cause of the gastroenteritis. In some instances, a lack of response to antibiotics may have occurred because EPEC isolated from cases was an incidental finding in disease caused by other agents, especially rotaviruses. When gastroenteritis occurs in a premature or full-term nursery and a causative role can be ascribed to EPEC, uncontrolled trials suggest that orally administered gentamicin, colistin, or neomycin for a 1-week course of treatment may be of value [7a]. Systemic antibiotics should also be given to all such patients if sepsis occurs in one or more affected infants. Since the isolation of EPEC in a sporadic case of gastroenteritis is presently of uncertain value in establishing the cause, such laboratory findings offer little or no guidance for the clinician; the clinical severity of the illness is the only factor useful in deciding whether to institute treatment.

Epidemiologic Considerations
Classification of Infections

Incubation periods for EPEC disease are commonly 24 to 48 hours, but they may occasionally be much longer. Children with onset of gastroenteritis 48 hours or longer after admission should be considered to have nosocomial infections, as well as all infants who develop EPEC disease at any time during hospitalization following birth in the hospital. Isolation of an enteropathogenic serotype of *E. coli* from a stool culture in the absence of clinical symptoms of gastroenteritis should not be reported as an infection. For consistency in surveillance, an infection should be reported when an EPEC strain is isolated from a patient with gastroenteritis in whom no other recognized pathogen is identified.

Transmissibility

The only known population at risk to develop nosocomial enteric infections due to *E. coli* strains are newborn infants and young children. When an enteropathogenic *E. coli* strain is introduced into a nursery, hospital personnel and community contacts may become asymptomatic carriers of the organism, especially during an episode of infantile diarrhea, and may serve as an important epidemiologic link in the transmission of the disease to the newborns [27]. Enteric disease caused by enterotoxigenic *E. coli* is only very rarely transmitted from person to person.

Incidence

EPEC is an unusual cause of infectious nosocomial diarrheal disease caused by bacteria in the NNIS data (see Chap. 27). At the present time, these organisms are identified by serotype analysis. Outbreaks ascribed to EPEC have become much less common over the last decade. Only a few outbreaks of nosocomial disease caused by enterotoxin-producing *E. coli* have been reported [28].

Sources and Modes of Acquisition

The most common source of EPEC infections is an infected child admitted to a newborn nursery or readmitted to a pediatric ward. The infant may have acquired the infection at the time of delivery or may have acquired the organism during hospitalization and had an onset of enteric disease in the early days after discharge from the hospital. Secondary spread of the infecting strain to other infants occurs on the hands of hospital personnel or from articles in the nursery that have been contaminated with the strain during an epidemic. Pharyngeal colonization of infants is common during epidemics and, although unproved, may be an important intermediate step in producing disease in some cases. Proliferation of organisms at this site might produce an inoculum that is capable of establishing infection in the lower gastrointestinal tract.

Epidemics of infantile EPEC diarrhea have occurred at times when the organism can be detected in the dust and fomites within the hospital environment. Asymptomatic carriers are probably important as a cause of epidemics among susceptible infants and include antepartum mothers, hospital staff, or other children without disease. During periods of infantile diarrhea outbreaks, approximately 5 percent of pediatric patients without intestinal infection and up to one-third of antepartum women have been shown to harbor EPEC organisms in their stool. Outbreaks in the nursery usually follow the introduction of a new serotype of EPEC by a newly admitted, infected child or by colonized hospital personnel. The infecting strain is transmitted among children, generally on the hands of attendants or through articles and equipment in communal use.

A single, large, protracted nosocomial outbreak caused by a strain of *E. coli* that produced heat-stable enterotoxin and did not belong to a recognized enteropathogenic serotype has been reported [28]. The disease appears to have been transmitted by means of cross-contamination of oral feedings. The epidemic strain did not colonize or produce disease in adults despite its presence in multiple environmental sites. Illness was mild and characterized by 3 to 5 days of watery diarrhea without pus or blood in the stools. Prophylactic oral colistin, to which the multiply drug-resistant strain was sensitive, was ineffective in preventing acquisition. Antibiotic resistance and enterotoxin production were colinked on a transmissible plasmid of the epidemic strain [35].

Control

Control measures mentioned earlier in this chapter and elsewhere [17] can be helpful in curtailing an EPEC outbreak. Such measures are not indicated, however, unless a causative role can be ascribed to an EPEC strain on the basis of the previously outlined criteria. Colonization of infants with an EPEC strain in the absence of enteric disease attributable to the strain is not an indication for control measures.

Enterotoxigenic *E. coli* strains are believed to be transmitted mainly by food and water, and prevention of disease from these sources can be accomplished by proper food handling and chlorination of water supplies

Shigella Infections
General Aspects
Clinical and Microbiologic Features
Shigellosis, or bacillary dysentery, often represents a distinct clinical entity. Fever develops in 50 percent of the patients, and mucus with or without blood can be documented in the stool within 1 or 2 days after the onset of diarrhea. Patients are usually more toxic and symptoms more severe with this form of enteric infection than with others.

When newborns are infected by a *Shigella* strain, the mortality is higher, and complications (e.g., intestinal perforation and septicemia) develop with a higher frequency than in other common bacterial causes of gastroenteritis [16, 37]. Although there is some evidence that breast-fed infants show an increased resistance to *Shigella*, nearly all hosts are extremely susceptible to these organisms.

Shigella sonnei and *S. flexneri* are the species principally responsible for disease in the United States. *S. sonnei* strains can be differentiated from one another by colicin typing, and *S. flexneri* strains by serotyping. Clinicians should be aware that *Salmonella-Shigella* agar, a popular medium for stool cultures in many clinical laboratories, is toxic to many *S. flexneri* strains. For optimal recovery of strains, specimens should not be placed in holding or transport media but should be plated directly onto blood or xylose, lysine, and deoxycholate (XLD) agar as soon as possible after collection.

Therapy
In bacillary dysentery, appropriate antimicrobial agents are clearly beneficial in decreasing the excretion of the pathogenic shigellae and improving clinical symptoms. Trimethoprim-sulfamethoxazole (TMP/SMX) is the treatment of choice for all cases of shigellosis when susceptibility testing is not available. A 3- to 5-day course is generally adequate. The dose for children is TMP 10 mg/kg/day plus SMX 50 mg/kg/day in two divided doses; for adults, it is TMP 160 mg and SMX 800 mg twice daily. For TMP-resistant strains, the quinolones are recommended for adults. Norfloxacin 400 mg, ciprofloxacin 500 mg, or ofloxacin 200 mg, given twice daily for 3 days, is advised. For children infected by TMP-resistant shigellae, nalidixic acid 55 mg/kg/day in four equally divided doses or, for mild to moderately severe cases, furazolidone 7.5 mg/kg/day in four equally divided doses for 5 days is recommended. Antibiotic therapy is associated with the emergence of multiple drug resistance in originally sensitive strains, which is presumably caused by R-factor transfer from endogenous gastrointestinal flora. Thus patients should remain in enteric isolation until posttreatment cultures are negative.

Epidemiologic Considerations
Classification of Infections
Incubation periods for shigellosis vary from 1 to 6 days. Patients with positive cultures and an onset of gastroenteritis 24 hours or more after admission should be considered to have nosocomial infections unless epidemiologic evidence of community-acquired infection is found (e.g., occurrence of shigellosis in family contacts before the onset of the patient's illness). Isolation of shigellae from a patient's stool in the absence of clinical symptoms of gastroenteritis should be reported as a nosocomial infection only if previous stool cultures during hospitalization were negative or isolation occurs during a documented hospital outbreak due to the recovered strain.

Transmissibility
Though *Shigella* strains represent the most potentially communicable of the bacterial pathogens, the striking clinical disease often helps the physician spot the illness early and promptly institute effective therapy and control measures. Such early detection partly explains the usual, surprising lack of spread within the normal hospital environment. Other patients, hospital personnel, and community contacts appear to be at risk of developing bacillary dysentery when exposed to an infected patient because of the very low dose

of organisms (less than 10^2) necessary to produce disease.

Incidence

Although any hospitalized patient is at risk of developing nosocomial shigellosis when a case is admitted, only rarely do outbreaks occur [30]. The only population at high risk is that of persons housed in residential institutions for the mentally retarded, where crowded living conditions, poor personal hygiene, and overworked nursing personnel all appear to be important causes of serious outbreaks.

Shigellosis was reported in only 1 of the 3,363 patients with nosocomial enteric infections during the 1986–1989 period in NNIS data [3a]. How many of the 10,000 to 13,000 cases of shigellosis reported each year in the United States come from hospitals is unknown. Between 10 and 20 percent of the cases of shigellosis reported each year, however, originate in residential institutions for the retarded.

Sources and Modes of Acquisition

The usual sources are short-term carriers of the organism who are either ill or in the convalescent stages of their disease. In custodial institutions, a few long-term carriers may be present and may serve as an important reservoir. Long-term carriage, however, is rare. On occasion, shigellosis develops when contaminated food is ingested that was prepared by a person carrying the organism following an episode of disease. The vast majority of cases, however, are secondary to person-to-person spread of infection. Infections are rarely acquired by indirect contact spread from inanimate environmental sources, since these organisms are only able to survive for short periods in the environment.

Control

Antibiotics are effective in eradicating sensitive strains of *Shigella* from the gastrointestinal tract but, as noted earlier, infecting strains have a propensity to develop multiple drug resistance in response to therapy. Thus treatment of culture-positive patients should be coupled with individual enteric isolation

procedures for each patient to prevent the potential emergence and continued spread of a strain that has acquired additional antibiotic resistances (see Chap. 11).

Streptomycin-dependent vaccine strains of *Shigella* have been tested as a control measure in mental institutions with high endemic rates of shigellosis. The duration of protection is short, however, as it is with the natural disease. Furthermore, multiple oral doses of vaccine must be given, vaccine strains can be transmitted to nonimmunized patients, and there is a potential risk of reversion of such strains to streptomycin-independent virulent organisms.

Viral Gastroenteritis

Rotaviruses have been shown to be important causes of nosocomial gastroenteritis [8, 13, 29]. Nosocomial transmission of rotavirus [6, 12, 13, 29], hepatitis A virus [15], and adenoviruses [12] has been documented. Nosocomial adenoviral gastroenteritis, which appears to be much less frequent than rotaviral infections and produces milder clinical illness, will not be discussed in this section.

Although the transmission of hepatitis A infection is rare in the hospital setting, it is mentioned here briefly because of the occasional presentation of patients with unexplained diarrhea caused by hepatitis A (see Chap. 38). The diarrhea may antedate the onset of clinical jaundice by several days, or jaundice may not occur. The high titers of infectious virus in the stool during the preicteric phase make these patients excellent sources of hepatitis A nosocomial infection in settings in which good hand-washing practices are not followed.

Incidence of Rotavirus Infections

Rotaviruses are the most frequent enteric pathogens found in persons younger than 5 years in the United States (see Chap. 38). They have also been established as the leading cause of nosocomial infectious gastroenteritis in pediatric patients. Prospective studies in hospital nurseries have shown 33 to 70 percent of the infants may shed rotavirus in the stool by the fifth day of life, with 8 to 28 percent of those shedding the virus demonstrating clinical symptoms [2, 19a, 22]. Similar studies in pediatric patients have shown rotaviruses to account for nearly one-half of all nosocomial infectious gastroenteritis [2, 13, 36]. As noted earlier, data from the NNIS System for the years 1986–1989 recorded rotavirus as the causative agent in 75 percent of pediatric patients with nosocomial infectious gastroenteritis and 51 percent of such patients in high-risk nurseries [3a]. When patients are stratified by age, rotavirus is far more likely to cause nosocomial infectious gastroenteritis in patients younger than 2 years [2]. Infection rates tend to follow the seasonal pattern observed in the general community, with peak incidence in the winter and spring and lowest incidence in the summer [2].

Though less common in adults, rotaviruses may be responsible for nosocomial infectious gastroenteritis in this age group. Yolken and colleagues [38] found rotaviruses to be the causative agent in 9 of 31 patients who experienced infectious diarrhea on a bone marrow transplant unit. Outbreaks of rotavirus infection have also been reported in hospitalized geriatric patients [20] and in elderly patients on a long-stay ward [5]. For the period 1986–1989, the NNIS System found rotavirus to account for 4 percent and 2 percent of the nosocomial infectious gastroenteritis on oncology services and general surgical services, respectively, but for less than 1 percent of such disease on other adult services.

Clinical Aspects

Illness begins with the sudden onset of fever, abdominal pain, and vomiting and continues with moderate or severe watery diarrhea that generally lasts approximately 3 to 8 days. Rotavirus disease severe enough to require hospitalization occurs in 2 percent of all children during their lifetime [3]. Rotavirus can be identified in the stool or rectal swab specimens from infected patients through direct or immune electron microscopy. Commercially available kits for the accurate and rapid identification of rotavirus are currently available. These kits make use of either a modified enzyme-linked immunosorbent assay (ELISA) or latex agglutination. Due to the high incidence of asymptomatic shedding of rotavirus in children younger than 2 years, positive assays in isolated cases must be interpreted with caution.

Sources and Modes of Acquisition

Rotavirus disease appears to be highly infectious, and it can be spread from patients with disease to susceptible persons by direct contact. The peak incidence in winter suggests that droplet spread from the upper respiratory tract may play a role in transmission, since respiratory spread is a common feature of most illnesses with seasonal peaks in the winter. Nosocomial transmission probably occurs indirectly from patient to patient on the hands of hospital personnel as well as by person-to-person spread from patients with disease to susceptible persons when such patients are inadequately isolated. Hospital personnel are generally immune and do not carry the virus.

Prevention and Control

Rotaviruses are highly immunogenic, and serologic studies indicate a high level of acquired immunity in persons more than 5 years of age. These findings raise the possibility of ultimate control of the disease by vaccine. Children with nosocomial nonbacterial gastroenteritis should be placed on enteric precautions; although not currently recommended in Centers for Disease Control guidelines, considerations should be given to the use of masks on older children to prevent potential droplet transmission when they are transported out of the isolation area.

Other Gastrointestinal Diseases

Clostridium difficile Colitis

It is now established that *C. difficile* is the major cause of the clinical syndrome previously called *antibiotic-associated colitis*, with pseudomembranous colitis being the most severe form of the disease. The organism is rapidly and efficiently transmitted to hospital staff and patients.

Incidence

C. difficile is a common cause of nosocomial infectious gastroenteritis in hospitalized adult patients. Prospective studies are rare, but one institution found that *C. difficile* accounted for 15 percent of the nosocomial diarrhea in adult patients admitted to an intermediate care unit [32]. For the period 1986–1989, NNIS participants found *C. difficile* to be the causative pathogen in 95 percent of general surgery patients and 97 percent of medical patients with nosocomial infectious gastroenteritis [3a]. The role of *C. difficile* as a pathogen in neonatal and pediatric patients has been difficult to determine due to the high rate of asymptomatic colonization in these patients and the inability to correlate toxin production with clinical illness.

Clinical Aspects

Characteristically, *C. difficile* produces profuse diarrhea and fever that are temporally related to a course of antimicrobial therapy. Stools often contain mucus and blood. The major antibiotics associated with the disease are clindamycin, cephalosporins, and ampicillin. Nearly all commonly used antibiotics have been implicated in the process. Diagnosis is based on the clinical setting (diarrhea in a patient receiving an antibiotic) plus the use of other diagnostic tests and procedures. Sigmoidoscopy reveals the characteristic white or yellow plaques of pseudomembranous colitis. The toxin of *C. difficile* is demonstrated by documenting a histotoxic effect in tissue culture cells that is inhibited by clostridial antitoxin or more commonly by serologic methods.

Therapy includes stopping the antibiotic, administering fluids and electrolytes, and instituting chemotherapy when appropriate. Those with mild disease who do not have documented pseudomembranous colitis should have antibiotics withdrawn for 48 to 72 hours before initiation of chemotherapy. Patients who continue to have diarrhea after this period of time, or patients who have pseudomembranous colitis on initial evaluation, should receive either oral vancomycin or oral metronidazole for 10 to 14 days. Relapse can be expected in approximately 10 percent of patients who initially respond to chemotherapy.

Sources and Modes of Acquisition

C. difficile can be cultured from the stool of many normal neonates and children. Adults have been found to have a gastrointestinal colonization rate of 1 to 4 percent on admission to the hospital. Approximately 20 percent of hospitalized adult patients will acquire asymptomatic carriage of *C. difficile* [25]. Most nosocomial acquisition of *C. difficile* occurs via the contaminated hands of health care personnel. This hand contamination may originate from direct contact with colonized or infected patients or from contact with contaminated environmental sources. Several authors have documented the heavy contamination of environmental surfaces in the rooms of patients with *C. difficile* and the persistence of *C. difficile* on these surfaces for months. Patients admitted into these rooms have an increased likelihood of becoming carriers [25].

Whereas previous antibiotic administration is associated with a greater likelihood of stool carriage and pseudomembranous colitis, it is not required. Antibiotic administration predisposes to *C. difficile* colonization by suppressing the normal bowel flora, allowing the *C. difficile* to proliferate.

Prevention and Control

As noted earlier, the major mode of transmission of *C. difficile* is via the hands of health care workers. Hands can become contaminated by direct contact with patients who are colonized or infected with *C. difficile* or by contact with spores contaminating the environmental surfaces. McFarland and co-workers [25] have recently shown that washing with a nondisinfectant soap is unlikely to eliminate hand carriage but that the use of gloves and disinfectant soap did eliminate hand carriage.

Staphylococcal Enterocolitis

In contrast to *C. difficile* colitis, staphylococcal enterocolitis is not transmissible from person to person; however, the disease may be an important source from which nosocomial strains of *Staphylococcus aureus* can be transmitted.

Incidence

The true incidence of such infections is unknown. Since the appreciation of *C. difficile* as the common cause of pseudomembranous colitis, the reported incidence of staphylococcal enterocolitis has dropped sharply. No cases were reported in the NNIS reporting period of 1986–1989 [3a]. Staphylococcal enterocolitis occurs sporadically, and epidemics have not been reported.

Clinical Aspects

In certain hosts in whom there is impaired resistance due to surgery, antimicrobial therapy, alcoholism or diabetes mellitus, staphylococci may grow to large numbers in the intestinal tract and be responsible for morphologic damage to the intestinal mucosa that results in diarrhea and fever of varying severity. Intestinal involvement varies widely from minimal and self-limiting enteritis to fulminating pseudomembranous enterocolitis [7]. Patients with enteritis have diarrhea of a variable nature, often mild and watery, and may have low-grade fever, but they are not extremely toxic. Pseudomembranous enterocolitis frequently presents with fulminating and dehydrating diarrhea; bloody, mucoid stools; fever; leukocytosis; and toxemia. The entire colon may be involved with the disease, and there may be some involvement of the small intestine. Mortality in such patients is high and ranges from 10 to 50 percent.

The diagnosis is established by documenting abundant polymorphonuclear leukocytes and sheets of gram-positive cocci in stool specimens, which on subsequent culture grow large numbers of *S. aureus*. Proctologic examination shows a white membrane that reflects areas of mucosal necrosis in those with pseudomembranous enterocolitis.

Patients should receive replacement fluid and electrolytes. Both oral vancomycin [21] and fecal retention enemas containing stool flora from a healthy person (the latter may have only historical significance) have been shown to be of value in treating patients with serious forms of the disease. Parenteral semisynthetic penicillinase-resistant penicillin treatment is advised for very toxic patients.

Sources and Modes of Acquisition

S. aureus can be cultured from the stool of approximately 10 percent of normal adults, but it is usually present in small numbers. Intestinal carriage of these organisms is twice as common in hospitalized patients as in persons outside the hospital environment. Most strains that cause staphylococcal enterocolitis are multiply drug-resistant, and some have been shown to produce an enterotoxin in laboratory tests. Pathogenic strains are probably acquired mainly from nosocomial sources, and they proliferate to displace normal flora when antibiotics to which they are resistant are administered. Staphylococcal enterotoxin is probably not important in the pathogenesis of the disease, since otherwise clinically identical pseudomembranous enterocolitis occurs following infection with nonenterotoxigenic strains. Destruction or replacement of normal endogenous flora is probably the principal inciting factor.

Prevention and Control

Prompt cessation of previously administered antibiotics and administration of oral vancomycin to patients with more serious staphylococcal enteritis may prevent the disease from progressing to pseudomembranous enterocolitis. Large numbers of *S. aureus* are often disseminated from patients with these diseases, and strict, rather than enteric, isolation procedures should be considered (see Chap. 11).

Neonatal Necrotizing Enterocolitis

Neonatal necrotizing enterocolitis (NEC) is a frequently fatal disease that usually affects low-birth-weight infants with preexistent perinatal complications. The disease is characterized by ischemic necrosis of the gastrointestinal tract and intramural gas (pneumatosis intestinalis), and it frequently results in intestinal perforation, peritonitis, and septicemia. NEC often occurs in epidemics within nurseries, which suggests an infectious cause. Three pathogenetic factors underlie the occurrence of disease: injury to the intestinal mucosa, due to relative ischemia from stress in newborns or other causes; the presence of intraluminal enteric bacteria; and enteral feedings that provide a metabolic substrate for the bacteria.

Most reports of NEC have not incriminated a particular bacterium as a cause of the disease, perhaps indicating that many strains of gram-negative bacteria or viruses may be involved in its pathogenesis. However, a particular strain of bacteria prevalent in the nursery has occasionally been linked with an epidemic of NEC [18]. The prophylactic use of systemic antibiotics does not prevent colonization of an infant's gastrointestinal tract with gram-negative bacteria, and most studies have shown no efficacy of such drugs in preventing NEC. The prophylactic use of oral kanamycin, however, appeared effective in one study [10], as did oral administration of IgA-IgG given to low-birth-weight infants [11].

Additional studies of sporadic and epidemic NEC cases, including careful aerobic and anaerobic culture studies of cases and controls, should assist in determining the role of microorganisms in this disease.

Yersinia enterocolitica Infections

Nosocomial transmission of infections caused by *Yersinia enterocolitica* has rarely been reported, but it probably occurs far more commonly than reports indicate. The organism, a gram-negative rod, can easily be misidentified, and sometimes prolonged cold enrichment is required for its optimal recovery from stool specimens. Early symptoms are usually those of fever and acute enterocolitis, and the abdominal pains are frequently so similar to those of appendicitis that appendectomies are performed. Mesenteric adenitis or ileitis is generally discovered. A wide variety of other features can be seen, including arthritis and erythema nodosum. Although the reservoir of the organism is in animals, person-to-person transmission also occurs, and nosocomial transmission has sometimes involved personnel [34].

A more deliberate search for this organism in otherwise unexplained nosocomial gastroenteritis outbreaks should be encouraged when clinical features suggest it is a possible causative agent. In addition to culture studies, serologic tests may be helpful in establishing the diagnosis of infection with this organism.

Other Pathogens

In addition to the enteropathogens discussed, outbreaks of nosocomial gastroenteritis have been caused by *Citrobacter freundii* [26], *Listeria monocytogenes* [22], and a variety of other agents. Although *Campylobacter jejuni* was encountered only rarely in the NNIS survey, it will undoubtedly prove to be an important cause of nosocomial gastroenteritis now that the organism can be readily identified in hospital laboratories. The ability of pathogens other than those normally associated with gastrointestinal disease to produce gastroenteritis must be remembered when evaluating an outbreak. One should be cautious not to dismiss lightly unusual pathogens recovered from stool cultures during the investigation of nosocomial enterocolitis.

References

1. Baine, W.B., Gangarosa, E.J., Bennett, J.V., and Barker, W.H., Jr. Institutional salmonellosis. *J. Infect. Dis.* 128:357, 1973.
2. Brady, M.T., Pacini, D.L., Budde, C.T., and Connell, M.J. Diagnostic studies of nosocomial diarrhea in children: Assessing their use and value. *Am. J. Infect. Control* 17:77, 1989.
3. Centers for Disease Control. Viral agents of gastroenteritis: Public health importance and outbreak management. *M.M.W.R.* 39 (No. RR-5): 1, 1990.
3a. Centers for Disease Control, National Nosocomial Infections Surveillance (NNIS) System, Hospital Infections Program, Atlanta, GA, 1986–1989.
4. Cravioto, A., Gross, R.J., Scotland, S.M., and Rowe, B. An adhesive factor found in strains of *Escherichia coli* belonging to the traditional

infantile enteropathogenic serotypes. *Curr. Microbiol.* 3:95, 1979.

5. Cubitt, W.D., and Holzel, H. An outbreak of rotavirus infection in a long-stay ward of a geriatric hospital. *J. Clin. Pathol.* 33:306, 1980.

6. Davidson, G.P., et al. Importance of a new virus in acute sporadic enteritis in children. *Lancet* 1:242, 1975.

7. Dearing, W.H., Baggenstoss, A.H., and Weed, L.A. Studies on the relationship of *Staphylococcus aureus* to pseudomembranous enterocolitis and to postantibiotic enteritis. *Gastroenterology* 38:441, 1960.

7a. DuPont, H.L., and Pickering, L.K. *Infections of the Gastrointestinal Tract: Microbiology, Pathophysiology, and Clinical Features.* New York: Plenum, 1980.

8. Echeverria, P., Blacklow, N.R., and Smith, D.H. Role of heat-labile toxigenic *Escherichia coli* and reovirus-like agent in diarrhea in Boston children. *Lancet* 2:1113, 1975.

9. Edes, T.E., Walk, B.E., and Austin, J.L. Diarrhea in tube-fed patients: Feeding formula not necessarily the cause. *Am. J. Med.* 88:91, 1990.

10. Egan, E.A., Mantilla, G., Nelson, R.M., and Eitzman, D.V. A prospective controlled trial of oral kanamycin in the prevention of neonatal necrotizing enterocolitis. *J. Pediatr.* 89:467, 1976.

11. Eibl, M.M., Wolf, H.M., Fürnkranz, H., and Rosenkranz, A. Prevention of necrotizing enterocolitis in low-birth-weight infants by IgA-IgG feeding. *N. Engl. J. Med.* 319:1, 1988.

12. Flewett, T.H., Boyden, A.S., and Davies, H. Epidemic viral enteritis in a long-stay children's ward. *Lancet* 1:4, 1975.

13. Ford-Jones, E.L., Mindorff, C.M., Gold, R., and Petric, M. The incidence of viral-associated diarrhea after admission to a pediatric hospital. *Am. J. Epidemiol.* 131:711, 1990.

14. Goldschmidt, M.C., and DuPont, H.L. Enteropathogenic *Escherichia coli:* Lack of correlation of serotype with pathogenicity. *J. Infect. Dis.* 133:153, 1976.

15. Goodman, R.A., et al. Nosocomial hepatitis A transmission by an adult patient with diarrhea. *Am. J. Med.* 73:220, 1982.

16. Haltalin, K.C. Neonatal shigellosis: Report of 16 cases and review of the literature. *Am. J. Dis. Child.* 114:603, 1967.

17. Harris, A.H., et al. Control of epidemic diarrhea of the newborn in hospital nurseries and pediatric wards. *Ann. N.Y. Acad. Sci.* 66:118, 1956.

18. Hill, H.R., Hunt, C.E., and Matsen, J.M. Nosocomial colonization with *Klebsiella*, type 26, in a neonatal intensive care unit associated with an outbreak of sepsis, meningitis, and necrotizing enterocolitis. *J. Pediatr.* 85:415, 1974.

19. Hirsch, W., et al. *Salmonella edinburg* infection in children: A protracted hospital epidemic due to a multiple drug resistant strain. *Lancet* 2:828, 1965.

19a. Jayashree, S., Bhan, M.K., Raj, P., et al. Neonatal rotavirus infection and its relation to cord blood antibodies. *Scand. J. Infect. Dis.* 20:249, 1988.

20. Kelly, T.W.J., Patrick, M.R., and Hillman, K.M. Study of diarrhea in critically ill patients. *Crit. Care Med.* 11:7, 1983.

21. Khan, M.Y., and Hall, W.H. Staphylococcal enterocolitis: Treatment with oral vancomycin. *Ann. Intern. Med.* 65:1, 1966.

22. Larsson, S., et al. *Listeria monocytogenes* causing hospital-acquired enterocolitis and meningitis in newborn infants. *Br. Med. J.* 2:473, 1978.

23. Lima, N., Searcy, M., and Guerrant, R. Nosocomial Diarrhea Rates Exceed Those of Other Nosocomial Infections on ICU and Pediatric Wards (abstr. 1050). In: *Proceedings of the Interscience Conference on Antimicrobial Agents and Chemotherapy.* Washington, DC: American Society of Microbiology, 1986.

24. Mackerras, I.M., and Mackerras, M.J. An epidemic of infantile gastro-enteritis in Queensland caused by *Salmonella bovis-morbificans* (Basenau). *J. Hyg.* (Camb.) 47:166, 1949.

25. McFarland, L.V., Mulligan, M.E., Kwok, R.Y.Y., and Stam, W.E. Nosocomial acquisition of *Clostridium difficile* infection. *N. Engl. J. Med.* 320:204, 1989.

25a. Oberhelman, R.H., et al. Efficacy of trimethoprim-sulfamethoxazole in treatment of acute diarrhea in a Mexican pediatric population. *J. Pediatr.* 110:960, 1987.

26. Parida, S.N., Verma, I.C., Deb, M., and Bhujwala, R.A. An outbreak of diarrhea due to *Citrobacter freundii* in a neonatal special care nursery. *Indian J. Pediatr.* 47, 81, 1980.

27. Rogers, K.B. The spread of infantile gastroenteritis in a cubicled ward. *J. Hyg.* (Lond.) 49:40, 1951.

28. Ryder, R.W., et al. Infantile diarrhea produced by heat-stable enterotoxigenic *Escherichia coli. N. Engl. J. Med.* 295:849, 1976.

29. Ryder, R.W., McGowan, J.E., Hatch, M.H., and Palmer, E.L. Reovirus-like agent as a cause of nosocomial diarrhea in infants. *J. Pediatr.* 90:698, 1977.

30. Salzman, T.C., Scher, C.D., and Moss, R. Shigellae with transferable drug resistance: Outbreak in a nursery for premature infants. *J. Pediatr.* 71:21, 1967.

31. Schroeder, S.A., Aserkoff, R., and Brachman, P.S. Epidemic salmonellosis in hospitals and institutions: A five-year review. *N. Engl. J. Med.* 279:674, 1968.

32. Silva, J., and Iezzi, C. *Clostridium difficile* as a

nosocomial pathogen. *J. Hosp. Infect.* 11 (Suppl. A): 378, 1988.

33. Taylor, J. Infectious infantile enteritis, yesterday and today. *Proc. R. Soc. Med.* 63:1297, 1970.

34. Toivanen, P., Toivanen, A., Olkkonen, L., and Aantaa, S. Hospital outbreak of *Yersinia enterocolitica* infection. *Lancet* 1:801, 1973.

35. Wachsmuth, I.K., Falkow, S., and Ryder, R.W. Plasmid-mediated properties of a heat-stable enterotoxin-producing *Escherichia coli* associ-ated with infantile diarrhea. *Infect. Immun.* 14: 403, 1976.

36. Welliver, R.C., and McLaughlin, S. Unique epidemiology of nosocomial infections in a children's hospital. *Am. J. Dis. Child.* 138:131, 1984.

37. Whitfield, C., and Humphries, J.M. Meningitis and septicemia due to *Shigellae* in a newborn infant. *J. Pediatr.* 70:805, 1967.

38. Yolken, R.H., et al. Infectious gastroenteritis in bone marrow transplant recipients. *N. Engl. J. Med.* 306:1009, 1982.

31

Puerperal Endometritis

William J. Ledger

Nature of Infections

Incidence

There is good evidence that the incidence of puerperal endometritis reported from individual hospitals with active surveillance of these infections (1 to 4 percent) is probably unchanged from the most accurate figures available from the preantibiotic decade of the 1920s. This statement is not an apology for modern obstetrics, for the status of puerperal endometritis and sepsis has dramatically changed in that same time interval. The number of cesarean sections has increased, and these have a higher risk of infection, whereas the most severe infections—those resulting in maternal death from sepsis—have virtually been eliminated from modern obstetrics.

The reported incidence of puerperal endometritis is higher than that noted in the National Nosocomial Infections Surveillance (NNIS) System (see Chap. 27), in which an incidence of less than 1 percent was found. Possible reasons for this lower incidence in the NNIS System are noted in the following sections.

Deficiencies in Reporting Infections

Obstetricians, who are surgically oriented physicians, tend to underestimate the incidence of nosocomial infections, including postpartum endometritis. This phenomenon of individual physician inaccuracy in assessing the frequency of infections reflects commonly observed patterns of clinical practice. Most patients with the early symptoms of a postpartum endometritis, such as temperature elevation, are first discovered at night and not during the traditional early-morning rounds of physicians (Fig. 31-1) [10]. In the majority of cases, these patients are placed on systemic antibiotics without prior culture studies. A nationwide evaluation of more

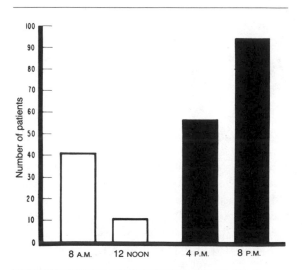

Fig. 31-1. The first temperature elevation of obstetric patients with postpartum morbidity. The majority of patients had initial rises in the late afternoon or evening hours.

than 12,000 women undergoing hysterectomy who were cared for by obstetrician-gynecologists revealed that more than 50 percent had received systemic antibiotics without prior culture tests [13]. A rapid response of the patient to the administered antibiotics with a quick return of temperature levels to normal may cause the attending physician to disregard the case as "true" morbidity. In addition, early discharge of patients from the hospital under the diagnosis-related group system means that many infections will be diagnosed outside of the hospital. In this context, the reader must be aware that any nationwide survey will detect only a portion of all cases of endometritis during the study interval. Despite the fact that some cases are inevitably missed by surveillance systems such as the NNIS System, pooled microbiologic data from cases that are reported do provide a good assessment of the major pathogens involved in postpartum endometritis.

Underestimates of the incidence of endometritis in modern obstetrics are also a result of continued dependence on a preantibiotic-era definition of morbidity based on temperature elevations. This definition was established by American obstetrician-gynecologists between the first and second world wars, and it is based on four separate oral temperature recordings each postpartum day; *morbidity* is defined as an oral temperature of 38°C (100.4°F) or greater on any 2 of the first 10 postpartum days, excluding the first 24 hours after delivery. This is in contrast to the early discharge system now in place, which precludes these observations over a 10-day period. Modern obstetric practice encourages in-house observation for 1 to 3 days after vaginal delivery and 3 to 5 days after cesarean section. The old definition excluded from consideration patients with one temperature elevation shortly after delivery as well as those who had a single temperature elevation later but no evidence of a postpartum pelvic infection. On a statistical basis, nearly all the women from the preantibiotic era who met these temperature criteria for morbidity had a pelvic infection, whether uterine or urinary tract. Appropriate microbiologic studies could be performed, and such patients could be isolated from other obstetric patients. Many of these patients now are being treated at home.

Another great barrier to a clear understanding of infectious disease in antibiotic-era obstetrics has been adherence to this old standard in the face of antibiotic use. Employment of powerful systemic antibiotics in postpartum patients with the first elevation of temperature may yield an immediate clinical response with rapid and persistent defervescence of fever. If the obstetric service adheres to traditional temperature-defined morbidity standards, the patient is not counted in morbidity statistics. This accounts in part for the frequent discrepancy between the low recorded morbidity figures and the high systemic antibiotic use in obstetric units.

Community-Acquired Versus Nosocomial Infections

All cases of postpartum endometritis should be considered nosocomial infections unless the amniotic fluid is infected at the time of admission or a patient was admitted 24 hours or more following rupture of the membranes. Some infections in the latter group are nosocomial, however, and available microbiologic, clinical, and epidemiologic data should be carefully reviewed to determine whether the infection is community-acquired or nosocomial.

Mechanisms of Infection

The uterus has excellent local defense mechanisms to protect itself against invasion by contaminating organisms from the lower genital tract. These defenses are present in the nonpregnant state, as is demonstrated by the rapid clearance of lower genital tract bacteria that are carried into the endometrial cavity during the insertion of an intrauterine device [19]. During pregnancy, Larsen and associates [11] have demonstrated inhibition of bacterial growth by the amniotic fluid. The stress of labor and delivery probably results commonly in uterine acquisition of organisms from the varied flora of the lower genital tract, but most postpartum patients remain free of symptoms as the uterus rapidly clears itself of the potentially pathogenic bacteria introduced from the vagina.

Postpartum endometritis occurs when these efficient uterine defense mechanisms are overcome by a combination of too many bacteria, the introduction of especially virulent bacterial strains, or local alterations (e.g., soft-tissue damage or the incomplete removal of the placenta) that provide a nidus for postpartum infection. The virulence of organisms is probably a more important factor than we have realized in the past. The increased risk for infection in women with bacterial vaginosis can reflect the greater risks with an overgrowth of anaerobic bacteria [23].

Postpartum pelvic infection follows a pattern of progression (Fig. 31-2), with ascension of the organisms into the endometrial cavity, invasion of the myometrium, extension into parametrial areas beyond the uterus, and bloodstream invasion in some instances [4]. If this progression is unchecked by the appropriate use of systemic antibiotics and anticoagulants when indicated, then myometrial, parametrial, or adnexal abscesses can occur with suppurative involvement of the pelvic

veins, septic pelvic thrombophlebitis, and even distant septic metastases to the liver and lung. In addition to the appropriate use of systemic medical agents, adequate uterine drainage must be ensured, and operative intervention for the drainage or removal of a pelvic abscess may be necessary for cure. This can occur even when what seem to be appropriate antibiotics are used. A subhepatic abscess has been reported after cesarean sections [8] and necrotizing fasciitis has been seen in postpartum patients [7]. These serious infections still occur.

Predisposing Host Factors
Host Susceptibility

The well-nourished pregnant patient with a middle-class background is far less likely to have infectious problems than her poorly nourished, anemic counterpart, a victim of her social class. This underclass has increased in numbers during the last decade, and drug abuse has also increased in this population. Drug abuse has an impact on maternal nutrition, and it exposes these women to potentially dangerous pathogens through prostitution and shared intravenous needles. In addition, risk of infection increases with prolonged rupture of the fetal membranes before delivery, increasing length of labor, and retention of fetal membranes or placental fragments after delivery.

Transvaginal Monitoring

In addition to reducing mortality, the availability of antibiotics has dramatically changed the practice of obstetrics-gynecology. Prolonged transvaginal monitoring of maternal intraamniotic pressures and transvaginal attachment of a fetal scalp electrode for electrocardiography could not have been considered if antibiotics were not available for postpartum use by obstetricians and neonatologists. However, these advances have been accompanied by enhanced infection risks. Among obstetric patients, the incidence of endometritis is relatively high in monitored patients as compared to unmonitored patients

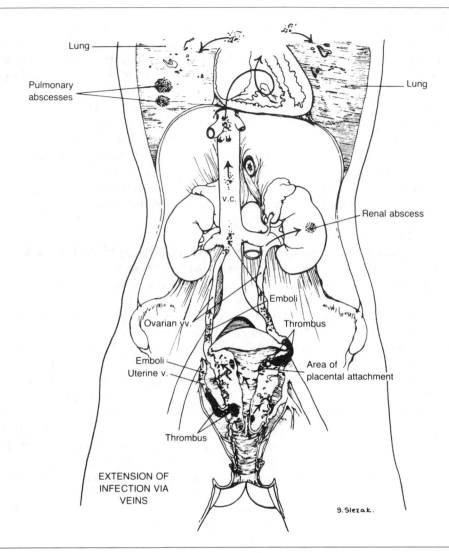

Labels within figure: Lung — Pulmonary abscesses — Lung — V.C. — Renal abscess — Emboli — Ovarian vv. — Thrombus — Emboli Uterine v. — Area of placental attachment — Thrombus — EXTENSION OF INFECTION VIA VEINS — S. Slezak.

Fig. 31-2. Potential spread of untreated postpartum endometritis.

[12]. In a clinic population, where there is a moderately high level of background infection, this difference is less apparent [6] (Figs. 31-3, 31-4).

Cesarean Section

Advances in the science of neonatology have increased fetal survival while also increasing the incidence of cesarean section for fetal indications in situations in which maternal risk of postpartum infection is above average. The frequency of infection following a cesarean section is ten times that following vaginal delivery. The obstetric service at the New York Hospital–Cornell Medical Center is now performing cesarean sections for infants estimated to weigh 500 g or more, instead of 700 g, the limit that previously existed. The result of this new criterion has been a dramatic reduction in perinatal mortality [21], but these results have been achieved at the cost of increased maternal risk of infection. Because cesarean sections are performed when there is evidence of fetal distress in these small infants, our own assessment is that the benefits to the fetus of this

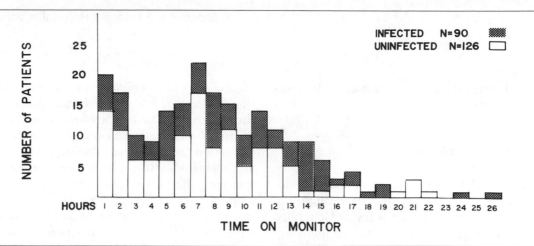

Fig. 31-3. The length of time of internal monitoring and the number of women with and without infection who delivered vaginally. Each bar represents the total number of women monitored for that time interval. (Reprinted with permission from C.B. Gassner and W.J. Ledger. The relationship of hospital-acquired maternal infection to invasive intrapartum monitoring techniques. *Am. J. Obstet. Gynecol.* 126:33, 1976.)

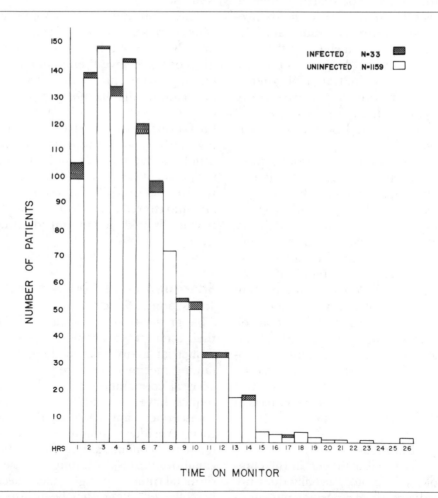

Fig. 31-4. The length of time of internal monitoring and the number of women with and without infection who delivered by cesarean section. Each bar represents the total number of women monitored for that time interval. (Reprinted with permission from C.B. Gassner and W.J. Ledger. The relationship of hospital-acquired maternal infection to invasive intrapartum monitoring techniques. *Am. J. Obstet. Gynecol.* 126:33, 1976.)

new obstetric philosophy outweigh the risks to the mother.

Diagnostic Criteria
Clinical Diagnosis
The clinical diagnosis of postpartum endometritis is based on a number of findings, the most significant of which is fever. Generally, affected women have an oral temperature elevation to approximately 38°C (100.4°F) and a tachycardia consistent with this rise. Patients usually have uterine tenderness and often have tenderness beyond the uterus in the parametrial and adnexal regions. A decrease in the normal postpartum uterine lochial flow is often noted 6 to 12 hours preceding the temperature elevation, and the lochial flow may be foul-smelling. If the physician makes a clinical diagnosis of endometritis and begins administration of systemic antibiotics with or without positive culture results, the patient should be included in all infection surveillance and postpartum morbidity statistics.

Attempts to assess the presence of a postpartum endometritis through evaluation of commonly employed, indirect hematologic measures of infection have not been successful. The phenomena of labor and delivery are accompanied by changes in the commonly employed parameters to measure the presence or absence of a bacterial infection. Thus a normal patient in labor or postpartum who has no evidence of an active bacterial infection may have an elevated white blood cell count (even exceeding 20,000), with an increase in the percentage of immature leukocytes and an elevated sedimentation rate. Bearing these facts in mind, practitioners should not depend on such laboratory tests to determine the diagnosis of infection.

Microbiologic Diagnosis
Isolation of a bacterial pathogen in the clinical microbiology laboratory usually does not establish the diagnosis of a postpartum endometritis. Exceptions are the discovery of a group A β-hemolytic streptococcus, *Neisseria*

gonorrhoeae, or *Chlamydia trachomatis*, which should trigger specific physician responses for treatment. The reasons for the usual lack of useful diagnostic, but not therapeutic, information from the microbiologic laboratory are manifold. Most culture techniques for sampling the postpartum endometrial cavity include a transcervical approach, which of necessity involves contamination by the abundant bacterial flora normally present in the endocervical canal of asymptomatic women. Also, the organisms recovered from the endometrial cavity of endometritis patients are usually the same as those normally inhabiting the vagina and endocervix of sexually active women.

These considerations do not mean that the laboratory will not be helpful, for it may indirectly contribute to the diagnosis or lack of diagnosis and give therapeutic guidance for treating postpartum endometritis. Assistance in excluding the diagnosis of postpartum endometritis may be provided, for example, in the febrile postpartum patient with no localizing uterine signs of infection when a significant bacterial colony count is obtained from a properly collected urine sample and the fever resolves successfully following therapy with an antibacterial agent (e.g., a nitrofurantoin) having limited action outside the urinary tract.

Specimen Collection and Transport
Transvaginal Specimens
The greatest difficulty facing clinicians in their attempts to sample the postpartum endometrial cavity microbiologically is in obtaining specimens that are free of vaginal and cervical contamination. To date, most techniques have stressed the transvaginal and transcervical approach to the endometrial cavity. Various techniques have been tried to decrease contamination from endocervical canal organisms, including the use of plastic or metal tubing through which specimens can be collected. There has been little physician enthusiasm for these more complicated diagnostic procedures. Also, there have been no

reports of attempts to quantitate the recovery of bacteria, similar to the methods of the colony counts of urine specimens, that might separate vaginal and endocervical contaminants from the more numerous pathogens at the site of infection.

Use of Blood Cultures

The most useful microbiologic technique, when it is positive, is the blood culture. A positive result focuses the clinician's attention on the most significant microorganisms in the infectious process. Those that invade the bloodstream are critical for the physician's therapeutic consideration. This diagnostic technique is positive in as many as 60 percent of febrile patients who deliver by cesarean section.

Transport

Significant changes in microbiologic sampling and the transportation of specimens have been brought about by the growing physician awareness of the importance of anaerobic microorganisms in postpartum infections. The recovery of anaerobes is crucially dependent on the clinician's efforts to reduce exposure of the specimens to atmospheric oxygen. Time is a critical factor, because exposure of a swab of the infection site to atmospheric oxygen for even a few minutes or less will reduce or eliminate certain anaerobic organisms. A number of alternative laboratory systems have been proposed to eliminate such exposure. Transport media—either liquid for primary culture or semisolid for transport to the laboratory and primary plating there—have been used. Alternatively, gassed tubes, free of oxygen, have been used for transport to a laboratory where primary plating and anaerobic incubation can be performed (see Chap. 9).

There is a major weakness in all these clinical schemes for the obstetrician-gynecologist. Figure 31-1 documents the first temperature elevation of obstetric patients with postpartum morbidity, which is the logical time for initial patient evaluation [16]. It is clear that the majority of microbiologic samples will be obtained late in the afternoon or in the early evening, when laboratory coverage, particularly by technicians with familiarity in anaerobic methods, will usually be inadequate.

General Control Measures
Patient Care Practices
Prenatal Care

The emphasis on the preventive aspects in patient care has been heavily weighted toward patient management during pregnancy, labor, and delivery. For the patient in labor, most obstetricians believe that the results of prenatal care culminating in delivery largely determine the frequency and severity of postpartum endometritis.

Rectal and Vaginal Examinations

One of the great changes in practice patterns in obstetrics in the past three decades has been the abandonment of the rectal examination during labor. Rectal examination was firmly established in the preantibiotic era and was predicated on the belief that it would avoid the introduction of exogenous organisms into the vagina. Since the most feared bacterial pathogens—the group A β-hemolytic streptococci—were often introduced into the vagina from personnel sources, prohibition of vaginal examination was undoubtedly beneficial. A number of studies demonstrated no differences in the postpartum endometritis rate when patients undergoing vaginal examination during labor were compared to those having rectal examination. These results probably reflect the low frequency of involvement of exogenous organisms such as group A β-hemolytic streptococci in postpartum endometritis. Both rectal and vaginal examinations, however, can result in the displacement of organisms from the lower genital tract to the uterus, and these manipulations, as well as other manipulations with similar risks (e.g., intrauterine placement of forceps or the physician's hand at delivery), should be limited to as few as necessary for good management of the patient.

Prophylactic Antibiotics

Prophylactic antibiotics for the patient in labor who needs a cesarean section (see Chap. 12) is the standard of care in the United States. Studies have shown diminished postpartum morbidity with their use [25]. The timing of the prophylactic dosage differs from that in gynecology. Postoperative administration delivers a therapeutic level of antibiotic to the fetus and can make evaluation for neonatal sepsis more difficult. The standard of care is administration after clamping of the cord. The use of antibiotic solution lavage in the operating room has had a variety of outcomes. In some studies, the results are not as good as with intravenous antibiotics [2].

Hand-Washing and Gloves

In the nineteenth century, Semmelweis recognized the importance of hand transfer of organisms from the postmortem room and the autopsy in the production of endometritis; physicians carried the bacterial pathogens from the autopsy room on their hands and clothing to the vagina and endocervix of the patient in labor, which led to the subsequent development of infection. Semmelweis's great achievement was to require hand-bathing in an antiseptic solution by physicians before the next patient was seen to break the chain of bacterial contamination and infection. Hand-washing and the use of sterile gloves for vaginal examinations remain important general control measures.

Environmental Factors

Environmental factors are infrequently involved in the development of postpartum endometritis. Indeed, the studies of the effect of ultraviolet irradiation on the rate of all postoperative wound infections [9] suggest that this would be true in the delivery room, because such studies demonstrated little impact on clinical results despite reductions in the bacterial contamination of air (see Chap. 22). The lack of importance of the environment is anticipated in the case of endometritis, because most of these infections derive from the patients' endogenous bacterial flora.

Therapy

The cornerstones of therapy in patients with postpartum endometritis are adequate uterine drainage and the use of appropriate antimicrobials. Uterine drainage must be ensured, and the maneuver of removing membranes at the time of pelvic examination provides the patient undergoing clinical examination the added benefit of an assessment of the extent of infection; a microbiologic specimen may also be obtained at this time.

Antibiotics are usually required for cure. They are prescribed before the results of culture susceptibility tests are known, and the initial choices reflect the individual physician's philosophy of antibiotic use, which should be based on past experiences with similar patients. At the New York Hospital–Cornell Medical Center, staff will frequently use a single antibiotic such as ampicillin or a cephalosporin to treat the patient who is not allergic to penicillin and who has had a vaginal delivery. This course usually results in cure, even in the patient with a concomitant bacteremia, because these agents provide coverage against most of the commonly recovered organisms. In patients who have had a cesarean section, there are a number of antibiotic choices available. Standard therapy has been a combination of clindamycin and an aminoglycoside, usually gentamicin [3]. This combination of antibiotics provides coverage against most of the commonly recovered aerobes and anaerobes and has shown superior results to the previously employed combination of penicillin and an aminoglycoside. A concern has been the maintenance of adequate levels of gentamicin on standard doses, based on body weights [26]. I have favored obtaining serum levels to correct low levels found in 40 percent of patients, but one recent study suggests that this is infrequently necessary [1]. Alternatively, a second cephalosporin such as cefoxitin or cefotetan, one of the newer broad-spectrum penicillins such as mezlocillin, or penicillins with a β-lactamase inhibitor can be used alone. A number of studies indicate the standard 10-day-long treatment regimen is not needed in these patients [5].

Endogenous Infections from Lower Genital Tract Flora

The microorganisms mainly responsible for postpartum endometritis are nearly always endogenous to the patient; that is, they normally reside in the gastrointestinal and lower genital tracts (vagina and endocervix) of asymptomatic, pregnant women. The stress of labor and delivery, rupture of the membranes, frequent vaginal examinations by the medical team caring for the patient, use of invasive monitoring devices in the vagina, and delivery by the intrauterine placement of forceps or physician's hands all introduce opportunities for uterine acquisition of lower genital tract flora. After introduction, these flora may find a suitable uterine environment where they can survive and invade.

The endogenous organisms that most frequently become pathogenic and result in an endometritis include certain aerobic streptococci (α-hemolytic streptococci, the group B β-hemolytic streptococci, and the enterococci); anerobic cocci (*Peptostreptococcus*); gram-negative aerobes (*Escherichia coli, Klebsiella* species, and *Hemophilus influenzae*); and finally, gram-negative anaerobic rods, *Bacteroides fragilis, B. bivius,* and *B. disiens.* There is evidence that nearly all patients with endometritis, particularly those with severe infections, have a mixed infection involving more than one organism.

Epidemics of endometritis caused by these endogenous organisms have not been recognized, and their control depends on avoiding predisposing factors, when possible, and adherence to general control measures.

Gram-Negative Aerobic Infections
Gram-negative aerobes are less frequently recovered from these women today than they were in the 1970s. The most frequently isolated organisms are *E. coli, Klebsiella* species, and *H. influenzae,* with an associated bacteremia. There are no distinctive clinical signs, however, to alert the clinician to the possibility that an associated bacteremia is present.

The low frequency of antimicrobial-resistant organisms is a major advantage to the clinician treating women with endometritis in which gram-negative aerobes are involved. Most postpartum obstetric patients have intact host defense mechanisms and usually have not had prolonged exposure to systemic antimicrobial therapy before labor and delivery or prolonged hospitalization before delivery. Effective first-line drugs include the aminoglycosides, gentamicin, and tobramycin. Since there are few resistant gram-negative aerobic organisms seen in these patients, we usually rely on gentamicin as our most frequently used aminoglycoside, with amikacin reserved for the patient who is suspected of having gram-negative aerobic bacterial sepsis or who had repeated exposure to antibiotics for urinary tract infections during pregnancy. The cephalosporins and broad-spectrum penicillins are highly effective against such gram-negative aerobes, and these are an acceptable alternative to aminoglycosides, as is aztreonam.

Gram-Negative Anaerobic Infections
Incidence
Recent studies show that *Bacteroides* species were frequently isolated from patients with postpartum endometritis [20]. Undoubtedly, the majority of these isolates are *B. bivius* or *B. disiens,* but *B. fragilis* has been isolated in patients with serious infection.

Clinical Features
Patients with postpartum endometritis due to *B. fragilis, B. bivius,* or *B. disiens* can be seriously ill, and they frequently have lochia with a fecal odor. Although most patients respond to antibiotics, pelvic abscess formation can occur and operative drainage or removal may be necessary for cure, despite the use of appropriate antibiotics in adequate dosages.

Septic thrombophlebitis can follow infections with *Bacteroides* species, but this is a much less frequently seen entity since physicians have used antibiotics effective against gram-negatative anaerobes from the beginning of therapy.

Therapy

Postpartum endometritis due to *B. fragilis, B. bivius,* or *B. disiens* requires specific antibiotic strategies. The current first-line drugs of choice are clindamycin and metronidazole. Clindamycin has been associated with pseudomembranous enterocolitis, a serious clinical entity that affects approximately 1 in 25,000 treated patients (see Chaps. 12, 30). Alternative drugs include the newer cephalosporins and broad-spectrum penicillins.

Operative removal and drainage of pelvic abscesses, treatment of septic pelvic thrombophlebitis with intravenous heparin therapy, and continued use of appropriate antibiotics may result in a rapid defervescence of fever in a patient with previously persisting temperature spikes.

Gram-Positive Anaerobic Infections
Incidence

There is a consistency in the bacterial causes of endometritis. Microbiologic studies of patients with postpartum endometritis in the preantibiotic era showed *Peptostreptococcus* to be the most commonly isolated organism [22], and it remains a common isolate today [20]. In surveillance studies of obstetric infections with proper anaerobic culture techniques, *Peptostreptococcus* and *Peptococcus* organisms are frequently recovered from the endometrium [20] and bloodstream [15] of patients with endometritis.

Clinical Features

A postpartum endometritis due to gram-positive anaerobic cocci can be suspected in a patient whose lochia has a putrid, fecal odor. Pelvic abscess formation rarely occurs but, when it does, operative drainage or removal may be necessary for cure, despite the use of appropriate antibiotics as judged by in vitro antibiotic susceptibility testing. The postpar-

tum retention of fetal membranes or placental fragments has frequently been observed with these infections.

Therapy

Peptostreptococcus is highly susceptible to clindamycin in serum levels that are easily achieved by frequently administering therapeutic doses of this agent. Other alternative antibiotics include the newer cephalosporins and penicillins.

Aerobic Infections
Incidence

There has been increasing evidence of group B β-hemolytic streptococcal maternal infections since the late 1980s [20]. Enterococci are also frequently encountered. Group A infections are rare but serious (see Chap. 37).

Clinical Features

Postpartum endometritis due to aerobic streptococci has no characteristic clinical findings that distinguish it from endometritis due to other organisms.

Therapy

The group-B β-hemolytic streptococci and α-hemolytic streptococci are susceptible to penicillin and clindamycin. The group D streptococci have unique antibiotic susceptibility patterns: In the laboratory, the organism is frequently not susceptible to penicillin or an aminoglycoside alone, but when both antibiotics are used together or when ampicillin is substituted for penicillin, there is both laboratory and clinical evidence of a response. In the penicillin-allergic patient with enterococcal endometritis, vancomycin is the antibiotic of choice, since the cephalosporins and clindamycin have little effect against this group of organisms.

Group A β-Hemolytic Streptococcal Infections

In contrast to the preceding category of infections, endometritis caused by group A streptococci commonly derives from exogenous sources, is highly invasive and transmissible, and has produced outbreaks requiring special measures for control.

General Aspects
Transmissibility

The group A β-hemolytic streptococci are highly contagious agents (see Chap. 37). For this reason, obstetricians justifiably fear the introduction of this organism into the labor room environment lest it will be transmitted to patients in labor and result in serious cases of postpartum endometritis. A patient with an active *Streptococcus pyogenes* infection can transmit these organisms to patients or medical personnel, resulting in colonization. Hospital personnel can be asymptomatic carriers of group A streptococci and transmit the organisms to patients in labor. Community contacts also may be important in the transmission of this organism to patients in labor, particularly in the modern obstetric setting that logically allows husband and wife to be together during all of labor and delivery. This practice can be a problem if the husband is a carrier of group A streptococci.

Incidence

The importance of group A β-hemolytic streptococcal infections is not based on a high frequency of infections but rather on the clinical invasiveness and epidemiologic virulence of such strains. The low frequency of isolation matches our surveillance experience with endometritis and the bacteremia associated with it.

Sources and Modes of Acquisition

Endogenous sources are probably mainly responsible for specific cases. The vagina of an affected patient is often asymptomatically colonized with group A streptococci when the patient is admitted to the delivery room, but the patient may also have an upper respiratory tract infection or skin lesion that harbors such organisms.

The most common method of spread of exogenous organisms involves direct transmission from personnel who are asymptomatic carriers to the patients. Clinically infected personnel may also be responsible (see Chaps.

33, 34, 37). Personnel may become colonized after providing care to a patient with postpartum endometritis; they may then transmit these organisms to patients in labor.

Clinical Considerations
Manifestations

There are a number of distinctive clinical features seen in the patient with group A β-hemolytic streptococcal endometritis. Historically, this entity has been called *puerperal fever, puerperal sepsis,* and *childbed fever.* The most striking feature is the early onset of high spiking fevers (Fig. 31-5) in the postpartum patient [14]. Patients appear critically ill, but abdominal and pelvic examinations reveal diffuse tenderness with no localizing signs. The cervical discharge is usually clear and watery, is not purulent, and contains many gram-positive cocci when the exudate is Gram-stained. Although this organism is very susceptible to penicillin and clindamycin, patients with endometritis frequently do not become afebrile for 48 hours or more (see Fig. 31-4).

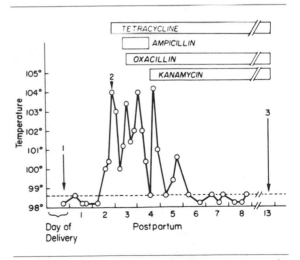

Fig. 31-5. The early onset of a high, spiking temperature pattern in a postpartum patient with group A β-hemolytic streptococcal endometritis. Despite the use of penicillin analogs (ampicillin and oxacillin), the patient required several days to become completely afebrile. The patient delivered at point 1 on the chart, was started on antibiotic treatment at point 2, and was discharged at point 3.

Therapy

The drug of choice for treating group A β-hemolytic streptococcal endometritis remains penicillin G; clindamycin is also effective against this organism. Tetracycline is not an acceptable alternative for treating patients with this infection because of the frequency of resistant strains.

Epidemic Infections

Reported Outbreaks

Since the introduction of antibiotics, sporadic outbreaks of group A β-hemolytic streptococcal endometritis epidemics have been reported in New York City [18] and Boston [10]. In the New York City outbreak, there were 9 confirmed cases, whereas in Boston there were 20 women in whom this diagnosis was made.

Sources

In the New York City outbreak, the source of the bacteria that were disseminated throughout the hospital was colonized, asymptomatic newborn infants [18]. In Boston, a common source was the cutaneous lesions of an anesthesiologist [10]. A preantibiotic-era study of this problem found many personnel colonized with such streptococci [24]. Colonization of medical personnel and subsequent transmission to patients in labor seem to be the crucial ingredients in the maintenance of an epidemic. Another outbreak of group A streptococcal infections affecting obstetric-gynecologic patients was ultimately traced to an anesthesiologist who was an asymptomatic rectal carrier of the organism [17]. Thus operating room sources of this type should be suspected in endometritis outbreaks that exclusively or primarily involve patients with cesarean sections.

Prevention and Control

Infections due to group A β-hemolytic streptococci are so serious that the discovery of one case of puerperal sepsis should be considered an epidemic. The patient needs to be placed on wound and skin isolation, and hospital personnel should don gown and gloves before providing personal care (see Chap. 11). All labor and delivery room personnel on duty during this patient's labor and delivery should be screened for possible infections by history and physical examination, and cultures should be obtained from the nose, throat, any suspected skin lesion, and rectum of each. Lochial culture specimens should be obtained from postpartum patients who were in the delivery room at the same time as the infected patient, and appropriate antibiotics should be given to those whose cultures are positive. If available on a timely basis, antibiotics can be limited to those positive for the same strain as the one isolated from the infected patient (which is established by M and T typing). If epidemiologically related to the case, colonized staff should be relieved of patient care responsibilities until appropriate antibiotic therapy has resulted in negative cultures. All culture-positive personnel should be treated if the typing of strains cannot be done expeditiously.

There were a number of significant differences between the preantibiotic-era epidemics and those recently reported. The preantibiotic-era study reported maternal deaths, and the outbreak was controlled only by closing the maternity service of the hospital until all infected patients had been discharged [24]. Recent epidemics have been controlled by the use of appropriate antibiotics, isolation of infected patients, epidemiologic identification of disseminating carriers, and eradication of carried strains by proper treatment of colonized or infected hospital personnel. If initial nose and throat cultures of personnel epidemiologically associated with the outbreak are negative, and careful physical examinations do not reveal a site of infection, then multiple culture specimens should be obtained, including ones from rectal and vaginal sites. In Boston, all admissions to the service in the midst of the epidemic were treated with penicillin or penicillinlike antibiotics [10]. Such broad-scale prophylaxis may be especially indicated at the time an outbreak is first recognized, because it may permit a maternity unit to remain open while epidemiologic and microbiologic investigations are undertaken. If such investigations are successful in identifying the sources and modes of spread, then attention focused on these areas should obviate the need for continued chemoprophylaxis of patients. Outbreaks should be promptly reported to local public health authorities.

Coagulase-Positive Staphylococci

Maternal infections due to coagulase-positive staphylococci do occur. They most frequently involve the breast and are discovered after patients have been discharged from the hospital. If these organisms are found in women with endometritis, the same control concerns as detailed elsewhere should be employed (see Chaps. 33, 37).

References

1. Briggs, G.G., Ambrose, P., and Nageotte, M.P. Gentamicin dosing in postpartum women with endometritis. *Am. J. Obstet. Gynecol.* 160:309, 1988.
2. Conover, W.B., and Moore, T.R. Comparison of irrigation and intravenous antibiotic prophylaxis at cesarean section. *Obstet. Gynecol.* 63:787, 1984.
3. DiZerega, G., et al. A comparison of clindamycin-gentamicin and penicillin-gentamicin in the treatment of post-cesarean section endomyometritis. *Am. J. Obstet. Gynecol.* 134:238, 1979.
4. Eastman, N.J., and Hellman, L.M. In: L.W. Williams (Ed.), *Obstetrics* (13th ed.). New York: Appleton-Century-Crofts, 1966.
5. Gall, S.A., Addison, W.A., and Hill, G.B. Moxalactam therapy for obstetric and gynecologic infections. *Rev. Infect. Dis.* 4:S701, 1982.
6. Gassner, C. B., and Ledger, W.J. The relationship of hospital-acquired maternal infections to invasive intrapartum monitoring techniques. *Am. J. Obstet. Gynecol.* 126:33, 1976.
7. Golde, S., and Ledger, W.J. Necrotizing fasciitis in postpartum patients: A report of four cases. *Obstet. Gynecol.* 50:670, 1977.
8. Harper, A.K., and Slocumb, J.T. Right subhepatic abscess for cesarean section: A case report. *J. Reprod. Med.* 34:376, 1989.
9. Howard, J.M., et al. Postoperative wound infections: The influence of ultraviolet irradiation of the operating room and of various other factors. *Ann. Surg.* 160(Suppl.): 1, 1964.
10. Jewett, J.F., Reid, D.E., Safon, L.E., and Easterday, C.L. Childbed fever—a continuing entity. *J.A.M.A.* 206:344, 1968.
11. Larsen, B., Snyder, I.S., and Galask, R.P. Bacterial growth inhibition by amniotic fluid. *Am. J. Obstet. Gynecol.* 119:492, 1974.
12. Larsen, J.W., Goldkrand, J.W., Hanson, T.M., and Miller, C.R. Intrauterine infection on an obstetric service. *Obstet. Gynecol.* 43:838, 1974.
13. Ledger, W.J., and Child, M. The hospital care of patients undergoing hysterectomy. *Am. J. Obstet. Gynecol.* 117:423, 1973.
14. Ledger, W.J., and Headington, J.T. The group A beta-hemolytic streptococcus. *Obstet. Gynecol.* 39:474, 1972.
15. Ledger, W.J., Norman, M., Gee, C., and Lewis, W. Bacteremia on an obstetric gynecologic service. *Am. J. Obstet. Gynecol.* 121:205, 1975.
16. Ledger, W.J., Reite, A.M., and Headington, J.T. A system for infectious disease surveillance on an obstetric service. *Obstet. Gynecol.* 37:769, 1971.
17. McIntyre, D.M. An epidemic of *Streptococcus pyogenes* puerperal and postoperative sepsis with an unusual carrier site—the anus. *Am. J. Obstet. Gynecol.* 101:308, 1968.
18. Mead, P.B., Ribble, J.C., and Dillon, T.F. Group A streptococcal puerperal infection. *Obstet. Gynecol.* 32:460, 1968.
19. Mishell, D.R., Bell, J.H., Good, R.G., and Moyer, D.L. The intrauterine device: A bacteriologic study of the endometrial cavity. *Am. J. Obstet. Gynecol.* 96:119, 1966.
20. Newton, E.R., Prihoda, T.J., and Gibbs, R. A clinical and microbiologic analysis of risk factors for puerperal endometritis. *Obstet. Gynecol.* 75:402, 1990.
21. Paul, R.H., and Hon, E.H. Clinical fetal monitoring v. effect on perinatal outcome. *Am. J. Obstet. Gynecol.* 118:529, 1974.
22. Schwarz, O.H., and Dieckman, W.J. Puerperal infection due to anaerobic streptococci. *Am. J. Obstet. Gynecol.* 13:467, 1927.
23. Watts, D.H., Krohn, M.A., Hillier, S.L., and Eschenbach, D. Bacterial vaginosis as a risk factor for post-cesarean endometritis. *Obstet. Gynecol.* 75:52, 1990.
24. Watson, B.P. An outbreak of puerperal sepsis in New York City. *Am. J. Obstet. Gynecol.* 16:157, 1928.
25. Wong, R., Gee, C.L. and Ledger, W.J. Prophylactic use of cefazolin in monitored obstetric patients undergoing cesarean section. *Obstet. Gynecol.* 51:407, 1978.
26. Zaske, D.E., Rapid gentamicin elimination in obstetric patients. *Obstet. Gynecol.* 56:559, 1980.

Nosocomial Central Nervous System Infections

Arthur L. Reingold
Claire V. Broome

Central nervous system (CNS) infections, including meningitis, ventricular shunt infections, ventriculitis, infected subdural hematomas, and intracranial abscesses, are among the least common but most serious hospital-acquired infections. CNS infections accounted for only 0.5 percent of the nosocomial infections reported through the National Nosocomial Infections Surveillance (NNIS) System during the time period October 1986–April 1990 [R. Gaynes and G. Emori, CDC: personal communication]. Due to a variety of factors, however, including the age of patients at highest risk, organisms frequently involved, and difficulty of achieving adequate concentrations of effective antimicrobials in the cerebrospinal fluid (CSF), nosocomial CNS infections are associated with a high death rate, as well as severe neurologic impairment among many survivors. Consequently, prevention of such infections assumes greater importance than might seem warranted by their incidence.

As in other infection sites, it is sometimes difficult to determine whether a CNS infection in a hospitalized patient began in the hospital or in the community. Part of the difficulty arises from uncertainty about the incubation period between antecedent head trauma and subsequent development of meningitis; this incubation period can range from a day to many weeks. There is also uncertainty regarding how long a period between the implantation of a device such as a ventricular shunt and the development of a shunt infection is consistent with nosocomial acquisition of infection. Infections in patients with ventricular shunts generally are considered nosocomial in origin if onset occurs within 60 days of implantation, revision, or manipulation of a shunt. With the exception of patients with ventricular shunts, most patients with meningitis following neurosurgery have onset of symptoms within 3 weeks of the procedure, and approximately 50 percent of patients develop symptoms within 1 week of surgery [46]. As a general rule, all infections that occur during the first postoperative month should be considered nosocomial.

Meningitis that develops in patients several days into their hospitalization, secondary to a community-acquired infection at another body site, should not be classified as a nosocomial infection [27]. Neonatal meningitis due to organisms acquired during passage through the birth canal is considered to be nosocomial when the baby is born in the hospital. However, the implications for hospital personnel may be very different from those generated by other types of nosocomial meningitis.

These definitions, although necessary and useful for surveillance purposes, may result in the misidentification of the place of acquisition of infection in an individual patient. When multiple patients in the same institution develop meningitis or other infections due to the same organism, however, it usually becomes apparent that the infections are nosocomial in origin. Under these circumstances, rapid determination of the source of infection and mode of spread is vital to prevention of additional cases.

Patients at Risk

Although any hospitalized patient is at risk of acquiring a nosocomial CNS infection, three occasionally overlapping groups of patients are at greatest risk: neurosurgery patients, both with and without ventricular shunts, particularly those with antecedent head trauma; neonates, particularly those in neonatal intensive care units; and patients undergoing diagnostic or therapeutic procedures that involve penetrating the CNS. In NNIS hospitals, more than 85 percent of the nosocomial CNS infections reported in 1986–1990 were from newborn nurseries and surgical services, with the highest rate of such infections seen in the newborn nursery (Table 32-1) [R. Gaynes and G. Emori, CDC: personal communication].

Table 32-1. Nosocomial CNS infections in NNIS hospitals with hospitalwide surveillance by hospital service, October 1986–April 1990

Service	Number of cases (%)	Infection rate/100,000 discharges
Surgery	304 (62)	42.0
Newborn nursery	119 (24)	45.0
Medicine	40 (8)	4.0
Pediatrics	21 (4)	14.0
Obstetrics	3 (<1)	1.0
Gynecology	1 (<1)	1.0
Total	488	

CNS = central nervous system; NNIS = National Nosocomial Infections Surveillance.
Source: R. Gaynes and G. Emori, CDC: personal communication.

Neurosurgery Patients
Patients undergoing neurosurgery are at risk of seeding of their CNS directly at the operative site at the time of surgery. In addition, they are at substantial risk of developing secondary CNS infections due to direct spread from an infected surgical wound or seeding of devitalized tissue during bacteremia caused by infection at another site, such as the urinary tract. Overall, the incidence of postoperative meningitis among approximately 7,000 neurosurgery patients in one hospital-based study was 0.5 percent [46].

It has been suggested that the risk of postoperative CNS infection increases with increasing operative time and with increasing number of operative procedures, although the available evidence is not convincing. Prophylactic antimicrobials have not been demonstrated to decrease the risk of nosocomial CNS infections in neurosurgery patients in general [46], although randomized prospective studies are lacking. Furthermore, outbreaks in neurosurgical units of CNS infections caused by multiply resistant organisms have resulted from injudicious use of antimicrobials in such patients [62] (see Chap. 12).

Ventricular Shunt Patients
Patients with ventricular shunts form a special subgroup of neurosurgery patients that merits separate discussion. The increased

risk of CNS infections, both hospital- and community-acquired, among these patients has been recognized for many years, and factors related to that risk have been studied [3, 54, 73, 75, 78]. Most investigators have reported that 10 to 20 percent of patients undergoing shunt insertion or revision develop shunt infections.

The fact that most shunt infections have onset within 2 months of surgery (70 percent in one large series) strongly suggests that the infecting organism is usually introduced during the perioperative period [73]. It has been suggested that the risk of infection is a function of the number of previous procedures and the number of therapeutic or diagnostic entries into the CNS, but a study of 289 shunt patients in one hospital has shown that the rate of infection is independent of the number of previous procedures and that multiple entries into the CNS need not be associated with an increased risk of CNS infection [73]. The same study failed to show any association between the rate of infection and underlying disease, type of shunt, presence or absence of a valve, type of valve, or depth of the catheter in the right atrium. Other studies have shown that the rate of infection varies with the neurosurgeon [48] and, in at least one cluster of shunt infections, with the use of shunt extension tubing [J.L. Ho: personal communication].

The role of prophylactic perioperative antimicrobials in ventricular shunt patients remains unsettled. Whereas some authors have noted a lower rate of shunt infections among patients given prophylactic antimicrobials [23, 68, 73], others have not [54, 77]. All of these studies have biases or include very small numbers of patients. A large, randomized, prospective controlled clinical trial of the efficacy of prophylactic antimicrobials in this setting is needed.

Neonates

Whereas neurosurgery patients are at increased risk of nosocomial CNS infections because of the disruption of the normal barriers against infection, neonates, in whom these barriers are in general not well developed, are at increased risk of developing secondary CNS infection whenever they become bacteremic. Thus the factors associated with an increased risk of nosocomial meningitis are the same as those associated with an increased risk of sepsis and, in outbreak settings, the cases of nosocomial meningitis are usually only a subgroup of the affected infant population. Cases of nosocomial meningitis in neonates occur predominantly in neonatal intensive care units, presumably due to the fact that patients requiring care in such units are more premature and of lower birth weight, more likely to have invasive therapeutic and diagnostic procedures, more likely to be exposed to broad-spectrum antimicrobials, more likely to be exposed to potentially contaminated life-support systems, and more likely to have extended hospital stays. Other important factors believed to be associated with the development of nosocomial meningitis in such units include crowding, decreased nurse-to-infant ratio, and poor hand-washing practices.

Other Patients

The last group of patients at increased risk of nosocomial meningitis includes persons undergoing diagnostic or therapeutic procedures that penetrate the CNS, such as lumbar puncture for removal of CSF or instillation of dyes or medications [21, 42, 57, 69], use of a CSF (Omaya) reservoir [65], and induction of spinal anesthesia [20, 41]. Though such infections are less common in the present-day era of presterilized, single-use needles, syringes, and other equipment, they do still occur.

Etiologic Agents

Almost three-fourths of nosocomial CNS infections are caused by gram-negative bacilli and staphylococci, although the distribution by etiologic agent depends on the hospital service (Table 32-2). In contrast, *Hemophilus influenzae* and *Neisseria meningitidis*, the two most common causes of community-acquired bacterial meningitis, account for less than 1 percent of reported nosocomial CNS infections [R. Gaynes and G. Emori, CDC: personal communication].

Table 32-2. Pathogens isolated from nosocomial CNS infections in NNIS hospitals by service, October 1986–April 1990*

Etiologic agent	Service				
	Newborn nursery	Pediatrics	Surgery	Medicine	Total
Bacteria					
Staphylococcus epidermidis	57	18	181	14	270
Gram-negative bacilli	45	12	155	14	226
Staphylococcus aureus	18	11	98	8	135
Other streptococci, excluding *S. pneumoniae*	24	7	47	8	86
Group B streptococci	28	1	4	1	34
Other	5	0	15	5	25
Anaerobes	2	1	12	1	16
Streptococcus pneumoniae	2	0	2	2	6
Hemophilus influenzae	1	0	2	2	5
Listeria monocytogenes	0	0	0	0	0
Neisseria meningitidis	0	0	0	0	0
Viruses	6	1	0	2	9
Fungi and yeast	10	2	18	9	39
Total	198	53	534	66	851

CNS = central nervous system; NNIS = National Nosocomial Infections Surveillance.
*Excludes 2 CNS infections due to "other streptococci" on obstetric services.
Source: R. Gaynes and G. Emori, CDC: personal communication.

Neurosurgery Patients

There have not been many reports that systematically analyze the etiologic agents responsible for CNS infections in neurosurgery patients. In one large hospital series, however, investigators found that 69 percent of proved cases of meningitis in the post-neurosurgical period were caused by gram-negative bacilli and an additional 19 percent by staphylococci [46]. Of the cases of gram-negative bacillary meningitis, approximately 70 percent were caused by *Escherichia coli* and *Klebsiella pneumoniae*. While the data from NNIS hospitals in Table 32-2 show that only 155 (29 percent) of 534 nosocomial CNS infections on surgical services were due to gram-negative bacilli, it should be noted that the proportion of these cases that came from neurosurgical services is unknown, as is the number of ventricular shunt patients [R. Gaynes and G. Emori, CDC: Personal communication].

Ventricular Shunt Patients

Unlike nosocomial CNS infections in other neurosurgical patients, infections in patients with ventricular shunts are primarily caused by staphylococci. *Staphylococcus aureus* and *Staphylococcus epidermidis* together accounted for 75 percent of shunt infections in one large series and 81 percent in a smaller series, with gram-negative bacilli causing most of the other infections [48, 73]. Additional analysis of the data from one series, however, revealed that gram-negative enteric organisms caused 35 percent of the shunt infections in patients with ventriculoureteral shunts [73].

Neonates

As shown in Table 32-2, no single organism or group of organisms accounts for a majority of the cases of neonatal meningitis, although gram-negative bacilli and *S. epidermidis* together were implicated in more than half of the cases. Whereas cases of neonatal meningitis due to group B streptococci and *Listeria monocytogenes* are usually believed to be the result of mother-to-infant spread of the causative organism during passage through the birth canal, well-documented instances of horizontal spread of these organisms within the hospital also have occurred [1, 16, 26, 43, 44, 56, 74, 80].

Outbreaks

Reported outbreaks or clusters of cases of meningitis in hospitalized neonates or neurosurgical patients have been caused predominantly by a wide variety of gram-negative genera, including *Escherichia, Klebsiella, Pseudomonas, Citrobacter, Serratia, Enterobacter, Acinetobacter, Proteus, Salmonella, Campylobacter,* and *Flavobacterium* [2, 5, 8, 10, 11, 13, 14, 29–31, 33–35, 39, 51, 59, 61–64, 67, 70, 81]. However, clusters of cases of nosocomial meningitis caused by gram-positive organisms, including groups A and B streptococci, *S. aureus,* and *L. monocytogenes,* have been described [1, 16, 18, 22, 26, 36, 43, 44, 56, 66, 74, 80], as have clusters of CNS infections caused by fungi and viruses [52, 55, 65] and clusters in which no etiologic agent could be identified [47].

Nosocomial spread of *H. influenzae* and *N. meningitidis* CNS infections appears to be very rare. A single cluster of cases of *H. influenzae* infections, including meningitis, has been reported in a chronic-care hospital for children [28]. Also, secondary spread of *H. influenzae* in an acute-care hospital was recently reported [7]. Whereas secondary spread of *N. meningitidis* among patients in the hospital may have been more common when the United States was still experiencing epidemic meningococcal disease, there is only one well-documented instance of such transmission in the recent medical literature [19].

Modes of Spread and Sources of Infection

The source of infection and mode of spread in cases of nosocomial meningitis are primarily a function of the organism involved and the affected patient population.

Neurosurgery Patients

As mentioned earlier, neurosurgery patients are at risk of seeding of their CNS both during and after surgery, with either incompletely eradicated endogenous local flora or exogenous bacteria. In the former situation, bacteria found on the skin, such as *S. epidermidis* and *S. aureus,* are not completely killed by preoperative scrubbing and are thus able to enter the CNS via the surgical incision. Alternatively, staphylococci or gram-negative bacilli can be transmitted to patients by hospital personnel, during either surgery or postoperative wound care, or as a result of care unrelated to the neurosurgical procedure, such as manipulation of a urinary tract catheter or performance of respiratory therapy. In one cluster of cases of meningitis due to a *Klebsiella* species, for example, the neurosurgical patients were found also to be colonized with the causative agent in the urinary and respiratory tracts [63]. Furthermore, in one large series, 70 percent of neurosurgical patients with meningitis had the same organism isolated from another site before or at the same time as the initial isolation from the CSF [46]. Among patients with previous head trauma, infection of the paranasal sinuses frequently precedes meningitis due to the same organism [38].

During the investigation of several outbreaks of gram-negative bacillary meningitis in neurosurgical units, inanimate objects such as respirators [11] and a shaving brush used for preoperative preparation of the scalp [5] have been found to harbor the epidemic strain. While isolation of the epidemic strain from the environment in such settings has led to speculation about the role of fomites in transmission, a statistically significant association between exposure to the inanimate object and risk of infection has not been established.

Ventricular Shunt Patients

Many ventricular shunt infections probably result from incomplete eradication of "normal" skin flora—particularly *S. epidermidis*—

from the operative site before surgery. One study that examined this question in detail found that *S. epidermidis* was recovered from cultures of the operative site before closure in 58 of 100 operations to insert or revise shunts [9]. In 32 (55 percent) of these patients, the same organism (determined by colicin typing) was present in the nose or ear, on the scalp, or at the operative site before the operation. Of 9 patients whose shunts became infected, 7 had the infecting organism present at the operative site at the time of surgery. The finding in another study, however, that 35 percent of shunt infections in patients with ventriculoureteral shunts were due to gram-negative enteric organisms suggests that other sources of infection may be important in patients having this type of shunt procedure [73].

Neonates

Clusters of cases of meningitis in neonates caused by gram-negative enteric organisms probably result from the introduction of the organism into the newborn nursery from the stool of an infant or mother, or from the stool, vagina, or hands of someone on the hospital staff, with subsequent spread between infants via the hands of hospital personnel or improperly sterilized equipment. Investigations in such settings frequently reveal that many more infants are colonized (particularly at the umbilical stump and in the stool) than are infected and that one or more members of the nursery staff carry the implicated organism on the hands or in the stool or vagina. In one such outbreak, continued carriage of the causative organism on the hands of a nurse was believed to be at least partially due to a chronic dermatitis of the hands [59].

The causative organism frequently can also be found on inanimate objects in the nursery. Equipment found to be contaminated in such outbreaks has included oxygen tubing, water bottles used to humidify inspired air, suctioning equipment, aspirator bottles, rubber stoppers and cleaned "teats" for milk bottles, and isolettes [2, 8, 10]. In one cluster of cases of *Flavobacterium* meningitis, contamination of the saline used to rinse the eyes of newborn

babies was suggested as the source of infection [61]. In most of these situations, exposure to the contaminated object or product has not been conclusively linked epidemiologically to the risk of developing meningitis, although in a recently described outbreak of bacteremia and meningitis due to *S. marcescens* there was an epidemiologic association between infection and exposure to intravenous fluids prepared on the ward [81].

Groups A and B streptococci, *S. aureus*, and *L. monocytogenes* are probably also introduced into nurseries by an infected infant, mother, or medical care provider and subsequently spread among infants via hospital personnel. As with gram-negative bacilli, the role of aerosols and fomites in the spread of these organisms remains unsettled. However, a recently described outbreak of *L. monocytogenes* infections found strong evidence that contaminated mineral oil used to bathe newborn infants was the source of infection [74].

Other Patients

In any patient undergoing procedures that invade the CNS, contaminated medications and medical devices are a potential source of infection. Nosocomial meningitis has been linked to the use of contaminated amphotericin B suspensions given intrathecally [69] and to contaminated saline used during induction of spinal anesthesia [20]. In addition, 5 cases of streptococcal meningitis following myelography have been described, and the possibility that contaminated contrast medium may have been responsible has been suggested [57]. Contaminated quaternary ammonium compounds used to sterilize the skin have been implicated as the source of meningitis due to *S. marcescens* [70]. Prior treatment with OKT3, a murine monoclonal antibody used for treating acute renal allograft rejection, was found to be associated with the development of aseptic meningitis of unknown cause in a recent cluster of such cases [47]. Finally, it is notable that cases of both community-acquired and nosocomial meningitis due to *L. monocytogenes* have been linked to consumption of various foods [36, 72].

Clinical Findings and Outcome

Nosocomial meningitis does not differ clinically from meningitis acquired elsewhere. The clinical manifestations are largely a function of the patient's age and the presence of associated infections. Prompt recognition of nosocomial meningitis can be difficult, however, both in patients who have undergone recent neurosurgical procedures or invasion of the CNS and in neonates.

Neurosurgery Patients

Meningitis following neurosurgery is characterized by fever, with 94 percent of patients having fever on the first day of illness [46]. Chills, headache, nausea and vomiting, irritability, malaise, cervical rigidity, coma, and a positive Kernig's sign are also common manifestations of postoperative meningitis. Many of these findings, however, are also present in uninfected neurosurgery patients during the postoperative period, due to the presence of blood or other foreign matter in the CNS and to the surgical trauma. Furthermore, changes in mental status in such patients can be difficult to assess.

The choice of antimicrobials for treatment is governed by the antimicrobial sensitivities of the infecting organism, while the route of administration (systemic or intrathecal) depends on the ability to achieve adequate levels of an effective antimicrobial in the CSF. The outcome for neurosurgical patients with meningitis is generally poor, but it is a function of the infecting organism and its antimicrobial sensitivities and of the underlying neurosurgical problem.

Ventricular Shunt Patients

Meningitis in patients with ventricular shunts is manifested by fever, nausea and vomiting, malaise, and meningeal signs [54, 73]. Shunt infections per se can also be accompanied by local erythema over the shunt course, splenomegaly, anemia, and glomerulonephritis. CNS infections in shunt patients can become apparent within a day or two after surgery, or many months later [54, 73, 75]. The time interval between surgery and onset of illness is in large part a function of the infecting organism, with infections due to *S. aureus* usually becoming apparent early and infections due to *S. epidermidis* usually becoming apparent late [73]. Similarly, infections in patients with ventricular shunts can have an acute, rapidly progressive course (more common with *S. aureus* infections) or can be more indolent (more common with *S. epidermidis* infections).

There is substantial controversy about the role of antimicrobials (parenteral or intraventricular) alone in treating shunt infections, compared with antimicrobials plus removal of the shunt. Although antimicrobials alone have been reported to cure 36 to 41 percent of patients [49, 71], many authors have reported poor results without the complete removal of the infected shunt [12, 15, 45, 73, 76]. Whether or not the infected shunt is removed, the outcome of meningitis in ventricular shunt patients tends to be better than in neonates and other neurosurgical patients.

Neonates

Meningitis in neonates is usually characterized by fever (although hypothermia also has been reported) and nonspecific findings such as poor feeding, decreased tone, lethargy, listlessness, a weak cry, irritability, dyspnea or apnea, and jaundice. Specific findings that point toward the CNS as the site of infection (e.g., bulging fontanelle, stiff neck) are frequently absent [58]. Since neonatal meningitis is usually associated with bacteremia, it is not surprising that the clinical findings are almost indistinguishable from those seen in neonatal sepsis without meningitis.

Onset of illness usually occurs 4 to 8 days after birth but can be as early as 1 day or as late as 6 weeks. Thus many cases of nosocomial meningitis in neonates do not become apparent until after discharge from the hospital. As in meningitis in neurosurgical patients, the choice of antimicrobials and the route of administration depend on the causative organism, its antimicrobial sensitivities, and the penetration of the antimicrobial agent into the CSF. The outcome of neonatal meningitis, while dependent on the causative organism, is generally poor; the fatality rate is 60 percent (approaching 100 percent in some outbreaks), and there is permanent neurologic damage in many survivors [58].

Laboratory Findings

The laboratory findings in patients with nosocomial bacterial meningitis do not differ from those seen in other patients with bacterial meningitis. The opening pressure may be normal or increased; the CSF contains an elevated number of white blood cells, with a predominance of polymorphonuclear leukocytes; the CSF protein level is increased; the CSF glucose level is decreased; and bacteria may be visible on Gram stain. On rare occasions, the CSF may be entirely normal [32, 50]. Because the CSF protein level and leukocyte count may be elevated due to neurosurgery alone, however, and because organisms are not visible on Gram stain in approximately 50 percent of cases, a low CSF glucose concentration may be the only reliable indicator of meningitis in a neurosurgery patient until the CSF culture results are available [46]. Though an elevated peripheral white blood cell count also is usually present in patients with meningitis, the frequent administration of corticosteroids to neurosurgery patients and the resultant leukocytosis can make these counts difficult to interpret.

Factitious Meningitis and Pseudo-Outbreaks

Although CSF Gram stain evidence of bacterial meningitis in several hospitalized patients over a short period of time is suggestive of a problem with nosocomial meningitis, it is worth keeping in mind that such findings can be spurious. False-positive CSF Gram stains can be caused by the presence of viable or nonviable organisms in the Gram stain reagents, in transport media used for swabs, in the tubes used to centrifuge the CSF, and on improperly cleaned glass slides [24, 37, 53, 60, 79]. False-positive CSF Gram stains also

have been attributed to the use of unoccluded needles in the performance of the lumbar puncture [40]. Problems such as these should be considered whenever CSF culture results fail to confirm positive CSF Gram stain results; they can largely be avoided by proper cleaning of glass slides before use, filtration of staining reagents, and thorough rinsing of slides after staining.

Risk to Hospital Personnel

Hospital personnel in contact with infected patients are not considered to be at increased risk of developing meningitis except when the patient has meningitis or other invasive disease caused by *N. meningitidis*. Even when the patient has a meningococcal infection, the risk to hospital personnel is low and appears to be limited to those with unusually intimate contact with the patient's respiratory tract secretions (e.g., someone who has given the patient mouth-to-mouth resuscitation or suctioned the patient). The number of reported secondary meningococcal infections among medical personnel since the disappearance of epidemic meningococcal disease from the United States has been small [4, 17, 25] despite the fact that more than 2,500 patients with meningococcal meningitis and meningococcemia are admitted to U.S. hospitals each year [6].

Current recommendations for prevention of such cases seem to be adequate to protect hospital personnel. Recommendations include keeping patients with meningococcal infections in respiratory isolation (private room, with face masks worn by staff and visitors) until 24 hours after initiation of effective therapy and prompt use of chemoprophylaxis among hospital staff with unusually intimate exposure to respiratory secretions (see Chap. 11). Chemoprophylaxis of close community contacts of patients with meningitis caused by *H. influenzae* or *N. meningitidis* also is indicated. Such cases should be promptly reported to the appropriate state or local health department so that chemoprophylaxis can be given. Before discharge from the hospital, the patients should also receive antimicrobial therapy directed at eradication of nasopharyngeal carriage of these organisms, as many of the antimicrobial agents used to treat bacterial meningitis do not reliably eradicate carriage.

Surveillance and Prevention

The prevention of nosocomial meningitis does not differ fundamentally from the prevention of other nosocomial infections. An awareness of the problem and a surveillance system focused on high-risk areas such as neurosurgical wards and neonatal intensive care units are the keys to spotting cases early and preventing additional ones (see Chap. 5). Avoiding colonization of patients by impeccable surgical wound and umbilical stump care and scrupulous attention to handwashing can probably prevent most cases of nosocomial meningitis.

The infection control practitioner should carefully monitor the occurrence of cases of meningitis in neonates and neurosurgery patients. Given the generally poor outcome in cases of nosocomial meningitis, 2 or more cases due to a single organism, even if they are scattered in time, should be cause for additional investigation. In light of the sometimes prolonged incubation period, particularly in patients with ventricular shunts, such an investigation must include the follow-up of patients at risk who were not ill at the time of discharge. Culturing of the hospital environment and of hospital personnel, if undertaken at all, should follow and be guided by a thorough epidemiologic investigation.

References

1. Aber, R.C., et al. Nosocomial transmission of group-B streptococci. *Pediatrics* 58:346, 1976.
2. Abrahamsen, T.G., Finne, P.H., and Lingaas, E. *Flavobacterium meningosepticum* infections in a neonatal intensive care unit. *Acta Paediatr. Scand.* 78:51, 1989.
3. Anderson, F.M. Ventriculocardiac shunts. *J. Pediatr.* 82:222, 1973.
4. Artenstein, M.S., and Ellis, R.E. The risk of exposure to a patient with meningococcal meningitis. *Milit. Med.* 133:474, 1968.
5. Ayliffe, G.A.J., et al. Hospital infection with *Pseudomonas aeruginosa* in neurosurgery. *Lancet* 2:365, 1965.
6. Band, J.D., et al. Trends in meningococcal disease, United States 1975–1980. *J. Infect. Dis.* 148:754, 1983.
7. Barton, L.L., Granoff, D.M., and Barenkamp, S.J. Nosocomial spread of *Haemophilus influenzae* type b infection documented by outer membrane protein subtype analysis. *J. Pediatr.* 102:820, 1983.
8. Bassett, D.C.J., Thompson, S.A.S., and Page, B. Neonatal infections with *Pseudomonas aeruginosa* associated with contaminated resuscitation equipment. *Lancet* 1:781, 1965.
9. Bayston, R., and Lari, J. A study of the sources of infection in colonized shunts. *Dev. Med. Child Neurol.* 16(Suppl. 32): 16, 1974.
10. Becker, A.H. Infection due to *Proteus mirabilis* in newborn nursery. *J. Dis. Child.* 104:69, 1962.
11. Berkowitz, F.E. *Acinetobacter* meningitis—a diagnostic pitfall: A report of 3 cases. *S. Afr. Med. J.* 61:448, 1982.
12. Bruce, A.M., Lorber, J., Shedden, W.I.H., and Zachary, R.B. Persistent bacteraemia following ventriculocaval shunt operations for hydrocephalus in infants. *Dev. Med. Child Neurol.* 5:461, 1963.
13. Burke, J.P., et al. *Proteus mirabilis* infections in a hospital nursery traced to a human carrier. *N. Engl. J. Med.* 284:115, 1971.
14. Cabrera, H.A., and Davis, G.H. Epidemic meningitis of the newborn caused by flavobacteria. *Am. J. Dis. Child.* 101:289, 1961.
15. Callaghan, R.P., Cohen, S.J., and Stewart, G.T. Septicaemia due to colonization of Spitz-Holter valves by staphylococci: Five cases treated with methicillin. *Br. Med. J.* 1:860, 1961.
16. Campbell, A.N., Sill, P.R., and Wardle, J.K. *Listeria* meningitis acquired by cross-infection in a delivery suite. *Lancet* 2:752, 1981.
17. Centers for Disease Control. Nosocomial meningococcemia—Wisconsin. *M.M.W.R.* 27:358, 1978.
18. Christie, C.D.C., Havens, P.L., and Shapiro, E.D. Bacteremia with group A streptococci in childhood. *Am. J. Dis. Child.* 142:559, 1988.
19. Cohen, M.S., et al. Possible nosocomial transmission of group Y *Neisseria meningitidis* among oncology patients. *Ann. Intern. Med.* 91:7, 1979.
20. Corbett, J.J., and Rosenstein, B.J. *Pseudomonas* meningitis related to spinal anesthesia: Report of three cases with a common source of infection. *Neurology* 21:946, 1971.
21. Cutler, M., and Cutler, P. Iatrogenic meningitis. *J. Med. Soc. N.J.* 50:510, 1953.

22. Dillon, H.C. Group A type 12 streptococcal infection in a newborn nursery. *Am. J. Dis. Child.* 112:177, 1966.

23. Djindjian, M., Fevrier, M.J., Otterbein, G., and Soussy, J.C. Oxacillin prophylaxis in cerebrospinal fluid shunt procedures: Results of a randomized open study in 60 hydrocephalic patients. *Surg. Neurol.* 25:178, 1986.

24. Ericsson, C.D., et al. Erroneous diagnosis of meningitis due to false-positive Gram stains. *South. Med. J.* 71:1524, 1978.

25. Feldman, H.A. Recent developments in the therapy and control of meningococcal infections. *Dis. Mon.* Feb. 1966, pp. 18–20.

26. Franciosi, R.A., Knostman, J.D., and Zimmerman, R.A. Group-B streptococcal neonatal and infant infections. *J. Pediatr.* 82:707, 1973.

27. Garner, J.S., et al. CDC definitions for nosocomial infections, 1988. *Am. J. Infect. Control* 16:128, 1988.

28. Glode, M.P., et al. An outbreak of *Hemophilus influenzae* type b meningitis in an enclosed hospital population. *J. Pediatr.* 88:36, 1976.

29. Goossens, H., et al. Nosocomial outbreak of *Campylobacter jejuni* meningitis in newborn infants. *Lancet* 2:146, 1986.

30. Graham, D.R., et al. Epidemic nosocomial meningitis due to *Citrobacter diversus* in neonates. *J. Infect. Dis.* 144:203, 1981.

31. Gross, R.J., Rowe, B., and Easton, J.A. Neonatal meningitis caused by *Citrobacter koseri. J. Clin. Pathol.* 26:138, 1973.

32. Gruskay, J., et al. Neonatal *Staphylococcus epidermidis* meningitis with unremarkable CSF examination results. *Am. J. Dis. Child.* 143:580, 1989.

33. Gwynn, C.M., and George, R.H. Neonatal *Citrobacter* meningitis. *Arch. Dis. Child.* 48:455, 1973.

34. Headings, D.L., and Overall, J.C., Jr. Outbreak of meningitis in a newborn intensive care unit caused by a single *Escherichia coli* Kl serotype. *J. Pediatr.* 90:99, 1977.

35. Hill, H.R., Hunt, C.E., and Matsen, J.M. Nosocomial colonization with *Klebsiella*, type 26, in a neonatal intensive-care unit associated with an outbreak of sepsis, meningitis, and necrotizing enterocolitis. *J. Pediatr.* 85:415, 1974.

36. Ho, J.L., et al. An outbreak of type 4b *Listeria monocytogenes* infection involving patients from eight Boston hospitals. *Arch. Intern. Med.* 146:520, 1986.

37. Hoke, C.H., et al. False-positive Gram-stained smears. *J.A.M.A.* 241:478, 1979.

38. Humphrey, M.A., Simpson, G.T., and Grindlinger, G.A. Clinical characteristics of nosocomial sinusitis. *Ann. Otol. Rhinol. Laryngol.* 96:687, 1987.

39. Jentsch, H.J., Guggenbichler, J.P., and Waltl, H. Salmonella meningitis in the newborn. *Monatsschr. Kinderheilkd.* 127:415, 1979.

40. Joyner, R.W., Idriss, Z.H., and Wilfert, C.M. Misinterpretation of cerebrospinal fluid Gram stain. *Pediatrics* 54:360, 1974.

41. Kilpatrick, M.E., and Girgis, N.I. Meningitis—a complication of spinal anesthesia. *Anesth. Analg.* 62:513, 1983.

42. Kremer, M. Meningitis after spinal analgesia. *Br. Med. J.* 2:309, 1945.

43. Larsson, S., et al. *Listeria monocytogenes* causing hospital-acquired enterocolitis and meningitis in newborn infants. *Br. Med. J.* 2:473, 1978.

44. Laugier, J., et al. Meningite du nouveaune a *Listeria monocytogenes* et contamination en maternite. *Arch. Fr. Pediatr.* 35:168, 1978.

45. Luthardt, T. Bacterial infections in ventriculoauricular shunt systems. *Dev. Med. Child Neurol.* 22(Suppl): 105, 1970.

46. Mangi, R.J., Quintiliani, R., and Andriole, V.T. Gram-negative bacillary meningitis. *Am. J. Med.* 59:829, 1975.

47. Martin, M.A., et al. Nosocomial aseptic meningitis associated with administration of OKT3. *J.A.M.A.* 259:2002, 1988.

48. McCarthy, M.F., Jr., and Wenzel, R.P. Postoperative spinal fluid infections after neurosurgical shunting procedures. *Pediatrics* 59:793, 1977.

49. McLaurin, R.L. Infected cerebrospinal fluid shunts. *Surg. Neurol.* 1:191, 1973.

50. Michael, M., Barrett, D.J., and Mehta, P. Infants with meningitis without cerebrospinal fluid pleocytosis. *Am. J. Dis. Child.* 140:851, 1986.

51. Morgan, M.E.I., and Hart, C.A. *Acinetobacter* meningitis: Acquired infection in a neonatal intensive care unit. *Arch. Dis. Child.* 57:557, 1982.

52. Muschner, V.K., et al. Meningitisepidemid durch Coxsackievirus typ B 5 auf einer sauglingsstaion. *Kinderarztl. Prax.* 7:290, 1972.

53. Musher, D.M., and Schell, R.F. False-positive Gram stains of cerebrospinal fluid. *Ann. Intern. Med.* 79:603, 1973.

54. Naito, H., et al. High incidence of acute postoperative meningitis and septicemia in patients undergoing craniotomy with ventriculoatrial shunt. *Surg. Gynecol. Obstet.* 137:810, 1973.

55. Nardi, G., et al. Epidemia da virus coxsackie di gruppo B in un reparto neonatale. *Ann. Sclavo* 18:793, 1976.

56. Nelson, K.E., et al. Transmission of neonatal listeriosis in a delivery room. *Am. J. Dis. Child.* 139:903, 1985.

57. Noiby, N., Schneibel, J., and Sebbesen, O. Streptococcal Meningitis After Myelography. In: *Communicable Disease Report*, Vol. 5. London: Public Health Laboratory Service, Communicable Disease Surveillance Center, 1982.

58. Overall, J.C., Jr. Neonatal bacterial meningitis: Analysis of predisposing factors and outcome

compared with matched control subjects. *J. Pediatr.* 76:499, 1970.

59. Parry, M.F., et al. Gram-negative sepsis in neonates: A nursery outbreak due to hand carriage of *Citrobacter diversus. Pediatrics* 65:1105, 1980.

60. Peterson, E., et al. Factitious bacterial meningitis revisited. *J. Clin. Microbiol.* 16:758, 1982.

61. Plotkin, S.A., and McKitrick, J.C. Nosocomial meningitis of the newborn caused by a flavobacterium. *J.A.M.A.* 198:194, 1966.

62. Price, D.J.E., and Sleigh, J.D., Control of infection due to *Klebsiella aerogenes* in a neurosurgical unit by withdrawal of all antibiotics. *Lancet* 2:1213, 1970.

63. Price, D.J.E., and Sleigh, J.D. *Klebsiella* meningitis—report of nine cases. *J. Neurol. Neurosurg. Psychiatry* 35:903, 1972.

64. Rance, C.P., et al. An epidemic of septicemia with meningitis and hemorrhagic encephalitis in premature infants. *J. Pediatr.* 61:24, 1962.

65. Ratcheson, R.A., and Ommaya, A.K. Experience with the subcutaneous cerebrospinal fluid reservoir: Preliminary report of 60 cases. *N. Engl. J. Med.* 279:1025, 1968.

66. Ravenholt, R.T., and LaVeck, G.D. Staphylococcal disease: An obstetric, pediatric, and community problem. *Am. J. Public Health* 46:1287, 1956.

67. Ribeiro, C.D., Davis, P., and Jones, D.M. *Citrobacter koseri* meningitis in a special care baby unit *J. Clin. Pathol.* 29:1094, 1976.

68. Salmon, J.H. Adult hydrocephalus: Evaluation of shunt therapy in 80 patients. *J. Neurosurg.* 37:423, 1972.

69. Sarubbi, F.A., Jr., Wilson, M.B., Lee, M., and Brokopp, C. Nosocomial meningitis and bacteremia due to contaminated amphotericin B. *J.A.M.A.* 239:416, 1978.

70. Sautter, R.L., Mattman, L.H., and Legaspi, R.C. *Serratia marcescens* meningitis associated with a contaminated benzalkonium chloride solution. *Infect. Control* 5:223, 1984.

71. Schimke, R.T., Black, P.H., Mark, V.H., and Swartz, M.N. Indolent *Staphylococcus albus* or *aureus* bacteremia after ventriculoatriostomy: Role of foreign body in its initiation and perpetuation. *N. Engl. J. Med.* 264:264, 1961.

72. Schlech, W.F., et al. Epidemic listeriosis: Evidence for transmission by food. *N. Engl. J. Med.* 308:203, 1983.

73. Schoenbaum, S.C., Gardner, P., and Shillito, J. Infections of cerebrospinal fluid shunts: Epidemiology, clinical manifestations, and therapy. *J. Infect. Dis.* 131:543, 1975.

74. Schuchat, A., et al. Outbreak of neonatal listeriosis associated with mineral oil. *Pediatr. Inf. Dis. J.* 10:183, 1991.

75. Sells, C.J., Shurtleff, D.B., and Loeser, J.D. Gram-negative cerebrospinal fluid shunt—associated infections. *Pediatrics* 59:614, 1977.

76. Shurtleff, D.B., Foltz, E.L., Weeks, R.D., and Loeser, J. Therapy of *Staphylococcus epidermidis* infections associated with cerebrospinal fluid shunts. *Pediatrics* 53:55, 1974.

77. Tsingoglou, S., and Forrest, D.M. A technique for the insertion of Holter ventriculo-atrial shunt for infantile hydrocephalus. *Br. J. Surg.* 58:367, 1971.

78. Venes, J.L. Control of shunt infection: Report of 150 consecutive cases. *J. Neurosurg.* 45:311, 1976.

79. Weinstein, R.A., et al. Factitious meningitis: Diagnostic error due to nonviable bacteria in commercial lumbar puncture trays. *J.A.M.A.* 233:878, 1975.

80. Winterbauer, R.H., Fortuine, R., and Eickhoff, T.C. Unusual occurrence of neonatal meningitis due to group B beta-hemolytic streptococci. *Pediatrics* 38:661, 1966.

81. Zaidi, M., et al. Epidemic of *Serratia marcescens* bacteremia and meningitis in a neonatal unit in Mexico City. *Infect. Control Hosp. Epidemiol.* 10:14, 1989.

Surgical Infections

N. Joel Ehrenkranz
Jonathan L. Meakins

Historical Background

Prior to 1885, wound infection was a common companion of any surgical procedure, and life-threatening infection was the anticipated outcome of major operations. Once a patient's major defense against infection, the intact skin, was breached by either trauma or the surgical knife, a broad avenue was opened to introduction of virulent bacteria. In hospitals, outbreaks of cellulitis and septicemia swept among postoperative patients, undoubtedly reflecting epidemic spread of virulent streptococci. It is difficult to conceive the terror such infections wrought in patients and hospital personnel alike. Minor skin trauma resulted in cellulitis, which rapidly progressed to lymphangitis, gangrene, bacteremia, and death. This was variously described as *streptococcal gangrene* or *hospital gangrene*. A relatively recent description from the 1940s serves to convey some of this terror: "[At times] the operations in the hospital suddenly became fatal. If a nurse scratched her finger with a pin, she died of septicemia. All the surgical patients died: An operation was an execution" [68] *Septicemia* was a term often employed to describe fulminating cellulitis that arose 2 to 4 days after a traumatic wound (especially a compound fracture or deep soft-tissue laceration) and before suppuration was evident. Death from uncontrolled bacteremia generally occurred in a week. In contrast to these rapidly fatal cellulitic-septicemic episodes, localized purulent infections were virtually welcomed by surgeons. The term *laudable pus,* no doubt characterizing staphylococcal infections, portrayed a cautious expectation of recovery of a patient despite a suppurating wound. However, local purulent wound infections did have the potential for dissemination, thereby causing death by "pyemia."

Lister Pioneers Research into Surgical Infection Prevention

Joseph Lister is appropriately honored as the surgeon who initiated the scientific process to abolish both the terror and the mystery of surgical infection [48a]. The profound impact of Lister on surgical and biologic thinking in relation to surgical infection lasts to the present. The events of his investigations were instructive. He made the great intellectual leap from Pasteur's concept of invisible environmental germs causing fermentation and putrefaction to the hypothesis that similar bacteria in the ambient air could cause wound infection if they gained access to tissues through broken skin. Beginning studies in 1865, Lister selected carbolic acid (phenol) as an agent to prevent sepsis (antiseptic). He employed an antiseptic as a chemical shield to maintain the sterility of the operative site. His objective was to prevent tissue invasion of ambient bacteria through an open wound and thus to prevent wound infection. This concept was distinct from that of Semmelweis, who advocated an antiseptic be used on unbroken skin of physicians' hands to prevent them from serving as a vehicle of contact transmission of contagion from cadavers to postpartum women. For Lister, prevention of infection was an all-consuming research objective. He systematically explored the use of carbolic acid in experimental animals to prevent infection following compound fractures and persevered despite initial failures. By 1885, Lister was able to use carbolic acid in humans to prevent infection by direct application to the wound site. Despite such successes, a number of contemporaries were loath to accept Lister's measures as a regular surgical practice. A French observer, commenting on a demonstration of the outcome of Lister's use of antisepsis in 1883, spoke for many contemporaries when he said "C'est magnifique, mais ce n'est pas la chirurgie" [73a]. Later, more vigorous in his efforts to promote a wider atmosphere of antisepsis, Lister nebulized carbolic acid during operations. These effects have been graphically described by George Bernard Shaw [68]:

[Lister] invented a donkey engine which spread a mist of carbolic spray through the operating room, and poisoned the microbes, the patient, and the surgeon simultaneously. He thought that what was needed to abolish disease and make the human race permanently healthy was the substitution of carbolic spray for the atmosphere by a donkey engine at every street corner. The *fin de siecle* stank of carbolic acid.

Although Lister conducted extensive laboratory studies based on Pasteur's germ theory, it would appear he was not abreast of contemporaneous scientific developments. To quote Block [12]:

[Lister] chose phenol because he had heard about the remarkable results produced by carbolic acid (phenol) for the town of Carlisle in preventing the odor of the sewage . . . used to irrigate pastures . . . He was unaware that phenol . . . had been used by Kuchenmeister . . . in 1860 as a dressing for wounds . . . [Lister] succeeded, because he had great confidence that his method would work, and he pursued it doggedly despite initial failure and opposition. It worked because phenol was indeed a germicide that killed vegetative bacteria, if not spores; because the way Lister literally poured it on, it reached all parts of the wound.

Lister's great contribution to science was to demonstrate, by sound laboratory and clinical research, a rational approach to understanding the causation of surgical infection based on Pasteur's demonstration of an unseen ambient microbiologic world. His revolutionary approach emphasized that microorganisms must be prevented from entering a wound during or after operation, and that if microorganisms were already present in a wound at the time of operation, they must be prevented from spreading. These remain basic concepts in present-day surgery. He also stressed that all instruments, dressings, and everything else in contact with the operative site, including the hands of surgeons and assistants, should be made antiseptic. Moreover, the success of Lister's research efforts permanently fixed the principle of prophylaxis of infection as a practical surgical goal. His focus on prevention through antisepsis eventually gave way to a new school of thought emanating from Germany; namely, that the careful surgeon with "surgically clean" hands and sterile instruments could prevent infection without need for chemical disinfection of the environment. Studies reported by Robert Koch in 1881 [43a, 43b], describing the relative merits of dry and moist heat as sterilizing agents, gave impetus to the use of first boiling water and then steam autoclaves to sterilize surgical instruments and surgical dressings. Thus modern surgical aseptic technique was born. Lister eventually agreed that his hypothesis that ambient airborne bacteria were the cause of sepsis was incorrect and that the primary reason for wound infection was the bacterial contamination arising from surgeons' dirty hands and instruments. In current practice, however, vestiges of Lister's antisepsis still remain in the use of antibacterial agents to prepare a patient's skin and in their administration for surgical prophylaxis.

Management of Contaminated and Infected Wounds

Lister's wound irrigations with phenol, in fact, damaged tissues and delayed wound healing. However, the use of a chemical for antiseptic treatment of contaminated traumatic wounds has been a subject long of interest to military surgeons. Iodine was used in war wounds as early as the 1861–1865 American Civil War [12] and sodium hypochlorite solution (Dakin's solution) was employed during World War I [54]. Both iodine compounds and Dakin's solution are now also known to damage tissues. Sulfonamides were employed for local and systemic prophylaxis of traumatic wounds in World War II. A United States National Research Council study conducted in the early 1940s, however, revealed that local use of sulfonamides had little effect on preventing infection following severe injuries [54]. The goal to eradicate bacteria from contaminated traumatic wounds by chemical measures has proved to be illusory and unattainable, as measured by the failure of such treatments to permit primary wound closure without a considerable risk of infection. What was learned by military surgeons in their studies of antiseptics was the importance of delayed wound closure. Carrell and Dakin popularized local antisepsis, debridement, and delayed closure of traumatic wounds during World War I [54]. Churchill extended these observations on wound closure during World War II and reemphasized the danger of primary closure of contaminated traumatic wounds after seemingly adequate debridement [18]. This lesson, unfortunately, has had to be relearned by subsequent generations of battlefield and trauma surgeons.

During World War II, the efficacy of penicillin treatment for established surgical infections seemed almost miraculous. A variety of life-threatening surgical infections, including cellulitic-septicemic ones, acute suppurative arthritis, and acute osteomyelitis, finally became amenable to drug therapy alone. For the first time in history, military surgeons were able to treat virulent infections without an overwhelming case fatality rate and without mutilation.

Multiple Bacterial Species Etiology of Necrotic Wound Infections

Studies of surgical wound infections caused by multiple bacterial species were pioneered by Meleney and Altemeier [5, 53]. They identified the potent synergy of mixed aerobic and anaerobic bacterial species in causing destructive infections in soft tissues and intra-abdominal sites. Altemeier [5] first reported on the almost invariable presence of *Bacteroides* species in peritonitis complicating perforated appendicitis. He defined the influence of necrotic tissues in promoting infection in biologic terms: The virulence of *Clostridium perfringens* was found to be increased by a factor of 10^3 in the presence of dead tissue and by 10^6 if both foreign body and dead tissue were present [7]. A biologic basis for debridement was established. In addition, the groundwork was laid for quantitative bacteriologic studies in elucidating mechanisms of surgical infection.

Antimicrobial Prophylaxis

Shortly after World War II, the efficacy of systemic antimicrobial drugs for preventing infections in elective operations was explored by a number of investigators, with contradictory findings. This was primarily due to variations in timing of administration of drugs in relation to the time of operation in the different studies. Burke [16], in precise animal studies, defined the narrow time period after surgical incision during which prophylactic antibiotics may prevent infection. This concept led to several well-conducted studies, including those of Bernard and Cole [11] and Polk and Lopez-Mayor [61], which provided unequivocal evidence of effectiveness of preoperative antibiotic prophylaxis in preventing infections after elective clean-contaminated operations. By contrast, antibiotics administered only postoperatively have no prophylactic effect.

Until recently, antimicrobial prophylaxis was not recommended for elective operations considered to carry very low risks of wound infection, such as breast operations, herniorrhaphy, and low-risk cesarean sections. However, it has now been demonstrated in multicenter studies involving large numbers of patients that prophylaxis does bring about a significant reduction of a variety of postoperative infections even in low-risk operations [31, 60], including those occurring beyond the immediate operative site. This expanded concept of prevention of postoperative infection reveals the need for additional research about perioperative uses of antibiotics to maximize the effectiveness of surgery.

Infection Surveillance and Control

Routine surveillance of surgical infections evolved from the great epidemics of *Staphylococcus aureus* infection in hospitals in the late 1940s and 1950s. The World War II vision of easy control of infections by antibiotics gave way to the reality of worldwide outbreaks of antibiotic-resistant *S. aureus*. In addition to antibiotic resistance, these staphylococci—generally of the 52/52A/80/81 phage-type complex—clearly possessed enhanced virulence, as manifested by epidemics of breast abscess in postpartum women, pustules in newborn infants, and rapid secondary spread of suppurative disease [19a]. A 1964 United States National Research Council and National Academy of Science (NRC/NAS) study at five university hospitals, conducted to evaluate the efficacy of ultraviolet light in operating rooms to prevent wound infection, did serve to emphasize the variety of host and operative conditions predisposing to infection [1]. A striking finding was the wide range of differences in frequency of wound infection at the different participating hospitals for similar classes of operations. Among clean-contaminated operations, for example, infection rates varied from 3.5 to 19.6 percent. Cruse and Foord [23] expanded the concept of surveillance from a research activity to one of ongoing assessment. Systematic surveillance of postoperative patients for infection has become a central activity in infection control programs and serves as a benchmark in evaluation of infection control programs by hospital regulatory and accrediting agencies. Especially useful now is the surveillance of specific clean and clean-contaminated operations, which provide a basis for meaningful comparisons. Surveillance of postoperative infection has further evolved into a quality assurance measure in many North American hospitals.

Biology of Surgical Infections

Surgical infections are almost always bacterial in origin. They usually arise as a result of intraoperative seeding of exogenous bacteria or as a consequence of dissemination of endogenous bacteria to the operative site. Exogenous bacteria are generally transmitted as a result of direct or indirect contact from fomites or operating room personnel. The latter include heavy droplets of bacteria-laden particles transmitted through the air for a short distance.

Infection developing as a result of bacterial

inoculation of the closed surgical wound is believed to be distinctly uncommon. Soon after closure of the incision, the surgical wound is regarded as being sealed. Resistance of the closed wound to infection appears to increase rapidly with healing [2]. Postoperative onset of operative site infection of a closed wound resulting from hematogenous or lymphatic bacterial dissemination, or by microbial invasion through a closed wound site, has been previously considered to be extremely rare. However, recent studies have demonstrated that in some critical care settings, postoperative initiation of both incisional and deep operative site infections can occur in clusters [32a, 49a]. Such demonstrations require unusual and intensive investigational efforts, which may not be easily performed in many hospitals [42a]. Thus, a postoperative causation of operative site infection may be more frequent than hitherto suspected.

Classification of Surgical Wounds and Rates of Infection

A widely used classification of surgical wounds is based on an estimate of likelihood of bacterial contamination of the operative site. In the 1964 NRC/NAS study, five general classes of operations were defined [1]:

1. *Refined-clean:* elective operations, not drained and primarily closed
2. *Other clean:* clean cases other than refined-clean
3. *Clean-contaminated:* gastrointestinal or respiratory tract entered without significant spillage, entrance of genitourinary tract in presence of infected urine, entrance of biliary tract in presence of infected bile or minor break in technique
4. *Contaminated:* major break in operative technique (e.g., surgical entrance of unprepared bowel without gross spillage of bowel contents); acute bacterial inflammation without pus; fresh, traumatic wound from a relatively clean source
5. *Dirty:* presence of pus or perforated viscus (prior to operation), old traumatic wound or traumatic wound from a dirty source

Currently, this classification has been condensed into four groups for general use, without a subdivision of the clean category [6]. The four categories are useful for describing expected infection rates in a crude (unadjusted) way. As the classification of surgical procedures progresses from clean to dirty, the rates of incisional infection progressively increase (Table 33-1). However, within a given category, rates of infection vary considerably according to the inherent characteristics of different operations and of risk factors of the surgical patient. In theory, if the technical abilities of individual surgeons are adequate, surgical technique should not be a factor in promoting postoperative infection. Obviously, this is a consideration that increases in importance in direct relation to increasing demands for technical skills in different operations. For epidemiologic purposes, it may be useful to consider more than

Table 33-1. Historical rates of wound infections

Wound classification	Infection rate (no./100 patients)			
	1960–62: 15,613 patients [1]	*1967–77: 62,939 patients [22]*	*1975–76: 59,353 patients [39]*	*1977–86: 25,919 patients [58]*
Clean	5.1	1.5	2.9	1.4
Clean-contaminated	10.8	7.7	3.9	2.8
Contaminated	16.3	15.2	8.5	8.4
Dirty or infected	28.0	40.0	12.6	—

four groups. For example, within the clean operation category, it would be meaningful to revive the refined-clean classification for a group of elective operations such as cataract extraction procedures, cosmetic operations, thyroidectomy, and certain other operations that generally have a lower rate of infectious complications than do femoropopliteal bypass, coronary artery bypass operations, and certain neurosurgical and orthopedic procedures.

Table 33-1 demonstrates how much progress has been made in controlling or, more appropriately, preventing wound infections since the 1964 NRC/NAS report [1]. Improvements have come primarily in the clean-contaminated, contaminated, and dirty procedures, reflecting operations with a progressive increase in probability of bacterial wound contamination. A variety of factors are responsible: improvements in anesthesia, surgical technique, selection and preoperative preparation of patients, control of nonsurgical diseases and, most important, the widespread and appropriate use of antibiotics for prophylaxis (see Chap. 12).

When the NRC/NAS study was reported in 1964, many of today's clean operations were not yet devised. With the narrowing of the differences in wound infection rates between groups, it is evident that a new way to identify who is at risk for wound infection must be developed. Many variables have been identified as being associated with wound infection [22, 51]. Davidson and colleagues [24] devised a weighted set of risk factors for wound infection to express the various conditions promoting infection in an integrated format. Bacterial contamination of the wound during operation was found to be the most important factor. Contributing to this was the degree of contamination inherent in the operation (dirty operation), duration of operations (more than 1 hour), and other environmental factors promoting bacterial hazards to a patient. This concept was expanded later in the 1970s in the Study on the Efficacy of Nosocomial Infection Control (the SENIC Project) [39]. Four independent variables, each having the same weight, were employed to identify patients at high risk of surgical wound infection: abdominal operation, operation lasting more than 2 hours, contaminated or dirty-infected operation, and three or more discharge diagnoses. The use of the SENIC simplified risk index (Table 33-2) permits greater refinement of estimation of patient risk to wound infection than does stratification based only on the probability of bacteria contaminating the surgical wound and defined by clean, clean-contaminated, contaminated, and dirty conditions. Since virtually all patients undergoing elective clean-contaminated and contaminated operations now receive prophylactic antibiotics, wound infections in these patients are generally uncommon. The usefulness of the SENIC index was that it better defined the patient at risk to infection in terms of specific patient-dependent variables rather than by consideration of only the probability of bacterial contamination of the wound. The multivariable analysis may appear to be more cumbersome than the traditional classifi-

Table 33-2. Comparison of wound classification systems: surgical wound infection rates among 59,352 randomly selected patients hospitalized in 1975–76

Traditional wound classification	SENIC risk index				
	Low	Medium	High 1	High 2	High 3
Clean	1.1	3.9	8.4	15.8	
Clean-contaminated	0.6	2.8	8.4	17.7	
Contaminated		4.5	8.3	11.0	23.9
Dirty-infected		6.7	10.9	18.8	27.4

Source: Modified from R.W. Haley et al., Identifying patients at high risk of surgical wound infection. *Am. J. Epidemiol.* 121:206, 1985.

cation, but it serves to identify patients for whom additional measures to reduce infection will need to be devised.

A newer and more sophisticated version of the SENIC index is the "patient risk index score." This method was derived from analyses of 1987–1990 findings of the National Nosocomial Infection Surveillance (NNIS) System [23a]. The patient risk index score is calculated as the sum of risk estimate points from (1) preoperative patient evaluation according to the American Society of Anesthesiologists' system of scores of 3 to 5, (2) operation class contaminated or dirty, and (3) duration of operation based on the 75th percentile for that category of procedures. This last is a novel approach that reflects the unique attributes of individual types of operations; for example, the 75th percentile duration for cesarean sections will be distinct from that of coronary bypass graft operations. It is noteworthy that in this 1990s version of the NNIS patient risk index there is no differentiation of risk between clean and clean-contaminated operations. In addition, a surgeon whose operating time consistently exceeds the 75th percentile for a procedure class may have an "acceptable" infection rate as determined from this index, but may nevertheless be increasing patients' risk of infection by being a slow operator. Thus, in use of this index, it may be important to determine a surgeon's distribution of patients among risk categories below and above the 75th percentile and, in the event of a consistently skewed distribution in excess of the 75th percentile, to obtain informed opinion as to possible reasons. Validation of this new methodology is eagerly anticipated.

Host Factors Influencing Infection Rates

A wide variety of preoperative host attributes have been identified as being associated with increased likelihood of infection. These include advanced age, extreme obesity, malnutrition, anemia, and diabetes mellitus. It is probable that some of these risk factors are markers for a diminished blood supply that in turn results in decreased tissue oxygenation and lessened phagocytic function. Anergy

[50] and hypoalbuminemia also appear to be indicators of increased susceptibility to postoperative infections, presumably reflecting yet other aspects of diminished host defenses.

Abnormal skin conditions or uncontrolled infection in the patient in an area remote from the operative site prior to operation may reflect heavy abnormal bacterial colonization that could readily contaminate the operative site. Patients with some abnormal skin conditions such as cellulitis, certain erythrodermas and dermatides, exudative dermatoses, pustular lesions, or psoriasis may be heavy carriers of virulent bacteria or fungi. A common misconception among surgeons is that if the skin at the planned incision site appears to be normal, other abnormal skin areas may either be disregarded or be dealt with merely by local application of antiseptic. This view is fraught with danger for serious postoperative infection. Bacteria colonizing abnormal skin sites may be readily transported to the operative site during operation by lymphatic routes as well as by direct or indirect contact spread. If 10^5 or more bacteria gain access to an operative site, infection is likely to occur [44]. Other areas of preexisting uncontrolled infection, remote to the operative site, may also be sources of postoperative infections [28]; these include the respiratory and urinary tracts.

The anatomic region of an operation is an important determinant of wound infection. Surgical procedures involving the scalp, face, arms, and upper body trunk have a lower frequency of complicating infection than do operations in lower body areas. These differences undoubtedly reflect variations in regional blood supply.

Trauma is important in causing infection as it leads directly to tissue necrosis, organ damage and, particularly, to contamination of sterile areas. Trauma-induced extravasation of body fluids or vascular collapse may lead to either regional hypoperfusion or general hypovolemia and, indirectly, to multiple organ dysfunctions. These events may set the stage for translocation of enteric bacteria [25]. During translocation, viable bacteria of the mucosa and submucosa penetrate the intact intestinal wall to gain access to peritoneal structures, abdominal organs, and the bloodstream. This may permit a variety of widespread infectious complications, even though the bowel wall has not been directly damaged by traumatic force.

Intraoperative Events Influencing Infection Rates

Certain intraoperative events are of paramount importance in relation to wound infection. The length of an operation correlates directly with risk of infection: The longer the operation, the greater the opportunity for intraoperative bacterial introduction. An operator's technical skills and dexterity should be reflected in an ability to minimize tissue trauma by gentle handling, conduct sharp anatomic dissections along tissue planes, contain bleeding in the surgical field, and eliminate dead spaces. Fluid collections—in seromas, hematomas, or large dead spaces—require but few bacteria to initiate infection. Other surgical factors promoting infection include overzealous use of electrocautery to coagulate and destroy blood vessels for hemostasis. This may allow infection to occur if more than a very small amount of necrotic tissue remains, by providing a site into which seeded bacteria may flourish. Differences in suture materials selected for closure of incised areas may influence the occurrence of infection [75]. Insertion of a foreign body, whether as a prosthesis or drainage conduit, may impede phagocytic function [27], thereby decreasing the number of bacteria required to establish infection.

Sound operative technique, rather than reliance on postoperative percutaneous drains, is the key to preventing postoperative hematoma. The indiscriminant use of drains by some surgeons in the hope of preventing infection paradoxically promotes infection. Such practices often reflect the uncritical continuation of old habits. In particular, open drains are two-way conduits that provide exogenous bacteria with an avenue of access to the operative site [56]. Open Penrose drains, for example, designed to diminish hematoma

formation in wounds, actually serve to increase wound infection occurrence [1, 48]; drains placed in the operative incisional wound are especially likely to increase wound infection frequency [22].

There are specific indications for use of postoperative drains: Following thoracotomy, chest tubes are placed to remove pleural effusions, reduce pneumothorax, and prevent mediastinal shift; after cardiac operations, mediastinal drains serve to prevent tamponade; and after certain orthopedic operations and such procedures as lymph node dissections in which fluid collections such as seroma or hematoma are virtually inevitable, drains prevent fluid accumulations at operative sites. In management of deep infections such as an abscess that cannot be readily left open (another form of drainage), drains provide an exit for pus. Under these circumstances, closed-suction surgical drainage should be employed through a dedicated incision [4, 22]. Draining intraabdominal operative sites is usually not necessary. Following cholecystectomy, patients without drains were found to have shorter hospital stays than those who were unnecessarily drained [66]. Routine drainage after splenectomy was abandoned when it became apparent that subphrenic infection occurrence increased [19, 41, 58]. Franco and colleagues [33] have reported excellent postoperative results in undrained patients after major hepatic operations. In summary, drains should not be *routinely* used in surgery but rather should have a specific and clear indication. Drains should be closed-suction in type and should not exit through the operative incisional wound.

In contrast to incisions in clean elective operations, in which wound margins are safely approximated by the surgeon on completion of the procedure and healing then occurs by primary intention, immediate surgical closure of an infected or contaminated wound will often lead to incisional infections, despite seemingly adequate debridement. In wound contamination with 10^5 commensal bacteria per gram of tissue, primary wound closure is to be avoided. Some wounds that can be cared for within 3 hours of trauma (e.g., dog bites) may have a lower level of contamination than this and may be safely closed after appropriate assessment [44]. On the other hand, human bite wounds, because of a very large bacterial transfer, generally contain a large number of bacteria at the outset and thus should not be primarily closed. Closure may be safely done on or after the fifth day in most instances, by which time wound contamination is minimal. The surface of clean incisional sites may become colonized with *S. aureus* [15], including methicillin-resistant species for prolonged periods after complete healing [49]. Reoperation through a scar as well as a recent clean wound that is colonized with *S. aureus* is likely to pose an increased risk of infection. Well-healed operative sites may be marked by growth of substantial amounts of scar tissue. Reoperation at such sites can result in considerable diffuse bleeding during or after operation, leading to persisting hematomas and subsequent infection.

Some operative procedures, particularly those necessitating lymph node dissections of the axilla or groin, destroy vascular and lymphatic channels and permit large residual areas of dependent edema to persist. Other operations that lead to considerable areas of dead space (mastectomy, for example) may be further complicated by persisting fluid collections (seromas, lymphoceles) or large hematomas. Since fluid collections may become infected, they should be carefully drained if they persist.

Commensal endogenous bacteria are the usual causes of postoperative infections in clean-contaminated, contaminated, and dirty classes of operations. In the latter two classes, the number of commensal bacteria at the operative site reflects the nature and extent of bacterial contamination in the existing disease process present at the time of surgery. An inoculum of 10^5 or more bacteria appears to be the infective dose required to establish peritoneal infection in association with a perforated or gangrenous appendix [64]. However, in the presence of a foreign body, the infective inoculum for a wound infection may be as few as 10 bacteria [27]. It is possible that certain virulent bacterial species, such as spe-

cific *Streptococcus pyogenes* strains, may initiate infection with very small numbers. In clean-contaminated operations, the bacterial species usually causing infection are the mucosal-associated organisms. These are a subset of the intraluminal microflora that adhere to epithelial surfaces and resist mechanical removal [38]. In clean operations that include placement of prosthetic devices, especially late infection may occur by means of hematogenous or lymphatic spread of bacteria originating from other infected sites remote to the operative field.

There is a direct relation between the total number of people in an operating room and the bacterial air count. Curiously, there is little dissemination of bacteria during surgical incision of pustular lesions [70]. In contrast, wide dispersal of bacteria occurs during dressing changes of contaminated wounds. Short-distance airborne transmission of resident body bacteria on desquamated particles from personnel present in the operating room leads to contamination of the operative site [47]. Such bacterial dissemination dramatically increases after bathing with bland soap [52] and does not occur if washing is done with an antiseptic. Very few personnel who are vaginal, rectal, or skin carriers of pathogenic bacteria actually transmit bacteria to patients during an operation. This type of transmission, occurring only at a close range, is a form of indirect contact and is to be distinguished from the putative ambient airborne contamination described by Lister and from true airborne droplet nuclei resulting in transmission of viral infections (see Chaps. 1, 38). When a member of the surgical team is an efficient bacterial disseminator, capable of being a source of patient infection, bacterial transmission to the operative site may take place in the absence of any demonstrable break in established operative technique. These disseminators may have no clinical findings of overt infection or skin colonization and can cause outbreaks of common types of *S. aureus* or *S. pyogenes* wound infections [10, 55]. It must be emphasized that colonized individuals who are uniquely able to spread infection in this manner are distinctly uncommon, as compared to colonized nondisseminating personnel. The former can be definitely identified only through methodical investigation (see Chap. 37).

Prevention of Surgical Infection

Prolongation of hospitalization prior to operation has been associated with an increase in surgical infection. However, it is likely that this marker reflects patients of a greater intrinsic susceptibility for reasons other than simply the time spent in the hospital. To the extent consistent with good care, however, shortening preoperative hospitalization stay is recommended in the hope it will serve to limit patient colonization with hospital bacteria.

Operating Room Environment
The operating room environment should be clean and safe. Procedures to accomplish this and architectural considerations are presented elsewhere (see Chap. 22). There are no systematic studies of the relative importance of various environmental factors in ensuring a safe operating room environment; however, it is known that contaminated fluids or equipment in the operating room may result in contamination of surfaces and lead to outbreaks of wound infection with *Pseudomonas aeruginosa* or *Serratia marcescens* [32, 72]. The ambient operating room air should be as dust- and lint-free as possible, as particulate foreign matter entering the operative site promotes infection. Although there are specifications for temperature and humidity control in an operating room, it is not known to what extent variations in these influence infection rates (see Chap. 22). The 1964 NAS/NRC study [1] did demonstrate that ultraviolet air irradiation in operating rooms decreased infection occurrence but only in the patients with ultraclean operations. British studies have also revealed that control of bacterial dispersion into ambient air will reduce infections in operations involving joint replacement [47]. Surgical wound contamination was reported to be reduced by 50 percent in these operations by use of turbulent

ventilation, when the surgical staff were wearing ordinary cotton scrub suits. However, the reducing effect of turbulent ventilation was less than 25 percent if the staff wore special clothing that retarded penetration by particulate matter. Infection rates were reduced to the greatest extent when ultraclean air–handling techniques and body exhaust surgical suits were combined.

Appropriate operating room attire is important for individuals during surgery, since body bacteria from the operating room staff are a potential source of wound contamination. Materials used for surgical gowns and for draping the patient to contain patient body bacteria should be impervious to transmission of microorganisms and have characteristics essential for comfort.

Preparation of Personnel and Patients
Patient hair need not be removed unless it will actually interfere with the operative procedure. If necessary, hair removal should be accomplished by clipping just before operation, employing a sterile clipper head. Shaving hair—either the night before or immediately preoperatively—may increase wound infections, in contrast to clipping hair [3].

The goal of preoperative preparation of the patient's skin is to reduce the numbers of normal skin bacteria throughout the operation and thereby decrease the opportunity for wound infection from this source. A preoperative antiseptic bath is not necessary if other prophylactic measures are correctly administered. In the presence of skin abnormalities or uncontrolled remote infection at any site prior to operation, specific preoperative evaluation of the patient is advisable, to seek measures that will effectively preclude contamination of the operative field by bacteria arising from the patient's colonized or infected body surfaces. This would include systemic antimicrobial therapy. Although chlorhexidine compounds appear to be more effective than iodophors in reducing resident body bacteria for preoperative preparation of a patient's skin [46], there is no evidence that any one antiseptic is more effective than others in decreasing postoperative wound infections. A variety of antiseptics are available for this purpose, and any one is acceptable for routine use depending on considerations of patient and staff allergy and cost.

A large number of studies have been reported on various antiseptic agents and techniques for preoperative hand scrubbing for the surgical staff. Whether any agent is more efficacious than 70% ethyl alcohol, for example, is not established [45]. Product acceptability by operating room staff after repeated usage is probably the most important criterion. The goal of the surgical hand scrub is to reduce numbers of resident skin bacteria and eliminate transient ones. Resident skin bacteria will regrow and increase in numbers under the glove during operation. Should a small unnoticed hole develop in a surgical glove, then the likelihood of bacterial contamination of the wound with skin bacteria would increase in relation to the time elapsed since the surgical scrub. This would become a consideration if skin flora such as *Corynebacterium* or coagulase-negative staphylococcal species were responsible for clusters of operative site infections. A 2-minute scrub (by the clock) is adequate if a brush is used to remove debris around the fingernails. Repeated use of chlorhexidine gluconate is recommended by some authorities because of a residual antibacterial effect, although repeated applications of ethyl alcohol may yield a similar effect [45]. Use of certain hand creams by operating room staff may reverse the residual chlorhexidine effect. Studies evaluating various agents for hand antisepsis have not shown a direct relationship to decreased operative site infection, though demonstrating such a relationship would be extraordinarily difficult given the amazing infrequency of operative site infections in clean operations conducted under adverse and grossly unsterile conditions [8]. That gloving actually has preventive efficacy is suggested by anecdotal reports of surgical wound infections resulting from failure to use gloves [71, 73].

Antimicrobial Prophylaxis
Approach to Prophylaxis in Various Operations

Prevention of surgical infection in patients with clean-contaminated, contaminated, and certain clean operations by means of antimicrobial prophylaxis is now an established surgical principle (Table 33-3). After incision, laboratory studies indicate a 4-hour time interval during which antimicrobials are decreasingly effective for infection prophylaxis [16]. The exact duration of the effective time period is a function of both the degree of bacterial contamination and the duration of antibacterial drug efficacy at the wound site. A generally accepted routine is to initiate parenteral prophylaxis within 30 minutes of an operation prior to incision and, in any event, no later than 2 hours afterward, but always prior to closure. For operations lasting more than 4 hours, or in the event of major hemorrhage, when serum levels will change, a second intraoperative antimicrobial dose is to be given. In clean and clean-contaminated operations, there is no evidence that additional doses administered postoperatively provide any benefit in preventing wound or operative site infections [9]; postoperative dosing is potentially harmful in selecting antibiotic-resistant bacteria as patient colonizers. However, in association with implantation of indwelling devices and prostheses, an empiric argument has been made for three postoperative prophylactic antibiotic doses administered over an 18-hour period [42]. In patients with contaminated and dirty operations, prophylaxis is not the sole consideration. The use of antimicrobials during these types of operations is for the purpose of controlling spread of infection at the time of surgery, with the object of curing the infection postoperatively. Judicious selection of antimicrobial treatment in these situations is based on knowledge of the likely infecting bacteria, preoperative culture results, and examination of infected material found at surgery.

In patients with clean-contaminated operations, the prophylactic goal is to diminish the number of mucosal-associated bacteria that may gain access to the operative site. For head and neck operations, *S. aureus* and various aerobic and anaerobic streptococcal species of the airway are the common causes of postoperative infection; clindamycin (with or without gentamicin) is currently recommended

Table 33-3.   Choice of prophylactic antimicrobial drug for prevention of surgical infections[a]

Clean operations

Cardiac: Cefazolin 1–2 gm preoperatively, 1–2 gm after completion of cardiopulmonary bypass, and 1–2 gm 8 hours later; for patients allergic to cephalosporins, vancomycin 15 mg/kg preoperatively and 10 mg/kg after completion of bypass. If renal function is compromised, the second vancomycin dose may be omitted.

Orthopedic operations with implanted devices or prostheses: Standard prophylaxis.[b] It is appropriate to delay the first dose of prophylactic antibiotic up to 2 hours after incision for intraoperative administration but always prior to closure, in order to obtain cultures at the operative site.

Vascular operations involving abdomen or lower extremities or both (including amputation) or with use of vascular prosthesis: Standard prophylaxis.

Other clean operations with placement of an implanted device: Prophylaxis is not routinely recommended in institutions at which surveillance reveals a low occurrence of infection but may be considered when infection frequency is increased. Standard prophylaxis.

Clean-contaminated operations

Major head and neck procedures with incision of oral or pharyngeal mucosa: Clindamycin 600 mg (with or without gentamicin 1.5 mg/kg) 30 minutes preoperatively and every 8 hours IV, for a total of 3 doses.

Gastroduodenal, according to surgical judgment of high-risk patient: Standard prophylaxis.

Percutaneous endoscopic gastrotomy and gastric bypass operation for obesity: Standard prophylaxis.

Biliary tract, according to surgical judgment of high-risk patient: Standard prophylaxis. In addition, it is appropriate to delay the first dose of prophylactic antibiotic up to 2 hours after incision for intraoperative administration but prior to closure, in order to obtain cultures at the operative site.

Colorectal elective (including elective appendectomy): Oral[c] plus standard prophylaxis.

Colorectal, urgent: Cefotaxime 1 or 2 gm IV and metronidazole 1 gm administered over 30–60 minutes immediately preoperatively.

Cesarean section, urgent or high-risk cases: Standard prophylaxis after clamping the cord.

Hysterectomy
  Vaginal: Standard prophylaxis.
  Abdominal, according to surgical judgment of high-risk patient: Standard prophylaxis.

Urologic
  Prostatectomy: If urine culture reveals bacteria, a course of preoperative treatment or a single dose

rather than a cephalosporin [69a]. For gastroduodenal operations, gastric acidity and bowel motility normally serve to inhibit bacterial growth in the stomach and duodenum. In conditions in which these defenses are lessened as a consequence of relative or absolute achlorhydria (as a result of aging, disease, or medical therapy), necrotic tissue, obstruction, or hemorrhage, bacterial colonization may occur in the stomach or duodenum with a variety of enteric species that may be readily inhibited by cefazolin. In persons having biliary tract surgery, antimicrobial prophylaxis is recommended for those at high risk for infection, including patients who are 70 years or older or who have recently experienced acute cholecystitis, obstruction, or common duct stones, conditions in which the usually limited bacterial population of the biliary tree is profoundly altered. Colonization with a variety of enteric bacteria likely to be inhibited by cefazolin is to be anticipated, and this drug is the recommended prophylactic choice. In patients with vaginal hysterectomy, prolonged abdominal hysterectomy, emergency cesarean section associated with premature membrane rupture or labor (see Chap. 31), clean operations in which a foreign body is being inserted (e.g., joint prosthesis [see Chap. 36]), or surgery of arteries of the abdomen or legs (including lower-extremity amputation because of ischemic necrosis [see Chap. 35]),

Table 33-3. (*continued*)

of antimicrobial administered immediately prior to operation is indicated, drugs to be selected on the basis of in vitro efficacy against urinary bacterial isolates. If an indwelling catheter is present prior to prostatectomy and no bacteriuria is detected, an antibiotic with efficacy against common aerobes likely to cause urinary tract infection may be administered in a single dose immediately prior to operation.

Genitourinary instrumentation: Prior treatment or prophylaxis immediately before procedure as above, directed against bacteria identified in urine culture.

Repeat clean procedure to be done at a recent operative site, and likely to be colonized with *S. aureus*, may be viewed as clean-contaminated operation: Standard prophylaxis.

Contaminated operations

Open extremity fractures within 6 hours of fracture: Cefazolin 1 or 2 gm IV immediately preoperatively and every 8 hours for a total of 3 doses.

Penetrating abdominal wound with prompt transfer of patient to hospital: Cefotaxime 2 gm IV immediately preoperatively followed by 2 gm IV every 8 hours for at least 2 days, along with metronidazole 1 gm preoperatively and 500 gm every 8 hours for 2 days; gentamicin 1.5 mg/kg every 8 hours IV may be added. Alternative program: Clindamycin 600–900 mg every 8 hours IV plus gentamicin 1.5 mg/kg IV every 8 hours.

[a]Other prophylactic regimens may be recommended in chapters concerned with the same sites of infection. The reader is advised to consult these for additional perspectives.

[b] *Standard prophylaxis:* Cefazolin 1 or 2 gm IV preoperatively within 30 minutes of incision and again every 4 hours of operating time or in association with massive hemorrhage. For persons allergic to cephalosporins, vancomycin or clindamycin may be substituted.

[c]*Oral prophylaxis:* Gastrointestinal lavage followed by erythromycin and neomycin 1 gm of each at 1 PM, 2 PM, and 11 PM on the day preceding surgery.

Notes. 1. Surgical antimicrobial prophylaxis is not designed to prevent bacterial endocarditis. For this, see standard recommendations [51].

2. Concurrent remote site infections or heavily colonized sites capable of contaminating the operative site should be effectively treated in patients scheduled for clean operations at the time of elective operation.

3. Repeated dosage of antimicrobials in contaminated operations may require changes in relation to body weight or renal function.

4. When a choice of cefazolin or cefotaxime dosage is indicated, the 2-gm dose is preferred for the initial treatment.

5. If colonization with methicillin-resistant *S. aureus* is likely [49], vancomycin is indicated for prophylaxis.

similar conditions of colonization may be anticipated, and prophylaxis with cefazolin or other agents is indicated.

In patients with large-bowel and rectal operations, effective antimicrobial prophylaxis is directed against anaerobic as well as aerobic species. Drug efficacy against species of the *Bacteroides fragilis* group is necessary for maximum success of prophylactic efforts. In experimental studies, oral erythromycin and neomycin together have been demonstrated to reduce the aerobic and anaerobic colonic mucosal-associated bacterial flora by 5 to 6 $\log_{10}$ and 6 to 7 $\log_{10}$ per milligram of mucosal tissue, respectively, to a level of bacteria that is considerably below that at which

wound contamination leads to infection [38]. Oral antimicrobial prophylaxis administered the day before elective operation of bowel and rectum, by itself, does not appear to be the most effective method. In three double-blind placebo-controlled studies, oral neomycin-erythromycin alone was compared with oral neomycin-erythromycin plus a first-generation cephalosporin administered parenterally immediately before operation [29]. In each study, wound infections were less frequent with addition of the cephalosporin, and in two studies the differences were statistically significant. Pooling the results of these studies in metaanalysis [29] has yielded a 7 percent rate of wound infection for the oral antimicrobials alone, in contrast to a 4 percent rate when the parenteral cephalosporin was added. Thus, in addition to oral prophylaxis the day before operation, a single dose of parenteral cefazolin administered at the time of incision is the most effective as well as the least costly antimicrobial prophylaxis program currently available. Obviously patients with partial or complete bowel obstruction or colostomies are likely to fail to benefit from use of oral agents for antimicrobial prophylaxis. Prophylactic programs in relation to urologic instrumentation and cardiac operations are discussed in Chapters 28 and 35.

In patients with contaminated conditions such as recent abdominal trauma, antimicrobials administered for a short period (48 hours or less) have demonstrated prophylactic efficacy [36]. Drugs that are effective against common enteric colonizing aerobic and anaerobic bacteria should be selected. In management of a recent open fracture, a 1-day course of a cephalosporin antibiotic appears effective [26].

Recommended Choices for Antimicrobial Prophylaxis

We believe cefazolin to be the agent of choice for prophylaxis in many operations in order to prevent *S. aureus* incisional infections. A single preoperative dose of 1 gm, or preferably 2 gm, administered in a timely fashion and repeated every 4 hours of operating time or following major hemorrhage, is a generally accepted routine. In the event that surveillance indicates that *S. aureus* infections are occurring despite the use of 2 gm cefazolin prophylaxis, use of an alternate drug less susceptible to β-lactamase hydrolysis is warranted [43]. Selection of cefazolin as a prophylactic antimicrobial agent for most operations in which antimicrobial prophylaxis is indicated derives from a considerable experience of efficacy. The success of cefazolin issues from its good tissue penetration and relatively long half-life during which growth of bacteria commonly causing surgical infection is inhibited. At this writing, there are at least 10 cephalosporins with approved indications

for surgical prophylaxis. Whether any has important advantages over cefazolin remains to be proved.

Cefoxitin is a widely used alternate to the regimen of oral neomycin-erythromycin plus cefazolin in abdominal and rectal operations and is frequently selected when a patient cannot be treated orally or when the patient cannot be prepared the day before. The short half-life of cefoxitin and the resultant need for multiple doses, along with a narrow attainable margin of bacterial inhibition in serum, are important limitations of this antibiotic. The manufacturer's recommended dose of cefoxitin for surgical prophylaxis in adults is 2 gm [59a], not 1 gm as is sometimes suggested. An alternate program of prophylaxis in this setting is a single dose of both cefotaxime and metronidazole.

For patients who are seriously allergic to penicillins or cephalosporins, or when there is a clear indication for prophylaxis against methicillin-resistant staphylococci, vancomycin is an alternate choice. For those allergic to erythromycin, oral metronidazole may be substituted for prophylaxis against anaerobic gram-negative colonizing species. For those allergic to oral neomycin, oral ciprofloxacin is likely to be equally effective in diminishing aerobic gram-negative colonizing species in the bowel.

In postoperative patients, the loss of oropharyngeal fibronectin, a substance that binds gram-positive bacteria to mucosa, allows for broad changes in the character of colonizing bacteria of the oropharynx (see Chaps. 13, 29). Loss of acidic pH in gastric contents as a result of histamine-blocking medication, gastric disease, or atony allows colonization with large numbers of aerobic gram-negative bacilli. Retrograde spread of gastric bacteria to the oropharynx and their subsequent aspiration sets the stage for lower respiratory infection with gram-negative bacteria; use of nasogastric tubes to manage gastric or bowel atony promotes repeated aspirations. Thus surgical techniques or procedures resulting in prolonged gastric atony or bowel ileus exacerbate the risk of postoperative pneumonia [21].

Selective Digestive Decontamination

Prevention of a variety of postoperative nosocomial infections other than those of the wound will have increasing importance as wound infections continue to decline to an irreducible minimum rate. A number of preventive techniques will bear scrutiny, including considerations of expanded use of antimicrobials for prophylaxis in clean cases [60] and use of the more controversial selective digestive decontamination (SDD) method [69]. SDD implies both gastrointestinal and oropharyngeal decontamination, in contrast to the other more limited measures. There may also be a role for decontamination of the oropharynx alone to prevent colonization with gram-negative bacteria and their consequent aspiration and the maintenance of gastric acidity to alter the bacterial reservoir in the achlorhydric stomach. The uses of SDD and oropharyngeal decontamination in critical care units are discussed elsewhere (see Chap. 42).

The use of SDD in surgical patients will likely be limited to the trauma patient; this is the setting in which it is often impossible to administer other prophylactic antiinfection measures prior to operation, and contamination from the traumatic event, including the unknown invasive microbial consequences of shock and the effects of regional hypoperfusion in abdominal viscera, may be countered by SDD. For routine use in prevention of nosocomial surgical wound infections, however, SDD cannot currently be recommended [20]. In one report, despite effectively curtailing a critical care outbreak of intestinal colonization and infection with multiresistant Enterobacteriaceae species, SDD had no significant effect on the occurrence of endemic nosocomial infections [13].

Other Considerations

Prevention of endocarditis following surgery is a separate issue. Standard prophylactic recommendations should be followed [63]. Prevention of infection in association with organ transplantation is a highly specialized subject and is covered in Chapter 41.

On some routine occasions, surgeons may choose antimicrobial agents for prophylaxis in the absence of data from clinical trials to support their choice. In the event of a poor outcome, there is a potential for adverse medicolegal implications of such decisions (see Chap. 26).

Systemic Surveillance of Postoperative Infection

The basic elements of a successful infection surveillance program include (1) a definition of specific types of postoperative infections, (2) a method for screening patients at risk, and (3) a reliable means of recording and retrieving information (see Chap. 5). The observer who records the presence or absence of infection (infection control practitioner or hospital epidemiologist) should have no conflict of interest in performing these duties. The surgical staff should be aware of methodology for screening and recording infection and should accept the criteria to define infections. It is useful for the observer to make rounds with several surgeons to ensure agreement on the use of definitions. The general criteria put forth by the Centers for Disease Control [35] are widely accepted; modifications may be made to individualize usage in different hospitals (Table 33-4). A common definition error is to equate infection with recovery of a certain bacterial species from the wound site. Bacteriologic findings do not distinguish between colonization and infection.

Surveillance objectives should be defined. All surgical infections are not necessarily equally important to identify. Highest priority is given to detecting infections in patients that lead to death, reoperation, increased acuity of services, and special diagnostic or therapeutic management (including parenteral administration of antimicrobials, prolongation of hospital stay, or hospital readmission). Lower priority is assigned to finding patients with superficial infections that do not lead to the outcomes just cited and that are readily managed on an ambulatory basis, without a major increase in therapeutic costs or delay in pa-

Table 33-4.   Criteria for surgical wound infection

1. *Superficial:* All criteria to be present. Manifestations within 30 days of operation, no prosthesis implanted.
   a. Minimal purulent drainage from incision site or drain located above fascial layer.
   b. Minimal cellulitis.
   c. No systemic findings of infection.
   d. No sinus tract.
   e. Management of infection can be done at bedside or in office.
   f. Infection does not prolong hospitalization, increase acuity of services, delay return to usual activities, result in readmission to hospital or death.
2. *Incisional:* Any one criterion to be present. Manifestations occurring within 30 days of operation, no prosthesis implanted.
   a. Moderate or extensive purulent drainage from incision or drain located above fascial layer.
   b. Moderate or extensive cellulitis.
   c. Partial wound dehiscence as a result of infection (or necessary opening of wound by surgeon to manage infection) without disruption of fascial approximation.
   d. Systemic findings of infection.
   e. Reoperation for control of infection.
   f. Hospital readmission for management of infection.
   g. Infection management prolongs hospitalization or increases acuity of care.
   h. Surgeon or consulting physician diagnosis.
3. *Operative site infection:* Any one criterion to be present. Manifestations occur within 30 days of operation or within 1 year if prosthesis implanted.
   a. Purulent drainage from beneath fascial layer.
   b. Extension of incisional infection beyond operative site (mediastinitis, peritonitis, osteomyelitis, cellulitis, abscess, necrotizing fasciitis, etc.) or new infection arising within the operative area ("leaking" anastomosis, cholangitis, fistula, empyema, etc.).
   c. Complete wound dehiscence including fascia as a result of infection (or necessary complete opening of wound to manage infection).
   d. Sinus tract extending beneath fascia.
   e. Surgeon or consulting physician diagnosis.
   f. Infection resulting in death.

Source: Modified from J.S. Garner et al. CDC definitions for nosocomial infection, 1988. *Am. J. Infect. Control.* 16:128, 1988.

tient return to regular activities. In the latter group are most patients whose infections arise only after hospital discharge.

There may be substantive differences in the impact of postoperative infections on patients undergoing various elective operations that are commonly performed. Infections, especially deep ones, complicating operations involving cardiac, vascular, and neurologic structures, bones, joints, stomach, bowel, or rectum are more likely to compromise patient well-being than are similar infections complicating hernia repair, uterus, gallbladder, or thyroid operations.

Postoperative infections occurring beyond the operative site may bring about considerable patient morbidity and should be included in routine systematic surveillance. This is particularly true for pneumonia. In special-care surgical units, particularly those devoted to trauma patients, surveillance of various infections caused by multiply drug-resistant bacteria may be especially useful to provide information to surgeons about possible inappropriate antibiotic usage and may serve as an indicator of personnel or environmental transmission of bacteria.

Hospitalwide outbreaks of infections due to methicillin-resistant *S. aureus* and clusters of diarrhea or colitis due to *Clostridium difficile* toxin may be manifest first among postoperative patients. Surveillance activities should be geared to identify them.

As a minimal surveillance program, occurrences of incisional wound and operative site infections and postoperative episodes of bacteremia, pneumonia, and symptomatic urinary tract infection should be identified for elective clean and clean-contaminated operations. Reports that originate from physicians' offices, are initiated spontaneously, or appear in response to requests can provide information about patients with onset of infection occurring after hospital discharge. These findings should be summarized, tabulated, and regularly presented to both the hospital Infection Control Committee and to the department of surgery, with an evaluation of trends. Once objectives are established and prior to initiating actual surveillance, it is advisable to prepare mock tables to demonstrate how data will be portrayed. This will also provide an opportunity to explore any theoretic concerns of the surgical staff. As the surveillance findings from patients undergoing specific types or groups of operations become large enough for meaningful interpretation, infection rates for various procedures may be established as a baseline. After a database has been collected, cluster definitions and threshold levels for outbreak investigation may be defined. It may not be possible, because of methodologic and interobserver differences as well as differences in patient populations, to compare directly infection rates complicating specific operations done at different hospitals. Infection rates reported from university or municipal hospitals are generally higher than those reported from nonteaching community hospitals.

The relative sensitivities of various methods for finding nosocomial infection have been reported [34] (see Chap. 5). A comprehensive method for surveillance of postoperative infections is a systematic program of active evaluation of postoperative patients during hospitalization along with passive reporting from surgeons' offices of infections arising after hospital discharge. This may be coupled with an independent review of medical records of infected patients and a sample of uninfected ones, to provide a measure of observer sensitivity and specificity. At the Florida Consortium for Infection Control (FCIC), an organization of nonteaching community hospitals, a combined program of concurrent active and passive observations along with retrospective chart review by independent medical records personnel has been found to be highly efficient for detecting postoperative infections. The expected infection control practitioner–observer sensitivity for detecting such infections is greater than 0.90.

A surveillance worksheet is useful to record important details about an infected patient, indicating the criteria used for definition. Only the minimum information necessary for further tabulation to identify clusters or outbreaks should be included. Patient demographic characteristics and details of operations are generally readily available in the medical record and need not be routinely recorded. However, in some hospitals it is not possible to determine the operating room in which surgery was done or the critical care bed that was utilized for postoperative care. On infrequent occasions, this information may be important to record, in order to determine assignments of patient care personnel or in relation to architectural considerations. Computer analysis of surveillance data is helpful only to the extent that the data output is consonant with the previously determined objectives (see Chap. 8).

Operation-specific surveillance has proved to be useful as an activity in which eventuation of infection may be evaluated in relation to the sequence of surgical care: preoperative (therapeutic and host factors), intraoperative, and postoperative. By identifying a specific operation as the point of selection, rather than an operator, a wide range of possible contributions to individual infection risks is likely to be fully explored. Ideally, all operations should be concurrently surveyed for postoperative infections at operative and nonoperative sites. As an ongoing activity, risk factors and other events associated with individual types of operations should be recorded (Fig. 33-1), and pertinent observations of possible infection sources should be routinely noted. Over time, the cumulative infection record for groups of similar operations will serve to establish a baseline of expected distribution of specific risk factors in relation to occurrence of various postoperative infections. These may be inspected to seek commonalities or clusters of events associated with,

Fig. 33-1.   Line list for collecting data about patients with postoperative infections.

Name of operation group ____   ICD-9-Codes ____   Class of operation: (ultra-clean, clean, clean-contaminated, contaminated, dirty)

Host Factors							*Intraoperative Factors*		
Patient name	Age	Sex	Admit date	ASA* class	Specific risk factors (e.g., remote infection, obesity, vascular insufficiency)	Perioperative antimicrobial therapy	Medical conditions coexisting (e.g., diabetes)	Attending surgeon	Date of operation	Duration of operation

but not necessarily causative of, specific infections, or may be further evaluated as outlined in the next section.

Analyses of Crude Data: Investigations of Outbreaks and Clusters

It is especially important to recognize the potentially pejorative implications of incorrectly interpreting crude data sets of postoperative infections. Dissemination of crude data to an uncritical audience has the power to cause damage to a surgeon or an institution. The limitations of crude findings of postoperative infections should be identified for those who review them. Access to crude data sets should be restricted to those who have an actual need to know about interval findings of work in progress. There should also be constant concern about disseminating interpretations of a single set of data indicating highly unusual findings, because of possible sampling bias or other biases and for type I error due to inadequate sample size. Failure to identify potential limitations in interpreting crude data and possible sampling errors in small clusters may result in a loss of credibility of the surveillance program, may

create a climate of suspicion and animosity among the surgical staff, and may jeopardize the success of any future efforts. Thus, sound epidemiologic methods and strict confidentiality of records are central to an effective program.

Clusters of infections may be sought by grouping infected patients according to characteristics such as time, place, person, infecting organisms, surgeons, types of operations, preoperative host and surgical risk factors, use of various devices, characteristics of critical care, preoperative duration of hospitalization, and postoperative intervals to onset of infection. In stratification, the analyst seeks to identify possible commonality in sources of infection. For example, a lengthened preoperative time period of hospitalization may be an indicator of patients with unusual or complex manifestations of disease. Relatively long periods from operation to onset of infection may suggest that a postoperative event has played a role in infection. In the latter instance, time periods especially in excess of 10 to 12 days raise the possibility of postoperative factors (including hematoma, seroma, remote site infection, prolonged or

Repeat procedure[‡] Yes _____ No _____ Elective _____ Non-Elective _____

	Postoperative Factors				Infection				Comments
Special factors (e.g., massive bleeding, implant, electrocautery, technical problems)	Drain (type, site, duration), hematoma, seroma	Duration of pharyngeal intubation	Vascular catheter (site, duration)	Duration of critical care	Onset date[†]	Site	Organism	Criteria	

Note: List only factors present *prior* to onset of infection.
[‡] Note: It is advisable to consider initial and repeat operations as separate groups, elective and non-elective operations as separate groups, and infections in operative and non-operative sites as separate groups.
*ASA = American Society of Anesthesiologists [23a]; other preoperative assessment of patient health may be employed.
[†] Onset of infection is the date of first clinical manifestation, not the first date of culture.

unnecessary use of surgical drains, or postoperative manipulation of the wound) aiding in the initiation of infection. An open conduit at the surgical site (e.g., Penrose drain) may also be a factor in permitting infection after operation. Recent studies have revealed additional mechanisms of postoperative onset of operative site infection [32a, 49a].

An important first step in stratification is segregating low- and high-risk patients into separate groups, to determine comparative rates of infection. For patients with a variety of clean and clean-contaminated elective operations commonly done in community hospitals, the FCIC low-risk definition may be useful and includes patients whose operations do not last longer than 4 hours and who do not have diabetes mellitus or remote site infections [30]. For patients with operations done in municipal or university hospitals, the SENIC low-risk criteria may be more appropriate. These include persons with fewer than three discharge diagnoses and operations lasting less than 2 hours. For the elective clean and clean-contaminated operations in FCIC community hospitals, low-risk patients had an overall wound infection rate of 1.5 percent, whereas the rate for high-risk patients was 3.7 percent [30]. For the lowest-risk clean and clean-contaminated patients in the SENIC study, the infection rate was in the 1.0 percent range [39]. Rates increased in a stepwise fashion as additional risk factors were added (see Table 33-2). In the absence of other risk factors, rates of infections in clean and clean-contaminated operations may be grouped together for initial (crude) comparisons of infection rates of operations at different hospitals; they have a similar infection risk [23a]. These studies, and those of others [1, 23, 57] (see Table 33-1) yield several important points in common: (1) The current expected rate of infection for low-risk patients with elective clean operations is approximately 1.5 percent; (2) the expected rate of infection in low-risk patients with elective clean-contaminated operations may be slightly higher but is less than 3 percent; and (3) these rates increase directly with additional patient or operative risk factors. In some pseudoepidemics, an apparent increase in postoperative infection occurrence is due to a change in patient risk characteristics with the introduction of a population having an increased susceptibility to infection.

In small clusters of surgical infections, chance alone may bring about a concatenation of unrelated events, giving the false appearance of a group of infections linked by common causation. Alternatively, a small cluster of serious postoperative infections in high-risk patients may be an indicator of a much larger outbreak with a wide array of disease manifestations. A systematic search for unreported infections, including those arising after hospital discharge, is usually necessary to determine the actual size of such clusters. Once all infections are identified, analysis according to various risk factors is useful to aid in formulating an hypothesis of causation.

Three scenarios, modified from actual occurrences, are presented to illustrate methods by which a hospital epidemiologist may explore apparent excesses of infection occurrence.

Hospital Remodeling and Concurrent Rise in Infection Rates

The obstetric operating rooms of a large community hospital are remodeled to deal with an expanding local patient population and an increasing number of staff obstetricians. Over a 3-year period after remodeling, the hospital epidemiologist finds rates of both endometritis and wound infection complicating cesarean sections to have risen progressively, although the annual number of cesarean sections performed has remained constant at approximately 400. Definitions of infection have remained unchanged. The crude findings of combined rates of both infections are 4.5 percent in year 1 after remodeling, 9.8 percent in year 2, and 13.3 percent in year 3. Patients of a number of different obstetricians

have experienced infection, and infections have been due to a variety of bacterial species. Some administrators express concern about possible environmental sources of patient contamination in the remodeled operating rooms.

The hospital epidemiologist stratifies the patient population according to whether operations were elective or urgent and whether women were having initial or repeat cesarean sections. He finds that the rate of combined infections for patients having elective repeat cesarean sections is constant at 1.0 percent for all 3 years and that the rate of infections for urgent primary cesarean sections also has been constant at 15 percent for all 3 years. The apparent increase in rate of infections has been due to a relative change in indications for cesarean section by the new staff obstetricians, with many fewer elective repeat cesarean sections and many more urgent primary ones being progressively done in the second and third years, as compared with the first year. The well-known greater frequency of postoperative infections in women with urgent primary cesarean section is assumed to account for the apparent increase in infections after cesarean section. No environmental investigation is undertaken. Efforts are made to identify additional risk factors among the infected women with urgent primary cesarean sections and to ensure appropriate use of antimicrobial prophylaxis to reduce their higher infection rates.

Increased Incisional Wound Infection Rate Associated with Specific Personnel

Multiple Bacterial Species Cluster A hospital epidemiologist finds that the incisional wound infection rate for patients having laminectomy operations is 3.5 percent for patients of an older surgeon, in contrast to 0.5 percent for patients of 3 younger surgeons. The older surgeon indicates that her practice includes patients who have had one or more previous laminectomy operations. The hospital epidemiologist stratifies the occurrences of infection in patients of the older surgeon according to the number of prior operations.

In patients with no prior laminectomy operation, the infection rate is also 0.5 percent, but the rate is much higher, 4 to 6 percent, in patients who have had multiple prior operations. The infections are due to a variety of bacterial species. It is postulated that the increased rate of infection is attributable to host risk factors in the patients with multiple prior operations. A number of patients with repeat laminectomy operations are examined, and persisting hematoma formation at the reincision (scar) site is found to be a frequent postoperative occurrence. This is considered to be the responsible factor that sets the stage for postoperative infection with different bacterial species. Efforts are made to reduce the occurrence of hematoma as a postoperative complication.

Single Bacterial Species Cluster Shortly after a young surgeon joins the medical staff of a community hospital, the rate of postoperative infection complicating elective herniorrhaphy operations increases markedly. Among this surgeon's first 20 elective herniorrhaphy operations, there are 5 episodes of *S. aureus* wound infections (25 percent). The rate of wound infection complicating herniorrhaphies done by other surgeons is 0.3 percent for the same time period. The hospital epidemiologist reviews the medical records of the young surgeon's patients to seek predisposing risk factors; none of his patients can be characterized as being at increased risk. The hospital epidemiologist then consults the chief of the department of surgery to request an impartial evaluation of the surgeon's operative technique. If the surgeon's technique is found to be satisfactory, a prospective bacteriologic study of newly infected patients and surgical personnel (including molecular methods of epidemiologic analysis) will be carried out to seek *S. aureus* carriers among all persons present at operations (See Chap. 37). If surgical technique is not satisfactory, this will be addressed by the chief of surgery along with selected peers in the department as a confidential issue, and the bacteriologic investigation will be deferred.

Case-Control Studies of Postoperative Infections

If analysis reveals that an excess infection rate has occurred in surgical patients, it may be instructive to do a case-control study to identify associated factors (Fig. 33-1) and to measure the relative strength of association for each factor by case, by calculating an odds ratio (See Chap. 7). A useful initial step in comparing cases and controls for analysis of possible events contributing to operative site infection is a line listing of specific risk factors (Fig. 33-1). Strong associations indicate a potential, but do not necessarily establish, etiologic relationships. Preoperative patient risk factors, intraoperative factors, environmental factors, surgical personnel, therapeutic events after operation, and postoperative critical care activities should all be considered for evaluation. Case-control analysis is especially useful when new equipment, a new procedure, or a new process has been introduced that may be a source of infection.

Following the outline of the 1964 NRC/NAS study [1], Cruse and Foord [23] devised a program of concurrent observation of surgical wounds in patients with clean operations to provide individual surgeons with infection rates. This study and others [57] have appeared to demonstrate that providing surgeon-specific infection rates results in a decreased occurrence of wound infection. These findings are consonant with the results of a large SENIC study [40], in which reduction of surgical infection occurrences was found to be associated with a strong infection control program that included an effective hospital epidemiologist and a system for reporting surgical wound infection rates to the surgical staff, but not necessarily on a surgeon-specific basis (see Chap. 4). The extent to which reporting surgeon-specific infection data is actually effective cannot be determined since all of the reported studies lacked concurrent controls. A temporal decline in surgical wound infections took place during the period of these investigations [17] that continues to the present (see Table 33-1). Nonetheless, the broad support of the surgical community and regulating agencies for this type of surveillance and its self-evident attractiveness have resulted in its adoption at a number of hospitals.

The goal of surgeon-specific surveillance is to reduce the occurrence of wound infection by making individual surgeons aware of excesses in infection rates and thereby promote adherence to accepted principles of operative care. Implicit in this approach is the assumption that, without additional inquiry, surgical infections may be entirely attributed to flaws in surgical techniques or judgment (including incorrect use of antibiotic prophylaxis), with no consideration of possible technical errors of others also present at operation (e.g., anesthesiologists [62]). Also implicit is the assumption that the reduction in surgical wound infection rates following the provision of information of excess rates to an individual surgeon results from improvement in faulty surgical technique or judgment.

To what extent is surgeon-specific surveillance likely to be useful? If the increase in infection is due to a surgeon's failure to use antimicrobial prophylaxis correctly, this practice may be identified and improved. If the increase is due to technical events that are readily apparent, including postoperative hematoma and seroma, prolonged or inappropriate usage of drains, or postoperative wound manipulations, these may be addressed. If the increase is due to shedding of an identifiable strain of bacteria by a specific surgeon or member of the surgical team, that too can be evaluated and altered. If the increase is due solely to a surgeon's selection of especially high-risk patients for operation, this may, in part, be both reassuring and laudable. However, some aberrations in surgical technique may be difficult for a surgeon to identify, let alone change, outside of a supervised surgical training program. These are thorny problems in community hospitals, especially in institutions in which only one surgeon performs a given type of operation. There are no current schemata for intraoperative observations of surgical technique as a surveillance activity, and the various aspects of surgical technique and other intraoperative activities are generally unknown to postoperative surveyors. Infection control surveyors are not able to identify poor surgical technique in patients who later experience infection. Assessment of surgical craft skills is often subjective. This is of particular concern in surveillance activities conducted in smaller community hospitals, in which access to objective assessments and systematic epidemiologic analyses are not immediately available. When it is deemed appropriate to assess a surgeon's technical skills, if possible it should be done by at least 2 surgical peers who evaluate technique according to a set of predetermined criteria.

Concerns about the dangers of inappropriate use of surgeon-specific surveillance have been voiced by some hospital epidemiologists [14, 67]. It has been suggested that surgeon-specific rates of infections should be calculated only for specific operations (or perhaps certain groups of similar operations) and in patients stratified by host risk factors according to a standard classification (e.g., that used by the American Society of Anesthesiologists). It is clearly inappropriate to determine the infection rate of a surgeon by combining rates of infections among widely disparate classes of operations or among patients with widely disparate risk factors [23a], including operations with different degrees of urgency. Further, it is inappropriate to attribute to one surgeon operative site infections that have a postoperative causation and are entirely due to events beyond the surgeon's control. It is also inappropriate to deny care to patients with increased risk for infection for fear that resulting infections will adversely affect a surgeon's or a hospital's infection rate. It is, however, appropriate to inform high-risk patients or their families of the expectation of increased occurrence of postoperative infection based on existing surveillance data.

New Directions in Surveillance
Operative Site Infection
As wound infection frequencies progressively decrease, new thinking is required to define the next step in improving patient care in relation to controlling postoperative infections.

Traditionally, incisional wound infection is defined as occurring between the skin and the fascia. In reality, the surgical wound extends from the skin incision to the limits of the operative field. In contrast to infection manifest at the incisional site, infection occurring initially at the operative site is likely to claim future priority for control efforts. An example is the patient with colon resection who has incisional wound healing *per primum* but develops an anastomotic leak and intra-abdominal abscess. With increasing numbers of complex operations involving implantation of foreign materials (vascular grafts, cardiac valves, orthopedic implants), there will be increasing concern for infection occurring throughout the entire operative field. Surveillance of these and other complex operations (e.g., pancreaticoduodenectomy and abdominoperineal resection) to seek deep infections will become a more important activity. Since acquisition of deep infections may occur as a result of hematogenous spread as well as by perioperative contamination, the methods of postoperatively managing these patients to prevent infection will bear scrutiny.

Viral Infections

Recent studies of patients receiving transplants have demonstrated viral infection as a surgical complication. The principal agents are transferred by human tissue—organs and blood. Cytomegalovirus, hepatitis B, hepatitis C, and coxsackieviruses are the viruses most frequently identified (see Chap. 38). Human immunodeficiency is most feared (see Chap. 39). Routine methods for surveillance of viral postoperative infections need to be developed.

Fungal Infections

Candida species are increasingly prominent causes of operative site infection. This is particularly true in surgical management of transplant patients, burned patients, and patients with prosthetic devices (see Chaps. 34–36, 41, 42). Intravenous catheters and urine cultures may yield fungi on culture prior to systemic involvement [65], and it is likely that patients are infected from such

sources by hematogenous spread. Improved methods to identify and control such infections will become more important as technical advances in surgery lead to management of more immunocompromised subjects.

The Costs of Surgical Infections

Postoperative infections in the surgical patient may prolong the length of hospitalization for substantial periods, depending on the type of operation, and thereby greatly increase the cost of patient care [37, 59]. Cardiothoracic, orthopedic, and gastrointestinal operations are likely to be especially costly in this regard, as a result of both pulmonary and operative site infections [59, 74]. In addition to increasing the direct costs of patient care, indirect costs are a consideration in calculating the consequences of postoperative infection. These include the time lost by the patient from gainful employment and the possible medicolegal actions that may be taken against a hospital or the surgical staff (see Chaps. 25, 26).

References

1. Ad Hoc Committee on Trauma, Division of Medical Sciences, National Academy of Sciences–National Research Council. Postoperative wound infections: The influence of ultraviolet irradiation of the operating room and of various other factors. *Ann. Surg.* 160:1, 1964.
2. Alexander, J.W., and Altemeier, W.A. Penicillin prophylaxis of experimental staphylococcal wound infections. *Surg. Gynecol. Obstet.* 120:243, 1965.
3. Alexander, J.W., et al. The influence of hair-removal methods on wound infections. *Arch. Surg.* 118:347, 1983.
4. Alexander, J.W., Korelitz, J., and Alexander, N.S. Prevention of wound infections—a case for closed suction drainage to remove wound fluids deficient in opsonic proteins. *Am. J. Surg.* 132:59, 1976.
5. Altemeier, W.A. The bacterial flora of acute perforated appendicitis with peritonitis. *Ann. Surg.* 107:517, 1938.
6. Altemeier, W.A., Burke, J.F., Pruitt, B.A., and Sandusky, W.R. (Eds.). Definitions and Classi-

fications of Surgical Infections. In: *Manual on Control of Infection in Surgical Patients* (2nd ed.). Philadelphia: Lippincott, 1984. Pp. 19–30.

7. Altemeier, W.A., and Furste, W.L. Gas gangrene. *Surg. Gynecol. Obstet.* 84:507, 1947.

8. Altemeier, W.A., and Todd, J. Studies on the incidence of infection following open chest cardiac massage for cardiac arrest. *Ann. Surg.* 158:596, 1963.

9. Antimicrobial prophylaxis in surgery. *Med. Lett. Drugs Ther.* 31:105, 1989.

10. Berkelman, R.L., et al. Streptococcal wound infections caused by a vaginal carrier. *J.A.M.A.* 247:2680, 1982.

11. Bernard, H.R., and Cole, W.R. The prophylaxis of surgical infection: The effect of prophylactic antimicrobial drug on the incidence of infection following potentially contaminated operations. *Surgery* 56:151, 1964.

12. Block, S.S. Historical Review of Chemical Disinfectants. In: *Proceedings of the Symposium on Chemical Germicides in the Health Care Field.* Washington, DC: American Society for Microbiology, 1987. Pp. 8–16.

13. Brun-Buisson, C., et al. Intestinal decontamination for control of nosocomial multiresistant gram-negative bacilli: Study of an outbreak in an intensive care unit. *Ann. Intern. Med.* 110:873, 1989.

14. Bryan, C.S. Surgeon-specific wound surveillance: The family or the bean counters? *Infect. Control Hosp. Epidemiol.* 10:376, 1989.

15. Burke, J.F. Identification of the sources of staphylococci contaminating the surgical wound during operation. *Ann. Surg.* 158:898, 1963.

16. Burke, J.F. The effective period of preventive antibiotic action in experimental incisions and dermal lesions. *Surgery* 50:161, 1961.

17. Centers for Disease Control. *National Nosocomial Infections Study Report, Annual Summary 1978* (issued 1981). HEW Publication (CDC) No. 81-8257. Atlanta, Ga: U.S. Public Health Service, 1981.

18. Churchill, E.D. The surgical management of the wounded in the Mediterranean theater at the time of the fall of Rome. *Ann. Surg.* 120:268, 1944.

19. Cohn, L.H. Local infections after splenectomy. *Arch. Surg.* 90:320, 1965.

19a. Colbeck, J.C. An extensive outbreak of staphylococcal infections in maternity units. *Can. Med. Assoc. J.* 61:557, 1949.

20. Condon, R.E. Selective bowel decontamination. *Arch. Surg.* 125:1537, 1990.

21. Craven, D.E., and Steger, K.A. Nosocomial pneumonia in the intubated patient; new concepts of pathogenesis and prevention. *Infect. Dis. Clin.* 3:843, 1989.

22. Cruse, P.J.E. Wound Infections: Epidemiology and Clinical Characteristics in Surgical Infectious Disease. In: R.J. Howard and R.L. Simmons (Eds.), *Surgical Infectious Disease* (2nd ed.). Norwalk, CT: Appleton and Lange, 1988. Pp. 324–325.

23. Cruse, P.J.E., and Foord, R. The epidemiology of wound infection: A 10-year prospective study of 62,939 wounds. *Surg. Clin. North Am.* 60:27, 1980.

23a. Culver, D.H., et al. Surgical wound infection rates by wound class, operative procedure, and patient risk index. *Am. J. Med.* 91(3B):1525, 1991.

24. Davidson, A.I.G., Clark, C., and Smith, G. Postoperative wound infection: A computer analysis. *Br. J. Surg.* 58:333, 1970.

25. Deitch, E.A. The role of intestinal barrier failure and bacterial translocation in the development of systemic infection and multiple organ failure. *Arch. Surg.* 125:403, 1990.

26. Dellinger, E.P., et al. Duration of preventive antibiotic administration for open extremity fractures. *Arch. Surg.* 123:333, 1988.

27. Edlich, R.F., et al. Physical and chemical configuration of sutures in the development of surgical infection. *Ann. Surg.* 177:679, 1973.

28. Edwards, L.D. The epidemiology of 2056 remote site infections and 1966 surgical wound infections occurring in 1865 patients: A four year study of 40,923 operations at Rush-Presbyterian-St. Luke's Hospital, Chicago. *Ann. Surg.* 184:758, 1976.

29. Ehrenkranz, N.J. Containing costs of antimicrobials in the hospital: A critical evaluation. *Am. J. Infect. Control* 17:300, 1989.

30. Ehrenkranz, N.J. Surgical wound infection occurrence in clean operations. Risk stratification for interhospital comparisons. *Am. J. Med.* 70:909, 1981.

31. Ehrenkranz, N.J., et al. Infections complicating low-risk cesarean sections in community hospitals: Efficacy of antimicrobial prophylaxis. *Am. J. Obstet. Gynecol.* 162:337, 1990.

32. Ehrenkranz, N.J., et al. Antibiotic-sensitive *Serratia marcescens* infections complicating cardiopulmonary operations: Contaminated disinfectant as a reservoir. *Lancet* 2:1289, 1980.

32a. Ehrenkranz, N.J., and Pfaff, S.J. Mediastinitis complicating cardiac operations: evidence of postoperative causation. *Rev. Infect. Dis.* 13:803, 1991.

33. Franco, D., et al. Hepatectomy without abdominal drainage: Results of a prospective study in 61 patients. *Ann. Surg.* 210:64, 1989.

34. Freeman, J., and McGowan, J.E. Methodological issues in hospital epidemiology: I. Rates, case finding and interpretation. *Rev. Infect. Dis.* 3:658, 1981.

35. Garner, J.S., et al. CDC definitions for nosocomial infections, 1988. *Am. J. Infect. Control* 16:128, 1988.

36. Gentry, L.O., et al. Perioperative antibiotic therapy for penetrating injuries of the abdomen. *Ann. Surg.* 200:561, 1984.

37. Green, J.W., and Wenzel, R.P. Postoperative wound infection: A controlled study of the increased duration of hospital stay and direct cost of hospitalization. *Ann. Surg.* 185:264, 1977.

38. Groner, J.I., et al. The efficacy of oral antimicrobials in reducing aerobic and anaerobic colonic mucosal flora. *Arch. Surg.* 124:281, 1989.

39. Haley, R.W., et al. Identifying patients at high risk of surgical wound infection. *Am. J. Epidemiol.* 121:206, 1985.

40. Haley, R.W., et al. The efficacy of infection surveillance and control. *Am. J. Epidemiol.* 121:182, 1985.

41. Hay, T. Infections of the Liver and Spleen. In: R.J. Howard and R.L. Simmons (Eds.), *Surgical Infectious Diseases* (2nd ed.). Norwalk, CT: Appleton and Lange, 1988. P. 674.

42. Kaiser, A.B. Antimicrobial Prophylaxis of Infections Associated with Foreign Bodies. In: A.L. Bisno and F.A. Waldvogel (Eds.), *Infections Associated with Indwelling Medical Devices.* Washington, DC: American Society for Microbiology, 1989. Pp. 277–287.

42a. Kaiser, A.B. Surgical-wound infection. *N. Engl. J. Med.* 324:123, 1991.

43. Kernodle, D.S., et al. Failure of cephalosporins to prevent *Staphylococcus aureus* surgical wound infections. *J.A.M.A.* 263:961, 1990.

43a. Koch, R., and Wolffhugel, G. Untersuchungen uber die Desinfektion mit heisser Luft. *Mitt. Kaiserl. Gesund.* 1:301, 1881.

43b. Koch, R., Gaffky, G., and Loeffler, F. Versuche uber die Verwerthbarkeit heisser Wasserdampfe zu Desinfektionszwecken. *Mitt. Kaiserl. Gesund.* 1:322, 1881.

44. Krizek, T.J., and Robson, M.C. Evolution of quantitative bacteriology in wound management. *Am. J. Surg.* 130:579, 1975.

45. Larson, E.L., Butz, A.M., Gullette, D.L., and Laughon, B.A. Alcohol for surgical scrubbing? *Infect. Control Hosp. Epidemiol.* 11:139, 1990.

46. Leclair, J.M., et al. Effect of preoperative shampoos with chlorhexidine or iodophor on emergence of resident scalp flora in neurosurgery. *Infect. Control Hosp. Epidemiol.* 9:8, 1988.

47. Lidwell, O.M. Air, antibiotics and sepsis in replacement joints. *J. Hosp. Infect.* 11:18, 1988.

48. Lidwell, O.M. Sepsis in surgical wounds: Multiple regression analysis applied to records of postoperative hospital sepsis. *J. Hyg.* 59:259, 1961.

48a. Lister, J. On a new method of treating compound fracture, abscess etc., with observations on the conditions of suppuration. *Lancet* 1:326, 1867.

49. Longfield, J.N., Townsend, T.R., and Cruess, D.F. Methicillin-resistant *Staphylococcus aureus* (MRSA): Risk and outcome of colonized vs. infected patients. *Infect. Control* 6:445, 1985.

49a. Lowery, P.W., et al. A cluster of *Legionella* sternal-wound infections due to postoperative topical exposure to contaminated tap water. *N. Engl. J. Med.* 324:109, 1991.

50. Meakins, J.L. Clinical importance of host resistance to infection in surgical patients. *Adv. Surg.* 15:225, 1981.

51. Meakins, J.L. Guidelines for the Prevention of Wound Infections. In: D.D. Wilmore et al. (Eds.), *Care of the Surgical Patient,* Vol. 2, Sec. 9. New York: Scientific American, 1988. Chap. 5, pp. 1–10.

52. Meers, P.D., and Yeo, G.A. Shedding of bacteria and skin squames after hand-washing. *J. Hyg.* (Camb.) 81:99, 1978.

53. Meleney, F.L. Bacterial synergism in disease processes. *Ann. Surg.* 94:961, 1931.

54. Meleney, F.L. The past 50 years in the management of surgical infections. *Surg. Gynecol. Obstet.* 100:1, 1955.

55. Nahmias, A.J., et al. Postsurgical staphylococci infections: Outbreak traced to an individual carrying phage strains 80/81 and 80/81/52/52A. *J.A.M.A.* 174:1269, 1960.

56. Nora, P.F., Vanecuo, R.M., and Bransfield, J.J. Prophylactic abdominal drains. *Arch. Surg.* 105:173, 1972.

57. Olson, M.M., and Lee, J.T. Continuous, 10-year wound infection surveillance; results, advantages and unanswered questions. *Arch. Surg.* 125:794, 1990.

58. Olson, W.R., and Beaudoin, D.E. Wound drainage after splenectomy: Indications and complications. *Am. J. Surg.* 117:615, 1969.

59. Penin, G.B., and Ehrenkranz, N.J. Priorities for surveillance and cost-effective control of postoperative infection. *Arch. Surg.* 123:1305, 1988.

59a. *Physicians' Desk Reference 1991.* Oradell, NJ: Medical Economics Co., 1991. Pp. 1454–1991.

60. Platt, R., et al. Perioperative antibiotic prophylaxis for herniorrhaphy and breast surgery. *N. Engl. J. Med.* 322:153, 1990.

61. Polk, H.C., and Lopez-Mayor, J.F. Postoperative wound infection: A prospective study of determinant factors and prevention. *Surgery* 66:97, 1969.

62. Postsurgical infections associated with an ex-

trinsically contaminated intravenous anesthetic agent—California, Illinois, Maine and Michigan, 1990. *M.M.W.R.* 39:426, 1990.

63. Prevention of bacterial endocarditis. *Med. Lett. Drugs Ther.* 31:112, 1989.

64. Raahave, D., et al. The infective dose of aerobic and anaerobic bacteria in postoperative wound sepsis. *Arch. Surg.* 121:924, 1986.

65. Richards, K.E., Pierson, C.L., Bucciarelli, L. and Feller, I. Monilial sepsis in the surgical patient. *Surg. Clin. North Am.* 52:1399, 1972.

66. Ross, F.P., and Quinlan, R.M. Eight hundred cholecystectomies, a plea for many fewer drains. *Arch. Surg.* 110:721, 1975.

67. Scheckler, W.E. Surgeon-specific wound infection rates—a potentially dangerous and misleading strategy. *Infect. Control Hosp. Epidemiol.* 9:145, 1988.

68. Shaw, G.B. The Collective Biologist. In: *Everybody's Political What's What?* New York: Dodd, Mead & Company, 1944. Pp. 234–244.

69. Stoutenbeek, C.P., et al. The effect of selective decontamination of the digestive tract on colonization and infection rate in multiple trauma patients. *Intensive Care Med.* 10:185, 1984.

69a. Swanson, D., et al. Cefonicid versus clindamycin prophylaxis for head and neck surgery in a randomized double-blind trial with pharmacokinetic implications. *Antimicrob. Agents Chemother.* 35:1360, 1991.

70. Thom, B.T., and White, R.G., The dispersal of organisms from minor septic lesion. *J. Clin. Pathol.* 15:559, 1962.

71. Thomas, M., and Hollins, M. Epidemic of postoperative wound infection associated with ungloved abdominal palpation. *Lancet* 1:1215, 1974.

72. Thomas, M.E.M., Piper, E., and Maurer, I.M. Contamination of an operating theatre by gram-negative bacteria. Examination of water supplies, cleaning methods and wound infections. *J. Hyg.* 70:63, 1972.

73. Walter, K.W., and Kundsin, R.B. The bacteriologic study of surgical gloves from 250 operations. *Surg. Gynecol. Obstet.* 129:949, 1969.

73a. Willis, A.T. History. In: S.M. Finegold and W.L. George (Eds.), *Anaerobic Infections in Humans.* San Diego: Academic Press, 1989.

74. Wenzel, R.P., Osterman, C.A., and Hunting, K.J. Hospital-acquired infections. *Am. J. Epidemiol.* 104:645, 1976.

75. Zimmerli, W., et al. Pathogenesis of foreign body infection: Description and characteristics of an animal model. *J. Infect. Dis.* 146:487, 1982.

Infections of Burn Wounds

Ronald G. Tompkins
John F. Burke

Survival from thermal injuries has significantly improved over the past years to the extent that younger adults and children routinely survive massive burn injuries involving more than 80 percent of the body surface area [4, 9, 22, 23]. In the past, survival after thermal injury was greatly hindered by the inevitable invasive microbial infection that was a consequence of the colonized necrotic soft tissues of the burn injury. Today, however, patients are more likely to have the necrotic tissue removed promptly after the injury and to have the burn wound closed with autologous skin or other skin replacement materials. This therapeutic approach has greatly diminished the likelihood of invasive burn wound infections. Nonetheless, the patient remains highly susceptible to other infectious processes, especially specific infections originating in the pulmonary system. It is either the infection in the burn wound or other foci or the host's inflammatory response to these processes that continues to contribute to the very significant morbidity and mortality resulting from thermal injury. Therefore, a thorough understanding of the associated infectious processes and their therapy remains the key to successful treatment of burn injuries.

Treatment of Burn Injuries

Using a therapeutic approach that incorporates prompt excision of the burn wound and the immediate closure of the resulting open wound with proper wound closure materials, survival rates in adults have significantly im-

The contributions of Bruce G. MacMillan, Ian Alan Holder, and J. Wesley Alexander from the previous edition are gratefully acknowledged.

proved during the last decade. Generally, in large treatment centers, current data indicate that young adults (younger than 30 years) have an 80 percent likelihood of surviving a thermal injury to 70 percent or more of the body's surface area (Fig. 34-1); even in the 50-year-old patient with a similar injury, the likelihood of survival is 50 percent. In nationally recognized pediatric burn treatment centers, dramatic improvement in survival has occurred with burns covering more than 50 percent of the body surface area. Since 1979, mortality has been essentially eliminated in children with burns covering less than 70 percent of the total body surface area (Fig. 34-2). During the period 1979–1986 at the Boston Unit of the Shriners Burns Institute, 29 of 37 patients (78 percent) survived a thermal injury to 80 percent or more of their total body surface area. To achieve these survival rates

requires a treatment approach that prevents burn wound infections and their sequelae, because it is the infection or the associated infectious processes that remain the major cause of complications and death in the thermally injured patient. Therefore, therapy should be directed toward prevention of burn wound infections and associated infectious processes.

The problem in burn injury is the large, open wound of necrotic tissue, the decreased host resistance that results from serious thermal trauma, and the body's inflammatory reaction to these processes. Basic science and clinical studies have shown that decreased host resistance after burn injury is more important in determining the seriousness of infection than is the virulence of the causative bacterium. Consequently, factors resulting in decreased host resistance must be minimized.

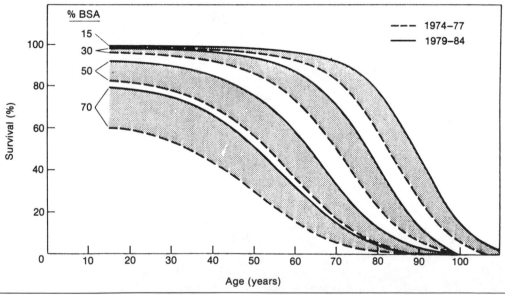

Fig. 34-1. Logistic regression curves of survival *versus* age for various burn sizes for the periods 1974–1977 and 1979–1984. The ordinate is survival and the abscissa is age. The continuous curves represent survival curves from the 1979–1984 mortality data modeled with logit for the indicated percent of body surface area (%BSA). The dotted curves represent survival curves from 1974–1977 mortality data modeled with logit for the indicated %BSA. The smooth curves are shifted upward and to the right, indicating a greater likelihood of survival for a given age and %BSA in 1979–1984 compared to the previous period of 1974–1977. Shifting to the right indicates that for a given %BSA, an older patient in 1979–1984 has the same likelihood of survival as did a younger patient in the 1974–1977 period. (Reprinted with permission from R.G. Tompkins et al., Prompt eschar excision: A treatment system contributing to reduced burn mortality. *Ann. Surg.* 204:272, 1986.)

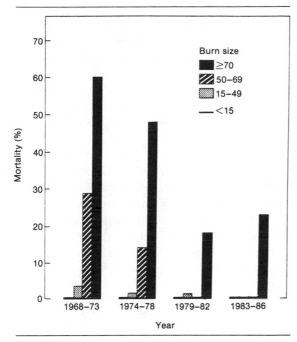

Fig. 34-2. Mortality *versus* time by burn size. Mortality has markedly declined in the massive burn size group (>70 percent of body surface area [%BSA]). Mortality has been essentially eliminated in moderate and large burn sizes of 15–69 %BSA during the most recent time period (1983–1986). (Reprinted with permission from R.G. Tompkins et al., Significant reductions in mortality for children with burn injuries through the use of prompt eschar excision. *Ann. Surg.* 208:577, 1988.)

Necrotic tissue that contributes to the depressed host's susceptibility must be promptly removed and the wounds closed. Secondary derangements in physiology and metabolism leading to caloric and protein starvation must also be corrected.

A reasonable treatment system to prevent burn wound infection can be summarized as follows:

1. Promptly excise the necrotic tissue of the burn injury and immediately close the wound with grafts.
2. Maintain the patient in a controlled, isolated environment such as a bacteria-controlled nursing unit (BCNU) to protect the burn wounds from cross-contamination.
3. Apply topical antibacterial agents such as 0.5% silver nitrate solution, 10% mafenide acetate cream (Sulfamylon), or silver sul-

fadiazine cream to reduce bacterial colonization of the burn wound.
4. Avoid the routine use of prophylactic antibiotics given with the idea of preventing burn wound infections with gram-negative organisms. These antibiotics do not prevent such infections, but they do lead to an emergence of antibiotic-resistant bacterial strains and so should be avoided.

Burn Wound Infections
Incidence

The overall incidence of invasive burn wound infections is decreasing as a result of the earlier attention to removal of the devitalized tissue. Although there is a decreased incidence of wound infections, colonization of the burn wound invariably occurs; wound colonization begins within days of the injury and is present by 7 to 10 days postinjury in nearly all burn wounds with necrotic or devitalized tissues remaining. Infections within partial-thickness burn wounds (injuries that have not completely destroyed both the epidermis and dermis) are particularly important because a burn wound infection can convert a partial-thickness injury to a full-thickness one.

To distinguish between extensive wound colonization and actual tissue invasion can be difficult and can only be accomplished by a combination of clinical observation and careful histologic evaluation. In a recent study from the U.S. Army Institute of Surgical Research at Fort Sam Houston in Texas, the initial tissue biopsies from 200 burned patients were both quantitatively cultured and examined histologically to distinguish between colonization of the wound and invasive tissue infection [4]. In these 200 burned patients, 39 invasive burn wound infections were found. A very high correlation was seen between low microbial counts and the absence of histologically documented invasive infection; microbiologic counts of 10^5 colony-forming units (cfu) or less were almost never seen with microbial invasion tissues. On the other hand, microbial counts in excess of 10^5 cfu were completely unpredictive of invasive wound infections. High microbial counts (greater than 10⁵) were not considered useful as a diagnostic substitute for histologic examination, because the high tissue counts very often did not correlate with histologic invasion of tissue. The principal value of quantitative wound biopsies is therefore to demonstrate the predominant flora resident in the burn wound and not to distinguish between colonization and invasive tissue infection.

The incidence of serious burn wound infection varies with the extent of the injury and the age of the patient. With current methods of topical treatments, serious infections are not expected in otherwise healthy patients with burns involving less than 30 percent of the body surface area. A progressive increase in the incidence of serious infection, however, is seen as the extent of the injury increases. Therefore, an increasing awareness of and vigilant attention to tissue invasion by the microbes of the burn wound must be assumed in larger injuries. Another strong relationship occurs between the risk of burn wound infection and age. This relationship has been emphasized by many others and was especially documented by Thomsen [21]. Therefore, in summary, the incidence of burn wound infection increases with age (dramatically in patients older than 60) and with the extent of injury (infection can occur in many patients with wounds over more than 40 percent of their body surface area).

Pathogens

The most common pathogens occurring within the first three days post injury are the gram-positive cocci, including β-hemolytic streptococci. However, 5 to 7 days postinjury, nearly all the burn wounds containing burn eschar have also become colonized with at least one, but usually multiple, species of gram-negative organisms. The most prominent of these facultative anaerobic bacilli are *Escherichia coli* and species of *Klebsiella, Enterobacter, Serratia, Proteus,* and *Pseudomonas.* Although relatively uncommon, the most prominent of the anaerobic bacilli are *Clostridium* species. The burn wound and other systemic foci occasionally become colonized by fungi, in particular, *Candida albicans.* With the

more recent extensive use of potent broad-spectrum antibiotics, it seems that systemic bacteremias are becoming increasingly more common with gram-positive organisms (especially *Staphylococcus aureus, S. epidermidis,* and enterococci) and the fungus *Candida albicans.*

Before the availability of penicillin and sulfonamides, β-hemolytic *Streptococcus pyogenes* was the pathogen most frequently recognized. The clinical course of such infections was often dramatic; an invasive streptococcal cellulitis would spread rapidly to become a fulminating infection with generalized toxicity, and early death of the patient would ensue. In 1933, Aldrich [1] reported that all severe burns at the Johns Hopkins Hospital were colonized with streptococci within the first day. Since proper antibiotics became available, common practice in many units has included preventive antibiotics at least during the first few days postinjury in order to prevent streptococcal infections.

Data collected by the National Nosocomial Infections Surveillance (NNIS) Systems for the years 1980–1982 revealed that gram-negative microorganisms are recovered from burns most frequently, with gram-positive organisims a close second (Table 34-1). Fungi and anaerobic bacilli constitute only a small percentage of total microorganisms isolated. The breakdown of these organisms by genera is presented in Table 34-2. *S. aureus* and *Pseudomonas aeruginosa* are the most frequently isolated gram-positive and gram-negative organisms, respectively. Enterococci constitute another major group of gram-positive isolates, whereas gram-negative organisms including *E. coli, Enterobacter cloacae, Serratia marcescens,* and *Klebsiella* species are also important in burn wound infections. *Candida albicans,* other *Candida* species, and other fungi account for a small percentage (usually less than 1 percent) of potentially dangerous burn wound infections. Recent concern has arisen over an increase in the incidence of infections resulting from a variety of viruses. Therefore, at present, it would appear that virtually any organism can become a lethal pathogen in the immunocompromised seriously burned patient.

The changing pattern of flora in the burn

Table 34-1. Distribution of groups of microorganisms recovered from infected burns

Group	Percentage of total
Gram-negative organisms	51.8
Gram-positive organisms	42.6
Fungi	4.4
Anaerobes	1.0

Source: From the National Nosocomial Infections Surveillance System, 1980–82.

Table 34-2. Distribution of 648 microorganisms recovered from infected burns

Organisms	Number recovered	Percentage of total
Staphylococcus aureus	157	24.2
Pseudomonas aeruginosa	135	20.8
Enterococci	76	11.7
Escherichia coli	50	7.7
Enterobacter cloacae	50	7.7
Serratia marcescens	39	6.0
Klebsiella species	22	3.4
Staphylococcus epidermidis	19	2.9
Candida albicans	14	2.3
Proteus species	12	1.9
Non-Enterococcus streptococci	12	1.9
Pseudomonas species	6	0.9
Anaerobes	6	0.9
Acinetobacter species	5	0.8
Aspergillus species	4	0.6
Candida (non-albicans)	3	0.5
Providencia species	2	0.3
Other bacteria	28	4.3
Other fungi	8	1.2

Source: National Nosocomial Infections Surveillance System, 1980–82.

wound often reflects changing methods of therapy more than any other factor and, although the ecology of the burn wound flora can be altered by therapy, the burn wound cannot be sterilized. All too often, the administration of antimicrobial agents merely provides environmental pressure for a change in the burn wound flora to the more antibiotic-resistant organisms. To complicate the picture further, there is ample evidence that depression of numerous immune resistance factors in seriously burned patients contrib-

utes significantly both to proliferation of microbes on the burn wound and to their systemic invasion.

The question of the origin of these pathogens and the method of their spread to the burn wound remains unsettled. One key point is that, in most instances, the burn wound flora is similar to the patient's own gastrointestinal flora. This suggests at least two possibilities: (1) The wound may become directly inoculated by fecal contamination or (2) the bacteria may be absorbed across the intestinal mucosa and spread systemically by the process of translocation, the extraintestinal dissemination of intestinal bacteria. The latter process of translocation is considered to be potentially important and has been reviewed recently by Steffen [20] and Wells [24] and their colleagues.

The distinction between whether the wound infections are nosocomial or community-acquired is made based primarily on the time that the infection was first recognized. Infections of burn wounds should be considered nosocomial if the onset of the infection occurs during hospitalization. Infection of burn wounds on initial admission should be classified as community-acquired; these are most likely to be encountered among persons with minor burns whose injury did not initially require hospital care.

Host Factors
Clinical Syndrome
Sepsis that is usually associated with an invasive bacterial, fungal, or viral infection needs to be further defined. Over the past decade, it has become apparent that the clinical state of fever, hyperdynamic metabolism, hyperdynamic cardiovascular physiology, and mental alterations including confusion can be the result of toxic factors from microbial organisms or inflammatory mediators from the host's own macrophages and does not necessarily indicate that a bacterial infection with systemic invasion is present. These toxic microbial products include endotoxin (gram-negative bacterial cell wall) and zymogen (fungal cell wall) and the protein secretion products of the patient's own inflammatory system including interleukin 1 (IL1), tumor necrosis

factor (TNF), and interleukin 6 (IL6). The important point about this febrile, metabolically and cardiovascularly hyperdynamic state is that high doses of potent, broad-spectrum antibiotics will not necessarily remedy this condition but will only select for more antibiotic-resistant organisms or facilitate colonization with fungi. Under these conditions, general supportive measures and a careful search for potential specific infectious foci are the best therapeutic approach.

Blood cultures frequently may be positive during the hospital course of a patient with a serious thermal injury. Both colonizing and invading bacteria may enter the lymphatics and traverse into the systemic circulation; direct invasion of bacteria into blood vessels can also occur. Thus when repeated blood culture specimens are taken on a routine basis on patients with large burns, it is not unusual to recover organisms. Recovery of organisms by blood culture in burn patients sometimes occurs without clinical evidence of systemic infection and, as mentioned earlier, septic death can occur without septicemia. Furthermore, bacteremia and septicemia in burn patients may derive from sites of infection other than the burn wound, and these may be caused by the same organisms as those isolated from the burn wound. Consequently, some burn centers have placed decreasing emphasis on monitoring burn sepsis by repeated blood cultures, but we find this pessimism unfounded. Although it is true that both false-negative and false-positive blood cultures can be obtained, there is nevertheless a very good correlation between clinical evidence of septicemia and the presence of positive blood cultures. It is our strong feeling that differentiation among bacteremia, septicemia, and burn wound sepsis should not be too rigid and that the entire clinical and bacteriologic picture must be taken into account in the frequent and critical reevaluation of infection in these patients.

It is apparent that the clinical manifestations of invasive infection of the burn wound associated with septicemia and bacteremia are not really much different from those that occur without bacteremia although, in our ex-

perience, the large majority of patients with burn wound sepsis have an associated bacteremia. The former deserve separate classification, however, because of the objective nature of the diagnosis. In cases of invasive burn wound sepsis with septicemia and bacteremia, it is not unusual to recover more than one organism from the blood culture, which indicates that such patients have a generalized lack of resistance to infection.

Apparent Deficiencies in Host Immune Function

Virtually every measurement of immune function has been found to be abnormal at some time following burn injury [8]. Some abnormalities are depression of circulating IgG and complement levels, especially in association with hemodilution and protein loss during the first week following injury; abnormalities of complement function; depressed response of circulating antibody to certain antigens, especially in large burns after the fifth postinjury day; a decrease in chemotactic activity of leukocytes; lymphoid depletion of both primary and secondary lymphoid organs, especially in relation to the T-cell population of lymphocytes; altered T-cell function; abnormal response to antigens that cause delayed hypersensitivity reaction (e.g., tuberculin and streptokinase); prolongation of allografts; depressed response to nonspecific stimuli; and abnormalities of the antibacterial function of neutrophils. Undoubtedly, any of these could contribute in a significant way to the development of nosocomial infection in burn patients. From clinical and laboratory evidence, abnormalities of neutrophil function and of the opsonic proteins may play the dominant role in infection in burn patients, whereas abnormalities of lymphoid function probably do not significantly influence the burned patient's clinical course.

Management
General Treatment Measures

Mortality following the burn injury is not related to the toxic biologic effect of thermally injured skin but to the metabolic and bacterial consequences of a large open wound, depletion of the patient's host resistance, and extensive malnutrition. These abnormalities set the stage for life-threatening bacterial infection originating from the burn wound. Systemic antibiotics and topical therapy have proved important but are only adjuncts to more definitive therapy of prompt wound closure and do not solve the problems presented by large open wounds and related protein and caloric deprivation. A more rational approach to the problem of extensive skin destruction from burns is the rapid excision of devitalized tissue and immediate closure of the wound following excision. This concept, coupled with strict protection of the patient from cross-infection and intensive nutritional support until wound closure in the clinical setting, may be easily employed as routine burn care for small and moderate burns that require hospitalization. For more extensive burns, the problem of wound closure is more difficult because of the lack of available autograft and the rejection of allograft in a short period of time which recreates the large open wound. Early and continuous attention to wound closure appears to be essential if a patient is to survive with massive (greater than 70 percent of body surface area) burns.

Prompt Excision and Immediate Wound Closure

Prompt excision and immediate wound closure removes devitalized tissue and replaces this tissue with either autograft or acceptable skin substitutes such as allograft or skin replacements. The plan of prompt excision and immediate wound closure consists of excision of all areas of burn that are judged to require more than 3 weeks to heal spontaneously. Separate surgical procedures begin as soon as possible after injury and are continued until all devitalized tissues have been excised. It is important to begin the operative procedures as soon after injury as possible, because the physiology of the patient is near normal immediately after injury. It is important to recognize that the physical state of the resuscitated patient does not recover after the injury but steadily deteriorates until the

wound is closed. Extensive operative procedures, therefore, are more safely carried out in the first week than in the third week following injury. It is equally important to harvest the autograft donor sites soon after injury. Since donor sites heal and may be reharvested as early as 2 weeks, the sites harvested on day 1 postinjury may usually be reharvested on approximately day 14. This plan minimizes the time required for autograft closure and hospital stay. In a large burn, the skin autograft supply is usually exhausted before all of the excised areas are covered. In such cases, temporary wound coverage until donor sites reepithelialize can be accomplished with allograft and, for definitive long-term coverage, artificial skin is the medium of choice.

Controlled Patient Environment

Because the burned patient's host resistance is defective during the time required to achieve wound closure clinically, the patient should be housed in a protective environment such as the BCNU [6]. This unit prevents bacterial contamination of the patient from staff and equipment, as well as cross-contamination from other patients. The protective environment not only provides a controlled bacterial area through the use of clear plastic walls and a continuous downflow of bacteria-free air, but also controls temperature and humidity to a level that provides the patient with maximum benefit. The unit temperature usually is held at 31°C (88°F), and relative humidity is maintained at 88 to 92 percent. These conditions markedly reduce the patient's energy expenditures. The BCNU provides environmental control of a 6×10−ft area that immediately surrounds the patient's bed. The controlled environment is effective in preventing bacterial cross-infection because it is possible to deliver medical care without entering the patient's environment and to maintain all monitoring, life support, and intravenous equipment outside the patient's environment.

The BCNU provides an environment that minimizes body heat loss and evaporative water loss, as well as reducing the energy required to maintain body heat. The patient's metabolic state is such that body temperature is often maintained above 37°C (98.6°F). Any attempt to lower the patient's body temperature by reducing environmental temperature is met with an increased energy expenditure by the patient. In a patient who is catabolic as a result of the injury, this added energy expenditure is another threat to survival.

The BCNU affords medical and nursing staff an additional advantage in that the temperature and humidity that are most effective for treating the patient can be maintained though they are above the range in which the staff can work effectively.

Nutrition

There are two critical problems for nutritional management of an injured patient in the early care of a burn injury: (1) What level of caloric intake will be required to allow the patient to meet caloric needs in response to his or her injury; and (2) what mixture of substrates (proteins, carbohydrates, and fats) will meet this patient's caloric requirements and optimally allow him or her to meet the body's metabolic needs without incurring a negative nitrogen balance? In answer to the first question, oxygen consumption studies have shown that the metabolic rate of burn patients does not exceed twice the patient's normal basal metabolic rate (BMR) as predicted by the Harris-Benedict table of correlations for adults and children older than 2 years. Prompt excision and immediate wound closure with grafting have contributed to lowering metabolic requirements below those reported in the past. The Harris-Benedict correlation considers age, sex, height, and weight as factors determining basal caloric requirements, because these variables normally control individual metabolic rates. Studies have demonstrated that, although the size of the open burn wound and body temperature contribute to hypermetabolism, their contribution is small and, for clinical purposes in the treatment of burn patients, they may be disregarded in determining daily caloric requirements. Since twice the BMR has been

shown to overestimate slightly even the largest burn, one may neglect burn size and body temperature to simplify the clinical calculation of caloric need.

The second question is more complex. The total caloric requirement is met with carbohydrate, protein, and fat. Carbohydrate at 5 mg/kg/min has been shown to provide enough calories to prevent amino acid breakdown as an energy source and to suppress endogenous glucose production via hepatic gluconeogenesis, which requires mobilization of amino acids as gluconeogenic precursors. This glucose infusion rate approximates the maximum rate of glucose oxidation for an injured patient at strict bed rest. Additional exogenous glucose delivered to a patient at rest is not used for adenosine triphosphate production but is converted to fat. At the infusion rate of 5 mg/kg/min, the respiratory quotient is slightly below unity, indicating the glucose is oxidized to carbon dioxide, water, and energy, and is not being stored as fat.

Protein is infused at 1.5 to 2.5 gm/kg/day, depending on the size of the injury and the presence or absence of sepsis. For moderate injuries, the lower rate is used and, for severe injuries or sepsis, the higher rate is used. Using nitrogen balance analysis and kinetic amino acid turnover studies, this rate of administration was shown to maintain a positive nitrogen balance in adults and in children. However, it is important to recognize that the exact protein requirements or the optimal mixture of amino acids for seriously injured patients remains unknown. Until synthesis rates of muscle protein, collagen components of host defense, and other proteins are accurately measured in vivo, this protein replacement rate can be only an estimate and is as accurate as estimates made by others. While burn wounds are open and healing, the nitrogen requirement is known to be higher than normal. Unfortunately, these nitrogen balance studies do not translate into exact information about the quantity and composition of the proteins required.

Earlier and more aggressive metabolic support, possibly beginning hours after the injury with amino acids, should be given to (1) patients with burns over greater than 20 percent of their body surface area, (2) patients with preinjury malnutrition, (3) patients with complications such as sepsis or associated injuries, and (4) patients admitted late in their burn course who have a weight loss in excess of 10 percent of their premorbid weight. Nutritional support is begun as soon as possible after the injury and not later than postburn day 1 on completion of the immediate resuscitation phase. This support is accomplished by oral feeding, tube feeding, or total parenteral nutrition (TPN), depending on the patient's ability to receive nutritional support. The enteral route is preferred because of fewer complications and lower cost associated with enteral feedings as compared to parenteral feedings. However, anorexia, facial burns, or dysphagia may make oral feeding difficult or impossible. If these are present but gastric motility and absorption is normal, then tube feedings are given; if gastric emptying is impaired but small-intestinal absorption is normal, then postduodenal enteral feedings may be employed. These tube feedings are given at a constant infusion rate, as either a supplement to oral feedings or a replacement of the oral feedings as the total caloric source. TPN is used if intestinal motility or absorption is abnormal or if multiple excision and grafting procedures are anticipated over the first week of the admission that will not allow the gastrointestinal tract to recover between operations.

Topical Wound Care

Before application of a topical agent, all grease, oil, and loose skin, burned clothing, and other contaminants are removed. At the Massachusetts General Hospital Burn Unit, a thick layer of wide mesh gauze dressing is placed on the wound and saturated with 0.5% silver nitrate. A 0.5% silver nitrate solution not only markedly decreases bacterial growth on the burn wound but also minimizes water evaporation and may be used for donor sites and newly grafted areas as well as the burn wound. Silver nitrate is not used in the peri-neum or on the face because of the mechanical problems of application. Dressings are soaked with the 0.5% solution every 2 hours to maintain a 0.5% concentration at the wound surface; a lesser concentration is not bacteriostatic, and a greater concentration may damage adjacent viable skin.

Two other frequently used topical agents are 10% mafenide acetate cream (Sulfamylon) and silver sulfadiazine. Each is supplied as a cream, applied directly to the burn wound after the initial removal of wound contaminants, and reapplied twice daily. Care must be taken to remove previous Sulfamylon or silver sulfadiazine before a fresh layer is applied.

Occasional side effects may occur with the use of these topical agents. Sulfamylon easily penetrates eschar and is systemically absorbed and excreted by the kidney. Since Sulfamylon is a carbonic anhydrase inhibitor, metabolic acidosis may develop in the presence of renal or respiratory failure. Allergic reactions and hemolysis in patients deficient in glucose-6-phosphate dehydrogenase (G6PD) may develop for both Sulfamylon and silver sulfadiazine. A rare reaction of methemoglobinemia may result when nitrates (including silver nitrate) are reduced by wound bacteria such as certain *E. coli* and *Klebsiella*.

Preventive Antibiotics

Infection of the burn wound is still a major cause of complications and death in burn patients. To prevent the sequelae of wound infection, by far the best approach is to prevent wound infection [5]. Preventive therapy includes the previously described prompt excision of the necrotic tissue of the burn injury and immediate closure of the wound with skin grafts. As described, protection of the wound from cross-contamination is promoted by maintaining the patient in a controlled, isolated environment such as a BCNU. An additional and important adjunct is the application of topical antibacterial agents, which reduce bacterial colonization of the burn wound. Finally, routine systemic antibiotics given throughout the burn illness with the objective of avoiding burn wound infection do not prevent such infection and should not be given. These routine antibiotics only lead to an emergence of bacterial strains that are resistant to the particular antibiotic used. However, antibiotics can, in specific instances and for short times, supplement the patient's natural ability to prevent invasive infection, as described later. The use of antibiotics for indiscriminate periods in a general attempt to avoid infection is an ineffective approach and applies environmental pressure resulting in alterations in the normal flora, allergic reactions, and wound colonization by antibiotic-resistant bacterial strains. Clearly, such use of prophylactic, potent, broad-spectrum antibiotics is not in the patient's best interest.

Antibiotics are of considerable importance for two general indications: established infection and prevention of infection during specific periods of reduced host resistance. There are two clinical states in which antibiotics may be used in a preventive mode with demonstrable therapeutic effect. One of these clinical states occurs immediately after injury when host defenses are seriously reduced. Penicillin is given parenterally or orally for 3 days after the burn injury in all serious second-degree and all third-degree burns for the prevention of β-hemolytic streptococcal wound cellulitis. In the case of penicillin allergy, erythromycin or vancomycin may be administered. A second clinical state occurs because of the high incidence of bacteremia during excision of colonized burn eschar. Perioperatively, antibiotics are administered immediately prior to the operation, during the operative procedure, and in the immediate postoperative period until normal cardiovascular hemodynamics are reestablished (usually within 24 hours) and other normal physiologic signs are present. The perioperative antibiotic is chosen on the basis of previous burn wound culture results and sensitivities of the organisms (see Chap. 33). If these are unavailable, general antimicrobial coverage for both gram-positive cocci and gram-negative rods is recommended. A preventive intravenous antibiotic directed against the commonly encountered *S. aureus* is nafcillin

or alternatively, in the presence of penicillin allergy, clindamycin or vancomycin. The common gram-negative bacilli encountered are *P. aeruginosa, E. coli,* and *Enterobacter, Klebsiella,* and *Proteus* species. The recommended intravenously administered aminoglycoside is gentamicin; more recently, other aminoglycosides have become available and generally have demonstrated a lower incidence of drug resistance. Other antibiotics, including second- and third-generation cephalosporins and monobactams, have an increased effectiveness against gram-negative bacilli, the latter group being particularly effective against *P. aeruginosa;* these two groups of antibiotics also have fewer side effects such as ototoxicity or nephrotoxicity. Both vancomycin and aminoglycoside serum levels should be obtained when these antibiotics are continued for more than 72 hours [7]. In addition to the use of a preventive systemic antibiotic as just described, Sulfamylon may be placed on the wound 5 to 6 hours before the operative procedure to reduce the eschar burden of bacteria.

Treatment of Invasive Infection

Identification of invasive infection requiring antibiotics is difficult because burn wounds are rarely sterile and it is often difficult to distinguish between wound colonization and wound invasion on wound bacteriologic studies alone. The established diagnosis of invasive infection, however, demands prompt systemic antibiotic therapy. Some indications for antibiotic treatment in burn patients include:

1. Deterioration of the patient's overall clinical condition together with a considerable increase in the number of bacteria cultured from the wound (from scant or moderate growth to abundant growth)
2. Signs or symptoms of bacteremia with or without positive blood cultures
3. Less specific findings of sepsis such as isolated cardiovascular failure, altered mental alertness, hypothermia, spiking fevers, or the onset of gastrointestinal ileus

The causative organism can usually be determined by referring to the recent surveillance cultures of the burn wound, urine, and respiratory tract secretions. In large burn injuries, surveillance cultures should be taken of body fluids on a regular basis at least weekly; for example, at the Massachusetts General Hospital Adult Burn Unit, surveillance cultures are performed each Wednesday. Often the last strain cultured from the burn wound is the strain responsible for the invasive infection. More definitive information can be obtained from blood cultures, which should be obtained at the first clinical indication of invasive infection. Since quantitative bacteriologic studies have been shown to be ineffective to distinguish gross colonization from infectious invasion, they are not used at Massachusetts General. In assessing methods giving evidence of wound invasion, the highest correlation with invasive burn wound infection was histologic evidence of bacterial invasion of viable tissue at the base of the wound [14]. Since the necrotic wounds are excised as early as possible during the hospital course, biopsies of the wound to determine microbial tissue invasion are unnecessary.

Gram-negative bacteria, especially *Pseudomonas*, *E. coli*, *Klebsiella*, and *Enterobacter* species, are often responsible for invasive infection. These organisms are best managed on the basis of sensitivity testing. When the involved pathogen cannot be identified, both an aminoglycoside and a penicillinase-resistant penicillin should be given for wide-spectrum coverage until more specific antibiotic therapy can be administered. Treatment can be initiated with the same antibiotics and dosages recommended in the previous section. For life-threatening infection with *Pseudomonas*, treatment is often enhanced with carbenicillin in addition to an aminoglycoside.

In patients with large, open wounds, especially children, drug leakage from the wound complicates accurate therapy, which anticipates serum levels based on body size [12]. Antibiotic levels are therefore often low in these patients, and serum levels obtained by peak and trough levels must be used for accurate therapy.

Review of Approaches to Burn Wound Treatment and Infection Management

Treatment of the massive burn injury is directed toward the metabolic and bacterial consequences of the large open wound, depletion of the patient's host resistance, and extensive malnutrition. The treatment plan is based on removal of the devitalized tissue and immediate closure of the wound. During the period of wound closure, the patient's physiology is maintained at near normal levels by the following measures:

1. Blood volume is restored with adequate initial fluid resuscitation, preventing complications of severe hypovolemia.
2. Open wounds not yet excised and closed are protected from cross-contamination, and unnecessary energy expenditures are avoided through the use of a controlled patient environment.
3. Metabolic requirements are met by delivering twice the BMR of calories, with careful attention to the protein and glucose proportion of those calories.
4. Preventive antibiotics are used for only brief periods for clinical states that are well defined, and antibiotics are not used routinely for prolonged periods with the objective of avoiding burn wound infection.
5. Established infection is treated with appropriate antibiotics and removal of the source of invasive infection in a manner similar to the treatment of infections in nonburned patients.

With regard to the use of antibiotics for established infections, the following general principles should be followed:

1. Use surveillance cultures to monitor the patient's microbial environment.
2. Avoid treating potential pathogens, but select antibiotics directed against specific pathogens as often as possible.
3. Regularly review antibiotic selections and

decide on the duration of administration. Usually, 5 to 7 days will be sufficient to achieve a clinical response, and this will generally be tolerated in terms of the development of antibiotic-resistant bacterial strains or fungi colonization (see Chap. 12).

4. We use high doses of oral nystatin and nystatin for bladder irrigations in patients on potent long-term antibiotics, to decrease the incidence of fungal colonization (see Chap. 28).

Group A *Streptococcus pyogenes*
General Aspects
Transmissibility
Group A *S. pyogenes* is a highly transmissible organism that can cause rapidly lethal infections in the burn patient.

Clinical Course
The clinical course is characterized by an abrupt deterioration in the wound that is associated with an increase in wound pain, redness, induration, and swelling. Redness extending from the margin of the burn wound is perhaps the most significant sign of streptococcal infections, which characteristically invade into normal tissues. Within hours of the onset of the more fulminant infections, systemic symptoms occur, characterized by a high, spiking fever, rapid tachycardia, and flushing of the face. Untreated, the condition can rapidly progress to death. Leukocytosis with a marked shift to the left is characteristic. Shock usually does not occur until the condition is terminal. Most streptococcal infections are seen within the first week following burn injury, and invasive infection of healthy granulation tissue by streptococci rarely occurs. It is for this reason that penicillin has been used so extensively in most burn units for prophylaxis during the early burn period (see Chap. 37).

Predisposing Host Factors
The predisposing host factors are not different from those of other types of bacterial infection in burn patients.

Therapy
Fortunately group A streptococcal infection almost always responds to penicillin therapy. For those individuals allergic to penicillin, alternative drugs include erythromycin, vancomycin, and the cephalosporins. Patients with penicillin allergy tend to be sensitive to cephalosporin as well, and cephalosporins should probably not be used in those with a history of severe penicillin reactions. Streptococci are exquisitely sensitive to vancomycin, and this is the drug of choice in treating life-threatening infection in a patient with penicillin allergy. It is well to remember that although gentamicin has a broad spectrum of activity against most staphylococcal organisms, it is relatively ineffective against streptococcal infections.

Endemic Infections
Incidence
Despite the high transmissibility, endogenous infections are much more common than exogenous infections in well-run burn units.

Sources
The major source of group A streptococci that cause endemic infection is the nasopharynx of the patient. The patient's wounds can also be an important source, however, particularly the small, chronically draining wounds in ulcerated burn scars or burn sites that are slow to heal. Fomites and other environmental sources do not seem to play a prominent role in endemic infections.

Modes of Spread
Spread is usually within the patient, either from the nasopharynx or from open areas to recently grafted sites. Less common but very important is spread by nursing and support staff from one patient to another by contaminated hands or possibly by colonization in the nares and dissemination to susceptible patients.

Prevention
Prevention of endemic infections with group A streptococci is best accomplished by bac-

teriologic monitoring of the patient and his or her wound. On admission to a burn unit, every patient should have a nasopharyngeal culture as well as cultures of all wounds. Such cultures should be repeated on a routine, periodic basis during the hospital stay as surveillance cultures. Patients who have or develop a positive culture for group A streptococci should be isolated immediately and treated with systemic penicillin therapy until the cultures are negative. Any patient with positive cultures in the recent past that required an operation or debridement should be given prophylactic penicillin therapy to protect against invasive infection by β-hemolytic streptococci.

Epidemic Infections
Incidence
With good environmental control and bacteriologic monitoring, epidemic infections should be exceedingly rare.

High-Risk Areas
Both open wards and intensive care units can pose high risks in hospitals that treat burns in such areas. The enhanced risk is related mostly to a high density of patients with susceptible wounds, which in turn results in inadequate protective isolation of the burn patient.

Sources
In epidemic infections, nursing and support personnel must be highly suspected, but initial infections may come from the patients or visitors (see Chaps. 33, 37).

Modes of Spread
In contrast to endemic infections, spread is usually by contact from carriers or from personnel who transmit the infection from patient to patient.

Control of Outbreaks
Strict isolation procedures should be used to control any acute group A β-hemolytic streptococcal burn infection. All patient care personnel and patients should have cultures of the nares, oropharynx, and wounds, and epidemiologic studies should be undertaken to identify potential disseminating carriers (see Chaps. 6, 33, 37). Patients with positive cultures should be isolated and treated with penicillin (see Chap. 11). Personnel with positive cultures must be removed from patient care duties until either they are treated and have negative cultures or their strains are shown to be different from the epidemic strain on the basis of M and T typing. Strict attention to "no-touch" technique is essential to the control and prevention of outbreaks, and gloves and masks should be worn anytime there is contact with the wound. One important aspect of the prevention of such outbreaks is to prohibit visitation by persons with upper respiratory tract infections.

Staphylococcus Aureus
General Aspects
Transmissibility
S. aureus is an organism of moderate virulence that is easily transmitted. The extremely large numbers of organisms that may colonize or infect burns are accompanied by significant risks of transmission by contact and airborne routes. Because they survive even in the dried state, staphylococci can become airborne on dust particles and desquamated epithelial cells, but contact is by far the most important mode of their transmission in burn patients.

Clinical Features
Patients who develop invasive infections of the burn wound with *S. aureus* have an insidious course; 2 to 5 days often elapse between the earliest symptoms and the full-blown infection. These patients have early dissolution of granulation tissue in the burn wound, become hyperpyretic with a leukocytosis, develop disorientation that is often severe, and often develop a prominent gastrointestinal ileus. Shock is not infrequent and is often accompanied by renal failure.

Predisposing Host Factors
The most important host factor that predisposes to staphylococcal infections appears

to be an abnormality of the antibacterial function of the neutrophils. Serum factors seem to be less important in the control of this microorganism than they are in other infections.

Therapy

Fortunately, many antimicrobial agents are effective against *S. aureus.* Although penicillin is effective against some strains, the high incidence of penicillin resistance makes it mandatory that other antibiotics be chosen as a primary agent. In our unit, systemic nafcillin has proved to be a valuable drug. The occasional strains that have been nafcillin-resistant have been uniformly susceptible to vancomycin. Antibiotics should be administered only when there is evidence of invasive infection of the burn wound. Because of the problem of superinfection, therapy should be restricted to relatively short time intervals. To reverse a tendency to administer the anti-staphylococcal drugs for too long a time, we recommend thorough reassessment of the need for their continuation after every 5 days of therapy. Generally, *S. aureus* cannot be eradicated completely from a burn wound until the wound is covered by graft.

Endemic Infections
Incidence

S. aureus is an important organism causing infection in burn patients. With the availability of effective antimicrobial agents for the treatment of systemic infection, mortality from staphylococcal infection is rare.

Sources

Environmental sources are probably much more important for *S. aureus* than for most of the organisms encountered in the burn unit. Indeed, the organism is almost ubiquitous. Furthermore, patients colonized in the anterior nares may spread the organisms to their burns. The greatest source of endemic spread is the nosocomial reservoir. For this reason, it is extremely important to develop rigid environmental control techniques, as mentioned previously.

Modes of Spread

Staphylococcal carriers among personnel can be an important source, but the most important mode of spread is usually via personnel from patient to patient in an environment that is not closely controlled. Fomites and even food are occasionally implicated.

Prevention

Environmental control is of utmost importance in preventing endemic infection by *S. aureus;* these measures have already been outlined. In addition, the restrictive use of systemic antibiotics favors easier control of this infection. Among the topical agents, povidone-iodine and mafenide acetate appear to give reasonably good control for *S. aureus* infection, and our strains have been uniformly susceptible to nitrofurazone.

Epidemic Infections

There is a low incidence of epidemic infections with *S. aureus* even in high-patient-density areas such as intensive care units. When they do occur, epidemiologic studies and bacteriologic surveys of personnel for carriers should be performed. If carriers are epidemiologically associated with the outbreak, they should be temporarily excused from duty, and attempts should be made to eradicate the colonizing strain (see Chaps. 33, 37).

Pseudomonas Aeruginosa
General Aspects
Transmissibility

P. aeruginosa is an organism of low pathogenicity that rarely causes infections in immunologically normal individuals. However, it grows well in moist environments, especially in open wounds; it is resistant to most commonly used antibiotics; and it invades frequently in immunodepressed individuals.

Clinical Features

Invasion of the burn wound by *P. aeruginosa* may occur either abruptly or slowly. In a typical case, the burn wound develops a heavy, green-pigmented, foul-smelling discharge over a period of 2 or 3 days. In rapidly advancing and invasive infections, the eschar may become dry, and previously healthy granulation tissues develop a shaggy, green exudate and later progress to form patchy, black areas of necrosis. *Pseudomonas* infections can have very adverse effects, including graft loss in freshly excised and grafted areas, though in certain cases, the affected areas may not show necrosis and may not have a greenish exudate. Gangrene in nonburned areas (ecthyma gangrenosum) is often seen before death in patients with septicemia. Patients usually become hypothermic and have a depressed white blood cell count, clinical ileus, and mental confusion suggestive of severe and overwhelming sepsis.

Predisposing Host Factors

Predisposing host factors are extremely important in the development of infections with *P. aeruginosa*. In burn patients, these factors are considered to be related both to abnormalities of the antibacterial function of neutrophils and to deficiencies in serum opsonins—that is, specific natural or immune antibody and components of the complement system.

Virulence Factors

In addition to host factors that predispose patients to *P. aeruginosa* infections, research in recent years has defined several virulence-associated factors for this microorganism, including elastase, alkaline protease, and exotoxin production and motility. It is the activity of these virulence-associated factors, alone or in concert, taken together with the predisposing host factors that make *P. aeruginosa* infections in burn patients the most devastating of the gram-negative infections.

Therapy

In the treatment of established septicemia in the burn patient, certain aminoglycosides—especially gentamicin, tobramycin, and amikacin—have been the antibiotics of choice in the treatment of *Pseudomonas* septicemia.

Simultaneous administration of carbenicillin has been useful in selected cases, especially in overwhelming infections. An alarming observation has been a marked increase in the numbers of bacteria in some hospitals that have been found to be resistant to gentamicin, carbenicillin, and even the newer aminoglycosides.

Some newer penicillins—piperacillin and azlocillin—show significant antipseudomonal activity in vitro, but resistance develops rapidly in patients when they are used alone. Newer third-generation cephalosporins and monobactam antibiotics have demonstrated very reasonable effectiveness against many gram-negative bacilli. In particular, the monobactam aztreonam is effective against *Pseudomonas*.

Monitoring Serum Aminoglycoside Levels

Gram-negative infections, particularly those due to *P. aeruginosa*, *Klebsiella pneumoniae*, and *Enterobacter* species, are frequently the cause of death of patients suffering from major burns. Septicemia and burn wound sepsis resulting from these pathogens have, in the past, produced an alarmingly high death rate. Because of the favorable antibacterial spectrum of gentamicin and other aminoglycosides, these agents have become widely used in the treatment of burn sepsis. Optimal treatment with these agents requires the careful establishment of dosage schedules.

In 1976, Zaske and co-workers [26], using a digital computer program nonlinear regression analysis of postinfusion serum concentration versus time analysis, calculated the estimated half-life of gentamicin in burn patients. They found that the recommended dosage of 5 mg/kg/day resulted in a shorter half-life in burned compared to nonburned patients and that this shortened half-life in burned patients led to extended periods of subtherapeutic serum antibiotic concentrations. Furthermore, it was determined that among adult burn patients, there was a wide variability of gentamicin half-lives and that younger burn patients eliminated gentamicin even more rapidly than older burn patients.

Dosages of 8 mg/kg/day to 20 mg/kg/day have been used, but each dosage is individualized to the specific patient based on data obtained from the initial clearance rate of the standard dosage. The established dosage schedule should be checked at frequent intervals in the early course of aminoglycoside therapy to ensure that levels are being adequately maintained and that half-lives are not changing during this time. This technique probably represents one of the major therapeutic advancements in delivering and assessing systemic antibiotic therapy.

Endemic Infections
Incidence
As indicated earlier, it is difficult to establish the incidence of infection by any one organism in burn patients because of the spectrum between colonization and frank sepsis.

Sources
A major source of *P. aeruginosa* in a patient's burn wound was the patient himself, predominantly via the gastrointestinal tract [13]. This observation has been emphasized by others [8, 19]. Nosocomial acquisition of *P. aeruginosa* in the gastrointestinal tract is common among seriously ill hospitalized patients. *P. aeruginosa* was found in a number of environmental areas, but these were not believed to be reservoirs for pathogenic organisms, since the organisms were invariably of the rough, nonpathogenic type not found on patients. Other reports relating to *Pseudomonas* in hospital environments, however, have indicated that fomites (including mop buckets, sink traps, faucet aerators, respirators, nebulizers, hospital food, contaminated oral medications, and flowers) may be reservoirs for *P. aeruginosa* [11, 12]. The first two items are probably of little or no importance as proximate sources of infective organisms.

Modes of Spread
The predominant mode of spread within burn units is transference by personnel who have direct patient contact. Another important mode of spread in some burn units is via whirlpool and Hubbard tank units; for this

and other reasons, the use of whirlpools and Hubbard tanks for burn patients is strongly discouraged.

Prevention
Colonization of the burn patient by *P. aeruginosa* is extremely difficult to prevent. General control measures are important in preventing the spread of this organism, and topical therapy has been beneficial in limiting its growth in colonized patients. Increases in antibiotic resistance patterns emphasize the need for an immunologic approach to therapy. A variety of immunologic approaches to *Pseudomonas* prophylaxis have been tried. Vaccines prepared against lipopolysaccharides, polysaccharides, ribosomes, exoproducts, outer membranes, and flagella have been used in experimental animals and, in some cases, clinical trials. Though some of these preparations appear to have limited merit, continued research is necessary before widespread use of antipseudomonal vaccines can occur. Passive immunization using IgG fractionated from the serum of volunteers immunized with *Pseudomonas* antigens appears to be a practical approach to immunotherapy and is closer to being available for clinical use than is active immunization [3].

Epidemic Infections
Epidemic infections with *P. aeruginosa* are practically nonexistent in a well-controlled environment. Outbreaks traced to contaminated hydrotherapy and respiratory equipment have occurred, and these sources should be carefully evaluated if an outbreak develops.

Other Organisms Causing Burn Infections
Candida albicans
Clinical Course
Invasive infection caused by *Candida albicans* is not frequently seen; it occurs commonly only in patients who have extensive and debilitating burn injuries. Such patients usually received broad-spectrum antibiotics for relatively long periods of time for the treatment of other infectious complications. Clinically,

the granulating wound usually becomes dry and flat with a yellow or orange color. There is a gradual downhill course, during which the patient's temperature and white blood cell count usually remain unchanged.

Predisposing Host Factors

The mechanisms for defense against *Candida* infections are essentially the same as those for bacterial infections, although delayed hypersensitivity mechanisms seem to be more important and antibody-mediated immune reactions less important for ridding the host of these pathogens. Such agents infrequently cause primary infections, but they are troublesome opportunistic invaders in patients with abnormalities of host resistance such as occur in some immunologic deficiency diseases or during immunosuppressive therapy. An improvement in the survival rate for the extensively burned patient has contributed to the rise in the incidence of serious yeast and fungal infections. *Candida* often becomes the predominant organism of mucosal surfaces and burn wounds when the usual bacterial flora have been destroyed by antibiotic therapy, and superinfections not infrequently follow successful treatment for systemic bacterial sepsis. Among mycotic agents, *C. albicans* is the most frequent cause of both local and systemic infections as a secondary invader, probably because of its normal occurrence in the gastrointestinal tract. Local and systemic infections from other mycotic agents, including *Aspergillus* and *Mucor* species, should be exceedingly rare. A report of any *Candida* species in the wounds or body fluids of a burned patient should be viewed with concern.

Although the presence of *Candida* on the burn wound only is of little clinical significance in the majority of cases, colonization may precede invasion, which can herald the occurrence of *Candida* septicemia and systemic mycosis. In this instance, biopsies of the burn wound can be helpful, because the demonstration of pseudohyphae deep in viable subcutaneous tissue by wound biopsy can alert the clinician to the danger of possible *Candida* septicemia and systemic candidiasis

[16]. However, these wounds should have been excised earlier under most circumstances. Systemic candidiasis may also be suspected by the demonstration of *Candida* organisms in the urine. Krause and co-workers [10] have demonstrated candiduria in a human promptly after swallowing a pure culture of *albicans*, and they have shown that invasion from the gastrointestinal tract can be effectively controlled by the use of oral nystatin (Mycostatin).

Colonization of the burn wound depends on several predisposing factors, including antibiotic therapy. Nash and associates [15] have shown a tenfold increase in the occurrence of fungi on burn wounds following the use of mafenide acetate cream as a topical antibacterial agent at the U.S. Army Institute of Surgical Research. Seelig [18] has noted the development of candidiasis in patients receiving multiple systemic broad-spectrum antibiotics. Williams and colleagues [25] have noted an increase in the incidence of candidiasis in association with certain therapeutic measures—that is, the use of blood transfusions, central venous pressure lines, and intravenous hyperalimentation therapy.

Therapy

Local colonization with *Candida* in the burn wound can be controlled by the incorporation of nystatin in the appropriate topical antibacterial agent. Systemic spread from the gastrointestinal tract can be effectively controlled by the use of oral nystatin. Early invasive candidiasis should be treated by the discontinuation of systemic antibiotic therapy whenever possible, the removal of intravenous and urinary catheters, and the intravenous administration of amphotericin B or the recently available fluconazole.

Endemic and Epidemic Infections

Endemic colonization of the wounds of burn patients with *C. albicans* can be minimized by the limited and selective use of antibiotic therapy, including, whenever possible, the avoidance of broad-spectrum agents. Consideration might also be given to the prophylactic use of oral nystatin in units experiencing high rates of *Candida* infection. Epidemic infections with candidal organisms are rarely seen in well-controlled burn units.

Other Aerobic Gram-Negative Bacteria
Pathogenic Agents
Gram-negative enteric bacteria other than *P. aeruginosa* have become increasingly important in infections occurring in burn patients. These organisms include *Escherichia, Klebsiella, Proteus, Enterobacter,* and *Acinetobacter* species. *Salmonella* and *Shigella* species do not seem to cause infections of the burn wound. The gram-negative organisms generally appear on a burn wound as a consequence of contamination from the endogenous flora of the patient or the environment, but the most important factor in their becoming pathogenic is the selective elimination of competing gram-positive organisms from the burn wound by antibiotic therapy. Another problem of special importance is that these organisms can be controlled on the burn wound, but they can rarely be eliminated by antibiotic therapy. When antibiotic-resistant strains begin to appear, the transfer of resistance (R) factors to nonresistant strains occurs (frequently even to different genera), which leads to the accumulation and proliferation of antibiotic-resistant organisms within the nosocomial environment of the burn unit [17] (see Chaps. 12, 14).

Transmissibility
Most of the gram-negative bacteria of enteric origin have low pathogenicity, and most infections occur because the host is immunologically compromised.

Clinical Features
Invasive infections may show deterioration of healthy granulation tissue, which becomes edematous and pale. Classic ecthyma gangrenosum is rare with gram-negative organisms other than *Pseudomonas,* but progressive thrombosis of extensively invaded vessels can occur and result in conversion of partial-thickness injuries to full-thickness injuries. The clinical picture of systemic infections with these gram-negative organisms in burn patients is similar to that of gram-negative septicemia in other patients. Systemic infection is usually heralded by an initial elevation in temperature, which may be followed by hypothermia in later stages. Hypotension is not uncommon. Either leukocytosis or leukopenia may be present, but there is usually a marked shift in the differential count to immature forms.

Predisposing Host Factors
Abnormalities of complement, natural antibody, and neutrophil antibacterial function have all been shown to be important in the development of systemic invasion with these organisms.

Therapy
Systemic gentamicin has been our drug of choice for initial treatment of gram-negative sepsis before specific antibiotic sensitivity patterns are established, but therapy should be altered if so indicated by specific sensitivities. Topical therapy can be determined based on the results obtained using an agar well diffusion topical antimicrobial test assay.

Prevention
Most infections caused by gram-negative bacteria are endemic, and there is a relatively high incidence of superinfections following therapy for infections with gram-positive organisms. The usual source of the gram-negative agents is the gastrointestinal tract of the patients themselves. Hyperendemic disease caused by one or more of the pathogens may occur from time to time within particular burn units, and this probably results from the establishment of a large reservoir of a particular strain. Such strains are usually multiply drug-resistant and are selected by the continuous use of particular popular antibiotic regimens. They are usually found in the patients and environment of the burn unit, and continual cross-colonization and infection of new admissions take place. Parenteral antibiotic therapy in burn patients should thus be restricted to situations with clear indications, and periodic shifts in popular drug regimens, when possible, might also

be considered. The prevention of such infections depends on excellent care of the burn wound and strict attention to the general control measures mentioned earlier in this chapter, including the use of the BCNUs.

Anaerobic Bacterial Infections

Anaerobic infections following burn injury are surprisingly infrequent, possibly because of the aerobic environment of the burn wound in most instances. However, early contamination with clostridial species, including *Clostridium perfringens* and *Clostridium tetani*, is relatively common. In very deep burns, such as can occur with electrical injuries in which muscle necrosis is often associated, prevention of gas gangrene and tetanus should be of great concern, and early debridement or excision of dead tissue is advisable. Tetanus in the burn patient is a potential hazard in almost every case, but it can be easily prevented by current active and passive immunization procedures. In present practice, both gas gangrene and tetanus are exceedingly rare. Other types of anaerobic infections, such as those caused by *Bacteroides* species, are also very uncommon and cause no particular problem.

Viral Infections

Viral infections have increasingly been reported in burn patients. Herpesvirus and cytomegalovirus are the agents most frequently found, either by serologic tests or by direct culture. The clinical significance of these findings is not clear at the present time.

References

1. Aldrich, R.H. The role of infection in burns: The theory and treatment with special reference to gentian violet. *N. Engl. J. Med.* 208: 299, 1933.
2. Alexander, J.W. Infections in the Patient with Severe Burns. In: H.J. Nahmis and R.J.
O'Reilly (Eds.), *Immunology of Human Infections*, Vol. 1. New York: Plenum (in press).
3. Alexander, J.W., and Fisher, M.W. Immunization against *Pseudomonas* in infection after thermal injury. J. Infect. Dis. 130:S152, 1974.
4. Bowser, B.H., Caldwell, F.T., Baker, J.A., and Walls, R.C. Statistical methods to predict morbidity and mortality: Self assessment techniques for burn units. *Burns* 9:318, 1983.
5. Burke, J.F. The effective period of preventive antibiotic action in experimental incisions and dermal lesions. *Surgery* 50:161, 1961.
6. Burke, J.F., et al. The contribution of a bacterially isolated environment to the prevention of infection in seriously burned patients. *Ann. Surg.* 186:377, 1977.
7. Glew, R.H., Moellering, R.C., and Burke, J.F. Gentamicin dosage in children with extensive burns. *J. Trauma* 16:819, 1976.
8. Haynes, B.W., Jr., and Hench, M.E. Hospital isolation system for preventing cross-contamination by staphylococcal and pseudomonas organisms in burn wounds. *Ann. Surg.* 162: 641, 1965.
9. Herndon, D.N., et al. Determinants of mortality in pediatric patients with greater than 70% full-thickness total body surface area thermal injury treated by early total excision and grafting. *J. Trauma* 27:208, 1987.
10. Krause, W., Matheis, K., and Wulf, K. Fungemia and funguria after oral administration of *Candida albicans. Lancet* 1:598, 1969.
11. Lowbury, E.J.L. Infection of burns. *Br. Med. J.* 1:994, 1960.
12. Lowbury, E.J.L., and Fox, J. The epidemiology of infection with *Pseudomonas pyocyanea* in a burns unit. *J. Hyg.* (Camb.) 52:403, 1954.
13. MacMillan, B.G., Edmonds, P., Hummel, R.P., and Maley, M.P. Epidemiology of *Pseudomonas* in a burn intensive care unit. *J. Trauma* 13: 627, 1973.
14. McManus, A.T., et al. Comparison of quantitative microbiology and histopathology in divided burn-wound biopsy specimens. *Arch. Surg.* 122:74, 1987.
15. Nash, G., et al. Fungal burn wound infection. *J.A.M.A.* 215:1664, 1971.
16. Nash, G., Foley, F.D., and Bruitt, B.A., Jr. *Candida* burn-wound invasion: A cause of systemic candidiasis. *Arch. Pathol.* 90:75, 1970.
17. Roe, E., and Jones, R.J. Effects of topical chemoprophylaxis on transferable antibiotic resistance in burns. *Lancet* 1:109, 1972.
18. Seelig, M. The role of antibiotics in the pathogenesis of *Candida* infections. *Am. J. Med.* 40:887, 1966.
19. Shooter, R.A., Fecal carriage of *Pseudomonas aeruginosa* in hospital patients: Possible spread from patient to patient. *Lancet* 2:1331, 1966.
20. Steffen, E.K., Berg, R.D., and Deitch, E.A.

Comparison of translocation rates of various indigenous bacteria from the gastrointestinal tract to the mesenteric lymph node. *J. Infect. Dis.* 157:1032, 1988.

21. Thomsen, M. The burns unit in Copenhagen: VI. Infection rates. *Scand. J. Plast. Reconstr. Surg.* 4:53, 1970.

22. Tompkins, R.G., et al. Prompt eschar excision: A treatment system contributing to reduced burn mortality. *Ann. Surg.* 204:272, 1986.

23. Tompkins, R.G., et al. Significant reductions in mortality for children with burn injuries through the use of prompt eschar excision. *Ann. Surg.* 208:577, 1988.

24. Wells, C.L., Maddaus, M.A., and Simmons, R.L. Proposed mechanisms for the translocation of intestinal bacteria. *Rev. Infect. Dis.* 10: 958, 1988.

25. Williams, R., Chandler, J., and Orloff, J.J. *Candida* septicemia. *Arch. Surg.* 103:8, 1971.

26. Zaske, D.E., Sawchuk, R.J., Gerding, D.N., and Strate, R.G. Increased dosage requirements of gentamicin in burn patients. *J. Trauma* 16:284, 1976.

Infections of Cardiac and Vascular Prostheses

John P. Burke

The development of synthetic materials that are chemically inert and durable enough to retain their geometric and other physical properties over many years has made possible the wide application of reconstructive operations on the heart and blood vessels. Devices that are commonly implanted in the cardiovascular system include cardiac valve prostheses, patches for repairing congenital heart defects, arterial grafts, permanent cardiac pacemakers, and arteriovenous shunts for performing hemodialysis. Ventriculoatrial shunts for treating hydrocephalus are discussed in Chapter 32 and will not be specifically addressed in this chapter.

All prosthetic devices have the propensity to fail because of mechanical, thromboembolic, or infectious complications. The risk of these complications continues throughout the life of the prosthesis. Operations to implant prostheses, therefore, should be viewed as palliative rather than curative. Fortunately, failure of the prosthesis need not be catastrophic because replacement is often feasible.

Although many varieties of cardiac valve substitutes have been developed, only several have achieved widespread use [31, 73]. Current heart valve prostheses may be classified as either mechanical or tissue valves. The caged ball, tilting disc, and bileaflet valves are the principal types of mechanical prostheses. Tissue valves may be of either human or animal origin. In recent years, the use of cryopreserved human homografts has increased. The various types of porcine xenografts that have been widely implanted in the past two decades are constructed of an aortic valve removed from a pig, treated with glutaraldehyde for sterilization and tanning, and mounted on a prosthetic support. Bovine pericardial xenografts are similar to the porcine valves but are no longer marketed in the

United States. All heart valve prostheses have similar and persistent risks of endocarditis, but late structural failure is more common with tissue than with mechanical valves [33, 34, 77].

Nature of Infections
Incidence
Patients who receive cardiovascular implants are predisposed to a variety of nosocomial infections. The overall frequency of infections following open-heart operations, for example, has ranged from 8 to 44 percent [17, 70]. The highest rates of infection have been found when special efforts have been made to identify minor and asymptomatic infections. The most common infections are of the respiratory tract, the sternal wound and mediastinum, and the bloodstream [7, 12, 24a, 63, 64, 66, 68].

The frequencies of intracardiac and other infections that occur in tissues adjacent to the prostheses vary widely and are lower in patients operated on in the 1970s than in those operated on in the 1960s (60). Insufficient data are available to determine whether further decreases occurred in the 1980s. Table 35-1 shows representative rates of infection according to actuarial methods of data analysis, if available, for each of the major groups of cardiac and vascular prostheses [10, 30, 50, 84]. The highest rates of infection are associated with devices such as external arteriovenous cannulas that are continuously

Table 35-1. Frequencies of cardiovascular prosthesis—associated infections

Type of prosthesis	Percentage of patients with infections
Cardiac valve [10]	
12 Months after surgery	3.1[a]
60 Months after surgery	5.7[a]
Vascular prosthesis	
Aortic graft [30]	0.77–2.6
Permanent pacemaker [84]	4.0
Hemodialysis fistula/graft [50]	1.3[b]

[a]Cumulative rates.
[b]Rate per 100 patient-months.

exposed to skin flora and with vascular grafts that require an incision involving the groin [30]. Endocarditis has occurred more often with aortic than mitral prostheses, although this has not been true in more recent reports [36, 45]. The risk does appear greater after multiple valve implantations than after single valve implantation. Similarly, the risk of infection appears greater with a prosthetic cardiac valve than with a patch repair of a congenital heart defect [76].

Infections at the site of a prosthetic implant account for a minuscule proportion of the entire spectrum of nosocomial infections. Nonetheless, the cost of these infections is high compared to that of many other types of nosocomial infection [65] and, for patients with infected cardiac valve prostheses, the mean case fatality rate was 54.6 percent in eight studies summarized in 1982 [60]. However, more effective antibiotic therapy and prompt aggressive replacement of infected prostheses in many instances have been associated with an overall survival rate that now approaches 70 percent [51].

The small numbers of reported cases, the anecdotal nature of many reports, and the lack of a centrally coordinated national surveillance of patients who receive prosthetic implants are each responsible for important gaps in epidemiologic information. Case report information is not reliably returned to the hospital or physician responsible for the implantation of the device, and surveillance of in-hospital events will miss prosthetic device—related infections that often appear at a distance both in time and place. It has recently been proposed that existing infection control units develop a system to return case data to the hospital of origin [40]. Computer-assisted reporting systems for the long-term follow-up of patients with prosthetic heart valves and uniform guidelines for reporting morbidity and mortality after cardiac valvular operations are beginning to appear and may help to establish baseline levels of endemic infections associated with these prostheses [23, 58]. One example of the benefits to a community hospital of surveillance of selected clean cardiac and vascular surgical procedures has been reported in which modest increases in wound infection rates led to the uncovering of possible problems in the cleaning of sternal saws and in the inappropriate timing of "on-call" prophylactic antibiotics [47].

Epidemics in cardiac surgery units have generally been recognized by the occurrence of infections due to an unusual pathogen rather than by an analysis of the overall infection rate. Two outbreaks of *Aspergillus* infections associated with cardiac prostheses and one "outbreak" with 2 cases of *Penicillium* endocarditis, for example, were traced to environmental contamination [28, 32, 61]. Organisms of the *Mycobacterium fortuitum* complex, including *Mycobacterium chelonei*, have been recognized as an intrinsic contaminant of porcine valve prostheses, a cause of epidemic sternal wound infections following cardiac surgery, and a cause of prosthetic valve endocarditis. Although modifications of the glutaraldehyde disinfection regimen used by a company to prepare porcine bioprostheses appear to have reduced the risk of such intrinsic contamination, the possible source of contamination in several outbreaks is still unidentified [39]. Nonsterile ice water used for cooling the cardioplegic solution was the possible environmental source in one outbreak [56].

A few experiences have raised the disturbing possibilities that outbreaks due to common organisms may also be insidious and protracted. Clustering of cases of prosthetic valve endocarditis caused by *Staphylococcus epidermidis* has been observed and, in one hospital, was associated with an attack rate of 10 percent over a 32-month period [21, 35]. In several outbreaks, methicillin-resistant *S. epidermidis* sternal wound infections and prosthetic valve endocarditis have been linked to chronic carriers of the epidemic strains [8, 59, 62, 79]. In another outbreak, the intensive care unit staff was the suspected source, with transient hand carriage being an important route of transmission [41].

Other recent investigations have identified previously unsuspected sources and pathways of infection. *Pseudomonas cepacia* and *Xanthomonas maltophilia* bacteremias after open-heart surgery have been linked to contaminated transducers used with intraarterial pressure-monitoring systems that became contaminated even though disposable transducer domes were used [25, 86]. *Serratia marcescens* bacteremia has similarly been associated with the use of intraaortic balloon pumps and re-usable pressure transducers that were not processed with high-level disinfection or sterilization between patient uses [82]. An outbreak of bacteremia with *Enterobacter cloacae* among aortic valve surgery patients was associated with nonsterile manometers used to measure the pressure of cardioplegia solution injected into the coronary arteries [11], and cardioplegia solution contaminated with *E. cloacae* has been recognized as a cause of a variety of septic complications [42]. *Legionella* sternal wound infection and endocarditis have been associated with postoperative bathing with contaminated tap water [57a].

Finally, outbreaks associated with the injudicious use of quaternary ammonium compounds as disinfectants have been a recurring problem in cardiovascular surgery units (see Chap. 15). In the early years of open-heart surgery, improper cleaning of cardiopulmonary bypass equipment with these agents was responsible for bacteremic infections. Recently, contaminated disinfectants used on various surfaces in the operating room were also associated with contamination of blood in extracorporeal circulators and with subsequent cases of sternal wound infection and endocarditis due to *S. marcescens* [24].

Pathogens

A wide variety of bacterial, mycobacterial, fungal, and rickettsial species has been identified from infections associated with cardiovascular prostheses. Although gram-negative bacilli are the most frequent isolates in many nosocomial infections, this has not been true of cardiac and vascular prosthesis-associated infections (Table 35-2). Gram-negative bacilli are especially common in retroperitoneal vascular prostheses contaminated from the gastrointestinal or genitourinary tract. Multiple organisms are often isolated in mixed culture from infections associated with arterial grafts

Table 35-2. Causative agents of infections associated with cardiac valve and aortofemoral vascular prostheses

Organism	No. (%) of cases with cardiac valve prosthesis[a]		No. (%) of cases with aortofemoral prosthesis[b]	
	≤12 mo[c]	>12 mo	≤4 mo	>4 mo
Coagulase-negative staphylococci	41 (56.9)	10 (22.7)		15 (55.5)
Staphylococcus aureus	5 (6.9)	5 (11.4)	1 (33.3)	2 (7.4)
Gram-negative bacilli	3 (4.2)	1 (2.3)	3 (100.0)	8 (29.6)
Streptococci (nonenterococcal)	1 (1.4)	12 (27.2)		2 (7.4)
Enterococci	2 (2.8)	4 (9.1)	1 (33.3)	
Diphtheroids	4 (5.6)	1 (2.3)		
Fungi	4 (5.6)	1 (2.3)		
Fastidious gram-negative coccobacilli	1 (1.4)	7 (15.9)		
Other	5 (6.9)	1 (2.3)		1 (3.7)
Culture negative	6 (8.3)	2 (4.5)		3 (11.1)
Total	72 (100.0)	44 (100.0)	3 (100.0)	27 (100.0)

[a] Multiple organisms reported in 2 cases (other). From S.B. Calderwood et al., Risk factors for the development of prosthetic valve endocarditis. *Circulation* 72:31, 1985.
[b] Multiple organisms reported in 5 cases. From D.F. Bandyk, G.A. Berni, B.L. Thiele, and J.B. Towne, Aortofemoral graft infection due to *Staphylococcus epidermidis.* *Arch. Surg.* 119:102, 1984.
[c] Time of onset after surgery.

[4] and cardiac pacemakers, especially from pulse-generator pocket abscesses [13, 84]. *Staphylococcus aureus* is the pathogen most often responsible for infections of vascular access sites for hemodialysis [50]; however, an appreciable number of cases are due to enteric gram-negative bacilli and *Pseudomonas* species [19]. Recent reports have documented hemodialysis fistula infections due to unusual causes such as *Legionella pneumophila* and *Cephalosporium* species [48, 67].

Organisms that have been judged to be of low virulence are often recovered from these infections and cannot be easily dismissed as contaminants in blood cultures. Staphylococci, especially *S. epidermidis,* are involved most often in prosthetic valve endocarditis and have also been recognized to have increasing importance in late arterial graft infection [30]. Streptococci (both α-hemolytic and group D), a variety of enteric gram-negative bacilli, diphtheroids, fastidious gram-negative coccobacilli (the so-called HACEK group), and *Candida* and *Aspergillus* organisms are also commonly found in prosthetic cardiac valve endocarditis. The relative frequencies of the different pathogens may vary in different centers; for example, *S. epidermidis* was found

in only 2 of 45 cases at the Mayo Clinic [87]. The patterns of microbial species reported from infections associated with patch repairs for congenital heart defects are similar to those from prosthetic valve infections, although staphylococci may be more frequent with prosthetic valve endocarditis [49].

Classification of Infections

The Centers for Disease Control's (CDC's) revised definitions for nosocomial infections are formulated as algorithms and now include criteria for cardiovascular system infection that can be applied to endocarditis of prosthetic heart valves and mediastinitis after open-heart surgery [29]. These definitions are not entirely satisfactory for nosocomial infections related to other intravascular prostheses and require additional interpretation. However, a physician's diagnosis of infection derived from direct observation during surgery or other diagnostic study, or based on clinical judgment, is recognized as an acceptable criterion unless there is compelling evidence to the contrary. Positive blood cultures alone are insufficient evidence of prosthesis-associated infection because patients may have bacteremia or fungemia from a focal infection without involvement of the prostheses [71]. In contrast, others with prosthesis-associated infection may not have positive blood cultures, as when subvalvular ring abscesses are present and direct communications with the bloodstream are absent [36].

The clinical onset of infection related to an intracardiac prosthesis may be delayed until weeks or months after the operative procedure and discharge from the hospital. The incubation period of postoperative infections related to prosthetic materials is often uncertain and probably varies within broad limits, perhaps depending on such factors as the virulence of the organism, size of the inoculum, prophylactic use of antibiotics, and host resistance. Infections related to prosthetic cardiac valves have been classified according to the time of onset of symptoms as either *early* (less than 60 days after the operation) or *late* (more than 60 days after). In recent studies, the similarities in the patterns of organisms causing prosthetic valve endocarditis throughout the initial 12 months after surgery (Table 35-2) and the association of these organisms with nosocomial acquisition have suggested that 12 months may be a better break point for defining nosocomial infection than the 60-day period [51]. For example, nearly all *S. epidermidis* infections in the first 12 months are methicillin-resistant, whereas only approximately 30 percent of those occurring later are methicillin-resistant (see Chap. 13) [10]. Infections throughout the initial 12-month period are considered to arise most commonly either from intraoperative contamination or from perioperative invasive devices and catheters, whereas the late-onset cases arise from bacteremias such as those associated with dental, urinary, or other medical procedures.

Infections associated with vascular prostheses may also be classified as either early or late in onset, although a 4-month break point is commonly suggested (see Table 35-2). Vascular grafts may be more susceptible to infection from bacteremias during the first 4 months postoperatively, but the majority of infections in both early and late groups are believed to arise from contamination at the time of implantation. Therefore, infections that become apparent within 12 months after placement of a cardiovascular prosthesis should be classified as nosocomial, even though some patients with community-acquired infections will be incorrectly classified. In addition, intravascular infections that are secondary to nosocomial infections in other sites, such as the urinary or respiratory tract, should be considered separate nosocomial infections even though their onset may occur after hospital discharge. A patient who enters the hospital with an intravascular infection for which he or she receives a vascular graft or prosthesis and who later develops postoperative infection with a new and different organism involving the implanted material should also be considered to have a nosocomial infection.

Diagnostic Criteria

The sudden appearance of a regurgitant murmur or cardiac failure, the disappearance of the distinct click of a mechanical prosthetic valve, an abnormal tilting motion of the valve demonstrated fluoroscopically, or evidence of a new vegetation seen on echocardiogram are each virtually diagnostic of endocarditis in patients with prosthetic cardiac valves and sustained bacteremia. Furthermore, bacteremia that is persistent after extracardiac sources of infection have been eliminated strongly supports a diagnosis of endocarditis. Criteria have been presented to categorize the diagnosis of endocarditis as *definite, probable,* or *possible* [83]. Varying combinations of findings that support a diagnosis of endocarditis in the presence of an intracardiac prosthesis are listed in the CDC definitions for nosocomial infection [29]. This surveillance definition requires that, in the absence of isolation of the organism from direct culture of the valve itself or a vegetation, the physician must have instituted appropriate antimicrobial therapy if the diagnosis was made antemortem.

Positive blood cultures are not as common in patients with vascular graft infections as in those with prosthetic valve endocarditis. Bleeding, clotting, or other evidence of malfunction of the graft are diagnostic of infection in the presence of purulent wound drainage, exteriorization of the graft, or systemic sepsis.

In the presence of clinical findings of infection, the discovery of microorganisms by microscopy or culture in vegetations or pus removed from completely intravascular prostheses at either repeat operations or autopsy is evidence of active infection. A positive culture from a removed arteriovenous cannula or an extruded cardiac pacemaker, in conjunction with the recovery of the same organism from a blood culture obtained from a different site, is also evidence of prosthesis infection. In most other instances, the diagnosis of infection at the site of a cardiovascular prosthesis is indirect and is based on the presence of either typical clinical findings or repeated positive blood cultures, or both.

Predisposing Factors

Postoperative endocarditis occurs more often following open-heart surgery that requires the implantation of foreign material than following other open-heart procedures. Foreign bodies may potentiate infection both by reducing the inoculum of bacteria required to induce inflammation and by promoting sequestration of bacteria in areas inaccessible to host defenses [20] (see Chap. 33). Bacterial adherence to the prosthetic device, conditioned by a layer of host substances known as *biofilm,* is also important in the genesis of foreign body–associated infections. Adherence to these host proteins appears to be responsible for the ability of *S. aureus* to cause device-related infections, whereas *S. epidermidis* commonly produces a slime layer that facilitates colonization of the device [15].

The risk of infection has generally been believed to be greater in procedures involving the placement of a prosthesis in a high-pressure system with turbulent blood flow, which might explain, in part, the higher infection rates with prosthetic valve implantations than with patch repairs of congenital heart defects. The risks of infection are similar for all available cardiac valve prostheses.

However, two recent reports document a significantly higher risk in the early months after valve replacement with mechanical prostheses than with bioprostheses [10, 44]. However, based on 5 years of follow-up, there appears to be no significant difference in the cumulative risk between mechanical and porcine valve recipients [10].

Cardiopulmonary bypass itself appears to reduce the defense mechanisms of patients as well as to increase the opportunities for operative contamination, and the deleterious hematologic consequences may be greater with bubble than with membrane oxygenators [43, 80, 81]. Concomitant infection in other sites, such as the urinary or lower respiratory tract, the surgical wound, and venous and arterial catheters, provides a source for direct contamination during the operative procedure and also predisposes to bacteremia with seeding of the prosthetic device. The risk of infection at the site of a femoral-popliteal arterial graft is increased by open, infected lesions on the legs at the time of the operation [37].

The most important single factor shaping the character of postoperative endocarditis and other infections related to cardiovascular prostheses is the use of antimicrobial agents before, during, and after operative procedures. The extensive preoperative use of antibiotics may increase the risk of postoperative endocarditis when an intracardiac prosthesis is implanted [57]. The reasons for this are not clear, but they may be related to the replacement of normal flora by antibiotic-resistant species and the overgrowth of certain microbial flora of the skin, mucous membranes, or gastrointestinal tract. The use of prophylactic antimicrobial agents during and after operations has been responsible for shifting the patterns of infecting agents to a more antibiotic-resistant group of pathogens including *S. epidermidis,* the diphtheroids, and various fungi [2].

The overall risk of infection is probably greater with longer than with shorter courses of chemotherapy, both preoperatively and postoperatively. When a major break in aseptic technique occurs during the operation, however, prophylaxis merges with early treatment, and a prolonged course of high-dose chemotherapy may be desirable (see Chap. 12).

Certain patients have other risk factors that are commonly associated with nosocomial infections. Serious underlying illnesses (e.g., congestive heart failure, rheumatoid arthritis, and diabetes mellitus) and the use of medications (e.g., steroids and nonsteroidal antiinflammatory drugs) are associated with decreased host resistance and often with defective inflammatory or immune responses, which thereby increase the risks of both prosthesis-associated infection and other focal infections. A high carriage rate of *S. aureus* in asymptomatic patients receiving hemodialysis has been suggested to be related to an increased incidence of shunt infections and bacteremia [54]. This is consistent with the observation that the risk of staphylococcal infections of incisional wounds in general is increased in patients who carry *S. aureus* in the anterior nares (see Chaps. 33, 37).

Specimens
Collection
Isolation of the pathogen from blood cultures is the essential laboratory procedure for the diagnosis and effective treatment of intravascular infections. The techniques for obtaining specimens are far more important than the use of special media or the ability of the laboratory to isolate unusual microbial species (see Chap. 9).

The bacteremias accompanying prosthetic valve endocarditis have not been studied with quantitative blood cultures during the untreated course of the disease, as were those of native valve endocarditis in the preantibiotic era. Patients with prosthetic valve endocarditis appear to have a slightly lower frequency of positive blood cultures than do patients with native valve endocarditis, and positive rates as low as 68 percent have been reported in prosthesis cases [83]. Nonetheless, when bacteremia occurs, it is usually continuous, and timing of blood cultures should not be critical. Blood cultures should be obtained at various intervals to document the *persistence* as well as the *presence* of bacteremia. Continuous bacteremia can be documented by requiring that two or more cultures be positive with the same organism.

The blood obtained from one venipuncture site defines a single blood culture, even though the blood is distributed between aerobic and anaerobic culture bottles at the time of collection. The volume of blood sampled is critically important since there is a direct relation between the volume and culture yield. In adults, a total blood sample of 50 to 60 ml should be sufficient to allow detection of low-density bacteremia. Therefore, four to six blood culture sets are usually recommended when endocarditis is suspected, with each set containing at least 10 ml blood; 1- to 2-ml samples are often taken from infants. However, some automated detection systems supply culture bottles that accommodate volumes of blood that are smaller than 10 ml, and so additional blood culture sets may be needed. The use of antimicrobials within the previous 2 weeks appears to lower the rate of blood culture positivity and may justify the collection of more than six blood culture sets.

The microorganisms that are the most common contaminants in blood cultures (e.g., *S. epidermidis* and diphtheroids) are also often responsible for infections associated with cardiac and vascular prostheses. Strict adherence to aseptic technique and avoidance of sampling from indwelling catheters can reduce the chance that contaminants introduced during blood collection will be assigned clinical importance. Between 1 and 4.5 percent of blood cultures have been reported to be falsely positive [3], and the rate of false-positive cultures depends on the aseptic precautions used in obtaining specimens.

Use of alcohol (70 to 95% isopropanol or 70% ethanol) for skin cleansing followed by tincture of iodine (2%) is preferred for preparing the skin for venipuncture to collect blood for culture. Solutions of benzalkonium chloride and other quaternary ammonium compounds should not be used for skin disinfection because these agents are relatively inactive against gram-negative bacilli and may become contaminated with such organisms. Outbreaks of pseudobacteremia caused by contaminated blood-drawing equipment [22], collection tubes [38], benzalkonium chloride [52], and povidone-iodine [18] have been reported.

The disinfecting agent should be allowed to act for approximately 1 minute, and the venipuncture site should not be probed with a finger unless it has been decontaminated or unless surgical gloves are worn. The diaphragm top of the culture bottle should be wiped with alcohol or tincture of iodine before the needle is inserted. Alcohol may be used to remove residual iodine on the skin after the blood culture is collected.

Evaluation and Special Procedures

Direct communication between the physician and laboratory personnel is necessary for evaluating these serious infections. The physician should be responsible for ensuring that a colony of any microorganism recovered is placed in a holding medium and not discarded by the laboratory as a contaminant. A separate colony from each positive culture should be preserved for later typing by biochemical reactions, antibiotic susceptibility patterns (antibiograms), phage typing, or serologic methods when these results may be useful for determining whether the organisms are pathogens or contaminants (see Chap. 9). If the isolates are clearly different, their probable clinical significance is reduced. Specimens of the isolated microorganism will also be necessary for tests to estimate the effectiveness of antibiotic treatment.

When the clinical findings suggest intravascular infection and the conventional blood cultures are negative, special procedures should be employed to recover potential pathogens. In patients receiving antimicrobials, the optimal blood-to-broth ratio of 1:5 to 1:10 dilutes out most antimicrobial agents to noninhibitory concentrations and also neutralizes the bactericidal effects of whole blood. Because of these antibacterial properties, blood for culture must be inoculated into the medium at the bedside or into collection tubes containing the anticoagulant sodium

polyanetholsulfonate. This substance inhibits phagocytosis, lysozyme, and complement as well as aminoglycoside antibiotics, and is included in many commercially available media. A commercial device for the removal of antibiotics from blood by using an absorbent resin has shown conflicting results in several trials [3].

In special instances, incubation of the cultures should be continued for 2 to 3 weeks so that organisms such as *Candida* species and fastidious gram-negative coccobacilli (*Hemophilus* species, *Actinobacillus actinomycetemcomitans*, *Cardiobacterium hominis*, *Eikenella corrodens*, and *Kingella* species) might be isolated. Nutritionally variant streptococci may fail to grow in routine culture media unless they are supplemented with pyridoxal hydrochloride. Special procedures for recognizing cell wall–defective bacterial variants (L forms) may be performed in research laboratories. The techniques of lysis filtration and lysis centrifugation may permit greater sensitivity for detecting bacteremia, and the use of biphasic media improves the yield of fungi.

Negative blood cultures may be found in patients with intravascular infections due to *Legionella*, *Chlamydia*, *Rickettsia*, *Aspergillus*, *Candida*, and certain other fungi. If embolism to a major artery occurs, the embolus should be removed and later examined and cultured to detect the presence of fungi. *Candida* and *Aspergillus* may be isolated more often from arterial blood than from venous blood. Blood cultures are also occasionally negative when bacterial infection involves the right side of the heart.

Clinical Aspects of Intravascular Infections
Manifestations
General Features

The symptoms and signs of intravascular infection related to prosthetic materials are similar to those of native valve infective endocarditis, with some important differences such as more frequent signs of valve dysfunction and myocardial invasion in prosthetic valve endocarditis. The intravascular location is the feature that all these infections have in common and that is responsible for their protean manifestations. The specific clinical features are determined by the type and location of the prosthesis, nature of the responsible microbial agent, and presence of underlying chronic illness, especially uremia.

The most common symptoms are nonspecific, such as fever, malaise, and weakness. Fever and other signs of infection may be suppressed by injudicious antibiotic treatment before the true nature of the infection is recognized, or they may not occur in the presence of chronic illness such as uremia. In patients whose illness begins early in the postoperative period, the dominant symptoms may be of associated infection, such as pneumonia and wound infection.

Valvular Prostheses

In patients with prosthetic cardiac valves, the occurrence of regurgitant murmurs and severe cardiac failure as a result of dehiscence of the prosthesis is highly suggestive of endocarditis, but valve dysfunction may be due to technical or mechanical problems rather than to endocarditis. Prosthetic valve endocarditis is frequently accompanied by embolic phenomena and paravalvular myocardial abscesses. The valve itself may become occluded by a thrombus. Other findings usually associated with endocarditis—such as anemia, hematuria (macroscopic or microscopic), Roth's spots, subungual hemorrhages, conjunctival petechiae, and enlargement of the spleen—help to direct attention to the possibility of intravascular infection. Acute fulminant presentation with hypotension may occur, especially with infections caused by *S. aureus* or *Streptococcus pyogenes* [51].

Fungal endocarditis with unusually large and friable vegetations is often complicated by embolic occlusion of the large arteries, especially those in the lower extremities. The complications of uveitis or endophthalmitis are especially suggestive of infection due to *Candida* species.

Other Vascular Prostheses

In endocarditis following repair of a congenital heart defect (e.g., ventricular septal defect), the only evidence of infection may be fever, either low-grade or spiking. Separation of the patch with or without subsequent embolism may occur.

Inflammation at the operation site may be found in patients with infected arterial grafts, subcutaneous cardiac pacemakers, and arteriovenous shunts. Common signs of infections related to arterial grafts are bleeding, clotting of the prosthesis, localized abscess, chronic draining sinus, and peripheral septic emboli with secondary abscesses. Arteriovenous shunts may also show instability of the cannula, oozing of blood, repeated clotting, or local abscess.

Management
Initial Treatment

The management of bacterial infections associated with intravascular prostheses requires the use of high doses of bactericidal antimicrobial agents intravenously and a consideration of the removal and possible replacement of the prosthesis. The principles of antimicrobial therapy are similar to those for the treatment of native valve endocarditis [5]. Full bacteriologic study of the susceptibility of the pathogen is necessary for optimal treatment of these intravascular infections. Nonetheless, chemotherapy is often begun before the results of the susceptibility tests are available. The selection of antimicrobial agents at that time is based on consideration of the usual sensitivities of the specific pathogen and the antimicrobial agents previously used for that patient. The pathogen should be assumed to be resistant to the prophylactic antibiotics used for open-heart surgery. Postoperative infections commonly occur, however, with organisms that are susceptible to the prophylactic antibiotics as determined by conventional laboratory tests, especially in infections due to *S. aureus* [53].

In fulminant prosthetic valve endocarditis, especially when complicated by hemodynamic instability due to prosthetic valve dysfunction, it is necessary to begin treatment promptly. Even in urgent circumstances, it is possible to obtain several blood cultures before treatment is begun. Initial treatment before culture results are available commonly includes vancomycin and gentamicin. Some experts also recommend that ampicillin or an expanded-spectrum cephalosporin be used as well to cover fastidious gram-negative coccobacilli when the onset is 6 or more months after surgery [51].

Treatment for Specific Pathogens

The details of antimicrobial therapy for the various pathogens reflect an evolving science that is beyond the scope of this discussion, but some general guidelines and comments are warranted. Antimicrobial treatment regimens for intravascular infection in the presence of prosthetic devices differ from those required for treatment of infections not associated with foreign bodies. The treatment of prosthetic valve endocarditis nearly always requires the use of a combination of two or more antibiotic agents, and treatment is generally continued for longer periods of time: 4 to 6 weeks for uncomplicated endocarditis due to penicillin-susceptible streptococci and 6 to 8 weeks for nonstreptococcal endocarditis. A penicillinase-resistant penicillin is used for infections due to *S. aureus*, although penicillin G can be used if the minimum inhibitory concentration of the organism is less than 0.1 μg/ml. The addition of an aminoglycoside for the initial 2 weeks of therapy has been advocated for more rapid killing of *S. aureus*, provided that the isolate is susceptible. Use of rifampin as part of a combination regimen is controversial because its use may result in either synergy or antagonism.

The majority of strains of coagulase-negative staphylococci are resistant to methicillin. Special care is required when disk susceptibility or microbroth dilution tests are used to detect resistance to penicillinase-resistant penicillins because the resistance is heterogeneic—that is, only a small subpopulation of organisms is highly resistant while the bulk of the population is susceptible. Apparent susceptibility should be confirmed using higher inocula on agar containing the antibiotic or other special tests (see Chap. 12).

Unless susceptibility to methicillin can be confirmed, coagulase-negative staphylococci should be assumed to be resistant to all β-lactam antibiotics, including cephalosporins. Optimal therapy for methicillin-resistant staphylococci (*S. epidermidis*) is provided by vancomycin combined with gentamicin (for the first 2 weeks of therapy) and rifampin. If the organism is resistant to gentamicin, another aminoglycoside to which it is susceptible should be used.

Intravascular prosthesis—associated infections due to viridans streptococci, enterocci, or diphtheroids may usually be treated with combined penicillin G and gentamicin. The American Heart Association currently recommends that gentamicin be given for at least the first 2 weeks of therapy, even for highly penicillin-susceptible viridans streptococci [5]. Nutritionally variant streptococci should be treated with this combination therapy for the full duration of treatment. Some strains of diphtheroids are resistant to the combination of penicillin and gentamicin, and other strains may be difficult to test for susceptibility because of their slow growth. Vancomycin with or without gentamicin appears to be an effective alternative.

Most patients with infections due to nonenterococcal streptococci or methicillin-sensitive staphylococci who are allergic to penicillin can be safely treated with first-generation cephalosporins. A cephalosporin can be used if the reaction to penicillin is mild or the history is vague. Vancomycin is a suitable alternative for patients with a history of a life-threatening reaction to either penicillin or a cephalosporin and should be used in most instances when there is a history of an anaphylactic reaction to penicillin therapy. In rare instances, the physician may wish to consult detailed protocols for penicillin desensitization.

Selection of antibiotics for treating infections due to gram-negative bacilli is based on in vitro susceptibility testing and, when available, studies of antibiotic synergy. Initial therapy must always include at least two antimicrobial agents that are likely to be effective against recent nosocomial isolates of that species in the hospital in which the patient was most likely infected. The newer expanded-spectrum cephalosporins and carbapenem antibiotics and the monobactam aztreonam are useful additions to the aminoglycosides and ureidopenicillins that have been the mainstays of treatment of serious gram-negative bacillary infections. Nonetheless, these infections nearly always require early operative intervention, and removal and replacement of the prosthesis may be lifesaving.

Yeast and fungal infections, which are usually due to *Candida* or *Aspergillus* species, require removal of the prosthesis and systemic treatment with amphotericin B. The value of combining amphotericin B with either 5-fluorocytosine or rifampin is unclear. The newer imidazoles, fluconazole and itraconazole, may be useful in *Candida* and *Aspergillus* prosthetic valve endocarditis, respectively, but they may antagonize amphotericin B.

The effectiveness of chemotherapy in bacterial infections is commonly monitored by determining the antibacterial activity of the patient's serum against the organism recovered from the blood (or from the prosthesis itself) with a serial, twofold dilution test. Numerous problems have been associated with such tests, including determing the most appropriate time for collection of the blood specimen (peak versus trough antibiotic levels), lack of standardized methods for performing the tests, and lack of evidence that the results are of prognostic value [85]. The test is especially likely to result in misleading information in assessing regimens that rely on combinations of antibiotics to produce bactericidal synergy.

Antibiotic assays are a suitable substitute for serial, twofold dilution tests of the patient's serum when the infecting organism is known to be susceptible, and such assays can assist in preventing toxicity from excessive drug levels. Assays are also preferable in monitoring therapy with antibiotics that are highly protein-bound or sensitive to pH changes, since erratic results sometimes occur with the serum dilution method.

Removal of Prostheses

Vigorous antibiotic therapy will cure some intravascular prosthesis infections; in others, antibiotics may suppress the systemic signs and symptoms while the infection persists at the site of the prosthesis. Antibiotic therapy of prosthetic valve endocarditis fails more often in cases with an early postoperative onset than in those with a late onset. To detect antibiotic failure at the earliest possible time, it is useful to obtain blood for culture periodically during treatment and once or twice in the 8 weeks after the completion of treatment.

Removal of an intracardiac prosthesis is necessary when antibiotic therapy has failed to clear the bacteremia or if fever persists for 10 days or more during appropriate antibiotic therapy. Other indications for the removal of a prosthetic valve, in addition to uncontrolled infection or resistance of the organism to available bactericidal chemotherapeutic agents, include moderate to severe heart failure due to prosthesis dysfunction; invasive and destructive paravalvular infection manifest by partial valve dehiscence, new or progressive conduction system disturbances, or purulent pericarditis; and recurrent arterial embolism.

Furthermore, it seems advisable to recommend removal of the prosthesis early in the course of prosthetic valve endocarditis complicated by other factors associated with an unfavorable outcome [9]. Such factors include infection caused by organisms not easily treated by antibiotics (e.g., fungi, *S. aureus,* and coagulase-negative staphylococci). In the presence of indications for the removal of the prosthesis, temporizing for more than 10 to 14 days with antibiotic therapy does not reduce the risk of relapse, and longer periods of antibiotic therapy before surgery do not correlate with the inability to recover bacteria from intraoperative cultures or with a more favorable outcome. The most important consideration in determining the time of cardiac surgery is the hemodynamic status of the patient.

Patients with culture-negative endocarditis and continued fever during empiric antibiotic therapy will often be found to have fungal endocarditis, and removal of the prosthesis is necessary for cure.

Epidemiologic Considerations
Sources and Prevention

In general, nosocomial infections at the site of a prosthetic implant may arise either from direct contamination at the time of the operation or from bacteremic seeding of the tissues adjacent to the prosthesis secondary to another focal infection. Appropriate preoperative care and aseptic surgical technique may lessen the risk of the former circumstance; practices described elsewhere in this book related to prevention of urinary, respiratory, wound, and vascular access device–related infections will assist in the control of the latter situation (see Chaps. 28, 29, 33, 40). In two reviews of nosocomial endocarditis, nearly one-half of the cases in both series had infection at the site of prosthetic cardiac valves or intracardiac prosthetic material, and half of the cases in both series were judged to be preventable by the application of currently accepted infection control procedures and practices, including the optimal insertion and care of invasive devices, aggressive early treatment of bacterial infections, and proper use of prophylaxis [27, 78].

An important preventive measure is routine surveillance of patients following surgery. Surveillance should be maintained not only during hospitalization but also after discharge and for the period during which nosocomial infection remains a potential threat.

Patient Care Practices

Many operative procedures to implant cardiac or vascular prostheses are semielective, thereby allowing for meticulous preoperative care. In one review, nearly half of the patients with prosthetic valve endocarditis had clinical evidence of extracardiac infection at the time of surgery [69]. Special attention should be given to the preoperative diagnosis and treatment of focal infections, especially periodontal, prostate, and urinary infections.

Some surgeons recommend washing the patient's skin daily with hexachlorophene- or chlorhexidine-containing soaps for 1 to 2 days before the operation [16]. Preoperative shaving is associated with increased infection rates; clipping immediately before the operation is the preferred method for hair removal (see Chap. 33).

Many procedures to implant a cardiovascular prosthesis are so complex and lengthy that eventual breaks in aseptic technique are almost inevitable. Punctured gloves, for ex-

ample, occur with nearly every sternotomy. Considering the many opportunities for contamination of the operative field, the low infection rates observed suggest that infections may be caused by uncommonly massive contamination, unusually virulent microorganisms, or especially dangerous personnel shedders. Firm discipline in the operating room, avoidance of unnecessary traffic and talking, and exclusion of personnel with overt skin infections should assist in the control of infection.

The development and maintenance of the professional skills of the nursing and technical staff are especially important. The Inter-Society Commission for Heart Disease Resources has recommended guidelines for the clinical and physical environment in which cardiac surgery may be performed most effectively [72].

The prompt recognition and treatment of other postoperative infections, especially those related to intravascular lines and catheters, could also have a role in preventing later prosthesis-associated infection. For example, from 31 to 91 percent of patients with early-onset prosthetic valve endocarditis have been found to have predisposing postoperative infections of other sites with the same bacterial species [51].

Measures for the prevention of arteriovenous shunt–associated infections are similar to those for the prevention of intravenous catheter–associated infections (see Chap. 40). Because the cannula is exposed on the surface of an extremity, the site is continually subject to microbial contamination from the patient's own flora as well as from external sources, including dialysis fluid and equipment. The surgically created subcutaneous arteriovenous fistula or graft is used more often than external cannulas in most hemodialysis centers, in part because there is a lower risk of infection with the internal fistula.

All access site punctures should be performed with meticulous aseptic technique. Disinfection of the site with a povidone-iodine solution appears to be satisfactory, and gloves (either sterile or nonsterile) should be worn as well as a face mask. A recent randomized study found no difference in infection rates between the use of sterile gloves and drapes and the use of so-called clean technique for skin preparation [50]. Efforts to further reduce the risk of infection in hemodialysis patients have focused on the use of newer topical and oral antimicrobial agents (such as mupirocin and rifampicin) for the prophylactic eradication of *S. aureus* from the nose [14].

Environmental Factors

The majority of infections associated with cardiovascular prostheses that occur in the initial 12 months after cardiac surgery are believed to be nosocomial in origin. Some of these infections, including those with a prolonged latent period, may occur as a result of operative field and bypass equipment contamination, whereas others may result from postoperative infections.

Conflicting data exist as to the relative importance of operative field versus bypass equipment contamination. In one study, the most common site of microbial contamination was the repaired area of the myocardium and the prosthesis just before wound closure, and the bypass equipment was infrequently contaminated [55]. In other reports, positive cultures of the pump-oxygenator blood have been associated with an increased risk of later infection. Contamination of the extracorporeal circuit has been found in 10 to 44 percent of patients after bypass [6, 26]. Blood in the operative field is returned by suction tubing to the pump oxygenator for recirculation. These suction lines may become contaminated from operating room air that is drawn through each suction unit at the rate of 1 to 2 cu ft/min. One possible means of partially reducing this source of contamination is clamping the suction tubing when it is not in use.

An additional potential source for contamination during cardiopulmonary bypass is the "cell-saver apparatus," a centrifuge for intraoperative autotransfusion that has been widely used in the past decade. However, positive cultures from the apparatus have not been linked to postoperative infections [74].

The instruments and equipment for bypass procedures should be thoroughly cleaned of debris, autoclaved, and assembled under aseptic conditions. The use of disposable membrane and bubble oxygenators has simplified the problems of sterilization. Many centers use a bacterial filter in the oxygen supply line, because the oxygen itself and the junction between the nonsterile oxygen tank and the oxygenator may be sources of potential contamination.

The operating room air should have a slightly positive pressure in relation to surrounding areas, and the doors must be kept closed. The American Institute of Architects Committee on Architecture for Health has published guidelines that require at least 15 complete changes of operating room air per hour and that describe other architectural requirements for rooms for cardiovascular surgery [1]. The development of clean-room technology and laminar (or unidirectional) airflow systems that are capable of reducing the microbial concentration to fewer than one organism per cubic foot has provided a research tool for the investigation of the relation of airborne microbes to wound infection [75] (see Chaps. 22, 33, 36). Conventional air-conditioning systems, however, are capable of reducing the microbial concentration in operating room air to between one and three organisms per cubic foot. Nonetheless, it seems advisable to protect prostheses from prolonged exposure to operating room air before their insertion in the patient.

A variety of other unproved measures has been recommended to reduce environmental contamination in the operating room. A few, such as regular cleaning of the operating room floor with a phenolic disinfectant and using disposable, waterproof, paper draping materials and surgical gowns, are reasonable and in widespread use; others, such as changing shoe covers at the entrance to the operating room and passing all traffic over disinfectant-soaked blankets, appear irrational and useless. All such measures should be secondary to proper aseptic techniques, hand-scrubbing, and reducing personnel and traffic in the operating room (see Chap. 22).

Inadequate sterilization of the prosthesis

before insertion has also been suspected as a cause of subsequent infection. Prosthetic materials that cannot be autoclaved are frequently sterilized with ethylene oxide. Intrinsic contamination is more likely for materials treated with ethylene oxide. Neither of these techniques is used for porcine valves, which are treated with glutaraldehyde. When sterilization is undertaken by a hospital, the process should be monitored with bacterial spore strips. Some surgeons have resorted to soaking the device in an antibiotic-containing solution just before insertion, with the hope of killing any surviving organisms in the interstices of the fabric of the prosthesis. Contamination of the prosthesis could occur from soaking in a nonsterile antibiotic solution, however, and patients allergic to the antibiotics used may be inadvertently exposed to serious reactions by this practice.

Prophylactic Antibiotics

The use of antibiotic prophylaxis has become standard practice during surgery involving the implantation of prosthetic devices and vascular grafts [46]. However, the benefits of such prophylaxis remain uncertain because placebo-controlled studies have ended prematurely, owing to the devastating consequences of implant infections among placebo recipients, or have yielded inconclusive results. No placebo-controlled study of antibiotic prophylaxis in cardiac valve replacement surgery has been performed in the past two decades, and there is no available information on infection rates in patients not receiving antibiotics. On the other hand, antibiotic prophylaxis was significantly associated with reduced wound infection rates in at least six placebo-controlled trials involving placement of vascular grafts. However, important caveats include the facts that infection of the prosthetic material itself was not shown to be significantly reduced in any of these studies and that the predominant pathogens causing infections in the prosthetic devices often differ substantially from those causing wound infections (see Chap. 12).

Antibiotic prophylaxis directed at specific pathogens known to be susceptible to the drug will probably be effective. Thus prophylactic use of penicillinase-resistant penicillins or first- and second-generation cephalosporins probably reduces the incidence of postoperative infection with *S. aureus* and other susceptible pyogenic cocci. Recent findings from controlled studies in cardiac surgery suggest that cefazolin may be inferior to either cefuroxime or cefamandole in preventing sternal infections due to methicillin-susceptible staphylococci [53]. In centers where methicillin-resistant staphylococci are frequently encountered, surgeons have often substituted vancomycin for cephalosporins.

The optimal timing and duration of prophylactic antibiotics is also an unsettled issue. Prophylactic antibiotics should be started no earlier than 2 hours before the operation, and intraoperative dosing should be used for a drug with a short half-life and with prolonged operative durations. Several studies have shown no benefit in their postoperative use beyond 2 days. Many surgeons insist on continuing them, however, until all possible sources of contamination, such as arterial catheters, have been removed.

Management of Outbreaks
Methods of Investigation

The identification of the source and mode of spread of the pathogen is the first goal of the epidemiologist and is a necessary basis for applying control measures for an outbreak (see Chap. 6). The first step is to prepare a line listing of the cases. Although only a few cases may have occurred, a detailed list of the clinical and epidemiologic circumstances of each case is made, and each feature shared by 2 or more cases is expressed as a ratio. The list should include the dates of onset and the outcomes of the infections. Additional factors might include the age and sex of each patient, underlying diseases that predispose to such infections, durations of preoperative hospitalization, dates of operations, types and suppliers of the prostheses, methods of sterilization and handling of prostheses before insertion, locations of the operating rooms, names of surgeons and other members of the surgical teams, results of cultures and antibiograms of isolates, prophylactic antimicrobial agents used, durations of anesthesia and pump time, proportions of emergency and nighttime procedures and of emergency reoperations, proportion of patients who experienced intraoperative problems such as bleeding and difficulty in weaning from the pump, and presence of other focal infections [7]. These data should also be collected from a group of patients who underwent comparable surgical procedures during the same time period but who did not develop infections associated with their prostheses. Analysis of these data may suggest factors associated with the cases that will determine directions for the investigation.

Recent operating room records should be reviewed to determine the total number of operative procedures of a similar nature that have been performed. These procedures should be tabulated separately for periods before and during the epidemic, for use in determining changes in the infection rate. At the same time that these data are being collected and analyzed, a review of aseptic techniques, methods for disinfecting equipment, and the mechanics of the ventilating system in the operating room may reveal a productive area for special bacteriologic study (see Chap. 22).

The pathogen recovered from each case should be saved whenever possible, both for serum inhibition tests to be used in evaluating treatment and for later laboratory study to characterize the epidemic strain. Review of the susceptibilities to antimicrobial agents of the pathogens will help to determine whether a single strain or multiple strains are involved, and such susceptibility data may lead the epidemiologist to recommend changes in prophylactic antibiotic use (see Chap. 9).

While the investigation is proceeding, the epidemiologist should recommend a protocol for collecting prospective data from new patients. For example, culture of blood from the bypass machine after each operation will help to establish the frequency of contamination from this source. If such cultures have been routinely performed, an immediate review of the results from preepidemic and epidemic periods may be useful. Prospective cultures of prostheses just before insertion might also be undertaken, especially when the epidemic

strain is an organism that is more likely than others to resist sterilization or the prostheses are subjected to disinfecting rather than sterilizing procedures. Diphtheroids, staphylococci, and spore-forming bacilli, for example, are more difficult to kill than gram-negative bacilli, and mycobacterial species appear to be relatively resistant to certain disinfectants. The temptation to obtain nasopharyngeal or other swabs for culture from personnel and environmental cultures from the operating room should be resisted until the foregoing tasks have been completed. Because the pathogens from these infections are ubiquitous, positive cultures from such human and environmental sites have limited meaning and may be misleading. Cultures from these sites should be obtained only when epidemiologic data suggest that one of these sites may be relevant to the outbreak, and isolates of appropriate identity should then be fully characterized and compared with isolates of the epidemic strain.

Control

The measures taken to control an epidemic are determined by the epidemiologic findings and the urgency of the problem. In an outbreak with a high attack rate that is recognized as a grave threat to the safe conduct of such operations, it may be necessary to close the operating room temporarily and suspend procedures. In less urgent circumstances— usually when the outbreak is insidious and protracted—thoughtful investigation may precede the application of control measures. Appropriate control measures should not be withheld pending completion of the investigation if there is a reasonable chance that additional cases of infection will be prevented by their institution (see Chap. 6).

Available data should be reported to local and federal health authorities. Pooled data from multiple institutions may be necessary to establish conclusively low-frequency, intrinsic contamination of commercially distributed prosthetic materials.

If the investigation fails to uncover the source of the outbreak, the operating room should be temporarily closed and thoroughly cleaned. The importance of hand-washing and aseptic technique should be stressed to personnel. In some circumstances, discontinuation of the use of ineffective prophylactic antibiotics may alone control the outbreak, even if the source is not found. Prompt removal or elimination of a possible source suggested by the epidemiologic investigation, even when the data are inconclusive, will allow the epidemiologist to evaluate a hypothesis through well-planned, continuing surveillance. Regardless of the solution to the problem, surveillance of patients on the involved services should continue, with the purpose of either evaluating the control and prevention measures or providing additional data that might help define the cause (see Chap. 5).

References

1. American Institute of Architects Committee on Architecture for Health. *Guidelines for Construction and Equipment of Hospital and Medical Facilities* (1987 ed.). Washington, DC: American Institute of Architects Press, 1987. Pp. 25–26, 47–52.
2. Archer, G.L., and Armstrong, B.C. Alteration of staphylococcal flora in cardiac surgery patients receiving antibiotic prophylaxis. *J. Infect. Dis.* 147:642, 1983.
3. Aronson, M.D., and Bor, D.H. Blood cultures. *Ann. Intern. Med.* 106:246, 1987.
4. Bandyk, D.F., Berni, G.A., Thiele, B.L., and Towne, J.B. Aortofemoral graft infection due to *Staphylococcus epidermidis*. *Arch. Surg.* 119:102, 1984.
5. Bisno, A.L., et al. Antimicrobial treatment of infective endocarditis due to viridans streptococci, enterococci, and staphylococci. *J.A.M.A.* 261:1471, 1989.
6. Blakemore, W.S., et al. Infection by air-borne bacteria with cardiopulmonary bypass. *Surgery* 70:830, 1971.
7. Bor, D.H., et al. Mediastinitis after cardiovascular surgery. *Rev. Infect. Dis.* 5:885, 1983.
8. Boyce, J.M., et al. A common source outbreak of *Staphylococcus epidermidis* infections among patients undergoing cardiac surgery. *J. Infect. Dis.* 161:493, 1990.
9. Calderwood, S.B., et al. Prosthetic valve endocarditis. Analysis of factors affecting outcome of therapy. *J. Thorac. Cardiovasc. Surg.* 92:776, 1986.
10. Calderwood, S.B., et al. Risk factors for the development of prosthetic valve endocarditis. *Circulation* 72:31, 1985.
11. Centers for Disease Control. Bacteremia among aortic-valve surgery patients—Boston. *M.M.W.R.* 31:88, 1982.
12. Cheung, E.H., et al. Mediastinitis after cardiac valve operations. *J. Thorac. Cardiovasc. Surg.* 90:517, 1985.
13. Choo, M.H., et al. Permanent pacemaker infections: Characterization and management. *Am. J. Cardiol.* 48:559, 1981.
14. Chow, J.W., and Yu, V.L. *Staphylococcus aureus* nasal carriage in hemodialysis patients. Its role in infection and approaches to prophylaxis. *Arch. Intern. Med.* 149:1258, 1989.
15. Christensen, G.D., et al. Microbial and Foreign Body Factors in the Pathogenesis of Medical Device Infections. In: A.L. Bisno and F.A. Waldvogel (Eds.), *Infections Associated with Indwelling Medical Devices.* Washington, DC: American Society for Microbiology, 1989. Pp. 27–59.
16. Clark, R.E., et al. Infection control in cardiac surgery. *Surgery* 79:89, 1976.
17. Conte, J.E., Jr., Cohen, S.N., Roe, B.B., and Elashoff, R.M. Antibiotic prophylaxis and cardiac surgery: A prospective double-blind comparison of single-dose versus multiple-dose regimens. *Ann. Intern. Med.* 76:943, 1972.
18. Craven, D.E., et al. Pseudobacteremia caused by povidone-iodine solution contaminated with *Pseudomonas cepacia*. *N. Engl. J. Med.* 305:621, 1981.
19. Dobkin, J.F., Miller, M.H., and Steigbigel, N.H. Septicemia in patients on chronic hemodialysis. *Ann. Intern. Med.* 88:28, 1978.
20. Dougherty, S.H., and Simmons, R.L. Infections in bionic man: The pathobiology of infections in prosthetic devices. Part I. *Curr. Probl. Surg.* 29:217, 1982.
21. Downham, W.H., and Rhoades, E.R. Endocarditis associated with porcine valve xenografts. *Arch. Intern. Med.* 139:1350, 1979.
22. DuClos, T.W., Hodges, G.R., and Killian, J.E. Bacterial contamination of blood-drawing equipment: A cause of false-positive blood cultures. *Am. J. Med. Sci.* 266:459, 1974.
23. Edmunds, L.H., Jr., et al. Guidelines for reporting morbidity and mortality after cardiac valvular operations. *J. Thorac. Cardiovasc. Surg.* 96:351, 1988.
24. Ehrenkranz, N.J., Bolyard, E.A., Wiener, M., and Cleary, T.J. Antibiotic-sensitive *Serratia marcescens* infections complicating cardiopulmonary operations: Contaminated disinfectant as a reservoir. *Lancet* 2:1289, 1980.
24a. Ehrenkranz, N.J., and Pfaff, S.J. Mediastinitis complicating cardiac operations: Evidence of postoperative causation. *Rev. Infect. Dis.* 13:803, 1991.
25. Fisher, M.C., et al. *Pseudomonas maltophilia* bacteremia in children undergoing open heart surgery. *J.A.M.A.* 246:1571, 1981.

26. Freeman, R., and Hjersing, N. Bacterial culture of perfusion blood after open-heart surgery. *Thorax* 35:754, 1980.

27. Friedland, G., et al. Nosocomial endocarditis. *Infect. Control* 5:284, 1984.

28. Gage, A.A., Dean, D.C., Schimert, G., and Minsley, N. *Aspergillus* infection after cardiac surgery. *Arch. Surg.* 101:384, 1970.

29. Garner, J.S., et al. CDC definitions for nosocomial infections, 1988. *Am. J. Infect. Control* 16:128, 1988.

30. Golan, J.F. Vascular graft infection. *Infect. Dis. Clin. North Am.* 3:247, 1989.

31. Grunkemeier, J.L., and Rahimtoola, S.H. Artificial heart valves. *Annu. Rev. Med.* 41:251, 1990.

32. Hall, W.J., III. *Penicillium* endocarditis following open heart surgery and prosthetic valve insertion. *Am. Heart J.* 87:501, 1974.

33. Hammermeister, K.E., et al. Comparison of outcome after valve replacement with a bioprosthesis versus a mechanical prosthesis: Initial 5 year results of a randomized trial. *J. Am. Coll. Cardiol.* 10:719, 1987.

34. Hammond, G.L., Geha, A.S., Kopf, G.S., and Hashim, S.W. Biological versus mechanical valves. *J. Thorac. Cardiovasc. Surg.* 93:182, 1987.

35. Hammong, G.W., and Stiver, H.G. Combination antibiotic therapy in an outbreak of prosthetic endocarditis caused by *Staphylococcus epidermidis. Can. Med. Assoc. J.* 118:524, 1978.

36. Heimberger, T.S., and Duma, R.J. Infections of prosthetic heart valves and cardiac pacemakers. *Infect. Dis. Clin. North Am.* 3:221, 1989.

37. Hoffert, P.W., Gensler, S., and Haimovici, H. Infection complicating arterial grafts: Personal experience with 12 cases and review of the literature. *Arch. Surg.* 90:427, 1965.

38. Hoffman, P.C., et al. False-positive blood cultures: Association with nonsterile blood collection tubes. *J.A.M.A.* 236:2073, 1976.

39. Hoffman, P.C., et al. Two outbreaks of sternal wound infections due to organisms of the *Mycobacterium fortuitum* complex. *J. Infect. Dis.* 143:533, 1981.

40. Hopkins, C.C. Recognition of endemic and epidemic prosthetic device infections: The role of surveillance, the hospital infection control practitioner, and the hospital epidemiologist. *Infect. Dis. Clin. North Am.* 3:211, 1989.

41. Houang, E.T., et al. Problems in the investigation of an apparent outbreak of coagulase-negative staphylococcal septicaemia following cardiac surgery. *J. Hosp. Infect.* 8:224, 1986.

42. Hughes, C.F., Grant, A.F., Leckie, B.D., and Baird, D.K. Cardioplegic solution: A contamination crisis. *J. Thorac. Cardiovasc. Surg.* 91:296, 1986.

43. Ide, H., et al. The effect of cardiopulmonary bypass on T cells and their subpopulations. *Ann. Thorac. Surg.* 44:277, 1987.

44. Ivert, T.S.A., et al. Prosthetic valve endocarditis. *Circulation* 69:223, 1984.

45. Jones, E.L., et al. Ten-year experience with the porcine bioprosthetic valve: Interrelationship of valve survival and patient survival in 1,050 valve replacements. *Ann. Thorac. Surg.* 49:370, 1990.

46. Kaiser, A.B. Antimicrobial Prophylaxis of Infections Associated with Foreign Bodies. In: A.L. Bisno and F.A. Waldvogel (Eds.), *Infections Associated with Indwelling Medical Devices.* Washington, DC: American Society for Microbiology, 1989. Pp. 277–287.

47. Kaiser, A.B. Effective and creative surveillance and reporting of surgical wound infections. *Infect. Control* 3:41, 1982.

48. Kalweit, W.H., Winn, W.C., Jr., Rocco, T.A., Jr., and Girod, J.C. Hemodialysis fistula infections caused by *Legionella pneumophila*. *Ann. Intern. Med.* 96:173, 1982.

49. Kaplan, E.L., Rich, H., Gersony, W., and Manning, J. A collaborative study of infective endocarditis in the 1970s: Emphasis on infections in patients who have undergone cardiovascular surgery. *Circulation* 59:327, 1979.

50. Kaplowitz, L.G., et al. A prospective study of infections in hemodialysis patients: Patient hygiene and other risk factors for infection. *Infect. Control Hosp. Epidemiol.* 9:534, 1988.

51. Karchmer, A.W., and Bisno, A.L. Infections of Prosthetic Heart Valves and Vascular Grafts. In: A.L. Bisno and F.A. Waldvogel, (Eds.), *Infections Associated with Indwelling Medical Devices.* Washington, DC: American Society Microbiology, 1989. Pp. 129–159.

52. Kaslow, R.A., Mackel, D.C., and Mallison Nosocomial pseudobacteremia: Positive cultures due to contaminated benp., and antiseptic. *J.A.M.A.* 236:2407, lghs to prevent *Staphylococcus aureus* infections. *J.A.M.A.* 263:9*occus aureus* car-

53. Kernodle, D.S., Classen, D.C., wound in-Kaiser, A.B. Failure of ceph6.

54. Kirmani, N., et al. St.ving long-term heriage rate of patients.*Ied.* 138:1657, 1978. modialysis. *Arch. In.*M., McLaughlin, J.S.,

55. Kluge, R.M., Ca.ources of contamination and Hornick, R.gery. *J.A.M.A.* 230:1415, in open hear. , et al. Sternal wound infections 1974. diti s due to organisms of the *My-*

56. Kuritsky,*fortuitum* complex. *Ann. Intern. Med.* and end cobacte. 1983.

98:.J.W., Jr., Imperato, A.M., Hackel, A.,

57. L. Doyle, E.F. Endocarditis complicating open-heart surgery. *Circulation* 23:489, 1961. a.Lowry, P.W., et al. A cluster of legionella sternal wound infections due to postoperative

topical exposure to contaminated tap water. *N. Engl. J. Med.* 324:109, 1991.

58. MacGregor, D.C., et al. Computer-assisted reporting system for the follow-up of patients with prosthetic heart valves. *Am. J. Cardiol.* 42:444, 1978.

59. Maki, D., et al. Methicillin-Resistant *Staph. epidermidis* Surgical Wound Infections Linked to a Chronic Carrier. In: *Program and Abstracts of the Twenty-Second Interscience Conference On Antimicrobial Agents and Chemotherapy* (abstr. 566). Washington, DC: American Society for Microbiology, 1982.

60. Mayer, K.H., and Schoenbaum, S.C. Evaluation and management of prosthetic valve endocarditis. *Prog. Cardiovasc. Dis.* 25:43, 1982.

61. Mehta, G. *Aspergillus* endocarditis after open heart surgery: An epidemiological investigation. *J. Hosp. Infect.* 15:245, 1990.

62. Mickelsen, P.A., et al. Instability of antibiotic resistance in a strain of *Staphylococcus epidermidis* isolated from an outbreak of prosthetic valve endocarditis. *J. Infect. Dis.* 152:50, 1985.

63. Miholic, J. Risk factors for severe bacterial infections after valve replacement and aortocoronary bypass operations: Analysis of 246 cases by logistic regression. *Ann. Thorac. Surg.* 40:224, 1985.

64. Nagachinta, T., Stephens, M., Reitz, B., and Polk, B.F. Risk factors for surgical wound infection following cardiac surgery. *J. Infect. Dis.* 156:967, 1987.

65. Nelson, R.M., and Dries, D.J. The economic implications of infection in cardiac surgery. *Ann. Thorac. Surg.* 42:240, 1986.

66. ...man, L.S., Szczukowski, L.C., Bain, R.P., ...erlino, C.A. Suppurative mediastinitis

67. Open heart surgery: A case control study analysis. *Chest* 94:546, 1988.

68. Parker, ...M., et al. Fungal infections of di... prosthetic... *Ann. Intern. Med.* 91:50, 1979. 147, 1982.

69. Quenzer, R.W. ...r., et al. Bacteremia following ...replacement. *Ann. Surg.* 197: A comparative ...24 prosthetic va... wards, L.D., and Levin, S. *Heart J.* 92:15, 197... of 48 host valve and ...docarditis cases. *Am.*

70. Rosendorf, L.J., Dar..., G., and Baer, H. Sources of gram-negativ... ...ection after open heart surgery. *J. Thorac....iovasc. Surg.* 67: 195, 1974.

71. Sande, M.A., Johnson, W.D., ...Hook, E.W., and Kaye, D. Sustained bacterer... in patients with prosthetic cardiac valves. *N.* ...l. J. Med. 286:1067, 1972.

72. Scannel, J.G. (Chairman). Report ... the Inter-Society Commission for Heart D...ase

Resources. Optimal resources for cardiac surgery: Guidelines for program planning and evaluation. *Circulation* 52:A-23, 1975.

73. Schoen, F.J. Cardiac valve prostheses: Review of clinical status and contemporary biomaterials issues. *J. Biomed. Mater. Res.: Appl. Biomater.* 21:91, 1987.

74. Schwieger, I.M., et al. Incidence of cell-saver contamination during cardiopulmonary bypass. *Ann. Thorac. Surg.* 48:51, 1989.

75. Soots, G., et al. Air-borne contamination hazard in open heart surgery: Efficiency of HEPA air filtration and laminar flow. *J. Cardiovasc. Surg.* 23:155, 1982.

76. Stanton, R.E., Lindesmith, G.G., and Meyer, B.W. *Escherichia coli* endocarditis after repair of ventricular septal defects. *N. Engl. J. Med.* 279:737, 1968.

77. Starr, A., and Grunkemeier, G.L. The expected lifetime of porcine valves. *Ann. Thorac. Surg.* 48:317, 1989.

78. Terpenning, M.S., Buggy, B.P., and Kauffman, C.A. Hospital-acquired infective endocarditis. *Arch. Intern. Med.* 148:1601, 1988.

79. van den Broek, P.J., et al. Epidemic of prosthetic valve endocarditis caused by *Staphylococcus epidermidis*. *Br. Med. J.* 291:949, 1985.

80. van Oeveren, W., Dankert, J., and Waldevuur, C.R.H. Bubble oxygenation and cardiotomy suction impair the host defense during cardiopulmonary bypass: A study in dogs. *Ann. Thorac. Surg.* 44:523, 1987.

81. van Oeveren, W., et al. Deleterious effects of cardiopulmonary bypass: A prospective study of bubble versus membrane oxygenation. *J. Thorac. Cardiovasc. Surg.* 89:888, 1985.

82. Villarino, M.E., et al. Epidemic of *Serratia marcescens* bacteremia in a cardiac intensive care unit. *J. Clin. Microbiol.* 27:2433, 1989.

83. von Reyn, C.F., et al. Infective endocarditis: An analysis based on strict case definitions. *Ann. Intern. Med.* 94(Part I):505, 1981.

84. Wade, J.S., and Cobbs, C.G. Infections in Cardiac Pacemakers. In: J.S. Remington and M.N. Swartz (Eds.), *Current Clinical Topics in Infectious Diseases 9*. New York: McGraw-Hill, 1988. Pp. 44–61.

85. Weinstein, M.P., et al. Multicenter collaborative evaluation of a standardized serum bactericidal test as a prognostic indicator in infective endocarditis. *Am. J. Med.* 78:262, 1985.

86. Weinstein, R.A., Emori, T.G., Anderson, R.L., and Stamm, W.E. Pressure transducers as a source of bacteremia after open heart surgery: Report of an outbreak and guidelines for prevention. *Chest* 69:338, 1976.

87. Wilson, W.R., et al. Prosthetic valve endocarditis. *Ann. Intern. Med.* 82:751, 1975.

Infections of Skeletal Prostheses

William Petty

Plastic and metal skeletal prostheses have been used by orthopedic surgeons in the treatment of many clinical problems—principally fracture repair and partial joint replacement—for several decades. In the past three decades, prostheses for replacing the hip, knee, shoulder, elbow, ankle, wrist, and finger joints have been used increasingly, while surgeons and engineers continue to develop total replacement prostheses for special purposes such as after resection for tumors [6, 21, 22, 24, 30, 33, 34, 35]. Patients who have been in constant pain and unable to walk or take care of themselves can now be successfully rehabilitated by the insertion of such prosthetic devices. Unfortunately, not all these efforts are successful. The most common complication following total joint replacement is loosening of the prosthetic components. Although infection is less common than loosening, it is more likely to cause permanent failure of the procedure. These infections lead to compromise or loss of function of the prostheses and rarely have led to loss of limb or death of the patient.

Since total hip replacement (THR) has been studied more extensively from the standpoint of infection than operations involving any other skeletal prosthesis, the ensuing discussion centers around this procedure and device. The principles, however, pertain to all implantable skeletal devices.

Classification of Infections
Early (Acute) Infections
Early infections are defined as those that occur during the first postoperative month. As a general rule, all such infections should be considered nosocomial. Early infections are subdivided according to whether they are superficial or deep to the fascia lata.

Suprafascial (superficial) infections, the most

common of all surgical infections in THR, possess the characteristics of incisional wound infections (see Chap. 33). Since superficial infections have a good prognosis compared to deep infections, they are omitted or mentioned only briefly in the majority of reports dealing with THR complications.

Deep wound infections include all infections extending deep to the fascia lata. These acute infections are much less common than late deep infections. This difference appears to be related to the stricter aseptic discipline in the operating room for joint replacement procedures.

Late Infections

Late infections present after the patient has resumed painless function. Such infections are deep wound infections that are noted months or even years after apparently successful THR, and they represent a mixture of nosocomial and hematogenously acquired infections, information is often insufficient to permit reliable differentiation, though an infection associated with a prosthetic joint due to the same organism as cultured previously from an infection in another site of the body is presumed to have seeded in the joint through the bloodstream.

Incidence

The incidence of surgical wound infections involving skeletal prostheses varies widely in different reports. In the early history of THR, without the use of antibiotics or environmental control, the infection rate was disturbingly high, up to 11 percent (Table 36-1). When antibiotics began to be administered shortly before and for a brief time after surgery, the average infection rate for several series was reduced to 1.3 percent (Table 36-2) [25]. In contemporary series, the infection rate was 0.7 percent with the use of "clean" rooms but no antibiotics, and 0.6 percent when antibiotics were added (Tables 36-3, 36-4) [25]. Infection rates are somewhat higher in prosthetic knee replacement [13] and correction of scoliosis with Harrington rod instrumentation [16]. This variation in

Table 36-1. Deep infection in regular operating room without use of prophylactic antibiotics

Study	No. of cases/ infections	Percentage
Charnley	190/13	6.8
Müller	683/27	4.0
Wilson et al.	100/11	11.0
Patterson and Brown	368/30	8.2
Benson and Hughes	321/17	5.3
Murray	126/5	4.0
Ritter et al.	92/6	6.5
Total	1,880/109	5.8

Source: Adapted from J.P. Nelson, The operating room environment and its influence on deep wound infections. In: *The Hip: Proceedings of the Fifth Open Scientific Meeting of the Hip Society.* St. Louis: Mosby, 1977. P. 129.

Table 36-2. Deep infection in regular operating room with use of prophylactic antibiotics

Study	No. of cases/ infections	Percentage
Eftekhar et al.	800/4	0.5
Fitzgerald	3,215/42	1.3
Murray	622/7	1.1
Lowell and Knudsen	621/19	3.1
Leinbach and Barlow	275/4	1.5
Welch et al.	150/0	0
Collis and Steinhaus	298/0	0
Irvine et al.	167/4	2.4
Bentley and Simmonds	117/2	1.7
Salvati	526/8	1.5
Total	6,791/90	1.3

Source: Adapted from J.P. Nelson, The operating room environment and its influence on deep wound infections. In: *The Hip: Proceedings of the Fifth Open Scientific Meeting of the Hip Society.* St. Louis: Mosby, 1977. P. 129.

infection rate is not completely understood but could be related to factors such as anatomic site, selection of patients, immunologic status of the patient, experience and technique of the surgeon, and characteristics of the implant.

Pathogens

The principle pathogenic organisms reported in a composite of publications on deep wound

Table 36-3. Deep infections in clean-air operating room without use of prophylactic antibiotics

Study	No. of cases/ infections	Percentage
Brady et al.	300/3	1.0
Charnley	2,152/12	0.6
Ritter et al.	278/3	1.1
Total	2,730/18	0.7

Source: Adapted from J.P. Nelson, The operating room environment and its influence on deep wound infections. In: *The Hip: Proceedings of the Fifth Open Scientific Meeting of the Hip Society.* St. Louis: Mosby, 1977. P. 129.

Table 36-4. Deep infections in clean-air operating room with use of prophylactic antibiotics

Study	No. of cases/ infections	Percentage
Nelson	243/0	0
Irvine et al.	107/1	0.9
Welch et al.	600/0	0
Leinbach and Barlow	425/3	0.7
Bentley and Simmonds	130/1	0.8
Salvati	1,249/12	1.0
Total	2,754/17	0.6

Source: Adapted from J.P. Nelson, The operating room environment and its influence on deep wound infections. In: *The Hip: Proceedings of the Fifth Open Scientific Meeting of the Hip Society.* St. Louis: Mosby, 1977. P. 129.

infections following THR are listed in Table 36-5. In practice, isolation of suspected microorganisms from an infected prosthetic hip is not always easy. In some large series of THR, the microbial cause of deep wound infection is not documented in at least 12 percent of cases [3]. Because of this problem, surgeons tend to consider the isolation of any organisms from deep tissue as conclusive evidence of infection. This situation is compounded by the fact that *Staphylococcus epidermidis*, which in the past was considered nonpathogenic, is one of the leading causes of wound infection in THR.

Staphylococcus aureus

Coagulase-positive *Staphylococcus aureus* causes approximately one-fifth of all deep in-

Table 36-5. Microorganisms isolated from specimens taken at the time of resection arthroplasty

Organism	No. of isolates
Staphylococcus epidermidis	37
Staphylococcus aureus	19
α-Hemolytic streptococci	10
Group D streptococci	7
Escherichia coli	4
Proteus mirabilis	3
Pseudomonas aeruginosa	6
Enterobacter species	4
Acinetobacter species	1
Peptococcus species	5
Bacillus species	3
Corynebacterium species	6
Bacteroides species	2
β-Hemolytic streptococci	2
Propionibacterium acnes	1
No organism isolated	2

Source: From D.J. McDonald, R.H. Fitzgerald, Jr., and D.M. Ilstrup, Two-stage reconstruction of a total hip arthroplasty because of infection. *J. Bone Joint Surg. [Am.]* 71(6):831, 1989. By permission of the journal.)

fections following THR (see Table 36-5). For additional microbiologic, clinical, and epidemiologic features, the reader should refer to Chapters 33 and 37.

Staphylococcus epidermidis

The term *coagulase-negative staphylococci* is used by most clinical laboratories to encompass all members of the family Micrococcaceae other than *S. aureus*. The majority of clinical microbiology laboratories do not distinguish *S. epidermidis* from other Micrococcaceae species; hence, the relative frequency of these two groups of organisms in reported infections is not known, and potentially important clinical and epidemiologic differences remain undisclosed. We will refer to coagulase-negative staphylococci as *S. epidermidis*.

S. epidermidis has assumed the role of a major pathogen in implant surgery; it causes approximately 33 percent of all infections following THR (see Table 36-5). Undoubtedly, *S. epidermidis* is a bona fide pathogen in late infections after THR operations; when these organisms are cultured from deep tissue, especially when cultured from several specimens, they should be considered causative agents of the infection.

Aerobic Gram-Negative Rods

Aerobic gram-negative rods are responsible for a smaller proportion of THR infections than other surgical wound infections (see Chaps. 27, 33). Gram-negative rods are isolated from approximately one-fifth of deep THR wound infections. Infections caused by this group of bacteria are especially difficult to eradicate.

Anaerobes

Although anaerobic surgical wound infections are receiving increasing attention, they have seldom been reported in THR patients, and anaerobes have been infrequently recovered from wounds at the time of surgery. Evidence is increasing that the lack of reported infections with anaerobic organisms is due to a lack of proper anaerobic culture techniques; the incidence of reported anaerobic infections has increased with improved culture techniques.

Less commonly, infections may be associated with atypical mycobacteria and fungi [8, 11]. *Mycobacterium tuberculosis* may cause infection of total joint prostheses, usually in patients with previous infection of the hip associated with the same organism. Recurrence of infection is reduced by appropriate chemotherapy at the time of and after the hip replacement [14, 32].

Microbiologic Diagnosis

Microbiologic findings can be considered only as supportive evidence in the diagnosis of hip infections. Clinical diagnosis clearly is of primary importance, but the identification of the pathogenic organisms involved is highly valuable, especially for choosing the appropriate antimicrobial therapy. The following points should be kept in mind when collecting specimens or interpreting the results of cultures [18].

Swabs and Liquid Specimens

A superficial (skin) swab of the wound is not a suitable specimen, because in most cases it is impossible to determine whether the isolates are members of the normal skin flora or the causative agents of the infection. These swab specimens also are not adequate for the recovery of anaerobic organisms (see Chap. 9).

When pus is present, it should be aspirated with a needle and immediately taken to the laboratory. This is the best specimen (short of a tissue biopsy) for recovering both anaerobic and aerobic organisms. If possible, such a specimen should be collected before antibiotic therapy is started.

Biopsy Specimens

When tissue from biopsy is sent to the laboratory for culture, deep tissue should be used to minimize contamination; the specimens should be handled as cautiously as possible to avoid contamination of the tissue with gloves, gown, and the like. The presence of one or two colonies in a tissue specimen must be interpreted with caution. *S. epidermidis,* diphtheroids, micrococci, and some streptococci are ubiquitous organisms in the surgical theater, hospital wards, and laboratory, and airborne contamination of biopsy specimens with these organisms is a possibility.

A negative Gram stain of a tissue section is not to be interpreted as indicating the absence of infection, but it must be remembered that the occurrence of some granulomatous tissue may be directly related to the presence of the acrylic cement, the prosthesis itself, or both. As a part of exploratory surgery in a clinically suspected infected hip without microbiologic evidence of infection, multiple specimens should be submitted to the laboratory, including pieces of deep tissue, cement, pseudocapsule, and so on. Recovery of the same organisms from several areas is important, because such data should rule out specimen contamination.

Specimens for Anaerobes

For the best recovery of anaerobic organisms, the laboratory must be provided with a proper specimen. All liquid specimens should be collected in syringes to maintain anaerobic conditions. Transport tubes for tissue or swabs must be oxygen-free; these tubes are commercially available. Finally, the laboratory must have appropriate anaerobic isolation and identification equipment (see Chap. 9).

Predisposing Factors
Operative Factors

It has long been recognized that bacteria produce necrosis of the bone, when an infection occurs, by destroying the tenuous blood supply in the marrow spaces or haversian canals. Bacteria in this environment are relatively inaccessible to host defense mechanisms and antibiotics. Thus the presence of necrotizing organisms in bone leads to persistent infection until the necrotic sequestrated bone is spontaneously extruded or removed.

The insertion of a prosthetic device compromises the blood supply of the microenvironment around the implant. Bleeding from bone cannot be controlled in the usual surgical fashion; therefore, all skeletal implants are surrounded by hematoma. The fact that both early and late infections of total joint replacements are often caused by organisms of low virulence has suggested that the implant materials, used because of either their chemistry or their structure, may inhibit the host's ability to deal effectively with contaminating organisms. There is both in vitro and in vivo experimental data suggesting that some implant materials are more likely than others to be associated with infection because of inhibition of normal immune mechanisms [7]. The bone cement polymethylmethacrylate has been most strongly incriminated in this respect. The bone necrosis surrounding a total joint replacement implant is probably caused by a combination of surgical insult, heat of polymerization, and toxicity of methylmethacrylate monomer. Other implant materials, particularly the ions of some metallic alloys, may also be toxic to mammalian tissues; this may become increasingly important due to the increased surface area present in implants designed for biologic fixation (bone ingrowth) [13]. The presence of necrosis and hematoma provides favorable growth conditions for microorganisms.

THR surgery is associated with the implantation of large foreign bodies. It has been established experimentally that fewer *S. aureus* organisms are needed to establish an infection in the presence of a foreign body (see Chap. 33).

Gristina and Costerton have shown that many bacteria produce a slimelike glycocalyx that protects the bacteria from humoral and cellular defenses (Fig. 36-1) [9]. Finally, a large wound may be exposed to contamination for a relatively long period of time (2 or 3 hours) in technically difficult cases or in the hands of inexperienced operators.

These factors conspire to produce a high risk of infection. This risk, coupled with the serious disability from infected implants, has led to major efforts to prevent postoperative sepsis associated with these procedures [10].

Previous Hip Surgery

A substantial portion of THR patients with infection have had previous hip operations. It is well known that the incidence of infection in primary, clean cases is lower than that in patients operated on previously [23]. Approximately one-third of THR operations are now being done after the failure of other types of implants. These "idiopathic" painful hips may be attributable to occult infection. Despite negative preoperative cultures, the incidence of infection in THR is twice as high in such cases compared to the incidence in previously unoperated hips. Under circumstances in which the surgeon strongly suspects infection, it may be preferable to remove the device, carefully obtain culture and biopsy specimens from the wound, and close it. If subsequent studies indicate that occult infection is not present and if the wound is well healed, subsequent THR might be contemplated with relative safety. Others prefer to rely on Gram-stained smears, frozen sections, and gross inspection to reach an intraoperative decision; the validity of these methods in determining whether infection is present has not been firmly established.

When clinically obvious occult deep infection compromises a previous implant, the safest management is implant removal, wound drainage or suction irrigation, appropriate antibiotic treatment, and a delay of a few weeks to many months with no signs of inflammation before undertaking a repeat THR. Some advocate implant excision, radical debridement, antibiotic lavage, and THR with massive antibiotic treatment. THR after only a short delay or immediate exchange of

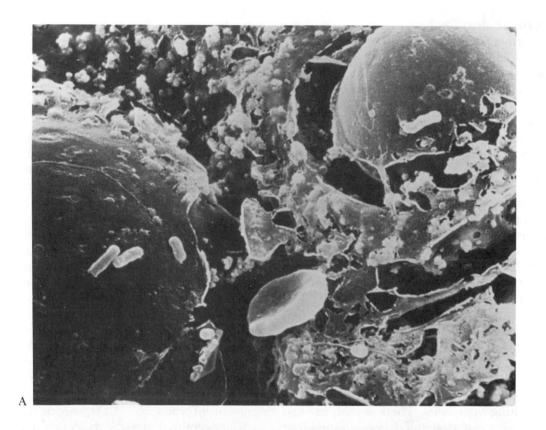

A

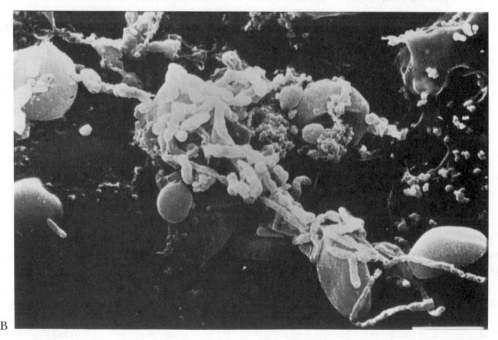

B

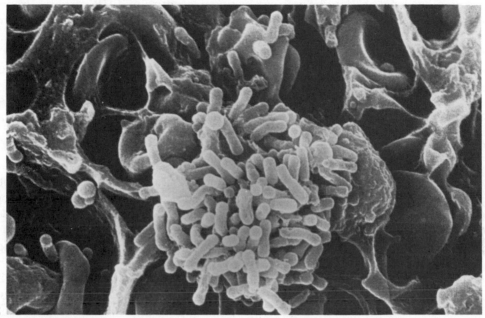

C

Fig. 36-1. Biofilm protecting bacteria. *A.* Scanning electron micrograph of intramedullary bone cement from infected and loosened total hip prosthesis, showing rod-shaped bacteria in association with and partly buried in extensive biofilm of surface of the cement. *Pseudomonas aeruginosa* was isolated from this specimen. *B.* Biofilm is incompletely formed in this area, and individual adherent bacterial microcolonies can be seen. *C.* Surface of bone from infected total hip joint, showing development of discrete adherent microcolonies in which bacteria of a single morphotype are partly surrounded by amorphous condensed material. (Reprinted with permission from A. G. Gristina and J. W. Costerton. Bacterial adherence to biomaterials and tissue. *J. Bone Joint Surg.* 67A: 264, 1985.)

an infected implant for a replacement implant is more likely to be successful with gram-positive organisms. Success is most likely for re-implantation of the prosthesis when 1 year elapses prior to reimplantation [19].

Immediate or early THR following the diagnosis of infection with gram-negative organisms has a high likelihood of failure and, even after a significant period of apparent quiescence of infection, infections with gram-negative organisms are more likely to be associated with recurrent infection when a new prosthesis is implanted [19].

Other Factors

Another factor that may contribute to infection is obesity. Conclusive data are not available, but circumstantial evidence points out that obese patients are more prone than non-obese patients to develop superficial wound infections. This difference appears to be re-

lated to the heavy retraction required on the subcutaneous tissue, which leads to necrosis and difficulty in closing the subcutaneous space in obese patients, and the often prolonged operative time.

A large number of patients receive steroid therapy for rheumatoid arthritis. It has been shown by Charnley [3] as well as others that these patients are at a slightly higher risk of infection than other candidates for total joint replacement.

General Control Measures

Orthopedic surgeons involved in THR operations have gone to great lengths to control surgical wound infections. The pioneers in THR experienced an initial infection rate of 8 to 10 percent. As noted in Tables 36-2, 36-3, 36-4, and 36-6, the infection rate has decreased to a low level. Although some surgeons have emphasized antibiotic prophylaxis, others are advocates of "clean-room" surgery, employing either a unidirectional airflow system (UAFS) or the use of ultraviolet (UV) lights.

Surgical Techniques

An awareness of the infection problem in THR has led to renewed emphasis on strict discipline in the operating room, with attention paid particularly to meticulous aseptic surgery, double gloving, double masking, and the use of hoods and body exhaust systems that employ relatively impermeable gowns. Such techniques have been accepted as routine procedure in THR surgery. Preparation of the skin before surgery is done meticulously because of the closeness of the surgical area to the perineum. Proper draping of the incision is important to avoid endogenous contamination. The use of self-sealing plastic drapes about the perineum has been of particular help in decreasing wound contamination with perineal flora.

Clean-Air Room System

The clean-air room has become popular among orthopedic surgeons, mainly because of the enthusiastic support of Charnley [3], Nelson [25], and others. The clean-air room usually has a UAFS installed in a Plexiglas or glass enclosure to which only the surgical personnel are allowed access (see Chap. 22). In many clean-air systems, the surgeons and supportive personnel inside the enclosure also wear body exhaust suits. Airflow systems of two major types—horizontal and vertical—are available. When horizontal airflow systems are used (Fig. 36-2), great care must be taken in setting up the operating room to avoid forcing bacteria into the area of the wound when personnel or other obstructions get between the source of airflow and the operative site (Fig. 36-3). It was demonstrated in one study that the infection rate is increased with the use

Table 36-6. Deep infections in ultraviolet-light operating room with use of prophylactic antibiotics

Study	No. of cases/ infections	Percentage
Lowell and Knudsen	665/5	0.8
Goldner et al.	700/8	1.1
Total	1,365/13	1.0

Source: Adapted from J.P. Nelson, The operating room environment and its influence on deep wound infections. In: *The Hip: Proceedings of the Fifth Open Scientific Meeting of the Hip Society.* St. Louis: Mosby, 1977. P. 129.

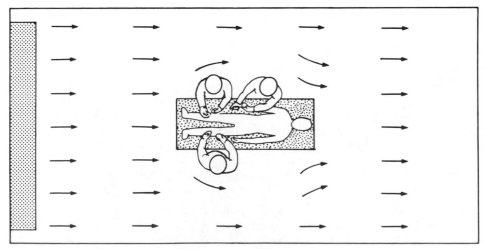

Fig. 36-2. Ultraclean-air-handling system. Horizontal flow system, without obstruction between air source and operative wound.

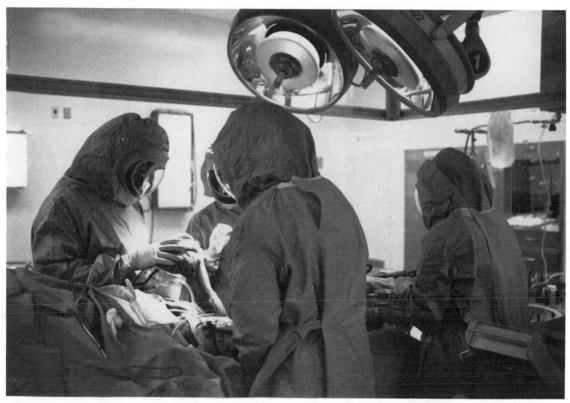

Fig. 36-3. Ultraclean-air-handling system. Obstruction of air source by operating room personnel, with potentially increased risk of infection.

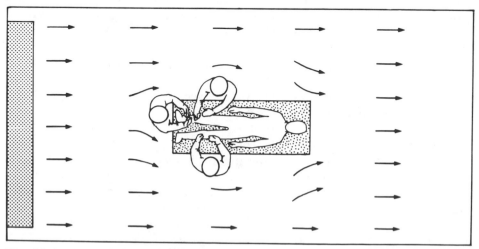

Fig. 36-4. A vertical unidirectional airflow system. Air enters from the ceiling of the enclosure through high-efficiency particulate air filters and flows downward to exit beneath the enclosing walls.

of horizontal airflow systems if this principle is ignored [31]. For similar reasons, body exhaust suits must be used with vertical airflow systems (Fig. 36-4).

UAFS equipment is capable of delivering a high volume of unidirectional air that has been filtered by high-efficiency particulate air (HEPA) filters capable of removing more than 99 percent of particles greater than 3 μm in size. This equipment provides an air volume sufficient to exchange the air of a room at a rate of up to 300 changes per hour.

Body exhaust suits consist of a helmet attached to a vacuum pump that is capable of sucking out all the expired air of the wearer, thus controlling the microbial fallout from the head, neck, and other body surfaces of the wearer.

The surgical enclosure unit usually consists of a series of transparent panels with dimensions of up to 10 × 20 ft. In addition to providing particulate-free air, the enclosure ensures restriction of traffic around the operating table. Furthermore, the body exhaust suits impose both discipline and close surgical teamwork. Many consider these additional benefits to be as significant as the clean air but believe they can be achieved without the inconvenience and expense of the system. The efficacy of such systems in reducing airborne particulate and microbial contamination at the periphery of the wound has been established in many studies. There is now strong evidence in a well-controlled study that this reduction in contamination results in a significant reduction of wound infection rates in total joint replacement operative procedures [15].

The question of whether a clean-air system is truly necessary for controlling sepsis in THR cannot be answered in absolute terms. It would appear that the wound infection rates under optimal conventional surgical conditions with thoughtful antibiotic therapy and proper patient selection are almost as low as they are when the surgical conditions are modestly improved with clean-air systems without antibiotics. Whether to use a clean room seems to require a judgment based on local conditions rather than a decision based on a universal rule.

Prophylactic Antibiotic Therapy

A national survey showed that 87 percent of orthopedic surgeons used antibiotic prophylaxis in total joint replacements [26]. This figure is not surprising, because the use of prophylactic antibiotics in THR has been widely advocated. Numerous studies strongly suggest a decrease in deep infection rates with appropriate use of perioperative antibiotics. Such antibiotic use is especially important when clean-air systems are not available or cannot be used to maximum efficiency. The literature abounds with reports of undesirable side effects following the use of prophylactic antibiotics, including the emergence of antibiotic-resistant organisms, alteration of the normal flora, allergic side effects, and so on, and the surgeon must be aware that the benefit from use of prophylactic antibiotics may be largely obviated by extended administration of antibiotic.

The timing of the dosage is critical (see Chap. 12). It has been established both clinically and experimentally that if optimal results are to be expected from prophylactic antibiotics, the antibiotic concentration in the tissues must be high at the time of surgery (when inoculation with organisms occurs) or very shortly thereafter [2]. Prophylactic antibiotics should be administered parenterally, at the time of anesthetic induction. In patients who are allergic to penicillins or cephalosporins, vancomycin is an excellent choice. There is no clinical evidence supporting the use of prolonged prophylactic antibiotics in THR, however, and experimental evidence indicates that prolonged treatment is unnecessary [1, 3]. Most authorities agree that under most circumstances administration of prophylactic antibiotics beyond 48 to 72 hours postoperatively is probably neither necessary nor beneficial, and even shorter duration may be effective.

Staphylococci are responsible for approximately half of infections in THR surgery. If prophylactic antibiotics are to be used to prevent staphylococcal infection, a semisynthetic, penicillinase-resistant penicillin (e.g., methicillin) or cephalosporin should be given. Cephalosporins have been used increasingly for prophylaxis in total joint replacement surgery; cefazolin should be considered the agent of choice. Although the second- and third-generation cephalosporin agents are often used, their efficacy against the staphylococci that most commonly cause infections after total joint replacement is not as good as that of the first-generation cephalosporins.

Early Deep Wound Infections
Clinical Features
Manifestations and Management
The prompt clinical diagnosis of postoperative wound infections following THR surgery is very important because the earlier the treatment is started, the better the chances are of salvaging the prosthesis.

Acute deep infections present within 2 to 4 weeks following surgery and are associated with fever, leukocytosis, and inflammation. Frequently, pus drains from the wound. Such infected patients should initially be treated vigorously with high doses of the appropriate antibiotics and incision and drainage of the wound. In most instances, subsequent removal of the device is required to achieve closure of the draining sinuses. As long as such preliminary steps contain the infection, the removal of the prosthesis should be delayed until it is certain that removal is inevitable. This state is manifested by recurrent dislocation, gross loosening of the device, or continued drainage. Cementless devices should be removed at the time of initial debridement for acute infection, because they are easier to remove before any biologic attachment has occurred and their removal allows more thorough debridement.

Once it is clearly established that an early acute infection is superficial in the fascia lata, it must be decompressed to prevent deep extension. These infections cause little systemic toxicity and, when evacuated, show no deep communication with the prosthesis. Should drainage persist an unusual length of time, extension deep to the fascia lata must be sought by fluoroscopy and contrast radiographic study.

Antibiotic Therapy
Therapy should be directed toward the organisms involved and should be based on the sensitivity studies of the pathogenic organisms. If an infection is suspected and the culture results are not available, antibiotic treatment should be started immediately to prevent involvement of the prosthesis. *S. aureus* is responsible for the majority of early deep wound infections; therefore, an anti-staphylococcal drug such as methicillin or a cephalosporin is the antibiotic of choice. *S. epidermidis* causes approximately 20 percent of acute deep infections, and methicillin will effectively treat sensitive strains. Resistance of *S. epidermidis* to methicillin and similar penicillins is frequently found in some hospitals, however, and vancomycin, rather than methicillin or cephalosporin, might be chosen for initial therapy in these circumstances (see Chap. 35). An aminoglycoside antibiotic should be given in addition, because many acute infections are caused by gram-negative organisms. As soon as the laboratory results are available, the antibiotic therapy should be adjusted according to the type of organisms found. Serum bactericidal levels against the specific organism causing the infection may be helpful, especially when dealing with infections caused by gram-negative organisms.

In the United States, England, and Germany, there are increasing problems with methicillin-resistant *S. aureus*, which points out the importance of performing adequate antibiotic susceptibility tests (see Chap. 12). If an antibiotic must be chosen in the absence of susceptibility testing, the physician should use antibiotics that are most effective against the organisms that have been isolated from acute deep infections in the hospital. Updated information regarding susceptibility patterns of organisms in the hospital should be routinely available through the clinical microbiology laboratory or the hospital epidemiologist (see Chap. 9).

Sources and Modes of Acquisition

The sources and modes of acquisition of organisms that produce surgical wound infections are systematically described in Chapter 33. Only features especially pertinent to infected THR prostheses are described in this section.

Glove Punctures

Direct contact spread by hands of personnel may play a role. Puncture holes in surgical gloves at the time of surgery are a common finding, especially in orthopedic surgery, in which surgeons handle hammers, saws, power tools, sharp wires, and bone with sharp edges (see Chap. 33). It has been shown by Wise and colleagues [37] that up to 1.8×10^5 organisms can be cultured from inside the gloves after a surgical procedure. Ninety-eight percent of the interior of gloves cultured were positive for microorganisms, and 14 percent of them were positive for *S. aureus;* the implication of this study is simply that when gloves are punctured during surgery by a surgeon who is a heavy carrier of *S. aureus,* the wound may be inoculated with a sufficiently large number of organisms to cause infection.

Postoperative Hand Transmission

Transmission from the hands of personnel after surgery (e.g., in wards or intensive care units) is a more controversial subject. It is doubtful that it plays a significant role in THR patients because the wound is covered at the time of surgery and the dressings are not usually removed for several days, allowing sufficient time for the skin to seal. The opportunity for infection to enter from the outside appears to be remote.

S. Aureus *Shedders*

S. aureus resides in the skin as well as in the anterior nares of many surgical personnel and patients. Desquamated skin loaded with *S. aureus* is released in the air and can settle into the open wound. It is conceivable that these organisms may cause a wound infection in these surgical procedures. It has been our experience that when personnel demonstrated to be shedders are present on a surgical team that is using clean-room techniques, *S. aureus* has not been recovered from the air, and no *S. aureus* infections attributable to such shedders have developed (see also Chap. 37).

Airborne Spread

Airborne spread from sources other than the patient and surgical personnel that leads to wound contamination and infections does not appear to be an important component in the epidemiology of early deep surgical wound infections. Filtration of the air and improved air-conditioning systems have controlled the spread of organisms from the outside as well as from adjacent wards.

Endogenous Sources

Endogenous sources are clearly a source of infection in many surgical wounds, and skeletal implants are no exception. The number of infections of endogenous origin, compared to other sources of contamination, has not been clearly established. It is highly probable that some of the acute implant infections and a larger proportion of the late infections are endogenous.

Prevention
Clean-Room System

Clearly, an institution with a high acute infection rate, in which surgical conditions are less than optimal and drug-resistant organisms are prevalent, would do well to consider seriously the use of a clean room. The system does not make up for poor surgical technique any more than do antibiotics. Of necessity, however, use of such a system does impose discipline on personnel who, in many hospitals, are not within the direct control of the surgeon. If a clean room is unavailable, infection rates can be reduced by the use of strict operating room and surgical techniques, which may be combined with appropriately selected and administered prophylactic antibiotics. The use of

UV light is another effective adjunct in reducing the incidence of infection associated with total joint replacement (see Table 36-6). It is less expensive than a clean-air installation, but care must be taken to protect the eyes and skin of the patient and all personnel within the operating room and the light source must be kept clean [12, 17].

Investigation and Attack of Causes

When the infection rate exceeds the expected range of 1 to 3 percent, the situation deserves a thoughtful approach. A blind rush to institute control measures should be avoided. Rather, attempts first should be made to determine why the infection rate is high. The first steps are to review the surgical techniques and conduct epidemiologic studies of the infections (see Chaps. 6, 33).

Carriers (i.e., shedders) that disseminate *S. aureus* into the environment may be responsible for surgical infections, but a carrier on the surgical team should not necessarily be considered a dangerous source of staphylococcal infections. If staphylococcal strains from a carrier have the same characteristics, including sensitivity profiles, as those recovered from infected wounds, this may then be sufficient to incriminate the carrier presumptively as a dangerous shedder (see Chaps. 1, 37). Epidemiologic incrimination of such a carrier requires the demonstration of a significantly higher risk of infections with the epidemic strain among patients whose THR operations are attended by the carrier than among patients whose THR procedures are not attended by the carrier. Such carriers should be managed as indicated in Chapter 33.

If surgical personnel are the sources of sporadic *S. aureus* infections, special efforts—such as the use of UAFS, body exhaust suits, and impermeable gowns—may be employed to minimize shedding. If the strains are usually traced to the patients (i.e., are endogenous), the method of preparation of the surgical area before surgery should be reviewed, and a change in antibiotic prophylaxis should be considered.

Late Deep Wound Infections
Clinical Features
Manifestations

It is necessary to emphasize the importance of the supplementary use of acrylics in implant fixation and its relation to late deep wound infections. The acrylic is used as a cement to fix the prosthesis to the bone. Loosening of the prosthesis is one of the universal symptoms of late infections. Bacteria causing bone resorption at the interface between the bone and the acrylic are sufficient to cause surgical failure. *S. epidermidis* is of special importance in this respect, since it is a frequent contaminant in surgical wounds. Even though these organisms are considered to be of relatively low virulence, they are capable of causing bone resorption with subsequent loosening of the prosthesis. *S. epidermidis* is nearly twice as common in late infections as in early infections, and it surpasses *S. aureus* as a cause of late deep infections. Gram-negative bacilli may also be associated with late infections.

Late deep wound infections present months or years after surgery. Due to their usually insidious nature, a high index of suspicion is necessary to establish the diagnosis at the earliest possible time. Early warnings are continuous pain in the hip area and an elevated erythrocyte sedimentation rate (ESR) or C-reactive protein value. Fever and leukocytosis are usually absent. The first sign suggestive of the presence of late infections is pain, which may or may not be associated with loosening of the prosthesis; loosening is usually detected radiographically. A lucency at the cement-bone or prosthesis-bone interface may be the initial sign of deep occult infection. Mechanical loosening of the prosthesis can also occur as a late complication in the absence of infection, and its appearance on radiograms is similar to that of infective loosening.

All late infections are not insidious, and some present with one or more of the typical characteristics of acute deep wound infections—that is, fever, leucocytosis, local inflammation, and abscess formation with or without sinus tracts.

Management

In general, late deep wound infections resolve only after the prosthesis is removed [28]. In a few instances, hip function may be salvaged by the removal of the loose device, debridement of the surrounding infected tissue, suction, irrigation, and the administration of antibiotics. Based on studies [36] in West Germany and elsewhere [27, 29], many surgeons recommend the insertion of a new prosthesis using antibiotics (e.g., gentamicin) mixed with the methylmethacrylate. There are insufficient data at the present time to determine the true efficacy of this approach. Experimental studies [36] have shown that the activity of gentamicin incorporated in methylmethacrylate is detectable for more than 70 weeks. Additional research in this area is needed to determine the usefulness of such an approach for the treatment and prevention of infection following THR surgery. In the United States, a two-stage exchange procedure, in which the surgeon delays from weeks to years between debridement of the infected prosthesis and placement of a new one, has been found more successful so it is the more popular treatment [18].

Antibiotic Therapy

Antibiotic treatment in patients with infections of insidious onset can be postponed until the microorganisms are identified and their antibiotic sensitivity patterns are established. This postponement is possible because by the time the infection is diagnosed, extensive involvement is present. When the culture reports are negative and a clinical diagnosis of infection is strongly suspected, the following factors should be taken into consideration in choosing an antibiotic: Late infections are usually due to staphylococci, either *S. aureus* or *S. epidermidis;* negative culture results may be obtained because of a failure to isolate strict anaerobic organisms; and Gram stains have been known to be positive, and wound cultures, negative. In such cases, guidance in choosing appropriate antibiotics may be provided by the morphologic and staining characteristics of the organisms.

In summary, an antistaphylococcal agent will usually be the drug of choice; preferably, one may be used that will be adequate for coagulase-negative staphylococci. When anaerobes are suspected, clindamycin seems to be a good choice, and *S. aureus* and *S. epidermidis* may also be susceptible to this drug. The choice of therapy for *S. epidermidis* infection should depend, whenever possible, on the sensitivity studies of the isolated pathogen. Vancomycin is the drug of choice for *S. epidermidis* in the absence of laboratory results.

Diagnostic Considerations

The following systematic approach is useful in evaluating the presence of latent deep infection about a skeletal prosthesis in a patient with a history of continuous pain accompanied by an elevated ESR or C-reactive protein level.

Radiography

X-ray films should be evaluated to determine whether the following indications of infection are present: Loosening of the prosthesis is a common sign, but it is not diagnostic of infection. This diagnosis may require both fluoroscopy and arthrography. The arthrograms are performed to determine whether the injected dye can be seen in the interface between the acrylic cement and the bone; this test is sometimes positive even when the x-ray shows no apparent loosening (Fig. 36-5). Arthrograms are also valuable to visualize abscess cavities and to determine whether sinus tracts communicate with the prosthesis. They also confirm the location of aspiration done for culture material. Periosteal reactive bone formation is another common finding in infection. Bone resorption about the cement or prosthesis, if present, will facilitate the diagnosis of osteomyelitis, and it is the most reliable radiographic sign of infection about a prosthesis (see Fig. 36-5).

Joint Aspiration

The aspiration of a prosthetic hip joint to obtain material for microbiologic examination is technically difficult but is of critical importance in evaluating the patient with suspected infection associated with total joint replace-

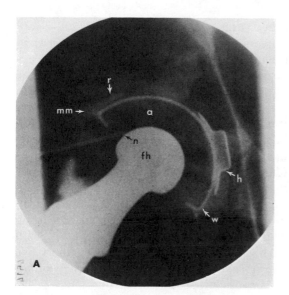

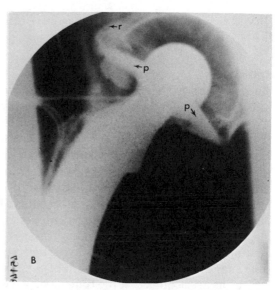

Fig. 36-5. Arthrogram of 67-year-old patient who had pain for 2 months following 14 months of pain-free function. After total hip replacement, there were no systemic or laboratory manifestations of infection. Cultures obtained during the procedure showed no growth. *A.* An anteroposterior view of the prosthesis. The tip of the needle (n) is in the articulation of the metallic prosthetic femoral head (fh) and the radiolucent polyethylene acetabular component (a). The methylmethacrylate used to bond the polyethylene socket to the adjacent bone is made radiodense by adding barium to it (mm). The circular wire (w) marks the junction between the plastic socket and the bonding methylmethacrylate. The wire "hat" (h) restrains methylmethacrylate from entering the pelvis. There is a distinct line of bone resorption (r) between the bone-methylmethacrylate interface that suggests loosening. *B.* After aspiration, an injection of opaque dye outlines the cavity about the prosthetic joint (p). Dye can be seen in the zone of resorption (r), which positively indicates loosening of the prosthesis and is highly suggestive of indolent infection. Culture of the aspirate yielded coagulase-negative staphylococci.

ment. Because the pseudocapsule must be entered with the needle, an arthrogram may be needed to confirm the position of the needle.

Radionuclide Scintimetry

The use of radionuclide scintimetry has been suggested in the diagnosis of hip infections [4]. Scintimetric results may be positive in the absence of positive radiographic findings. Scintimetry may also occasionally sharply delineate whether the acetabular component, the femoral component, or both are involved. Care should be taken in the interpretation of bone scintimetric results, however, because high scintimetric values may be due to periarticular bone formation rather than infection. Loosening of the prosthetic components, which is much more common than infection, will also be associated with increased uptake of radionuclides. Several investigators have suggested that the gallium scan can be effectively used in differentiating septic from aseptic component loosening. However, the efficacy of this technique has recently been questioned. Another technique that may be helpful in differentiating between septic and aspetic loosening of components is radionuclide scanning of indium-labeled white blood cells [20].

Biopsy

Frequently, the definitive diagnosis of infection requires examination of a biopsy specimen from the periprosthetic tissues. Biopsy specimens are usually obtained as part of the surgical procedure to remove the prosthetic device when it must be removed because of loosening. The material obtained should be from the deep tissue or bone to minimize contamination. The membrane between the bone and prosthetic material is an especially important tissue to culture. The material should be sent for microbiologic culture and histologic examination.

Sources and Modes of Acquisition

The sources of organisms that cause late infections are puzzling. Some are probably acquired at the time of surgery and remain dormant and undetected until the symptoms begin. Alternatively, the organisms may be seeded into the area via the bloodstream from distant foci.

Charnley [3] and Ericson and associates [5] have shown a reduction in the incidence of late infections when control measures were instituted in the surgical theater. Their results suggest that at least a portion of the late infections are acquired at the time of surgery. Additional evidence against a principal role for endogenous sources of late infections may be provided by the profile of causative agents, since this profile differs markedly from that of naturally occurring bacterial endocarditis (mainly viridans streptococci), and the latter infections clearly derive from bacteremic seeding.

There are convincing reports in the literature of infections of total joint replacements following infection elsewhere in the body. These may be infections with either grampositive or gram-negative organisms; several deep gram-negative infections have been reported following infections of the urinary tract with the same organism. There is not enough evidence at this time to determine whether late infections are due most often to surgical contamination or to late hematogenous spread. It seems clear, however, that endogenous sources and acquisition by direct and indirect contact at the time of surgery are each responsible for some infections.

Regarding endogenous infection, it is worth pointing out that many patients become colonized with *S. aureus* after admission. This colonization may be the source of a subsequent endogenous infection. Persistent colonization may be important, because a number of THR patients require bilateral hip replacements involving one or two periods of hospitalization.

Prevention

Prevention of infections with *S. epidermidis,* the most common cause of late infections, appears to be a very difficult task because of the large numbers of *S. epidermidis* organisms in the environment. The number of such organisms needed to establish a wound infection in a system including acrylics, polyethylene, metal, and bone is not known. If a large inoculum is needed to initiate an infection (more than 100 organisms), then preventive measures such as clean-air systems may be helpful in reducing the number of organisms settling in the wound during THR operations; with UAFS, it is calculated that fewer than five microorganisms per hour settle in the wound.

The use of prophylactic antibiotics to reduce the likelihood of endogenous contamination may be important if there is a significantly large number of endogenous infections. Prophylactic antibiotic administration for THR patients undergoing procedures likely to result in transient bacteremia might well be justified, and a controlled study of the effectiveness of this approach might provide insights into the relative importance of endogenous sources (see Chap. 42).

For infections that are acquired at the time of surgery, remain dormant, and subsequently cause late wound infection, all the preventive measures described previously for the prevention of early infections should be used. Clean rooms, prophylactic antibiotics, or both at the time of surgery should be effective in the prevention of such infections.

References

1. Bowers, W.H., Wilson, F. C., and Green, W. B. Antibiotic prophylaxis in experimental bone infections. *J. Bone Joint Surg. [Am.]* 55:795, 1973.
2. Burke, J. F. The effective period of preventative antibiotic action in experimental incision and dermal lesions. *Surgery* 50:161, 1961.
3. Charnley, J. Postoperative infections after total hip replacement with special reference to air contamination in the operating room. *Clin. Orthop.* 87:162, 1972.
4. Collie, L. P., Fitzgerald, R. H., and Brown,

M. L. In vivo localization of technetium and gallium radionuclides in infected bone. In: *Transactions of the Twenty-Ninth Annual Meeting of the Orthopedic Research Society*, 1983. P. 301.

5. Ericson, C., Lidgren, L., and Lindberg, L. Cloxacillin in the prophylaxis of postoperative infections of the hip. *J. Bone Joint Surg. [Am.]* 55:808, 1973.

6. Ewald, E. C., et al. Capitellocondylar total elbow arthroplasty. *J. Bone Joint Surg.* 62-A: 1259, 1980.

7. Fitzgerald, R. H., Jr., et al. Bacterial colonization of wounds and sepsis in total hip arthroplasties. *J. Bone Joint Surg. [Am.]* 55:1242, 1973.

8. Goodman, J. S., Seibert, D. G., Reahl, G. E., Jr., and Geckler, R. W. Fungal infection of prosthetic joints: A report of two cases. *J. Rheumatol.* 10(3):494, 1983.

9. Gristina, A. G., and Costerton, J. W. Bacterial adherence and the glycocalyx and their role in musculoskeletal infection. *Orthop. Clin. North Am.* 15:517, 1984.

10. Hill, C., Flamant, L., Mazar, F., and Evrard, J. Prophylactic cefazolin versus placebo in total hip replacement: Report of a multicenter double-blind randomized trial. *Lancet* 1:795, 1981.

11. Horadam, V. W., Smilack, J. D., and Smith, E. C. *Mycobacterium fortuitum* infection after total hip replacement. *South. Med. J.* 75(2): 244, 1982.

12. Howard, J. M., et al. Post-operative wound infections: The influence of ultraviolet irradiation of the operating room and of various other factors. *Am. Surg.* 160(Suppl.):1, 1964.

13. Kettlekamp, D. B., and Leach, R. B. Total knee replacement. *Clin. Orthop.* 94:2, 1973.

14. Kim, Y. Y., et al. Charnley low friction arthroplasty in tuberculosis of the hip. An eight to 13-year follow-up. *J. Bone Joint Surg. [Br.]* 70(5):756, 1988.

15. Lidwell, O. M., et al. Effect of ultraclean air in operating rooms on deep sepsis in the joint after total hip or knee replacement: A randomized study. *Br. Med. J.* 285:10, 1982.

16. Lonstein, J., Winter, R., Moe, J., and Gaines, D. Wound infection with Harrington instrumentation and spine fusion for scoliosis. *Clin. Orthop.* 96:222, 1973.

17. Lowell, J. D. Use of Ultraviolet Radiation in Total Joint Replacement Surgery. In: N. Eftekhar (Ed.), *Infections in Total Joint Replacement.* St. Louis: Mosby, 1984. Pp. 1979–185.

18. McDonald, D. J., Fitzgerald, R. H., Jr., and Ilstrup, D. M. Two-stage reconstruction of a total hip arthroplasty because of infection. *J. Bone Joint Surg. [Am.]* 71(6):828, 1989.

19. McElfresh, E. C., and Coventry, M. B. Femoral and pelvic fractures after total hip arthroplasty. *J. Bone Joint Surg.* 56A:483, 1971.

20. Merkel, K. D., Fitzgerald, R. H., Jr., Brown, M. L., and Dewanjel, M. K. Comparison of indium-WBC and sequential technetium-gallium imaging in suspected low-grade osteomyelitis. In: *Transactions of the Twenty-Ninth Annual Meeting of the Orthopedic Research Society,* 1983. P. 204.

21. Missenard, G., et al. Total Knee Prosthesis After Upper Tibia Resection for Tumors. In: T. Yamamuro (Ed.), *New Developments for Limb Salvage in Musculoskeletal Tumors.* Berlin: Springer-Verlag, 1989. Pp. 591–604.

22. Mutschler, W., Burri, C., and Kiefer, H. Functional Results After Pelvic Resection with Endoprosthetic Replacement. In. W. F. Enneking (Ed.), *Limb Salvage in Musculoskeletal Oncology.* New York: Churchill Livingstone, 1987. Pp. 156–166.

23. National Academy of Sciences, National Research Council. Postoperative wound infections: The influence of ultraviolet irradiation of the operating room and of various other factors. *Ann. Surg.* 160(Suppl.):1, 1964.

24. Neer, C. S., II, Watson, K. C., and Stanton, F. J. Recent experience in total shoulder replacement. *J. Bone Joint Surg.* 64-A:319, 1982.

25. Nelson, J. P. The operating room environment and its influence on deep wound infections. In: *The Hip: Proceedings of The Fifth Open Scientific Meeting of The Hip Society.* St. Louis: Mosby, 1977. P. 129.

26. Operating-Room Survey. Operating-room survey finds most orthopaedic surgeons use antibiotics regularly. *Orthop. Rev.* 3:156, 1974.

27. Petty, R. W. The effect of methylmethacrylate on phagocytosis and bacterial killing by human polymorphonuclear leucocytes. *J. Bone Joint Surg.* 60-A:752, 1978.

28. Petty, R. W., and Goldsmith, S. Resection arthroplasty following infected total hip arthroplasty. *J. Bone Joint Surg.* 62-A:889, 1980.

29. Petty, R. W., Spanier, S., and Silverthorne, C. Influence of skeletal implant materials on infection. In: *Transactions of the Twenty-Ninth Annual Meeting of the Orthopedic Research Society,* 1983. P. 137.

30. Ross, A. C., Wilson, J. W., and Scales, J. T. Endoprosthetic replacement of the proximal humerus. *J. Bone Joint Surg.* 69B:656, 1987.

31. Salvati, E. A., et al. Infection rates after 3,175 total hip and total knee replacements performed with and without a horizontal unidirectional filtered airflow system. *J. Bone Joint Surg.* 64-A:525, 1982.

32. Santavirta, S., et al. Total hip replacement in old tuberculosis. A report of 14 cases. *Acta Orthop. Scand.* 59(4):391, 1988.

33. Sim, F. H., and Chao, E. Y. S. Prosthetic replacement of the knee and large segment of the femur or tibia. *J. Bone Joint Surg.* 61A:887, 1979.

34. Sim, F. H., and Chao, E. Y. S. Segmental prosthetic replacement of the hip and knee. In: E. Y. S. Chao and J. C. Ivins (Eds.), *Tumor Prostheses for Bone and Joint Reconstruction.* New York: Thieme-Stratton, 1983. Pp. 247–266.

35. Stinchfield, F. E. Statistics on total hip replacement. *Clin. Orthop.* 95:2, 1973.

36. Wahlig, H., Hameister, W., and Grieben, A. Uber die freisetzung von gentamycin aus polymethylmethacrylat. I. Experimentelle untersuchungen in vitro. *Langenbecks Arch. Chir.* 331:169, 1972.

37. Wise, R. I., Sweeney, F. J., Jr., Haupt, G. J., and Waddell, M. A. The environmental distribution of *Staphylococcus aureus* in an operation suite. *Ann. Surg.* 149:30, 1958.

Epidemiology of Staphylococcus aureus and Group A Streptococci

Donald A. Goldmann

Historical Context

A review of staphylococcal and streptococcal epidemiology leads directly to the historical roots of infection control. Epidemics of puerperal sepsis first suggested that hospital-acquired infections could be a major cause of morbidity and mortality and might require an organized approach to control. Modern-day hospital infection control programs have developed largely in response to outbreaks of staphylococcal disease in the 1950s and 1960s. Thus it is not surprising that the early infection control literature was dominated by studies concerning the epidemiology of streptococcal and staphylococcal infection, and a rich and varied literature it is. More recently, other pathogens, particularly gram-negative bacilli, appeared to be supplanting gram-positive cocci on hospital wards, and the emphasis of the infection control literature changed accordingly. In the last few years, however, the field has come full circle as the emergence of methicillin-resistant *Staphylococcus aureus* and *Staphylococcus epidermidis* (see Chaps. 13, 27) has rekindled interest in staphylococcal epidemiology.

Epidemiology of Group A Streptococcal Infections
Transmission

Although streptococci have been a scourge of obstetric wards and surgical services for centuries, group A streptococcal nosocomial infection is relatively rare today. Group A streptococci are recovered from fewer than 1 percent of all surgical wound infections in hospitals participating in the National Nosocomial Infections Surveillance (NNIS) System. Thus the occurrence of even 1 group A streptococcal infection is reason for concern, and 2 or more cases in a short period of time should alert the infection control team that a full-scale epidemic investigation is warranted to determine the source of the outbreak.

Perhaps because streptococcal epidemics occur sporadically and unpredictably in hospitals, much of what we know about the transmission of group A streptococci comes from a series of remarkably careful studies in military populations performed by Rammelkamp and Wannamaker and their colleagues [67, 68, 70, 104]. It had already been demonstrated that streptococcal infections could be spread by contact with infected cutaneous lesions. Furthermore, it had been established that streptococcal disease could be transmitted to susceptible volunteers by inoculating the pharynx with secretions from patients with streptococcal pharyngitis. Thus it was known that transmission could occur by direct contact with the skin or secretions of infected individuals. The military studies were designed to answer two pivotal questions: (1) Could streptococci be transmitted by droplet nuclei generated from the respiratory tract of infected or colonized individuals, and (2) could dust and other environmental fomites serve as reservoirs for the airborne spread of streptococci? These studies therefore addressed one of the fundamental issues in infection control—the relative importance of airborne and contact transmission of infection.

To obtain a rough assessment of the relative significance of airborne transmission via dust or droplet nuclei versus direct contact spread via large droplets or respiratory secretions, Rammelkamp's group studied the incidence of streptococcal disease among susceptible soldiers as a function of the distance of their bunks from the beds of colonized or infected recruits [72]. If the risk of infection were increased only among soldiers whose bunks were very close to those of the index cases, the direct contact theory would be supported. On the other hand, if the incidence of infection were independent of location in the barracks, airborne spread would be the most likely explanation. In fact, the risk of a recruit acquiring group A streptococci turned out to be inversely proportional to the distance between

his bunk and that of a carrier (Fig. 37-1). At a distance of 30 ft, the acquisition rate was no higher than the background incidence of streptococcal acquisition among recruits in a control population. If the beds were located right next to each other, the risk more than tripled.

Although this study suggested that most streptococcal disease is transmitted by direct contact with large droplets, the possibility remained that some infections could be spread by contaminated dust or other environmental reservoirs. It seemed particularly important to rule out airborne transmission, since it was known that soldiers who carry streptococci in their throat or nose expel a prodigious number of bacteria onto their clothes, blankets, and other personal articles. Moreover, dust collected from barracks housing colonized or infected soldiers routinely yields enormous numbers of streptococci, and streptococci can remain viable in the environment for days. To find out whether contaminated dust or blankets could spread group A streptococcal infections among susceptible individuals, the following experiments were performed.

The initial studies were made possible by a bizarre but routine military procedure. Each new recruit was issued a set of wool blankets

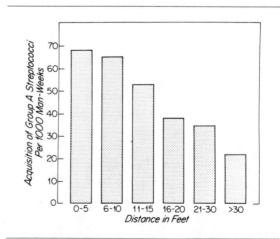

Fig. 37-1. Acquisition rates for group A streptococci according to bed distance from the nearest carrier. (Reprinted with permission from C.H. Rammelkamp et al., Transmission of streptococcal and staphylococcal infections. *Ann. Intern. Med.* 60:756, 1964.)

that he used until he was transferred to another unit or was admitted to a hospital. Unless these blankets were grossly soiled, they were reissued to a new recruit without cleaning. Thus it was common practice to issue blankets heavily contaminated with streptococci to susceptible soldiers. In the clinical study, blankets were donated by 83 colonized soldiers, including 15 who had just been hospitalized because of streptococcal disease. The blankets were stored for either 24 hours or 6 days and then reissued. Recipients were followed closely for acquisition of streptococci and clinical disease. A control group received laundered blankets that were shown not to harbor streptococci. Acquisition rates turned out to be slightly lower in soldiers issued the contaminated blankets (Fig. 37-2), although this difference was not statistically significant. Six recruits who received a contaminated blanket did develop streptococcal disease, but in only 2 cases did the serotype isolated from the throat of the soldier match the serotype from the contaminated blanket.

In the next experiment, 5 volunteers were placed in a small enclosure while approximately 50 to 100 gm of contaminated dust were blown in. The soldiers were asked to

sweep the floor for 10 minutes and to rest in a chair for 10 additional minutes. Air samples taken during the study period contained 100 to 1,600 streptococci per cubic foot. It was obvious that the volunteers had inhaled a considerable amount of contaminated dust since dust could be seen easily in mucus expelled by coughing or nose blowing for as long as 6 hours after exposure. No infections were observed, even though none of the volunteers had antibody to the streptococcal serotypes found in the dust.

To document additionally the inability of contaminated dust to transmit streptococcal infections, dust was sprinkled on the pharynx of 13 volunteers. Six other volunteers had dust containing 1,800 to 42,000 streptococci blown into the mouth. Streptococci could be recovered from the pharynx only transiently, and there were no infections.

Finally, 37 airmen were placed in a barracks while 50 to 150 gm of contaminated dust were blown into the room. The airmen lived in the barracks for 18 to 24 hours before sweeping it clean. No infections occurred.

These experiments suggest that airborne streptococci are not very infectious and rarely, if ever, produce pharyngitis in susceptible persons. Rather, it appears that close contact with respiratory secretions or droplets from colonized or infected patients is critical for transmission to occur.

Although airborne streptococci seem to be virtually incapable of producing pharyngitis, it does not necessarily follow that streptococci falling into a wound from contaminated air would be unable to initiate a streptococcal wound infection. Only a few streptococcal surgical wound infection outbreaks have been reported in the modern nosocomial infection literature, so data concerning the transmission of these infections are scarce. It is worth noting that the literature is virtually devoid of descriptions of outbreaks traced to a nasopharyngeal carrier on the medical or nursing staff, and outbreaks involving personnel with streptococcal skin lesions or extensive patient-to-patient transmission via hands (or, in a recent case, forearms) of personnel have been reported rarely in the last few decades [13].

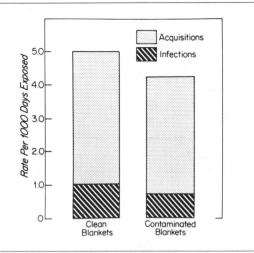

Fig. 37-2. Acquisition and infection rates with eight types of streptococci of men with clean or contaminated blankets. (Reprinted with permission from W.D. Perry et al., Transmission of group-A streptococci: I. The role of contaminated bedding. *Am. J. Epidemiol.* 66:89, 1957.)

Several reported epidemics have been attributed to vaginal or anal carriers among operating personnel. It is possible that this reflects a reporting bias: Anal or vaginal carriers may be perceived as unusual and therefore worthy of documentation [112], whereas epidemics caused by nasopharyngeal carriers may be seen as too mundane to warrant publication. Regardless, the reported outbreaks provide reasonably strong evidence that streptococci may reach operative wounds via the air [5, 62, 63, 66, 77, 81, 87].

Streptococci have been recovered from settling plates placed in operating rooms occupied by carriers who were linked epidemiologically to the surgical wound infections, and it has been suggested that streptococci are aerosolized by flatus or shed during exercise. As emphasized previously, mere dissemination of bacteria into the environment does not prove that these organisms actually were responsible for the observed infections. However, the carriers in some of the reported outbreaks had no direct contact with the infected patients. It is not known why airborne streptococci disseminated by carriers apparently can cause wound infections but not pharyngitis. Perhaps the open surgical wound is much more susceptible than the pharynx to airborne streptococci.

Epidemic Investigation

As soon as an outbreak of group A streptococcal nosocomial infection is recognized, the infection control team should immediately initiate a search for a carrier on the hospital staff (see Chap. 6). Of course, the possibility of person-to-person transmission via the hands of personnel cannot be ignored, particularly in the newborn nursery and on other non-surgical services, but streptococcal operative wound infections are generally inoculated in the operating room and can virtually always be traced to a carrier. As noted earlier, the recent literature suggests that the carrier is more likely to be colonized with streptococci in the anus or vagina than in the throat, but the prudent epidemiologist will not begin an investigation by indiscriminately culturing a particular anatomic site. Rather, a formal epi-

demiologic investigation should be undertaken to ascertain whether infected patients had a significantly greater exposure to individual members of the staff. Personnel identified by the epidemiologic investigation should be questioned closely about recent sore throats, skin infections, or vaginal or anal symptomatology. Although perineal disseminators may be totally asymptomatic, most of the carriers reported in the literature have had mild symptoms that could easily be missed by a casual investigation. For example, the surgeon responsible for the outbreak reported by Richman and colleagues [77] suffered from external hemorrhoids to which he applied corticosteroid ointment daily. The circulating nurse implicated in the epidemic described by Berkelman and associates [5] had chronic bouts of diarrhea complicated by shallow perineal ulcers.

Isolation of streptococci from anal or vaginal cultures taken from someone who has been linked epidemiologically to an outbreak is strong evidence pointing to the source of the problem, particularly since group A streptococci are rarely found at these sites in healthy adults. However, it is usually desirable to obtain additional laboratory data to prove that the carrier is colonized or infected with the same strain of group A streptococci that was recovered from the nosocomial infections. First, serogrouping should be performed to confirm that the organism is indeed group A, since streptococci of groups B, C, and G can also be both β-hemolytic and bacitracin-susceptible. Serogrouping occasionally yields surprises. Goldmann and Breton [33] found that the β-hemolytic streptococci recovered from a small cluster of orthopedic infections were of group C, and group C streptococci were subsequently isolated from the anus of a member of the surgical staff. If additional microbiologic confirmation is required, group A streptococci can be classified by reference laboratories according to their M and T antigens and by their serum opacity reaction [59]. Occasionally, the symptom complex caused by the streptococci is so distinctive that it is clear that all the cases are associated with the same strain. For example, Richman and co-workers [77] recognized their outbreak when 2 cases of scarlet fever occurred on the orthopedic service within a short period of time.

Nasopharyngeal carriers of group A streptococci can usually be treated successfully with penicillin or erythromycin. If streptococci are not eradicated by these regimens, amoxicillin–clavulanic acid or a penicillinase-resistant cephalosporin may be effective. The addition of a 4-day course of rifampicin to the standard penicillin regimen may be advisable [17, 92]. Vaginal and anal carriers pose a greater challenge. Oral penicillin may fail to eradicate anal carriage. Oral vancomycin, which is not absorbed from the bowel, has been advocated as a supplement to penicillin therapy. Other regimens may have to be tried empirically. Even if it appears that anal or vaginal carriage has been eliminated, vigilance should be maintained. In one outbreak [5], vaginal carriage recurred with a different strain of *Streptococcus*, leading to a renewed outbreak of streptococcal disease that received considerable attention in the national press. In another outbreak [66], a persistent anal carrier was associated with widely separated cases of endometritis and bacteremia occurring over more than a year, despite treatment with various regimens of penicillin, rifampicin, and oral vancomycin.

Increased Virulence of Group A Streptococci

In recent years, there has been an apparent increase in the virulence of group A streptococci, as well as in the incidence of nonpyogenic streptococcal sequelae. The implications of these developments for hospital infection control programs are not yet clear, but public alarm has been so great that hospital epidemiologists can expect publicity and scrutiny if group A streptococcal infections occur in their institution.

There has been a resurgence in rheumatic fever in several regions of the United States [18, 41, 99–101, 107], and military installations, many of which had become complacent during years of relatively low disease activity, have experienced dramatic outbreaks of streptococcal infection and rheumatic fever [101]. Although the sudden appearance of these geographically defined problems has not been fully explained, some investigators have suggested an association between rheumatic fever and the circulation of specific mucoid M types of streptococci, particularly M18. Of even greater potential concern to hospital epidemiologists is the reported increase in the severity of group A streptococcal infections [3, 89, 90]. These fulminant, potentially fatal infections have been dubbed *streptococcal toxic shock* [90] or *toxic shock–like* [89]. Although a pyrogenic (erythrogenic) toxin produced by some of the strains recovered from severely ill patients [50, 89] does resemble the toxin associated with *S. aureus* toxic shock [50], it is important to note that most of the patients reported to date have not presented with the classic staphylococcal syndrome. For example, in the report of 20 patients from the Rocky Mountain region that prompted initial public concern, none had diffuse erythema or a scarlatina-form eruption on admission [89]. Rather, severe soft-tissue infections, including cellulitis and necrotizing fasciitis, were common, often accompanied by bacteremia, shock, acute respiratory distress syndrome, and renal failure.

Epidemiology of *Staphylococcus aureus* Nosocomial Infections
Transmission

Group A streptococcal nosocomial infections gave the advocates of airborne and direct contact theories of transmission an excuse to have a skirmish; the epidemics of *S. aureus* infection in the 1950s and 1960s provided an opportunity to start a war. British investigators performed a vast number of detailed microbiologic studies to demonstrate how carriers of staphylococci could heavily contaminate the air. This extensive literature is not well known in the United States, and Americans with an interest in staphylococcal epidemiology have largely ignored the careful work of Hare, Ridley, Shooter, Nobel, Davies, Blowers, Lidwell, and many other British colleagues. Indeed, with the exception of Walter and Kundsin [103], who elaborated on the principles developed by Wells [106], the concept of airborne transmission of staphylococci has had few advocates in the United States. Among the many investigators who have sought to put airborne spread in perspective are Rammelkamp in the United States [72] and Williams in Great Britain [111]. The issues have been summarized succinctly by Williams, who wrote in 1966: "It is a characteristic of the airborne route of infection. . . that whenever there is the possibility of aerial transfer there is almost always the possibility of transfer by other routes. This is perhaps especially true of the forms of staphylococcal infection that have been most extensively studied, namely, those occurring in hospitals" [111]. This debate between proponents of airborne and contact spread is of more than historical interest; those who enthusiastically promote the performance of surgery in laminar airflow operating rooms [53] or under ultraviolet lights [70] are merely reflecting their continued belief in the importance of airborne spread of staphylococci and other bacteria.

Since most of the outbreaks of staphylococcal disease in the 1950s and 1960s were caused by a single phage type (often referred to as 80/81, although these strains were generally also lysed by other phages), early British investigators naturally concentrated on identifying carriers who might be disseminating the epidemic strain on wards and in the operating room. Had they been faced with the kinds of outbreaks that we tend to see today, which generally are caused by more than one phage type, it is possible that their research would have focused on the role of the patient's endogenous staphylococcal flora and the importance of transmission of staphylococci on the hands of personnel. Instead, they doggedly pursued staphylococcal carriers and shedders.

The principal site of staphylococcal colonization is the anterior nares. If repeated cultures are performed, up to 80 percent of adults are found to harbor *S. aureus* in the nose at one time or another [108]. In most persons, the carrier state is transient, but 20 to 40 percent of adults remain colonized for months or even years. Often the same strain remains in residence for prolonged periods of time and, if it is eradicated, a new strain of *Staphylococcus* tends to take its place. The factors that predispose to stable colonization are unknown. Hospital personnel and patients tend to have higher colonization rates than persons outside the hospital environment, particularly during nosocomial staphylococcal outbreaks.

Increased nasal colonization rates have also been noted in insulin-dependent diabetics [97], individuals on hemodialysis [113] and continuous ambulatory peritoneal dialysis [58], intravenous drug abusers [98], and even in patients receiving routine allergy injections [47]. Thus, percutaneous injections or catheterization may predispose to colonization, although the pathogenesis of this phenomenon is unclear. It has also been suggested that patients with symptomatic human immunodeficiency virus infection have an increased colonization risk [73].

When it was recognized that hospital personnel could be carriers of staphylococci, some hospitals required routine nasal cultures of personnel so that they could be treated before they transmitted their staphylococci to patients. This practice never gained widespread acceptance for a number of reasons:

1. Many carriers do not disseminate staphylococci during normal breathing.
2. Staphylococci are most efficiently liberated directly from the nose of a healthy carrier when air is forcefully expelled, creating a loud snorting sound [37].
3. Many carriers may be present on hospital wards without any infections occurring in patients.
4. Even if there is an outbreak of staphylococcal infection on a ward, personnel who become nasal carriers may be innocent bystanders rather than the cause of the problem.
5. Routine nasal cultures are expensive, and the resulting reams of data are generally uninterpretable.

6. Eradication of the nasal carrier state may be difficult.

Although the nose itself probably is not important in the direct dispersal of staphylococci, shedding is more likely to occur in nasal carriers who have a heavy growth of staphylococci on nasal swab cultures [25]. Moreover, the nose is the site that supports colonization of the entire skin surface of most carriers. Eradication of staphylococci from the nose is generally accompanied by elimination of *S. aureus* from the entire body. In some staphylococcal carriers, however, the perineum is the primary site of colonization, and staphylococci may not be found on repeated cultures of the nose [105].

Both nasal and perineal carriers continually shed staphylococci on skin squames—aptly called *rafts* by British investigators. Because of their size, shape, and weight, these contaminated squames may be carried along on currents of air in the hospital, resulting in airborne dispersal of staphylococci (see Chap. 1). Fortunately, most colonized hospital personnel shed modest numbers of squames, and the relatively small number of staphylococci dispersed into the environment are quickly diluted by conventional air-handling systems and washed away by standard housekeeping practices. A small percentage of colonized persons disperse much larger numbers of staphylococci into their immediate environment, however, and are referred to as *heavy shedders*. High concentrations of airborne staphylococci may result, and staphylococci contaminating the environment may remain viable for long periods of time. Dermatologic disorders, such as eczema and psoriasis, clearly predispose to skin scaling and shedding but, in most cases, the reason for heavy shedding is not readily apparent. Carriers who have a heavy growth of staphylococci on culture of the anterior nares tend to colonize body sites more readily than carriers with scant nasal colonization [110], but this observation does not explain the phenomenon of heavy shedding per se.

Some insight into staphylococcal shedding patterns has been gained by studying the dispersion of staphylococci from volunteers confined to a small enclosure. The test chamber may be either rudimentary or very elaborate (Fig. 37-3), but the basic principle involves collecting and quantitatively culturing the air in the chamber for staphylococci while the subject wears various types of clothing and moves about as instructed. Using this experimental technique, it has been demonstrated repeatedly that men are more likely than women to be heavy shedders [6, 40]. If a male heavy shedder is placed in a chamber clothed only in polyethylene or tightly woven cloth underpants, dispersal of staphylococci is practically eliminated, indicating that most bacteria are shed from the perineum of carriers [40]. However, subsequent studies demonstrated that there was little value in subjecting carriers to the discomfort of wearing plastic underwear since staphylococcus-bearing skin squames were liberated from other body sites when the shedder was fully clothed, presumably due to the friction of fabric against the skin [64]. Skin staphylococci readily escaped from street clothing and standard operating room garb [86], but dispersion could be reduced somewhat by clothing made of tightly woven fabric [7]. Taken to the extreme, efforts to eliminate shedding in the operating room have led to the development of total body suits with individual ventilation and exhaust systems. Although these suits are a logical extension of the staphylococcal shedding experiments just mentioned, it is important to emphasize that such radical and costly measures should rarely be necessary since very few hospital personnel actually shed significant numbers of staphylococci. Nosocomial outbreaks of staphylococcal infection, whether in the operating room or on the wards, have seldom been traced to a shedder on the hospital staff or to environmental contamination. For this reason, most hospital epidemiologists discourage extreme measures to eliminate shedding and concentrate instead on good aseptic surgical technique, careful hand-washing, and other measures designed to reduce direct contact transmission.

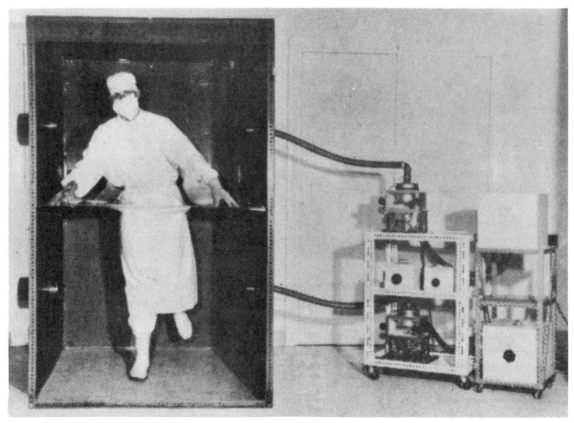

Fig. 37-3. Test chamber with door removed showing waistline division, air-inlet filters, and air-sampling equipment. (Reprinted with permission from D.W. Bethune et al., *Lancet* 27:4, 1965.)

Epidemic Investigation

The key to detecting the presence of a staphylococcal shedder lies not in surveillance cultures but in careful surveillance for nosocomial staphylococcal infections (see Chap. 5).

If an increasing incidence of infection is noted, phage typing should be requested to determine whether a single epidemic strain is responsible (see chap. 9). However, many strains are not typable with routine phage panels, and even strains with similar phage patterns may be unrelated epidemiologically. Capsular serotyping is of limited practical utility because most clinical strains fall within the same few serotypes [29, 44]. Occasionally, antibiotic resistance profiles may be helpful, particularly if the isolates are resistant to methicillin or specific aminoglycosides. However, multiply resistant strains may be epidemiologically distinct, and plasmid-mediated resistance patterns (see Chap. 14) may change in the course of an outbreak due to selective antibiotic pressure and the gain or loss of plasmids [48]. When plasmids are present in the staphylococcal isolates of interest, electrophoretic analysis of whole-plasmid DNA and restriction endonuclease digests of plasmid DNA can provide additional information, particularly in identifying the common origin of plasmids and their acquisition or loss [1, 48, 52, 61, 76, 114]. These techniques should be more than adequate for the vast majority of outbreak investigations, but occasionally even more sophisticated expertise will be needed to dissect the spread of *S. aureus* through the hospital population over time. Multilocus enzyme (esterase) electrophoresis has already been applied to the epidemiologic study of *S. aureus* [8, 10], and Western blots of whole staphylococcal cell lysates using pooled serum from patients who have had *S. aureus* infections has shown promise [91]. Molecular genetic techniques such as pulsed gel electrophoresis of chromosomal DNA and detection of specific staphylococcal genes by DNA probes also deserve further investigation. One recent cluster of postoperative wound infections, for example, was linked to a neurosurgeon by DNA blot-hybridization using DNA probes specific for chromosomal determinants of β-lactamase production and erythromycin and spectinomycin resistance [49]. Since the affected patients also had manifestations of the toxic shock syndrome, the outbreak strains were also probed with a toxic shock toxin gene probe and were found to have identical hybridization patterns.

When an epidemic strain is identified, personnel should not be cultured indiscriminately. Rather, the microbiologic investigation should focus on persons who appear to be associated epidemiologically with infected patients (see Chap. 6). These persons should be inspected carefully for signs of infection and questioned regarding recent infections or skin problems. Cultures of the nose, perineum, and sites of possible skin infection or dermatitis should be obtained, and any resulting *S. aureus* isolates should be phage-typed. Of course, it is difficult to know whether a staff member is colonized because of his or her contact with infected patients or vice versa. Formal shedding studies are cumbersome unless the infection control team happens to be in possession of a shedding chamber, but a rough measure of the intensity of shedding can be obtained by quantitatively culturing the carrier's clothing or by asking the carrier to exercise in a small, poorly ventilated room in which settling plates have been placed.

Staphylococcal epidemics caused by heavy shedders definitely are the exception rather than the rule, and most hospital epidemiologists probably will never be confronted by such an outbreak. At some point in the workup of almost all staphylococcal outbreaks, however, the infection control team will be forced at least to consider the possibility that a carrier is at the heart of the problem. Understandably, staff members tend to become apprehensive as the investigation proceeds, particularly if the investigators seem to be interested in their contact with the infected patients. Thus it is extremely important to proceed in a frank and forthright manner, to eschew premature conclusions based on incomplete data, and to avoid capricious culturing forays. If the epidemiologic study clearly implicates one person, the infection control team must expect to encounter guilt and fear. A surgeon, for example, may have justifiable anxiety about possible litigation and damage to his or her career. Depending on the tact and skill of the investigators, the implicated staff member may be fully cooperative or may display the hostility and defensiveness of someone accused. It is essential for the infection control team to speak with one voice and to follow a rational plan of action that has been discussed fully with the directors of the appropriate services.

If the epidemiologic evidence is very strong, it is prudent to remove the presumed carrier from patient care activities while cultures are obtained. If staphylococci are recovered on culture, treatment is generally begun before phage typing results are available, since reference laboratories may be unwilling to perform typing on an urgent basis. Because the carrier will usually want to return to work as soon as possible, the infection control team will be under considerable pressure to expedite treatment and issue work clearance. Unfortunately, there are no universally accepted criteria for determining when it is safe to send a carrier back to the wards. Certainly work should not be permitted until cultures of at least the nose and perineum are negative, although it must be realized that negative cultures while still undergoing therapy may indicate that the carrier state is suppressed but not eradicated. When treatment is concluded, therefore, the carrier should again be removed from work until follow-up cultures are performed and the results are available. Alternatively, some infection control teams may elect to take a more conservative approach and to suspend patient care activities for the entire period of treatment until follow-up cultures are negative. In either case, careful surveillance should be carried out after the carrier returns to work, since the carrier state and shedding may recur. Some authorities advocate placing settling plates in the immediate work environment for a period of several months as an additional, but untested, security measure.

A staggering array of systemic and topical antimicrobial regimens has been used in an effort to eradicate nasal carriage of staphylococci [108]. Systemic agents have included cephalosporins, semisynthetic penicillins, erythromycin, tetracycline, and fusidic acid. All these agents temporarily suppress the carrier state during therapy, but when adequate follow-up cultures are performed, staphylococci reappear in the majority of persons. Rifampicin, given in combination with another systemic agent, such as trimethoprim or trimethoprim-sulfamethoxazole, to retard emergence of rifampicin resistance, is a promising alternative to previously available regimens [27, 28, 56, 65, 79, 102, 105, 109]. Alternatively, some investigators have attempted to prevent resistance by combining rifampicin with an intranasal topical agent, such as bacitracin [75, 102], but this strategy may fail if there are extranasal sites of colonization [102]. If the staphylococci acquire resistance to the antibiotic being administered, staphylococcal shedding may actually increase, perhaps reflecting suppression of competing nasal flora. Most topical antimicrobials, including lysostaphin, gentamicin, neomycin, chlorhexidine, vancomycin, and bacitracin, have been equally unsuccessful in eradicating the carrier state. However, topical mupirocin (pseudomonic acid) has shown considerably greater promise when applied intranasally two to three times daily for 5 to 7 days [2, 15, 16, 40]. Recent reports have suggested that 8 doses given over 48 hours is sufficient to eliminate carriage, and that carriers may return to work within 24 hours of commencing therapy [14a]. Although mupirocin has been used primarily in the treatment of carriers of methicillin-resistant *S. aureus* (MRSA; see under the heading Methicillin-Resistant *S. aureus*), there is no compelling reason to believe that it would be less effective against methicillin-susceptible strains. Some investigators have noted the emergence of mupirocin resistance [85], but resistance remains rare even in the face of intensive use of this antimicrobial agent [19]. Unfortunately, in the United States, mupirocin is available only in a propylene glycol base that can be irritating to mucous membranes. In England, mupirocin is formulated in a paraffin base.

In addition to administering antibiotics and applying antimicrobial ointments to the nose, the infection control team may try other strategies that have not been tested systematically in staphylococcal carriers. Although suppression of nasal staphylococci eventually leads to elimination of staphylococci from other sites, it seems logical to try to hasten this process along by prescribing daily hexachlorophene showers during the treatment period. This approach is especially appealing in carriers who have colonization of the perineum or other sites in the absence of nasal colonization. Since other members of the carrier's family may also be colonized with the outbreak strain, thus providing a reservoir for recolonization of the shedder, it seems reasonable to treat them if nasal cultures yield staphylococci. In refractory cases, it may be advisable to recommend laundering of clothing and bedding as well as a thorough housecleaning to reduce the burden of staphylococci in the household.

Rarely, persistent or recurrent shedding of staphylococci may jeopardize a health professional's career. When all else fails, it is reasonable to consider trying bacterial interference. In the 1960s, Shinefield and co-workers [82] discovered that implantation of *S. aureus* strain 502A in the umbilicus and nose of neonates could prevent—or interfere with—colonization and infection with more virulent staphylococcal strains, such as phage type 80/81. Bacterial interference with strain 502A was subsequently tried in adults suffering from recurrent furunculosis; it showed considerable success provided the carrier state was first suppressed with antibiotics [88]. Although the implantation of strain 502A in neonates occasionally resulted in 502A infections, this complication has not been noted in adults and presumably would not cause problems for otherwise healthy carriers. Of course, it is unknown whether successfully recolonized carriers would become heavy shedders of 502A, which might then produce infections in susceptible patients.

The vast literature concerning staphylococcal carriers and shedders tends to obscure the fact that the patients themselves frequently serve as reservoirs for staphylococci and that staphylococci are transmitted from patient to patient on the hands of personnel. Thus prompt isolation of patients with documented staphylococcal infections is extremely important. When drainage is slight or easily contained by a dressing, it is sufficient to wear gloves when touching infectious material (see Chap. 11). Full contact precautions [30] are indicated for more extensive infections, and a private room and mask are generally recommended for patients with staphylococcal pneumonia or widespread cutaneous disease, such as infected dermatitis or burn wounds. Fear of airborne transmission is at the root of the single-room recommendation—transmission by skin squames in the case of cutaneous infections and by droplet nuclei in the case of pneumonia. Indeed the rooms of these patients quickly become contaminated with large numbers of staphylococci, so a single room may be reasonable despite the apparent rarity of airborne spread. Masks are recommended to protect personnel from colonization with nosocomial staphylococcal strains. Again, this may be logical but, even if a member of the attending staff is colonized, it is exceedingly unlikely that he or she will become a heavy shedder.

Staphylococcal Disease in the Nursery

Over the years, the nursery has provided numerous opportunities to study the acquisition and transmission of *S. aureus*. Newborns seldom acquire staphylococci from their mothers at the time of birth but rapidly become colonized if they are admitted to a nursery where many babies are already colonized. The umbilicus is usually the initial site of colonization [43], but staphylococci quickly spread to the nose and other skin sites. Spread from infant to infant undoubtedly occurs

via the hands of the doctors and nurses who care for colonized babies; airborne transmission almost never occurs. These principles, which are widely accepted today, were hotly disputed before Rammelkamp and his colleagues [72] performed their classic studies of nursery staphylococcal epidemiology in the 1950s.

Rammelkamp's studies were carried out in a small ward containing seven bassinets (Fig. 37-4) [72]. A baby known to be colonized with staphylococci was placed in one of these beds. Newborns were then admitted directly to the ward and placed either right next to the index baby or 4.5 or 11 ft away. The 3 nurses who cared for the noncolonized newborns wore double masks and washed their hands with hexachlorophene after each patient contact; the index patient was cared for by separate personnel. Nasal cultures were obtained from the babies every other day. Of the 91 newborns brought onto this special ward, only 3 became colonized with the index baby's staphylococcal strain. During 2 weeks of this study, one of the nurses, who was colo-

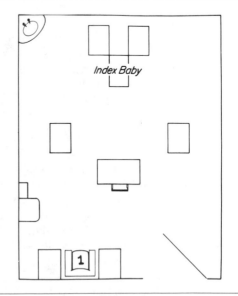

Fig. 37-4. Results of exposure of infants to carriers of staphylococci. (Reprinted with permission from C.H. Rammelkamp et al., Transmission of streptococcal and staphylococcal infections. *Ann. Intern. Med.* 60:756, 1964.)

nized with *S. aureus,* sat for 8 hours per day in the chair between the two bassinets in position 1 of Figure 37-4. Although she did not wear a mask, none of the babies in the room acquired her strain of *Staphylococcus.* This is hardly surprising since the probability that she was a heavy shedder was very small. More interesting results were obtained by allowing this nurse and another colonized nurse to handle the noncolonized babies in a routine fashion. Approximately 20 percent of the babies cared for by these nurses acquired their caretakers' staphylococcal strains.

A subsequent study revealed that these staphylococci were transferred to the babies by direct contact with organisms on the nurses' hands. In this study, the same 2 nurses and a third carrier handled 37 infants for 10 minutes each through the ports of an Isolette incubator. Fifty-four percent of these babies acquired staphylococci from their nurse, as determined by phage typing of organisms recovered from cultures of the nose and umbilicus. This study demonstrated that so-called Isolettes do not effectively shield newborns from the most important route of staphylococcal cross-infection in the nursery—transmission via the hands.

Even in spacious, well-staffed nurseries, spread of staphylococci may be difficult to control (see Chap. 21). Transmission occurs much more readily in crowded, hectic nurseries. Staffing appears to be a particularly critical factor. Haley and Bregman [36] were able to demonstrate that clusters of staphylococcal infections occur significantly more frequently when patient-staff ratios are highest.

Control of nursery staphylococcal outbreaks is facilitated by prompt recognition, but detection is not always easy. Most well babies spend only 2 or 3 days in the nursery, so hospital-acquired staphylococcal infections may not become manifest clinically until the baby is at home. Moreover, the majority of infections are mild and do not require readmission to the hospital. Therefore, community pediatricians must be encouraged to report all staphylococcal infections to the infection control office. Seemingly trivial infections, such as pustulosis, omphalitis, circumcision wound infection, and conjunctivitis, have just as much epidemiologic significance as infant mastitis, septic arthritis, or osteomyelitis. Community obstetricians should also participate in the reporting process, since a single case of maternal mastitis may be the initial sign of a nursery problem.

In an effort to predict when a staphylococcal outbreak is imminent, some nurseries routinely monitor staphylococcal colonization rates by culturing the umbilicus and nose when babies are discharged. Such surveillance cultures are expensive and rarely helpful. Although there is a rough correlation between the number of babies colonized with staphylococci and the incidence of staphylococcal infections [32], many nurseries routinely find high colonization rates without experiencing an outbreak [55, 82]. Surveillance cultures may be more informative when performed to determine the impact of specific control measures on transmission of staphylococci in the nursery or to verify that a particular epidemic strain has been eradicated.

The severe outbreaks of staphylococcal disease that struck nurseries in the 1950s and 1960s led to the introduction of a variety of infection control measures. Perhaps the simplest and most effective was routine bathing of neonates with 3% hexachlorophene [31]. Hexachlorophene, with its excellent and persistent activity against gram-positive bacteria, drastically reduced staphylococcal colonization and subsequent infection. By eliminating the normal gram-positive cutaneous flora along with the *S. aureus,* hexachlorophene paved the way for colonization by nosocomial gram-negative bacilli such as *Pseudomonas* [54], but this appeared to be a minor disadvantage at the time since the importance of neonatal gram-negative infections had not yet been recognized. Of greater concern were reports of hexachlorophene toxicity. Patients with burns or extensive dermatitis who were bathed with large amounts of hexachlorophene developed a convulsive disorder associated with cystic degenerative changes in the white matter. Similar neuropathologic changes were seen in infant animal models treated with topical hexachlorophene [46], as well as in human neonates, particularly premature infants [71, 84]. The human studies were retrospective, and there has been no convincing evidence that bathing full-term infants with hexachlorophene is hazardous. Nonetheless, in 1972 the Food and Drug Administration recommended against routine use of hexachlorophene in nurseries. This recommendation resulted in a sharp decline in hexachlorophene bathing and a significant increase in the number of outbreaks of nursery staphylococcal disease in the United States [45]. Balacing the potential risks and benefits of hexachlorophene use, it seems reasonable to avoid routine bathing of newborns. However, hexachlorophene may be a valuable adjunct to other control measures during a staphylococcal outbreak. As an added measure of safety, some investigators suggest diluting the hexachlorophene 1:4 or 1:5 and omitting baths for premature infants, although it is possible that these compromises could reduce efficacy. The safety and efficacy of alternative antiseptic agents, such as chlorhexidine gluconate and mupirocin, have not been adequately studied.

Since the umbilicus is one of the initial sites of staphylococcal colonization in the neonate, a variety of topical antiseptics have been applied to it in an effort to abort colonization without washing the entire body surface. The basic validity of this approach has been demonstrated by studies using triple dye, an aqueous mixture of brilliant green, proflavine hemisulfate, and crystal violet [69], but the safety of this agent has not been evaluated extensively. Other topical antiseptics such as bacitracin, alcohol, and iodophors may be as effective as triple dye and more acceptable aesthetically, but none has been studied adequately.

Recently, an outbreak of methicillin-resistant *S. aureus* in a special-care nursery for low-birth-weight infants apparently was controlled in part by applying mupirocin in a *paraffin* base to the umbilicus and nose twice daily for 7 days, coupled with a dusting of 0.3% hexachlorophene powder over the umbilicus, axillae, and perineum [23]. These results must

be considered preliminary. The safety of mupirocin in a propylene glycol base (the preparation available in the United States) has not been documented in newborns.

When topical antiseptics and conventional infection control measures failed to halt epidemics of severe staphylococcal disease in the 1960s, Shinefield and colleagues [83] tried the more radical approach of bacterial interference (see previous discussion). In general, implantation of *S. aureus* 502A in the nose and umbilicus was highly successful in preventing colonization by nosocomial staphylococcal strains. Although this strategy fell into disfavor when epidemics of staphylococcal disease abated and reports of occasional serious disease due to 502A appeared, bacterial interference remains a possible approach in difficult-to-control nursery epidemics.

The emphasis in the medical literature on topical antiseptics and bacterial interference tends to obscure the fact that adherence to standard infection control routines is of primary importance in limiting the transmission of staphylococci in the nursery. Thorough hand-washing after contact with infants is imperative (see Chap. 11). Hexachlorophene may be used for routine hand-washing when a staphylococcal problem is recognized in the nursery but probably should be avoided at other times because its use may encourage transmission of gram-negative bacilli on the hands. Infants with staphylococcal infections should be placed on contact precautions [30]. Consideration should be given to placing babies with intercurrent viral respiratory infections on more stringent precautions (mask when close to the patient and single room required), because such babies tend to aerosolize large numbers of staphylococci into the environment—the so-called cloud baby phenomenon described by Eichenwald and colleagues [26]. Colonized babies may be segregated with infected babies in a separate part of the nursery and, if possible, assigned separate nursing staff (see Chap. 21). Some nursery staffs have elected to use a cohort admissions system to reduce the opportunity for person-to-person spread. In a typical system, all infants admitted in a 48-hour period are placed in a single room, and traffic of personnel from this room to other rooms is minimized or avoided altogether. After 48 hours, the room is closed to additional admissions and not reopened until the entire cohort has been discharged and the room cleaned thoroughly. Clearly, the success of cohorting depends on the availability of separate nursery areas and sufficient personnel. In nurseries with inadequate facilities and insufficient staff, elegant cohorting and isolation arrangements may be impossible, and the only way to cope with an escalating rate of staphylococcal infection is to close the units temporarily to new admissions.

Outbreaks of nursery staphylococcal disease frequently are caused by multiple phage types and presumably result from lapses in technique rather than the presence of a carrier on the obstetric or neonatal staff. Unfortunately, as noted previously, phage typing results are seldom available immediately, and pressure may mount to treat all nasal carriers. This is understandable and perhaps unavoidable since there may be few epidemiologic clues in a busy nursery in which most of the staff have contact with most of the infants. Since few nursery staphylococcal outbreaks have been shown to be caused by shedders on the staff, however, it may be more prudent to stress good aseptic technique and other standard infection control measures than to jump immediately to wholesale treatment of nasal carriers.

Methicillin-Resistant *S. aureus*

S. aureus resistant to methicillin and a number of other frontline antibiotics has emerged as a major nosocomial pathogen over the past two decades. Data from the NNIS System indicate that the incidence of MRSA infections continues to increase progressively; MRSA has penetrated hospitals of virtually all sizes and types, except perhaps for the smallest community hospitals [R. Gaynes, Centers for Disease Control: unpublished data]. The result has been a resurgence of interest in staphylococcal epidemiology, as literally hundreds of published papers and several recent comprehensive reviews attest [9, 12, 14]. These inten-

sive studies have yielded few epidemiologic surprises, but it has been interesting to watch a new crop of epidemiologists reaffirming the observations made by their mentors who investigated methicillin-sensitive staphylococci years ago. Nonetheless, control (or preferably eradication) of MRSA is a high priority for hospital epidemiologists, since these strains are just as virulent as their more susceptible relatives but much more difficult and expensive to treat. In hospitals with major methicillin resistance problems, vancomycin, a relatively expensive and toxic agent that requires costly monitoring, has become the antibiotic of choice for empiric coverage of *S. aureus,* as well as for therapy of documented infections. Other agents—for example, trimethoprim-sulfamethoxazole, the quinolones, and new glycopeptides such as teicoplanin—may have therapeutic potential, but vancomycin is the last commercially available antibiotic that both has activity against all strains of *S. aureus* isolated to date and has demonstrated efficacy in animal models and patients.

Once MRSA has become established in a hospital, it is exceedingly difficult to eradicate. Accurate laboratory identification of methicillin resistance is therefore of paramount importance not only to the physician treating the patient but to the hospital epidemiologist as well. Appropriate susceptibility testing methods, including increased salt concentration, lower incubation temperature, and longer incubation times, are available in standard laboratory references and recent reviews [9]. Particular caution is required when using certain automated microdilution instruments, although some of these systems perform satisfactorily when appropriate media and cations are employed. As an additional screening measure, it may be advisable to inoculate isolates on Mueller-Hinton agar dilution plates containing 4% sodium chloride plus 6 μg/ml of oxacillin [95]. These antibiotic-containing plates can also be used to screen patients rapidly and efficiently for colonization with MRSA. In the author's experience, sensitivity of skin cultures can be enhanced by incubating the swab in broth media and then inoculating the plate directly with an aliquot of this overnight culture. Similar findings have been reported by others [20].

In the last few years, it has become clear that there are several types of methicillin resistance in *S. aureus*, and these developments have added further complexities to an already confusing field (see Chaps. 12 through 14). The strains of MRSA that have caused nosocomial headaches throughout the world are highly resistant to methicillin and related agents because they have altered penicillin-binding proteins (PBPs) with reduced affinity for these antibiotics. Specifically, these intrinsically resistant strains contain a 78-kilodalton PBP 2a or 2' [38] and a genetic determinant that can be detected with a *mec*-specific DNA probe. They are often called *heteroresistant* because only a small fraction of bacterial cells in a culture population actually expresses methicillin resistance. In addition to these highly methicillin-resistant strains of *S. aureus*, other strains have been recognized that have borderline resistance to methicillin, with minimum inhibiting concentrations in the range of 4 μg/ml [96]. Some of these isolates have the typical characteristics of heteroresistant strains in that they contain PBP 2a and are positive with the *mec* probe. Others do not react with the *mec* probe, do not have PBP 2a, and do not have any highly resistant subpopulations on culture. It has been hypothesized that the apparently normal PBPs of these isolates have decreased affinity for methicillin and related compounds [96]. Finally, some borderline resistant strains express large amounts of β-lactamase, particularly when grown under the high salt concentrations used to enhance detection of heteroresistance [60]. Since these β-lactamases can be inhibited by sulbactam and clavulanic acid, they can be recognized easily in vitro and may be amenable to therapy with currently available agents, such as amoxicillin–clavulanic acid and ampicillin-sulbactam. The dilemma for hospital epidemiologists is whether these borderline resistant *S. aureus* isolates, regardless of their specific resistance mechanism, require the same vigorous isolation and control measures as the classic MRSA hetero-

resistant strains. A conservative approach seems appropriate at this time until further data concerning the nosocomial importance and proper therapy of borderline resistant *S. aureus* are forthcoming.

The initial introduction of MRSA into a hospital population usually goes undetected, but in many cases the organism is brought in by a patient transferred from another institution in which MRSA already is endemic [35, 56]. Nursing homes and other chronic-care facilities are major reservoirs for MRSA, and the transfer of chronically colonized patients to acute-care settings requires particular vigilance [42, 93]. Colonized hospital personnel can also be responsible for interhospital spread of MRSA [21, 75, 105], although this probably occurs relatively rarely. In one outbreak, transmission was traced to a member of the surgical house staff who developed nasal colonization following a paronychia [105]. In another, a pediatric resident introduced a strain of rifampicin-resistant MRSA into a special-care nursery [21]. This physician had previously worked in a hospital where rifampicin-susceptible MRSA was endemic and had subsequently been treated with rifampicin for pulmonary tuberculosis, presumably leading to the selection of rifampicin resistance in the strain of MRSA he had acquired. Finally, when MRSA is endemic in the community, as it is in the intravenous drug–abusing populations of some inner cities, hospitalization of colonized individuals can trigger nosocomial transmission [80]. Hospitalized patients are at greater risk of becoming colonized with MRSA if they have prolonged hospital stays, have received a large number of antibiotics or lengthy antibiotic courses, or have invasive devices [35, 51, 56, 57, 78, 105]. Colonized patients, particularly those with chronic diseases, tend to remain carriers following discharge, so they must be screened on readmission to avoid reintroduction of MRSA into the hospital [35, 51, 56, 57, 78, 105].

In general, MRSA is transmitted in the hospital by personnel who have contaminated their hands while providing direct care for colonized patients [20]. Patients with tracheostomies, contaminated wounds or decubitus ulcers, and extensive skin disease or burns tend to be colonized with exceptionally large numbers of staphylococci and are especially likely to contribute to the cycle of person-to-person transmission. The role of carriers on the hospital staff in the nosocomial dissemination of MRSA is less clear. Personnel appear to be less likely to become persistent nasal carriers of MRSA than of methicillin-susceptible strains [12]. Carrier rates as low as 0.4 percent have been reported, even after extensive contact with colonized patients [94]. In a review of 49 studies involving 7,129 patients, Reboli and colleagues [74] found an average colonization rate of only 2.5 percent. Nonetheless, much higher carrier rates have been noted in some studies [75], and nasal carriers have been implicated in a few outbreaks [21, 75, 105]. Environmental contamination probably plays a minor role in most institutions, and it is difficult to recover MRSA outside of the immediate environment of most patients [20]. However, patients with colonized or infected burn wounds can heavily contaminate their environment [22, 94], and other colonized individuals, such as those with extensive skin lesions or endotracheal tubes or tracheostomies, probably require special consideration as well. To determine whether patients are likely to be heavy dispersers, settling plates may be placed in the room as a simple and inexpensive screening procedure, although the reproducibility and predictive value of this technique have not been validated.

Hospitals faced with the daunting task of trying to contain MRSA have adopted a wide variety of strategies, but almost all have found the effort inordinately expensive, both in terms of time and resources. The proper approach to take is a matter of considerable controversy. Recently, a working party of the Hospital Infection Society and the British Society for Antimicrobial Chemotherapy has issued [34] and revised [39] extraordinarily tough, comprehensive, and expensive recommendations for MRSA control [34]. In essence, these guidelines suggest isolation of known carriers or patients admitted from hos-

pitals where MRSA is endemic until screening culture results are available. If only a single colonized patient is present in the hospital, he or she should be discharged as soon as possible. If this patient was in a critical care area, all patients and staff who cared for the patient should be cultured; in other areas of the hospital, only patients in the vicinity of the colonized individuals need be screened. Suggested sites for screening cultures include nose, perineum (since some carriers may be culture-positive at this site without having MRSA in the nose [75]), fingers, and axilla, with the addition of wounds, tracheostomy sites, intravenous catheter sites, and so on for patients. If more than 1 case is detected, the net should be widened to include screening of all staff caring for colonized patients, including domestic staff and phlebotomists, and the ward may have to be closed to new admissions. Antiseptic hand-washing agents are recommended, and the use of agents other than chlorhexidine gluconate should be considered, since some MRSA strains seem to have reduced susceptibility to this antiseptic [11, 74]. Hospitalization in a customized isolation unit is suggested, but single rooms at negative pressure are second best; barrier precautions are considered inadequate. Terminal cleaning of rooms with a phenolic disinfectant is recommended. Carriers among patients and staff should be treated vigorously as discussed previously, and application of mupirocin to colonized lesions, or even total body bathing with an agent such as triclosan [4, 24], is considered an adjunct to the treatments for nasal colonization discussed earlier. Carriers are not considered cured until three sets of screening cultures are negative. Personnel with MRSA confined to the nose may return to clinical work after 1 day of intranasal mupirocin, but those with more widespread colonization are kept off the wards until treatment is completed and three cultures are negative.

These measures seem draconian and may not be necessary or feasible in all hospitals. Nonetheless, they do provide a framework for approaching this vexing problem, especially when considered in context with the isolation guidelines issued by the Centers for Disease Control [30].

References

1. Archer, G.L., and Mayhall, C.G. Comparison of epidemiological markers used in the investigation of an outbreak of methicillin-resistant *Staphylococcus aureus* infections. *J. Clin. Microbiol.* 18:395, 1983.
2. Barrett, S.P. The value of mupirocin in containing an outbreak of methicillin-resistant *Staphylococcus aureus* in an orthopaedic unit. *J. Hosp. Infect.* 15:137, 1990.
3. Barrter, T., Dascal, A., Carroll, K., and Curley, F.J. 'Toxic strep syndrome.' A manifestation of Group A streptococcal infection. *Arch. Intern. Med.* 148:1421, 1988.
4. Bartzokas, C.A., et al. Control and eradication of methicillin-resistant *Staphylococcus aureus* on a surgical unit. *N. Engl. J. Med.* 311:1422, 1984.
5. Berkelman, R.L., et al. Streptococcal wound infections caused by a vaginal carrier. *J.A.M.A.* 247:2680, 1982.
6. Bethune, D.W., Blowers, R., Parker, M., and Pask, E.A. Dispersal of *Staphylococcus aureus* by patients and surgical staff. *Lancet* 1:480, 1965.
7. Blowers, R., and McCluskey, M. Design of operating room dress for surgeons. *Lancet* 2:681, 1965.
8. Bouvet, A. Epidemiologic markers for epidemic strain and carrier isolates in an outbreak of nosocomial oxacillin-resistant *Staphylococcus aureus*. *J. Clin. Microbiol.* 28:1338, 1990.
9. Boyce, J.M. Methicillin-resistant *Staphylococcus aureus:* Detection, epidemiology, and control measures. *Infect. Dis. Clin. North Am.* 3:901, 1989.
10. Branger, C., and Goullet, P.H. Genetic heterogeneity in methicillin-resistant strains of *Staphylococcus aureus* revealed by esterase electrophoretic polymorphism. *J. Hosp. Infect.* 14:125, 1989.
11. Brumfitt, W., Dixson, S., and Hamilton-Miller, J.M.T. Resistance to antiseptics in methicillin and gentamicin resistant *Staphylococcus aureus*. *N. Engl. J. Med.* 320:1188, 1989.
12. Brumfitt, W., and Hamilton-Miller, J. Methicillin-resistant *Staphylococcus aureus*. *N. Engl. J. Med.* 320:1188, 1989.
13. Burnett, I.A., and Norman, P. *Streptococcus pyogenes:* An outbreak on a burns unit. *J. Hosp. Infect.* 15:173, 1990.
14. Casewell, M.W. Epidemiology and control of the "modern" methicillin-resistant *Staphylococcus aureus*. *J. Hosp. Infect.* 7 (Suppl. A):1, 1986.
14a. Casewell, M.W., and Hill, R.L.R. Minimal dose requirements for nasal mupirocin and its role in the control of epidemic MRSA. *J. Hosp. Infect.* 19 (Suppl. B):35, 1991.
15. Casewell, M.W., and Hill, R.L. The carrier state: Methicillin-resistant *Staphylococcus aureus*. *J. Antimicrob. Chemother.* 18 (Suppl A):1, 1986.
16. Cederna, J.E., et al. *Staphylococcus aureus* nasal colonization in a nursing home: Eradication with mupirocin. *Infect. Control Hosp. Epidemiol.* 11:13, 1990.
17. Chaudhary, S., Bilinsky, S.A., and Hennessey, J.L. Penicillin V and rifampin for the treatment of group A streptococcal pharyngitis: A randomized trial of 10 days penicillin *vs* 10 days penicillin with rifampin during the final 4 days of therapy. *J. Pediatr.* 106:481, 1985.
18. Congeni, B., Rizzo, C., Congeni, J., and Sreenvisasan, V.V. Outbreak of acute rheumatic fever in northeast Ohio. *J. Pediatr.* 111:176, 1987.
19. Cookson, B.D., et al. Mupirocin-resistant *Staphylococcus aureus*. *Lancet* 335:1095, 1990.
20. Cookson, B.D., et al. Staff carriage of epidemic methicillin-resistant *Staphylococcus aureus*. *J. Clin. Microbiol.* 27:1471, 1989.
21. Coovadia, Y.M., et al. A laboratory-confirmed outbreak of rifampin-methicillin resistant *Staphylococcus aureus* (RMRSA) in a newborn nursery. *J. Hosp. Infect.* 14:303, 1989.
22. Crossley, K., Landesman, B., and Zaska, D. An outbreak of infections caused by strains of *S. aureus* resistant to methicillin and aminoglycosides II. Epidemiological studies. *J. Infect. Dis.* 139:280, 1979.
23. Davies, E.A., et al. An outbreak of infection with methicillin-resistant *Staphylococcus aureus* in a special care baby unit: Value of topical mupirocin and of traditional methods of infection control. *J. Hosp. Infect.* 10:120, 1987.
24. Denning, D.W., and Haiduven-Griffiths, D. Eradication of low-level methicillin-resistant *Staphylococcus aureus* skin colonization with topical mupirocin. *Infect. Control Hosp. Epidemiol.* 9:261, 1988.
25. Ehrenkranz, N.J. Person-to-person transmission of *Staphylococcus aureus:* Quantitative characterization of nasal carriers spreading infection. *N. Engl. J. Med.* 271:225, 1964.
26. Eichenwald, H.F., Kotsevalov, O., and Fasco, L.A. The "cloud baby": An example of bacterial viral interactions. *Am. J. Dis. Child.* 100:161, 1960.
27. Ellison, R.T., III, et al. Oral rifampin and

trimethoprim/sulfamethoxazole therapy in asymptomatic carriers of methicillin-resistant *Staphylococcus aureus* infections. *West. J. Med.* 140:735, 1984.

28. Fekety, R. The Management of the Carrier in Methicillin-resistant *Staphylococcus aureus.* In J.S. Remington and M.N. Swartz (Eds.), *Current Clinical Topics in Infectious Diseases,* Vol. 8. New York: McGraw-Hill, 1987. P. 169.

29. Fournier, J.M., et al. Predominance of capsular polysaccharide type 5 among oxacillin-resistant *Staphylococcus aureus. J. Clin. Microbiol.* 25:1932, 1987.

30. Garner, J.S., and Simmons, B.P. Guidelines for isolation precautions in hospitals. *Infect. Control* 4:247, 1983.

31. Gezon, H.M., et al. Hexachlorophene bathing in early infancy: Effect on staphylococcal disease and infection. *N. Engl. J. Med.* 270:379, 1964.

32. Gillespie, W.A., Simpson, K., and Tozer, R.C. Staphylococcal infection in maternity hospital: Epidemiology and control. *Lancet* 2:1075, 1958.

33. Goldmann, D.A., and Breton, S.J. Group-C streptococcal surgical wound infections transmitted by an anorectal and nasal carrier. *Pediatrics* 61:235, 1978.

34. Report of a combined working party of the Hospital Infections Society and the British Society for Antimicrobial Chemotherapy. Guidelines for the control of epidemic methicillin-resistant *Staphylococcus aureus. J. Hosp. Infect.* 7:193, 1986.

35. Guiguet, M., et al. Effectiveness of simple measures to control an outbreak of nosocomial methicillin-resistant *Staphylococcus aureus* infections in an intensive care unit. *Infect. Control Hosp. Epidemiol.* 11:23, 1990.

36. Haley, R.W., and Bregman, D.A. The role of understaffing and overcrowding in recurrent outbreaks of staphylococcal infection in a neonatal special care unit. *J. Infect. Dis.* 145:875, 1982.

37. Hare, R., and Thomas, C.G.A. The transmission of *Staphylococcus aureus. Br. Med. J.* 2:840, 1956.

38. Hartman, B.J., and Tomasz, A. Low affinity penicillin-binding protein associated with beta-lactam resistance in *Staphylococcus aureus. J. Bacteriol.* 158:513, 1984.

39. Report of a combined working party of the Hospital Infection Society and the British Society for Antimicrobial Chemotherapy, prepared G. Duckworth. Revised guidelines for the control of epidemic methicillin-resistant *Staphylococcus aureus. J. Hosp. Infect.* 16:351, 1990.

40. Hill, R.L.R., Duckworth, G.J., and Case-well, M.W. Elimination of nasal carriage of methicillin-resistant *Staphylococcus aureus* with mupirocin during a hospital outbreak. *J. Antimicrob. Chemother.* 22:377, 1988.

41. Hosier, D.M., Craenen, J.M., Teske, D.W., and Wheller, J.J. Resurgence of acute rheumatic fever. *Am. J. Dis. Child.* 141:730, 1987.

42. Hsu, C.C.S., Macaluso, C.P., and Special, L. High rate of methicillin resistance in *Staphylococcus aureus* isolated from hospitalized nursing home patients. *Arch. Intern. Med.* 148:569, 1988.

43. Jellard, J. Umbilical cord as reservoir of infection in maternity hospital. *Br. Med. J.* 1:925, 1957.

44. Karakawa, W.W., et al. Method for serological typing of the capsular polysaccharides of *Staphylococcus aureus. J. Clin. Microbiol.* 22:445, 1985.

45. Kaslow, R.A., et al. Staphylococcal disease related to hospital nursery bathing practices: A nationwide epidemiologic investigation. *Pediatrics* 51 (Suppl.):418, 1973.

46. Kimbrough, R.D., and Gaines, T.B. Hexachlorophene effects on the rat brain: Study of high doses by light and electron microscopy. *Arch. Environ. Health* 23:114, 1971.

47. Kirmani, N., Tuazon, C.V., and Alling, D. Carriage rate of *Staphylococcus aureus* among patients receiving allergy injections. *Ann. Allergy* 45:235, 1980.

48. Kosarsky, P.E., Rimland, D., Terry, P.M., and Wachsmuth, K. Plasmic analysis of simultaneous nosocomial outbreaks of methicillin-resistant *Staphylococcus aureus. Infect. Control* 7:577, 1986.

49. Kreisworth, B.N., Kravitz, G.R., Schlievert, P.M., and Novick, R.P. Nosocomial transmission of a strain of *Staphylococcus aureus* causing toxic shock syndrome. *Ann. Intern. Med.* 105:704, 1986.

50. Lee, P.K., and Schlievert, P.M. Quantification and toxicity of Group A streptococcal pyrogenic exotoxins in an animal model of toxic shock syndrome—like illness. *J. Clin. Microbiol.* 27:1890, 1989.

51. Lentino, J.R., Hennein, H., and Krause, S. A comparison of pneumonia caused by gentamicin, methicillin-resistant and gentamicin, methicillin-sensitive *Staphylococcus aureus:* Epidemiologic and clinical studies. *Infect. Control* 6:267, 1985.

52. Licitra, C.M., et al. Use of plasmid analysis and determination of aminoglycoside-modifying enzymes to characterize isolates from an outbreak of methicillin-resistant *Staphylococcus aureus. J. Clin. Microbiol.* 27:2535, 1989.

53. Lidwell, O.M., et al. Effect of ultraclean air in

operating rooms on deep sepsis in the joint after total hip or knee replacement: A randomized study. *Br. Med. J.* 285:10, 1982.

54. Light, I.J., and Sutherland, J.M. What is the evidence that hexachlorophene is not effective? *Pediatrics* 51:345, 1973.

55. Light, I.J., Sutherland, J.M., Cochran, M.L., and Scitorius, J. Ecological relationship between *Staphylococcus aureus* and *Pseudomonas* in a nursery population. *N. Engl. J. Med.* 278:1243, 1968.

56. Locksley, R.M., et al. Multiply antibiotic-resistant *Staphylococcus aureus:* Introduction, transmission and evolution of nosocomial infection. *Ann. Intern. Med.* 97:317, 1982.

57. Longfield, J.N., et al. Methicillin-resistant *Staphylococcus aureus* (MRSA): Risk and outcome of colonized vs infected patients. *Infect. Control* 6:445, 1985.

58. Luzar, M.A., et al. *Staphylococcus aureus* nasal carriage and infection in patients on continuous ambulatory peritoneal dialysis. *N. Engl. J. Med.* 322:505, 1990.

59. Maxted, W.R., and Widdowson, J.P. The Protein Antigens of Group-A Streptococci. In: L.W. Wannamaker and S.M. Matsen (Eds.), *Streptococci and Streptococcal Diseases*. New York: Academic, 1972. P. 251.

60. McDougal, L.K., and Thornsberry, C. The role of B-lactamase in staphylococcal resistance to penicillinase-resistant penicillins and cephalosporins. *J. Clin. Microbiol.* 23:832, 1986.

61. McGowan, J.E., Jr., et al. Nosocomial infections with gentamicin-resistant *Staphylococcus aureus:* Plasmid analysis as an epidemiologic tool. *J. Infect. Dis.* 140:864, 1979.

62. McIntyre, D.M. An epidemic of *Streptococcus pyogenes* puerperal and postoperative sepsis with an unusual carrier site—the anus. *Am. J. Obstet. Gynecol.* 101:308, 1968.

63. McKee, W.M., Di Caprio, J.N., Roberts, C.E., Jr., and Sherris, J.C. Anal carriage as the probable source of a streptococcal epidemic. *Lancet* 1:1007, 1966.

64. Mitchell, N.J., and Gamble, D.R. Clothing design for operating-room personnel. *Lancet* 2:1133, 1974.

65. Murray-Leisure, K.A., et al. Control of methicillin-resistant *Staphylococcus aureus. Infect. Control Hosp. Epidemiol.* 11:343, 1990.

66. Viglionese, A., Nottebart, V.F., Bodman, H., and Platt, R. Recurrent group-A streptococcal carriage in a health care worker associated with widely separated nosocomial outbreaks. *Am. J. Med.* 91 (Suppl. B):3B, 1991.

67. Perry, W.D., et al. Transmission of group-A streptococci I. The role of contaminated bedding. *Am. J. Hyg.* 66:85, 1957.

68. Perry, W.D., Siegel, A.C., and Rammelkamp, C.H., Jr. Transmission of group-A streptococci II. The role of contaminated dust. *Am. J. Hyg.* 66:96, 1957.

69. Pildes, R.S., Ramamurthy, R.S., and Vidyasagar, D. Effect of triple dye on staphylococcal colonization in the newborn infant. *J. Pediatr.* 82:907, 1973.

70. Postoperative wound infections: The influence of ultraviolet irradiation of the operating room and of various other factors. *Ann. Surg.* 160(Suppl.):1, 1964.

71. Powell, H., Swarner, O., Gluck, L., and Lampert, P. Hexachlorophene myelinopathy in premature infants. *J. Pediatr.* 82:976, 1973.

72. Rammelkamp, C.H., Jr., Mortimer, E.A., Jr., and Wolinsky, E. Transmission of streptococcal and staphylococcal infections. *Ann. Intern. Med.* 60:753, 1964.

73. Raviglione, M.C., et al. High *Staphylococcus aureus* nasal carriage rate in patients with acquired immunodeficiency syndrome or AIDS-related complex. *Am. J. Infect. Control* 18:64, 1990.

74. Reboli, A.C., John, J.J., Jr., and Levkoff, A.H. Epidemic methicillin-gentamicin-resistant *Staphylococcus aureus* in a neonatal intensive care unit. *Am. J. Dis. Child.* 143:34, 1989.

75. Reboli, A.C., John, J.F., Platt, C.G., and Cantey, J.R. Methicillin-resistant *Staphylococcus aureus* outbreak at a veteran's affairs medical center: Importance of carriage of the organism by hospital personnel. *Infect. Control Hosp. Epidemiol.* 11:291, 1990.

76. Rhinehart, E., et al. Nosocomial clonal dissemination of methicillin-resistant *Staphylococcus aureus* infections. *Arch. Intern. Med.* 147:521, 1987.

77. Richman, D.D., Breton, S.J., and Goldmann, D.A. Scarlet fever and group A streptococcal surgical wound infection traced to an anal carrier. *J. Pediatr.* 90:387, 1977.

78. Rimland, D. Nosocomial infections with methicillin and tobramycin resistant *Staphylococcus aureus.* Implications of physiotherapy in hospital-wide dissemination. *Am. J. Med. Sci.* 290:91, 1985.

79. Roccaforte, J.S., Bittner, M.J., Stumpf, C.A., and Preheim, L.C. Attempts to eradicate methicillin-resistant *Staphylococcus aureus* colonization with the use of trimethoprim-sulfamethoxazole, rifampin, and bacitracin. *Am. J. Infect. Control* 16:141, 1988.

80. Saravolatz, L.D., Pohlod, D.J., and Arking, L.M. Community-acquired methicillin-resistant *Staphylococcus aureus* infections: A new source for nosocomial outbreaks. *Ann. Intern. Med.* 97:325, 1982.

81. Schaffner, W., Lefkowitz, L.B., and Good-

man, J.S. Hospital outbreak of infections with group-A streptococci traced to an asymptomatic anal carrier. *N. Engl. J. Med.* 280: 1224, 1969.

82. Shinefield, H.R. Staphylococcal Infections. In: J.S. Remmington and J.O. Klein (Eds.), *Infectious Diseases of the Fetus and Newborn Infant* (3rd ed.). Philadelphia: Saunders, 1990. P. 866.

83. Shinefield, H.R., Ribble, J.C., and Boris, M. Bacterial interference between strains of *Staphylococcus aureus*, 1960–1970. *Am. J. Dis. Child.* 121:148, 1971.

84. Shuman, R.M., Leech, R.W., and Alvord, E.C. Neurotoxicity of hexachlorophene in the human. I. A clinicopathologic study of 248 children. *Pediatrics* 54:689, 1974.

85. Smith, G.E., and Kennedy, C.T.C. *Staphylococcus aureus* resistant to mupirocin. *J. Antimicrob. Chemother.* 21:141, 1988.

86. Speers, R., Jr., Bernard, H., O'Grady, F., and Shooter, R.A. Increased dispersal of skin bacteria into the air after shower baths. *Lancet* 1:478, 1965.

87. Stamm, W.E., Feeley, J.C., and Facklam, R.R. Wound infections due to group-A streptococcus traced to a vaginal carrier. *J. Infect. Dis.* 138:287, 1978.

88. Steele, R.W. Recurrent staphylococcal infection in families. *Arch. Dermatol.* 116:189, 1980.

89. Stevens, D.L., et al. Severe Group A streptococcal infections associated with a toxic shock–like syndrome and scarlet fever toxin A. *N. Engl. J. Med.* 321:1, 1989.

90. Stollerman, G.H. Changing Group A streptococci: The reappearance of streptococcal toxic shock. *Arch. Intern. Med.* 148:1268, 1988.

91. Stolz, S.M., and Maki, D.G. The use of Western blotting to subtype nosocomial isolates of methicillin-resistant *Staphylococcus aureus* (abstr. A25). Presented at the Third Decennial International Conference on Nosocomial Infections, Atlanta, GA, July 31–August 3, 1990.

92. Tanz, R.R., et al. Penicillin plus rifampin eradicates pharyngeal carriage of Group A streptococci. *J. Pediatr.* 106:876, 1985.

93. Thomas, J.C., et al. Transmission and control of methicillin-resistant *Staphylococcus aureus* in a skilled nursing facility. *Infect. Control Hosp. Epidemiol.* 10:106, 1989.

94. Thompson, R.L., Cabezudo, I., and Wenzel, R.P. Epidemiology of nosocomial infections caused by methicillin-resistant *Staphylococcus aureus. Ann. Intern. Med.* 97:309, 1982.

95. Thornsberry, C., and McDougal, L.K. Successful use of broth microdilution in susceptibility tests for methicillin-resistant (heteroresistant) staphylococci. *J. Clin. Microbiol.* 18:1084, 1983.

96. Tomasz, A., et al. New mechanisms for methicillin resistance in *Staphylococcus aureus:* Clinical isolates that lack the PBP 2a gene and contain normal penicillin-binding proteins with modified penicillin-binding capacity. *Antimicrob. Agents Chemother.* 33:1869, 1989.

97. Tuazon, C.V., Perez, A., Kishaba, T., and Sheagren, J.N. *Staphylococcus aureus* among insulin-injecting diabetic patients: An increased carrier rate. *J.A.M.A.* 231:1272, 1975.

98. Tuazon, C.V., and Sheagren, J.N. Increased risk of carriage of *Staphylococcus aureus* among narcotics addicts. *J. Infect. Dis.* 129:725, 1974.

99. Veasy, L.G., et al. Resurgence of acute rheumatic fever in the intermountain area of the United States. *N. Engl. J. Med.* 316:421, 1987.

100. Wald, E.R., et al. Acute rheumatic fever in western Pennsylvania and the tri-state area. *Pediatrics* 80:371, 1987.

101. Wallace, M.R., Garst, P.D., Papadimos, T.J., and Oldfield, E.C., III. The return of acute rheumatic fever in young adults. *J.A.M.A.* 262:2557, 1989.

102. Walsh, T.J., et al. Prospective microbiologic surveillance in control of nosocomial methicillin-resistant *Staphylococcus aureus. Infect. Control* 8:7, 1987.

103. Walter, C.W., and Kundsin, R.B. The airborne component of wound contamination and infection. *Arch. Surg.* 107:588, 1973.

104. Wannamaker, L.W. The Epidemiology of Streptococcal Infections. In: M. McCarthy (Ed.), *Streptococcal Infections.* New York: Columbia University Press, 1954. P. 157.

105. Ward, T.T., Winn, R.E., Hartstein, A.I., and Sewell, D.L. Observations relating to an interhospital outbreak of methicillin-resistant *Staphylococcus aureus:* Role of antimicrobial therapy in infection control. *Infect. Control* 2:453, 1981.

106. Wells, W.F. *Airborne Contagion and Air Hygiene.* Cambridge: Harvard University Press, 1955.

107. Westlake, R.M., Graham, T.P., and Edwards, E.M. An outbreak of acute rheumatic fever in Tennessee. *Pediatr. Infect. Dis. J.* 9:97, 1990.

108. Wheat, L.J., Kohler, R.B., and White, A. Treatment of Nasal Carriers of Coagulase-Positive Staphylococci. In: H.I. Maibach and R. Aly (Eds.), *Skin Microbiology: Relevance to Clinical Infection.* New York: Springer, 1981. Pp. 50–58.

109. Wheat, L.J., Kohler, R.B., White, A.L., and White, A. Effect of rifampin on nasal carriers of staphylococci. *J. Infect. Dis.* 144:177, 1981.

110. White, A. Relation between quantitative nasal cultures and dissemination of staphylococci. *J. Lab. Clin. Med.* 58:273, 1961.

111. Williams, R.E.O. Epidemiology of airborne staphylococcal infection. *Bacteriol. Rev.* 30:660, 1966.

112. Willson, R., Bollinger, C.C., and Ledger, W.J. *Am. J. Obstet. Gynecol.* 90:726, 1964.

113. Yu, V.L., Goetz, A., and Wagener, M. *Staphylococcus aureus* nasal carriage and infection in patients on hemodialysis: Efficacy of antibiotic prophylaxis. *N. Engl. J. Med.* 315:91, 1986.

114. Zuccarelli, A.J., Roy, I., Harding, G.P., and Couperus, J.J. Diversity and stability of restriction enzyme profiles of plasmid DNA from methicillin-resistant *Staphylococcus aureus. J. Clin. Microbiol.* 28:97, 1990.

Selected Viruses of Nosocomial Importance

William M. Valenti

Viral infections probably account for more nosocomial infections than previously realized; at least 5 percent of all nosocomial infections are due to viruses [151], and this is probably an underestimate. Although much of the data on nosocomial viral infections comes from pediatric services [71, 111, 152], adults—especially the elderly and chronically ill—appear to be at risk as well [99, 151, 153].

Health care facilities bring together a great variety of workers of all ages with a wide range of educational and ethnic backgrounds, which complicates the implementation of infection control procedures. In addition, the numbers of pregnant women working in health care facilities are probably greater than in any other workplace, which adds to the complexities of protecting workers from developing infections. Medical facilities are a challenge in terms of prevention of infection in both patients and personnel. Infection control personnel must be familiar with the potential for nosocomial transmission of viruses and must be aware of their modes of transmission and possible methods of control and prevention. Health care workers are an integral part of the chain of transmission of viral infections in health care facilities. Vaccination programs for personnel and the widespread adoption of precautions systems, such as universal precautions and body substance isolation, are important ways of interrupting this chain of transmission.

With the continued development of rapid viral diagnostic methods, new and improved vaccines, and antiviral chemotherapy, virology has become an increasingly important component of the infection control program in health care facilities (see Chap. 4).

The significant contributions of Paul F. Wehrle in preparing the chapters on nosocomial viral infections for the previous editions are gratefully acknowledged.

Respiratory Viruses

Transmission of respiratory viruses in health care facilities is an annual event in temperate climates (see Chap. 29). Both patients and personnel are at special risk during the winter season, and large numbers of health care personnel with acute respiratory illnesses become a major concern. In addition to pediatric patients [71], patients who seem to be at greatest risk of acquiring nosocomial viral respiratory disease are patients in closed or semiclosed populations such as psychiatric units [151] and patients in extended-care facilities [99].

The two major mechanisms of transmission of respiratory viruses are by means of droplet nuclei (small-particle aerosol) and droplets (large-particle spread). Droplet nuclei aerosols (median diameter less than 10 μm) containing infectious virions are produced by coughing, sneezing, or talking and are capable of transmitting infectious virus over considerable distances (greater than 6 ft). Smallpox provided the classic example of this type of spread, but influenza virus and perhaps varicella and measles viruses also exhibit patterns of spread compatible with this mechanism. With droplet spread, other viral agents may be transmitted over shorter distances by mechanisms requiring close person-to-person contact, generally at a distance of less than 3 ft separating 2 persons. This method of transmission may occur when droplets produced by coughing or sneezing either directly infect the susceptible host (e.g., mucous membranes of the eye or nose) or contaminate the donor's hands or a fomite transferring infectious virus indirectly to the skin or mucous membranes of a susceptible host. Infection in the susceptible host may also result from autoinoculation, with transfer of virus from hands to mucous membranes of the eye or nose. Rhinoviruses and respiratory syncytial virus have patterns of spread compatible with close-contact transmission.

In the absence of viral diagnostic facilities, it may be possible to establish a presumptive viral diagnosis based on the predominant site of involvement in the respiratory tract, epidemiologic data such as season of the year, geographic location, type of patient population, and data from area surveillance activity.

Influenza Virus

Influenza A and B viral infections are among the most communicable diseases of humans. They are characterized by explosive epidemics, and nosocomial transmission of influenza A [43, 99] and B [153] has been well documented. Person-to-person transmission is believed to take place primarily by droplet nuclei. These aerosols may account for the explosive nature of influenza outbreaks, since, in a closed environment, one infected person can potentially infect large numbers of susceptible persons. During an outbreak of influenza A at the New York Hospital during the pandemic of 1957–1958, 15 of 29 patients and 15 of 30 personnel on one hospital floor became infected, possibly from a single index case [43]. Influenza A viral infection may result in significant morbidity (e.g., primary influenza pneumonia, secondary bacterial pneumonia) and mortality. It may also pose a significant risk to elderly or chronically ill institutionalized patients [99], to patients in closed or semiclosed populations such as psychiatric patients [151], and to pediatric patients [72, 151, 159, 161].

Precautions

Respiratory isolation with masks for hospital personnel, private room, and care in handling secretions and secretion-soiled articles are the most reasonable precautions for patients with proved or suspected influenza viral infection. However, the Centers for Disease Control's (CDC's) *Guidelines for Isolation Precautions in Hospitals* [59] do not recommend these precautions (see Chap. 11), presumably due to the delay in diagnosis of influenza because diagnostic laboratories for viral isolation are not available to many health care facilities. Nonetheless, because influenza virus is transmitted by small-particle aerosols, patients who are admitted to the hospital with febrile respiratory illness at a time when influenza is prevalent in the community should be considered to have influenza until proved otherwise and should be placed on appropriate precautions including mask use and private room. In hospital outbreaks involving large numbers of people, patients with influenza should be cohorted in the same room or on the same hospital floor [72]. Shedding of virus may persist for as long as 5 days after the onset of symptoms in adults [43] and for 7 days or longer in children [72]. At the present time, we maintain respiratory precautions for patients with influenza viral infection for 7 days or the duration of clinical illness, whichever is longer.

Immunization

Vaccination in the fall of each year of patients with chronic underlying illnesses, including immunodeficiency states such as infection with the human immunodeficiency virus (HIV), and persons older than 65 years should result in 60 to 90 percent protection against influenza A and B infections for many hospitalized patients [20, 22, 122, 123]. Additionally, vaccine appears to reduce mortality in those who acquire infection.

Although influenza viral infection in healthy, young hospital workers is often benign and self-limited, hospital staff who have contact with patients should be vaccinated because of their high degree of exposure to influenza and subsequent high risk of transmission of infection to hospitalized patients. Attempts at vaccinating hospital personnel are often unrewarding. Influenza vaccination programs directed at health care workers should include an intensive educational effort; we have found that large numbers of hospital personnel are reluctant to be vaccinated because of misinformation regarding vaccine efficacy and its side effects, including Guillain-Barré syndrome [90]. While a significant association between A/New Jersey/swine influenza vaccines and Guillain-Barré syndrome was noted, similar association has not been noted with previous or subsequent vaccine formulations [83].

Chemoprophylaxis

O'Donoghue and colleagues [121] have shown that amantadine hydrochloride is 80 percent effective in preventing clinical nosocomial in-

fluenza A viral disease. In addition, there is evidence to suggest that the effects of prophylactic amantadine plus vaccination are additive [115]. During periods of high prevalence of influenza viral infection in the hospital or community, amantadine may be used in unvaccinated hospital patients and personnel. Vaccination of susceptible persons should also be considered in the presence of an epidemic, in addition to amantadine administration, until an adequate serologic response to vaccine occurs—generally 2 weeks or so after vaccination. The usual dose of amantadine is 200 mg/day in either a single or divided dose. If susceptible personnel are not vaccinated, amantadine must be continued for the duration of the outbreak. Amantadine is not effective prophylactically for influenza B infection. In view of the problems with compliance when large numbers of people are taking amantadine, vaccination against influenza remains the best preventive measure against the disease.

Special Considerations

During documented influenza outbreaks, measures other than vaccination and amantadine chemoprophylaxis should be considered, depending on the severity of the outbreak: (1) curtailment or elimination of elective surgery and other elective admissions; (2) restriction of cardiovascular and pulmonary surgery; (3) restriction of hospital visitors, especially those with respiratory illnesses; and (4) work restriction for medical personnel with acute respiratory disease. Controlled studies to evaluate these measures have not been done. In addition, items 3 and 4 may be difficult to implement. It is often necessary to appeal to the common sense and good judgment of hospital personnel and visitors in restricting their contact in the hospital. If personnel recovering from influenza must work, it is advisable to assign them to areas of the hospital where influenza viral infections are prevalent.

Respiratory Syncytial Virus

Respiratory syncytial virus (RSV) is the most frequent cause of lower respiratory tract disease in children younger than 2 years [71]. In recent years, RSV infections have accounted for approximately 45 percent of all acute hospital admissions for respiratory disease in children younger than 2 years [70]. It is also the most common nosocomial infection on pediatric wards [74, 151]. In addition, people in all age groups are potentially susceptible to RSV infection and, because immunity is incomplete and not permanent, reinfections may occur throughout life [77]. RSV infections have also been documented in hospital personnel [74] and in elderly chronically ill patients [99]. Generally, RSV infections occur in annual epidemics of 2 to 3 months' duration, often beginning in late December. Early studies by Chanock and colleagues [29] showed that approximately 59 percent of children admitted to the hospital with nonviral diseases showed serologic conversion to RSV while hospitalized during periods of RSV prevalence in the community.

The primary mode of transmission of RSV appears to be by close person-to-person contact. Studies by Hall and co-workers [70, 73] have demonstrated that patients infected with RSV shed large amounts of virus in their respiratory secretions, with a mean duration of shedding of 6 to 7 days and a range of 1 to 21 days. The virus can be recovered from the immediate environment of infected patients for prolonged periods of time. For example, RSV in nasal secretions from infected infants can be recovered for up to 30 minutes from contaminated skin, gowns, or paper tissues [73]. The virus appears to survive best on nonporous surfaces such as countertops and has been recovered for up to 6 hours from these surfaces [73]. Infectious virus can then be transferred from these environmental surfaces to hands and from hand to hand [73]. Studies in volunteers have also demonstrated that infection can be initiated by instillation of RSV-containing fluid into the mucous membranes of the eyes or nose but not the mouth. Therefore, spread by direct inoculation of drops or large particles or by self-inoculation after touching contaminated surfaces such as skin or fomites seems feasible. Spread by small-particle aerosols seems less likely since

nosocomial outbreaks are not as explosive as those due to influenza virus, and studies in volunteers show that only persons cuddling infected infants and touching contaminated surfaces became infected with RSV. Persons did not become infected if kept more than 6 ft from an infected baby, suggesting that small-particle aerosol transmission is not a major route of transmission of RSV.

The risk of nosocomial RSV infection has been correlated with the duration of hospitalization; the risk increases with each subsequent week of hospitalization. In one study, RSV infection was acquired by 45 percent of contact infants hospitalized for 1 week or more. The rate of RSV acquisition increased with each subsequent week of hospitalization until all infants hospitalized 4 weeks or more became infected. The rate of infection was not related to underlying illness or age of the patient. In addition, the role of hospital personnel in the transmission of RSV is becoming increasingly important. Each year, approximately 50 percent of adult staff working on the pediatric service (nurses, house staff, and medical and nursing students) become infected with RSV. Conventional infection control measures such as hand-washing, gowns, isolation or cohorting of infected infants, and cohorting of staff to infants have decreased the rate of nosocomial acquisition of RSV in patients but not in hospital personnel [74].

Precautions
During periods of increased RSV prevalence in the community, infants with respiratory illness who are admitted to the hospital should be placed in single rooms or cohorted with other infants with RSV illness (see Chap. 11). A clean gown should be worn for each contact with an infected infant, and the gown should be changed after each contact. To prevent cross-infection, hospital personnel caring for infected infants should not care for infants who do not have respiratory illness, if at all possible. The need for a mask is not as clear, since the risk of droplet-nuclei aerosol transmission of RSV is small. However, masks, or possibly goggles, may prevent droplet

spread and thus prevent transmission of RSV via close contact [24, 29, 64, 65, 71]. The importance of careful hand-washing is evident.

Immunization
There is no effective vaccine for RSV.

Special Considerations
Attempts to reduce nosocomial transmission of RSV should be directed toward hospital personnel. Education of patient care staff should include special emphasis on both the mode of transmission of RSV and the role of personnel in the chain of infection.

Efforts should be made to curtail visits from family and friends who have respiratory illness, especially during periods of increased RSV prevalence in the community. In the absence of locally generated data on RSV prevalence, one can assume its occurrence during December through March in the United States and Europe. Children visiting pediatric services should be screened for present histories of respiratory illness of any kind and should be discouraged from visiting on the ward if there is any clinical respiratory disease.

Parainfluenza Virus
Nosocomial transmission of parainfluenza types 1, 3, and 4a on pediatric services has been documented [114]. Mufson [114] reports that 18 percent of infants who are well or infected with another respiratory pathogen at the time of admission to a children's hospital subsequently acquired nosocomial infections with parainfluenza type 3. Infections in hospitals have also been reported in adult renal transplant patients [39] and in elderly institutionalized patients [17]. Details of transmission of parainfluenza virus have not been fully elucidated, but transmission is believed to occur by contact spread, either direct (person-to-person) or indirect (person-to-fomite-to-person) [17]. Infections with parainfluenza types 1 and 2 are seasonal, with the greatest activity occurring during the fall months. Community epidemics with types 1 and 2 occur approximately every 2 years, whereas infections with parainfluenza virus type 3 tend to occur throughout each year.

Isolation Precautions
The importance of careful hand-washing cannot be overemphasized, especially in view of the proposed mechanism of transmission of parainfluenza virus. Precautions are similar to those used for RSV, with patients placed in a private room or cohorted together (see Chap. 11). Careful hand-washing and gown changes after each contact have been suggested as the most effective means of minimizing nosocomial transmission of parainfluenza viruses [17]. Precautions should be maintained for the duration of illness.

Rhinovirus
Although rhinovirus infections are ubiquitous during the winter and spring months, they have not been recognized as important nosocomial pathogens [151, 159, 161]. Rhinovirus may be a cause of significant morbidity in premature infants, as shown by an outbreak of rhinovirus infection in premature infants in an intensive care nursery [152]. The affected infants had significant respiratory distress related to rhinovirus infections, and one of them required intubation.

Large quantities of virus are present in nasal secretions and readily contaminate the hands of the infected person. Virus transmission appears to take place directly from hand to hand or indirectly via fomites. Virus may be inoculated from the recipient's hands via touching of the mucous membranes of the nose and eyes [69, 79].

Careful hand-washing appears to be the most effective way of minimizing transmission of rhinovirus. Dilute solutions containing 1% iodine have been shown to be effective skin antiseptics [78]. Since rhinoviruses are remarkably resistant to drying and survive for long periods of time on hard surfaces and plastic and synthetic fabrics [79], iodinated compounds may also be considered for use as disinfectants on surfaces contaminated with rhinovirus-containing secretions (see Chap. 15).

Generally, precautions other than hand-washing are not recommended for patients with rhinovirus infection (see Chap. 11). However, cohorting of patients with rhinovirus infection in nurseries may sometimes be indicated.

Adenovirus

Adenovirus infections occur in the general population throughout the year. These viruses are highly stable and can be transmitted via a number of routes and cause a variety of illnesses. Adenoviruses are associated with conjunctivitis, keratoconjunctivitis, pharyngoconjunctival fever, pneumonia, and a pertussislike syndrome. Respiratory transmission via aerosols occurs in all age groups [52], and volunteer studies have shown that inhalation of small doses of virus can initiate acute respiratory illness, including pneumonia [52]. Fecal-oral transmission occurs but probably is more important in children than in adults [52].

Hospital-acquired adenovirus infection has been reported in both patients and personnel [15, 139]. Infections in neonates [48] and in pediatric patients [139] account for many of the reported cases of nosocomial adenovirus infections. Although adenovirus pneumonia has been reported more frequently in military recruits, adenovirus can be the cause of sporadic pneumonia in up to 10 percent of pediatric patients admitted with pneumonia [52]. Transmission of adenovirus from patients with pneumonia to hospital personnel has occurred in these situations, with personnel developing conjunctivitis and pharyngoconjunctival fever. Recently, the role of adenovirus infections in immunocompromised hosts has led to speculation that adenoviruses, like herpesviruses, may be reactivated after primary infection [161]. Adenovirus has also been implicated as a cause of diffuse interstitial pneumonia in a renal transplant recipient [105] (see Chap. 41). All of these infections may have resulted from endogenous reactivation of adenovirus. Nosocomial transmission from staff with mild upper respiratory illness to immunocompromised patients may also have been involved.

An outbreak has been reported of epidemic keratoconjunctivitis due to adenovirus type 8, originating in an ophthalmology clinic, where 63 patients became infected in 1 month [16].

Health care workers served as a major source of virus, with transmission to susceptible patients occurring by direct transfer of virus from hands and by indirect transfer of the virus via a Schiötz tonometer. A similar outbreak of keratoconjunctivitis was associated with a contaminated ophthalmic solution in an industrial health clinic [137].

Adenoviruses called *noncultivable adenoviruses* (NCAV) are a frequent cause of sporadic diarrhea in children [110]. Outbreaks of diarrhea among young children living at a Royal Air Force station in the United Kingdom and in a long-stay orthopedic ward suggest that these viruses can cause epidemic diarrhea and can act as nosocomial pathogens in addition to causing sporadic disease [128]. Adenovirus type 3 associated with diarrhea has also been transmitted in premature nurseries [48].

Precautions

Patients with adenovirus infection should be in private rooms if possible (see Chap. 11). Personnel should wear gowns and gloves when direct contact with skin and mucous membranes is anticipated. A mask for personnel is also recommended at all times; this is because available evidence suggests that airborne transmission of adenovirus takes place easily in closed populations and because of the apparent susceptibility of most adults to infection. Care must also be taken when handling secretions, contaminated articles, and contaminated linens. Because shedding of adenovirus may be highly variable and prolonged, these precautions should be maintained for the duration of clinical illness.

Immunization

A live, attenuated trivalent vaccine containing adenovirus types 3, 4, and 7 has been used in military personnel and has been found to be safe and effective. However, this vaccine is not available for routine civilian use.

Special Considerations

Adenoviruses are very stable and survive for long periods of time. Special care must be given to the decontamination and sterilization of contaminated instruments such as tonometers (see Chap. 15). Thorough cleaning followed by steam sterilization consisting of 15 pounds per square inch (psi) for 15 minutes at 121°C (250°F), or 15 psi for 10 minutes at 126°C (259°F), or 29 psi for 3 minutes at 134°C (273°F) is recommended. The use of a disposable tonofilm to cover and preserve sterility of the tonometer has also been suggested [85]. Equipment now available for ocular pressure measurement without direct contact may be considered for use as well.

Once again, scrupulous hand-washing between contacts cannot be overemphasized. Personnel with conjunctivitis present a hazard to patients; it is recommended that personnel with infectious conjunctivitis have no contact with patients in nurseries, obstetric units, or operating rooms until all drainage ceases.

Herpesviruses

The members of the family Herpesviridae include varicella-zoster virus (VZV), herpes simplex virus (HSV) types I and II, cytomegalovirus (CMV), and Epstein-Barr virus (EBV). Herpesvirus infections become latent or inactive after primary infection and can reactivate at a time remote from the primary infection. Infectious virus can be isolated in both primary and reactivated infections due to herpesviruses. Often primary infection is symptomatic, whereas reactivation infection often is asymptomatic [158]. In the United States, most persons have come in contact with all the human herpesviruses (except herpesvirus II) by age 50 [158]. Thus nosocomial infection occurs relatively infrequently.

Transmission of the herpesviruses occurs primarily by direct-contact spread (person to person) and, except for VZV, requires close personal contact. Of the herpesviruses, VZV is the most capable of nosocomial transmission because of its direct-contact spread or airborne transmission. In addition, because of immunosuppression due to underlying diseases or chemotherapy, many hospitalized patients are susceptible to reactivation of

herpesvirus infections. When herpesviruses are transmitted in the hospital, however, nosocomial transmission may be difficult to establish since all but HSV I and II have prolonged incubation periods, and illness often develops after discharge.

In a 17-month period of careful viral surveillance, 20 cases of reactivation infection with herpesviruses were documented based on clinical criteria [151]. These infections were classified as endogenous nosocomial infections because signs and symptoms of infection were not apparent at the time of admission. During this same period, only one episode of primary CMV infection was detected; this was associated with virus from a transplanted kidney [151].

Varicella-Zoster Virus

VZV, the most communicable of the herpesviruses, is the causative agent of chickenpox and herpes zoster (shingles). Nosocomial transmission of chickenpox is well recognized [68, 94, 108] and is a cause of mortality and serious morbidity in immunocompromised patients [108, 112] (see Chap. 41). The primary mechanism of transmission of varicella is probably via direct contact with infectious lesions. However, nosocomial spread by the airborne route is also documented [94]. Epidemiologic evidence suggests that patients shed varicella virus in respiratory secretions as early as 2 days before the onset of rash [63], but this has never been proved by virus isolation.

Whenever possible, patients with uncomplicated chickenpox should not be admitted to the hospital because they present a hazard to susceptible patients and personnel. In addition, patients who develop chickenpox or are exposed to chickenpox while hospitalized should be discharged, if possible. Of course severely ill patients are exceptions to these rules.

Precautions

Nonimmune patients exposed to chickenpox or patients with chickenpox should be isolated in a private room or cohorted (see Chap. 11). Precautions that prevent contact with both respiratory secretions and secretions from patients' vesicles are required. Although the duration of contagion is variable, the period of contagion of varicella virus from vesicles appears to decrease approximately 5 days after the onset of rash. Because this period is somewhat variable, isolation precautions should be continued until all skin lesions are completely dried and crusted.

The susceptible patient exposed to chickenpox who cannot be discharged from the hospital often presents a difficult problem regarding restriction of activity and isolation precautions. Because of the high degree of communicability of chickenpox, personnel and patients in the same unit as a patient with chickenpox should be considered exposed [76]. Furthermore, patients with negative or unknown histories of chickenpox should be considered susceptible and will require isolation precautions beginning 10 days after exposure and continuing until 21 days after the last exposure. Since communicability of disease before the onset of the rash is not accurately predictable, precautions or cohorting of exposed persons should be initiated on the tenth day after exposure. Unless immunity can be proved, these patients should remain isolated until discharged from the hospital or for 21 days, whichever occurs first.

Hospital workers who have negative or unknown histories of previous varicella infection and who are exposed to persons with active varicella should not work with susceptible patients from the tenth to the twenty-first day after exposure [163]. If employee immunity to varicella can be proved, employees need not be sent home from work. If large numbers of employees are involved, these precautions may result in a significant expense to the hospital in time lost from work. In general, a history of previous chickenpox or herpes zoster in an adult or child is a reliable indication of immunity. In an attempt to control nosocomial transmission of chickenpox, the immune status in exposed persons with negative or unknown histories of chickenpox should be determined. The complement fixation (CF) antibody test is inexpensive and easy to perform,

but this antibody does not persist indefinitely, and false-negative results occur [61, 166]. Newer tests include the fluorescent antibody to membrane antigen test (FAMA) and the immune adherence hemagglutination test (IAH); both tests are more reliable than CF since these antibodies are believed to persist indefinitely [166].

Prophylaxis

Varicella-zoster immune globulin (VZIG) is intended primarily for passive immunization of susceptible immunocompromised children after significant exposure to chickenpox or herpes zoster [24]. Available evidence suggests that if VZIG is administered within 96 hours of exposure, chickenpox can be prevented or modified in children with impaired immunity. VZIG has been licensed by the U.S. Food and Drug Administration and is readily available [24]. The criteria for use of VZIG are shown in Tables 38-1 and 38-2. VZIS is not recommented routinely for susceptible workers who have been exposed to VZV.

Table 38-1.   Indications for use of varicella-zoster immune globulin: patient factors*

1. Susceptibility to varicella-zoster (see text)
2. Significant exposure.
3. Age of <15 years, with administration to immunocompromised adolescents and adults and to other older patients on an individual basis (see text)
4. One of the following underlying illnesses or conditions:
   a. Leukemia or lymphoma
   b. Congenital or acquired immunodeficiency
   c. Immunosuppressive treatment
   d. Newborn of mother who had onset of chickenpox within 5 days before delivery or within 48 hours after delivery
   e. Premature infant (≥28 weeks' gestation) whose mother lacks a previous history of chickenpox
   f. Premature infants (<28 weeks' gestation or ≤1,000 gm) regardless of maternal history

*Patients should meet all four criteria.
Source: From Centers for Disease Control, Recommendation of the Immunization Practices Advisory Committee (ACIP). Varicella-zoster immune globulin for the prevention of chickenpox. *M.M.W.R.* 33:84, 1984.

Table 38-2. Indications for use of varicella-zoster immune globulin: exposure factors*

1. One of the following types of exposure to persons with chickenpox or zoster:
   a. Continuous household contact
   b. Playmate contact (generally >1 hour of play indoors)
   c. Hospital contact (in same two- to four-bed room or adjacent beds in a large ward or prolonged face-to-face contact with an infectious staff member or patient)
   d. Newborn contact (newborn of mother who had onset of chickenpox 5 days or less before delivery or within 48 hours after delivery)

   and

2. Time elapsed after exposure is such that varicella-zoster immune globulin can be administered within 96 hours but preferably sooner

*Patients should meet both criteria.
Source: From Centers for Disease Control, Recommendation of the Immunization Practices Advisory Committee (ACIP), Varicella-zoster immune globulin for the prevention of chickenpox. *M.M.W.R.* 33:84, 1984.

Herpes Zoster Virus

Transmission of virus from patients with herpes zoster to produce chickenpox has occurred [9] but occurs less frequently than transmission of virus from patients with chickenpox. This may be due to the lower frequency of VZV in oral secretions of patients with herpes zoster than of patients with chickenpox.

Localized herpes zoster requires secretion precautions to guard against acquisition of infection by direct contact with secretions from vesicles and from secretion-contaminated articles (see Chap. 11). A private room is desirable but not required.

Patients with disseminated herpes zoster should be cared for in the same way as patients with chickenpox. They require strict isolation precautions in a private room with negative air pressure.

Hospital personnel with negative or unknown histories of chickenpox should avoid contact with patients with either localized or disseminated herpes zoster.

Gershon and colleagues [61] have shown that more than 95 percent of American-born women of childbearing age have detectable antibody to VZV. Ross [130] noted an 8 percent attack rate in historically susceptible adults with household exposure to chickenpox. A negative or unknown history of chickenpox in adults is often unreliable. These data suggest that the risk to hospital personnel for varicella acquisition from patients is small but measurable. The pool of susceptible persons, however small, represents a potential hazard for transmission of varicella to both susceptible patients and personnel.

Identification of persons with negative or unknown histories using reliable screening tests (FAMA or IAH) at the time of employment is an ideal infection control measure. Since these tests may not be readily available, selective screening should be done as quickly as possible after exposure to minimize the disruption of patient services.

Herpes Simplex Virus

Reaction of HSV type I infection frequently occurs spontaneously in healthy patients or personnel as well as in immunocompromised hosts (see Chap. 41). Persons with reactivated HSV I infection rarely have intraoral lesions and often do not have labial lesions. Therefore, asymptomatic personnel potentially can transmit HSV I to susceptible patients. Recently, it has been shown that individuals with herpes simplex labialis (fever blisters) do not transmit virus efficiently in respiratory secretions [149]. However, the same investigators were able to recover virus from the hands of two-thirds of the patients with herpes labialis [149]. This transmission may explain the clusters of infections that have been described in burned patients [51] and in immunocompromised patients [118]. Transmission of infection from hospital patients to personnel is well documented. Direct inoculation of HSV I on fingers of personnel after contact with the infected patient's mouth can result in herpetic whitlow [66]. Herpetic whitlow can easily be mistaken for pyogenic paronychia and is often quite disabling to hospital personnel [66]. Herpetic whitlow can occur in immune or nonimmune persons [10]. In addition, primary herpes simplex stomatitis and pharyngitis can occur in hospital personnel

[96]. A cluster of cases of primary HSV stomatitis and pharyngitis has occurred due to transmission of HSV I to patients in a dental office from a dental hygienist with herpetic whitlow [97].

HSV II and its potential for transmission from mother to newborn infant has long been a concern on obstretic and newborn services (see Chap. 21). When genital herpes is present in a mother at term, 40 to 60 percent of vaginally delivered infants will have clinically apparent infection with HSV II [117]. Approximately 50 percent of these infants will have severe or fatal illness. The risk of neonatal infection can be minimized, but not eliminated, if delivery is by cesarean section *and* membranes remain unruptured or have been ruptured for less than 6 hours [117]. The risk of infection at birth is also less if the mother's infection is reactivated rather than primary [117].

Although transmission of infection from mother to infant at the time of birth is well documented, evidence for transmission in the postpartum period is only indirect. Infection control policies under these circumstances are often ambiguous and confusing, and there is lack of uniformity from one institution to another [88, 132]. It is generally agreed, however, that certain precautions may be indicated, depending on the clinical status of the mother.

Precautions

Infection control recommendations for mothers with known, suspected, or inactive HSV have been described in detail [150] (see Chap. 11).

Women with Proved or Clinically Suspected Genital Herpes Simplex at Term Such women may transmit virus postnatally to their offspring as well as to other close contacts. Therefore, personnel should observe precautions, using gowns and gloves for direct contact with lesions containing virus. Perineal pads, dressings, and linen should be double-bagged. The mother may care for her baby, but she should be out of bed, wash hands thoroughly before

contact with the baby, and wear a clean cover gown. The infant should be observed after birth for signs and symptoms of illness, and personnel should follow drainage/secretion precautions for direct contact with the infant. Currently, there are no data regarding use of the observation or isolation nursery for such infants after birth. The value of such a nursery for use in these cases is controversial, and nursery outbreaks of herpes simplex infection are uncommon. However, an observation nursery for these infants is recommended, and good technique, including thorough hand-washing, should be emphasized. These precautions do not restrict mother-baby contact yet offer some degree of protection for other infants in the nursery.

Women with Active Nongenital Herpes Simplex at Term Wound and skin precautions similar to those recommended for women with genital herpes simplex are reasonable for these women. A private room is not indicated. Mothers may care for their infants using the same precautions as noted for mothers with known or suspected genital herpes simplex, with the addition of a mask or dressing to cover the lesions. The infant may be kept in the general newborn nursery without isolation after birth if there has been no maternal contact. After the first contact with the mother, the infant should be placed in the suspect or isolation nursery, using precautions noted previously for babies born to mothers with active genital herpes simplex.

Women with Clinically Inactive Herpes Simplex at Term No special precautions are necessary for either the mother or infant.

Special Considerations

The issue of work restrictions is raised frequently. When assessing the need for work restrictions for employees with herpes simplex infection, it is useful to distinguish between covered and uncovered active lesions of herpes simplex. Personnel who have uncovered or active lesions of herpes simplex should not work with newborn infants (term or preterm), burned patients, or immuno-compromised hosts until all lesions have dried and crusted. Personnel with herpetic whitlow should be excluded from any patient care until the lesions are dried and crusted. Wearing a glove on the involved hand has been suggested as an alternative, but it is not known if this is a truly effective barrier to disease transmission. Early treatment with acyclovir may shorten the period of contagion and restriction. Personnel who have active genital herpes simplex or covered lesions of herpes simplex are not restricted from patient contact, but strict hand-washing is required before and after patient contact.

Measures to prevent herpetic whitlow include wearing gloves on *both hands* if direct contact with oral or pharngeal secretions is anticipated [66, 150]. Gloves are especially important when suctioning patients and should be worn routinely during this procedure. Also, patients with proved or suspected herpes simplex labialis who require intensive nursing care should be placed on precautions that require the use of gloves whenever contact with these lesions is anticipated [66, 150].

Frequently, concerns arise over the possibility of acquiring genital herpes simplex infections from inanimate surfaces, such as toilet seats. Though the virus has been found to survive for short periods of time outside the human body, the geometric mean titer of virus on plastic and skin surfaces decreases rapidly during the first hour (Fig. 38-1) [149]. Transmission of herpes simplex from inanimate surfaces such as plastic and cloth has not been documented. The general consensus of viral epidemiologists is that such transmission is rare or nonexistent and that HSV is usually transmitted via direct contact with infectious lesions.

Cytomegalovirus

CMV, like other herpesviruses, requires direct contact for spread. CMV infection is most often a sexually transmitted disease. The virus is found in cervical and vaginal secretions and in semen. In addition, the prevalence of CMV antibody has been found to be greater in ho-

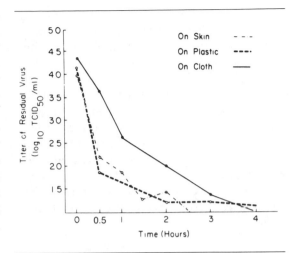

Fig. 38-1. Geometric mean titers of residual herpesvirus in saliva. TCID = tissue culture infective dose. (Reprinted with permission from R. Turner et al., Shedding and survival of herpes simplex virus from "fever blisters." *Pediatrics* 70:547, 1982.

mosexual (96 percent) than in heterosexual (57 percent) men [44]. It has also been shown to increase with years of sexual activity and is higher in prostitutes than in nuns [157].

In-hospital transmission of CMV has long been a concern of hospital personnel because of its role in congenital malformations. Yeager [164] showed a slight excess of antibody conversion in pediatric nurses working with children who were shedding CMV compared to personnel without patient contact. These differences, however, were not statistically significant. In another setting, dialysis personnel failed to show any seroconversion after 2 years of follow-up [147]. More recently, it has been shown that pediatric health care workers are not at increased risk of acquiring CMV infection compared to women in the community [5, 46]. Case reports have also demonstrated lack of transmission of CMV from patients to health care personnel by using restriction endonuclease techniques [162, 165].

CMV can also be transmitted via blood transfusion. This risk is reduced with leukocyte-poor blood and virtually eliminated if washed frozen red blood cells are used [92]. It can also be eliminated by screening potential blood donors for antibody to CMV and by eliminating those with antibody. Patients undergoing renal transplanation are an important source of CMV [80] (see Chap. 41). The majority of such patients have reactivation of endogenous CMV as a result of the transplant process or from associated immunosuppressive therapy. We have classified these infections as endogenous nosocomial infections [151]. A small number of transplant patients acquire CMV exogenously from the transplanted kidneys or from circulating cells present in the transplanted kidney.

Precautions

We suggest hand-washing as the most important infection control precaution for patients with congenital or acquired CMV infection. Because the risk of transmission of CMV to hospital personnel appears low, hospital personnel are not screened for CMV antibody. Personnel should be educated regarding the mode of transmission of CMV, but pregnant personnel need not be discouraged from having contact with patients with known or suspected CMV infection, nor is transfer to an alternative assignment necessary. Even though many patients with HIV infection and the acquired immunodeficiency syndrome (AIDS) also shed CMV, it is not necessary to restrict pregnant health care workers from caring for these patients.

Special Considerations

At the present time, routine screening for antibody to CMV of personnel on newborn, pediatric, or dialysis-transplant services is not recommended. Patients undergoing renal transplantation and their donors or donor kidneys are tested for antibody to CMV before transplantation [81]. Whenever possible, kidneys from antibody-negative donors are transplanted to antibody-negative recipients.

Epstein-Barr Virus

EBV is shed in high concentration from the oropharynx of infected patients. Although nosocomial transmission is relatively rare, infection has occurred through blood transfu-

sion [148] and from blood contamination of dialysis equipment [37] (see Chap. 41). Since transmission of EBV from the respiratory tract has not been documented in hospitals, isolation precautions for patients with EBV infections are not indicated.

Hepatitis
Hepatitis A

Nosocomial hepatitis A has been known for many years to occur in institutions for the mentally retarded [100]. Crowded conditions and poor hygienic practices on the part of many patients in these institutions appear to be predisposing factors. Up to 80 percent of susceptible institutionalized patients may develop hepatitis A virus (HAV) infection as measured by seroconversion of antibody to HAV within 3 years of admission [143]. This rate of seroconversion is considerably higher than the rate of seroconversion in noninstitutionalized adults or in child controls.

Transmission of HAV in general hospitals is relatively uncommon. Nosocomial transmission from personnel to patient has rarely been reported. Transmission of HAV infection from patients to personnel has occurred infrequently [16]. Foodborne outbreaks have also occurred, involving hospital workers primarily but also small numbers of patients [109].

Precautions

Current recommendations avoid the all-or-none phenomenon of past guidelines, allowing for more flexibility based on known or anticipated contact with infectious material [46] (see Chap. 11). Dienstag and colleagues [41] have shown that maximum fecal shedding of HAV occurs before the onset of symptoms. Because of these data, some experts have recommended that no precautions be taken: Once the symptomatic patient is admitted to the hospital, the time for maximal shedding should have passed. On the other hand, because viral shedding can be variable, isolation precautions should emphasize the importance of care and handling of feces, bedpans, and equipment or instruments contaminated with feces. Measures such as gowns, gloves, and masks are not required routinely but should be used whenever necessary to minimize contact with feces or material contaminated with feces. A private room is not required unless the patient is incontinent of feces.

Prophylaxis

Immune serum globulin (IG) is effective in preventing or modifying hepatitis A both before exposure and early in the incubation period. If given within 2 weeks of exposure, IG will prevent 80 to 90 percent of HAV infections.

Hepatitis B

Nosocomial transmission of hepatitis B virus (HBV) is believed to occur most often by parenteral exposure to blood positive for hepatitis B surface antigen (HBsAg). Transmission can occur from an acutely ill patient or, more likely, from an asymptomatic person who is positive for HBsAg and is unaware of it. The HBsAg carrier state accounts for the prolonged period of potential HBV infectivity of some patients even after the acute infection has resolved. The infectivity of blood is best correlated with the presence of either DNA polymerase or hepatitis B e antigen (HBeAg). For infection control purposes, however, all blood positive for HBsAg should be considered infectious. Although HBsAg has been detected in all body fluids, the frequency with which fluids other than blood contribute to hospital infection is probably low. The mechanisms of transmission are listed here in descending order of probability [51]:

1. *Overt parenteral.* Direct percutaneous inoculation by needles contaminated with serum or plasma (e.g., transfusion of contaminated blood or blood products, contaminated needle stick)
2. *Inapparent parenteral*
   a. Percutaneous inoculation of infective serum or plasma without overt needle puncture (e.g., contamination of cutaneous cuts, abrasions, or lacerations)
   b. Contamination of mucosal surfaces by infected serum or plasma (e.g., pipet-

ting accidents, accidental ingestion, other direct contact with mucous membranes of the eye or mouth)
   c. Contamination of mucosal surfaces by infective secretions other than serum or plasma (e.g., sexual activity)
   d. Transfer of infective material via fomites (e.g., toothbrushes, toys, drinking cups, horizontal surfaces in hospitals)

Clearly, ample opportunity exists for transmission of hepatitis B in the hospital to both patients and personnel.

Dienstag and Ryan [42] have reviewed the prevalence of hepatitis B markers in hospital personnel by job category. Emergency room nurses were found to have the highest prevalence of markers of previous HBV infection (30 percent), followed by surgical intensive care unit nurses, phlebotomists, chemistry laboratory technicians, and surgical house officers. While this survey reflects the HBV state of employees in a large urban hospital, it also serves to underscore the fact that health care workers are at higher risk of HBV infection than the general population. In a large survey reported by Denes and colleagues [40], evidence of previous HBV infection was higher among physicians practicing in urban communities, increased with the number of years in practice, and was highest among pathologists and surgeons. Dentists and physicians have a similar overall rate of positivity [135].

The issue of work restrictions for the HBsAg-positive worker is a controversial one (see Chap. 3). The *CDC Guidelines for Infection Control in Hospital Personnel* states that employees who are chronic carriers of HBsAg need not be restricted from patient contact unless they have been implicated in disease transmission [163]. Though this recommendation may seem paradoxical, it points out the difficult and sensitive nature of the problem. All available evidence suggests that the greatest risk of nosocomial transmission of HBV takes place from patients to personnel [163]. Transmission of HBV from personnel to patients is not as clear. Epidemiologic data are available that show both transmission [57,

129] and lack of transmission of hepatitis B [60, 107] from HBsAg-positive personnel to their patients. Factors contributing to transmission of HBV from personnel to patients are probably the level and duration of antigenemia in the employee and the type of contact the employee has with the patient. From the available data, it appears that routine patient care that does not afford contact with blood of infected personnel does not present a risk to patients [60, 107]. The physician-surgeon or dental surgeon who is HBsAg-positive may present a different degree of risk to patients when performing surgical procedures. It is not possible to make general recommendations regarding restrictions for these personnel in the operating room as this type of evaluation should be made on an individual basis. It is hoped that as more high-risk personnel are vaccinated with the hepatitis B vaccine, the dilemma of the HBsAg-positive health care worker can be avoided.

Isolation Precautions

A private room is not required routinely for acute hepatitis B patients (see Chap. 11), although the patient who is incontinent of feces or is bleeding is managed best in a private room. While routine use of gowns, gloves, and masks is not required, any or all of these precautions should be used if patient contact may also involve contact with blood or other body fluids. Gloves should be used for direct contact with blood or blood-contaminated equipment such as intravenous catheters, drains, or soiled dressings. Precautions should also be taken to avoid contact with feces or body fluids that have been contaminated with blood (see Chap. 11).

Prophylaxis

Preexposure Prophylaxis The hepatitis B vaccine should be used as preexposure prophylaxis for hepatitis B in high-risk individuals. The vaccine is also recommended for certain health care workers such as dialysis workers, nurses in emergency rooms and intensive care units, and other personnel at high risk due to regular contact with blood [12, 42, 163] (see Chap. 3). The high-risk groups should be se-

lected based on frequency of contact with blood or needles. Other data sources from the facility include results of serologic screening done on an ongoing basis in some institutions, prevalence studies of hepatitis B markers in certain groups of employees, and records of needle punctures. Once the high-risk groups are identified in an institution, prevaccination screening for all vaccinated persons may not be necessary and will depend on the expected prevalence of hepatitis B markers and the cost of screening [12]. Groups of workers who are screened periodically due to the high risk of hepatitis B exposure (e.g., dialysis and laboratory workers) are automatically candidates for vaccination. In these cases, the vaccine is more cost-effective than routine screening because it offers the additional benefit of protection from hepatitis B and makes further screening unnecessary in those who respond with hepatitis B surface antibody (anti-HBs).

The Occupational Safety and Health Administration (OSHA) has developed a standard for protection of health care workers from bloodborne pathogens, which includes free hepatitis B vaccine for health care workers who have blood contact. Points for consideration when developing a hepatitis B vaccination program are [2]:

1. Mandatory vaccination of high-risk employees may be a condition of employment. This may be desirable but may be difficult to enforce, especially for employees who are currently working. The legal ramifications of such a policy also need to be assessed in light of the OSHA standard.
2. Voluntary vaccination of high-risk individuals is an option under the OSHA rules. However, employees must sign a waiver if they choose not to be vaccinated. They may be vaccinated at a later time if they choose.
3. The vaccine has been shown to be immunogenic and effective in preventing hepatitis B [141]. Clinical trials in large numbers of homosexual men have shown that the vaccine is 100 percent effective in preventing hepatitis B infection in those

who respond with anti-HBs [141]. The rates of seroconversion have not been as high in the experience of most hospital infection control programs. The site of injection has been suggested as one reason for variable response rates, and the deltoid muscle is now the recommended site of injection [28]. Even with response rates of 80 to 85 percent, however, vaccination clearly offers protection against hepatitis B in the majority of people who receive it and is a worthwhile infection control and employee health activity. The safety of the vaccine has been questioned by some as a result of the occurrence of AIDS in certain high-risk groups whose serum may have been used to manufacture the original plasma-derived vaccine. The vaccine-manufacturing process has been shown to inactivate HIV, the cause of AIDS [12]. The plasma-derived vaccine is no longer in widespread use because of the availability of two recombinant vaccine preparations.

Postexposure Prophylaxis Hepatitis B immune globulin (HBIG) and the hepatitis B vaccine are recommended for use as postexposure prophylaxis for hepatitis B. Current guidelines from the Advisory Committee on Immunization Practices (ACIP) [21] state that these agents should be used together for the following types of contact: (1) parenteral inoculation of HBsAg-containing material, such as a needle stick or contamination of open skin with a large inoculum of HBsAg-positive blood; or (2) accidental ingestion of HBsAg-positive blood (e.g., pipetting accident); or (3) accidental splash of HBsAg-positive blood on the mucous membranes of the eye or mouth. Ideally, prophylaxis should be given as soon as possible but within 7 days of exposure. HBIG is given once at a dose of 0.06 ml/kg at the same time as the first dose of hepatitis B vaccine. Additional doses of vaccine are given 1 and 6 months after the first dose. A second dose of HBIG is not given with this regimen. Workers who refuse the hepatitis B vaccine should be given two doses of HBIG (0.06 ml/kg each dose) 1 month apart (see Chaps. 3, 18).

One of the most difficult aspects of postexposure hepatitis B prophylaxis is to determine whether the exposure was significant—that is, whether it involved parenteral inoculation of HBsAg-positive material. It is also important that the HBsAg status of the source be determined as soon as possible. Infection control and employee health personnel should try to apply uniform and consistent criteria when evaluating the need for prophylaxis after a hepatitis B exposure. However, the final evaluation may need to be done on an individual basis in some cases.

Infants born to mothers who are HBsAg-positive at the time of delivery should also be given hepatitis B prophylaxis to prevent development of the HBsAg carrier state. Both HBIG and the hepatitis B vaccine should be given at the time of birth. One dose of HBIG (0.5 ml) should be given along with the first dose of vaccine (0.5 ml). The additional doses of vaccine should be given 1 month and 6 months after the first [21, 144].

Special Considerations
One of the most important infection control measures for all forms of hepatitis involves the education of hospital personnel. Health care workers must be aware of the modes of transmission of hepatitis viruses, the importance of appropriate precautions in the care of such patients, and of the availability of hepatitis B vaccine. Obtaining blood from patients with HBsAg presents one of the greatest hazards to hospital personnel. In some cases, large numbers of personnel may be exposed to blood containing HBsAg before the patient is known to be HBsAg-positive. For this reason, and because patients may have detectable HBsAg before the onset of illness, blood from all patients should be considered infectious and handled in the manner of universal precautions or body substance isolation. Special emphasis should be placed on avoiding contamination of skin and mucous membranes by blood spills from acutely ill patients who are HBsAg-positive. Since it is not possible to recommend specific precautions for each instance, employees should be encouraged to use universal precautions or

body substance isolation that will minimize contact with blood or blood-contaminated body fluids at all times (see Chaps. 3, 18).

Hepatitis B in Hemodialysis Units

Infection with HBV has been an infection control hazard to both patients and personnel in many units [21] (see Chaps. 19, 41). Hepatitis B was often introduced into the dialysis unit by HBsAg-positive patients, who probably acquired their infection from transfusion of HBsAg-positive blood. Screening of blood for HBsAg, use of hepatitis B vaccine, and adoption of universal precautions have changed the approach to hepatitis B in dialysis settings [21]. In a study of 65 dialysis units conducted by the CDC from 1967–1970, 82 percent of the units surveyed had patients, staff, or both with hepatitis B [140]. In 1974, Szmuness and associates [140] reported overall rates of seropositivity (HBsAg- and anti-HBs-positive) in 15 U.S. dialysis units of 51 percent in patients and 34 percent in staff members. By 1980, the incidence of hepatitis B had decreased to 1 percent of patients and 0.7 percent of staff [1]. Transmission of HBV infection from hemodialysis personnel to patients has not been reported. Transmission to personnel from either HBsAg-positive patients or contaminated equipment or environmental surfaces, on the other hand, is well documented. The greatest risk in such instances has been shown to be contact with blood or blood-contaminated materials and instruments.

Regular hepatitis screening for dialysis patients and staff has been an important component of hepatitis B prevention programs in dialysis units for many years. However, this activity has served only to monitor the introduction or transmission of HBV in dialysis settings (see Chaps. 3, 19). Ideally, all dialysis candidates should be screened for hepatitis B markers (HBsAg, anti-HBs, and anti-HBc) prior to admission to the dialysis unit [21]. Similarly, all dialysis workers should be screened for hepatitis B markers prior to their employment in the unit. The use of the hepatitis B vaccine, however, has changed the approach to screening after admission or employment in dialysis centers. Vaccina-

tion can be a more cost-effective activity than screening alone because it will obviate the need for hepatitis B screening in those who respond to the vaccine with protective levels of anti-HBs. Vaccination rather than screening offers the added advantage of providing immunity to infection rather than merely monitoring the introduction of hepatitis B into the hemodialysis unit [142].

Once dialysis patients and personnel have been vaccinated, those who respond with protective levels of anti-HBs can be screened less frequently (e.g., yearly) to check for persistence of antibody.

Non-A, Non-B Hepatitis

Non-A, non-B hepatitis is caused by more than one agent [21, 113]. Available data suggest that transmission in the United States is primarily parenteral, through transfusions of blood or blood products [106]. Recently, hepatitis C has been characterized [49] and is believed to be the most common form of posttransfusion hepatitis since the advent of routine screening of donor blood for HBsAg and elimination of HBsAg-positive donors. The recently developed assay for hepatitis C antibody appears to detect a substantial number of persons with chronic infection and has also been instituted as a part of the screening process for blood donors [21].

Isolation Precautions

Isolation precautions for patients with non-A, non-B hepatitis are similar to those for patients with hepatitis B, with emphasis on precautions in handling blood or blood-contaminated articles.

Prophylaxis

Preliminary data suggest that IB (0.06 ml/kg) may be useful in prophylaxis of non-A, non-B hepatitis [21], but additional study is required.

Rubella

The introduction of rubella vaccine in 1969 has resulted in a marked decrease in the number of cases of rubella in school-aged children.

The vaccine has not decreased the incidence of rubella in older age groups as dramatically, however [20, 26]. From 1976 to 1979, more than 70 percent of reported cases occurred in persons 15 years of age or older [26], and in 1980 46.6 percent of patients were older than 15 years [80]. Overall seronegativity among hospital employees has been reported to be as high as 14 percent [44]. Outbreaks of rubella in hospitals have also been reported [27, 102, 124–126]. These outbreaks emphasize the potential for transmission of rubella in institutional settings and underscore the importance of immunity against rubella to protect patients and personnel. In general, efforts to vaccinate susceptible hospital personnel on a voluntary basis, especially physicians, have been disappointing [126].

Isolation Precautions
Congenital Rubella
In congenitally acquired infection, virus may persist in pharyngeal secretions for many months after birth and may be shed for up to 4 years [133]. In general, these infants are not believed to be hazardous to others after approximately 2 to 3 years of age because little virus is present [75]. Infants with congenital rubella syndrome should be in private rooms and remain on precautions for the duration of hospitalization (see Chap. 11). Until additional data are available, we recommend that infants with congenital rubella who are less than 2 years of age be placed on precautions when readmitted to the hospital.

Acquired Rubella
Patients with acquired rubella or susceptible patients who have been exposed to rubella should be isolated for 21 days after exposure or for 5 days after the onset of rash.

Screening and Immunization
The current rubella strategy in the United States involves elimination of the congenital rubella syndrome, replacing an earlier narrower approach to rubella, which involved only vaccination of women of childbearing age. A rubella program should be designed to prevent the introduction and spread of rubella in health care facilities [156]. Screen-

ing for immunity is not enough. All health care workers, male or female, should be immune to rubella. Immunity to rubella is defined as laboratory evidence of a protective titer for rubella or evidence of vaccination with live rubella vaccine after 12 months of age [163]. Previous history of disease is not acceptable since many exanthematous diseases can be confused with rubella [20, 163]. Also, the trivalent mumps-measles-rubella (MMR) vaccine should be used whenever possible. Vaccination with MMR of persons who are already immune to one of its components is not associated with significant adverse effects [20].

Special Considerations
To prevent the transmission of rubella in outbreaks, those susceptible should be vaccinated promptly [20]. It is not recommended, however, that pregnant women be vaccinated [20]. McLaughlin and Gold [102] have outlined restrictions for use during outbreaks. Personnel with rubella should not work in any area of the hospital because of the risk of transmitting disease to susceptible persons. Immune or nonexposed staff should care for pregnant patients in their first trimester and, whenever possible, for all pregnant patients regardless of gestational stage [102]. Immune serum globulin may modify the disease in exposed persons, but its use is generally not recommended during pregnancy [102].

Measles (Rubeola)

Large hospital outbreaks of measles have been uncommon in recent years. Susceptible young health care workers are another potential reservoir of measles infection [125, 134]. Measles has the potential to become a nosocomial pathogen again if programs are not in place to ensure immunity of health care workers.

The most significant change in measles control involves new recommendations to help achieve the goal of measles elimination. The goal of measles eradication has not been reached because of (1) failure to implement the previous vaccination strategy and (2) vaccine failure. Despite the previous recommendation of universal vaccination with one dose of live measles vaccine at 15 months of age, there remain large numbers of young people susceptible to measles [47].

Overall, the great majority of vaccines appear to have long-term, probably lifelong, immunity. In recent years, however, measles outbreaks have occurred in the United States among the following groups: unvaccinated preschool-aged children, previously vaccinated school-aged children, and students and personnel on college campuses.

Isolation Precautions

A single room (or cohorting) is required, and all personnel should observe respiratory precautions (see Chap. 11). Maintain precautions until 7 days after onset of rash in known cases. When exposure to measles has occurred, the patient should be isolated from the fifth to the twenty-first day after exposure. If clinical disease occurs, isolation should continue for 7 days after the appearance of the rash.

Screening and Immunization

The currently recommended immunization schedule, an attempt to increase the pool of immune individuals, calls for two doses of live measles vaccine, the first at 15 months of age for most children and the second at the time the child enters school.

As with rubella, health care facilities should adopt policies that require immunity to measles: evidence of two live measles vaccinations, documentation of physician-diagnosed measles disease, or laboratory evidence of measles immunity for staff who will have direct patient contact. Personnel who were born before 1957 can be considered immune. Personnel who were born in 1957 or later who have no documentation of immunity should be vaccinated at the time of employment and revaccinated 1 month later. Trivalent MMR vaccine for both injections will ensure adequate immunity to all three viruses. However, to contain costs when large numbers of personnel are vaccinated, the first injection could be given as MMR, and the second dose can be given as monovalent measles.

Special Considerations
"Modified Measles"

Measles modified by IG may be overlooked or result in delays in diagnosis. Respiratory shedding of virus does occur in patients given IG, and the isolation precautions mentioned previously should be instituted and maintained.

Atypical Measles

The atypical measles syndrome occurs after exposure to wild measles virus in persons who have been vaccinated with the inactivated measles vaccine used before 1965 [116]. The illness is characterized by fever; an *unusual skin rash* that, like the measles rash, is maculopapular but is more likely to become petechial or hemorrhagic; and pulmonary manifestations. It appears to be caused by an altered immune response in a previously sensitized host [54]. The illness has also been recorded in persons vaccinated after 1965 with live attenuated vaccine [31]. Measles virus has not been isolated from patients with atypical measles. These patients are not believed to be infectious, and special isolation precautions are not recommended.

Outbreak Management

In the event of an outbreak of measles in a health care facility, employees born in or after 1957 should be vaccinated if they have direct patient contact and do not have proof of immunity to measles. Susceptible personnel who have been exposed should be relieved from direct patient contact from the fifth to the twenty-first day after exposure or, if they become ill, for 7 days after the onset of the rash.

Mumps

Mumps virus is less communicable than either measles or varicella (chickenpox), and infections in compromised hosts have not been associated with the serious consequences that may follow measles or varicella [50]. Although nosocomial transmission has been documented [136, 160], outbreaks are usually confined to families, schools, and military personnel.

The use of the more expensive trivalent MMR vaccine for either the rubella or measles prevention programs in health care workers, as noted earlier, also has its advantages in mumps prevention.

Respiratory isolation and a private room are recommended. Presently, we maintain precautions until 9 days after the onset of parotitis, at which time infectiousness appears to decrease (see Chap. 11).

Parvovirus B19

Parvovirus B19 has been associated with five clinical entities: (1) erythema infectiousum (EI), (2) adult arthritis, (3) aplastic crisis in patients with diseases of increased red cell turnover (e.g., sickle cell anemia and hereditary spherocytosis), (4) chronic anemia in immunocompromised patients, and (5) fetal death in pregnant women. Most parvovirus B19 infections occur in children older than 5 years. By age 18, 30 to 60 percent of adults demonstrate B19 antibodies in their serum.

Parvovirus B19 transmission is not completely understood. The virus has been detected in respiratory secretions of patients with EI, and close contact seems to transmit the virus effectively. Spread may occur via large-particle aerosols, fomites (secretion-contaminated objects), or direct contact [35]. For example, teachers and other day-care providers were shown to be at highest risk of acquiring B19 infection during a recent outbreak in Connecticut [62].

Parvovirus B19 infection usually produces a mild, self-limited illness with no serious long-term side effects in normal children and adults. The disease generally consists of a viremic phase with constitutional symptoms (myalgias, pyrexia, headache, malaise). This phase occurs 5 to 6 days after exposure and continues for 2 to 3 days. An asymptomatic period lasting 5 to 10 days follows, after which the second stage of infection occurs. This second phase continues for 1 to 2 weeks more and consists of rash and joint pains. By the

time the rash occurs, viremia has resolved and the patient is no longer considered infectious. The incidence of secondary transmission among health care workers may be as high as 50 percent.

Currently, there is no diagnostic test available for parvovirus B19. The diagnosis is made primarily by having a high index of suspicion. EI is the classic B19 illness, characterized in children by a flulike illness followed by a maculopapular or erythematous macular eruption on the face, torso, and extremities. The facial rash has been described as resembling a slapped cheek.

Parvovirus B19 infection in pregnancy has been a concern because of potential risk to the fetus. In actuality, infants born to B19-infected women have not shown an increase in congenital malformations [4].

In health care and day-care settings, parvovirus B19 is of concern for pregnant health care workers. In contrast to other viral illnesses, it has been recommended that pregnant health care workers not care for patients with known B19 infection [33]. The problem with this type of restriction, of course, is that most patients will be identified during the second or rash phase of the illness, after the period of maximum contagion.

The best approach to prevention of B19 transmission involves universal precautions and the body substance isolation approach, which emphasizes frequent hand-washing and use of gloves and other protective clothing when needed. Restriction of pregnant health care workers may be possible or warranted in situations where patients are known to be infected with B19, such as an outbreak. Otherwise, a higher level of infection control practice remains the best means of prevention [25].

Creutzfeldt-Jakob Disease

Creutzfeldt-Jakob disease (CJD) is believed to be of viral origin with a long incubation period for 15 to 24 months. It is not contagious in the usual sense and does not appear to present excessive risks to hospital personnel.

Sufficient concern dealing with the transmission of CJD in hospitals has arisen in the past few years, because the diagnosis has been proved or suspected in more patients. The disease has been reported to occur following corneal transplantation [45], as well as in 2 patients through contaminated sterotactic electrodes used in previous neurosurgical procedures [8]. CJD has also occurred as a nosocomial surgical infection subsequent to allogeneic dura mater graphs [98] and from injections of growth hormone of human pituitary gland origin [53].

Isolation Precautions

Precautions are recommended for patients with suspected CJD until the diagnosis has been ruled out [55, 67] (see Chap. 11). If a diagnosis is established by brain biopsy, patients are maintained on precautions that emphasize care in handling of all body fluids and tissue, especially blood, cerebrospinal fluid, and brain tissue [55, 67]. To facilitate understanding by hospital personnel, it should be stressed that these precautions are similar to those used for patients with hepatitis B. Once a diagnosis of CJD has been confirmed, precautions are maintained for the duration of hospitalization and for subsequent hospitalizations.

Special Considerations

A policy should be established to ensure additional precautions for specimens from CJD patients, equipment, and instruments used for patients with CJD [52]. The infection control practitioner (ICP) should be notified of the admission of a CJD patient to the hospital. The ICP should then notify staff in other involved hospital departments and service areas, who should make the necessary arrangements for disposal and handling of specimens and sterilization of equipment and instruments. The details of such a policy have been described previously [55, 67].

Gastroenteritis Viruses

The two major causes of viral gastroenteritis were identified in the 1970s using immune electron-microscopic examination of stool and by electron-microscopic analysis of infected intestinal mucosa. The rotaviruses are a major cause of viral diarrhea in infants and children [145]. The caliciviruslike agents (Norwalk gastroenteritis–like agents) generally cause gastroenteritis in older children and adults [38].

Rotavirus

The human rotavirus (HRV; human reoviruslike agent, or infantile gastroenteritis virus) is a major case of gastroenteritis in infants and children during the winter in temperate climates [87, 93] (see Chap. 30). Kapikian and co-workers [87] showed that approximately half of all children admitted to hospitals in the winter months because of gastroenteritis are afflicted with HRV. Infants often are admitted to the hospital because of diarrhea and dehydration that may have been preceded by vomiting. Children 6 to 24 months of age are the most susceptible to HRV infection, and serum antibodies are rapidly acquired during this period. The majority of adults have such antibodies. The presence of serum antibodies does not protect completely against reinfection, however, and natural and experimental infections in adults do occur [89, 104]. Although adults may serve as a reservoir of infection despite the presence of preexisting antibody, the amount of virus shed is less than that shed by infectious children [89]. Approximately 55 percent of adult contacts of children with rotavirus infection develop serologic evidence of infection [89]. Asymptomatic shedding also occurs. Using electron microscopy, Bolivar and colleagues [11] showed that while 25 percent of symptomatic students had rotavirus in their stool, 12 percent of asymptomatic students also had rotavirus in their stool.

Transmission is by the fecal-oral route. Although nosocomial infection affects newborn infants most frequently [89, 138], infections in older children, adults, and hospital personnel have also been documented [37].

Isolation Precautions

Isolation precautions should emphasize care in handling articles contaminated with feces (see Chap. 11). Patients with rotavirus are maintained on these precautions for the duration of hospitalization, because the duration of shedding is highly variable.

Special Considerations

Rotaviruses are not readily isolated from tissue culture. The diagnosis is made by electron-microscopic examination of stool or by serologic methods (complement fixation [CF], enzyme-linked immunosorbent assay [ELISA], or counterimmunoelectrophoresis [CIE]). Because these tests may not be available in some institutions, the ICP should suspect rotavirus infection in infants who are admitted to the hospital for or who become ill with vomiting, diarrhea, dehydration, and fever during the winter months.

It is recommended that all infants with diarrhea be maintained on isolation precautions pending the results of culture for bacterial pathogens and serologic study for rotavirus. When rotaviral and bacterial causes are ruled out, patients with presumed nonbacterial gastroenteritis are maintained on precautions for 48 hours after they become asymptomatic.

Norwalk Gastroenteritis Virus and Related Agents

Included in this group are the Norwalk, Hawaii, W, and Montgomery County agents. These agents are major causes of viral gastroenteritis in children and adults and are associated with school, family, and community outbreaks; they probably are transmitted by fecal-oral spread. Although nosocomial transmission has not been documented, it probably occurs in a manner similar to that of rotavirus.

Isolation Precautions

Precautions for Norwalk gastroenteritis–like agents should be the same as for rotavirus. Isolation in these cases, however, is maintained for 72 hours after symptoms have ceased, because the period of shedding appears to be somewhat shorter than that of rotavirus [146].

Special Considerations

Like rotavirus, the Norwalk gastroenteritis–like agents cannot be isolated on viral culture.

The only laboratory test presently available for identifying infected materials is immune electron microscopy, which is tedious and not widely available. When rotavirus and nonbacterial pathogens have been ruled out, patients may be classified as having nonbacterial gastroenteritis other than rotavirus. Other agents, such as coronaviruslike agents, astrovirus, and mini-reovirus agents, also may be involved.

Picornaviruses

Of the three genera of the Picornaviridae family (enterovirus, rhinovirus, and calcivirus), the enteroviruses are the most frequent causes of nosocomial infection. Included in the enterovirus group are coxsackieviruses A and B, echoviruses, polioviruses, and enterovirus types 68 to 71.

Enteroviruses cause sporadic disease throughout the year but are most prevalent in the community during the summer and fall in temperate climates [103, 123, 124]. Transmission of the virus is via the fecal-oral route, but droplet transmission has been described for coxsackie A21 and probably occurs with other enteroviruses as well [103]. Virus can be recovered easily from the oropharynx and rectum and may be shed for 1 month or more after infection. Transmission occurs in hosts with or without preexisting antibody [103].

Nonpolio Enteroviruses

Infection is common in the general population, particularly among children, and results in a variety of illnesses. Patients may be asymptomatic or have mild illness with fever, rash, and upper respiratory or gastrointestinal symptoms. Symptomatic and severe disease occurs in newborn infants, particularly in full-term infants who may develop meningitis, encephalitis, myocarditis, or pericarditis in addition to the other symptoms mentioned. In older children, infection often is asymptomatic or benign. For these reasons, most of the reported nosocomial enterovirus infections have been outbreaks in neonatal units [30, 36, 86, 91, 101], whereas nosocomial enterovirus acquisition among older children often is undetected.

Most nursery outbreaks involve the non-polio enteroviruses. Often the virus is introduced into the nursery by an infected infant, and transmission occurs by indirect contact (i.e., from infant to infant via the hands of personnel). Infection also has been found in nursery personnel, suggesting that they may serve as sources of infection [30].

The most consistent mode of acquisition of nonpolio enteroviruses in infants is transmission from the mother [30]. Transmission may take place before, during, or after delivery. In a study of 27 newborn infants with symptomatic infection, 30 percent had onset of symptoms within the first 3 days of life, and 60 percent of the mothers were symptomatic at the time of delivery [91]. In a prospective study done during enterovirus season, Cherry and colleagues [32] demonstrated that 2 of 55 women were shedding virus at the time of delivery, and 1 of these 2 transmitted virus to her child. Others have reported the endemic occurrence of enterovirus infection in nurseries [30]. Additional epidemiologic studies are needed, however, to determine the frequency with which infected infants are introduced into the nursery and the risk they pose to other babies and personnel.

Precautions

Because of the potentially serious consequences of enterovirus infection in newborn infants, precautions for the control of nosocomial enterovirus infection in the nursery are especially important. Infants with suspected or proved infection should be isolated in a private room or cohorted together (see Chap. 11). The cohort method of isolation may be useful in situations involving several infants and has proved to be an effective control measure in containing nursery outbreaks [36] (see Chap. 21). Enteric precautions for isolating infants, using gowns and gloves for direct contact, should be maintained. Gowns should be changed after each patient contact. The decision to close a nursery to new admissions is always difficult but may be necessary, especially with prolonged outbreaks, or if adequate cohort programs cannot be maintained. Rigorous and strict hand-washing before and after each patient contact clearly is required, and its importance cannot be overemphasized.

Unless a particularly virulent enterovirus has been identified in the community (e.g., poliovirus or certain strains of enterovirus-71), such rigorous isolation precautions generally are not necessary for adults or for children beyond the neonatal period. Careful handling of feces and secretions and soiled objects and instruments should be the rule for all patients with enterovirus infection.

Prevention

Often a thorough maternal history is the best way to identify the infant at risk during the enterovirus season, and a mild febrile illness in the mother during the summer may warn of infection in the infant. Any infant born to a mother who is known to have had a recent febrile illness should be placed in an observation nursery rather than the main nursery area (see Chap. 21).

In addition, nursery personnel should be aware of their potential for infecting the newborn. Though it may not be possible or necessary to identify employees with these nonspecific illnesses, the importance of reporting febrile, respiratory, or diarrheal illnesses to the employee health service and the necessity for careful hand-washing as part of an inservice program for nursery personnel must be emphasized (see Chap. 3).

The attenuation of enterovirus disease by passive immunization has been suggested. Antibody does not protect against infection but appears to reduce the severity of disease and duration of virus shedding. The administration of IG in the setting of a sudden and particularly virulent nursery outbreak has been suggested by Cherry [30].

Polioviruses

Poliovirus infection has become rare since the institution of widespread immunization programs, and nosocomial transmission of poliovirus is no longer a problem. Virus shedding may follow vaccination with live oral polio vaccine (OPV) for a brief period of time. In general, paralytic poliovirus infection today is associated with the use of live OPV, but this is rare [7, 20, 131]. Cases occur in recipients of live vaccine (recipient cases) or in their contacts (contact cases). The incidence of vaccine-induced paralysis in recipients is estimated to be 0.44 per million vaccinated and, in contacts, 1.5 per million vaccinated [119]. Several community outbreaks of paralytic polio among groups of nonimmunized persons were described recently [18], and seroligic surveys have demonstrated that an unacceptably high proportion of the population remains at risk [120].

Isolation Precautions
Children identified as having unspecified enterovirus infections should be isolated using precautions that minimize contact with secretions and excretions pending identification of the specific agent. Asymptomatic children subsequently found to be shedding poliovirus present a potential risk to certain high-risk patients, especially children with congenital immunodeficiency diseases (e.g., agammaglobulinemia, hypogammaglobulinemia, combined immunodeficiency states). It is recommended that, as a precaution, unimmunized children or children with congenital or acquired immunodeficiency states not be placed in the same room as children who are known to be shedding poliovirus. However, routine screening of hospitalized children for poliovirus is not recommended.

Immunization
Because of the persistence of wild and vaccine strains of poliovirus, adequate immunity against polioviruses is essential for both pediatric patients and hospital personnel. Routine vaccination of adults currently is not recommended [20].

Special Considerations
Enteroviruses are unusually stable and resist many commonly used disinfectants (e.g., 70% alcohol, 5% Lysol, and 1% quaternary ammonium compounds). The most effective virucidal agent is 5% sodium hypochlorite solution, which may be used for surface decontamination but is corrosive to metal, including stainless steel (see Chap. 15).

Rhabdovirus: Rabies

Although nosocomial rabies is uncommon, 2 cases have been documented in human-to-human transmission of rabies from corneal transplantation [14, 82]. Both donors had obscure neurologic illnesses, one resembling Guillain-Barré syndrome and the other flaccid paralysis. Because of this atypical presentation, the diagnosis of rabies was not suspected before the death of either donor, and their tissues were considered acceptable for transplantation.

Hospital personnel also are theoretically at risk when exposed to patients with rabies in whom the diagnosis may not be suspected before death [13]. In an investigation of hospital personnel exposed to one such patient, many employees were unable to recall the extent of exposure 15 to 43 days earlier. Because of this and because of the long duration of hospitalization of the index case, 198 of 371 hospital employees were believed to have had significant rabies exposure and were advised to receive postexposure rabies prophylaxis [13].

Laboratory personnel working with bat colonies and other potentially rabid animals also are at increased risk of this disease. Laboratory-associated rabies, presumably transmitted by aerosolization of laboratory virus strains, has been reported, resulting in revised safety recommendations for laboratory personnel working with rabies virus [23].

Isolation Precautions
Strict isolation precautions are recommended for the duration of illness in patients with proved or suspected rabies (see Chap. 11).

Immunization
Human diploid cell rabies vaccine (HDCV) is recommended in the following situations [19, 23]:

1. Individuals with documented rabies exposure
2. Individuals with probable or possible exposure
3. Laboratory workers working with bats or

other potentially rabid animals, for pre-exposure prophylaxis

Postexposure prophylaxis of hospital personnel should be handled according to established recommendations [23]. In addition, local wounds should be cleansed with soap and water [4]. Preexposure prophylaxis of laboratory workers at high risk also should be undertaken. Personnel should not work with potentially rabid animals until a complete series of vaccine has been administered.

Special Considerations

The potential for transmission of rabies and other viral pathogens in transplanted tissues presents problems in evaluating potential donors. In general, corneas from individuals who have died with a diagnosis of dementia, encephalopathy, undiagnosed neurologic illness, multiple sclerosis, conjunctivitis, or other viral diseases including hepatitis B, rabies, or Creutzfeldt-Jakob disease should not be utilized for the purposes of corneal transplantation. Corneas in such cases may be accepted for research purposes if they are labeled *biohazard.*

Arenaviruses

Lymphocytic choriomeningitis (LCM) has been implicated as a cause of outbreaks of flu-like illness with aseptic meningitis in laboratory workers and other hospital personnel [154]. It is not known to be transmitted from person to person in hospital settings other than after contact with laboratory animals. No special isolation precautions are required for patients with LCM infection.

Papillomaviruses

The human papillomaviruses (HPVs) are small, double-stranded DNA viruses. HPVs affect the skin and mucous membranes and cause warts and other benign tumors. The natural history of these tumors is variable, with some regressing spontaneously whereas others become malignant. There is good evidence to show that HPVs are sexually transmitted viruses. There is also a high prevalence of HPV-associated malignancies in the male sexual partners of women with genital cancers [6]. Other studies have shown an association between squamous cell carcinomas and genital warts [84, 127]. Clinically, these associations point to the importance of early detection and treatment of HPV-associated genital lesions.

Laser therapy or vaporization has become a popular way of treating HPV condyloma, warts, and associated growths. Patients with laryngeal, cervical, and skin lesions may benefit from carbon dioxide laser therapy. The carbon dioxide laser generates a vapor or plume as it destroys these HPV-associated growths, and intact viral DNA has been shown to be liberated into the air with the vapor of laser-treated warts [56]. The nosocomial significance of this is not clear at this time, although there are a few anecdotal reports of health care workers using lasers who have developed warts on their hands and fingers, raising the possibility of work-related transmission.

Therefore, as a first step, infection control and employee health personnel need to become involved with laser safety programs in operation in their facilities. With the recent widespread availability of the laser, current safety practices are probably variable. The most practical solution for now is proper maintenance of equipment, including suction and exhaust apparatus. Until additional information is available, it also makes sense for laser operators to wear masks, gowns, gloves, and protective eyewear in the universal precautions mode, as they would for any procedure that generated an aerosol [56].

Methods of Preventing Spread of Viruses
Cohort Isolation Precautions

In hospital epidemiology, a *cohort* is a group of individuals kept together to minimize contact between members of the cohort and other patients or personnel to decrease opportunities for transmission of infectious agents. Cohort isolation programs have proved effective in controlling some nursery outbreaks of *Staphylococcus aureus* [95] as well as those due to enteroviruses (see Chap. 21) [36]. Cohort isolation programs also have been used outside of nurseries during hospital outbreaks of influenza.

Cohort isolation generally consists of two groups of people, an *infected* group and an *uninfected* group, that are separated from one another. Occasionally a third group, an *exposed* group, is separated from the uninfected group and cared for separately from both of the other groups. This method of separation may involve the use of geographically distinct rooms or, if not available, physical separation in the same room. To ensure complete separation of cohorts, geographically separate rooms are preferable and should be used whenever possible. The separation of hospital staff often is overlooked, but this also is essential to a successful cohort program. Although it is not always possible to separate house staff and support personnel, the nursing staff caring for infected and noninfected cohorts should be separated as much as possible without disrupting services to patients. If possible, those caring for infected patients should be immune to the disease in question or receiving prophylactic treatment or vaccine. This immunity may be determined by previous infection or vaccination and may be identified by appropriate history of illness, vaccination, or antibody testing. In cohort programs for viral illness, especially respiratory viruses, the same groups of personnel ideally should care for the same cohort for the duration of isolation. This plan minimizes the risk of transmission of infection to the uninfected cohort. Personnel who have recently recovered from the viral illness under consideration also may care for the infected cohort. In other cohort programs (e.g., staphylococcal outbreaks in nurseries), personnel may work with different cohorts on different days but not during the same day. In many instances, groups of personnel such as house staff and support personnel cannot be restricted as easily. In these situations, person-

nel should see patients in the "clean" area first, then go to the "dirty" area.

It is also important to remember that separation of groups on the basis of symptoms alone will not guarantee that all members of the cohort have the same illness. It is desirable, therefore, to take appropriate steps to confirm the suspected diagnosis as quickly as possible to ensure proper cohorting of patients. More detailed guidelines for the use of cohort programs are presented in Table 38-3.

The cohort method of isolation may involve small numbers of patients or hospital

Table 38-3. General guidelines for use of cohort isolation

1. Patients should be separated into cohorts of infected ("dirty") and noninfected ("clean") patients.
2. Only persons with proved or suspected infection should be admitted to the infected cohort.
3. All exposed (potentially infected) individuals should be included with the cohort of infected patients; in some instances, the potentially infected cohort may be separated into a third cohort.
4. The infected cohort should be closed to new, uninfected admissions, and all new, uninfected admissions should be placed with the uninfected cohort.
5. Personnel working with the infected cohort should be immune to the illness in question by either previous history of illness or vaccination *whenever possible.*
6. Personnel should be assigned so that separate groups work with the infected and uninfected cohorts *whenever possible;* crossover between cohorts should be discouraged to minimize the risk of cross-infection of the uninfected cohort.
7. Ideally, personnel should be separated for the duration of the cohort program, especially when viral illnesses are proved or suspected.
8. When personnel must work in both areas, they should work in the "clean" area first, then work in the "dirty" area.
9. The infected cohort area should be closed as patients are discharged from the hospital and may be used for new uninfected admissions after thorough cleaning of the area and its equipment.

Source: Reproduced from W.M. Valenti et al., Nosocomial virus infections IV: Guidelines for cohort isolation and the communicable disease survey. *Infect. Control* 2: 236, 1980, with permission.

staff, such as in clusters of infections in intensive care units. Other uses of the cohort method may involve restriction of larger groups of patients and personnel; for example, outbreaks of viral respiratory infections, such as RSV, are approached in this way [74]. In general, however, cohort programs using geographically separate areas of the same room are not recommended for the control of viral respiratory infections.

Communicable Disease Survey

The purpose of the communicable disease survey (contagion check) is to screen pediatric patients and visitors quickly to determine whether they are currently infected or have been exposed to and are incubating any communicable diseases. The main concern of the survey is to prevent the introduction of varicella into the hospital, but other illnesses such as measles, mumps, and viral respiratory illnesses also should be considered. A contagion check should be done for every pediatric patient and child visitor and is especially important during periods of peak virus activity in the community.

Before the admission of a pediatric patient to the hospital, information regarding the child's immunization history, susceptibility to chickenpox, and history of recent exposure to chickenpox should be obtained. Questions that may yield additional helpful information, shown in Table 38-4, may be included in the communicable disease survey, especially for child visitors. This survey is relatively uncomplicated and assists in screening patients who present potential hazards to susceptible patients and personnel. Susceptible pediatric patients who have been exposed to proved or suspected viral illnesses are placed on precautions as previously noted.

Infection Control and the Pregnant Health Care Worker

Employee health personnel and infection control personnel are often consulted by the pregnant employee regarding contact with patients who have various infectious diseases (see Chap. 3). In these situations, the concern

Table 38-4. Items to include in a communicable disease survey

Essential components
  Immunization history
    Measles, mumps, rubella
    Polio
    Diphtheria, pertussis, tetanus
  Has the child had or recently been exposed to chickenpox?
Other considerations, especially for child visitors
  Has the child had or recently been exposed to the following?
    Measles
    Mumps
    German measles
    Hepatitis
  Does the child have any of the following now or has the child had any of the following recently?
  Streptococcal infection
  Cough, cold, or upper respiratory infection of any kind
  Diarrhea
  Vomiting
  Fever
  Rash
  Infection of any kind

Source: Reproduced from W.M. Valenti et al., Nosocomial virus infections IV: Guidelines for cohort isolation and the communicable disease survey. *Infect. Control* 2: 236, 1980, with permission.

is not only for the pregnant employee but also for the fetus, who may be at risk of developing infection in the perinatal period. To counsel patients effectively in these matters, employee health personnel should be familiar with the mode of transmission of the various infectious agents as well as their risk to the pregnant employee. The educational gain from these visits may be all that is required to resolve the employee's concerns.

The infectious processes that generate the most concern among pregnant employees include viral agents such as CMV, HSV, hepatitis B, rubella, and VZV.

Work Restrictions for the Pregnant Employee

It may sometimes be advisable to restrict particular types of contact between infected patients and pregnant personnel. However, the transfer of pregnant employees to other areas of the hospital or other positions is probably not necessary in most situations. A practical approach should be developed to deal with the issue of the pregnant health care worker in much the same way that the ICP deals with work restriction in other infection control problems, taking into consideration the rights of the employee as well as the protection of the patient.

It should be kept in mind that pregnancy by itself does not usually make an employee more susceptible to acquiring infectious diseases from patients. Transferring employees during pregnancy may not be realistic since the same infectious hazards may be present throughout the health care facility. In addition, routine movement of personnel may create an unnecessary burden on the departments involved. Recommendations for work restriction for pregnant employees are noted in Table 38-5 and discussed in detail by Votra and colleagues [155].

Special Considerations

It is important to emphasize that some viral agents are more easily transmitted than others. Personnel may respond with extraordinary concern when caring for patients with CMV infection, whereas influenza vaccination programs and precautions for other more highly contagious viruses are often overlooked. Table 38-6 reviews briefly the relative risk of transmission to hospital personnel and patients of commonly seen viruses.

The relationship of virology to infection control has only recently been appreciated; viral infections have traditionally been an enigma to infection control personnel. The health care facility presents a unique challenge to virologists and infection control personnel as they attempt to develop comprehensive programs for the control and prevention of nosocomial viral infections. Certainly, the next few years should help clarify this relationship as additional developments in anti-

Table 38-5. Recommendations for work restriction for pregnant employees

| | Restriction | | |
Disease	No contact	Follow isolation precautions	Comment
Cytomegalovirus			
Congenital		X	Risk of transmission very low in health care settings
Acquired		X	
Herpes simplex			
Genital		X	
Other		X	
Varicella-zoster virus	X*	If immune	If history of chickenpox is negative or unknown, employee should not have contact with patients with chickenpox or herpes zoster
Parvovirus	X		
Rubella	X*	If immune	Ideally, employee should be immune to rubella according to testing at employment or via vaccination
Hepatitis B			
Dialysis units		X	Employees of hemodialysis units should be vaccinated against hepatitis B
Other areas		X	

*Until immunity is proved by serologic testing.

Table 38-6. Interaction of factors in nosocomial transmission of viruses

Virus	*Transmissibility*	*Susceptibility of staff or other patients*	*Resultant nosocomial risk*
Respiratory viruses			
Influenza	High	Variable[a]	High
Respiratory syncytial	High	High	High
Rhinovirus	Moderate	Moderate[a]	Moderate
Other (e.g., adenovirus, coronavirus)	Moderate	Moderate[a]	Moderate
Hepatitis B			
Needle sticks	High	High	High
Other exposure	Low	High	Low
Herpesviruses			
Herpes simplex I	Low	Moderate[a]	Low
Herpes simplex II	Very low	Moderate[a]	Very low[b]
Varicella (chickenpox) or disseminated zoster	High	Very low[a]	Low[a]
Herpes zoster (localized)	Moderate	Very low[a]	Very low
Epstein-Barr virus	Very low	Very low[a]	Very low
Cytomegalovirus	Low	Moderate[a]	Very low[c]
Parvovirus	Moderate	Moderate	Moderate
Rubella	High	Moderate[a]	High

[a] High in pediatric age groups.
[b] Except to newborn during delivery or after rupture of membranes.
[c] Except for blood transfusion or organ transplantation.
Source: Reproduced from W.M. Valenti et al., Nosocomial virus infections IV: Guidelines for cohort isolation and the communicable disease survey. *Infect. Control* 2:236, 1980, with permission.

viral chemotherapy and rapid viral diagnostic techniques occur.

References

1. Alter, M.J., et al. National surveillance of dialysis-associated hepatitis and other diseases 1976 and 1980. *Dialysis Transp.* 12:860, 1983.
2. Amendment of part 1910 of Title 29 of the Code of Federal Regulations. *Fed. Reg.* Dec. 6, 1991. P. 64175.
3. Anderson, L., and Hurwitz, E. Human parvovirus B19 infection and pregnancy. *Clin. Perinatol.* 15:273, 1988.
4. Anderson, L.J., and Winkler, W.G. Aqueous quaternary ammonium compounds and rabies treatment. *J. Infect. Dis.* 139:494, 1979.
5. Balcarek, K.B., et al. Cytomegalovirus infection among employees of a children's hospital: No evidence for increased risk associated with patient care. *J.A.M.A.* 263:840, 1990.
6. Barrasso, R., et al. High prevalence of papillomavirus-associated penile intraepithelial neoplasia in sexual partners of women with cervical intraepithelial neoplasia. *N. Engl. J. Med.* 317:916, 1987.
7. Basilico, F.C., and Bernat, J. Vaccine-associated poliomyelitis in a contact. *J.A.M.A.* 239:2275, 1978.
8. Benoulli, C., et al. Danger of accidental person-to-person transmission of Creutzfeldt-Jakob disease by surgery. *Lancet* 1:478, 1977.
9. Berlin, B.S., and Campbell, T. Hospital-acquired herpes zoster following exposure to chickenpox. *J.A.M.A.* 211:1831, 1970.
10. Blank, H., and Haines, H.G. Experimental reinfection with herpes simplex virus. *J. Invest. Dermatol.* 61:223, 1973.
11. Bolivar, R., et al. Rotavirus in travelers' diarrhea: Study of an adult student population in Mexico. *J. Infect. Dis.* 137:324, 1978.
12. Centers for Disease Control. Hepatitis B vaccine: Evidence confirming lack of AIDS transmission. *M.M.W.R.* 33:685, 1984.
13. Centers for Disease Control. Human rabies—Pennsylvania. *M.M.W.R.* 28:75, 1979.
14. Centers for Disease Control. Human-to-human transmission of rabies via a corneal transplant. *M.M.W.R.* 29:25, 1980.
15. Centers for Disease Control. Epidemic keratoconjunctivitis in an ophthalmology clinic—California. *M.M.W.R.* 39:598, 1990.
16. Centers for Disease Control. Outbreak of viral hepatitis in the staff of a pediatrics ward—California. *M.M.W.R.* 26:77, 1977.

17. Centers for Disease Control. Parainfluenza outbreaks in extended-care facilities. *M.M.W.R.* 27:475, 1978.

18. Centers for Disease Control. Poliomyelitis—Pennsylvania, Maryland. *M.M.W.R.* 28:49, 1978.

19. Centers for Disease Control. Rabies prevention. *M.M.W.R.* 29:265, 1980.

20. Centers for Disease Control. Recommendation of the Immunization Practices Advisory Committee (ACIP). Adult immunization. *M.M.W.R.* 33 (Suppl. 1S):1, 1984.

21. Centers for Disease Control. Recommendation of the Immunization Practices Advisory Committee (ACIP). Protection against viral hepatitis. *M.M.W.R.* 39:1 (52), 1990.

22. Centers for Disease Control. Recommendation of the Immunization Practices Advisory Committee (ACIP). Prevention and control of influenza. *M.M.W.R.* 39:1 (RR-7), 1990.

23. Centers for Disease Control. Recommendation of the Immunization Practices Advisory Committee (ACIP). Rabies prevention—United States. *M.M.W.R.* 40:1 (RR-3), 1991.

24. Centers for Disease Control. Recommendation of the Immunization Practices Advisory Committee (ACIP). Varicella-zoster immune globulin for the prevention of chickenpox. *M.M.W.R.* 33:84, 1984.

25. Centers for Disease Control. Risks associated with human parvovirus B19 infection. *M.M.W.R.* 38:81, 1989.

26. Centers for Disease Control. Recommendations of rubella prevention. *M.M.W.R.* 39:1 (RR-15), 1990.

27. Centers for Disease Control. Rubella in hospitals in California. *M.M.W.R.* 32:37, 1983.

28. Centers for Disease Control. Suboptimal response to hepatitis B vaccine given by injection into the buttock. *M.M.W.R.* 34:105, 1985.

29. Chanock, R.M., et al. Respiratory syncytial virus: I. Virus recovery and other observations during the 1960 outbreak of bronchiolitis, pneumonia, and respiratory diseases in children. *J.A.M.A.* 176:647, 1961.

30. Cherry, J.D. Non-Polio Enteroviruses. In: R.D. Feigin and J.D. Cherry (Eds.), *Pediatric Infectious Diseases*. Philadelphia: Saunders, 1981. Pp. 1316–1365.

31. Cherry, J.D., et al. Atypical measles in children previously immunized with attenuated measles virus vaccine. *Pediatrics* 50:712, 1973.

32. Cherry, J.D., Soriano, F., and Jahn, C.L. Search for perinatal virus infection: A prospective, clinical, virologic, and serologic study. *Am. J. Dis. Child.* 116:245, 1968.

33. Committee on Infectious Diseases 1989–1990. Parvoviruses, erythema infectiosum and pregnancy. *Pediatrics* 85:131, 1990.

34. Corey, L., et al. HBsAg-negative hepatitis in a hemodialysis unit: Relation to Epstein-Barr virus. *N. Engl. J. Med.* 293:1273, 1975.

35. Cossart, Y.E., Field, A.M., Cant, B., and Widdows, D. Parvo-like particles in human sera. *Lancet* 1:72, 1975.

36. Cramblatt, H.B., et al. Nosocomial infection with echovirus type 11 in handicapped and premature infants. *Pediatrics* 51:602, 1973.

37. Crystei, I.L., et al. Rotavirus infections in a maternity unit. *Lancet* 2:79, 1975.

38. Davidson, G.P. Importance of a new virus in acute sporadic enteritis in children. *Lancet* 1:242, 1975.

39. DeFabritis, A.M., et al. Parainfluenza type 3 in a transplant unit. *J.A.M.A.* 241:384, 1979.

40. Denes, A.E., et al. Hepatitis B infection in physicians: Results of a nationwide seroepidemiologic survey. *J.A.M.A.* 239:210, 1978.

41. Dienstag, J.L., et al. Fecal shedding of hepatitis A antigen. *Lancet* 1:765, 1975.

42. Dienstag, J.L., and Ryan, D.M. Occupational exposure to hepatitis B virus in hospital personnel: Infection or ummunization? *Am. J. Epidemiol.* 115:26, 1982.

43. Douglas, R.G., Jr. Influenza in Man. In: E.D. Kilbourne (Ed.), *The Influenza Viruses and Influenza*. New York: Academic, 1975.

44. Drew, W.L., et al. Prevalence of cytomegalovirus infection in homosexual men. *J. Infect. Dis.* 143:188, 1981.

45. Duffy, P., et al. Possible person-to-person transmission of Creutzfeldt-Jakob disease (letter). *N. Engl. J. Med.* 290:692, 1974.

46. Dworskey, M.E., Welch, K., Cassady, G., and Stagno, S. Occupational risk for primary cytomegalovirus infection among pediatric health care workers. *N. Engl. J. Med.* 309:950, 1983.

47. Edmonson, M.B., et al. Mild measle and secondary vaccine failure during a sustained outbreak in a highly vaccinated population. *J.A.M.A.* 263:2467, 1990.

48. Eichenwald, H.F., McCracken, G.H., and Kindberg, S.J. Virus infections of the newborn. *Prog. Med. Virol.* 9:35, 1967.

49. Esteban, J.I., Gonzalez, A., Hernandez, J.M., and Viladomiu, L. Evaluation of antibodies to hepatitis C virus in a study of transfusion-associated hepatitis. *N. Engl. J. Med.* 323:1107, 1990.

50. Feldman, H.A. Mumps. In: A.S. Evans (Ed.), *Viral Infections of Humans: Epidemiology and Control*. New York: Plenum, 1976. Pp. 317–332.

51. Foley, F.D., Greenwald, K.A., Nash, M.C., and Pruitt, B.A. Herpes virus infection in burned patients. *N. Engl. J. Med.* 282:652, 1970.

52. Foy, H.M., and Grayston, J.T. Adenoviruses.

In: A.S. Evans (Ed.), *Viral Infections of Humans: Epidemiology and Control.* New York: Plenum, 1976. Pp. 53–69.

53. Fradkin, J.E., et al. Creutzfeldt-Jakob disease in pituitary growth hormone recipients in the United States. *J.A.M.A.* 265:880, 1991.

54. Fulginiti, V.A., and Arthur, J.M. Altered reactivity to measles virus: Skin test reactivity and antibody response to measles virus antigens in recipients of killed measles virus vaccine. *J. Pediatr.* 75:604, 1979.

55. Gradjusek, D.C., et al. Precautions in medical care of and in handling materials from patients with transmissible virus dementia (Creutzfeldt-Jakob disease). *N. Engl. J. Med.* 297:1253, 1977.

56. Garden, J.M., et al. Papillomavirus in the vapor carbon dioxide laser-treated verrucae. *J.A.M.A.* 259:1199, 1988.

57. Garibaldi, R.A., et al. Hospital-acquired serum hepatitis: Report of an outbreak. *J.A.M.A.* 219:1577, 1972.

58. Garibaldi, R.A., et al. Hemodialysis-associated hepatitis. *J.A.M.A.* 225:384, 1973.

59. Garner, J.S., and Simmons, B.P. Guidelines for isolation precautions in hospitals. *Infect. Control* 4 (Suppl.):24S, 1983.

60. Gerber, M.A., et al. The lack of transmission of type B hepatitis in a special care nursery. *J. Pediatr.* 91:120, 1977.

61. Gershon, A.A., Kalter, Z.G., and Steinberg, S. Detection of antibody to varicella-zoster virus by immune adherence hemagglutination. *Proc. Soc. Exp. Biol. Med.* 151:762, 1976.

62. Gillespie, S., et al. Occupational risk of human parvovirus B19 infection for school and day-care personnel during an outbreak of erythema infectiousum. *J.A.M.A.* 263:2061, 1990.

63. Gordon, J.E. Chickenpox: An epidemiological review. *Am. J. Med. Sci.* 244:362, 1962.

64. Graman, P.S., and Hall, C.B. Epidemiology and control of nosocomial infections. *Infect. Dis. Clin. North Am.* 3:815, 1989.

65. McCarthy, C.A., and Hall, C. Prevention of nosocomial respiratory syncytial virus in the pediatric patient. *Infect. Med.* 7:4, 1990.

66. Greaves, W.L., et al. The problem of herpes whitlow among hospital personnel. *Infect. Control* 1:381, 1980.

67. Greenlee, J.E. Containment precautions in hospitals for cases of Creutzfeldt-Jakob disease. *Infect. Control* 3:222, 1982.

68. Gustafson, J.L. An outbreak of nosocomial airborne varicella. *Pediatrics* 70:550, 1982.

69. Gwaltney, J.M., Mosalski, P.B., and Hendley, J.O. Hand-to-hand transmission of rhinovirus. *Ann. Intern. Med.* 88:453, 1978.

70. Hall, C.B. The shedding and spreading of respiratory syncytial virus. *Pediatr. Res.* 11:236, 1977.

71. Hall, C.B. Nosocomial viral respiratory infections: Perennial weeds on pediatric wards. *Am. J. Med.* 70:670, 1981.

72. Hall, C.B., and Douglas, R.G., Jr. Nosocomial influenza as a cause of intercurrent fever in infants. *Pediatrics* 55:673, 1975.

73. Hall, C.B., Douglas, R.G., Jr., and Geiman, J.M. Possible transmission by fomites of respiratory syncytial virus. *J. Infect. Dis.* 141:98, 1980.

74. Hall, C.B., Geiman, J.M., Douglas, R.G., Jr., and Meagher, M.P. Control of nosocomial respiratory syncytial virus infections. *Pediatrics* 62:728, 1978.

75. Hanshaw, J.B., Dadgeon, J.A., and Marshall, W.C. (Eds.). Congenital Cytomegalovirus. In: *Major Problems in Clinical Pediatrics.* Philadelphia: Saunders, 1985. P. 92.

76. Hayden, C.F., Meyers, J.D., and Dixon, R.E. Nosocomial varicella: Part II. Suggested guidelines for management. *West. J. Med.* 130:300, 1979.

77. Henderson, F.W., et al. Respiratory syncytial virus infections, reinfections, and immunity: A prospective longitudinal study in young children. *N. Engl. J. Med.* 300:530, 1979.

78. Hendley, J.O., Mika, L.A., and Swaltney, J.M. Evaluation of virucidal compounds for inactivation of rhinovirus on hands. *Antimicrob. Agents Chemother.* 14:690, 1978.

79. Hendley, J.P., Wenzel, R.P., and Gwaltney, J.M. Transmission of rhinovirus colds by self-inoculation. *N. Engl. J. Med.* 288:1362, 1973.

80. Hethcote, H.W. Measles and rubella in the United States. *Am. J. Epidemiol.* 117:2, 1983.

81. Ho, M., et al. The transplanted kidney as a source of CMV infection. *N. Engl. J. Med.* 293:1109, 1975.

82. Houff, S.A., et al. Human-to-human transmission of rabies virus by corneal transplant. *N. Engl. J. Med.* 300:603, 1979.

83. Hurwitz, E.G., et al. Guillain-Barré syndrome and the 1978–79 influenza vaccine. *N. Engl. J. Med.* 304:1557, 1981.

84. International Agency for Research on Cancer. Human papillomavirus and cervical cancer. *Lancet* 1:756, 1988.

85. Jawetz, E., et al. Laboratory infection with adenovirus type 8: Laboratory and epidemiologic observations. *Am. J. Hyg.* 69:13, 1979.

86. Jones, M.J., et al. Intrauterine echovirus type 11 infections. *Mayo Clin. Proc.* 55:509, 1980.

87. Kapikian, A.Z., et al. Human reovirus-like agent as the major pathogen associated with "winter" gastroenteritis in hospitalized infants and young children. *N. Engl. J. Med.* 294:965, 1976.

88. Kibrick, S. Herpes simplex infection at term: What to do with mother, newborn, and nursery personnel. *J.A.M.A.* 243:157, 1980.

89. Kim, H.W., et al. Human reovirus-like agent infection occurrence in adult contacts of pediatric patients with gastroenteritis. *J.A.M.A.* 238:404, 1977.

90. Kuenz, J.C., and Valenti, W.M. An attitudinal study of an influenza vaccination program (abstr. 26). Presented at the Eighth Educational Conference of the Association for Practitioners in Infection Control, Atlanta, GA, May 28, 1981.

91. Lake, A.M., Lauer, B.A., and Clark, J.C. Enterovirus infections in neonates. *J. Pediatr.* 89:787, 1976.

92. Lang, D.J., et al. Reduction of post-transfusion cytomegalovirus infections following use of leukocyte-depleted blood. *Transfusion* 17:391, 1977.

93. Le Baron, C.W., et al. Annual rotavirus epidemic patterns in North America. *J.A.M.A.* 264:983, 1990.

94. LeClair, J.M., et al. Airborne transmission of chickenpox in a hospital. *N. Engl. J. Med.* 302:450, 1980.

95. Light, I.J., Brackvogel, M.S., Walton, R.L., and Sutherland, J.M. An epidemic of bullous impetigo arising from a central admission-observation nursery. *Pediatrics* 49:15, 1972.

96. Linneman, C.C., Jr., et al. Transmission of herpes simplex virus type I in a nursery for the newborn: Identification of viral isolates by DNA fingerprinting. *Lancet* 1:964, 1978.

97. Manzella, J., et al. An outbreak of herpes simplex virus stomatitis in a dental practice. *J.A.M.A.* 252:2019, 1984.

98. Marx, R.E., and Carlson, E.R. Creutzfeldt-Jakob disease from allogeneic dura: A review of risks and safety. *J. Oral Maxillofac. Surg.* 49:272, 1991.

99. Mathur, U., Bentley, D.W., and Hall, C.B. Concurrent respiratory syncytial virus and influenza A infections in the institutionalized elderly and chronically ill. *Ann. Intern. Med.* 93:49, 1980.

100. Matthew, E.B., et al. A major epidemic of infectious hepatitis in an institution for the mentally retarded. *Am. J. Epidemiol.* 98:199, 1973.

101. McDonald, L.L., St. Geme, J.W., and Arnold, B.H. Nosocomial infection with ECHO virus type 31 in neonatal intensive care unit. *Pediatrics* 47:995, 1971.

102. McLaughlin, M.C., and Gold, L.H. The New York rubella incident: A case for changing hospital policy regarding rubella testing and immunization. *Am. J. Public Health* 69:287, 1979.

103. Melnick, J.L. Enteroviruses. In: A.S. Evans (Ed.), *Viral Infections in Humans: Epidemiology and Control.* New York: Plenum, 1976. Pp. 163–201.

104. Meurman, O.H., and Laine, M.J. Rotavirus epidemic in adults. *N. Engl. J. Med.* 296:1289, 1977.

105. Meyerowitz, R.L., et al. Fatal disseminated adenovirus infection in a renal transplant recipient. *Am. J. Med.* 59:591, 1975.

106. Meyers, J.D., et al. Parenterally transmitted non-A, non-B hepatitis: An epidemic reassessed. *Ann. Intern. Med.* 87:57, 1977.

107. Meyers, J.D., et al. Lack of transmission of hepatitis B after surgical exposure. *J.A.M.A.* 240:1725, 1978.

108. Meyers, J.D., MacQuarrie, M.B., Merigan, T.C., and Jennison, M.H. Nosocomial varicella. Part 1: Outbreak in oncology patients at a children's hospital. *West. J. Med.* 130:196, 1979.

109. Meyers, J.D., Romm, F.J., Then, W.S., and Bryan, J.A. Food-borne hepatitis A in a general hospital. *J.A.M.A.* 231:1049, 1975.

110. Middleton, P.J., Azymanski, M.T., and Petric, P.J. Viruses associated with acute gastroenteritis in young children. *Am. J. Dis. Child.* 131:233, 1977.

111. Mintz, L., et al. Nosocomial respiratory syncytial virus infections in an intensive care nursery: Rapid diagnosis by immunofluorescence. *Pediatrics* 64:149, 1979.

112. Morens, D.M., et al. An outbreak of varicella-zoster virus infection among cancer patients. *Ann. Intern. Med.* 93:414, 1980.

113. Mosley, J.W., et al. Multiple hepatitis viruses in multiple attacks of acute viral hepatitis. *N. Engl. J. Med.* 296:75, 1977.

114. Mufson, M.A., Mocega, H.E., and Krause, H.E. Acquisition of parainfluenza 3 virus infection by hospitalized children: I. Frequencies, rates, and temporal data. *J. Infect. Dis.* 128:141, 1973.

115. Muldoon, R.L., Stanley, E.D., and Jackson, G.G. Use and withdrawal of amantadine chemoprophylaxis during epidemic influenza A. *Am. Rev. Respir. Dis.* 133:487, 1976.

116. Nadar, P.R., Horowitz, M.S., and Rousseau, J. Atypical exanthem following exposure to natural measles: Eleven cases in children previously inoculated with killed vaccine. *J. Pediatr.* 72:22, 1968.

117. Nahmias, A.N., et al. Perinatal risk associated with maternal genital herpes simplex virus infection. *Am. J. Obstet. Gynecol.* 110:825, 1971.

118. Naragi, S., Jackson, G.G., and Jonasson, O.M. Viremia with herpes simplex type 1 in adults. *Ann. Intern. Med.* 85:165, 1976.

119. Nathanson, N., and Martin, J.R. The epidemiology of poliomyelitis: Enigmas surrounding its appearance, epidemicity and disappearance. *Am. J. Epidemiol.* 110:672, 1976.

120. Nightingale, E.O. Recommendations for a national policy on poliomyelitis vaccination. *N. Engl. J. Med.* 297:249, 1977.

121. O'Donoghue, J.M., et al. Prevention of nosocomial influenza with Amantadine. *Am. J. Epidemiol.* 97:276, 1973.

122. Orenstein, W.A., Heseltine, P.N.R., LeGagnoux, S.J., and Portnoy, B. Rubella vaccine and susceptible hospital employees. *J.A.M.A.* 245:711, 1981.

123. Parkman, P.D., Galasso, G.H., Top, F.H., and Noble, G.R. Summary of clinical trials of influenza vaccines. *J. Infect. Dis.* 134:100, 1976.

124. Phillips, C.A., et al. Enteroviruses in Vermont, 1969–1978: An important cause of illness throughout the year. *J. Infect. Dis.* 141:162, 1980.

125. Poland, G.A., and Nichol, K. Medical students as sources of rubella and measles outbreaks. *Arch. Intern. Med.* 150:44, 1990.

126. Polk, B.F., White, J.A., DeGirolami, P.C., and Modlin, J.F. Outbreak of rubella among hospital personnel. *N. Engl. J. Med.* 303:541, 1980.

127. Rando, R. Human papillomaviruses: Implications for clinical medicine. *Ann. Intern. Med.* 108:628, 1988.

128. Richmond, S.J., et al. An outbreak of gastroenteritis in young children caused by adenoviruses. *Lancet* 1:1178, 1979.

129. Rimland, D., et al. Hepatitis B traced to an oral surgeon. *N. Engl. J. Med.* 296:953, 1977.

130. Ross, A.H. Modification of chickenpox in family contacts by administration of gamma globulin. *N. Engl. J. Med.* 267:369, 1962.

131. Schonberger, L.B., McGowan, J.E., and Gregg, M.B. Vaccine-associated poliomyelitis in the United States, 1961–1972. *Am. J. Epidemiol.* 104:202, 1976.

132. Schreiner, R.L., Kleinman, M.B., and Gresham, E.L. Maternal oral herpes: Isolation policy. *Pediatrics* 63:247, 1979.

133. Shewmon, D.A., Cherry, J.D., and Kirby, S.E. Shedding of rubella virus in a 4½-year-old boy with congenital rubella. *Pediatr. Infect. Dis.* 1:342, 1982.

134. Sienko, D.G., et al. A measles outbreak at university medical settings involving health care providers. *Am. J. Public Health* 77:1222, 1987.

135. Smith, J.L., et al. Comparative risk of hepatitis B among physicians and dentists. *J. Infect. Dis.* 6:705, 1976.

136. Sparling, D. Transmission of mumps (letter). *N. Engl. J. Med.* 280:276, 1979.

137. Sprague, J.B., et al. Epidemic keratoconjunctivitis. *N. Engl. J. Med.* 289:1341, 1977.

138. Steinhoff, M.C., and Gerber, M.A. Rotavirus infection of neonates. *Lancet* 1:775, 1978.

139. Straube, R.C., et al. Adenovirus type 7b in a children's hospital. *J. Infect. Dis.* 147:814, 1983.

140. Szmuness, W., et al. Hepatitis B infection: A point prevalence study in 15 U.S. hemodialysis centers. *J.A.M.A.* 227:901, 1974.

141. Szmuness, W., et al. Hepatitis B vaccine: Demonstration of efficacy in a controlled clinical trial in a high risk population in the United States. *N. Engl. J. Med.* 303:833, 1980.

142. Szmuness, W., et al. Hepatitis B vaccine in medical staff of hemodialysis units: Efficacy and subtype cross protection. *N. Engl. J. Med.* 307:4181, 1982.

143. Szmuness, W., Purcell, R.H., Dienstag, J.L., and Stevens, C.E. Antibody to hepatitis A antigen in institutionalized mentally retarded patients. *J.A.M.A.* 237:1702, 1977.

144. Tada, H., et al. Combined passive and active immunization for preventing perinatal transmission of hepatitis B virus carrier state. *Pediatrics* 70:613, 1982.

145. Tallett, S., et al. Clinical, laboratory and epidemiologic features of a viral gastroenteritis in infants and children. *Pediatrics* 60:217, 1977.

146. Thornhill, T.S., et al. Pattern of shedding of Norwalk particle in stools during experimentally induced gastroenteritis in volunteers as determined by immune electronmicroscopy. *J. Infect. Dis.* 132:28, 1975.

147. Tolkoff-Rubin, N.E., et al. Cytomegalovirus infection in dialysis patients and personnel. *Ann. Intern. Med.* 89:625, 1978.

148. Turner, A.R., MacDonald, R.N., and Cooper, B.A. Transmission of infectious mononucleosis by transfusion of pre-illness serum. *Ann. Intern. Med.* 77:751, 1972.

149. Turner, R., et al. Shedding and survival of herpes simplex virus from "fever blisters." *Pediatrics* 70:547, 1982.

150. Valenti, W.M., et al. Nosocomial viral infections: II. Guidelines for prevention and control of respiratory viruses, herpesviruses, and hepatitis viruses. *Infect. Control* 1:165, 1980.

151. Valenti, W.M., et al. Nosocomial viral infections: I. Epidemiology and significance. *Infect. Control* 1:33, 1980.

152. Valenti, W.M., et al. Concurrent outbreaks of rhinovirus and respiratory syncytial virus in an intensive care nursery: Epidemiology and associated risk factors. *J. Pediatr.* 100:722, 1982.

153. VanVoris, L.P., Belshe, R.B., and Shaffer, J.L. Nosocomial influenza B in the elderly. *Ann. Intern. Med.* 96:153, 1982.

154. VanZee, B.E., et al. Lymphocytic choriomeningitis in University Hospital personnel. *Am. J. Med.* 58:803, 1975.

155. Votra, E.M., Rutala, W.A., and Sarubbi, F.A. Recommendations for pregnant employee interaction with patients having communicable infectious diseases. *Am. J. Infect. Control* 11:10, 1983.

156. Weiss, K.E., et al. Evaluation of an employee health service as a setting for a rubella screening and immunization program. *Am. J. Public Health* 69:281, 1979.

157. Weller, T.H. The cytomegaloviruses: Ubiquitous agents with protean manifestations. *N. Engl. J. Med.* 285:203, 1971.

158. Wentworth, B.B., and Alexander, E.R. Seroepidemiology of infections due to members of the herpes virus group. *Am. J. Epidemiol.* 94:496, 1971.

159. Wenzel, R.P., Deal, E.C., and Hendley, J.O. Hospital-acquired viral respiratory illness on a pediatric ward. *Pediatrics* 60:367, 1977.

160. Wharton, M., et al. Mumps transmission in hospitals. *J.A.M.A.* 150:47, 1990.

161. Wigger, H.F., and Blank, W.A. Fatal hepatic and bronchial necrosis in adenovirus infection with thymic alymphoplasia. *N. Engl. J. Med.* 275:870, 1977.

162. Wilfert, C.M., Huang, E., and Stagno, S. Restriction endonuclease analysis of cytomegalovirus deoxyribonucleic acid as an epidemiologic tool. *Pediatrics* 70:717, 1982.

163. Williams, W.W. *CDC Guidelines for Infection Control in Hospital Personnel.* Springfield, VA: National Technical Information Service (NTIS), July 1983.

164. Yeager, A.S. Longitudinal serological study of cytomegalovirus in nurses and personnel without patient contact. *J. Clin. Microbiol.* 2:448, 1975.

165. Yow, M.D., et al. Use of restriction enzymes to investigate the source of primary cytomegalovirus infection in a pediatric nurse. *Pediatrics* 70:713, 1982.

166. Zaia, J.A., and Oxman, M.N. Antibody to varicella-zoster-virus–induced membrane antigen: Immunofluorescence assay using monodisperse glutaraldehyde target cells. *J. Infect. Dis.* 136:519, 1977.

Human Immunodeficiency Virus Infection

David M. Bell
James W. Curran

In this chapter, we review available data on the risk of human immunodeficiency virus (HIV) transmission in health care settings (including from patients to health care workers [HCWs], HCWs to patients, and patients to patients), current strategies to reduce this risk, and some of the unresolved issues and prospects for the future.

Transmission from Patients to HCWs

Information on occupationally acquired HIV infection in HCWs in the United States is available from surveillance data and risk assessment studies.

Surveillance Data

Surveillance data provide information on HCWs with the acquired immunodeficiency syndrome (AIDS) and, in a newly developed surveillance system, on persons who may have acquired HIV infection from occupational exposure. AIDS surveillance data are reported to the Centers for Disease Control (CDC) by all state and territorial health departments in the United States. Reports must meet the CDC surveillance case definition for AIDS and, hence, do not include asymptomatic HIV infections or other HIV-related illnesses. Case report forms include a question as to whether the case-patient has worked in a health care or clinical laboratory setting since 1978 [47].

As of September 30, 1991, the CDC's National AIDS Case Surveillance System had received reports of 192,406 cases of AIDS in adults in the United States. Of 151,942 patients for whom information is available, 7,250 (4.8 percent) reported a history of employment in a health care or clinical laboratory setting [C. Ciesielski, CDC: personal communication]. In comparison, approximately 5.7 percent of the U.S. labor force is employed in health services [16].

Of the 7,250 HCWs with AIDS, 3 seroconverted and subsequently developed AIDS after a documented occupational exposure to HIV-infected blood. Of the remaining 7,247, 94 percent fall within one or more well-recognized nonoccupational transmission categories, and 6 percent have an undetermined risk. In contrast, 3 percent of the 144,692 non-HCWs with AIDS have an undetermined risk. Possible reasons for the higher proportion of cases with undetermined risk among HCWs with AIDS may include an unrecognized or unreported occupational exposure to HIV in these workers, as well as failure of HCWs to recognize or report behavioral risks. Of the 424 HCWs in the undetermined risk group, 55 percent are still under investigation; 25 percent have died or refused to be interviewed or were lost to follow-up; and 20 percent (84 HCWs) had no identified risk after follow-up investigation [C. Ciesielski, CDC].

Compared with the 6.9 million HCWs in the United States, the 84 investigated HCWs with no identified risk were more likely to be men (71 percent versus 23 percent) and more likely to be black (30 percent versus 13 percent). Thus, in terms of gender and race, they resemble other AIDS cases more closely than other HCWs. The 84 include 11 physicians (1 of whom is a surgeon), 3 dental workers, 12 nurses, 5 paramedics, 15 aides or attendants, 2 therapists, 11 technicians, 12 hospital maintenance workers, 3 embalmers, and 10 persons in other occupations. Of 76 of these 84 HCWs who responded to a standardized questionnaire, 44 (58 percent) retrospectively recalled needle-stick, mucous membrane, or nonintact skin exposures to the blood or body fluids of patients during the 10 years before their diagnosis of AIDS. However, none of the source patients was known to be infected with HIV at the time of exposure, and none of the HCWs were evaluated at the time of exposure to document seroconversion to HIV. Thus the proportion of these workers who acquired infection due to occupational exposure cannot be determined [25].

As of September 30, 1991, through a separate surveillance system for occupationally acquired HIV infection, the CDC is aware of 28 HCWs in the United States who have been documented as having seroconverted to HIV after an occupational exposure; 3 of these HCWs have developed AIDS. Twenty-seven workers were exposed to HIV-infected blood, and 1 worker was exposed to concentrated virus. Of the 28 HCWs, 23 had percutaneous exposures, 4 mucocutaneous, and 1 both a percutaneous and a mucocutaneous exposure. Twelve of the seroconverters are laboratory workers (11 in clinical laboratories and 1 in a nonclinical facility), 11 are nurses, 3 are physicians (none of whom is a surgeon), and 2 have other health care occupations [C. Ciesielski, CDC].

The CDC is also aware of 18 other HCWs in the United States with HIV infection (without AIDS) who have been reported through the occupationally acquired HIV infection surveillance system. These 18 HCWs have not reported other risk factors for HIV infection, but seroconversion after exposure was not documented [C. Ciesielski, CDC]. At least 11 published cases of occupationally acquired HIV infection have been reported from outside the United States [111]. Transmission due to occupational exposure to a body fluid other than blood has not been documented in a clinical setting, except in 1 case due to exposure to visibly bloody pleural fluid [126]. It is essential that suspected cases of occupational HIV infection be reported to appropriate health authorities so that the frequency and circumstances of these infections can be assessed and appropriate preventive measures developed.

Risk Assessment Studies

Risk assessment data are available from HIV seroprevalence surveys and from prospective studies of exposed workers. Crude estimates of the risk to an uninfected HCW may also be derived from studies of the HIV seroprevalence in patients, the risk of infection transmission after a single blood contact, and the nature and frequency of blood contacts.

Seroprevalence Surveys Among HCWs

Available HIV seroprevalence data from selected HCW groups are summarized in Table 39-1. Among 3,420 orthopedic surgeons who participated in a voluntary, anonymous HIV serosurvey conducted by the CDC at the annual meeting of the American Academy of Orthopaedic Surgeons in 1991, 2 were HIV-seropositive (0.06 percent; upper limit of 95 percent confidence interval [CI] = 0.18 percent) and 1 was indeterminate [29]. Each of the 2 HIV-seropositive participants reported nonoccupational risk factors for HIV; among the 108 surgeons reporting such risk factors, HIV seroprevalence was 1.8 percent (upper limit of 95 percent CI = 5.7 percent). Among the 3,267 participants not reporting nonoccupational HIV risk factors, none was HIV-positive (upper limit of 95 percent CI = 0.092 percent). Of the 45 participants who did not respond to the question on risk factors, none was HIV-positive. The 1 surgeon whose serum tested indeterminate for HIV antibody did not report a nonoccupational risk.

Both of the HIV-positive participants were male and reported having performed surgery on patients with risk factors for HIV infection. One of the 2 surgeons reported performing surgery on patients with known HIV infection or AIDS. Although they had both sustained percutaneous injuries in the previous year, neither reported an injury from a sharp object contaminated with the blood of a patient known to have HIV infection or AIDS. The surgeon with an indeterminate result, a man who had retired from clinical practice, reported never having operated on a patient with known HIV infection or AIDS or on a patient with risk factors for HIV infection or AIDS.

Although participants may not have been representative of all orthopedic surgeons, preliminary analyses suggest that the likelihood of occupational HIV exposure was at least as high for serosurvey participants as for more than 10,000 orthopedic surgeons in the United States and Canada who responded to a mailed questionnaire survey conducted by the American Academy of Orthopedic Sur-

geons [29]. In comparison with this larger group, serosurvey participants were more likely to be in residency or fellowship training (18 percent versus 14 percent), to have trained or practiced in one or more areas of high AIDS incidence since 1977 (75 percent versus 69 percent), to have operated on one or more patients with known HIV infection (49 percent versus 43 percent), to have had a patient's blood contact their skin in the previous month (87 percent versus 83 percent), and to have sustained a percutaneous injury (e.g., needle stick, cut) from a sharp object contaminated with a patient's blood in the previous month (39 percent versus 34 percent). Thus, although these results may not be generalizable to all orthopedic surgeons, no evidence was found to suggest a high rate of previously undetected HIV infection among a large group of these surgeons, including those who train or practice in areas of high HIV or AIDS incidence.

A number of studies of dentists [61, 67, 74, 81, 95, 146] and two studies of dental hygienists and dental chairside assistants [67, 95] have found low rates of infection among persons without community risk factors. In the most detailed report, Klein and colleagues [95] tested 1,309 dental workers, including 1,132 dentists and 177 dental hygienists and assistants, most of whom practiced in AIDS-endemic areas. Of those tested, 15 percent reported treating patients known to have AIDS and 72 percent reported treating patients with known risk factors for HIV infection. The workers' median reported frequency of self-injury with a sharp instrument was once per month, with a range of up to twenty-five times per month. Only one dentist without behavioral risk factors was HIV-seropositive (seroprevalence rate 1/1,309 = 0.08 percent). In contrast, 21 percent of the 767 dentists who had not received hepatitis B vaccine were positive for markers of previous infection with hepatitis B virus.

In a testing program conducted among physicians, surgeons, and dentists in the U.S. Army Reserve, who normally spend 90 percent of their time in civilian life, the HIV

Table 39-1. Human immunodeficiency virus seroprevalence in selected groups of health care workers

Worker group	No. tested	No. positive (%)	No. positive with non-occupational risk	Percent prevalence excluding seropositives with non-occupational risk	Reference
Orthopedic surgeons, U.S.A. and Canada (1991 annual meeting)	3,420	2 (0.06)	2	0.00	[29]
Physicians and dentists in U.S. Army Reserve	3,347	3 (0.09)	NA	NA	[54]
Dentists					
San Francisco	304[a]	0 (0)	0	0	[74]
Sacramento	89	0 (0)	0	0	[67]
U.S.A.—1986 annual meeting and New York City	1,132[a]	1 (0.09)	0	0.09	[95]
U.S.A.—1987 annual meeting	1,195	0 (0)	0	0	[146]
U.S.A.—1988 annual meeting	1,165	1 (0.09)	0	0.09	[81]
U.S.A.—1989 annual meeting	1,480	0 (0)	0	0	[81]
Denmark	961	0 (0)	0	0	[61]
Dental hygienists, New York City and Sacramento	167	0 (0)	0	0	[67, 95]
Dental assistants, New York City and Sacramento	176	0 (0)	0	0	[67, 95]
Hemodialysis staff, New York, Paris, Chicago, Brussels, Florence	356	0 (0)	0	0	[10, 48, 53, 79, 130]
Health care worker blood donors, U.S.A.—20 urban regions	9,449	3	2[b]	—[b]	[46]

NA = not available.

[a] Persons with community risk not included.

[b] Two health care workers had nonoccupational risks; the third health care worker was lost to follow-up.

seroprevalence was 0/263 among women and 3/3,084 among men [54]. No further information is available concerning these 3 seropositive men (e.g., possibility of behavioral risk factors, nature or location of practice, and history of exposure to blood).

HCWs in hemodialysis units have also been studied because of the recognized high risk of hepatitis B virus infection in such workers in the past. Among 356 hemodialysis staff in five cities, none was seropositive [10, 48, 53, 79, 130].

In a study conducted by the CDC in cooperation with the American Red Cross and several regional blood centers in the United States, the prevalence of HIV infection was determined in blood donors at hospital or health facility blood drives who indicated on a questionnaire that they were HCWs. Of 9,449 HCW blood donors evaluated in six urban regions between March 1990 and May 1991, 3 (0.03 percent) were HIV-seropositive; 2 of the 3 had nonoccupational risk factors for HIV infection, and 1 was lost to follow-up [46].

In several serosurveys among health care and laboratory workers of mixed occupations, personnel with widely varying degrees of contact (minimal to extensive) with patients with AIDS have had similar HIV seroprevalence rates [54, 64, 94, 97, 106, 122, 155]; suggesting that such contact was not a major risk for HIV infection. However, the power of these studies to detect increased HIV seroprevalence among subgroups of HCWs with potentially frequent exposure to HIV-infected blood was often limited.

A major limitation of HIV seroprevalence studies in HCWs to date is that the extent of occupational or community exposure to HIV of most workers tested is not known. Also, some of these rates may be underestimates if workers who knew or suspected that they might be positive declined to be tested.

HIV Seroprevalence Among Patients

The likelihood that an HCW will be exposed to the blood of a patient with HIV infection depends in part on the prevalence of HIV in the patient population. Among 89,547 specimens tested at 26 hospitals in the United States in the CDC sentinel hospital study from January 1988 to June 1989, seroprevalence rates ranged from 0.1 to 7.8 percent, depending on the hospital location [149]. Patients were excluded from this study if they were admitted for diagnoses possibly associated with HIV, such as pneumonia and certain other infections, unexplained fever, neuropsychiatric conditions, neoplasms, and gunshot or knife wounds. Thus the rate of HIV infection was quite high in some areas; these represent minimum estimates because of the exclusion criteria.

Studies of HIV seroprevalence have also been conducted in emergency department patients [92, 93, 107, 139, 148]. In a CDC study of patients presenting to emergency departments in three pairs of hospitals (one inner city and one suburban hospital in each of three cities in the United States with a high AIDS incidence), seroprevalence rates were 4.1 to 8.9 per 100 patient visits in the inner cities; 6.1 per 100 patient visits in one suburban hospital; and 0.2 to 0.7 per 100 patient visits in the other two suburban hospitals. Rates were highest among patients in the 15- to 44-year age group, in men, in blacks, and among patients presenting with pneumonia [107].

Kelen and co-workers [93] at Johns Hopkins Hospital in Baltimore found 5.2 percent of patients presenting to the emergency department were infected with HIV in 1987; the rate had increased to 6.0 percent in 1989. At Charity Hospital in New Orleans, 2 percent of emergency department patients' sera were HIV-seropositive [139].

Among childbearing women, hospital-based HIV seroprevalence rates have been 0 to 5 percent nationally, with the highest rates observed in certain inner city hospitals [96, 99, 124].

Studies among dialysis patients have revealed HIV seroprevalence rates ranging from 0 to 39 percent, depending on the city and the patient population treated. Centers that treated a large proportion of intravenous drug users had higher rates of HIV infection among the patients [109].

Several studies have found that many

patients' HIV infection is unrecognized. In the CDC multicenter emergency department study, the percentage of patients whose HIV infection was unknown to the emergency department staff was 66 to 70 percent for the inner city emergency departments, 40 percent in the suburban emergency department with the highest seroprevalence, and 76 and 91 percent in the other two suburban emergency departments [107]. Studies of consecutive admissions to the Department of Veterans Affairs Hospital in Washington, DC, and of emergency department visits at the Johns Hopkins Hospital in Baltimore have also found that the infection status of approximately two-thirds of HIV-infected patients was unknown to the health care providers at the time of presentation [80, 93].

In the United States, data are also available from seroprevalence surveys among patients at clinics for sexually transmitted diseases, drug treatment, women's health, tuberculosis, college students, and primary care outpatients [27]. Collectively, these patient seroprevalence studies demonstrate that the prevalence of HIV infection varies by geographic area and patient diagnosis, as well as the patient's age, sex, and race (ethnicity), and that the infection status of patients is often unknown. The results of these studies reveal variable rates of HIV prevalence, with many infections unrecognized, and so emphasize the need for observing universal precautions.

Risk of HIV Infection After Exposure

The risk of HIV infection after a documented exposure to the blood of an HIV-infected patient has been estimated in prospective studies conducted by the CDC and others.* The risk of HIV transmission to an HCW due to a single percutaneous exposure to HIV-infected blood is approximately 0.3 percent (upper limit of 95 percent CI = 0.6 percent) [75, 84, 108]. Most HCWs enrolled in these

---

*Health care institutions in the United States are encouraged to enroll HCWs exposed to HIV-infected blood in the CDC Prospective Surveillance Project. Information and a solicitation packet may be obtained by contacting the Hospital Infections Program, National Center for Infectious Diseases, CDC, at (404) 639-1547.

studies had a needle-stick exposure to the blood of a patient with AIDS. There are likely to be subgroups of percutaneous exposures for which the risk of transmission is higher than 0.3 percent and subgroups for which it is lower; however, there are currently insufficient epidemiologic data to identify such subgroups. For example, as of November 1991, all reported cases of occupational HIV transmission due to a documented needle-stick exposure have involved hollow-bore needles, but few HCWs exposed to HIV-infected blood as a result of injury with a solid-bore needle have been enrolled in prospective studies to estimate the risk of infection transmission. The possible influence of stage of disease in the source patient (i.e., AIDS vs. asymptomatic HIV infection) has not been determined. Preliminary data from in vitro studies suggest that the volume of blood transferred in a needle-stick injury is greater with increased depth of penetration, is somewhat greater for hollow-bore than solid-bore needles, and is reduced at least 50 percent with glove use [112].

Transmission of HIV after a mucous membrane or skin exposure to HIV-infected blood has also been reported [42], although no seroconversions have been detected in cohort studies of HCWs after mucous membrane and skin contact with HIV-infected blood [75, 84, 108]. In these prospective studies of exposed HCWs, the observed rate of HIV transmission after a mucous membrane or skin contact with HIV-infected blood is zero; the upper limits of the 95 percent confidence interval are 0.3 percent and 0.04 percent, respectively. Although the risk of transmission after such exposures is not precisely known, it is clearly much lower than that due to percutaneous exposures. In these studies, no HCWs seroconverted after exposure to fluids other than blood.

Several investigators have used the polymerase chain reaction (PCR) to examine specimens from HIV antibody–negative HCWs greater than 6 months after exposure to HIV-infected blood [77, 84, 86, 158]. Of a total of 237 seronegative workers, 3 were positive by PCR in one study. In these 3 cases, enzyme-linked immunosorbant assay (ELISA) and Western blot antibody studies, p24 antigen, and viral culture were negative. Subsequently, PCR testing on 2 of these workers was negative, casting additional doubt on the significance of the initial positive test. The remaining HCW has continued to be positive by the PCR test but has no other laboratory evidence of HIV infection [77]. The significance of this isolated positive PCR result is unknown. These data, combined with data on several hundred HCWs who have remained seronegative when tested 2 or more years after exposure [77, 84, 108], suggest that seroconversion beyond 6 months after an occupational exposure, if it occurs, is uncommon.

Epidemiology of Blood Contact

Studies of the epidemiology of blood contact among HCWs and patients have begun to describe the nature and frequency of exposures, to define risk factors, and to evaluate preventive measures. A number of prospective studies have assessed the frequency of blood contact (defined as a percutaneous injury, mucous membrane, or skin contact) among HCWs during surgical and obstetric procedures [60, 73, 88, 118, 127–129, 134, 143, 150, 151, 159]. The percentage of operations in which 1 or more members of the surgical team sustained any blood contact and the percentage in which 1 or more team members sustained a percutaneous injury are summarized in Table 39-2 for six studies in which observers recorded episodes of blood contact and one study in which surgeons themselves recorded these data. The rates in Table 39-2 do not apply to an individual worker, since several workers are normally involved in one operation. The range of results may be attributable to differences in study methods, definition of blood contact, procedures observed, and the use of precautions by the surgical team. Studies in which gloves were examined after surgery have also noted an appreciable rate of glove perforation, although it is often unclear in these studies whether the perforations were due to percutaneous injuries or other causes [15, 51, 57, 113, 116, 143].

The CDC has conducted prospective studies in areas of the United States with a high AIDS incidence in which HCWs in surgical, obstetric, and hospital emergency departments were observed while performing procedures, to ascertain the frequency and preventability of blood contact. Blood contact rates appeared to be higher for obstetricians, for surgeons, and for emergency department workers who did not wear gloves while performing procedures. Considerably lower rates were observed in surgical scrub personnel and emergency department workers who did wear gloves. Sharps injury rates were higher for surgeons and obstetricians than for emergency department workers (Table 39-3) [107, 127, 151].

Table 39-2. Prospective studies of blood contact among operating and delivery room personnel

Location	*No. of procedures*	*Percent of procedures with ≥1 blood contact*	*Percent of procedures with ≥1 sharp injury*	*Reference*
San Francisco	1,307*	6.4	1.3	[73]
Atlanta				
Surgery	206	30.1	4.9	[128]
Obstetrics	230*	32.2	1.7	[127]
Albuquerque	684*	27.8	3.1	[134]
Milwaukee	234	50.4	15.4	[150]
Saudi Arabia	2,016	NA	5.6	[88]
New York, Chicago	1,382	46.6	6.9	[151]

*Includes procedures not involving an incision.
NA = not available.

Table 39-3.   Blood contact rates observed in HCWs: Preliminary results of CDC studies

Occupation	No. of HCW-procedures observed	Blood contact rate per 100 HCW-procedures	Sharp injury rate per 100 HCW-procedures	Reference
Surgeon (5 specialties)*	3,510	27.0	2.5	[151]
Scrub person (5 specialties)*	2,080	2.3	0.2	[151]
Obstetrician	353	15.3	0.8	[127]
Hospital emergency department worker				
Gloved	8,098	1.6	} 0.07	[107]
Not gloved	1,690	13.4		

HCWs = health care workers; CDC = Centers for Disease Control.
*General, orthopedic, gynecologic, cardiac, and trauma surgery.

Table 39-4.   Estimates of blood contact frequency in health care workers

Occupation	No. of procedures per year	No. of blood contacts per year	No. of sharp injuries per year	Reference
Surgeon (5 specialties)*	500	135.0	12.5	[151]
Scrub person (5 specialties)*	500	11.5	1.0	[151]
Obstetrician	500	76.5	4.0	[127]
Hospital emergency department worker	625	24.2	0.4	[107]
Physician on medical ward	NA	31.2	1.8	[157]
Dentist	NA	NA	12.0	[95]

NA = not available
*General, orthopedic, gynecologic, cardiac, and trauma surgery.

In Table 39-4, the estimated number of procedures done per year by a member of each occupational group in these studies and data on the frequency of blood contact per HCW-procedure have been used to estimate the frequency of blood contact per year for an individual HCW in the locations studied. Other investigators have collected prospective data on blood exposure frequency among physicians on medical wards [157], dentists [95], and personnel in a university hospital [114]. These figures should be viewed as crude estimates that may not be applicable to every worker in each occupational group. Furthermore, not all exposures may be comparable. For example, injuries during surgical procedures tend to occur with solid-bore suture needles, which may be less likely to transmit infection than hollow-bore needles that might inject blood.

Additional prospective studies of the epidemiology of blood contacts are needed. Interpretation of data is facilitated if sharps exposures are clearly separated from other blood contacts and frequency data are expressed per individual worker per unit of time. When combined with information on patient seroprevalence, data such as these may be used to estimate the cumulative risk of HIV infection in groups of workers [115]. For example, Gerberding and co-workers [73] have estimated that one occupational HIV infection may occur among surgical personnel at San Francisco General Hospital every 8 years. Such calculations are most likely to be accurate at institutions where patient seroprevalence and blood contact epidemiology are well defined.

Exposure Prevention
General Principles
Exposure prevention involves a triad of strategies—(1) engineering controls that do not depend on worker compliance (e.g., self-sheathing needles); (2) safe work practices and techniques; and (3) personal protective equipment (e.g., gloves)—as well as training of workers in the use of these preventive measures. New devices, work practices, and personal protective equipment must be scientifically evaluated for efficacy in protecting HCWs from injuries and other exposures to patient blood and body fluids without compromising patient care. Students should receive instruction in exposure prevention beginning at the earliest stages of their professional training; such instruction should also be a prominent feature of continuing inservice training and employee education programs.

Universal Precautions
To reduce the occupational risk of infection with bloodborne pathogens (including HIV, hepatitis B and C viruses, human T-cell lymphotropic viruses [HTLVs], and other pathogens), the CDC recommends that blood and certain body fluids of all patients be considered potentially infectious: These recommendations are known as *universal precautions* [34, 45] (see Chap. 11). The term *universal* refers to all *patients*, not to all body fluids or to all pathogens. The purpose of universal precautions is to prevent transmission of bloodborne pathogens from patient to HCW, HCW to patient, and patient to patient. Universal precautions are intended to supplement, rather than replace, long-standing recommendations for control of nonbloodborne pathogens [71]. Universal precautions apply to blood, fluids containing visible blood, semen, vaginal secretions, tissues, and to cerebrospinal, synovial, pleural, peritoneal, pericardial, and amniotic fluid. Universal precautions do not apply to tears, nasal secretions, saliva, sputum, sweat, urine, feces, or vomit unless visible blood is present. In excluding these fluids, universal precautions is different from a system of infection control known as *body substance isolation* [104], in which barrier precautions are recommended for contact with all body fluids (see Chap. 11). Unlike body substance isolation, universal precautions apply only to fluids and tissues that may transmit bloodborne pathogens. If additional infections are suspected, additional precautions are indicated (e.g., enteric precautions for a patient with an enteric infection) (see Chap. 30). Infection control programs that incorporate the principles of universal precautions (i.e., appropriate use of hand-washing, protective barriers, and care in the use and disposal of sharp instruments) should be maintained rigorously in all health care settings. Proper application of these principles will assist in minimizing the risk of transmitting HIV and other bloodborne pathogens from patient to HCW, HCW to patient, or patient to patient. Universal precautions and body substance isolation are discussed further in Chapter 11.

To prevent skin and mucous membrane exposures, appropriate barrier precautions should be used routinely when contact with blood or the other body fluids previously listed may be anticipated. Although the risk of HIV transmission to HCWs after skin or mucous membrane exposure to HIV-infected blood is lower than that due to percutaneous exposure, HIV transmission to HCWs after such exposures has occurred [42], and the number of (particularly skin) contacts with blood among HCWs is large, prompting the CDC recommendations for barrier precautions. Appropriate barriers may include gloves, masks, gowns, or eye protection but may also include something as simple as a pad of gauze to wipe up a small spot of blood, for example, provided that the gauze is thick enough to prevent the blood from soaking through and contacting the skin. In addition, hand-washing has long been recommended after contact with patients or their blood or body fluids and still remains one of the most important measures for preventing the transmission of infection and for general hygiene.

Intact skin is one of the body's most important defenses against infection with microbial agents. However, skin is not always intact, particularly on the hands. The CDC recommends barrier precautions to prevent contact of skin, whether intact or not, with blood or other body fluids requiring universal precautions. Skin exposures to these fluids may be considered occupational exposures to HIV (see p. 836) [33].

Prevention of percutaneous injuries primarily requires engineering controls and careful work practices, since these injuries are not readily prevented with currently available barriers. Safe handling and disposal of needles and other sharp objects is important, including avoiding recapping by hand and disposal in conveniently located impervious containers. Development of safer medical devices and improved protective equipment, such as new glove materials that resist needle puncture yet preserve tactile sensation, is needed. Procedures requiring sharp instruments and techniques of handling them should be periodically reevaluated to determine whether any procedures or techniques could be modified or new instruments used to reduce the risk of injury without compromising patient care. On hospital wards, self-sheathing needles and other design improvements may be helpful in reducing injuries [62, 89]. Also, unnecessary needle use, such as in connecting pieces of tubing together or transferring liquids from one container into another, should be avoided.

In surgical and obstetric settings, injury prevention presents an even greater challenge, owing to the ubiquity of sharp objects and their potential for use in conditions of urgency or poor visibility. Recommendations have been made to reduce blood exposures during surgery [2, 12, 14, 137, 142]. Suggestions for preventing percutaneous injuries have included (1) preoperative discussion of exposure prevention with the surgical team; (2) establishment of a "one wound, one surgeon" policy whenever possible (i.e., only one person at a time has his or her hands in a wound when sharp instruments are in use); (3) coordination of roles, including identification of which team member will deal with emergencies such as unexpected bleeding; (4) the importance of slow, deliberate, and well-choreographed movements intraoperatively; (5) avoidance of gloves that are too large, as the protruding glove finger tips may snag a sharp instrument; (6) use of forceps to load or adjust a needle in a needle holder or a scalpel blade in a handle; (7) storage of loaded needle holders with the needle point downward; (8) taking care that sharp instruments do not extend beyond the edge of the Mayo stand; (9) use of an intermediate tray to pass instruments; (10) announcement that a sharp instrument is being passed; (11) increased use of staples, electrocautery, instrument ties, and other nontouch suturing and sharp instrument techniques when possible; (12) use of instruments, rather than fingers, to handle, stabilize, or retract tissue; (13) use of forceps to retrieve a needle during suturing; (14) not tying a suture with the needle in hand; (15) disposal of sharp instruments in impervious containers; (16) not recapping, bending, or breaking needles prior to disposal; and (17) particularly for orthopedic surgery, covering exposed internal wires or pins with catheter tubing or cork stoppers and using three pairs of gloves (latex-cotton-latex) for palpating sharp fracture fragments and working with multiple exposed wires or sharp instruments such as osteotomes, drill bits, or saws.

Saliva

HIV transmission via contact with saliva and respiratory secretions has not been demonstrated in epidemiologic studies among household contacts of persons with HIV infection [19, 68, 69, 101, 140, 145] or in (a relatively small number of) HCWs after exposure to saliva of infected patients [78, 84, 108, 141, 145, 152]. Nevertheless, certain precautions are indicated for HCWs whose exposures to saliva may exceed simple casual contact. The CDC has long-standing recommendations that HCWs wear gloves for contact with mucous membranes of all patients, especially during dental and oropharyngeal procedures, when contamination of saliva with blood is predictable. Gloves may also protect the patient from contact with the HCW's blood, which may occur from breaks in the skin of the HCW's hands. Additional barrier precautions, such as surgical masks, protective eyewear, or face shields should be worn by the HCW during procedures in which splashing or spattering of blood, saliva, or gingival fluids is likely [38].

Cardiopulmonary Resuscitation

The greatest risk of bloodborne pathogen transmission to HCWs performing cardiopulmonary resuscitation (CPR) is due to injuries with large-bore needles that are used in a sometimes hectic setting and then may be disposed of improperly. In the CDC's prospective study of HCWs exposed to HIV, two of the three seroconversions were attributable to needles handled by co-workers during CPR, illustrating the importance of handling needles carefully even during emergencies [108].

No case of HIV infection acquired by performing mouth-to-mouth resuscitation has been documented. Instances have been reported of rescuers performing mouth-to-mouth resuscitation on patients with AIDS or HIV infection without becoming infected with HIV [78, 141]. However, in health care settings, where the need for CPR is predictable, mechanical respiratory assist devices (e.g., bag-valve devices) should be widely available, and personnel should be trained in their proper use. Guidelines for the performance of mouth-to-mouth resuscitation have been published [39, 63].

Glove Materials

Studies of the fragility of various glove materials under conditions of use and the penetrability of these materials to various test probes, including viral particles, blood, and water, have been difficult to interpret owing to variations in test methods [55]. The U.S. Food and Drug Administration regulates the quality of medical gloves and has established standards for medical gloves marketed in the United States. Gloves do not offer absolute protection against blood contact but, when combined with other measures, including hand-washing after removing the gloves, they greatly reduce the frequency of blood contact and, hence, infection transmission.

Efficacy of Precautions in Preventing Blood Contact

The efficacy of barrier precautions in preventing blood contact has been assessed in a number of settings. In a prospective study in which physicians on medical wards completed a daily questionnaire, Wong and associates [157] found that implementation of universal precautions resulted in a decrease in the rate of exposure to blood and body fluids from 5.07 to 2.66 per physician per patient care month, primarily due to a reduced rate of skin contact with blood because of glove use. In this study, the needle-stick injury rate also declined from 0.39 to 0.15 per physician per patient care month, a change that the authors speculated may have been due to the presence of a sharps disposal unit in every patient room [157]. Surveys using a pair of questionnaires completed by HCWs in a variety of (predominantly nonsurgical) hospital settings before and after implementation of universal precautions also found a reduction of approximately 50 percent in estimated annual rates of nonparenteral exposure to blood and other body substances [65]. In a study in which trained observers monitored more than 9,000 procedures in six hospital emergency departments, blood contact rates were considerably lower for HCWs who wore gloves (Table 39-5) [107]. These data strongly support the efficacy of universal precautions in preventing blood contact by workers on medical wards and in hospital emergency departments.

In studies in surgical and obstetric settings, most skin and mucous membrane contacts could also have been prevented with additional barriers [127, 128]. However, the greatest risk of HIV transmission comes from percutaneous injuries, which are generally not preventable by currently available barriers. It is essential to learn more about the circumstances of percutaneous injuries and

Table 39-5. Efficacy of gloves in preventing blood contact with skin: CDC study in hospital emergency department workers

Procedure	Blood contact rate per 100 procedures		Relative risk of blood contact for ungloved vs. gloved (95% CI)
	Ungloved	Gloved	
Obtaining arterial blood gas specimen	10.1	0.5	19.8 (4.6–85.3)
Starting intravenous line	16.3	1.2	13.0 (8.5–19.9)
Phlebotomy	5.7	1.0	5.4 (3.1–9.4)
Equipment disposal	22.3	1.2	19.1 (9.3–39.0)
Wound care	15.9	2.4	6.6 (4.2–10.6)

CDC = Centers for Disease Control; CI = confidence interval.
Source: Adapted from R. Marcus et al., Contact with blood of patients infected with HIV among emergency care providers (abstr. Th.C. 604). In: *Proceedings of the Sixth International Conference on AIDS, San Francisco, 1990.*

the devices and circumstances with which they are associated.

In a CDC study in four hospitals, 99 sharp injuries were observed during 1,382 operations [151]. In 34 injuries (34 percent), the surgeon was holding the tissue being sutured with his or her fingers. In 7 (7 percent), the surgeon retrieved the suture needle with his or her fingers while suturing. Five injuries (5 percent) occurred while the suture needle was being adjusted in the needle holder. Seven injuries (7 percent) were related to unanticipated movements of co-workers, such as unannounced instrument passes. These data suggest that some injuries during surgery might be preventable by changes in technique. Additional needs include development of puncture-resistant gloves and changes in instrument design. All such changes must be carefully evaluated to document that they enhance worker safety without compromising patient care.

Sterilization, Disinfection, and Waste Disposal

Recommendations for sterilization, disinfection, waste disposal, and other aspects of environmental control have been published [66, 70] and are discussed more fully elsewhere (see Chap. 15). Standard sterilization and disinfection procedures for patient care equipment currently recommended for use in a variety of health care settings are adequate to sterilize or disinfect instruments, devices, or other items contaminated with blood or other body fluids from persons infected with bloodborne pathogens, including HIV. Environmental surfaces such as walls, floors, and other surfaces are not associated with transmission of HIV infection to patients or HCWs. Therefore, extraordinary attempts to disinfect or sterilize these environmental surfaces are not necessary. However, cleaning and removal of soil should be done routinely. All spills of blood and blood-contaminated fluids should be promptly cleaned up by a person wearing gloves and using an Environmental Protection Agency–approved disinfectant or a 1:100 solution of household bleach. Visible material should first be removed with disposable towels or other appropriate means that will ensure against direct contact with blood. If splashing is anticipated, protective eyewear should be worn along with an impervious gown or apron that provides an effective barrier to splashes. The area should then be decontaminated with an appropriate disinfectant.

Specialized Settings

Detailed recommendations have also been published for laboratory workers [20], dental workers [38], home HCWs and others (e.g., friends and relatives) who provide health care in the home [21, 147], and first responders who provide emergency medical care

[23]. Workers in psychiatric health care facilities may need to be familiar with appropriate procedures for dealing with assaultive patients [23, 105], in addition to the infection control principles outlined earlier.

Aerosols

Aerosols should not be confused with droplets and splashes. The CDC recommends barrier precautions (face shields, masks, gowns, etc.) to prevent contact with droplets and splashes [34]. Aerosols are not droplets; rather, they are tiny invisible particles called *droplet nuclei* which, unlike droplets, remain suspended in air for extended periods of time. Whereas inspired particles 10 to 100 μm in diameter may be deposited in the upper airway or in bronchi, true respirable aerosols capable of reaching alveoli consist of particles less than 5 to 10 μm in diameter. Aerosols require considerable mechanical energy (e.g., power equipment) to generate and are not likely to be present in most clinical settings. There are no known instances of transmission of a bloodborne pathogen by aerosol in a clinical setting. In studies conducted in dental operatories and hemodialysis centers, hepatitis B surface antigen could not be detected in the air during the treatment of hepatitis B carriers, including during procedures known to generate aerosols [131]. This suggests that detection of HIV in aerosols in clinical settings would also be uncommon, since the concentration of HIV in blood is generally lower than that of hepatitis B virus. HIV has been detected in a laboratory aerosol [90], but this does not necessarily mean that HIV-containing aerosols are produced in clinical settings or that HIV is transmissible by aerosol in a clinical setting. The CDC is sponsoring research to assess the potential for aerosolization of blood and tissue during a variety of surgical procedures and to assess possible resulting hazards to surgical personnel.

Routine Testing of Patients for HIV Antibody

The Public Health Service (PHS) has recommended that routine voluntary testing of hospitalized patients be considered (for the benefit of the patients) in groups with a high prevalence of HIV infection [32]. The medical benefits of early HIV detection include therapy for persons with HIV infection with CD4 lymphocyte counts of less than 500 per millimeter [121]. An estimated 58 to 64 percent of the approximately 1 million persons with HIV infection in the United States have CD4 lymphocyte counts in this range [24]. Thus hospitalized patients in high-prevalence areas are increasingly likely to be offered voluntary testing for their own medical benefit.

Personnel in some hospitals have also advocated testing of patients to protect HCWs in settings where exposure of HCWs to large amounts of patients' blood may be anticipated. Specific patients for whom testing has been advocated include those undergoing major operative procedures and those undergoing treatment in critical care units, especially if they have conditions involving uncontrolled bleeding. For surgical patients who test positive, additional precautions have been advocated [2, 137] (e.g., use of stapling instruments rather than hand suturing to perform tissue approximation, use of electrocautery devices and scissors rather than scalpels as cutting instruments, use of gowns that totally prevent seepage of blood onto the skin of operative team members, use of "space suits" or respirators with an air filter or self-contained air supply to prevent inhalation of aerosols, and exclusion of inexperienced personnel from the operating team). The efficacy of these and other measures in protecting workers and their effect on patient care are unknown.

At present, it is unclear whether testing patients, in addition to implementing universal precautions, is helpful in protecting HCWs. Although the issue requires further study, there is some evidence that knowledge that a patient has HIV infection or risk factors for HIV infection may not necessarily influence the likelihood of blood exposure by operative personnel [72, 73, 127, 151]. If personnel routinely follow universal precautions, knowledge of a patient's HIV serostatus should not make a difference. One group of investigators who evaluated the practical aspects of a voluntary HIV admission screening program in a large private hospital concluded that the benefit of the program appeared to be greater for the patient than for the hospital or HCW [82].

Decisions regarding the need to establish routine voluntary testing programs for patients should be made by individual institutions in consultation with public health authorities and based, in part, on the HIV seroprevalence in patients in their institutions. In addition, when deemed appropriate, testing of individual patients may be performed on agreement between the patient and the physician providing care. Patient testing should include provisions for (1) obtaining informed consent, (2) providing appropriate counseling, (3) ensuring confidentiality of results, and (4) providing optimal care for infected patients. Testing programs should be evaluated to determine whether they reduce the frequency of adverse exposures and to determine their effect on patient care [34].

HCWs whose infection control practices are based on a patient's HIV test result risk a false sense of security, since patients with a negative HIV test result may nevertheless be infected with HIV or with another bloodborne pathogen. Focusing on a patient's HIV test result may divert attention from the need for HCWs to recognize that blood is a potentially hazardous substance. There are a number of other bloodborne pathogens, among them hepatitis C virus and HTLV-I. The best way for HCWs to protect themselves from occupational acquisition of a bloodborne infection is to assume that all blood may be infectious and to observe infection control measures incorporating the principles of universal precautions.

Management of an Occupational Exposure to HIV

An occupational exposure that may place a worker at risk of HIV infection has been defined by the CDC [33] as follows:

. . . A percutaneous injury (e.g., a needle stick or cut with a sharp object), contact of mucous membranes, or contact of skin (especially when the exposed skin is chapped, abraded, or afflicted with dermatitis or the contact is prolonged or involving an extensive area) with blood, tissues, or other body fluids to which universal precautions apply including: (a) semen, vaginal secretions, or other body fluids contaminated with visible blood, because these substances have been implicated in the transmission of HIV infection; (b) cerebrospinal fluid, synovial fluid, pleural fluid, peritoneal fluid, pericardial fluid, and amniotic fluid, because the risk of transmission of HIV from these fluids has not yet been determined; and (c) laboratory specimens that contain HIV (e.g., suspensions of concentrated virus), during the performance of job duties.

Detailed recommendations for management of occupational exposures to blood and bloodborne pathogens have been published [30, 33]. These include prompt reporting to receive appropriate counseling and management, evaluation of the need for hepatitis B postexposure prophylaxis, and testing of the patient (with consent) for hepatitis B surface antigen (HBsAg) and for HIV antibody. Routine measures for the local treatment of minor wounds should be followed; extraordinary measures (e.g., application of caustic agents) may be harmful and have not been shown to be of value in preventing the transmission of bloodborne pathogens.

After an exposure has occurred, the source patient should be informed of the incident and tested for serologic evidence of HIV infection after consent is obtained. If the source individual has AIDS, is known to be HIV-seropositive, or refuses testing, the worker should be evaluated clinically and serologically for evidence of HIV infection as soon as possible after the exposure (baseline) and, if seronegative, should be restested periodically for a minimum of 6 months after exposure (e.g., at 6 weeks, 12 weeks, and 6 months after exposure) to determine whether HIV infection has occurred. The worker should be advised to report and seek medical evaluation for any acute illness that occurs during the follow-up period. Such illness, particularly if characterized by fever, rash, myalgia, fatigue, malaise, or lymphadenopathy, may be indicative of acute HIV infection, drug reaction, or another medical condition. During the follow-up period, especially the first 6 to 12 weeks after the exposure, when most infected persons are expected to seroconvert, exposed workers should follow PHS recommendations for preventing transmission of HIV [33]. These include refraining from blood, semen, or organ donation and abstaining from, or using measures to prevent HIV transmission during, sexual intercourse. In addition, in countries such as the United States where safe and effective alternatives to breastfeeding are available, exposed women should not breastfeed infants during the follow-up period, in order to prevent possible exposure of the infant to HIV in breast milk. *During all phases of follow-up, it is vital that the confidentiality of the worker and the source patient be protected.*

If the source individual is HIV-seronegative and has no clinical manifestations of AIDS or HIV infection, no further HIV follow-up of the exposed worker is necessary unless there is epidemiologic evidence to suggest that the source individual may have recently been exposed to HIV or if testing is desired by the worker or recommended by the health care provider. In this case, the worker may be followed as just described.

If the source individual cannot be identified, decisions regarding appropriate follow-up should be individualized, based on factors such as whether potential sources are likely to include an individual at increased risk of HIV infection.

Serologic testing should be made available by the employer to all workers who may be concerned that they have been infected with HIV through an occupational exposure. Appropriate psychologic counseling may be indicated as well.

Available data from animal and human studies are inadequate to establish the efficacy or safety of zidovudine (AZT) for postexposure prophylaxis of HIV infection [33, 144]. In the absence of conclusive data, there are diverse opinions among physicians regarding the use of AZT for this purpose [83, 85]. HCWs who may be at risk for occupational exposure to HIV should be aware of the considerations that pertain to the use of AZT after exposure. These include the postexposure risk of HIV infection and the factors that have been postulated to influence this risk, the apparent need to begin prophylaxis promptly if prophylaxis is given, the limitations of current knowledge of efficacy and toxicity of AZT, and the need for postexposure follow-up, regardless of whether AZT is taken. Ideally, HCWs should be familiarized with these considerations *prior to* exposure, to facilitate prompt and rational decision making after exposure. Some hospitals have found that a 24-hour "needle-stick hotline" to provide *confidential* counseling and, if desired, starter doses of AZT is effective in managing exposures, in counseling workers, and in bolstering HCW morale by demonstrating institutional support [76].

A prospective, randomized, double-blind, placebo-controlled trial begun by the Burroughs-Wellcome Company to evaluate AZT postexposure use in HCWs was terminated prematurely because of low enrollment [98]. However, this and several other prospective studies have provided preliminary information on short-term toxicity among HCWs after occupational exposure to HIV (Table 39-6). In these studies, the most commonly reported symptoms and signs of acute toxicity have included nausea, vomiting, headache, malaise, fatigue, anemia, and granulocytopenia [33, 76, 83, 98, 136, 110]. No HCW enrolled in these studies who took AZT after exposure seroconverted to HIV, but that is not unexpected since the risk of HIV transmission after a needle-stick exposure to infected blood is, on average, approximately 0.3 percent.

Failure of AZT to prevent HIV infection postexposure has been reported in at least seven instances. One case involved a transfusion of HIV-infected blood [33], one involved suicidal self-injection of several milliliters of infected blood [59], and one was an assault on

Table 39-6. Zidovudine use in health care workers after occupational exposure to human immunodeficiency virus

Institution	Zidovudine regimen	No. of qualifying exposures	No. (%) treated with zidovudine	No. (%) discontinuing zidovudine before course completed	No. (%) reporting side effects	Reference
CDC Surveillance Project	Median: 1,000 mg/day (for 42 days)[a]	630[b]	166 (26)	40 (30)[c]	96 (72)[c]	[110]
San Francisco General Hospital	200 mg 5x daily for 6 weeks	12	9 (75)	3 (33)	2 (17)	[76]
NIH—Clinical Center	200 mg q4h for 6 weeks	27	20 (76)	6 (24)	10 (50)	[83]
Burroughs-Wellcome clinical trial	200 mg q4h for 6 weeks	48	48	17 (35)	14 (29)	[98]
Italian study group	100 mg/day for 3 days to 1,250 mg/day for 42 days[a]		48	2 (4)	16 (33)	[136]

CDC = Centers for Disease Control; NIH = National Institutes of Health.
[a] Participants in the CDC and Italian multicenter surveillance projects received a variety of regimens.
[b] All exposures reported to the CDC during this period; the number offered zidovudine by their institution is unknown.
[c] Percent of the 133 health care workers taking zidovudine for whom follow-up information at 6 weeks is available.
Source: Modified from D.K. Henderson, Post-exposure chemoprophylaxis for occupational exposure to HIV-1. *Am. J. Med.* 91 (Suppl. 3B): 312S, 1991.

a prison guard with a needle-syringe containing HIV-infected blood [91]. In the fourth and fifth cases, HIV infection occurred after inadvertent intravenous injection of HIV-infected blood into a patient during a nuclear medicine procedure [100, 133]. In the fourth case, the amount of blood injected was estimated at 100 to 200 μl [100]. These five incidents involved circumstances very different from most needle-stick exposures that an HCW might experience; these circumstances (e.g., injection of a larger volume of blood than would be expected from most needle sticks [112, 120]) might have accounted for the failure of AZT to prevent infection.

In 2 additional cases, AZT failed to prevent HIV infection in an HCW after a needle-stick exposure to HIV-infected blood. In one episode, AZT was begun within 6 hours after a deep needle-stick injury at a dose of 250 mg every 6 hours for 8 weeks [102]. In another case, AZT was begun within 8 hours after an intramuscular injury with a 16-gauge needle

at a dose of 1,000 mg/day for 1 week [C. Ciesielski, CDC: personal communication]. The regimens of AZT used in these latter 2 cases are somewhat less intensive and were begun later than has been recommended at some institutions, where if an HCW wishes to receive AZT, efforts are made to begin therapy within 1 hour after an eligible exposure at a dose of 200 mg five to six times per day for 4 to 6 weeks [85]. These more intensive regimens were adopted because of their efficacy in delaying progression of disease in HIV-infected patients; it is not known whether they are effective as postexposure prophylaxis.

The Role of the Occupational Safety and Health Administration

Statutory authority to regulate workplaces to protect the health of workers rests with the Occupational Safety and Health Administration (OSHA), an agency of the U.S. Department of Labor. OSHA regulations are issued in the form of a *standard,* which requires employers to take specific measures to protect workers exposed to a particular hazard. In all cases, it is the employer, rather than the worker, who is held responsible by OSHA for ensuring that the regulations are enforced. Employees who violate OSHA regulations may be subject to disciplinary action by the employer. Standards are issued after a lengthy rule-making process, in which public review and comment is solicited at several stages. On December 6, 1991, an OSHA standard for occupational exposure to bloodborne pathogens, based largely on CDC recommendations regarding universal precautions and the use of hepatitis B vaccine, was published in the *Federal Register* [125].

HIV Transmission to Patients During Invasive Procedures
Risk Assessment
Recognition in the mid-1980s that HIV, like hepatitis B virus (HBV), was potentially transmissible from patients to HCWs due to occupational blood exposure led to recognition of the possibility that HIV, like HBV (see Chap. 38), might also be transmissible from an infected HCW to a patient [34, 37]. In 1990, investigation of a patient with AIDS with no identified risk for HIV infection strongly suggested that this patient had acquired HIV infection while receiving care in the practice of a dentist who had AIDS [28]. Subsequently, 4 additional cases of HIV transmission associated with dental care in this practice were detected among approximately 1,000 patients whose test results are known [44]. Evidence that the 5 patients acquired their infections during dental care came from a careful epidemiologic investigation, which did not reveal a recognized risk for HIV infection in the patients, and also from a novel laboratory technique, which demonstrated a high degree of similarity between genetic sequences of HIV isolated from the patients and from the dentist. The mechanism of transmission of HIV from the dentist to the patients is not known. Although it has been speculated that inadequate sterilization or

disinfection of instruments may have been responsible, evidence of breaches in recommended sterilization or disinfection practice sufficient to allow transmission of HIV to 5 patients was not identified [28, 43, 44].

Discovery of this cluster of cases highlighted the need for additional data on the risk of HIV transmission from an infected HCW to a patient during an invasive procedure; this risk appears to be very low but has not been well quantified to date. Well-designed retrospective investigations of patients who have had invasive procedures performed by an infected HCW offer an opportunity to evaluate patient risk. In the largest and most systematic study of patients of an infected surgeon to date, testing was offered to patients who had been operated on by a general surgeon within 7 years prior to his receiving a diagnosis of AIDS [119]. Of 1,340 patients contacted, 616 (46 percent) were tested. One patient, a known intravenous drug user who may already have been infected at the time of surgery, was HIV positive. Excluding this patient, the observed transmission rate was 0/615 patients tested (upper limit of 95 percent CI = 0.5 percent) [119].

As of November 15, 1991, the CDC is aware of 5 HIV-infected HCWs, including the surgeon just cited and 2 other surgeons, for whom retrospective patient investigations have been completed. Of 1,200 patients tested, only the patient of the general surgeon cited earlier has tested seropositive for HIV [8, 52, 56, 119, 135].

Other investigations are still ongoing, including that of the Florida dental practice in which 5 patients were infected. To the CDC's knowledge, as of November 15, 1991, approximately 9,000 additional patients of HIV-infected HCWs have been tested. Although no additional cases of HIV transmission from HCW to patient have been documented, these preliminary results must be interpreted carefully. First, approximately 60 patients have tested HIV-positive. Investigation of most of these 60 patients for possible risk factors for HIV infection has not been completed. Most resided in areas of high HIV seroprevalence;

determination of their source of infection will be difficult, will take considerable time, and may be inconclusive. Second, the procedures undergone by most of these patients have not been characterized. Many of these patients did not undergo invasive procedures and therefore should not be included in the risk assessment [M.E. Chamberland, CDC: unpublished data].

Difficulties in conducting and interpreting retrospective studies include confidentiality issues involving both HCWs and patients, difficulties in assessing infection control practices and behavioral risk exposures retrospectively and, given the low risks involved, the need to evaluate a large number of patients to obtain precise estimates of risk for specific categories of invasive procedures. Finally, if positive patients are identified, it may not be technically possible to conduct a satisfactory epidemiologic investigation of the patients or to compare viral isolates from patients and HCWs using genetic sequencing techniques. Thus it may not be possible to ascertain whether infection was acquired from a particular surgeon or dentist during a particular invasive procedure. For all of these reasons, it seems unlikely that precise estimates of patient risk from specific invasive procedures performed by infected surgeons or dentists will become available through such studies in the near future.

Patient risk has been estimated by using modeling techniques. The CDC has estimated the average risk of sporadic HIV transmission from an HIV-infected surgeon to a patient during an invasive procedure as 2.4 to 24 per million procedures [13, 22]. This is similar to estimates by Rhame [138] of 1 to 10 per million procedures and by Lowenfels and Wormser [103] of 2 to 36 per million per hour of surgery. These estimates place the average risk one order of magnitude lower than the risk of anesthesia-associated mortality (100 per million [49]) and in the same order of magnitude as the risk of HIV infection from a transfusion of blood in the United States that has been screened as negative for HIV antibody (6.7 to 25 per million [17, 156]). The CDC's estimate for the risk of HBV trans-

mission to a patient of a surgeon positive for hepatitis B e antigen is 100-fold higher (240 to 2,400 per million) [13, 22]. However, since eventual mortality due to HBV infection (fulminant liver failure in acute infection or liver cancer or cirrhosis in chronic infection in 1 to 2 percent of cases [11, 117]), the risk of death due to infection transmission is comparable for HBV and HIV. The theoretical models used to derive these patient risk estimates have several limitations, including the fact that they are broad averages that do not account for variations in practice or technique by individual surgeons. Also, the models are not applicable during *outbreaks* (i.e., unpredictable clusters of patients infected by a single surgeon), in which the risk is much higher.

Additional well-designed studies are needed to quantitate risk more precisely and to determine the mechanism(s) of transmission. By analogy with HBV, it is most likely that the mechanism(s) involve exposure of the patient, either directly or indirectly, to the blood of the infected HCW. Few data are available on the proportion of surgical or dental procedures in which such exposures may occur. Possible circumstances might include (1) injury of an HCW with a sharp object, followed by percutaneous inoculation of the patient or contact of the object with a patient's open wound or body cavity; (2) injury of the HCW by a sharp wire or bone fragment that is affixed inside a patient's body; (3) laceration or puncture of the HCW's skin with a sharp instrument, resulting in bleeding into a patient's open wound or body cavity; (4) contact of a patient's open wound wtih exudate from an HCW's exudative dermatitis; and (5) contact with the blood of an HCW (or of another patient) through inadequate sterilization or disinfection of reusable devices used in invasive procedures.

In a prospective CDC observational study conducted in two inner-city and two suburban hospitals in areas of high AIDS incidence in the United States, preliminary data indicate that a percutaneous injury occurred among surgical personnel during 96 (6.9 percent) of 1,382 operative procedures on the general surgery, gynecology, orthopedic, cardiac, and trauma services [151]. In this study, trained observers noted the mean rate of blood exposure due to percutaneous injury per 100 procedures was 2.5 for a surgeon and 0.2 for a scrub nurse. The observers noted that the sharp object causing the injury recontacted the patient's open wound, resulting in a potential percutaneous exposure of the patient to the HCW's blood, in 28 (32 percent) of the 88 observed injuries in surgeons (range among surgical specialties, 8 to 57 percent; range among hospitals, 24 to 42 percent). Of these 28 injuries, 21 (75 percent) were caused by suture needles, 3 (11 percent) were caused by surgical wires, and 1 each was caused by a bone fragment, scissors, a staple gun, and a retractor [158]. Although these data document the potential for exposure of surgical patients to their surgeon's blood, the risk of HIV transmission from an infected surgeon to a patient as a result of such an exposure is unknown.

Strategies to Prevent HCW-to-Patient Transmission of HIV and Other Bloodborne Pathogens

Documentation of HIV transmission from an infected HCW to a patient during invasive procedures has led to considerable controversy over appropriate preventive strategies. In 1987, the CDC recommended that the patient care duties of HCWs infected with HIV be determined on an individual basis by the HCW's personal physician(s), in conjunction with the medical directors and personnel health service staff of the institution or hospital [34]. During the late 1980s, an increasing number of requests were made to the CDC for more specific guidance. In addition, reports of cases in which HCWs who posed no risk to patients were removed from patient care duties led to increasing awareness that additional recommendations were needed.

In July 1991, the CDC published recommendations for preventing transmission of HIV and HBV to patients during exposure-prone invasive procedures [35]. These recommendations were based on information indicating that for some invasive procedures,

standard infection control practices (including universal precautions) may not reliably prevent transmission of a bloodborne pathogen from an HCW to a patient. These data come from two sources: (1) investigations of HBV transmission from HCWs to patients that occurred despite compliance with the principles of universal precautions and (2) studies demonstrating that sharp injuries continue to occur among surgeons in the era of universal precautions and that some of these injuries potentially expose the patient to the surgeon's blood [35].

After publication of this document, the CDC received additional input from many professional organizations of physicians, dentists, and other health care providers. Many organizations recommended that the determination of whether a particular procedure has a potential for exposure of the patient to the HCW's blood include consideration of the HCW's technique, skill, and medical status as well as the specific procedure. Revision of the CDC recommendations is currently under discussion [36].

Several professional societies and other organizations have also developed recommendations for the management of HIV-infected HCWs, including the American Medical Association [6, 7], American Dental Association [4], Association for Practitioners in Infection Control, Society of Hospital Epidemiologists of America [9], American College of Obstetricians and Gynecologists [3], American Academy of Orthopaedic Surgeons [1], American Hospital Association [5], California Medical Association [18], New York State Department of Health [123], and the British Department of Health [153].

Notification of Patients of Infected HCWs

Hospital officials who become aware that an HCW on their staff who has performed invasive procedures is infected with HIV have faced the difficult decision as to whether previous patients should be notified. These decisions will remain difficult until the risk and risk factors for transmission to patients are better defined. Such decisions should be made on an individual, case-by-case basis in consultation with state public health officials. Factors that may be considered in assessing possible patient risk include whether (1) the HCW performed procedures that have been associated with hepatitis B transmission from an HCW to patients or other procedures in which injury to the HCW may have led to exposure of the patient to the HCW's blood (e.g., digital palpation of a needle tip inside a body cavity); (2) the HCW practiced proper infection control technique, including appropriate use of gloves and care in handling sharp instruments; (3) the HCW had exudative skin lesions in exposed areas that may have facilitated transmission of infection; (4) the HCW had neurologic complications that may have resulted in decreased manual dexterity and increased risk of self-injury while performing invasive procedures; and (5) reusable instruments used by this HCW in invasive procedures were sterilized or disinfected appropriately. State health officials can assist in evaluating the complex confidentiality and liability issues, which may vary from state to state, and the possibility of conducting a carefully designed investigation to collect additional scientific data on transmission risk. Notification of state professional licensing boards may also be required by state law.

If a decision to notify patients is made, state and local public health departments can potentially assist in the notification process and in dealing with the public response. They may also be able to provide counseling and testing and to coordinate the collection and reporting of test results. If an HIV-seropositive patient is identified, these departments will normally bear the responsibility for further investigation, including epidemiologic investigation of the patient for other risks. The CDC can provide consultation and, if appropriate, technical assistance to state health departments on request.

Patient-to-Patient Transmission

Since HIV is not transmitted by casual contact or fomites, patient-to-patient transmission in health care settings should be entirely preventable, assuming there is adequate disinfection or sterilization of reusable instruments used in invasive procedures (see Chap. 15). When reusable needles were not properly sterilized between patients, nosocomial outbreaks of HIV transmission have occurred [87, 132]. Data supporting the lack of nosocomial transmission of HIV between patients when standard infection control procedures are followed are available from a prospective study of patients undergoing chronic hemodialysis [109]. At the onset of the study, the prevalence of HIV infection among 1,324 patients in 28 hemodialysis centers was 0.98 percent, with infection generally confined to patients having a history of blood transfusion before the 1986–1988 study period or a history of sharing needles for the injection of drugs. On retesting 1 year later, no seroconversions occurred among 667 initially seronegative patients who were available for follow-up, including 254 who were dialyzed at centers with known HIV-infected patients. In contrast to HBV, for which a well-documented risk of transmission among patients and staff in hemodialysis centers has led to recommendations for screening and cohorting of infected patients (see Chap. 19), standard infection control procedures in hemodialysis settings, including compliance with the principles of universal precautions, appear to be effective in preventing HIV transmission.

Patient-to-patient nosocomial HIV transmission has been reported during a nuclear medicine procedure in the Netherlands, due to inadvertent use of a syringe containing HIV-infected blood in a procedure on a different patient [100]. Similar incidents have occurred in the United States: In 1990, the CDC investigated two episodes in hospital nuclear medicine departments in which patients were inadvertently injected with HIV-contaminated material from previous patients [133]. These incidents emphasize the need for review of procedures that involve withdrawal and subsequent reinjection of blood or other body fluids, in order to minimize the likelihood of inadvertent substitution of syringes or other contaminated material.

HIV transmission via blood transfusion,

artificial insemination, and bone and organ donation has been documented. Recommendations for preventing such transmission include screening potential donors for HIV antibody and for a history of risk factors for HIV infection [26, 31, 40, 41]. As a result of these preventive measures, the risk of HIV transmission in a unit of screened blood has been reduced to approximately 1 in 60,000 or less [17, 50, 58, 154].

Future Trends

Much has been learned about the risk and prevention of HIV transmission in health care settings, but additional data are needed. Future directions include more systematic surveillance of occupationally acquired HIV infection; additional HIV seroprevalence and incidence studies among workers with frequent blood exposures; better definition of the epidemiology of blood contact and the efficacy of preventive measures; development and evaluation of new devices and protective barriers; evaluation of postexposure prophylaxis; and assessment of the risk to patients undergoing invasive procedures by HIV-infected HCWs. A sustained commitment will ensure maximum protection for HCWs and patients and the availability of optimal medical care for all who need it.

References

1. American Academy of Orthopaedic Surgeons. *Advisory Statement: HIV-Infected Orthopaedic Surgeons.* Park Ridge, IL: American Academy of Orthopaedic Surgeons, 1991.
2. American Academy of Orthopaedic Surgeons Task Force on AIDS and Orthopaedic Surgery. *Recommendations for the Prevention of Human Immunodeficiency Virus (HIV) Transmission in the Practice of Orthopaedic Surgery.* Park Ridge, IL: American Academy of Orthopaedic Surgeons, 1989.
3. American College of Obstetricians and Gynecologists, Committee on Ethics. Human immunodeficiency virus infection: Physician's responsibilities. *Obstet. Gynecol.* 75 : 1043, 1990.
4. American Dental Association. *Interim Policy on HIV-Infected Dentists.* Chicago, IL: American Dental Association, 1991.
5. American Hospital Association. *Management of HIV Infection in the Hospital* (3rd ed.). Chicago, IL: American Hospital Association, 1988.
6. American Medical Association, Council on Ethical and Judicial Affairs. Ethical issues in the AIDS crisis: The HIV-positive practitioner. *J.A.M.A.* 260 : 790, 1988.
7. American Medical Association, Council on Ethical and Judicial Affairs. Ethical issues involved in the growing AIDS crisis. *J.A.M.A.* 259 : 1360, 1988.
8. Armstrong, F., Miner, J., and Wolfe, W. Investigation of a health care worker with symptomatic human immunodeficiency virus infection: An epidemiologic approach. *Milit. Med.* 152 : 414, 1987.
9. Association for Practitioners in Infection Control, Society of Hospital Epidemiologists of America. Position paper: The HIV-infected healthcare worker. *Infect. Control Hosp. Epidemiol.* 11 : 647, 1990.
10. Assogba, U., et al. Prospective study of HIV 1 seropositive patients in hemodialysis centers. *Clin. Nephrol.* 29 : 312, 1988.
11. Beasley, R. P. Hepatitis B virus: The major etiology of hepatocellular carcinoma. *Cancer* 10 : 1942, 1988.
12. Beck, W.C., and Meyer, K.K. Barrier Protection Technology. In: R.J. Howard (Ed.), *Infectious Risks in Surgery.* Norwalk, CT: Appleton and Lange, 1991. Pp. 125–137.
13. Bell, D.M., et al. Risk of endemic HIV and hepatitis B virus transmission to patients during invasive procedures (abstr. M.D. 59). Presented at the Seventh International Conference on AIDS, Florence, Italy, 1991.
14. Bessinger, C.D., Jr. Preventing transmission of human immunodeficiency virus during operations. *Surg. Gynecol. Obstet.* 167 : 287, 1988.
15. Brough, S.J., Hunt, T.M., and Barrie, W.W. Surgical glove perforations. *Br. J. Surg.* 75 : 317, 1988.
16. Bureau of Labor Statistics. *Employment and Earnings,* Vol. 35. Washington, DC: U.S. Department of Labor, Bureau of Labor Statistics, 1988. P. 13.
17. Busch, M.P., Eble, B., Heilbron, D., and Vyas, G. Risk associated with transfusion of HIV-antibody-negative blood. *N. Engl. J. Med.* 322 : 850, 1990.
18. California Medical Association. *Protection of Patients from the Blood-Borne Infections of Health Care Workers.* San Francisco: California Medical Association, 1989.
19. Castro, K.G., et al. Transmission of HIV in Belle Glade, Florida: Lessons for other com-

munities in the United States. *Science* 239: 193, 1988.

20. Centers for Disease Control. 1988 Agent summary statement for human immunodeficiency virus and report on laboratory-acquired infection with human immunodeficiency virus. *M.M.W.R.* 37 (Suppl. S4): 1, 1988.

21. Centers for Disease Control. *Caring for Someone with AIDS: Information for Friends, Relatives, Household Members, and Others who Care for a Person with AIDS at Home.* Rockville, MD: National AIDS Information Clearinghouse, 1990.

22. Centers for Disease Control. *Draft: Estimates of the Risk of Endemic Transmission of Hepatitis B Virus and Human Immunodeficiency Virus to Patients by the Percutaneous Route During Invasive Surgical and Dental Procedures.* Atlanta: Centers for Disease Control, January 30, 1991.

23. Centers for Disease Control. Guidelines for prevention of transmission of human immunodeficiency virus and hepatitis B virus to health-care and public safety workers. *M.M.W.R.* 38(S-6): 1, 1989.

24. Centers for Disease Control. HIV prevalence estimates and AIDS case projections for the United States: Report based on a workshop. *M.M.W.R.* 39(RR-16): 10, 1990.

25. Centers for Disease Control. HIV/AIDS Surveillance Report. Atlanta: Centers for Disease Control, Oct. 1991. P. 16.

26. Centers for Disease Control. Human immunodeficiency virus infection transmitted from an organ donor screened for HIV antibody. *M.M.W.R.* 36:306, 1987.

27. Centers for Disease Control. *National HIV Seroprevalence Surveys: Summary of Results* (2nd ed.). Atlanta: Centers for Disease Control, 1990. Pp. 1–26.

28. Centers for Disease Control. Possible transmission of human immunodeficiency virus to a patient during an invasive dental procedure. *M.M.W.R.* 39:489, 1990.

29. Centers for Disease Control. Preliminary analysis: HIV serosurvey of orthopedic surgeons, 1991. *M.M.W.R.* 40:309, 1991.

30. Centers for Disease Control. Protection against viral hepatitis: Recommendations of the Immunization Practices Advisory Committee (ACIP). *M.M.W.R.* 39(RR-2): 1, 1990.

31. Centers for Disease Control. Provisional Public Health Service inter-agency recommendations for screening donated blood and plasma for antibody to the virus causing acquired immunodeficiency syndrome. *M.M.W.R.* 34:1, 1985

32. Centers for Disease Control. Public Health Service guidelines for counseling and antibody testing to prevent HIV infection and AIDS. *M.M.W.R.* 36:509, 1987.

33. Centers for Disease Control. Public Health Service statement on management of occupational exposure to human immunodeficiency virus, including considerations regarding zidovudine postexposure use. *M.M.W.R.* 39 (RR-1): 1, 1990.

34. Centers for Disease Control. Recommendations for prevention of HIV transmission in health-care settings. *M.M.W.R.* 36(Suppl. 25): 1, 1987.

35. Centers for Disease Control. Recommendations for preventing transmission of human immunodeficiency virus and hepatitis B virus to patients during exposure-prone invasive procedures. *M.M.W.R.* 40(RR-8): 1, 1991.

36. Centers for Disease Control. Office of Public Affairs Statement. Atlanta, GA, Dec. 4, 1991.

37. Centers for Disease Control. Recommendations for preventing transmission of infection with human T-lymphotropic virus type III/ lymphadenopathy-associated virus during invasive procedures. *M.M.W.R.* 35:221, 1986.

38. Centers for Disease Control. Recommended infection control practices for dentistry. *M.M.W.R.* 35:237, 1986.

39. Centers for Disease Control. Safety in training for and providing CPR. *J.A.M.A.* 255: 2926, 1986.

40. Centers for Disease Control. Testing donors of organs, tissues, and semen for antibody to human T-lymphotropic virus type III/ lymphadenopathy associated virus infection. *M.M.W.R.* 35:448, 1986.

41. Centers for Disease Control. Transmission of HIV through bone transplantation: Case report and public health recommendations. *M.M.W.R.* 37:597, 1988.

42. Centers for Disease Control. Update: Human immunodeficiency virus infections in health-care workers exposed to blood of infected patients. *M.M.W.R.* 36:285, 1987.

43. Centers for Disease Control. Update: Transmission of HIV infection during an invasive dental procedure—Florida. *M.M.W.R.* 40: 21, 1991.

44. Centers for Disease Control. Update: Transmission of HIV infection during invasive dental procedures—Florida. *M.M.W.R.* 40:377, 1991.

45. Centers for Disease Control. Update: Universal precautions for prevention of human immunodeficiency virus, hepatitis B virus, and other bloodborne pathogens in health-care settings. *M.M.W.R.* 37:377, 1988.

46. Chamberland, M.E., et al. Health-care workers who donate blood: Surveillance for occupationally acquired HIV-1 infection (abstr. 7). In: *Program and Abstracts of the Thirty-First Interscience Conference on Antimicrobial Agents and Chemotherapy, Chicago, 1991.* Washing-

ton, DC: American Society for Microbiology, 1991.

47. Chamberland, M.E., et al. Health-care workers with AIDS: National surveillance update. *J.A.M.A.* 266:3459, 1991.

48. Chirgwin, K., Rao, T.K.S., and Landesman, S.H. HIV infection in a high prevalence dialysis unit. *AIDS.* 3:731, 1989.

49. Cohen, M.M., Duncan, P.G., and Tate, R.B. Does anesthesia contribute to operative mortality? *J.A.M.A.* 260:2859, 1988.

50. Cohen, N.D., et al. Transmission of retrovirus by transfusion of screened blood in patients undergoing cardiac surgery. *N. Engl. J. Med.* 320:1172, 1989.

51. Cole, R.P., and Gault, D.T. Glove perforation during plastic surgery. *Br. J. Plast. Surg.* 42:481, 1989.

52. Comer, R.W., et al. Management considerations for an HIV positive dental student. *J. Dent. Educ.* 55:187, 1991.

53. Comodo, N., et al. Risk of HIV infection in patients and staff of two dialysis centers: Seroepidemiological findings and prevention trends. *Eur. J. Epidemiol.* 4:171, 1988.

54. Cowan, D.N., et al. HIV infection among members of the US Army Reserve Components with medical and health occupations. *J.A.M.A.* 265:2826, 1991.

55. Cyr, W.H., and Lytle, C.D. Investigation of defects in barriers using virus probes (abstr. C/33). Presented at the Third International Conference on Nosocomial Infections, Atlanta, 1990.

56. Danila, R.N., et al. A look-back investigation of patients of an HIV-infected physician: Public health implications. *N. Engl. J. Med.* 325:1406, 1991.

57. Dodds, R.D.A., et al. Surgical glove perforation. *Br. J. Surg.* 75:966, 1988.

58. Donahue, J.G., et al. Transmission of HIV by transfusion of screened blood. *N. Engl. J. Med.* 323:1709, 1990.

59. Durand, E., Le Jeunne, C., and Hugues, F.C. Failure of prophylactic zidovudine after suicidal self-inoculation of HIV-infected blood. *N. Engl. J. Med.* 324:1062, 1991.

60. Duthie, G.S., Johnson, S.R., Packer, G.J., and Mackie, I.G. Eye protection, HIV, and orthopaedic surgery. *Lancet* 1:481, 1988.

61. Ebbesen, P., et al. Lack of antibodies to HTLV-III/LAV in Danish dentists. *J.A.M.A.* 256:2199, 1986.

62. ECRI. Needlestick-prevention devices. *Health Devices* 20:154, 1991.

63. Emergency Cardiac Care Committee of the American Heart Association. Risk of infection during CPR training and rescue: Supplemental guidelines. *J.A.M.A.* 262:2714, 1989.

64. Evans, R., and Shanson, D.C. Serological studies on health care workers caring for patients with human immunodeficiency virus. *J. Hosp. Infect.* 12:85, 1988.

65. Fahey, B.I., Koziol, D.E., Banks, S.M., and Henderson, D.K. Frequency of nonparenteral occupational exposures to blood and body fluids before and after universal precautions training. *Am. J. Med.* 90:145, 1991.

66. Favero, M.S., and Bond, W.W. Sterilization, Disinfection, and Antisepsis in the Hospital. In: *Manual of Clinical Microbiology* (5th ed.). Washington, DC: American Society for Microbiology, 1991. Pp. 183–200.

67. Flynn, N.M., et al. Absence of HIV antibody among dental professionals exposed to infected patients. *West. J. Med.* 146:439, 1987.

68. Friedland, G.H., et al. Lack of transmission of HTLV-III/LAV infection to household contacts of patients with AIDS or AIDS-related complex with oral candidiasis. *N. Engl. J. Med.* 314:344, 1986.

69. Friedland, G.H., and Klein, R.S. Transmission of the human immunodeficiency virus. *N. Engl. J. Med.* 317:1125, 1987.

70. Garner, J.S., and Favero, M.S. *Guideline for Handwashing and Hospital Environmental Control, 1985.* Atlanta: Department of Health and Human Services, Public Health Service, Centers for Disease Control (HHS publication no. [CDC] 99-1117), 1985.

71. Garner, J.S., and Simmons, B.P. CDC guideline for isolation precautions in hospitals. *Infect. Control* 4 (Suppl.): 245, 1983.

72. Gerberding, J.L. Does knowledge of HIV infection decrease the frequency of occupational exposures to blood? *Am. J. Med.* 91 (Suppl. 3B): 308S, 1991.

73. Gerberding, J.L., et al. Risk of exposure of surgical personnel to patients' blood during surgery at San Francisco General Hospital. *N. Engl. J. Med.* 322:1788, 1990.

74. Gerberding, J.L., et al. Risk to dental professionals from occupational exposure to human immunodeficiency virus: Follow-up (abstr. 698). In: *Program and Abstracts of the Twenty-Seventh Interscience Conference on Antimicrobial Agents and Chemotherapy, New York, 1987.* Washington, DC: American Society for Microbiology, 1987.

75. Gerberding, J.L., et al. Risk of transmitting the human immunodeficiency virus, cytomegalovirus, and hepatitis B virus to health care workers exposed to patients with AIDS and AIDS-related conditions. *J. Infect. Dis.* 156:1, 1987.

76. Gerberding, J.L., et al. Zidovudine postexposure chemoprophylaxis for health care workers exposed to HIV at San Francisco

General (abstr. 977). In: *Program and Abstracts of the Thirty-First Interscience Conference on Antimicrobial Agents and Chemotherapy, Chicago, 1991.* Washington, DC: American Society for Microbiology, 1991.

77. Gerberding, J.L., Littell, C., Brown, A., and Raniro, N. Cumulative risk of HIV and hepatitis B (HBV) among health care workers (HCW): Longterm serologic followup & gene amplification for latent HIV infection (abstr. 959). In: *Proceedings of the Thirtieth Interscience Conference on Antimicrobial Agents and Chemotherapy,* Atlanta, 1990. Washington, DC: American Society for Microbiology, 1990.

78. Goebel, F.D., Zoller, W.G., Erfle, V., and Hehlmann, R. Resuscitation of patients with AIDS: Risk of HIV transmission. *AIDS Forschung* 5:277, 1988.

79. Goldman, M., et al. Markers of HTLV-III in patients with end stage renal failure treated by hemodialysis. *Br. Med. J.* 293:161, 1986.

80. Gordin, F.M., Gibert, C., Hawley, H.P., and Willoughby, A. Prevalence of human immunodeficiency virus and hepatitis B virus in unselected hospital admissions: Implications for mandatory testing and universal precautions. *J. Infect. Dis.* 161:14, 1990.

81. Gruninger, S.E., et al. Hepatitis B, C, and HIV infection among dentists (abstr. 2131). *J. Dent. Res.* 70, 1991.

82. Harris, R.L., Boisaubin, E.V., Salyer, P.D., and Semands, D.F. Evaluation of a hospital admission HIV antibody voluntary screening program. *Infect. Control Hosp. Epidemiol.* 11: 628, 1990.

83. Henderson, D.K. Post-exposure chemoprophylaxis for occupational exposure to HIV-1. *Am. J. Med.* 91 (Suppl. 3B): 312S, 1991.

84. Henderson, D.K., et al. Risk for occupational transmission of human immunodeficiency virus type 1 (HIV-1) associated with clinical exposures: A prospective evaluation. *Ann. Intern. Med.* 113:740, 1990.

85. Henderson, D.K., and Gerberding, J.L. Prophylactic zidovudine after occupational exposure to the human immunodeficiency virus: An interim analysis. *J. Infect. Dis.* 160: 321, 1989.

86. Henry, K., et al. Long-term follow-up of health care workers with work site exposure to human immunodeficiency virus. *J.A.M.A.* 263:1765, 1990.

87. Hersch, B.S., et al. Acquired immunodeficiency syndrome in Romania. *Lancet* 338: 645, 1991.

88. Hussain, S.A., Latif, A.B.A., and Choudhary, A.A.A.A. Risk of surgeons: A survey of accidental injuries during operations. *Br. J. Surg.* 75:314, 1988.

89. Jagger, J., Hunt, E.H., Brand-Elnaggar, J., and Pearson, R.D. Rates of needlestick injury caused by various devices in a university hospital. *N. Engl. J. Med.* 319:284, 1988.

90. Johnson, G.K., and Robinson, W.S. Human immunodeficiency virus-1 (HIV-1) in the vapors of surgical power instruments. *J. Med. Virol.* 33:47, 1991.

91. Jones, P.D. HIV transmission by stabbing despite zidovudine prophylaxis. *Lancet* 338: 884, 1991.

92. Jui, J., et al. Multicenter HIV and hepatitis B seroprevalence study. *J. Emerg. Med.* 8:243, 1990.

93. Kelen, G.D., et al. Human immunodeficiency virus infection in emergency patients: Epidemiology, clinical presentations and risk to health-care workers. The Johns Hopkins experience. *J.A.M.A.* 262:516, 1989.

94. Kelley, P.W., et al. Human immunodeficiency virus seropositivity among members of the active duty US Army 1985–89. *Am. J. Public Health* 80:405, 1990.

95. Klein, R.S., et al. Low occupational risk of human immunodeficiency virus infection among dental professionals. *N. Engl. J. Med.* 318:86, 1988.

96. Krasinski, K., Borkowsky, W., Bebenroth, D., and Moore, T. Failure of voluntary testing for human immunodeficiency virus to identify infected parturient women in a high risk population. *N. Engl. J. Med.* 318:185, 1988.

97. Kuhls, T.L., et al. Occupational risk of HIV, HBV, and HSV-2 infections in health care personnel caring for AIDS patients. *Am. J. Public Health* 77:1306, 1987.

98. LaFon, S.W., et al. A double-blind, placebo-controlled study of the safety and efficacy of Retrovir (Zidovudine, ZDV) as a chemoprophylactic agent in health care workers exposed to HIV (abstr. 489). In: *Proceedings of the Thirtieth Interscience Conference on Antimicrobial Agents and Chemotherapy, Atlanta, 1991.* Washington, DC: American Society for Microbiology, 1991.

99. Landesman, S., et al. Serosurvey of human immunodeficiency virus infection in parturients. *J.A.M.A.* 258:2701, 1987.

100. Lange, J.M.A., et al. Failure of zidovudine prophylaxis after accidental exposure to HIV-1. *N. Engl. J. Med.* 322:1375, 1990.

101. Lifson, A.R. Do alternate modes for transmission of human immunodeficiency virus exist? *J.A.M.A.* 259:1353, 1988.

102. Looke, D.F.M., and Grove, D.I. Failed prophylactic zidovudine after needlestick injury. *Lancet* 335:1280, 1990.

103. Lowenfels, A.B., and Wormser, G. Risk of transmission of HIV from surgeon to patient (lett.). *N. Engl. J. Med.* 325:888, 1991.

104. Lynch, P., Jackson, M.M., Cummings, M.J., and Stamm, W.E. Rethinking the role of isolation precautions in the prevention of noso-

comial infections. *Ann. Intern. Med.* 107: 243, 1987.

105. Management of Assaultive Behavior Task Force. *Management of Assaultive Behavior: Staff Manual.* Sacramento: California Department of Mental Health, 1991. P. 107.

106. Mann, J.M., et al. HIV seroprevalence among hospital workers in Kinshasa, Zaire: Lack of association with occupational exposure. *J.A.M.A.* 256:3099, 1986.

107. Marcus, R., Bell, D.M., Culver, D., and Cooperative Emergency Department Study Group. Contact with blood of patients infected with HIV among emergency care providers (abstr. Th.C. 604). In: *Proceedings of the Sixth International Conference on AIDS, San Francisco, 1990.*

108. Marcus, R., and CDC Cooperative Needlestick Study Group. Surveillance of healthcare workers exposed to blood from patients infected with the human immunodeficiency virus. *N. Engl. J. Med.* 319: 1118, 1988.

109. Marcus, R., et al. Prevalence and incidence of human immunodeficiency virus among patients undergoing long-term hemodialysis. *Am. J. Med.* 90:614, 1991.

110. Marcus, R., et al. Zidovudine use after occupational exposure to HIV-infected blood (abstr. 979). In: *Program and Abstracts of the Thirty-First Interscience Conference on Antimicrobial Agents and Chemotherapy, Chicago, 1991.* Washington, DC: American Society for Microbiology.

111. Marcus R., Kay, K., and Mann, J. Transmission of human immunodeficiency virus (HIV) in health-care settings worldwide. *Bull. W.H.O.* 67:577, 1989.

112. Mast, S.M., and Gerberding, J.L. Factors predicting infectivity following needlestick exposure to HIV; an in vitro model. *Clin. Res.* 39:58A, 1991.

113. Matta, H., Thompson, A.M., and Rainey, J.B. Does wearing two pairs of gloves protect operating theatre staff from skin contamination? *Br. Med. J.* 297:597, 1988.

114. McCormick, R.D., et al. Epidemiology of hospital sharps injuries: A 14-year prospective study in the pre-AIDS and AIDS eras. *Am. J. Med.* 91 (Suppl. 3B): 301, 1991.

115. McKinney, W.P., and Young, M.J. The cumulative probability of occupationally acquired infection: The risks of repeated exposures during a surgical career. *Infect. Control Hosp. Epidemiol.* 11:243, 1990.

116. McLeod, G.G. Needlestick injuries at operations for trauma: Are surgical gloves an effective barrier? *J. Bone Joint Surg.* 71-B: 489, 1989.

117. McMahon, B.J., et al. Acute hepatitis B virus infection: Relation of age to the clinical expression of disease and subsequent develop-

118. McNicholas, A., Jones, D.J., and Sibley, G.N.A. AIDS: The contamination risk in urological surgery. *Br. J. Urol.* 63:565, 1989.

119. Mishu, B., et al. A surgeon with AIDS: Lack of evidence of transmission to patients. *J.A.M.A.* 264:467, 1990.

120. Napoli, V.M., and McGowan, J.E. How much blood is in a needlestick? *J. Infect. Dis.* 155: 828, 1987.

121. National Institute of Allergy and Infectious Diseases. Recommendations for zidovudine: Early infection. *J.A.M.A.* 263:1606, 1990.

122. N'Galy, B., et al. Human immunodeficiency virus among employees in an African hospital. *N. Engl. J. Med.* 319:1123, 1988.

123. New York State Department of Health. *Policy Statement and Guidelines: Health Care Facilities and HIV-Infected Medical Personnel.* Albany: New York State Department of Health, 1991.

124. Novick, L.F., et al. HIV seroprevalence in newborns in New York State. *J.A.M.A.* 261: 1745, 1989.

125. Occupational Safety and Health Administration. Occupational exposure to bloodborne pathogens. *Fed. Reg.* 56:64004, 1991.

126. Oksenhendler, E., et al. HIV infection with seroconversion after a superficial needlestick injury to the finger. *N. Engl. J. Med.* 315:582, 1986.

127. Panlilio, A., et al. Blood and amniotic fluid contact during obstetrical procedures (abstr. Th.C. 603). In: *Proceedings of the Sixth International Conference on AIDS, San Francisco, 1990.*

128. Panlilio, A.L., et al. Blood exposures during surgical procedures. *J.A.M.A.* 265:1533, 1991.

129. Pate, J.W. Risks of blood exposure to the cardiac surgical team. *Ann. Thorac. Surg.* 50:248, 1990.

130. Peterman, T.A., et al. HTLV-III/LAV infection in hemodialysis patients. *J.A.M.A.* 255:2324, 1986.

131. Petersen, N.J. An assessment of the airborne route in hepatitis B transmission. *Ann. N.Y. Acad. Sci.* 353:157, 1980.

132. Pokrovsky, V.V., and Eramova, E.U. Nosocomial outbreak of HIV infection in Elista, USSR (abstr. W.A.O.5). Presented at the Fifth International Conference on AIDS, Montreal, Canada, 1989.

133. Polder, J., et al. Investigation of inadvertent injection of HIV-contaminated material during nuclear medicine procedures (abstr. M.C. 3324). Presented at the Seventh International Conference on AIDS, Florence, Italy, June 1991.

134. Popejoy, S.L., and Fry, D.E. Blood contact

and exposure in the operating room. *Surg. Gynecol. Obstet.* 172 : 480, 1991.

135. Porter, J., et al. Management of patients treated by a surgeon with HIV infection. *Lancet* 335 : 113, 1990.

136. Puro, V., et al. Zidovudine prophylaxis after occupational exposure to HIV in health care workers (abstr. S.C. 767). In: *Proceedings of the Sixth International Conference on AIDS, San Francisco, 1990.*

137. Quebbeman, E.J., Telford, G.L., and Condon, R.E. Should Patients or Health Care Workers Be Screened for Human Immunodeficiency and Hepatitis Viruses? In: R.J. Howard (Ed.), *Infectious Risks in Surgery.* Norwalk, CT: Appleton and Lange, 1991. Pp. 117–123.

138. Rhame, F.S. The HIV-infected surgeon. *J.A.M.A.* 264 : 507, 1990.

139. Risi G.F., et al. Human immunodeficiency virus: Risk of exposure among health care workers at a southern urban hospital. *South. Med. J.* 82 : 1079, 1989.

140. Rogers, M.F., et al. Lack of transmission of human immunodeficiency virus from infected children to their household contacts. *Pediatrics* 85 : 210, 1990.

141. Saviteer, S.M., White, G.C., Cohen, M.S., and Jason, J. HTLV-III exposure during cardiopulmonary resuscitation. *N. Engl. J. Med.* 313 : 1606, 1985.

142. Schecter, W.P. Precautions in the Operating Room for HIV-Infected Patients and Patients with Hepatitis. In: R.J. Howard (Ed.), *Infectious Risks in Surgery.* Norwalk, CT: Appleton and Lange, 1991. Pp. 97–109.

143. Serrano, C.W., Wright, J.W., and Newton, E.R. Surgical glove perforation in obstetrics. *Obstet. Gynecol.* 77 : 525, 1991.

144. Shih, C.C., et al. Postexposure prophylaxis with zidovudine suppresses human immunodeficiency virus type 1 infection in SCID-hu mice in a time-dependent manner. *J. Infect. Dis.* 163 : 625, 1991.

145. Shirley, L.R., and Ross, S.A. Risk of transmission of human immunodeficiency virus by bite of an infected toddler. *J. Pediatr.* 114 : 425, 1989.

146. Siew, C., Gruninger, S.E., and Hojvat, S. Screening dentists for HIV and hepatitis B. *N. Engl. J. Med.* 318 : 1400, 1988.

147. Simmons, B., et al. Infection control for home health. *Infect. Control Hosp. Epidemiol.* 11 : 362, 1990.

148. Soderstrom, C.A., et al. HIV infection rates in a trauma center treating predominantly rural blunt trauma victims. *J. Trauma* 29 : 1526, 1989.

149. St. Louis, M.E., et al. Seroprevalence rates of human immunodeficiency virus infection at sentinel hospitals in the United States. *N. Engl. J. Med.* 323 : 213, 1990.

150. Quebbeman, E.J., et al. Risk of blood contamination and injury to operating room personnel. *Ann. Surg.* 214 : 614, 1991.

151. Tokars, J.I., et al. Percutaneous injuries during surgical procedures (abstr. Th.D. 108). Presented at the Seventh International Conference on AIDS, Florence, Italy, June 1991.

152. Tsoukas, C.M., et al. Lack of transmission of HIV through human bites and scratches. *J. A.I.D.S.* 1 : 505, 1988.

153. United Kingdom Health Departments. *AIDS-HIV Infected Health Care Workers: Occupational Guidance for Health Care Workers, Their Physicians, and Employers.* London: Department of Health, Dec. 1991.

154. Ward, J.W., et al. Transmission of human immunodeficiency virus (HIV) by blood transfusions screened as negative for HIV antibody. *N. Engl. J. Med.* 318 : 473, 1988.

155. Weiss, S.H., et al. Risk of human immunodeficiency virus (HIV-1) infection among laboratory workers. *Science* 239 : 68, 1988.

156. Ward, J.W., et al. Transmission of human immunodeficiency virus (HIV) by blood transfusions screened as negative for HIV antibody. *N. Engl. J. Med.* 318 : 473, 1988.

157. Wong, E.S., et al. Are universal precautions effective in reducing the number of occupational exposures among health care workers? A prospective study of physicians on a medical service. *J.A.M.A.* 265 : 1123, 1991.

158. Wormser, G.P., et al. Polymerase chain reaction for seronegative health care workers with parenteral exposure to HIV-infected patients. *N. Engl. J. Med.* 321 : 1681, 1989.

159. Wright, J.G., et al. Mechanisms of glove tears and sharp injuries among surgical personnel. *J.A.M.A.* 266 : 1668, 1991.

Infections Due to Infusion Therapy

Dennis G. Maki

Reliable intravascular access for administration of fluids and electrolytes, blood products, drugs, nutritional support, and hemodynamic monitoring is now one of the most essential features of modern medical care (Table 40-1). Each year in the United States, approximately 150 million intravascular devices are purchased by hospitals and clinics. The vast majority are peripheral venous catheters and needles; however, more than 5 million central venous devices of various types are sold in the United States annually.

Unfortunately, infusion therapy has substantial and generally underappreciated potential for producing iatrogenic disease, particularly septicemia originating from the percutaneous device used for vascular access or from contamination of the infusate administered through the device. More than one-half of all epidemics of nosocomial bacteremia or candidemia reported in the world literature between 1965 and 1991 derived from vascular access in some form [128, 132]. Nosocomial intravascular device-related bacteremia or candidemia in hospitalized patients is associated with a twofold to threefold increase in attributable mortality [1, 114, 155, 230].

Infusion-related sepsis is often unrecognized, in large part owing to its relative infrequency. The percentage of infusions identified as producing bloodstream infection is sufficiently low—less than 1 percent on average—that most physicians or nurses are unlikely to encounter more than an occasional case. However, even a low incidence of infection applied to the estimated 30 million patients who receive infusion therapy in U.S. hospitals annually translates to an estimated 50,000 to 100,000 septicemias nationwide each year [128, 132]. Because neither the de-

Table 40-1.   Applications of infusion therapy in the 1990s

Fluid and electrolyte replacement
Transfusion therapy
  Blood products
  Exchange transfusion
  Plasmapheresis and apheresis
Intravenous drug administration
  Immediate circulatory access for critically ill
    patients
  High blood and tissue levels
  Drugs that cause tissue necrosis
Hemodialysis
Hemodynamic monitoring
  Central venous catheters
    Central venous pressure
  Pulmonary artery flow-directed (Swan-Ganz)
    catheters
    Pulmonary artery pressure
    Pulmonary artery occlusion (left atrial filling)
      pressure
    Thermodilution cardiac output
  Arterial catheters
    Continuous arterial blood pressure
Total parenteral nutrition
  Hyperalimentation (central venous catheters)
  Peripheral parenteral nutrition (peripheral IV
    catheters)
  Special nutritional support regimens for
    Sepsis
    Acute renal failure
    Hepatic failure
    Cardiac cachexia
    Pancreatitis
    Acquired immunodeficiency syndrome
Intraarterial cancer chemotherapy

vice nor the infusate is cultured, the source of the bloodstream infection in a large proportion of cases is never identified.

Intravascular device-related sepsis is largely preventable. Therefore, the primary goal must not be simply to identify and treat these iatrogenic infections but to prevent them. By critically scrutinizing existent knowledge of the pathogenesis and epidemiology of device-related infection—the reservoirs of nosocomial pathogens and modes of transmission to patients' infusions—rational and effective guidelines for prevention can be formulated.

Sources and Forms of Infusion-Related Inflammation and Sepsis

There are two major sources of bloodstream infection associated with any intravascular device: infection of the cannula* wound or contamination of the fluid (infusate) administered through the cannula. Cannulas, which cause most *endemic* device-related infections, produce septicemia far more frequently than contaminated infusate, the source of most *epidemics* of infusion-associated sepsis [132].

It is important to understand the different stages and forms of device-related inflammation or infection, which range from infusion phlebitis (usually unrelated to infection) to asymptomatic colonization of the intravascular device (usually by skin commensals with little intrinsic virulence) to overwhelming septic shock originating from an infected thrombus in a cannulated great central vein or from infusate heavily contaminated by gram-negative bacilli.

Infusion Phlebitis

Infusion phlebitis, defined as inflammation of the cannulated vein—pain, erythema, tenderness, or an inflamed, palpable, thrombosed vein—is a common cause of pain and discomfort to the millions of patients who receive infusion therapy through peripheral cannulas each year in U.S. hospitals. Most investigators have concluded that infusion phlebitis is primarily a physicochemical phenomenon, and prospective studies have shown that the cannula material, length, and bore size, operator skill on insertion, the anatomic site of cannulation, duration of cannulation, frequency of dressing changes, character of the infusate, and host factors such as patient age, race, and gender, and the presence of underlying diseases significantly influence the risk of infusion phlebitis (Table 40-2).

In a recent prospective clinical study of

Cannula is a generic term that refers to all types of percutaneous devices used for vascular access, including small steel (scalp-vein or butterfly) needles and plastic catheters of numerous forms and sizes.

Table 40-2. Risk factors for infusion phlebitis in peripheral intravenous therapy identified in prospective studies by multivariate discriminant analysis or in prospective, randomized, controlled trials*

Catheter material	*Infusate*
Polypropylene > Teflon	Low pH solutions (e.g., dextrose-containing)
Silicone elastomer > polyurethane	Potassium chloride
Teflon > polyetherurethane	Hypertonic glucose, amino acids, lipid for par-
Teflon > steel needles	enteral nutrition
Catheter size	*Antibiotics* (especially beta-lactams, vancomycin,
Large bore > smaller bore	metronidazole)
8-inch > 2-inch Teflon	High rate of flow of intravenous fluid
Insertion in emergency room > inpatient units	(>90 ml/hr)
Disinfection of skin with antiseptic prior to cathe-	Disinfection of insertion site prior to catheter in-
ter insertion	sertion: none > chlorhexidine-alcohol
Experience, skill of person inserting catheter	Frequent intravenous site dressing changes: daily
House officers, nurses > hospital intravenous	> every 48 hr
team	*Catheter-related infection*
House officers, nurses > decentralized unit in-	Host factors
travenous nurse educator	"Poor-quality" peripheral veins
Increasing duration of catheter placement in site	Insertion site: *upper arm, wrist > hand*
Subsequent catheters beyond the first	Age
	Children: older > younger
	Adults: younger > older
	Sex: *female > male*
	Race: whites > blacks
	Underlying medical disease
	Individual biologic vulnerability

*Denotes significantly greater risk of phlebitis. Factors found to be significant predictors of risk in a recent prospective study of 1,054 peripheral IV catheters in the University of Wisconsin Hospital and Clinics are indicated by italic type.
Note: Factors shown not to increase risk in well-controlled, prospective randomized trials include catheters made of polyethylene versus siliconized elastomer or of Teflon versus siliconized elastomer; type of antiseptic solutions used for cutaneous disinfection; use of topical antimicrobial ointment or spray on catheter insertion sites; type of dressing (e.g., gauze versus transparent polyurethane dressing); dressing change every 48 hours versus not at all; administration of infusate by gravity flow versus pump; administration of intravenous antibiotics by slow infusion versus intravenous push over 2 minutes; maintenance of heparin locks with saline versus heparinized saline); frequency of routine change of intravenous delivery system.
Source: D.G. Maki and M. Ringer, Risk factors for infusion-related phlebitis with small peripheral venous catheters. A randomized controlled study. *Ann. Intern. Med.* 114:845, 1991.

1,054 peripheral IV catheters inserted in patients in our university hospital, we found that the Kaplan-Meier risk for phlebitis exceeded 50 percent by the fourth day after catheterization [149]. Intravenous antibiotics (relative risk [RR], 2.0), female gender (RR, 1.9), prolonged catheterization longer than 48 hours (RR, 1.8), and catheter material (polyetherurethane [Vialon] vs. tetrafluoroethylene-hexafluoropropylene [Teflon], RR, 0.7) were strong predictors of phlebitis in a Cox proportional hazards model (each, *p* <.003) [149]. The best-fit model for severe

phlebitis identified the same predictors in addition to catheter-related infection (RR, 6.2), phlebitis with the previous catheter (RR, 15), and anatomic site (hand-forearm, RR, 0.7; wrist-forearm, RR, 0.6).

Although not all studies have identified an association between phlebitis and catheter-related infection [81, 98], this large, prospective study [149] showed a strong statistical association, as have other studies [2, 49, 118, 151, 229]. In our study, local catheter-related infection was associated with a twofold to sixfold increased risk for severe phlebitis by proportional hazards modeling. Phlebitis can also be produced by contaminated infusate. Patients with septicemia from intrinsically contaminated fluid in a large nationwide epidemic traced to the contaminated products of one U.S. manufacturer in 1970–1971 had a much higher incidence of phlebitis than patients receiving intravenous fluids who did not develop sepsis [146].

Clearly, only a small proportion of patients with IV cannula–associated peripheral vein phlebitis have infusion-related infection, and fewer than one-half of patients with peripheral IV catheter–related septicemia show phlebitis; however, the presence of phlebitis connotes a substantially increased risk of infection and indicates the need for immediate removal of the catheter to reduce the severity of phlebitis and to prevent local catheter-related infection from progressing to septicemia.

Cannula-Related Infections

Between 5 and 25 percent of intravascular devices are colonized by skin organisms at the time of removal, as reflected by semiquantitative or quantitative cultures showing large numbers of organisms on the intravascular portion of the removed catheter or its tip. Colonization, which in most instances is asymptomatic, provides the biologic setting and is necessary for systemic infection to occur and can be considered synonymous with local infection. However, colonized cannulas are more likely than noncolonized ones to show phlebitis or local inflammation, especially purulence (pus spontaneously draining or expressable from the insertion site), and are far more likely to cause systemic infection (e.g., cannula-related bacteremia or fungemia) [6, 151, 184].

One of the most serious forms of intravascular device–related infection occurs when intravascular thrombus surrounding the cannula becomes infected, producing septic (suppurative) thrombophlebitis with peripheral IV cannulas [106, 250] or septic thrombosis of a great central vein with centrally placed catheters [243, 259, 260]. With

suppurative phlebitis, the vein becomes an intravascular abscess, discharging myriad microorganisms into the bloodstream, even after the cannula has been removed. The clinical picture is predictable: overwhelming sepsis with high-grade and often unremitting septicemia. This syndrome is most likely to be encountered in burned patients or other intensive care unit (ICU) patients who have heavy cutaneous colonization and who develop cannula-related infection that goes unrecognized, permitting microorganisms to proliferate to high levels within the intravascular thrombus (see Chap. 34). The catheter insertion site is devoid of signs of inflammation more than half the time, and the clinical picture may not present until several days after the catheter has been removed. *In any patient with an intravascular catheter who develops high-grade bacteremia or candidemia, persisting* after *an infected cannula has been removed, it is likely the patient has infected thrombus in the recently cannulated vein and may even have developed secondary endocarditis or seeding to other distant sites.*

The microorganisms most frequently implicated in suppurative phlebitis are the same organisms that cause uncomplicated cannula-related septicemia: *Staphylococcus aureus*, nosocomial aerobic gram-negative bacilli and, especially in recent years, *Candida* species [106, 243, 250, 260]. Suppurative phlebitis of peripheral IV catheters is now rare, and the syndrome of intravenous suppuration is predominantly a complication of central venous catheters, characteristically catheters that have been left in place for many days in heavily colonized ICU patients.

Sepsis from Contaminated Infusate

It is important to recognize that the infusate—parenteral fluid, blood products, or intravenous medications—administered through an intravascular device can also become contaminated and produce infusion-related septicemia, which is more likely than cannula-related infection to culminate in frank septic shock. Studies [13, 34, 85, 108, 138, 235] indicate that contaminated fluid is a rare cause of endemic infusion-related infection with most intravascular devices, with the exception of arterial infusions used for hemodynamic monitoring and, possibly, surgically implanted cuffed Hickman or Broviac catheters. Most nosocomial epidemics of infusion-related septicemia, however, have been traced to contamination of infusate by gram-negative bacilli, introduced during its manufacture (*intrinsic contamination*) or during its preparation and administration in the hospital (*extrinsic contamination*) [128, 132].

Diagnosis of Infusion-Related Septicemia
Clinical Features

Although meticulous aseptic technique during cannula insertion and good follow-up care will greatly reduce the risk of device-related septicemia, sporadic cases and even epidemics can still be expected to occur occasionally because of human error, intrinsically contaminated products, or the undue susceptibility to infection of many patients. If affected patients are to survive, the causal relationship between an infusion and a picture of sepsis must be recognized as early as possible.

The general clinical features of infusion-related septicemia are nonspecific and indistinguishable from bloodstream infections arising from any local site of infection, such as urinary tract or an infected surgical wound (Table 40-3). Infusion-related sepsis occurring in ICU patients can be particularly insidious: Bacteremia or fungemia is usually identified by positive blood cultures but is attributed to nosocomial pneumonia or urinary tract or surgical wound infection or is simply accepted as "cryptogenic" and treated empirically. More than one-half of all outbreaks of infusion-related bloodstream infection have occurred in ICUs [128, 132].

Certain clinical, epidemiologic, and microbiologic findings can be extremely helpful to the clinician evaluating a hospitalized patient with a picture of nosocomial sepsis or cryptogenic bacteremia or candidemia, and then point toward an intravascular device as the source (see Table 40-3):

1. The patient is an unlikely candidate for sepsis, being healthy and without underlying predisposing diseases [146, 163].

Table 40-3. Clinical, epidemiologic, and microbiologic features of intravascular device–related sepsis

Nonspecific	*Suggestive of Device-Related Etiology*
Fever	Patient unlikely candidate for sepsis (e.g., young, no underlying diseases)
Chills, shaking rigors[a]	
Hypotension, shock[a]	Source of sepsis inapparent
Hyperventilation, respiratory failure	No identifiable local infection
Gastrointestinal[a]	Intravascular device in place, especially central venous catheter
Abdominal pain	
Vomiting	Inflammation or purulence at insertion site
Diarrhea	Abrupt onset, associated with shock[a]
Neurologic[a]	Sepsis refractory to antimicrobial therapy or dramatic improvement with removal of cannula and infusion[a]
Confusion	
Seizures	Septicemia caused by staphylococci (especially coagulase-negative staphylococci), *Corynebacterium* (especially JK-1) or *Bacillus* species, or *Candida, Trichophyton, Fusarium,* or *Malassezia* species[b]

[a]Commonly seen in overwhelming gram-negative sepsis originating from contaminated infusate, peripheral suppurative phlebitis, or septic thrombosis of a central vein.
[b]Conversely, septicemia caused by streptococci, aerobic gram-negative bacilli, or anaerobes is unlikely to derive from an intravascular device [163].

2. There is no local infection to account for a picture of sepsis [146, 163].

3. An intravascular device, *especially a central venous catheter,* is in place at the outset of sepsis [163].

4. Local inflammation [6, 12, 151, 184], especially purulence at the insertion site [12, 184], though present in only a minority of cases, is strongly suggestive of catheter-related infection.

5. Abrupt onset, associated with fulminant shock, is suggestive of a massively contaminated infusate [133].

6. Nosocomial bloodstream infection caused by staphylococci [163], especially coagulase-negative staphylococci, *Corynebacterium* (especially JK-1) or *Bacillus* species, or *Candida* [163], *Fusarium, Trichophyton,* or *Malassezia* species suggests an intravascular device is involved. (In contrast, bacteremia caused by streptococci, aerobic gram-negative bacilli [especially *Pseudomonas aeruginosa*], or anaerobes is very unlikely to have originated from an infected intravascular device [163].)

7. Sepsis is refractory to antimicrobial therapy or dramatic improvement with removal of the cannula or discontinuation of the infusion strongly suggests an intravascular device as the point of origin [146, 163].

During a large nationwide outbreak of infusion-related septicemia in 1970–1971 due to intrinsic contamination of one U.S. manufacturer's products, patients treated with antibiotics to which the epidemic organisms were susceptible remained clinically septic, continued to have positive blood cultures after 24 hours or more of appropriate therapy, and did not improve clinically until their infusions were serendipitously or intentionally removed [146].

Focal retinal lesions (cotton-wool spots) are commonly seen in patients with deep *Candida* infection deriving from central catheters, even in those without positive blood cultures [93]. Careful ophthalmologic examination should be a routine feature of the evaluation of patients with central venous catheters with suspected catheter-related sepsis, especially patients receiving total parenteral nutrition (TPN). Septicemia from arterial catheters may be heralded by embolic lesions that manifest as tender, erythematous papules, 5 to 10 mm in diameter, appearing in the distal distribution of the involved artery, usually in the palm or sole (Osler's nodes) [46, 145]. Arterial bleeding from the insertion site is often the harbinger of septicemia caused by an infected arterial catheter and may denote an infective pseudoaneurysm [8, 145]. Endocarditis, particularly right-sided, is a rare but well-documented complication of flow-directed pulmonary artery catheters [64, 210].

Blood Cultures

Blood cultures are essential to the diagnosis of device-related bloodstream infection and, in any patient suspected of infusion-related infection, two or three separate 10-ml blood cultures should be drawn [9, 261], ideally from peripheral veins by separate venipunctures (see Chap. 9). If the patient is receiving antimicrobial therapy, blood cultures obtained immediately before a dose is due to be administered, when blood antibiotic levels are likely to be low, may provide a higher yield. Use of resin-containing media to adsorb and remove any antibiotic present in the blood specimen may also increase the yield [245]. The use of a biphasic system, such as the Isolator (E.I. DuPont, Nemours and Co., Wilmington, DE), appears to enhance the laboratory detection of fungemia significantly [89].

The volume of blood cultured is critical to maximize the yield of cultures for diagnosis of bacteremia or candidemia: In adults, obtaining at least 20 ml (but ideally 30 ml) per drawing, with each specimen containing 10 or 15 ml and inoculated into aerobic and anaerobic media, significantly improves the yield as compared to obtaining only 5 ml at each drawing and culturing a smaller total volume [101, 115, 263]. It is rarely necessary to obtain more than two 15-ml cultures or three 10-ml cultures in a 24-hour period. If at least 30 ml of blood is cultured, 99 percent of detectable bacteremias should be identified [263].

It is common practice in many ICUs to draw blood cultures through central venous or arterial catheters or, in neonates, through umbilical catheters. Comparative studies of standard blood cultures drawn through central venous or arterial catheters in adults have generally shown good concordance with cultures drawn by percutaneous peripheral venipuncture [102, 189, 266], but rates of false-positive (contaminated) cultures can be considerably higher with catheter-drawn specimens [30]. The practice of drawing blood cultures through indwelling vascular catheters probably ought not to be encouraged because of the risk of introducing contamination during the manipulation [142, 180]. If, however, to preserve dwindling superficial veins it is considered unavoidable to use a vascular catheter to obtain blood cultures, an attempt should be made to use a newly inserted catheter [102, 189, 266] and to draw at least every other specimen by percutaneous venipuncture.

If the laboratory is prepared to do pour-plate blood cultures or has available an automated quantitative system for culturing blood, such as the Isolator system, catheter-drawn blood cultures can permit the diagnosis of device-related septicemia to be made with reasonable sensitivity and specificity (both in the range of 90 percent) without removing the catheter [18, 72, 200, 254, 262]. With infected catheters, a quantitative blood culture drawn through the catheter usually shows a marked step-up (more than tenfold) in the concentration of organisms as compared with quantitative blood cultures drawn at the same time percutaneously through a peripheral vein. Quantitative catheter-drawn blood cultures probably have their greatest utility in the diagnosis of device-related infection with surgically implanted cuffed Hickman or Broviac catheters and subcutaneous central venous ports [18, 72, 200, 262].

Microbiology of Device-Related Sepsis
The microbiologic profile of bloodstream infection can strongly suggest an infusion-related source (Table 40-4). Cryptogenic staphylococcal bacteremia (particularly with coagulase-negative staphylococci), bacteremia caused by *Bacillus* or *Corynebacterium* (especially JK-1) species or *Enterococcus,* or fungemia caused by *Candida, Fusarium, Trichophyton,* or *Malassezia* species, especially in a patient with a central venous catheter, is most likely to reflect catheter-related infection [128, 132, 163].

Bacteremias caused by members of the tribe Klebsielleae—*Enterobacter cloacae* or especially *Enterobacter agglomerans*—or by non-*aeruginosa* pseudomonads, particularly *Pseudomonas cepacia* or *Pseudomonas maltophilia,* or *Citrobacter* species, in the setting of infusion therapy may signal an epidemic and should prompt studies to rule out contaminated infusate [129]. A cluster of cases should mandate a full-scale investigation, which may include culturing of large numbers of in-use infusions and informing the local, state, and federal public health authorities. Such actions averted a large nationwide epidemic in 1973 when, prompted by five unexplained bacteremias in three hospitals, intrinsic contamination of one U.S. company's products was identified and a recall put into effect so rapidly that the outbreak was limited to the five initially recognized cases [39]. It must be emphasized, however, that for surveillance of bacteremias to be maximally effective, all blood isolates must always be fully speciated. Failure to do so during the 1970–1971 nationwide epidemic traced to the contaminated products of one U.S. manufacturer resulted in preeminent hospitals experiencing large numbers of cases that were recognized as infusion-related only in retrospect [146].

Cryptogenic nosocomial bacteremia caused by psychrophilic (cold-growing) organisms, such as non-*aeruginosa* pseudomonads, *Achromobacter, Flavobacterium, Enterobacter,* or *Serratia* species [25, 185], or by *Salmonella* [92] or *Yersinia* species [40], with a picture of overwhelming sepsis, may indicate a contaminated blood product.

Cultures of Intravascular Devices
Many laboratories still culture vascular catheters qualitatively, amputating the tip aseptically and immersing it in liquid media.

Table 40-4. Microorganisms most frequently encountered in various forms of intravascular line–related infection

Source	Pathogens
Catheter-related	
Peripheral IV catheter	Coagulase-negative staphylococci
	Staphylococcus aureus
	Candida species
Central venous catheters	Coagulase-negative staphylococci
	S. aureus
	Candida species
	Corynebacterium species (especially JK-1)
	Klebsiella and *Enterobacter* species
	Mycobacterium species
	Trichophyton beiglii
	Fusarium species
	Malassezia furfur*
Contaminated intravenous infusate	Tribe Klebsielleae
	Enterobacter cloacae
	Enterobacter agglomerans
	Serratia marcescens
	Klebsiella species
	Pseudomonas cepacia, X. maltophilia, P. acidivorans, P. pickettii
	Citrobacter freundii
	Flavobacterium species
	Candida tropicalis
Contaminated blood products	*E. cloacae*
	S. marcescens
	Achromobacter species
	Flavobacterium species
	Pseudomonas species
	Salmonella species
	Yersinia species

*Also seen with peripheral IV catheters in association with the administration of lipid emulsion for parenteral nutritional support.

Unfortunately, a positive culture by this technique is diagnostically nonspecific since a single organism picked up from the skin as the catheter is removed can produce a positive (false-positive) culture. Most catheter-related septicemias derive from local infection of the transcutaneous cannula tract (vide infra). Culture of the external surface of the withdrawn cannula should reflect the microbiologic status of the wound, and quantitative culture should more accurately distinguish infection from contamination. We have developed a standardized semiquantitative method for culturing vascular cannulas in solid media [151]. That technique is as follows:

Before removing the cannula, the skin about the insertion site is first cleansed with an alcohol-impregnated pledget, to reduce contaminating skin flora and remove any residual antimicrobial ointment. After the alcohol dries, the cannula is withdrawn, taking care to avoid contact with the surrounding skin. If pus can be expressed from the cannula wound, it should be Gram-stained and cultured separately. For short catheters and steel needles, the entire length of the cannula is amputated at the former skin surface–catheter junction, using sterile scissors and breaking the steel needle off with a sterile hemostat; for longer catheters, two 1-inch segments (the tip and the intracutaneous segment) are cultured (Fig. 40-1). The segments are transported to the laboratory in sterile

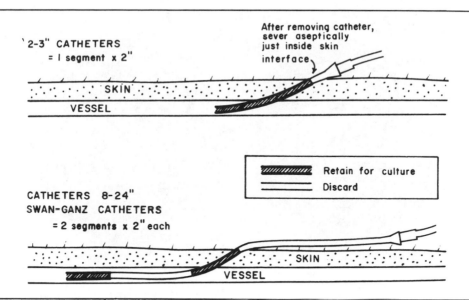

Fig. 40-1. Segments of vascular cannulas cultured semiquantitatively. (Reproduced with permission from D.G. Maki et al., A semiquantitative culture method for identification of catheter-related infection in the burn patient. *J. Surg. Res.* 22:513, 1977.)

transport tubes (Culturette, American Scientific Products). The segments should be cultured as soon as possible after removal, ideally within 2 hours.

In the laboratory, using a flamed forceps, the segment is transferred onto the surface of a 100-mm 5% sheep blood agar plate and is rolled back and forth at least four or five times across the agar surface to ensure adequate surface-to-surface contact (Fig. 40-2). Plates are incubated aerobically at 37°C for at least 72 hours. It is unnecessary to culture intravascular devices anaerobically.

Colony counts on semiquantitative cultures are bimodally distributed as they are in quantitative urine cultures. The method provides excellent discrimination between infection and insignificant contamination acquired during catheter removal (Fig. 40-3). Fifteen or more colony-forming units (cfu) growing on a semiquantitative plate is regarded as a positive culture, denoting local cannula-related infection [143A, 151]. Based on experience with more than 10,000 devices, positive cultures found using this technique have shown a 15 to 40 percent association with concordant bloodstream infection. Cannulas posi-

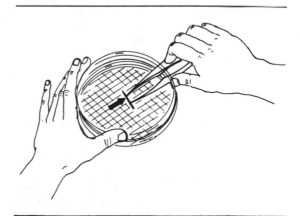

Fig. 40-2. Semiquantitative method for culturing vascular cannulas. It is important to maintain downward pressure on the segment as it is rolled (or, for bent or twisted segments, smeared) back and forth at least four or five times across the surface of the blood-agar plate, to ensure adequate surface-to-surface contact. (Reproduced with permission from D.G. Maki et al., A semiquantitative culture method for identification of catheter-related infection in the burn patient. *J. Surg. Res.* 22:513, 1977.)

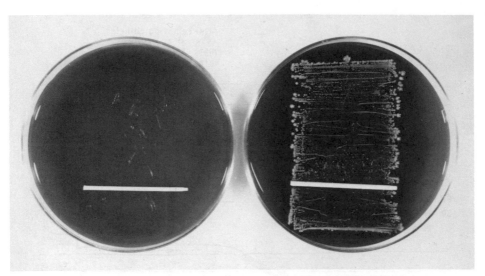

Fig. 40-3. Typical negative (left) and positive (right) semiquantitative cultures of catheter segments. The two catheters were removed at the same time from a patient with *Staphylococcus aureus* septicemia originating from the semiquantitative culture-positive catheter. (Catheter segments are left on the plates for perspective only.) (Reproduced with permission from D.G. Maki et al., A semiquantitative culture method for identification of catheter-related infection in the burn patient. *J. Surg. Res.* 22:513, 1977.)

tive on semiquantitative culture are also strongly associated with local inflammation [151], further affirming the validity of considering a positive semiquantitative culture (more than 15 cfu) as representative of local infection.

Studies in many centers have shown that culturing catheter segments semiquantitatively on solid media [47, 51, 73, 233, 234] or culturing the intravascular segment quantitatively in liquid media—removing organisms from the catheter by sonication [29, 219]—both provide excellent sensitivity and specificity for diagnosis of vascular catheter-related infection, with good correlation between high colony counts and catheter-related bloodstream infection. Not surprisingly, direct Gram stains [51] or acridine orange stains [272] of intravascular segments of removed catheters also show excellent correlation with quantitative techniques for culturing catheters and can permit rapid diagnosis of catheter-related infection.

Given the strong evidence implicating cutaneous microorganisms in the genesis of most bacteremias caused by short-term, noncuffed intravascular catheters, a number of studies have shown that a quantitative culture [21, 41, 69, 71, 117, 139, 144, 159] or Gram stain [159] of skin at the insertion site can also identify infected catheters with reasonable sensitivity and specificity, greatly exceeding an assessment based solely on clinical signs of infection. The combination of culturing both skin at the insertion site and the catheter hub has been reported to provide even better sensitivity for diagnosis of catheter-related infection, without removing the catheter [41, 69, 117].

To diagnose infection caused by contaminated infusate reliably requires a sample of fluid to be aspirated from the line and cultured quantitatively [129]. A variety of techniques are now available for culturing or processing parenteral admixtures and fluid medications in the laboratory for microbial contamination [5, 91, 122, 157]. Since there is no evidence that anaerobic bacteria can grow in parenteral crystalloid admixtures, anaerobic culture techniques are not necessary unless blood or another biologic product is involved (see Chap. 9).

Definitions for Infusion-Related Infection

Using the results of semiquantitative or quantitative culture of the catheter and cultures of the hub of the catheter and of infusate aspirated from the line at the time the catheter is removed, and concomitant blood cultures, it is possible to formulate rigorous definitions for intravascular device–related infection [136, 139, 164]:

Local catheter-related infection A positive semiquantitative (or quantitative) culture of the catheter, considered synonymous with colonization of the catheter

Catheter-related septicemia (1) Semiquantitative (or quantitative) catheter culture and blood cultures positive for the same species, with a negative culture of infusate; (2) no other clear-cut source for the septicemia disclosed by clinical and microbiologic data

Septicemia due to a contaminated hub (1) Isolation of the same species from the catheter hub and from separate percutaneously drawn blood cultures, with semiquantitative (or quantitative) culture of the catheter negative for the infecting organism; (2) no other identifiable source for the septicemia

Septicemia due to contaminated infusate (1) Isolation of the same species from infusate and from separate, percutaneously drawn blood cultures with semiquantitative (or quantitative) culture of the catheter negative for the infecting organism; (2) no other identifiable source for the septicemia

These definitions, which have served us well for research purposes, may be unnecessarily rigorous for use in clinical nosocomial infection surveillance because very few clinicians obtain cultures of catheter hubs or infusate, even if the cannula is cultured. Moreover, patients with disseminated candidiasis originating from an infected catheter often have negative blood cultures. The Centers for Disease Control (CDC), Atlanta, has used the following definitions for vascular device-related infection for the purposes of nosocomial infection surveillance [82]:

Organism isolated from culture of arteries or veins [of access site] removed during surgery

or

Evidence of infection at involved [vascular access] site seen during surgery or by histopathologic examination

or

One of the following: fever (higher than 38°C) or pain, erythema, or heat at involved vascular [access] site *and* more than 15 colonies cultured from intravascular cannula tip using semiquantitative culture method

with or without

Recognized pathogen isolated from blood culture that is not related to [local] infection at another [extravascular] site

or

One of the following: fever (greater than 38°C), chills, or hypotension *and* any of the following:

1. Common skin contaminant isolated from two blood cultures drawn on separate occasions *and* organism is not related to infection at another site

2. Common skin contaminant isolated from blood cultures from patient with intravascular access device *and* physician institutes appropriate antimicrobial therapy

or

Patient younger than 12 months has one of the following: fever (exceeding 38°C), hypothermia (less than 37°C), apnea, or bradycardia *and* any of the following:

1. Common skin contaminant isolated from two blood cultures drawn on separate occasions *and* organism is not related to infection at another site

2. Common skin contaminant isolated from blood cultures from patient with intravascular device *and* physician institutes appropriate antimicrobial therapy

Cannula-Associated Infection
Incidence of Cannula-Related Septicemia
Intravascular device–related sepsis is perhaps the least frequently recognized nosoco-

mial infection. The true incidence of vascular catheter–related bloodstream infection is underestimated in most centers because a catheter is often not suspected as a source of the patient's clinical picture of nosocomial sepsis and is not cultured. Prospective studies in which every device enrolled is cultured at the time of removal indicate clearly that every type of intravascular device carries some risk of causing bacteremic infection, but the magnitude of risk per device varies greatly, depending on its type [128].

Table 40-5 shows representative rates of infection for various types of intravascular devices. The lowest rates are now with small peripheral intravenous (IV) steel needles and Teflon or polyurethane catheters: Large prospective studies have shown rates of infection of approximately 0.2 bacteremias per 100 peripheral IV catheters [49, 52, 81, 98, 118, 147, 149, 244, 248, 252, 265]; two large comparative trials have shown that if IV cannulas are inserted under conditions of scrupulous asepsis, plastic catheters probably pose no greater risk of device-related bacteremia or candidemia than steel needles [252, 265]. Peripheral venous catheters inserted by surgical cutdown are now rarely used, which is probably desirable, because older studies reported

rates of complicating septicemia in the range of 6 percent [168]. Recent prospective studies of arterial catheters used for hemodynamic monitoring have found rates of infusion-related bacteremia in the range of 1 percent [56, 148, 222, 246].

The device that poses the greatest risk of iatrogenic septicemia today is the central venous catheter in its many forms [27, 175, 251, 264]. Numerous prospective studies of short-term noncuffed single-lumen or multilumen catheters inserted percutaneously into the subclavian or internal jugular vein have found rates of catheter-related septicemia in the range of 3 to 5 percent, and rates of 7 to 10 percent have not been uncommon in some hospitals [7, 21, 51, 71, 139, 144, 175, 206, 228]. Percutaneously inserted, noncuffed central venous catheters used for hemodialysis have been associated with the highest rates of bacteremia, in the range of 10 percent [43, 182, 218]. Notably, recent studies suggest that peripherally inserted central venous catheters (PICCs) pose a substantially lower risk of catheter-related bloodstream infection [60, 87] and bear closer study. Swan-Ganz pulmonary artery catheters used for hemodynamic monitoring have been associated with rates of infection in the range of 1 to 3 percent [23,

Table 40-5. Approximate risks of septicemia associated with various types of devices for intravascular access

Type of Device	Representative Rate	Range
Short-term temporary access (no. septicemias per 100 devices)		
Peripheral IV cannulas		
Winged steel needles	<0.2	0–1
Peripheral IV catheters		
Percutaneously inserted	0.2	0–1
Cutdown	6	—
Arterial catheters	1	0–1
Central venous catheters		
All-purpose, multilumen	3	1–7
Swan-Ganz	1	0–5
Hemodialysis	10	3–18
Long-term indefinite access (no. septicemias per 100 device-days)		
Peripherally inserted central venous catheters	0.20	—
Cuffed central catheters (e.g., Hickman, Broviac)	0.20	0.10–0.53
Subcutaneous central venous ports (e.g., Infusaport, Port-a-cath)	0.04	0.00–.10

Source: Based on data from recently published prospective studies.

100, 164]. The lowest rates of infection with central venous devices have been with surgically implanted Hickman or Broviac catheters that incorporate a Dacron cuff, which have been associated with rates of infection in the range of 0.2 bacteremias per 100 catheter-days [80, 195, 268], and surgically implanted subcutaneous central venous ports, associated with rates of bacteremia in the range of 0.04 per 100 device-days [28, 42, 121].

It is estimated that 50,000 to 100,000 patients in U.S. hospitals develop a nosocomial intravascular device–related bloodstream infection each year, 90 percent of which originate from central venous catheters of various types [128]. Data from the National Nosocomial Infections Surveillance Study of the CDC have shown that the incidence of secondary bloodstream infections, deriving from identifiable local infections such as of the urinary tract, postoperative surgical wounds, or pneumonias, has remained stable over the past decade. In contrast, the incidence of primary nosocomial bloodstream infections, the largest proportion of which derive from in-

travascular devices, has increased more than twofold over this same period [14, 128], reflecting the great increase in the use of infusion therapy and, especially, the use of central venous devices of all types. It seems clear that the greatest hope for reducing the risk of intravascular device–related sepsis will come from better understanding of the pathogenesis of infection with central venous catheters, which will form the basis for more effective strategies for prevention.

Epidemiology

The first and perhaps most important question that must be addressed in order to develop effective strategies for prevention is to determine the major source or sources of microorganisms that can colonize a percutaneous intravascular device (Fig. 40-4) and cause invasive infection leading to bacteremia or candidemia. An intravascular catheter can easily become colonized extraluminally by organisms from the patient's cutaneous microflora. Microorganisms can also contaminate the catheter hub where the administration set attaches to the catheter or can gain access to

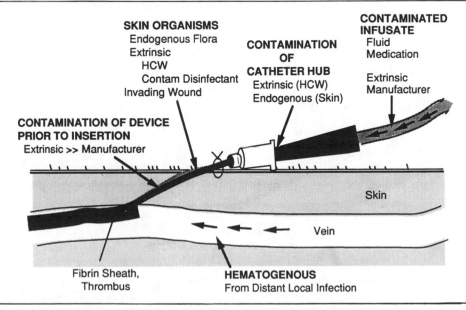

Fig. 40-4. Sources of intravascular cannula–related infection. The major sources are the skin flora, contamination of the catheter hub, contamination of infusate, and hematogenous colonization of the intravascular device and its fibronectin-fibrin sheath. (*HCW* = health care worker.)

the fluid column and be infused directly into the patient's bloodstream. The device can also become infected hematogenously from remote sources of local infection, or the device might even be contaminated during its manufacture, which, fortunately, is very rare.

A large body of clinical and microbiologic data indicate that most intravascular device–related septicemias caused by short-term, percutaneously inserted, noncuffed catheters are caused by extraluminal microorganisms of cutaneous origin that invade the transcutaneous insertion wound at the time the catheter is inserted or in the days following insertion:

Numerous prospective studies of intravascular device–related infection have shown that coagulase-negative staphylococci, the predominant aerobic species on the human skin [126], is now the most common agent of catheter-related bacteremia [7, 14, 23, 28, 42, 43, 52, 56, 60, 80, 87, 100, 121, 128, 132, 147, 148, 168, 175, 182, 195, 206, 218, 222, 228, 244, 246, 248, 251, 252, 265, 268]. The vast majority of vascular catheter–related bloodstream infections are caused by microorganisms that colonize the skin of hospitalized patients: staphylococci, both coagulase-negative and coagulase-positive (*Staphylococcus aureus*); *Candida*, *Corynebacterium*, and *Bacillus* species; and, to a much lesser degree, aerobic gram-negative bacilli (see Table 40-4).

● Prospective studies have shown strong concordance between organisms present on skin surrounding the catheter wound and organisms recovered from central venous catheters producing septicemia [21, 41, 43, 69, 71, 73, 117, 139, 144, 159, 164, 233]. There appears to be a direct parallel between the level and profile of cutaneous colonization at the insertion sites of short-term central venous, arterial, and peripheral IV catheters and the risk of catheter-related bloodstream infection [131].

● Hemodialysis patients with cutaneous colonization by *S. aureus* experience sixfold higher rates of vascular access–related bacteremia [270]. Similarly, use of recombinant interleukin-2, with or without lymphokine-activated killer (LAK) cells for cancer immunotherapy, which is associated with frequent dermatotoxicity (desquamation) and heavy cutaneous colonization by *S. aureus,* has been associated with a prohibitively high incidence of venous catheter–related *S. aureus* bacteremia [232].

● Burned patients, who have huge populations of microorganisms on the skin surface, experience very high rates of catheter-related sepsis [73, 143, 196] (see Chap. 34).

● Numerous outbreaks of intravascular catheter–related sepsis have been traced to contaminated cutaneous antiseptics [61, 74, 109] (see Chap. 15).

● High counts of microorganisms on semiquantitative culture of the external surface of a removed catheter are strongly associated with bacteremia caused by the catheter [6, 7, 47, 51, 71, 73, 87, 139, 143, 144, 151, 164, 175, 206, 228, 233, 234].

● Microscopic examination of infected central venous catheters has shown microorganisms primarily on the external surface [51, 272].

● A recent prospective study has shown that use of a more effective cutaneous disinfectant, such as chlorhexidine, for disinfection of the insertion site at the time of catheter insertion and in follow-up care of the catheter greatly reduces the risk of infusion-related septicemia [136].

● Prospective trials have shown that antiseptics or antimicrobials applied topically to the intravascular catheter insertion site can also reduce the risk of catheter-related septicemia [96, 119, 137].

● Surgically implanted Broviac or Hickman catheters, which have a subcutaneous Dacron cuff that becomes ingrown by tissue and poses a mechanical barrier against invasion of the tract by skin organisms, have been associated with considerably lower rates of catheter-related bacteremia (approximately 0.20 cases per 100 catheter-days) [80, 195, 268] than short-term, noncuffed central venous catheters (approximately 0.6 to 1.0 per 100 catheter-days) [7, 23, 43, 51, 100, 139, 144, 164, 175, 182, 206, 218, 228] (see Table 40-4). In clinical trials, a subcutaneous silver-impregnated cuff that can be attached to a short-term central venous catheter at the time of insertion has proved capable of reducing the risk of catheter-related septicemia [71, 139]. In addition, recent studies have shown that novel central venous catheters with an external antimicrobial [110] or antiseptic [152] coat greatly reduce the risk of catheter-related infection, including bacteremia [152].

Studies by Sitges-Serra and his co-workers [120, 226, 227] have shown that the hubs of intravascular catheters can also become con-taminated, particularly by coagulase-negative staphylococci, and can cause catheter-related bacteremia, but contaminated hubs do not appear to be as important in the pathogenesis of intravascular device–related sepsis with most short-term, noncuffed venous cathe-ters as do microorganisms on the skin surface that invade the intracutaneous catheter tract (Tables 40-6, 40-7) [41, 43, 73, 136, 139, 147,

Table 40-6. Sources of central venous catheter–related infection, based on a prospective study of 234 central venous catheters

Potential Source	No. of Catheter-Related Infections Associated with the Source*	
	Local (> 15 cfu) [n = 40]	With Bacteremia [n = 6]
Colonization of skin of insertion site	36	6
Contamination of catheter hub	4	2
Contaminated intravenous fluid	1	1
Hematogenous colonization from remote site of infection	4	0
Unknown	1	0

cfu = colony-forming units.
*Based on finding bacteriologic concordance between the potential source (or sources) and the colonized catheter (> 15 cfu on semiquantitative culture). These were six catheters with more than one source of the organisms causing catheter-related infection: skin and hub, 3 (including 1 bacteremia); skin, hub, and fluid, 1 (including 1 bacteremia); skin and hematogenous source, 2.
Source: D.G. Maki et al., An attachable silver-impregnated cuff for prevention of infection with central venous cathe-ters. A prospective randomized multi-center trial. *Am. J. Med.* 85:307, 1988.

Table 40-7. Sources of organisms causing Swan-Ganz catheter–related infection, based on a prospective study of 297 catheters using molecular subtyping

Potential Source (showing > 10 cfu)	Concordance with Infected Catheter by:		
	Species, Antibiogram[a] (n = 65)	Plasmid Profile[b] (n = 24)	Projected Source(s)[c] (n = 65)
Skin	45 (69%)	19 (79%)	52 (80%)
Hub(s)	11 (17%)	3 (16%)	11 (17%)
Infusate	4 (6%)	—	2 (3%)
Extravascular portion of pulmo-nary artery catheter beneath external protective sleeve	5 (8%)	5 (21%)	12 (18%)
Hematogenous colonization from remote, unrelated infection	2 (3%)	—	2 (3%)
Indeterminate	—	3 (12%)	10 (15%)

cfu = colony-forming units.
[a] By speciation and antibiogram for bacteria, speciation for yeasts.
[b] With strains of coagulase-negative staphylococci from infected catheters similar by antibiogram.
[c] Based on extrapolation of the results of plasmid profile analysis to all 59 catheters infected with coagulase-negative staphylococci, combined with the results obtained with the six catheters infected by other organisms.
Source: L. Mermel, R. McCormick, and D.G. Maki, Epidemiology and pathogenesis of infection with Swan-Ganz catheters. A prospective study utilizing molecular subtyping. *Am. J. Med.* 91(3B):197S, 1991.

164]. However, with surgically implanted cuffed (Hickman or Broviac) catheters, microorganisms colonizing the hub may be the most important source of bloodstream infection deriving from these long-term devices [72, 262].

Central venous and arterial catheters can also become colonized hematogenously, from remote unrelated sites of infection [12, 142, 143A], but the evidence suggests that this occurs relatively infrequently [136, 139, 147, 148] (see Tables 40-6, 40-7).

Whereas infusate not infrequently becomes contaminated by small numbers of organisms—mainly skin commensals such as coagulase-negative staphylococci—with the exception of arterial catheters used for hemodynamic monitoring [136, 148], endemic bacteremic infections originating from contaminated infusate appear to be rare [136, 139, 147]. In contrast, contaminated infusate is the single most common identified cause of epidemic nosocomial bacteremia [128, 132], caused predictably by microorganisms ca-

pable of multiplying in parenteral glucose-containing admixtures, members of the tribe Klebsielleae (*Klebsiella, Enterobacter,* and *Serratia* species), non-*aeruginosa* pseudomonads (such as *Pseudomonas cepacia* or *Pseudomonas pickettii*), or *Citrobacter* species [129]. Nearly 100 epidemics of infusion-related septicemia since 1965 have been traced to contaminated infusate or intravenous medications, with microorganisms most frequently introduced during preparation or administration in the hospital (*extrinsic* contamination) or during its manufacture (*intrinsic* contamination).

In a prospective study of the mechanisms of catheter-related infection of 234 central venous catheters inserted in patients in 3 ICUs (see Table 40-6), it was found that the most common source of organisms colonizing 40 catheters and accounting for all 6 catheter-related bacteremias was skin of the insertion site. Four colonized catheters were also associated with concordant contamination of the hub; however, skin of the insertion site in both cases of septicemia and also intravenous

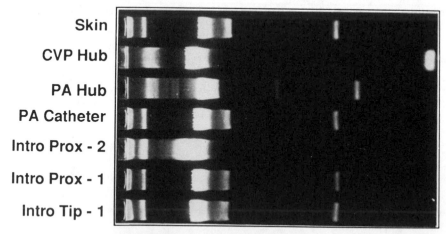

Skin
CVP Hub
PA Hub
PA Catheter
Intro Prox - 2
Intro Prox - 1
Intro Tip - 1

Fig. 40-5. Plasmid profiles of eight isolates of coagulase-negative staphylococci from potential sources of infection with an infected Swan-Ganz catheter that caused bacteremia. Isolate I from the proximal segment and tip of the introducer (and blood) shows concordance (three plasmids) with isolates from skin of the insertion site and from the infected introducer and pulmonary artery (PA) catheter. The second isolate from the introducer and the strains isolated from the PA catheter hub and the central venous pressure line (CVP) hub differ from the infecting strain. Presumed pathogenesis: skin → introducer [→ PA catheter] → blood. (*Intro Prox-1* and *Intro Prox-2* = isolates 1 and 2 from proximal introducer segment; *Intro Tip-1* = isolate from introducer tip; *CVP Hub* = isolate from hub of the central venous lumen of the PA catheter; *PA Hub* = isolate from hub of PA lumen of the PA catheter.) (Reproduced with permission from L. Mermel, R. McCormick, and D. G. Maki, Epidemiology and pathogenesis of infection with Swan-Ganz catheters. A prospective study using molecular epidemiology. *Am. J. Med.* 91(3B):197S, 1991.)

fluid in one were concordantly colonized. Four catheters exposed to candidemia or bacteremia from a distant and unrelated site of infection became hematogenously colonized, although none later produced septicemia, probably because the catheter had been removed shortly after the septicemia had been identified [139].

In a similar but larger recent study of the pathogenesis and epidemiology of catheter-related infection with Swan-Ganz pulmonary artery catheters, utilizing molecular subtyping of coagulase-negative *Staphylococcus* isolates by plasmid profile analysis (Fig. 40-5), it was found that 80 percent of the infected Swan-Ganz catheters showed concordance with organisms cultured from skin of the insertion site, 17 percent with a contaminated hub, and 18 percent with organisms contaminating the extravascular portion of the

pulmonary artery catheter beneath the external protective sheath (see Table 40-7); only 1 percent of infected catheters showed concordant contamination of infusate [164].

Analysis of risk factors predisposing to intravascular catheter–related infection by stepwise logistic regression of data from large prospective studies done in our center of peripheral IV catheters [147], arterial catheters used for hemodynamic monitoring [148], multilumen central venous catheters used in ICU patients [131], and Swan-Ganz pulmonary artery flotation catheters [164] shows that heavy cutaneous colonization of the insertion site is the single most powerful predictor of catheter-related infection with all types of short-term, percutaneously inserted catheters (Table 40-8). With central venous catheters in ICU patients, exposure to bacteremia or fungemia from a remote source or cathe-

Table 40-8. Risk factors for intravascular catheter–related infection based on multivariate analysis of data from large prospective studies in the University of Wisconsin Hospital and Clinics

Type of Catheter [Study]	*Catheters Studied (no.)*	*Risk Factors*	*Approximate Magnitude of Increased Risk[a]*
Peripheral IV [147]	2,050	Cutaneous colonization of site >10^2 cfu	3.9
		Contamination of catheter hub	3.8
		Moisture on site, under dressing	2.5
		Placement >3 days	1.8
		Systemic antimicrobial therapy	0.5
Arterial [148]	491	Cutaneous colonization of site >10^2 cfu	10.0
		Second catheter in site, placed over guide wire	—[b]
Central venous [273]	345	Exposure of catheter to unrelated bacteremia	9.4
		Cutaneous colonization of site >10^2 cfu	9.2
		Placement >4 days	—[b]
Pulmonary artery Swan-Ganz [164]	297	Cutaneous colonization of site >10^3 cfu	5.5
		Internal jugular vein cannulation	4.3
		Duration >3 days	3.1
		Placement in operating room under less stringent barrier precautions	2.1

cfu = colony-forming units.
[a] Relative risk or odds ratio (all p <.05, most p <.01).
[b] Indeterminate (e.g., zero incidence).

terization in the same site exceeding 4 days was also shown to be significant risk factors. With Swan-Ganz catheters, insertion into an internal jugular vein rather than the subclavian vein, catheterization exceeding 3 days, and insertion in the operating room using less stringent barrier precautions were each associated with significantly increased risk of catheter-related infection.

Pathogenesis

Examination of an infected intravascular device by scanning electron microscopy characteristically shows the surface covered by an amorphous film, presumably representing host proteins, with microcolonies of the infecting organism encased in a thick matrix of glycocalyx (slime), all comprising a biofilm (Fig. 40-6) [75, 154]. Studies of the pathobiology of prosthetic device–related infection have shown considerable differences in the capacity of microorganisms to adhere to various prosthetic materials in vitro and in vivo. In vitro, catheters made of Teflon or poly-

urethane are more resistant to bacterial adherence, especially by staphylococci, than catheters made of polyethylene, polyvinylchloride or, especially, silicone [10, 11, 16, 209, 220]. These differences diminish greatly, however, if the experiments are done with implanted catheters [16] or catheters precoated with specific plasma proteins [179, 256].

Adherence appears to be promoted by surface exoglycocalyx [44, 45, 57, 68, 116, 208, 214, 255] and hydrophobicity [11, 179, 214] of the infecting strain; however, the importance of glycocalyx in mediating adherence [68] or contributing materially to pathogenicity [116] is not yet completely resolved. Host factors may play the most important role of all in modulating microbial adherence to foreign bodies, such as intravascular catheters: It is now clear that following insertion or implantation of a device, the surface becomes coated by plasma and tissue proteins—albumin, fibrinogen-fibrin, fibronectin, laminin, collagen, and immunoglobulins [256]. Al-

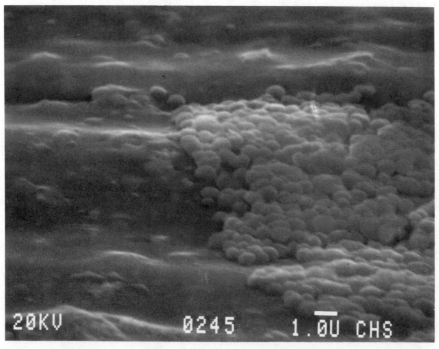

Fig. 40-6. Scanning electron micrograph of an infected central venous catheter (×6,000). The amorphous matrix encasing the microcolonies of *Staphylococcus epidermidis* is glycocalyx (slime).

bumin inhibits adherence whereas fibronectin and, to a lesser degree, fibrinogen-fibrin and laminin, promote adherence in vivo [94, 211, 255, 256, 258]. Thrombosis on the catheter surface also appears to promote adherence and catheter-associated infection [26, 241]. Whereas subtherapeutic levels of antibiotics reduce microbial adherence [179, 214], once microorganisms such as coagulase-negative staphylococci colonize a prosthetic surface, most defenses become secondarily impaired and are unable to eradicate the infection spontaneously [62, 88, 257]. Moreover, once associated with a foreign surface, microorganisms exhibit increased resistance to antimicrobials [65, 221]. It should be no surprise that most infections of prosthetic implants cannot be reliably cured by antimicrobial therapy alone, even with prolonged administration of high doses of bactericidal drugs.

Sepsis from Contaminated Infusate

It took more than 10 years after the initial introduction of intravascular plastic catheters before they were recognized as an important source of serious iatrogenic infection. However, it required more than 40 years and the occurrence of epidemic gram-negative bacteremias in hospitals across the United States in 1970 and 1971 [146] to bring about awareness that fluid given in intravascular infusions (infusage) also was vulnerable to contamination. It has become clear that whereas the vast majority of intravascular device–related bloodstream infections derive from infection of the percutaneous infection wound or contamination of the catheter hub, contamination of infusate is the most common cause of epidemic device-related bloodstream infection [132]. From 1965 to 1978, 28 (85 percent) of the 30 reported epidemics of infusion-related bacteremia were traced to contaminated infusate, organisms introduced during its manufacture (intrinsic contamination, which accounted for 7 of the 20 epidemics) or during its preparation and administration in the hospital (extrinsic contamination, which accounted for the remaining 21 outbreaks) [128, 132].

Growth Properties of Microorganisms in Parenteral Fluids

The pathogens implicated in nearly all reported septicemias linked to contaminated infusate have been aerobic gram-negative bacilli capable of rapid growth at room temperature (25°C) in the solution involved [129] (e.g., certain members of the family Enterobacteriaceae in 5% dextrose in water, pseudomonads, or *Serratia* species in distilled water). It must be emphasized that microbial growth in most parenteral solutions—the exception being lipid emulsion—is actually very limited.

In 1970, we evaluated the ability of 105 clinical isolates from human nosocomial infections, representing 9 genera and 13 species, to grow at room temperature (25°C) in 5% dextrose in water, the most frequently used commercial parenteral solution [143]. Of 51 strains of the tribe Klebsielleae (*Klebsiella, Enterobacter,* and *Serratia* species), 50 attained concentrations of 100,000 cfu/ml or more within 24 hours, beginning with washed organisms at an initial concentration of 1 cfu/ml. In contrast, only 1 of 54 strains of other bacteria, including staphylococci, *Escherichia coli, P. aeruginosa,* and *Acinetobacter* and *Candida* organisms, showed any growth in 5% dextrose in water. With most microorganisms, even with a level of contamination exceeding 10^6 cfu/ml fluid, evidence of microbial growth was not visible to the unaided eye.

A review of studies of the growth properties of microorganisms in various commercial parenteral products has shown [129] that rapid multiplication in 5% dextrose in water appears limited mainly to the tribe Klebsielleae and *P. cepacia;* in distilled water, to *P. aeruginosa, P. cepacia,* and *Acinetobacter* and *Serratia* species; and in lactated Ringer's solution, to *P. aeruginosa* and *Enterobacter* and *Serratia* species. Normal (0.9%) sodium chloride solution allows growth of most bacteria while supporting the growth of *Candida* rather poorly. *Candida* species can grow in the synthetic amino acid–25% glucose solutions used for TPN but only very slowly; most bacteria are greatly inhibited [84]. Most microorganisms grow rapidly in commercial 10% lipid emulsion for infusion (Intralipid) [53,

130]: In a study of 57 strains, we found that 12 of 13 bacterial species tested and *Candida* multiplied in Intralipid almost as rapidly as in bacteriologic media [130].

The growth properties of most microorganisms in commercial parenteral admixtures and the vast aggregate experience with epidemics and endemic bloodstream infections traced to contaminated infusate have shown that the identity of an organism causing nosocomial bloodstream infection can point strongly toward contaminated fluid as a plausible source: *Enterobacter* species, particularly *E. agglomerans* or *E. cloacae, Serratia marcescens, P. cepacia,* or *Citrobacter* cultured from the blood of a patient receiving infusion therapy should prompt strong suspicion of contaminated infusate (parenteral fluid or an intravenous drug) (see Table 40-4). Conversely, recovery of organisms such as *E. coli, Proteus* or *Acinetobacter* species, or staphylococci, all of which grow poorly, if at all, in parenteral admixtures, suggests strongly that the septicemia is unlikely to be due to contaminated infusate.

Mechanisms of Fluid Contamination

As noted, the vast majority of nosocomial bloodstream infections traced to contaminated infusate and reported in the literature occurred in an epidemic setting [128, 132]. Parenteral fluids do, however, commonly become contaminated during administration in the hospital. Recent culture surveys of in-use intravenous fluids in the hospital have shown contamination rates in the range of 1 to 2 percent [85, 108, 138, 235]. However, most of the organisms recovered from positive in-use cultures are common skin commensals that are generally considered of low virulence and grow poorly, if at all, in the parenteral admixture; the level of contamination (less than 10 cfu/ml) is usually far too low to produce clinical illness, even in the most compromised host. When contamination occurs with gramnegative bacilli capable of proliferation in the product to concentrations exceeding 10^2 to 10^3 cfu/ml, however, the risk of septicemia and even septic shock becomes substantial.

The likelihood of fluid becoming contaminated during use is directly related to the duration of uninterrupted infusion through the same administration set and the frequency with which the set is manipulated. Microorganisms gain access from air entering bottles as they evacuate, from entry points into the administration set (during injections into the line or aspiration of blood specimens from the intravascular device through the line), or at the junction between the administration set and the catheter hub. Microorganisms capable of growth in fluid, once introduced into a running infusion, may persist in an administration set for many days despite multiple replacements of the bottle or bag and high rates of flow [146, 166]; it appears more likely, however, that the majority of introduced contaminants are rapidly cleared from the running infusion by the continuous flow [13, 34, 108, 138, 235], especially if the organisms grow poorly in the fluid.

Occasionally a health care worker may encounter a filmy cloud within a glass intravenous bottle. Microscopic examination of the material reveals it is a filamentous fungus, such as *Penicillium* or *Aspergillus*. Molds usually gain access into glass intravenous bottles through microscopic cracks long before the bottle is hung for use and, over the course of weeks or months, grow to produce visible cloudiness or filmy precipitates. Fortunately, "fungus balls" in intravenous bottles have rarely resulted in systemic infection in patients receiving a mold-contaminated infusion [55].

The incidence of endemic nosocomial bacteremia caused by extrinsically contaminated intravenous fluid is not precisely known but, based on studies of the pathogenesis of device-related infection (see Tables 40-6, 40-7), is five- and tenfold lower than the incidence of endemic cannula-related septicemia. Moreover, prospective studies of the optimal interval for periodic replacement of administration sets (Table 40-9) [13, 34, 85, 108, 138, 235], which have involved cultures of infusate from large numbers of in-use infusions in an institution, have shown low rates of contamination and a very low risk of related septicemia. Metaanalysis of 5 studies in which more than

Table 40-9. Studies of replacing intravenous administration sets at periodic intervals as an infection control measure

Study	Location of Patients	Type of Infusions	No. of Sets Cultured	Prevalence of Contamination in Sets Changed at Intervals				Concordant Bacteremias
				24 Hr	48 Hr	72 Hr	Indefinite	
Buxton et al., 1979 [34]	Ward	Mainly peripheral[c]	2,537	0.4	0.6	—	—	0
Band and Maki, 1979 [13]	Ward, ICU	Peripheral	694	0.5	1.0	0.7	—	0
		Central, access[a,b] plus TPN	119	0	0	0	—	0
Gorbea et al., 1984 [85]	ICU	Peripheral (62%) plus central, access (38%)[a]	676	2.0	4.0	—	—	0
Josephson et al., 1985 [108]	Ward	Peripheral	219	—	0.8	—	0.8	0
Snydman et al., 1985 [235]	ICU	Peripheral plus central, access[a]	1,194	—	5.0	4.4		0
Maki et al., 1987 [138]	Ward, ICU	Peripheral	878	—	0.2	1.0		0
		Central, access	331	—	1.9	1.2		0
		Central, TPN	165	—	2.7	4.4		0
	Ward	All types	1,168	—	0.5	1.4		0
	ICU	All types	204	—	3.2	1.8		0

ICU = intensive care unit; TPN = total parenteral nutrition.

[a] Infusions for TPN excluded; contamination rates with different types of infusions not given.

[b] Access refers to a central venous infusion used for administering fluids, blood products, delivery of drugs, or hemodynamic monitoring, but not TPN.

Source: D.G. Maki, J.T. Botticelli, M.L. LeRoy, and T.S. Thielke, Prospective study of replacing administration sets for intravenous therapy at 48- vs 72-hour intervals: 72 hours is safe and cost effective. *J.A.M.A.* 258:1777, 1987.

6,000 infusions in 5 hospitals were prospectively cultured, with no associated septicemias identified, yields a confidence interval for the incidence of endemic septicemia due to contaminated infusate of less than 1 case per 2,000 intravenous infusions. It must be emphasized, however, that intravenous infusate can be identified as the source of septicemia only if it is cultured. Because this rarely occurs in most hospitals, unless a cluster of cases (an epidemic) occurs, it is likely that most sporadic (endemic) septicemias caused by contaminated fluid go unrecognized or are attributed to the intravascular cannula.

A recent study in our center has shown that approximately one-half of the septicemias caused by arterial infusions used for hemodynamic monitoring stem from contamination of fluid within the infusion [148], perhaps because these infusions consist of a stagnant column of fluid subjected to frequent manipulations, including frequent drawing of blood specimens. Over the past 20 years, there have been more than 25 epidemics of nosocomial bloodstream infection traced to contaminated fluid within arterial infusions used for hemodynamic monitoring [162]. Nearly all of these epidemics have involved gram-negative bacilli, particularly *Serratia marcescens,* pseudomonads, or *Enterobacter* species that are able to multiply rapidly within the 0.9% saline commonly used in these infusions.

Between less than 1 percent and 6 percent of blood units can be shown to contain small numbers of microorganisms [103, 267], yet endemic septicemias deriving from transfusion of contaminated blood products have been rare, presumably because most blood products are routinely refrigerated, because contamination is low-level, and because of universal awareness that blood products must be used promptly after removal from refrigeration. Sepsis from contaminated whole blood is often associated with overwhelming shock and a high mortality because of the massive numbers of psychrophylic (cold-growing) organisms such as *Serratia,* pseudomonads other than *P. aeruginosa,* and other

uncommon nonfermentative gram-negative bacilli, such as *Flavobacterium* species, in the contaminated unit [25, 90, 92, 185]. Bacteria have often been visible on a direct Gram-stained smear of the product. Blood products should be infused immediately after they are removed from refrigeration. On completion of the transfusion, the entire delivery system should be replaced. If sepsis is suspected of being related to a contaminated blood product, the entire infusion should be removed. Aliquots of the remaining product should be cultured aerobically *and* anaerobically on solid media at both 35° to 37°C and 16° to 20°C [129].

The most important measures for preventing rare sporadic septicemias from contaminated in-use infusate are stringent asepsis during the preparation and compounding of admixtures in the hospital central pharmacy or on individual patient care units and good aseptic technique when infusions are handled during use, such as during injections of medications or changing bags or bottles of fluids. It also appears that replacing the administration set at periodic intervals can prevent the buildup of dangerous introduced contaminants and further reduce the risk of related septicemia: During the large nationwide U.S. epidemic in 1971 due to the contaminated products of one manufacturer, the empiric recommendation that the entire delivery system be routinely changed every 24 hours and, at every change of the cannula, all equipment be totally replaced resulted in a substantial reduction in epidemic septicemias [146]. Since that time, routinely replacing the delivery system at periodic intervals has been practiced in most North American hospitals as an important measure for reducing the hazard of contaminated infusate.

Epidemic Infusion-Related Septicemias

Whereas 10 percent of all endemic nosocomial bloodstream infections in American hospitals are considered to be infusion-related,

more than one-half of all epidemics of hospital-acquired bacteremia derive from infusion
therapy in some form [128, 132].

Outbreaks due to Intrinsic Contamination

Since 1970, there have been more than a
dozen reported epidemics of infusion-related
septicemia caused by intrinsically contaminated infusate—blood products, intravenous
drugs, or Vacutainer tubes (Table 40-10)—illustrating the potential iatrogenic hazards of
infusion therapy. The frequency and size of
these outbreaks has declined in recent years
[128], reflecting appreciation for the importance of stringent quality control during the
manufacturing process.

The first and largest epidemic, and the outbreak that more than any other factor brought
about wide-scale appreciation of the iatrogenic hazards of infusion therapy, had its
onset in mid-1970 when one U.S. manufacturer of large-volume parenterals began
to distribute bottles of fluid with a new
elastomer-lined screw cap closure [146]. By
early 1970, the first cases of infusion-related
septicemia caused by biologically characteristic strains of *E. cloacae* and *E. agglomerans*
(designated *Erwinia* at the time) were reported to the CDC, although retrospective review subsequently showed that numerous
hospitals had been experiencing epidemic
bacteremias for a number of months. Although it was established very early (virtually
at the outset of the investigation), that epidemic bacteremias derived from contaminated intravenous fluids, the ultimate source
of contamination—*intrinsic* contamination of
the new closures—was not conclusively established until March 1971. Between July 1970
and April 1971, 25 U.S. hospitals reported to
the CDC nearly 400 cases of infusion-related
septicemia (Fig. 40-7). It is likely that there
were more than 10,000 cases nationwide.
More than 20 microbial species, including *E.
agglomerans,* were isolated from the closures
of previously unopened bottles. Organisms
were readily dislodged from the cap liner
and introduced into intravenous fluid when
bottles were handled under conditions du-

Table 40-10. Reported sources of epidemics of
intravascular device–related septicemia

Extrinsic contamination

Antiseptics or disinfectants

Arterial pressure–monitoring infusate
  Disinfectants
  Transducers
  Heparin
  Ice for chilling blood gas syringes
  Anaeroid pressure-calibration device
  Hand carriage by medical personnel

Hemodialysis-related
  Inadequate decontamination of reused dialyzer
    coils
  Contaminated dialysate water
  Contaminated disinfectants

Parenteral crystalloid solutions

Lipid emulsion

Hyperalimentation solutions in central pharmacy

Intravenous medications, multidose vials

Theft of fentanyl and replacement by (contaminated) distilled water

Blood products
  Whole blood, platelet packs
  Blood donor with silent transient bacteremia

Intravenous radiologic contrast media

Sclerosing solution for injecting esophageal
  varices

Central venous catheter hubs

Leaking catheter hub–administration set
  connections

Adhesive tape used in intravenous site dressings

Warming bath for blood products

Green soap

Hand carriage by medical personnel

Heart-lung machines

Intraaortic balloon pumps

Inordinately prolonged intravascular catheterization in intensive care unit patients

Intrinsic (manufacturer-related) contamination

Commercial intravenous crystalloid solutions,
  container closures

Blood products
  Platelet packs
  Human albumin
  Plasma protein fraction (PPF)

Intravenous drugs

Vacutainer tubes

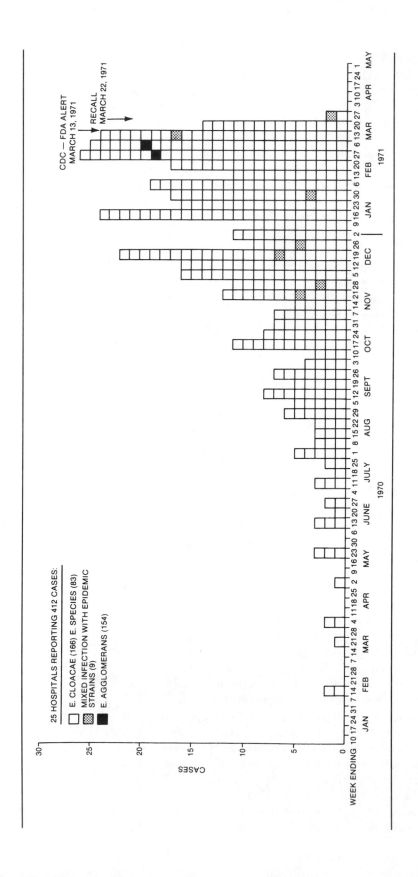

plicating normal in-hospital use. The appearance of epidemic septicemias within individual hospitals paralleled the distribution of the company's product with the new closures, and the epidemic was terminated only by a nationwide product recall in early April 1971.

Since 1971, numerous additional outbreaks have been reported from U.S. or European hospitals, all involving gram-negative bacilli and parenteral products shown to have become contaminated during manufacture [31, 36, 39, 104, 109, 129, 156, 161, 178, 183, 203, 207, 224, 239, 240]. Most have been of national scope. A large outbreak in Greece in 1981 [156] reaffirmed the findings of the large 1970–1971 U.S. outbreak [146] that screw-cap closures are not microbiologically safe for fluids used in medical care that must remain sterile. Outbreaks of pyrogenic reactions [240] and epidemic *Pseudomonas* septicemia [239] have been traced to intrinsically contaminated normal serum albumin, and epidemics of *E. cloacae* [178], *Salmonella* [92, 203], and *Yersinia* [40] septicemia have been traced to organisms from intrinsically contaminated platelet concentrates (which are maintained at 25°C to enhance viability). Most notable during the past decade have been outbreaks of *Pseudomonas* infection traced to intrinsic contamination of 10% povidone-iodine [36, 104, 178], the most widely used chemical antiseptic in North American hospitals.

All these outbreaks illustrate how subtle

Fig. 40-7. Nationwide outbreak of nosocomial bacteremias due to intrinsic contamination of one U.S. manufacturer's large-volume parenteral products. Three hundred ninety-seven cases of intravenous infusion–associated septicemia in 25 tabulated U.S. hospitals, occurring between July 1, 1970, and April 27, 1971, fulfilled criteria for epidemic cases. The epidemic was curtailed immediately within individual hospitals and nationally by a nationwide recall of the manufacturer's products. (*CDC* = Centers for Disease Control; *FDA* = Food and Drug Administration.) (Reproduced with permission from D.G. Maki et al., Nationwide epidemic of septicemia caused by contaminated intravenous products. *Am. J. Med.* 60:47, 1976.)

and insidious the factors that influence sterility can be. In many instances, there was no documented failure of the sterilization process. Instead, seemingly minor alterations in the manufacturing process resulted in contamination of individual units in the manufacturing plant after the sterilization stage [124].

Although intrinsic contamination is, fortunately, exceedingly rare, its potential for producing harm is great because of the large numbers of patients in multiple hospitals who may be affected. Also, direct contamination of infusate at the manufacturing level gives contaminants an opportunity to proliferate to dangerously high concentrations.

It seems likely that intrinsic contamination is a continuous source of infusion-related sepsis but of such low magnitude that the resulting septicemias are never identified as related to intrinsic contamination. Only when infusion-associated septicemias occur in epidemic numbers is intrinsic contamination likely to be suspected and proved. A substantial increase in the incidence of cryptogenic infusion-associated septicemia, particularly with *Enterobacter* species, pseudomonads, or *Citrobacter*, should prompt immediate and in-depth studies to exclude intrinsic contamination. There are no clinical clues to differentiate intrinsic from extrinsic contamination reliably. Bacteremia from contaminated fluid has the same manifestations and signs as catheter-related sepsis and other nosocomial septicemias. The few clues to infusion-related septicemia—absence of an obvious source of infection, its common occurrence in patients without a predilection to systemic infection, and the dramatic clinical response to discontinuing the infusion (see Table 40-3)—do not differentiate between intrinsic and extrinsic sources of contamination. The distinction must be made epidemiologically. *If intrinsic contamination of a commercially distributed product is identified or even strongly suspected, especially if clinical infections have occurred as a consequence, the local, state, and federal (CDC and Food and Drug Administration) public health authorities must be immediately contacted.* Unopened samples of the suspect lot or lots should be quarantined and saved for their analysis.

Outbreaks due to Extrinsic Contamination

Even when commercially manufactured products are sterile on arrival in the hospital, circumstances of hospital use can compromise that initial sterility. As previously noted, most sporadic infections deriving from infusion therapy, whether due to the cannula or contaminated infusate, are of extrinsic origin. Similarly, most reported epidemics have originated from exposure of multiple patients' infusions to a common source of contamination in the hospital [104, 128, 132].

Numerous outbreaks of infusion-related bacteremia have been caused by use of unreliable chemical antiseptics or antiseptics such as aqueous benzalkonium in the United States and aqueous chlorhexidine in the United Kingdom, for cutaneous disinfection [61, 74, 109] or, in recent years, for decontaminating transducer components employed in hemodynamic monitoring [162] (see Table 40-10).

Despite the numerous reports of epidemic gram-negative septicemias deriving from contaminated disinfectants used for decontaminating reusable transducer components in hemodynamic monitoring during the 1970s [37], one-third of all outbreaks of nosocomial bacteremia investigated by the CDC between 1977 and 1987 were traced to contamination of infusions used for arterial pressure monitoring [17]. Since 1980, there have been at least 12 outbreaks of associated nosocomial septicemia reported in the world literature, nearly all caused by gram-negative bacilli, most frequently *S. marcescens* and non-*aeruginosa* pseudomonads [162]. Two-thirds of all these epidemics were linked to failed decontamination of reusable transducer components, particularly the continued use of unreliable chemical disinfectants, such as aqueous benzalkonium in the United States or dilute solutions of aqueous chlorhexidine in the United Kingdom (see Chap. 42). Epidemic organisms were most commonly found on metal transducer heads, in the interface between transducers and disposable chamber domes. Eight epidemics were traced to introduction of organisms into closed monitoring systems from external sources of contamination in the hospital, such as contaminated ice used to chill syringes for drawing arterialized blood for blood gas measurements, heparinized saline from multidose vials, and contaminated external devices used to calibrate pressure-monitoring systems. The epidemic organisms were found on the hands of health care providers in at least nine outbreaks; however, most of the reports do not provide sufficient data to establish clearly the precise mechanism of fluid contamination.

With all forms of infusion therapy, the connection between the administration set and the catheter must be secure. This is especially important with central venous catheters, where accidental disconnections can result in exsanguination or life-threatening air embolus or blood loss. In TPN, a faulty connection may also increase the risk of iatrogenic infection. Deitel and colleagues [58] reported an outbreak of 23 catheter-related septicemias caused by different strains of coagulase-negative staphylococci, linked to a manufacturing defect that resulted in hyperalimentation solution leaking from administration set–catheter connections and seeping under dressings, where it resulted in heavy bacterial overgrowth.

During the 1970s, numerous outbreaks of gram-negative septicemia, particularly with pseudomonads other than *P. aeruginosa*, were traced to contamination of dialysate within patients' hemodialysis machines [127]. However, improved quality control, the decontamination of reused dialyzer coils, and the wide-scale practice of using disposable dialyzers has resulted in a marked decline in the incidence of nosocomial outbreaks traced to contaminated dialysate [128] (see Chap. 19).

Compounding of admixtures is another important means by which contamination can be introduced [63, 127, 187, 237]. The greatest concern about this mode of contamination, especially if it occurs in the central pharmacy, is that a large number of patients may be exposed. Moreover, the delay between compounding and use provides opportunity for proliferation of introduced microorganisms to levels that can cause overwhelming septic shock when administered [63]. Two large outbreaks of candidemia have been traced to contaminated solutions used for intravenous hyperalimentation [187, 237]: In each outbreak, a vacuum system in the hospital's pharmacy, used to evacuate fluid from bottles before introducing other admixture components, was shown to be heavily contaminated by the epidemic strain of *Candida*. Presumably, organisms refluxed into bottles during compounding of the admixtures. In outbreaks traced to contaminants introduced during compounding, after compounding bottles were permitted to stand at room temperature for up to 48 hours before use. The necessity for stringent attention to asepsis in central admixture programs cannot be overemphasized. Fluid admixtures should be used within 6 hours of admixing or should be immediately refrigerated.

Investigations of more than 100 epidemics over the past two decades [128, 132] have documented contamination of in-use infusate or contamination of cannula insertion sites, deriving from a myriad of extrinsic sources within the hospital (see Table 40-10). In many outbreaks, the hospital reservoir of the epidemic pathogen and even the mode of transmission eluded detection, but the microorganism was found in large numbers on the hands of health care providers caring for patients receiving infusion therapy and handling their infusions. Manipulations of the delivery system, especially the administration set, appear to provide a highly effective means for access of microorganisms to in-use infusate, as illustrated by a spate of nosocomial outbreaks across the United States traced to in-use contamination of a newly released intravenous anesthetic, propofol (Diprivan): The solution provides an almost uniquely rich medium for rapid microbial proliferation. Outbreaks of primary bacteremia or surgical wound infection with a variety of skin organisms, especially *S. aureus*, were traced to in-use contamination of propofol,

given by infusion pump in the operating room, because of poor aseptic technique [38]. Similarly, a veritable explosion of hospital outbreaks of nosocomial candidemia in the past decade [32, 33, 38, 187, 201, 237, 238], primarily within ICUs, has been linked to carriage of the epidemic strain on the hands of nurses handling vulnerable patients' intravascular devices and infusions.

Approach to an Epidemic

If an epidemic is suspected, the epidemiologic approach must be methodical and thorough yet expeditious. It is directed toward establishing the bona fide nature of the putative epidemic infections [134] and existence of an epidemic, defining the reservoirs and modes of transmission of the epidemic pathogens and, most importantly, controlling the epidemic quickly and completely. Control measures are obviously predicated on accurate delineation of the epidemiology of the epidemic pathogen (see Chap. 6).

The essential steps in dealing with a suspected outbreak of nosocomial bloodstream infection have been reviewed by the author in a previous publication [127] (Table 40-11). To illustrate the approach to an epidemic of infusion-related bacteremia, the epidemiologic investigation of an extraordinary outbreak that recently occurred in the University of Wisconsin Hospital and Clinics is recounted [140].

During a 2-week period in late March 1985, 3 patients in our university hospital developed primary nosocomial bacteremia with a similar nonfermentative gram-negative bacillus. All 3 patients had had open-heart surgery between March 11 and March 25 (Fig. 40-8) and became bacteremic 48 to 148 hours following operation.

The bloodstream pathogen in each case was shown to be *Pseudomonas pickettii* biovariant 1. The organism was also cultured from the intravenous fluid of 2 of the patients at the time because, serendipitously, during the outbreak most adult patients in the hospital receiving intravenous fluids were participating in a study of IV catheter dressings [147]: As part of the study protocol, specimens were routinely obtained

Table 40-11.   Evaluation of a suspected epidemic of nosocomial bloodstream infections

---

Administrative preparedness

Immediately retrieve putative epidemic blood isolates for confirmation of identity through spaces and subtyping by one or more methods

    Biotyping

    Antimicrobial susceptibility pattern (antibiogram)

    Antiseptic and chemical susceptibility profile (resistogram)

    Serotyping

    Phage typing

    Bacteriocin typing

    SDS-PAGE protein electrophoresis

    Immunoblot

    Multifocus enzyme electrophoresis

    Restriction enzyme digestion and restriction fragment polymorphism patterns

    DNA probes

Preliminary evaluations and control measures

    Identify and characterize individual cases in time, place, risk factors

    Strive to identify source of bloodstream infections

    Ascertain whether cases represent true bloodstream infections rather than pseudo-bacteremias

    Ascertain whether cases represent a true epidemic rather than a pseudoepidemic

    Provisional control measures

    Intensify surveillance, to detect every new case

    Review general infection control policies and procedures

    Determine need for assistance, especially extramural (local, state, Centers for Disease Control [CDC])

Epidemiologic investigations

    Clinical-epidemiologic studies, especially case-control studies

    Microbiologic studies

Definitive control measures

Confirm control of epidemic by intensified follow-up surveillance

Report the findings

    Intramurally, state health department, CDC

    Publish report

---

from patients' intravenous fluid when the catheter was removed. Review of nearly 1,000 cultures of intravenous fluid from the infusions of participants in the study since its outset 3 months earlier showed that 3 additional surgical patients operated on in March had had intra-

venous fluid cultures positive for *P. pickettii* biovariant 1 (see Fig. 40-7), even though none had shown clinical signs of bacteremia. Molecular subtyping by restriction enzyme digestion and pulsed-field electrophoresis to delineate restriction polymorphism patterns showed all six isolates to be the same. Three more patients who had been operated on in January had had intravenous fluid cultures positive for a similar nonfermentative gram-negative bacillus; although the three isolates were no longer available, the results of screening by AP-20E biochemical panel (API Analytab Inc, Plainville, NY) at the time were identical to those of the 6 patients with *P. pickettii* contamination of intravenous fluid, with or without associated bacteremia.

All of the patients had had multiple positive blood cultures and were clinically floridly septic. *Pseudomonas pickettii* had not been isolated from any local site of infection, such as the urinary tract, lower respiratory tract, or surgical wound, in any of the patients.

Review of nosocomial bacteremias over the past 7 years showed that *P. pickettii* had not previously been identified in blood cultures from our institution, indicating that the cluster of 3 cases and 6 instances of contaminated infusate without bactermia represented a true epidemic, and based on the results of the subtyping, a common-source epidemic.

The CDC and the manufacturer were contacted. None of more than 70 National Nosocomial Infection Surveillance Study hospitals had reported *P. pickettii* bacteremias in the past year.

A case-control study comparing the 9 case patients, all of whom had had recent surgery, and 19 operated patients who had had negative intravenous fluid cultures in the intravenous dressing study, showed that all 9 case patients but only 9 of the 19 operated control patients had received fentanyl intravenously in the operating room (Table 40-12; $p = .05$); the mean total dose given to the 9 case patients was far greater than that given to control patients who received the drug (3,080 μg versus 840 μg; $p < .001$).

The manufacturer had never identified contamination with *P. pickettii* in its quality control microbiologic sampling of its fentanyl prior to distribution, nor had it received any complaints from users about suspected contamination of this product. Moreover, survey of surrounding hospitals that also used the manufacturer's fen-

Table 40-12. Case-control analysis of risk factors for bacteremia or contaminated intravenous fluid with *Pseudomonas pickettii*

Risk Factor	Cases (n = 9)	Controls[a] (n = 19)	p Value
Age (mean)	50 yr	46 yr	NS
Duration of surgery (mean)	4.0 hr	3.07 hr	NS
Type of surgery			
Cardiovascular	5 (55%)	3 (16%)	NS
General	4 (45%)	16 (84%)	
Intravenous fluids			
Lactated Ringer's	8 (89%)	11 (58%)	NS
Dextrose in Ringer's lactate	5 (55%)	14 (74%)	NS
Saline 0.9%	6 (67%)	4 (21%)	NS
Blood products	7 (78%)	4 (21%)	NS
Albumin, fresh frozen plasma	4 (44%)	2 (10%)	NS
Intraoperative intravenous medications			
Thiopental	4 (45%)	13 (68%)	NS
Lidocaine	5 (55%)	5 (26%)	NS
Pancuronium	5 (55%)	4 (21%)	NS
Heparin	5 (55%)	0 (0%)	<.001
Cefazolin	9 (100%)	10 (53%)	NS
Fentanyl	9 (100%)	9 (47%)	.05
Volume of intravenous fentanyl (mean)	61.6 ml	16.8 ml[b]	<.001

NS = not significant at $p < .05$.
[a] Patients randomly selected who had had surgery on the same day as case patients but who had negative cultures of intravenous fluid from their infusion begun in the operating room.
[b] For the 9 control patients who received fentanyl.
Source: D.G. Maki et al., Nosocomial *Pseudomonas pickettii* bacteremias traced to narcotic tampering. A case for selective drug screening of health care personnel. *J.A.M.A.* 265:981, 1991.

tanyl revealed that none experienced nosocomial bacteremias with *P. pickettii*.

In our hospital at the time, fentanyl was used only in the operating rooms as part of balanced anesthesia. The drug was received in 20-ml ampules from the manufacturer, and each week 1 of 3 pharmacy technicians, by rotation, predrew into sterile syringes all fentanyl likely to be needed the following week in the operating rooms. Each day, one of the technicians delivered enough predrawn syringes to the operating rooms to meet the needs of the cases being done that day. Cultures of predrawn fentanyl in syringes in the central pharmacy, prompted by the findings of the case-control study, showed that twenty (40 percent) of fifty 30-ml syringes sampled were contaminated by *P. pickettii* in a concentration of more than 10^4 cfu/ml; none of thirty-five 5-ml or 2-ml syringes showed contamination ($p < .001$).

Extensive culturing within the central pharmacy was negative for evidence of environmental contamination by *P. pickettii* with one

exception: *P. pickettii* biovariant 1, with an identical antimicrobial susceptibility pattern and restriction enzyme fragment pattern to the epidemic strain recovered from blood cultures or patients' intravenous infusions, was cultured in a concentration of 28 to 80 cfu/ml from 5 specimens of distilled water drawn from a tap in the central pharmacy. The epidemic strain was shown to multiply well in the fentanyl solution, attaining concentrations exceeding 10^4 cfu/ml within 48 hours.

A second case-control study suggested strongly that the epidemic was caused by theft of fentanyl from 30-ml syringes by a pharmacy staff member and replacement by distilled water that the individual believed was sterile but that, unfortunately, was serendipitously contaminated by *P. pickettii*. The pharmacy member resigned early in the investigation and no longer works in our hospital. On April 29, the hospital's system for providing fentanyl and other narcotics to the operating rooms was changed: Narcotics are no longer predrawn into syringes in the central pharmacy but are delivered to the operating rooms in unopened vials or ampules. Anesthesiologists' orders for narcotics are filled by a staff pharmacist assigned to the operating room. There have been no further bacteremias with *P. pickettii* since March 25, 1985 (Fig. 40-8), and cultures of more than 6,000 samples of hospitalized patients' intravenous fluid in research studies since that time have shown no further contamination by *P. pickettii*.

This outbreak illustrates the power of case-control analyses to identify the probable cause of an epidemic (see Chap. 6). It further illustrates the potential for contamination of parenteral drugs or admixtures and the extraordinary range of epidemiologic mechanisms of nosocomial bloodstream infection deriving from such contamination.

Strategies for Prevention
Aseptic Technique
To accord it due respect, any device for vascular access must be considered a direct conduit

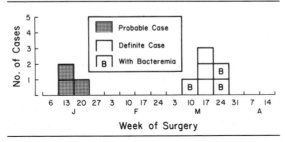

Fig. 40-8. Epidemic curve for outbreak of *Pseudomonas pickettii* bacteremias and contaminated intravenous infusions traced to contaminated fentanyl given intravenously. The isolates from blood or intravenous fluid of the 6 definite cases (March 1985) were available for reconfirmation and subtyping as *P. pickettii* biovariant 1. The isolates from intravenous fluid of the 3 probable cases (January 1985) were not available for retesting but are considered very likely to have also been *P. pickettii* biovariant 1 on review of the results of 20 biochemical tests common to these 3 and the 6 confirmed isolates. (Reproduced with permission from D.G. Maki et al., Nosocomial *Pseudomonas pickettii* bacteremias traced to narcotic tampering. A case for selective drug screening of health care personnel. *J.A.M.A.* 265:981, Copyright 1991, American Medical Association.)

between the external world and its myriad of microorganisms and the bloodstream of the patient. Vigorous hand-washing, ideally with an antiseptic-containing preparation, must always precede the insertion of a peripheral IV cannula and should also precede later handling of the device or the administration set [135]. It is further recommended that sterile gloves be used routinely during the insertion of peripheral IV cannulas in high-risk patients, such as leukemics. Sterile gloves are strongly recommended for placement of all other types of intravascular devices—specifically arterial and all central venous catheters—that are associated with a 1 percent or higher risk of septicemia. In the United States, sterile gloves are generally considered mandatory for insertion of arterial and central venous catheters.

Although there has been considerable controversy as to the level of barrier precautions necessary during insertion of a central venous catheter, in a recent study of the pathogenesis and epidemiology of Swan-Ganz pulmonary artery catheters, it was found that the use of maximal barrier precautions—sterile gloves, a long-sleeved sterile surgical gown, a surgical mask, and a large sterile sheet drape (as contrasted with the use of sterile gloves, a surgical mask, and a very small fenestrated drape)—was associated with a twofold lower risk of infection [164]. Despite the facts that Swan-Ganz catheters inserted in the ICU using maximal barrier precautions (1) remained in place an average of 22 hours longer than catheters inserted in the operating room (inserted with lesser barrier precautions), (2) were more frequently placed in infected patients, and (3) were used more frequently for TPN, such catheters were much less likely to be contaminated under the external protective sheath or infected than catheters inserted in the operating room by anesthesiologists using lesser barrier precautions (Table 40-13). Considering that, of all intravascular devices, central venous catheters are most likely to produce nosocomial bloodstream infection, a strong case can be made for mandating maximal barrier precautions during the insertion

Table 40-13.   Comparability of Swan-Ganz catheters inserted in an ICU (unless less stringent barrier precautions) versus in the operating room (using maximal barrier precautions)

Features	*ICU (n = 86)*	*Operating Room (n = 211)*
Location of catheter (%)		
Internal jugular	44	93*
Subclavian	42	6
Femoral	13	1
Use of catheter for total parenteral nutrition (%)	55*	3
Number catheter in the site (%)		
First	81*	100
Second	19	0
Duration introducer in place (mean hours)	92 hr*	70 hr
Infection unrelated to the catheter (%)	53*	5
Contamination of pulmonary artery catheter, beneath external protective sleeve (no.)	1 (1.2%)	11 (5.2%)*
Infection of Swan-Ganz catheter (no.)	13 (15.1%)	52 (24.6%)*

ICU = intensive care unit.
*p <.01.
Source: L. Mermel, R. McCormick, and D.G. Maki, Epidemiology and pathogenesis of infection with Swan-Ganz catheters. A prospective study using molecular epidemiology. *Am. J. Med.* 91(3B):197S, 1991.

of such devices, particularly the use of a long-sleeved surgical gown and large sterile sheet drape (to minimize touch contamination) in addition to sterile gloves, which should be routine.

Studies have shown that the use of special intravenous therapy teams consisting of trained nurses or technicians, to ensure a high level of aseptic technique during catheter insertion and in follow-up care of the catheter, have been associated with substantially lower rates of catheter-related infection [19, 70, 76, 113, 170, 172, 212, 236, 248] (Table 40-14). Tomford and Hershey [249] have reported a cost-benefit analysis indicating that a team can prove highly cost-effective, reducing the costs of complications of infusion therapy nearly tenfold. In many U.S. hospitals, all central venous catheters, particularly those dedicated to TPN, are cared for by such teams. However, even if they do not have an intravenous team, institutions can greatly reduce their rate of catheter-related sepsis by scrutinizing catheter-care protocols and more intensively educating and training nurses and physicians [48, 197, 253].

Cutaneous Antisepsis

Given the evidence for the important role of cutaneous microorganisms in the genesis of many intravascular device–related infections, measures to reduce cutaneous colonization of the insertion site would appear to be the highest priority, particularly through the use of chemical antiseptics for disinfection of the site. In the United States, an iodophor such as 10% povidone-iodine is used most widely.

The lack of published comparative trials of cutaneous antiseptics to prevent catheter-related infection recently prompted us to study this question prospectively: Central venous and arterial catheters in 668 patients in a surgical ICU were randomized to 10% povidone-iodine, 70% alcohol, or 2% aqueous chlorhexidine for disinfection of the site before insertion and site care every other day thereafter [136]. Chlorhexidine was associated with the lowest incidence of local catheter-related infection and catheter-related bacteremia; of the 14 infusion-related bacteremias identified in the study, 1 was in the chlorhexidine group and 13 were in the other two groups (odds ratio, 0.16; p = .04; Table

Table 40-14. Impact of a dedicated intravenous team on the rate of catheter-related septicemia

Type and Author of Study	Type of Catheter	Care Provider	No. of Catheters	Incidence of IV Catheter–Related Septicemia (per 100 catheters)	p Value
Concurrent but not randomized					
Bentley and Leper [19]	PIV	House officers	4,270	0.40	
		IV team	470	0.04	<.001
Freeman et al. [76]	CVC-TPN	Ward nurses	33	21.2	
		IV nurses	78	2.3	<.001
Nehme [170]	CVC-TPN	Ward nurses	391	26.2	
		IV team	284	1.3	<.001
Faubion et al. [70]	CVC-TPN	Ward nurses	179	24.0	
		IV team	377	3.5	<.001
Nelsen et al. [172]	CVC-TPN	House officers	45	28.8	
		IV nurses	30	3.3	<.001
Historical controls					
Sanders and Sheldon [212]	CVC-TPN	Ward nurses	335	28.6	
		IV team	172	4.7	<.001
Keohane et al. [113]	CVC-TPN	Ward nurses	51	33.0	
		IV nurses	48	4.0	<.001
Randomized, concurrent controls					
Tomford et al. [248]	PIV	House officers	427	2.1	
		IV team	433	0.2	<.05
Tomford and Hershey [249]	PIV	House officers	453	1.5	
		IV team	412	0.0	<.02

IV = intravenous; PIV = peripheral IV catheter; CVC = central venous catheter; TPN = total parenteral nutrition.

Table 40-15. Results of a prospective randomized trial of three cutaneous antiseptics for prevention of intravascular device–related septicemia

Source of Septicemia	10% Povidone-Iodine (n = 227)	70% Alcohol (n = 227)	2% Chlorhexidine (n = 214)
Catheter-related	6	3	1
Contaminated infusate	—	3	—
Contaminated hub	1	—	—
All sources (%)	7 (3.1)	6 (2.6)	1 (0.5)*

*Compared with the other two groups combined: odds ratio, 0.16, $p = .04$.
Source: D.G. Maki, C.J. Alvarado, and M. Ringer, A prospective, randomized trial of povidone-iodine, alcohol and chlorhexidine for prevention of infection with central venous and arterial catheters. *Lancet* 338:339, 1991.

40-15). This study suggests that the use of 2% chlorhexidine, rather than 10% povidone-iodine or 70% alcohol, for cutaneous disinfection before insertion of an intravascular device and in postinsertion site care can substantially reduce the incidence of device-related infection (see Chap. 15).

In an historical analysis of the impact on the incidence of catheter-related sepsis of using different antiseptics for site care and disinfecting tubing connections in a home TPN program, Rannem and co-workers [199] recently reported a rate of 0.58 cases per catheter-year during use of 10% povidone-iodine as contrasted with 0.26 to 0.28 cases per catheter-year during use of 0.5 to 2% tincture of iodine or 0.5% tincture of chlorhexidine.

"Defatting" the skin with acetone is still widely practiced in many centers as an adjunctive measure for disinfecting central venous catheter sites, especially in TPN. However, it was found to be of no benefit whatsoever in a prospective randomized trial [144]. Rather, the use of acetone was associated with greatly increased inflammation and discomfort to the patient.

Topical Antimicrobial Ointments

In theory, application of topical antimicrobial agents to the catheter insertion site should confer some protection against microbial invasion. Clinical trials of topical polyantibiotic ointments (polymyxin, neomycin, and bacitracin) on peripheral venous catheters have shown only moderate or no benefit [137, 173, 271], and the use of polyantibiotic ointments

has been associated with an increased frequency of *Candida* infections [71, 137]. Study of the new topical antibacterial mupirocin, which is active primarily against gram-positive organisms, applied to internal jugular catheters showed a significant reduction in catheter colonization, without colonization by *Candida*, but there were no catheter-related septicemias in either treatment group in the trial [96].

There have been two prospective studies of topical povidone-iodine ointment applied to central venous catheter sites. One large randomized trial in a surgical ICU showed no benefit [194], but a recent comparative trial with subclavian hemodialysis catheters showed a fourfold reduction in the incidence of hemodialysis catheter–related septicemia [119].

Dressings

The importance of the cutaneous microflora in the pathogenesis of device-related infection might suggest that the dressing applied to the catheter insertion site could have considerable influence on the incidence of catheter-related infection. The purpose of an intravenous site dressing is to prevent trauma to the catheter wound and the cannulated vessel as well as to prevent extrinsic contamination of the wound. Unfortunately, few studies prospectively examined the specific aspects of site care of intravascular catheter sites until polyurethane transparent films for dressing vascular catheters became available a decade ago. When used on vascular catheters, transparent dressings permit continuous inspection of the site, secure the device reliably, and are generally more comfortable than gauze and tape. Moreover, transparent dressings permit patients to bathe and shower without saturating the dressing. Clinical trials of these dressings have been prompted by the knowledge that cutaneous occlusion with tape or impervious plastic films results in an explosive increase in cutaneous microflora, with overgrowth of gram-negative bacilli and yeasts [3, 165]. Although polyurethane dressings are semipermeable—impervious to extrinsic microbial contaminants and liquid-phase moisture, and variably permeable to oxygen, carbon dioxide, and water vapor—and studies in healthy volunteers have shown little effect of these dressings on the cutaneous flora [204], clinical reports have raised concern that these dressings could increase cutaneous colonization and the risk of catheter-related infection [59, 111, 169, 191].

At the present time, many manufacturers produce and market a polyurethane transparent dressing. Whereas these products are almost indistinguishable from one another on gross inspection, there are substantive differences in physical properties, particularly moisture vapor transmission rate (MVTR), oxygen transmission, and cutaneous adherence [99, 198, 247], that may influence cutaneous floral populations beneath the dressings.

Transparent polyurethane dressings are more expensive than gauze and tape and, to obviate the issue of greater cost as well as for convenience, many users leave transparent dressings on for prolonged periods (up to 7 days or even longer). It has been questioned whether transparent dressings left on for prolonged periods might increase the risk of catheter-related infection. Most of the studies of polyurethane dressings have been relatively small and have not had adequate statistical power to allow meaningful conclusions to be drawn. However, there is a handful of larger studies from which it is possible to draw conclusions. The reported trials of polyurethane dressings compared with gauze and tape on peripheral venous catheters have ranged in size from 77 to 737 catheters [4, 52, 81, 98, 107, 112, 147, 158, 205]. Trials by Andersen and associates [4], Kelsey and Gosling [112], and Joseph and Marzouk [107]

found significantly higher rates of local catheter-related infection with transparent dressings left on indefinitely. Craven and colleagues [52] also found a higher rate of infection in catheters dressed with a transparent dressing, but only during the summer months. Other studies, however, did not find significant differences [81, 98, 147, 158, 205]. Rates of local catheter-related infection in all of these trials have been low with all dressings, in the range of 1.6 to 8.5 percent. Only 3 catheter-related bacteremias were identified among the nearly 4,000 catheters studied in all of the reported trials.

In a prospective randomized trial of various dressings used with 2,088 Teflon peripheral IV catheters [147], the transparent polyurethane dressing (Tegaderm, 3M Medical Products), left on for the lifetime of the catheter, was not associated with increased cutaneous colonization under the dressing or an increased rate of catheter-related infection as compared with the control gauze and tape dressing (Fig. 40-9). There were no cases of catheter-related bacteremia. Cutaneous colonization was not heavier under transparent dressings during the spring and summer months, as reported by Craven and coworkers [52], perhaps because our hospital is air-conditioned. Multivariate analysis showed cutaneous colonization of the insertion site (RR, 3.9) and moisture under the dressing (RR, 2.5) to be significant risk factors for catheter-related infection (see Table 40-8). These data indicate that it is probably not cost-effective to redress peripheral intravenous catheters at periodic intervals and that, for most patients, either sterile gauze or a transparent dressing can be used and left on until the catheter is removed.

Studies of transparent dressings on short-term, noncuffed central venous catheters have yielded conflicting results [50, 153, 171, 177, 192, 193, 205, 215, 269], in part reflecting differences in study protocols (such as the use of topical antimicrobial ointments under the dressing in the control gauze group but not in the transparent dressing group) and different dressings studied. Powell and coworkers [192] reported a threefold increase in infectious complications with subclavian

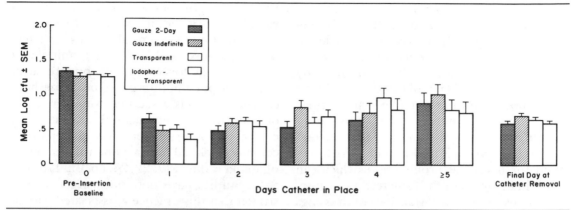

Fig. 40-9. Density of cutaneous colonization of catheter insertion sites in the 4 dressing groups in a prospective comparative randomized trial of 2 transparent dressings and gauze and tape with 2,088 peripheral IV catheters. Cutaneous colonization of the insertion site under the dressing was very low level (approximately $10^{0.65}$ cfu/10 cm²) and comparable with all 4 dressings. Moreover, it increased only marginally with increasing lengths of catheter placement, indicating that with the small peripheral IV catheters now used, for most patients either gauze or a transparent dressing with a high moisture vapor transmission rate can be used and left on indefinitely. (Reproduced with permission from D.G. Maki and M. Ringer, Evaluation of dressing regimens for prevention of infection with peripheral intravenous catheters. *J.A.M.A.* 258:2396, Copyright 1987, American Medical Association.)

catheters dressed with Opsite (Smith and Nephew, United Kingdom) for up to 7 days as compared with gauze replaced three times weekly, but the difference did not achieve statistical significance. A recent trial by Conly and associates [50] found a much higher rate of catheter-related septicemia with catheters dressed with Opsite than catheters dressed with gauze and tape (16 percent versus 0 percent). In a very similar trial done in our center, in ICU patients, we found that Tegaderm (3M) adhered well and that there were no significant differences in catheter-related infection with transparent dressings as compared to gauze dressings when the transparent dressing was changed every 2 days [153]; however, in these high-risk ICU patients, we observed a significant buildup of skin flora, associated with a 50 percent increase in catheter-related infection, when transparent dressings were left on for up to 7 days between changes. This finding suggests that, if used on central venous catheters in ICU patients, the dressing studied should be routinely replaced every other day, as is done in most U.S. hospitals with gauze and tape. Other prospective trials, which in aggregate studied hundreds of central venous catheters in high-risk patients, many of whom were receiving TPN through the catheter, did not find an increased risk of catheter-related infection associated with transparent dressing left on for up to 7 days, as compared to gauze and tape replaced every second or third day [171, 177, 193, 205, 215, 269].

There have been only two reported randomized studies of the use of transparent dressings on surgically implanted cuffed Hickman or Broviac catheters in which microbiologic data were provided [153, 223]. In both trials, one in renal transplant patients [153] and the other in bone marrow transplant recipients [223], the transparent dressing studied provided satisfactory cover and, even when left on for prolonged periods (up to 5 to 7 days), was not associated with a significantly increased risk of exit site or tunnel infection or catheter-related bacteremia.

There have also been only two reported studies of transparent polyurethane dressings with arterial catheters [98, 153]. In a prospective study of Tegaderm on arterial catheters used for hemodynamic monitoring in a surgical ICU, we found the use of the transparent dressing, even replaced every other day, to be associated with a fivefold increased incidence of catheter-related bacteremia as compared with gauze and tape [153]. We believe that the greatly increased risk of infection associated with transparent dressings used on arterial catheters found in this study may reflect the presence of macroscopic blood in the puncture wound, under arterial pressure, which is common under transparent dressings on arterial catheters; if the blood cannot be cleared, it may provide a rich medium for microbial proliferation, which can result in infection of the catheter. As a consequence, we believe that transparent dressings should not be used on arterial catheters unless future studies confirm their safety.

From our study showing a strong association between increased moisture on the site and greater cutaneous colonization and risk of peripheral IV catheter-related infection [147], it would seem desirable that a transparent dressing have a high MVTR to prevent the buildup of moisture. A new Opsite IV3000 dressing (Smith and Nephew) has an MVTR five to eight times greater than that of other transparent dressings currently available (3,000 versus 839 gm/m²/d MVTR) [247]. The promise of such a dressing is based on pilot studies showing much less accumulation of liquid moisture, and lower levels of cutaneous colonization, beneath the dressing [198], which in theory should reduce the risk of catheter-related infection. The interim results of a prospective study in our center comparing gauze and tape, Tegaderm, and Opsite IV3000 on 211 Swan-Ganz pulmonary artery catheters show that cutaneous colonization under the Opsite IV3000 dressing was comparable to gauze and tape and significantly lower than with Tegaderm [150]; there have been no differences in the rate of catheter-related infection between the groups.

Changing Catheters over a Guide Wire

The Seldinger technique, in which the vessel is identified and entered percutaneously with a fine-gauge needle and cannulated with a guide wire passed through the needle, following which the cannula is guided into the vessel over the guide wire, has been a major advance, permitting vessels to be cannulated with large catheters with much less risk of vascular injury and, in the case of subclavian or internal jugular central venous catheters, pneumothorax, and with less manipulation and potential for contamination. To avoid iatrogenic pneumothorax and other mechanical complications associated with percutaneous insertion of a new cannula, particularly a central venous catheter, new catheters are commonly placed over a guide wire in the site of an old catheter [7, 22, 24, 86, 97, 176, 188, 228]. Studies have not conclusively demonstrated that this practice is associated with an increased (or decreased) risk of infection [7, 22, 24, 35, 66, 83, 86, 95, 97, 174, 176, 181, 188, 190, 228, 231], and the issue has not been resolved satisfactorily by a sufficiently large, prospective, randomized trial. Six groups have examined this issue in randomized trials, but none of the trials had adequate statistical power to allow detection of a difference in the rate of catheter-related septicemia of as much as 50 percent between the two groups [83, 95, 174, 181, 190, 231].

If it is considered desirable to replace a central venous or arterial catheter because it has been in place for a prolonged period and there is suspicion of infection (e.g., unexplained fever) or the catheter has cracked and may be leaking, it is not unreasonable to replace the catheter in the same site over a guide wire *if* the patient has limited sites for new access or would be at high risk for the percutaneous puncture required for placement of a new catheter in a new site (e.g., has coagulopathy or is morbidly obese). However, it is imperative that the same meticulous aseptic technique that should be mandatory during insertion of any new catheter be employed, including the routine use of sterile gloves and a sterile drape and, for central venous catheters, a sterile gown as well. After vigorously cleansing the site and the old catheter with the antiseptic solution, inserting the guide wire, removing the old catheter, and cleansing the guide wire and site once more with the antiseptic solution, the operator should *reglove and redrape the site,* as the original gloves and drapes are likely to be contaminated from manipulation of the old catheter. After regloving and reprepping the site, the new catheter can be inserted over the guide wire.

It is also important to culture the old catheter routinely and, if the patient is febrile or shows other signs of sepsis, to obtain blood cultures. If these cultures demonstrate that the old catheter was infected, the new catheter just placed in the old site should be immediately removed to prevent progression to catheter-related septicemia (or perpetuation of ongoing catheter-related septicemia) as the new catheter has been inserted into an infected tract. Need for continued access would mandate placement of a new catheter in a new site. If, on the other hand, culture of the old catheter is negative, it has been possible to preserve access and to examine the initial catheter microbiologically and exclude it as the cause of fever or sepsis without subjecting the patient to the hazards associated with percutaneous insertion of a new catheter.

If the old insertion site is inflamed at the outset, and especially if it is purulent, or the patient shows signs of full-blown sepsis that might be originating from the catheter, or the catheter has been recently shown to be infected by quantitative blood cultures recently drawn through the catheter, it is strongly recommended that a new catheter *not* be inserted over a guide wire into an old, potentially infected site.

Measures Aimed at the Delivery System

Numerous studies have shown that most infusion-related bacteremias are caused by infection of the device used for vascular access [128, 132]. However, as we have seen, infusate can occasionally become contaminated and cause endemic bacteremia [43, 136, 139, 148, 164]. If an infusion runs continuously for an extended period, the cumulative risk of contamination increases and, further, there is increased risk that the contaminants can grow to dangerously high concentrations that will result in septicemia in the recipient of the fluid. For nearly 20 years, most U.S. hospitals have routinely replaced the entire delivery system of patients' intravenous infusions at 24- or 48-hour intervals [128, 132], to reduce

the risk of sepsis from extrinsically contaminated fluid. Recent studies (see Table 40-9), however, now indicate that intravenous delivery systems do not need to be replaced more frequently than every 72 hours, including infusion sets used for TPN or any infusions in ICU patients [108, 138, 235]. Extending the duration of use allows considerable cost savings to hospitals [138].

Four clinical settings might be regarded as exceptions to using the 72-hour interval for routine set change: (1) during administration of blood products, (2) during administration of lipid emulsions, (3) with arterial pressure monitoring, and (4) if an epidemic of infusion-related septicemias is suspected. In these circumstances, it is most prudent that administration sets be changed routinely at 24- or 48-hour intervals. Minute amounts of blood buffer acidic solutions and provide organic nutrients that greatly enhance the ability of most microorganisms to grow in parenteral fluids [143, 202]. Moreover, most hospital pathogens, including coagulase-negative staphylococci, grow rapidly in commercial lipid emulsion [53, 130], and sporadic epidemic septicemias [160] and outbreaks [105] have been traced to contaminated lipid emulsion.

As previously noted, arterial infusions used for hemodynamic monitoring appear to be considerably more vulnerable to becoming contaminated during use and produce endemic [142, 148] or epidemic infusate-related septicemia [162], usually caused by gram-negative bacilli. Recent studies suggest that if the infusion for hemodynamic monitoring is set up so that it flows continuously through the chamber dome, eliminating a blind stagnant column of fluid, extrinsic contamination is greatly reduced, and it also may be unnecessary to replace the administration set, chamber dome, and other components of the delivery system at 24- or 48-hour intervals [123, 186, 222]. If disposable transducers and chamber domes are used, there appears to be no need to replace the transducer assembly and other components of the delivery system more frequently than every 4 days [123].

If infusion-related septicemias occur in epidemic numbers, especially caused by gram-negative bacilli, such as *Enterobacter, Serratia,* or *Pseudomonas* species, contaminated infusate must be suspected, and it might be most prudent to reduce the interval for routine set change to every 24 or 48 hours.

Unless a hospital detects frequent contamination of intramurally compounded TPN solutions or experiences a high rate of cryptogenic primary bacteremia associated with TPN, there seems little basis for changing the delivery sets of infusions for TPN more frequently than every 72 hours [138]. Institutions with long-standing policies of replacing sets even less frequently have reported low rates of complicating infection [77, 213].

Terminal in-use membrane filters continue to be advocated as a means of reducing the hazard of contaminated infusate. However, filters must be changed at periodic intervals and can become blocked, leading to added manipulations of the system and, paradoxically, greater potential for contamination [77, 167]. Moreover, most commercial in-line filters permit the passage of endotoxin [15]. Studies suggest that the increased risk for phlebitis that is associated with the administration of intravenous antibiotics can be reduced by removing the microparticulates that are associated with compounding these drugs with 0.22-μm or 0.44-μm in-line filters [20, 67]. However, not all randomized trials have shown a substantial reduction in phlebitis with the use of in-line filters [125]. Moreover, filters are expensive and must be replaced at periodic intervals, and their use adds substantially to the costs of phlebitis from microparticulates. Controlled clinical studies establishing their cost-effectiveness are needed before their routine use can be advocated [79, 225], especially as a control measure for prevention of rare sporadic septicemias deriving from extrinsic contamination of infusate.

Innovative Technologic Advances

The development and application of novel technologic devices holds the greatest promise for a quantum reduction in the risk of infusion-related sepsis, especially that due to the percutaneous device used for intravas-cular access. Innovations in the design or construction of the infusion apparatus that implicitly deny access of microorganisms into the system or that prevent organisms which might gain access from proliferating to high concentrations or colonizing the implanted cannula can obviate the effects of poor aseptic technique or undue patient vulnerability.

Studies of incorporating an antiseptic, namely povidone-iodine, into a transparent catheter dressing to suppress cutaneous colonization under the dressing have been disappointing [147]. However, in light of the superiority of chlorhexidine over povidone-iodine for cutaneous disinfection of vascular catheter sites [136], incorporating chlorhexidine into a dressing's adhesive might prove more effective.

Recently, a tissue-interface barrier (Vita-Cuff, Vitafore Corporation, San Carlos, CA) was developed to incorporate aspects of the technology of Hickman and Broviac catheters. The device consists of a detachable cuff made of biodegradable collagen to which silver ion is chelated (Fig. 40-10). The cuff can be attached to any short-term central ven-

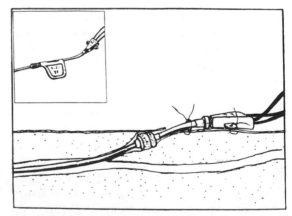

Fig. 40-10. Schematic depiction of a silver-impregnated, tissue-barrier cuff (VitaCuff) and the cuff attached to a central venous catheter in situ. It is important for the cuff to be positioned at least 0.5–1.0 cm below the surface of the skin and for the catheter to be well immobilized, preferably with a skin suture, to prevent extrusion. (Reproduced with permission from D.G. Maki et al., An attachable silver-impregnated cuff for prevention of infection with central venous catheters. A prospective randomized multi-center trial. *Am. J. Med.* 85:307, 1988.)

ous catheter immediately prior to insertion. After insertion, subcutaneous tissue grows into the collagenous matrix, anchoring the catheter and creating a barrier against invasive organisms from the skin. The silver ion provides an additional chemical barrier against introduced contamination, augmenting the mechanical barrier. In a prospective, randomized multicenter trial of the cuff, designed to prevent invasion of the catheter tract by microorganisms of skin origin, we found that catheters inserted with the cuff were three times less likely to be colonized on removal than were control catheters and were nearly four times less likely to produce bacteremia (Table 40-16) [139]. Adverse effects from the cuff were not seen. The cuff did not confer protection, however, against infection with catheters inserted over a guide wire to old sites. A similar comparative trial by Flowers and co-workers [71] also found a threefold reduction in catheter-related infections with central venous catheters inserted with the cuff. Although the cuff costs approximately $35, cost-benefit analysis shows that if an institution's rate of central venous catheter–related bacteremia is in the range of 2 to 3 percent, use of the cuff should prove cost-effective [139]. In addition, use of the cuff can permit high-risk temporary central venous catheters to be left safely in place for considerably longer periods.

Given the multiple potential sources for infection of an intravascular device and the importance of adherence of microorganisms to the catheter surface in the pathogenesis of infection, it would seem logical that the best strategy for prevention might be to develop a catheter material implicitly resistant to colonization. Binding a nontoxic antiseptic or antimicrobial to the catheter surface or incorporating such a substance into the catheter material itself might prove to be the most effective technologic innovation for preventing device-related infection. In a recent prospective randomized clinical trial of central venous and arterial catheters in a surgical ICU, catheters coated with cefazolin bonded to the surface with a cationic surfactant were associated with a sevenfold reduction in colonization of the catheter; however, there were no catheter-related bacteremias identified in the study population [110]. We have recently studied a novel central venous catheter in which the catheter material itself, polyurethane, is impregnated with minute quantities of silver-sulfadiazine and chlorhexidine. In a randomized comparative trial in 402 patients in a surgical ICU, antiseptic catheters were two times less likely to be colonized and four times less likely to produce bacteremia [152]. Adverse effects from the test catheter were not seen.

A novel closed system (utilizing a dia-

Table 40-16. Comparative randomized trial of a silver-impregnated cuff for prevention of infection with short-term central venous catheters

Features	*Controls* *(n = 135)*	*Cuffed Catheters* *(n = 99)*
Catheter-related infection (no.)		
Local (≥15 cfu)	33 (28.9%)	7 (9.1%)[a]
With bacteremia	5 (3.7%)	1 (1.0%)[b]
Infecting organisms (no.) [bacteremias]:		
Coagulase-negative staphylococci	23 [5]	5
Staphylococcus aureus	—	1
Enterococci	2	—
Gram-negative bacilli	8 [3]	2 [1]
Candida species	4 [2]	—

cfu = colony-forming units.
[a]*p* = .002, compared with value for control catheters.
[b]*p* = .12.
Source: D.G. Maki et al., An attachable silver-impregnated cuff for prevention of infection with central venous catheters. A prospective randomized multi-center trial. *Am. J. Med.* 85:307, 1988.

phragm) for obtaining blood specimens from arterial infusions used for hemodynamic monitoring has recently been studied in a comparative trial [54]. Use of the diaphragm for obtaining specimens was associated with a sixfold lower rate of contamination of fluid in the system than use of standard stopcocks. However, no infusion-related bacteremias were identified during the study.

Use of a novel catheter hub engineered to reduce the risk of central venous catheter hub contamination was shown by Stotter and associates [242] to reduce significantly the rate of central venous catheter—related septicemia. Segura and co-workers [216, 217] have also developed a contamination-resistant hub but have not confirmed its effectiveness in a clinical trial. The addition of a nontoxic, biodegradable or easily metabolized antiseptic to intravenous fluid [78] or intravenous admixtures might eliminate the hazard of fluid contamination altogether and further reduce the risk of hub contamination, obviating the need for periodic replacement of the delivery system.

Past Accomplishments, Future Goals

The future appears very promising for continued progress in the prevention of device-related infection. Great strides have been made over the past decade, with studies showing reduced rates of infection with the use of more stringent barrier precautions during insertion of central venous catheters [164], intravenous teams (see Table 40-14), more effective cutaneous antiseptics [136] (see Table 40-15), and topical povidone-iodine [119] or mupirocin [96] on central venous catheter insertion sites. Results of the first studies of innovative technologies such as contamination-resistant hubs [216, 217, 242], attachable cuffs [71, 139], and catheters with antimicrobial, colonization-resistant surfaces [110, 152] are also promising. I believe that by the year 2,000, intravascular devices will be highly resistant to thrombosis and infection and that it will be possible to allow per-

cutaneously inserted catheters to remain safely in place nearly indefinitely in high-risk patients.

References

1. Ada, N., et al. One-year historic prospective series of central venous catheter infections in a children's hospital (abstr.) *Clin. Res.* 39: 842A, 1991.
2. Adams, S.D., Killien, M., and Larson, E. Inline filtration and infusion phlebitis. *Heart Lung* 15:134, 1986.
3. Aly, R., et al. Effect of prolonged occlusion on the microbial flora, pH, carbon dioxide and transepidermal water loss on human skin. *J. Invest. Dermatol.* 71:378, 1978.
4. Andersen, P.T., Herlevsen, P., and Schaumburg, H. A comparative study of 'Op-site' and 'Nobecutan gauze' dressings for central venous line care. *J. Hosp. Infect.* 7:161, 1986.
5. Anderson, R.L., Highsmith, A.K., and Holland, B.W. Comparison of the standard pour plate procedure and the ATP and *Limulus* amebocyte lysate procedures for the detection of microbial contamination in intravenous fluids. *J. Clin. Microbiol.* 23:465, 1986.
6. Armstrong, C.S., et al. Clinical predictors of infection of central venous catheters used for total parenteral nutrition. *Infect. Control Hosp. Epidemiol.* 2:71, 1990.
7. Armstrong, C.W., et al. Prospective study of catheter replacement and other risk factors for infection of hyperalimentation catheters. *J. Infect. Dis.* 154:808, 1986.
8. Arnow, P.M., and Costas, C.O. Delayed rupture of the radial artery caused by catheter-related sepsis. *Rev. Infect. Dis.* 10:1035, 1988.
9. Aronson, M.D., and Bor, D.H. Blood cultures. *Ann. Intern. Med.* 106:246, 1987.
10. Ashkenazai, S. Bacterial adherence to plastics. *Lancet* 1:1075, 1984.
11. Ashkenazi, S., Weiss, E., and Drucker, M.M. Bacterial adherence to intravenous catheters and needles and its influence by cannula type and bacterial surface hydrophobicity. *J. Lab. Clin. Med.* 107(2):136, 1986.
12. Band, J.D., and Maki, D.G. Infections caused by indwelling arterial catheters for hemodynamic monitoring. *Am. J. Med.* 67:735, 1979.
13. Band, J.D., and Maki, D.G. Safety of changing intravenous delivery systems at longer than 24-hour intervals. *Ann. Intern. Med.* 91:173, 1979.
14. Banerjee, S.N., et al. Secular trends in nosocomial primary bloodstream infections in

the United States, 1980–1989. *Am. J. Med.* 91(Suppl. 3B):86S, 1991.

15. Baumgartner, T.G., et al. Bacterial endotoxin retention by inline intravenous filters. *Am. J. Hosp. Pharm.* 43:681, 1986.

16. Barrett, S.P. Bacterial adhesion to intravenous cannulae: Influence of implantation in the rabbit and of enzyme treatments. *Epidemiol. Infect.* 100:91, 1988.

17. Beck-Sague, C.M., and Jarvis, W.R. Epidemic bloodstream infections associated with pressure transducers: A persistent problem. *Infect. Control Hosp. Epidemiol.* 10:54, 1989.

18. BenEzra, D., et al. Prospective study of infections in indwelling central venous catheters using quantitative blood cultures. *Am. J. Med.* 85:495, 1988.

19. Bentley, D.W., and Lepper, M.H. Septicemia related to indwelling venous catheter. *J.A.M.A.* 206:1749, 1968.

20. Bivins, B.A., et al. Final inline filtration: A means of decreasing the incidence of infusion phlebitis. *Surgery* 85:388, 1979.

21. Bjornson, H.S., et al. Association between microorganism growth at the catheter site and colonization of the catheter in patients receiving total parenteral nutrition. *Surgery* 92:720, 1982.

22. Blewett, J.K., Jr., Kyger, E.R., III, and Patterson, L.T. Subclavian vein catheter replacement without venipuncture. *Arch. Surg.* 108:241, 1974.

23. Boyd, K.D., Thomas, S.J., Gold, J., and Boyd, A.D. A prospective study of complications of pulmonary artery catheterizations in 500 consecutive patients. *Chest* 84:245, 1983.

24. Bozzetti, F., et al. Prevention and treatment of central venous catheter sepsis by exchange via a guidewire. A prospective controlled trial. *Ann. Surg.* 198:48, 1983.

25. Braude, A.I., Carey, F.J., and Siemienski, J. Studies of bacterial transfusion reactions from refrigerated blood: The properties of cold-growing bacteria. *J. Clin. Invest.* 34:311, 1955.

26. Brismar, B., and Malmborg, A-S. Prophylaxis against microbial colonization of venous catheters. *J. Hosp. Infect.* 2:37, 1981.

27. Bross, J., Talbot, G.H., Maislin, G., and Hurwitz, S. Risk factors for nosocomial candidemia: A case-control study in adults without leukemia. *Am. J. Med.* 87:614, 1989.

28. Brothers, T.E., et al. Experience with subcutaneous infusion ports in three hundred patients. *Surg. Gynecol. Obstet.* 166:295, 1988.

29. Brun-Buisson, C., et al. Diagnosis of central venous catheter–related sepsis. Critical level of quantitative tip cultures. *Arch. Intern. Med.* 147:873, 1987.

30. Bryant, J.K., and Strand, C.L. Reliability of blood cultures collected from intravascular catheter versus venipuncture. *Am. J. Clin. Pathol.* 88:113, 1987.

31. Buchholz, D.H., et al. Bacterial proliferation in platelet products stored at room temperature. Transfusion-induced *Enterobacter* sepsis. *N. Engl. J. Med.* 285:429, 1971.

32. Burnie, J.P., et al. Four outbreaks of nosocomial systemic candidiasis. *Epidemiol. Infect.* 99:201, 1987.

33. Burnie, J.P., et al. Outbreak of systemic *Candida albicans* in an intensive care unit caused by cross infection. *Br. Med. J.* 290:746, 1985.

34. Buxton, A.E., et al. Contamination of intravenous fluid: Effects of changing administration sets. *Ann. Inter. Med.* 90:764, 1979.

35. Carlisle, E.J.F., et al. Septicemia in long-term jugular hemodialysis catheters; eradicating infection by changing the catheter over a guidewire. *Int. J. Artif. Organs* 14:150, 1991.

36. Centers for Disease Control. Contaminated povidone-iodine solution—Texas. *M.M.W.R.* 38:133, 1989.

37. Centers for Disease Control. Guideline for prevention of infections related to intravascular pressure-monitoring systems. *Infect. Control* 3:61, 1982.

38. Centers for Disease Control. Postsurgical infections associated with an extrinsically contaminated intravenous anesthetic agent—California, Illinois, Maine, and Michigan, 1990. *M.M.W.R.* 39:426, 1990.

39. Centers for Disease Control. Septicemias associated with contaminated intravenous fluids. *M.M.W.R.* 22:99, 1973.

40. Centers for Disease Control. *Yersinia enterocolitica* bacteremia and endotoxin shock associated with red blood cell transfusion. *M.M.W.R.* 37:577, 1988.

41. Cercenado, E., et al. A conservative procedure for the diagnosis of catheter-related infections. *Arch. Intern. Med.* 150:1417, 1990.

42. Champault, G. Totally implantable catheters for cancer chemotherapy: French experience on 325 cases. *Cancer Drug Delivery* 3:131, 1986.

43. Cheesbrough, J.S., Finch, R.G., and Burden, R.P. A prospective study of the mechanisms of infection associated with hemodialysis catheters. *J. Infect. Dis.* 154:579, 1986.

44. Christensen, G.D., et al. Adherence of coagulase-negative staphylococci to plastic tissue culture plates: A quantitative model for the adherence of staphylococci to medical devices. *J. Clin. Microbiol.* 22(6):996, 1985.

45. Christensen, G.D., Simpson, W.A., Bisno, A.L., and Beachey, E.H. Adherence of slime-producing strains of *Staphylococcus epidermidis*

to smooth surfaces. *Infect. Immun.* 37:318, 1982.

46. Cohen, A., Reyes, R., Kirk, B., and Fulks, R.M. Osler's nodes, pseudoaneurysm formation, and sepsis complicating percutaneous radial artery cannulation. *Crit. Care Med.* 12:1078, 1984.

47. Collignon, P.J., Soni, N., and Pearson, I.Y. Is semiquantitative culture of central vein catheter tips useful in the diagnosis of catheter-associated bacteremia? *J. Clin. Microbiol.* 24:532, 1986.

48. Collignon, P.J., Sorrell, T.C., and Uther, J.B. Prevention of sepsis associated with the insertion of intravenous cannulae. The experience in a coronary care unit. *Med. J. Aust.* 142:346, 1985.

49. Collin, J., Collin, C., Constable, F.L., and Johnston, I.D. Infusion phlebitis and infection with various cannulas. *Lancet* 2:150, 1975.

50. Conly, J.M., Grieves, K., and Peters, B. A prospective, randomized study comparing transparent and dry gauze dressings for central venous catheters. *J. Infect. Dis.* 159:310, 1989.

51. Cooper, G.L., and Hopkins, C.C. Rapid diagnosis of intravascular catheter-associated infection by direct gram staining of catheter segments. *N. Engl. J. Med.* 18:1142, 1985.

52. Craven, D.E., et al. A randomized study comparing a transparent polyurethane dressing to a dry gauze dressing for peripheral intravenous catheter sites. *Infect. Control* 6:361, 1985.

53. Crocker, K.S., et al. Microbial growth comparisons of five commercial parenteral lipid emulsions. *J.P.E.N.* 8:391, 1984.

54. Crow, S., Conrad, S.A., Chaney-Rowell, K., and King, J.W. Microbial contamination of arterial infusions used for hemodynamic monitoring: A randomized trial of contamination with sampling through conventional stopcocks versus a novel closed system. *Infect. Control Hosp. Epidemiol.* 10:557, 1989.

55. Daisy, J.A., Abrutyn, E.A., and MacGregor, R.R. Inadvertent administration of intravenous fluids contaminated with fungus. *Ann. Intern. Med.* 91:563, 1979.

56. Damen, J. The microbiological risk of invasive hemodynamic monitoring in adults undergoing cardiac valve replacement. *J. Clin. Monit.* 2:87, 1986.

57. Davenport, D.S., et al. Usefulness of a test for slime production as a marker for clinically significant infections with coagulase-negative staphylococci. *J. Infect. Dis.* 153(2):332, 1986.

58. Deitel, M., et al. An outbreak of *Staphylococcus epidermidis* septicemia. *J.P.E.N.* 7:569, 1983.

59. Dickerson, N., Horton, P., Smith, S., and Rose, R., III. Clinically significant central venous catheter infections in a community hospital: Association with type of dressing. *J. Infect. Dis.* 160(4):720, 1989.

60. Dietrich, K.A., and Lobos, J.G. Use of a single Silastic IV catheter for cystic fibrosis pulmonary exacerbations. *Pediatr. Pulmonol.* 4:181, 1988.

61. Dixon, R.E., et al. Aqueous quaternary ammonium antiseptics and disinfectants. Use and misuse. *J.A.M.A.* 236:2415, 1976.

62. Dougherty, S.H. Pathobiology of infection in prosthetic devices. *Rev. Infect. Dis.* 10(6):1102, 1988.

63. Edwards, K.E., et al. *Enterobacter aerogenes* primary bacteremia in pediatric patients. *Pediatrics* 62:304, 1978.

64. Ehrie, M., Morgan, A.P., Moore, E.D., and O'Connor, N.E. Endocarditis with the indwelling balloon-tipped pulmonary artery catheter in burn patients. *J. Trauma* 18:664, 1978.

65. Evans, R.C., and Holmes, C.J. Effect of Vancomycin hydrochloride on *Staphylococcus epidermidis* biofilm associated with silicone elastomer. *Antimicrob. Agents Chemother.* 31(6):889, 1987.

66. Eyer, S., et al. Catheter-related sepsis: Prospective, randomized study of three methods of long-term catheter maintenance. *Crit. Care Med.* 18:1073, 1990.

67. Falchuk, K.H., Peterson, L., and McNeil, B.J. Microparticulate-induced phlebitis. Its prevention by in-line filtration. *N. Engl. J. Med.* 312:78, 1985.

68. Falcieri, E., et al. Role of bacterial expolymers and host factors on adherence and phagocytosis of *Staphylococcus aureus* in foreign body infection. *J. Infect. Dis.* 155(3):524, 1987.

69. Fan, S.T., et al. Predictive value of surveillance skin and hub cultures in central venous catheter sepsis. *J. Hosp. Infect.* 12(3):191, 1988.

70. Faubion, W.C., Wesley, J.R., Khalidi, N., and Silva, J. Total parenteral nutrition catheter sepsis: Impact of the team approach. *J.P.E.N.* 10(6):642, 1986.

71. Flowers, R.H., III, et al. Efficacy of an attachable subcutaneous cuff for the prevention of intravascular catheter–related infection. *J.A.M.A.* 261:878, 1989.

72. Flynn, P.M., Shenep, J.L., Stokes, D.C., and Barrett, F.F. *In situ* management of confirmed central venous catheter-related bacteremia. *Pediatr. Infect. Dis. J.* 6:729, 1987.

73. Franceschi, D., Gerding, R.L., Phillips, G., and Gratianne, R.B. Risk factors associated with intravascular catheter infections in

burned patients: A prospective, randomized study. *J. Trauma* 29(6):811, 1989.

74. Frank, M.J., and Schaffner, W. Contaminated aqueous benzalkonium chloride. An unnecessary hospital infection hazard. *J.A.M.A.* 236:2418, 1976.

75. Franson, T.R., Sheth, N.K., Rose, H.D., and Sohnle, P.G. Scanning electron microscopy of bacteria adherent to intravascular catheters. *J. Clin. Microbiol.* 20(3):500, 1987.

76. Freeman, J.B., Lemire, A., and MacLean, L.D. Intravenous alimentation and septicemia. *Surg. Gynecol. Obstet.* 135:708, 1972.

77. Freeman, J.B., and Litton, A.A. Preponderance of gram-positive infections during parenteral alimentation. *Surg. Gynecol. Obstet.* 139:905, 1974.

78. Freeman, R., et al. Addition of sodium metabisulfite to left atrial catheter infusate as a means of preventing bacterial colonization of the catheter tip. *Thorax* 37:142, 1982.

79. Friedland, G. Infusion-related phlebitis—is the in-line filter the solution (edit.)? *N. Engl. J. Med.* 312:113, 1985.

80. Fuchs, P.C., Gustafson, M.E., King, J.T., and Goodall, P.T. Assessment of catheter-associated infection risk with the Hickman right atrial catheter. *Infect. Control* 5:226, 1984.

81. Gantz, N.M., Presswood, G.M., Goldberg, R., and Doern, G. Effects of dressing type and change interval on intravenous therapy complication rates. *Diagn. Microbiol. Infect. Dis.* 2:325, 1984.

82. Garner, J.S., et al. CDC definitions for nosocomial infections, 1988. *Am. J. Infect. Control* 16:128, 1988.

83. Gayo, D.S., Richey, H.M., and Matthews, J.I. Safety and efficacy of guidewire exchange technique for central venous catheters in the ICU. *Chest* 92(Suppl.):101S, 1987.

84. Goldmann, D.A., Martin, W.T., and Worthington, J.W. Growth of bacteria and fungi in total parenteral nutrition solutions. *Am. J. Surg.* 126:314, 1973.

85. Gorbea, H.F., et al. Intravenous tubing with burettes can be safely changed at 48-hour intervals. *J.A.M.A.* 251:2112, 1984.

86. Graeve, A.H., Carpenter, C.M., and Schiller, W.R. Management of central venous catheters using a wire introducer. *Am. J. Surg.* 142:752, 1981.

87. Graham, D.R., et al. Infectious complications among patients receiving home intravenous therapy with peripheral, central, or peripherally placed central venous catheters. *Am. J. Med.* 91(Suppl. 3B):95S, 1991.

88. Gristina, A.G. Biomaterial-centered infection: Microbial adhesion versus tissue integration. *Science* 237:1588, 1987.

89. Guerra-Romnero, L., et al. Comparison of Du Pont Isolator and Roche Septi-Chek for detection of fungemia. *J. Clin. Microbiol.* 25:1623, 1987.

90. Habibi, B., et al. Le Choc transfusionnel par contamination bacterienne du sang conserve. Analyse de 25 observations. *Rev. Fr. Transfus.* 16:41, 1973.

91. Hanson, A.L., and Shelley, R.M. Monitoring contamination levels of in-use intravenous solutions using "total sample" techniques. *Am. J. Hosp. Pharm.* 31:733, 1974.

92. Heal, J.M., Jones, M.E., Chaudry, A., and Stricop, R.L. Fatal *Salmonella* septicemia after platelet transfusion. *Transfusion* 27:2, 1987.

93. Henderson, D.K., Edwards, J.E., and Montgomerie, J.Z. Hematogenous *Candida* endophthalmitis in patients receiving parenteral hyperalimentation fluids. *J. Infect. Dis.* 143:655, 1981.

94. Herrmann, M., et al. Fibronectin, fibrinogen, and laminin act as mediators of adherence of clinical staphylococcal isolates to foreign material. *J. Infect. Dis.* 158(4):693, 1988.

95. High, K.P., et al. A randomized controlled trial of scheduled central venous catheter (CVC) replacement (abstr. 1080). In: *Proceedings and Abstracts of the Thirtieth Interscience Conference on Antimicrobial Agents and Chemotherapy,* Atlanta: American Society of Microbiology, 1989.

96. Hill, R.L.R., et al. Mupirocin for the reduction of colonization of internal jugular cannulae—a randomized controlled trial. *J. Hosp. Infect.* 15:311, 1990.

97. Hilton, E., et al. Central catheter infections: Single- versus triple-lumen catheters. Influence of guide wires on infection rates when used for replacement of catheters. *Am. J. Med.* 84:667, 1988.

98. Hoffman, K.K., et al. Bacterial colonization and phlebitis-associated risk with transparent polyurethane film for peripheral intravenous site dressings. *Am. J. Infect. Control* 16:101, 1988.

99. Holland, K.T., Davis, W., Ingham, E., and Gowland, G. A comparison of the in-vitro antibacterial and complement activating effect of 'OpSite' and 'Tegaderm' dressings. *J. Hosp. Infect.* 5:323, 1984.

100. Hudson-Civetta, J.A., Civetta, J.M., Martinez, O.V., and Hoffman, T.A. Risk and detection of pulmonary artery catheter-related infection in septic surgical patients. *Crit. Care Med.* 15:29, 1987.

101. Ilstrup, D.M., and Washington, J.A., II. The importance of volume of blood cultured in the detection of bacteremia and fungemia. *Diagn. Microbiol. Infect. Dis.* 1:107, 1983.

102. Isaacman, D.J., and Karasic, R.B. Utility of collecting blood cultures through newly in-

serted intravenous catheters. *Pediatr. Infect. Dis. J.* 9:815, 1990.

103. James, J.D. Bacterial contamination of reserved blood. *Vox Sang.* 4:177, 1959.

104. Jarvis, W.R., et al. Nosocomial outbreaks: The Centers for Disease Control's Hospital Infections Program experience, 1980–1991. *Am. J. Med.* 91(Suppl. 3B):101S, 1991.

105. Jarvis, W.R., et al. Polymicrobial bacteremia associated with use of lipid emulsion in a neonatal intensive care unit. *Pediatr. Infect. Dis. J.* 2:203, 1983.

106. Johnson, R.A., Zajac, R.A., and Evans, M.E. Suppurative thrombophlebitis: Correlation between pathogen and underlying disease. *Infect. Control* 7:582, 1986.

107. Joseph, P., and Marzouk, J. Transparent vs. dry gauze dressings for peripheral IV sites (abstr. 378). In: *Program and Abstracts of the Annual Meeting of the American Society for Microbiology.* Las Vegas: American Society for Microbiology, 1985.

108. Josephson, A., et al. The relationship between intravenous fluid contamination and the frequency of tubing replacement. *Infect. Control* 6(9):367, 1985.

109. Kahan, A., et al. Nosocomial infections by chlorhexidine solution contaminated with *Pseudomonas pickettii* (biovar VA-I). *J. Infect.* 7:256, 1983.

110. Kamal, G.D., Pfaller, M.A., Rempe, L.E., and Jebson, P.J.R. Reduced intravascular catheter infection by antibiotic bonding. *J.A.M.A.* 265(18):2364, 1991.

111. Katich, M., and Band, J. Local infection of the intravenous-cannulae wound associated with transparent dressings. *J. Infect. Dis.* 151:971, 1985.

112. Kelsey, M.C., and Gosling, M. A comparison of the morbidity associated with occlusive and non-occlusive dressings applied to peripheral intravenous devices. *J. Hosp. Infect.* 5:313, 1984.

113. Keohane, P.P., et al. Effect of catheter tunnelling and a nutrition nurse on catheter sepsis during parenteral nutrition. A controlled trial. *Lancet* Dec. 17: 1388, 1983.

114. Komshian, S.V., Uwaydah, A.K., Sobel, J.D., and Crane, L.R. Fungemia caused by *Candida* species and *Torulopsis glabrata* in the hospitalized patient: Frequency, characteristics, and evaluation of factors influencing outcome. *Rev. Infect. Dis.* 3:379, 1989.

115. Koontz, F.P., Flint, K.K., Reynolds, J.K., and Allen, S.D. Multicenter comparison of the high volume (10 ml) NR *Bactec Plus* system and the standard (5 ml) NR *Bactec* system. *Diagn. Microbiol. Infect. Dis.* 14:111, 1991.

116. Kotilainen, P. Association of coagulase-negative staphylococcal slime production and

adherence with the development and outcome of adult septicemias. *J. Clin. Microbiol.* 28:2779, 1990.

117. Kristinsson, K.G., Burnett, I.A., and Spence, R.C. Evaluation of three methods for culturing long intravascular catheters. *J. Hosp. Infect.* 14:183, 1989.

118. Larson, E., and Hargiss, C. A decentralized approach to maintenance of intravenous therapy. *Am. J. Infect. Control* 12:177, 1984.

119. Levin, A., et al. The value of topical povidone-iodine (PV-I) ointment in the prevention of hemodialysis related sepsis (abstr. 1078). In: *Program and Abstracts of the Twenty-Ninth Interscience Conference on Antimicrobial Agents and Chemotherapy.* Houston: American Society for Microbiology, 1989.

120. Linares, J., et al. Pathogenesis of catheter sepsis: A prospective study with quantitative and semiquantitative cultures of catheter hub and segments. *J. Clin. Microbiol.* 21:357, 1985.

121. Lokich, J.J., et al. Complications and management of implanted venous access catheters. *J. Clin. Oncol.* 3:710, 1985.

122. Longfield, J.N., Charache, P., Diamond, E.L., and Townsend, T.R. Comparison of broth and filtration methods for culturing of intravenous fluids. *Infect. Control* 3:397, 1982.

123. Luskin, R.L., et al. Extended use of disposable pressure transducers: A bacteriologic evaluation. *J.A.M.A.* 255:916, 1986.

124. Mackel, D.C., et al. Nationwide epidemic of septicemia caused by contaminated intravenous products: Mechanisms of intrinsic contamination. *J. Clin. Microbiol.* 2:486, 1975.

125. Maddox, R.R., John, J.F., Jr., Brown, L.L., and Smith, C.E. Effect of inline filtration on postinfusion phlebitis. *Clin. Pharm.* 2:58, 1983.

126. Maibach, H.I., and Hildick-Smith, G. *Skin Bacteria and Their Role in Infection.* New York: McGraw-Hill, 1965.

127. Maki, D.G. Epidemic Nosocomial Bacteremias. In: Wenzel, R.R. (Ed), *Handbook of Hospital Infection.* West Palm Beach, FL: CRC Press, 1981. Pp. 371–512.

128. Maki, D.G. The epidemiology and prevention of nosocomial bloodstream infections (abstr. 3). In: *Program and Abstracts of the Third International Conference on Nosocomial Infections.* Atlanta: Centers for Disease Control, The National Foundation for Infectious Diseases and the American Society for Microbiology, 1990.

129. Maki, D.G. Growth Properties of Microorganisms in Infusion Fluid and Methods of Detection. In: Phillips, I. (Ed.), *Microbiologic Hazards of Intravenous Therapy.* Lancaster, Engl.: MTP Press, 1977. Pp. 13–47.

130. Maki, D.G. Growth properties of microorganisms in lipid for infusion and implications for infection control. In: *Program and Abstracts of the Twentieth Interscience Conference on Antimicrobial Agents and Chemotherapy*, New Orleans: Amer. Soc. Microbiology, Sep., 1980.

131. Maki, D.G. Marked differences in insertion sites for central venous, arterial and peripheral IV catheters. The major reason for differing risks of catheter-related infection (abstr. 712)? In: *Program and Abstracts of the Thirtieth Interscience Conference on Antimicrobial Agents and Chemotherapy*. Atlanta: American Society for Microbiology, Oct., 1990.

132. Maki, D.G. Nosocomial bacteremia. *Am. J. Med.* 70:183, 1981.

133. Maki, D.G. Sepsis Arising from Extrinsic Contamination of the Infusion and Measure for Control. In: Phillips, I. (Ed), *Microbiologic Hazards of Infusion Therapy*. Lancaster, Engl.: MTP Press, 1977. Pp. 99–141.

134. Maki, D.G. Through a glass darkly. Nosocomial pseudoepidemics and pseudobacteremias (edit.). *Arch. Intern. Med.* 140:26, 1980.

135. Maki, D.G. The use of antiseptics for handwashing by medical personnel. *J. Chemother.* 1(Suppl. 1):3, 1989.

136. Maki, D.G. Alvarado, C.J., and Ringer, M. A prospective, randomized trial of povidone-iodine, alcohol and chlorhexidine for prevention of infection with central venous and arterial catheters. *Lancet* 338:339, 1991.

137. Maki, D.G., and Band, J.D. A comparative study of polyantibiotic and iodophor ointments in prevention of catheter-related infection. *Am. J. Med.* 70:739, 1981.

138. Maki, D.G., Botticelli, J.T., LeRoy, M.L., and Thielke, T.S. Prospective study of replacing administration sets for intravenous therapy at 48- vs 72-hour intervals. *J.A.M.A.* 258:1777, 1987.

139. Maki, D.G., et al. An attachable silver-impregnated cuff for prevention of infection with central venous catheters. A prospective randomized multi-center trial. *Am. J. Med.* 85:307, 1988.

140. Maki, D.G., et al. Nosocomial *Pseudomonas pickettii* bacteremias traced to narcotic tampering. A case for selective drug screening of health care personnel. *J.A.M.A.* 265:981, 1991.

142. Maki, D.G., and Hassemer, C.H. Endemic rate of fluid contamination and related septicemia in arterial pressure monitoring. *Am. J. Med.* 70:733, 1981.

143. Maki, D.G., and Martin, W.T. Nationwide epidemic of septicemia caused by contaminated infusion products. IV. Growth of microbial pathogens in fluids for intravenous infusion. *J. Infect. Dis.* 131:267, 1975.

143A. Maki, D.G., Jarrett, F., and Safarin, H.W. A semiquantitative culture method for identification of catheter-related infection in the burn patient. *J. Surg. Res.* 22:513, 1977.

144. Maki, D.G., and McCormack, K.N. Defatting catheter insertion sites in total parenteral nutrition is of no value as an infection control measure. *Am. J. Med.* 83:833, 1987.

145. Maki, D.G., McCormick, R.D., Uman, S.J., and Wirtanen, G.W. Septic endarteritis due to intra-arterial catheters for cancer chemotherapy: I. Evaluation of an outbreak. II. Risk factors, clinical features and management. III. Guidelines for prevention. *Cancer* 44:1228, 1979.

146. Maki, D.G., Rhame, F.S., Mackel, D.C., and Bennett, J.V. Nationwide epidemic of septicemia caused by contaminated intravenous products. *Am. J. Med.* 60:471, 1976.

147. Maki, D.G., and Ringer, M. Evaluation of dressing regimens for prevention of infection with peripheral intravenous catheters. *J.A.M.A.* 258:2396, 1987.

148. Maki, D.G., and Ringer, M. Prospective study of arterial catheter–related infection: Incidence, sources of infection and risk factors (abstr. 1075). In: *Proceedings of the Twenty-Ninth Interscience Conference on Antimicrobial Agents and Chemotherapy*. Houston: American Society for Microbiology, 1989.

149. Maki, D.G., and Ringer, M. Risk factors for infusion-related phlebitis with small peripheral venous catheters. *Ann. Intern. Med.* 114(10):845, 1991.

150. Maki, D.G., Stolz, S., and Wheeler, S. A Prospective, Randomized, Three-Way Clinical Comparison of a Novel, Highly-Permeable, Polyurethane Dressing with 206 Swan Ganz Pulmonary-Artery Catheters: OpSite IV3000 vs Tegaderm vs Gauze and Tape. I. Cutaneous Colonization Under the Dressing, Catheter-Related Infection. In: Maki, D.G., (Ed.), *Improving Catheter Site Care*. London: Royal Society of Medicine Services, 1991.

151. Maki, D.G., Weise, C.E., and Sarafin, H.W. A semiquantitative culture method for identifying intravenous-catheter infection. *N. Engl. J. Med.* 296:1305, 1977.

152. Maki, D.G., Wheeler, S.J., Stolz, S.M., and Mermel, L.A. Clinical trial of a novel antiseptic central venous catheter (abstr. 461). In: *Program and Abstracts of the Thirty-First Interscience Conference on Antimicrobial Agents and Chemotherapy*. Chicago: American Society for Microbiology, 1991.

153. Maki, D.G., and Will L. Colonization and infection associated with transparent dressings for central venous, arterial, and Hickman catheters: A comparative trial (abstr. 991). In: *Program and Abstracts of the Twenty-Fourth*

Interscience Conference on Antimicrobial Agents and Chemotherapy. Washington, DC: American Society for Microbiology, 1984.

154. Marrie, T.J., and Costerton, J.W. Scanning and transmission electron microscopy of in situ bacterial colonization of intravenous and intraarterial catheters. *J. Clin. Microbiol.* 19(5):687, 1984.

155. Martin, M.A., Pfaller, M.A., and Wenzel, R.P. Coagulase-negative staphylococcal bacteremia. Mortality and hospital stay. *Ann. Intern. Med.* 110:9, 1989.

156. Matsaniotis, N.S., et al. *Enterobacter* sepsis in infants and children due to contaminated intravenous fluids. *Infect. Control* 5:471, 1984.

157. Mayhall, C.G., Pierpaoli, P.G., Hall, G.O., and Thomas, R.B. Evaluation of a device for monitoring sterility of infectable fluids. *Am. J. Hosp. Pharm.* 38:1148, 1981.

158. McCredie, K.B., Lawson, M., Marts, K., and Stern, J. A comparative evaluation of transparent dressings and gauze dressings for central venous catheters (abstr.). *J.P.E.N.* 8:96, 1984.

159. McGeer, A., and Righter, J. Improving our ability to diagnose infections associated with central venous catheters: Value of Gram's staining and culture of entry site swabs. *Can. Med. Assoc. J.* 137:1009, 1987.

160. McKee, K.T., et al. Gram-negative bacillary sepsis associated with use of lipid emulsion in parenteral nutrition. *Am.J.Dis.Child.* 133:649, 1979.

161. Meers, P.D., Calder, M.W., Maxhar, M.M., and Lawrie, G.M. Intravenous infusion of contaminated dextrose solution: The Devonport incident. *Lancet* 2:1189, 1973.

162. Mermel, L.A., Maki, D.G. Epidemic bloodstream infections from hemodynamic pressure monitoring: Signs of the times. *Infect. Control Hosp. Epidemiol.* 10(2):47, 1989.

163. Mermel, L.A., Velez, L.A., Zilz, M.A., and Maki, D.G. Epidemiologic and microbiologic features of nosocomial bloodstream infection (NBSI) implicating a vascular catheter source: A case-control study of 85 vascular catheter-related and 101 secondary NBSIs (abstr. 454). In: *Program and Abstracts of the Thirty-First Interscience Conference on Antimicrobial Agents and Chemotherapy.* Chicago: American Society for Microbiology, 1991.

164. Mermel, L., McCormick, R., and Maki, D.G. Epidemiology and pathogenesis of infection with Swan-Ganz catheters. A prospective study using molecular epidemiology. *Am. J. Med.* 91(3B):197, 1991.

165. Mertz, P.M., and Eaglestein, W.H. The effect of a semiocclusive dressing on the microbial population in superficial wounds. *Arch. Surg.* 119:287, 1984.

166. Michaels, L., and Ruebner, B. Growth of bacteria in intravenous infusion fluids. *Lancet* 1:722, 1953.

167. Miller, R.C., and Grogan, J.B. Incidence and source of contamination of intravenous nutritional infusion systems. *J. Pediatr. Surg.* 8:185, 1973.

168. Moran, J.M., Atwood, R.P., and Rowe, M.I. A clinical bacteriologic study of infections associated with venous cut downs. *N. Engl. J. Med.* 272:554, 1965.

169. Mumford, F., Grossman, A., and Hilton, E. An outbreak of intravascular site infections (abstr.). *Am. J. Infect. Control* 13:140, 1985.

170. Nehme, A.E. Nutritional support of the hospitalized patient: The team concept. *J.A.M.A.* 243:1906, 1980.

171. Nehme, A.E., and Trigger, J.A. Catheter dressings in central parenteral nutrition: A prospective randomized comparative study. *Nutritional Support Services* 4:42, 1984.

172. Nelson, D.B., et al. Dressing changes by specialized personnel reduce infection rates in patients receiving central venous parenteral nutrition. *J.P.E.N.* 10(2):220, 1986.

173. Norden, C.W. Application of antibiotic ointment to the site of venous catheterization—a controlled trial. *J. Infect. Dis.* 120:611, 1969.

174. Norwood, S., and Jenkins, G. An evaluation of triple-lumen catheter infections using a guidewire exchange technique. *J. Trauma* 30:706, 1990.

175. Nyström, B., et al. Bacteraemia in surgical patients with intravenous devices: A European multicentre incidence study. *J. Hosp. Infect.* 4:338, 1983.

176. Padberg, F.T., Jr., Ruggiero, J., Blackburn, G.L., and Bistrian, B.R. Central venous catheterization for parenteral nutrition. *Ann. Surg.* 193:264, 1981.

177. Palidar, P.J., et al. Use of OpSite as an occlusive dressing for total parenteral nutrition catheters. *J.P.E.N.* 6(2):150, 1982.

178. Parrott, P.L., et al. *Pseudomonas aeruginosa* peritonitis associated with contaminated poloxamer-iodine solution. *Lancet* 2:683, 1982.

179. Pascual, A., Fleer, A., Westerdaal, N.A.C., and Verhoef, J. Modulation of adherence of coagulase-negative staphylococci to Teflon catheters in vitro. *Eur. J. Clin. Microbiol.* 5(5):518, 1986.

180. Perceval, A. Infection from intravenous delivery systems (lett.). *Ann. Intern. Med.* 93:376, 1980.

181. Pettigrew, R.A., et al. Catheter-related sepsis in patients on intravenous nutrition: A prospective study of quantitative catheter cultures and guidewire changes for suspected sepsis. *Br. J. Surg.* 72:52, 1985.

182. Pezzarossi, H.E., et al. High incidence of sub-clavian dialysis catheter-related bacteremias. *Infect. Control* 7(12):596, 1986.

183. Phillips, I., and Eykyn, S. *Pseudomonas cepacia* (multivorans) septicaemia in an intensive care unit. *Lancet* Feb. 20:375, 1971.

184. Pittet, D., Churad, C., Rae, A.C., and Auck-enthaler, R. Clinical diagnosis of central ven-ous catheter line infections: A difficult job (abstr. 453). In: *Program and Abstracts of the Thirty-First Interscience Conference on Anti-microbial Agents and Chemotherapy.* Chicago: American Society for Microbiology, 1991.

185. Pittman, M. A study of bacteria implicated in transfusion reactions and of bacteria isolated from blood products. *J. Lab. Clin. Med.* 42:273, 1953.

186. Platzner, N., et al. Eliminating the cul-de-sac from pressure cone infusion systems reduces fluid contamination (abstr. 931). In: *Proceed-ings of the Twenty-Second Interscience Conference on Antimicrobial Agents and Chemotherapy.* New Orleans: American Society for Microbiology, 1982.

187. Plouffe, J.F., et al. Nosocomial outbreak of *Candida parapsilosis* fungemia related to intra-venous infusions. *Arch. Inter. Med.* 137:1686, 1977.

188. Porter, K.A., Bistrian, B.R., and Blackburn, G.L. Guidewire catheter exchange with triple culture technique in the management of catheter sepsis. *J.P.E.N.* 12:628, 1988.

189. Pourcyrous, M., et al. Indwelling umbilical arterial catheter: A preferred sampling site for blood culture. *Pediatrics* 81:821, 1988.

190. Powell, C., et al. Effect of frequent guide-wire changes on triple-lumen catheter sepsis. *J.P.E.N.* 12:462, 1988.

191. Powell, C., et al. Increased catheter sepsis with use of semipermeable membrane dress-ings system (Opsite®) in total parenteral nu-trition (abstr.) *J.P.E.N.* 3:515, 1979.

192. Powell, C., Regan, C., Fabri, P.J., and Ruberg, R.L. Evaluation of Opsite catheter dressings for parenteral nutrition: A prospective, ran-domized study. *J.P.E.N.* 6:43, 1982.

193. Powell, C.R., et al. Op-site dressing study: A prospective randomized study evaluating povidone iodine ointment and extension set changes with 7-day Op-site dressings applied to total parenteral nutrition subclavian sites. *J.P.E.N.* 9:443, 1985.

194. Prager, R.L., and Silva, J. Colonization of central venous catheters. *South. Med. J.* 77:458, 1984.

195. Press, O.W., et al. Hickman catheter infec-tions in patients with malignancies. *Medicine* 63:189, 1984.

196. Pruitt, B.A., Jr., McManus, W.F., Kim, S.H., and Treat, R.C. Diagnosis and treatment of cannula-related intravenous sepsis in burn patients. *Ann. Surg.* 191:546, 1980.

197. Puntis, J.W.L., et al. Staff training: A key fac-tor in reducing intravascular catheter sepsis. *Arch. Dis. Child.* 65:335, 1990.

198. Quinlan, A. *In vivo* assessment of microbial proliferation under OpSite IV 3000, Tega-derm and Tegaderm Plus, with and without serum (abstr.). In: *Proceedings and Abstracts of the Third International Meeting of the Hospital Infection Society.* London: Hospital Infection Society, 1990.

199. Rannem, T., et al. Catheter-related sepsis in long-term parenteral nutrition with Broviac catheters. An evaluation of different disin-fectants. *Clin. Nutr.* 9:131, 1990.

200. Raucher, H.S., et al. Quantitative blood cultures in the evaluation of septicemia in children with Broviac catheters. *J. Pediatr.* 104(1):29, 1984.

201. Reagan, D.R., Pfaller, M.A., Hollis, R.J., and Wenzel, R.P. Characterization of the sequence of colonization and nosocomial candidemia using DNA fingerprinting and a DNA probe. *J. Clin. Microbiol.* 28:2733, 1990.

202. Reier, D., Rhame, F.S., and Vesley, D. Growth of microorganisms in IV solutions containing blood (abstr.). *Am. J. Infect. Control* 12:346, 1984.

203. Rhame, F.S., et al. *Salmonella* septicemia from platelet transfusions. Study of an outbreak traced to a hematogenous carrier of *Salmo-nella cholerae-suis. Ann. Intern. Med.* 78:633, 1973.

204. Rhame, F.S., et al. Transparent adherent dressings (TADs) do not promote abnormal skin flora (abstr.). *Am. J. Infect. Control* 11:152, 1983.

205. Ricard, P., Martin, R., and Marcoux, J.A. Protection of indwelling vascular catheters: Incidence of bacterial contamination and catheter-related sepsis. *Crit. Care Med.* 13:541, 1985.

206. Richet, H., et al. Prospective multicenter study of vascular-catheter-related complica-tions and risk factors for positive central-catheter cultures in intensive care unit patients. *J. Clin. Microbiol.* 28:2520, 1990.

207. Roberts, L.A., et al. An Australia-wide epi-demic of *Pseudomonas pickettii* bacteraemia due to contaminated "sterile" water for injec-tion. *Med. J. Aust.* 152:652, 1990.

208. Rotrosen, D., Calderone, R.A., and Edwards, J.E., Jr. Adherence of *Candida* species to host tissues and plastic surfaces. *Rev. Infect. Dis.* 8:73, 1986.

209. Rotrosen, D., Gibson, T.R., and Edwards, J.E., Jr. Adherence of *Candida* species to in-travenous catheters. *J. Infect. Dis.* 147(3):594, 1983.

210. Rowley, K.M., Clubb, K.S., Smith, G.J.W., and Cabin, J.S. Right-sided infective endocarditis as a consequence of flow-related pulmonary-artery catheterization. A clinicopathologic study of 55 autopsied patients. *N. Engl. J. Med.* 311:1152, 1984.

211. Russell, P.B., Kline, J., Yoder, M.C., and Polin, R.A. Staphylococcal adherence to polyvinyl chloride and heparin-bonded polyurethane catheters is species dependent and enhanced by fibronectin. *J. Clin. Microbiol.* 25(6):1083, 1987.

212. Sanders, R.A., and Sheldon, G.F. Septic complications of total parenteral nutrition. A five year experience. *Am. J. Surg.* 132:214, 1976.

213. Sanderson, I., and Deitel, M. Intravenous hyperalimentation without sepsis. *Surg. Gynecol. Obstet.* 136:577, 1973.

214. Schadow, K.H., Simpson, W.A., and Christensen, G.D. Characteristics of adherence to plastic tissue culture plates of coagulase-negative staphylococci exposed to subinhibitory concentrations of antimicrobial agents. *J. Infect. Dis.* 157:71, 1988.

215. Schwartz-Fulton, J., Colley, R., Valanis, B., and Fischer, J.E. Hyperalimentation dressings and skin flora. *NITA* 4:354, 1981.

216. Segura, M., et al. Assessment of a new hub design and the semiquantitative catheter culture method using an in vivo experimental model of catheter sepsis. *J. Clin. Microbiol.* 28(11):2551, 1990.

217. Segura, M., et al. In vitro bacteriological study of a new hub model for intravascular catheters and infusion equipment. *J. Clin. Microbiol.* 27(12):2656, 1989.

218. Sheretz, R.J., et al. Infections associated with subclavian Uldall catheters. *Arch. Intern. Med.* 143:52, 1983.

219. Sheretz, R.J., et al. Three-year experience with sonicated vascular catheter cultures in a clinical microbiology laboratory. *J. Clin. Microbiol.* 28(1):76, 1990.

220. Sheth, N.K., et al. *In vitro* quantitative adherence of bacteria to intravascular catheters. *J. Surg. Res.* 34:213, 1983.

221. Sheth, N.K., Franson, T.R., and Sohnle, P.G. Influence of bacterial adherence to intravascular catheters on in-vitro antibiotic susceptibility. *Lancet* 2:1266, 1985.

222. Shinozaki, T., et al. Bacterial contamination of arterial lines. *J.A.M.A.* 249:223, 1983.

223. Shivnan, J.C., et al. Comparison of transparent adherent and dry sterile gauze dressings for long-term central catheters in patients undergoing bone marrow transplant. *Oncol. Nurses Forum* 18:1349, 1991.

224. Siboni, K., et al. *Pseudomonas cepacia* in 16 non-fatal cases of postoperative bacteremia derived from intrinsic contamination of the anaesthetic Fentanyl. *Scand. J. Infect. Dis.* 11:39, 1979.

225. Simmons, B. Alternative to i.v. filter usage (lett.). *Infect. Control* 6:342, 1985.

226. Sitges-Serra, A., et al. Hub colonization as the initial step in an outbreak of catheter-related sepsis due to coagulase negative staphylococci during parenteral nutrition. *J.P.E.N.* 8:668, 1984.

227. Sitges-Serra, A., Linares, J., and Garau, J. Catheter sepsis: The clue is the hub. *Surgery* 97:355, 1985.

228. Sitzmann, J.V., Townsend, T.R., Siler, M.C., and Bartlett, J.G. Septic and technical complications of central venous catheterization. A prospective study of 200 consecutive patients. *Ann. Surg.* 202:766, 1985.

229. Smallman, L., Burdon, D.W., and Alexander-Williams, J. The effect of skin preparation on the incidence of infusion thrombophlebitis. *Br. J. Surg.* 67:861, 1980.

230. Smith, R.L., Meixler, S.M., and Simberkoff, M.S. Excess mortality in critically ill patients with nosocomial bloodstream infections. *Chest* 100:164, 1991.

231. Snyder, R.H., et al. Catheter infection. A comparison of two catheter maintenance techniques. *Ann. Surg.* 208:651, 1988.

232. Snydman, D.R., et al. Nosocomial sepsis associated with Interleukin-2. *Ann. Intern. Med.* 112:102, 1990.

233. Snydman, D.R., et al. Predictive value of surveillance skin cultures in total parenteral nutrition–related infection. *Lancet* 2:1385, 1982.

234. Snydman, D.R., et al. Total parenteral nutrition–related infections. Prospective epidemiologic study using semiquantitative methods. *Am. J. Med.* 73:695, 1982.

235. Snydman, D.R., Reidy, M.D., Perry, L.K., and Martin, W.J. Safety of changing intravenous (IV) administration sets containing burettes at longer than 48 hour intervals. *Infect. Control* 8:113, 1987.

236. Soifer, N.E., Edlin, B.R., Weinstein, R.A., and MRH IV Study Group. A randomized IV team trial (abstr. 1076). In: *Program and Abstracts of the Twenty-Ninth Interscience Conference on Antimicrobial Agents and Chemotherapy*, Houston: American Society for Microbiology, 1989.

237. Solomon, S.L., et al. An outbreak of *Candida parapsilosis* bloodstream infections in patients receiving parenteral nutrition. *J. Infect. Dis.* 149:98, 1984.

238. Solomon, S.L., et al. Nosocomial fungemia in neonates associated with intravascular pressure-monitoring devices. *Pediatr. Infect. Dis.* 5:680, 1986.

239. Steere, A.C., et al. *Pseudomonas* species bac-

teremia caused by contaminated normal human serum albumin. *J. Infect. Dis.* 135:729, 1977.

240. Steere, A.C., et al. Pyrogenic reactions associated with the infusion of normal serum albumin (human). *Transfusion* 18:102, 1978.

241. Stillman, R.M., Soliman, F., Garcia, L., and Sawyer, P.N. Etiology of catheter-associated sepsis. Correlation with thrombogenicity. *Arch. Surg.* 112:1497, 1977.

242. Stotter, A.T., Ward, H., Waterfield, A.H., and Sim, A.J.W. Junctional care: The key to prevention of catheter sepsis in intravenous feeding. *J.P.E.N.* 11:159, 1987.

243. Strinden, W.D., Helgerson, R.B., and Maki, D.G. *Candida* septic thrombosis of the great veins associated with central catheters. Clinical features and management. *Ann. Surg.* 202:653, 1985.

244. Tager, I.B., et al. An epidemiologic study of the risks associated with peripheral intravenous catheters. *Am. J. Epidemiol.* 118:839, 1983.

245. Tegtmeier, B.R., and Vice, J.L. Evaluation of the BACTEC® 16B medium in a cancer center. *Am. J. Clin. Pathol.* 81:783, 1984.

246. Thomas, F., et al. The risk of infection related to radial vs. femoral sites for arterial catheterization. *Crit. Care Med.* 11:807, 1988.

247. Thomas, S., Loveless, P., and Hay, N.P. Comparative review of the properties of six semipermeable film dressings. *Pharm. J.* 241:785, 1988.

248. Tomford, J.W., et al. Intravenous therapy team and peripheral venous catheter–associated complications. A prospective controlled study. *Arch. Intern. Med.* 144:1191, 1984.

249. Tomford, J.W., and Hershey, C.O. The I.V. therapy team. Impact on patient care and costs of hospitalization. *NITA* 8:387, 1985.

250. Torres-Rohas, J.R., et al. Candidal suppurative peripheral thrombophlebitis. *Ann. Intern. Med.* 96:431, 1982.

251. Trilla, A., et al. Risk factors for nosocomial bacteremia in a large Spanish teaching hospital: A case-control study. *Infect. Control Hosp. Epidemiol.* 12:150, 1991.

252. Tully, J.L., Friedland, G.H., Baldini, L.M., and Goldmann, D.A. Complications of intravenous therapy with steel needles and Teflon catheters. A comparative study. *Am. J. Med.* 70:702, 1981.

253. Vanherweghem, J-L., et al. Infections associated with subclavian dialysis catheters: The key role of nurse training. *Nephron* 42:116, 1986.

254. Vanhuynegem, L., Parmentier, P., and Potvliege, C. In situ bacteriologic diagnosis of total parenteral nutrition catheter infection. *Surgery* 103(2):174, 1987.

255. Vaudaux, P., et al. Fibronectin is more active than fibrin or fibrinogen in promoting *Staphylococcus aureus* adherence to inserted intravascular catheters. *J. Clin. Invest.* (in press).

256. Vaudaux, P., et al. Host factors selectively increase staphylococcal adherence on inserted catheters: A role for fibronectin and fibrinogen or fibrin. *J. Infect. Dis.* 160:865, 1989.

257. Vaudaux, P., Lew, D., and Waldvogel, F.A. Host-dependent pathogenic factors in foreign body infection. A comparison between *Staphylococcus epidermidis* and *S. aureus*. *Zbl. Bakt.* Suppl. 16:183, 1987.

258. Vaudaux, P.E., Waldvogel, F.A., Morgenthaler, J.J., and Nydegger, U.E. Adsorption of fibronectin onto polymethylmethacrylate and promotion of *Staphylococcus aureus* adherence. *Infect. Immun.* 45(3):768, 1984.

259. Verghese, A., Widrich, W.C., and Arbeit, R.D. Central venous septic thrombophlebitis—the role of medical therapy. *Medicine* 64:394, 1985.

260. Warden, G.D., Wilmore, D.W., and Pruitt, B.A. Central venous thrombosis: A hazard of medical progress. *J. Trauma* 13:620, 1973.

261. Washington, J.A., II, and Ilstrup, D.M. Blood cultures: Issues and controversies. *Rev. Infect. Dis.* 8(5):792, 1986.

262. Weightman, N.C., et al. Bacteraemia related to indwelling central venous catheters: Prevention, diagnosis and treatment. *Eur. J. Clin. Microbiol. Infect. Dis.* 7(2):125, 1988.

263. Weinstein, M.P., et al. The clinical significance of positive blood cultures: A comprehensive analysis of 500 episodes of bacteremia and fungemia in adults. I. Laboratory and epidemiological observations. *Rev. Infect. Dis.* 5:35, 1983.

264. Wey, S.B., et al. Risk factors for hospital-acquired candidemia. A matched case-control study. *Arch. Intern. Med.* 149:2349, 1989.

265. Williams, D.N., Gibson, J., Vos, J., and Kind, A.C. Infusion thrombophlebitis and infiltration associated with intravenous cannulae: A controlled study comparing three different cannula types. *N.I.T.A.* 5:379, 1982.

266. Wormser, G.P., et al. Sensitivity and specificity of blood cultures obtained through intravascular catheters. *Crit. Care Med.* 18:152, 1990.

267. Wrenn, J.E., and Speicher, C.E. Platelet concentrates: Sterility of 400 single units stored at room temperature. *Transfusion* 14:171, 1974.

268. Wurzel, C.L., Halom, C., Feldman, J.G., and Rubin, L.G. Infection rates of Broviac-Hickman catheters and implantable venous devices. *Am. J. Dis. Child.* 142:536, 1988.

269. Young, G.P., Alexeyeff, M., Russell, D.M., and Thomas, R.J.S. Catheter sepsis during

parenteral nutrition: The safety of long-term OpSite dressings. *J.P.E.N.* 12(4):365, 1988.

270. Yu, V.L., et al. *Staphylococcus aureus* nasal carriage and infections in patients on hemodialysis. Efficacy of antibiotic prophylaxis. *N. Engl. J. Med.* 315:91, 1988.

271. Zinner, S.H., et al. Risk of infection with intravenous indwelling catheters: Effect of application of antibiotic ointment. *J. Infect. Dis.* 120:616, 1969.

272. Zufferey, J., Rime, B., Francioli, P., and Bille, J. Simple method for rapid diagnosis of catheter-associated infection by direct acridine orange staining of catheter tips. *J. Clin. Microbiol.* 26(2):175, 1988.

273. Maki, D.G., and Will, L. Risk factors for central venous catheter-related infection within the ICU. A prospective study of 345 catheters. In: *Program and Abstracts of the Thirtieth Intersciences Conference on Antimicrobial Agents and Chemotherapy.* October, 1990.

41

Infection in Transplant Recipients

Patricia L. Hibberd
Robert H. Rubin

There are few areas of medicine that have progressed to the extent that transplantation has over the past three decades—from an interesting experiment in human immunobiology to the best possible means of rehabilitation of patients with end-stage kidney, liver, lung, and heart disease as well as an increasing number of malignant conditions. Two closely linked processes, rejection and infection, remain the major barriers to successful transplantation. Rejection and infection are linked in a number of ways. First, it is clear that the allogeneic reaction (which is the basis of both allograft rejection in organ transplant recipients and graft-vs-host disease (GVHD) in bone marrow transplant recipients) will reactivate and potentiate such infections as those due to herpes viruses. Second, it is becoming increasingly evident that the converse is also true: Infection, particularly with these same viruses, can play a significant role in the pathogenesis of both allograft injury and GVHD. Finally, the very immunosuppressive therapy administered to control rejection is a major driving force in the occurrence of all forms of infection in this patient population. Thus it is no surprise that despite all the successes and advances that have occurred over the past 30 years, clinically significant infection occurs in at least three-fourths of all transplant recipients and is still the leading cause of death. An important truism pervades both research in transplantation and clinical practice: Any manipulation or intervention that decreases the risk of infection will then permit the use of more intensive immunosuppression; conversely, any manipulation or intervention that decreases the risk of rejection and thus permits the use of lesser amounts of immunosuppression will decrease the risk of infection [83, 88].

The combination of rejection, lifelong immunosuppressive therapy, and exposures to a variety of potential microbial pathogens creates a unique set of challenges to the infectious disease clinician responsible for the care of the transplant recipient. These challenges include the following [83]:

1. The potential sources of infection are vast, including endogenous organisms, the allograft itself, and the very air, water, and food the patient encounters. The immunosuppressive therapy being administered to prevent or treat rejection renders the transplant recipient susceptible to microbial species and inoculum sizes that would have little impact on the normal host.

2. Chronic immunosuppressive therapy, persistent infection with such organisms as cytomegalovirus (CMV), Epstein-Barr virus (EBV), and the hepatitis viruses, and the presence of an allograft bearing histocompatibility antigens different from those of the host all combine to produce an array of clinical syndromes hitherto unknown to clinical medicine.

3. Although the clinical presentation of infection in these patients is often greatly blunted by their impaired inflammatory response, the cornerstone of effective therapy is early diagnosis and treatment. Thus, in this patient population, even seemingly innocuous physical or radiologic findings, as well as symptom complexes, must be evaluated aggressively.

4. The nature of the infections that occur, particularly those due to fungi, viruses, protozoans, and such bacteria as *M. tuberculosis* and *Nocardia asteroides,* renders treatment difficult, in that prolonged courses of toxic antimicrobial therapy are usually required. This challenge has been made even greater by the advent of cyclosporine-based immunosuppressive programs, because the risk of adverse interactions between cyclosporine and antimicrobial programs is great (Table 41-1).

5. Because the clinical impact of infection in these patients is so protean, and diagnosis and curative therapy so difficult, prevention of infection is a high priority.

Table 41-1. Drug interactions occurring between cyclosporine and commonly used antimicrobial agents

I. Upregulation of hepatic cytochrome P450 function, resulting in increased cyclosporine metabolism, lower blood levels, and an increased incidence of rejection. Example: rifampicin[a]

II. Inhibition or downregulation of hepatic cytochrome P450 function, resulting in decreased cyclosporine metabolism, higher blood levels, cyclosporine toxicity, and increased immunosuppression. Examples: erythromycin, ketoconazole[a]

III. Unexplained interaction with cyclosporine to produce synergistic nephrotoxicity. Examples: amphotericin B, aminoglycosides, vancomycin, high-dose trimethoprim-sulfamethoxazole[b]

[a] Both of these types of interaction may be monitored by serial measurements of cyclosporine blood levels and, when necessary, appropriate adjustments to cyclosporine dosage may be made.
[b] Serial measurements of cyclosporine blood levels have not been of value in preventing this form of drug interaction.

Factors Determining the Risk of Infection

The risk of infection, particularly opportunistic infection, in the transplant recipient, is due to the interaction between two major factors: *the net state of immunosuppression* and the *epidemiologic exposures* that the patient encounters. Thus overly immunosuppressed individuals are at risk for life-threatening infection after the most trivial exposure to ordinarily nonvirulent microorganisms, and even minimally immunosuppressed individuals may be seriously compromised if the exposure is great enough. This simple relationship is of great practical importance to both the epidemiologist and the clinician: The occurrence of infection in a patient whose net state of immunosuppression is minimal should trigger an epidemiologic investigation into the source of the infectious agent, usually within the hospital environment. The occurrence of infection that is not explained by epidemiologic factors suggests that there is a greater degree of host defense compromise than had been previously recognized and that there is a need for a modification of the prescribed immunosuppressive therapy [83, 88, 91].

Net State of Immunosuppression
The net state of immunosuppression is a complex function determined by a number of factors: the dose, duration, and temporal sequence of immunosuppressive therapy; the presence or absence of neutropenia; the presence or absence of a disrupted primary mucocutaneous barrier to infection by recent surgery, indwelling catheters, and the like; metabolic factors such as the state of nutrition and the presence of hyperglycemia or uremia; and the presence of infection with one of the immunomodulating viruses—CMV, EBV, the hepatitis viruses, and the human immunodeficiency virus (HIV). The importance of viral infection in determining the net state of immunosuppression is emphasized by the following observation: Over a 5-year period of careful observation of renal transplant patients at the Massachusetts General Hospital, virtually all cases of opportunistic infection occurred among patients with immunomodulating viral infection. The only exceptions were patients exposed to excessive challenges with microorganisms in their environment [83, 97].

Epidemiologic Exposures
The epidemiologic exposures of importance for the transplant recipient can be divided into two general categories—those taking place within the community and those occurring in the hospital. Community-acquired exposures of importance that should be sought, evaluated and, when possible, treated prior to transplantation and the initiation of immunosuppressive therapy include the following: *M. tuberculosis,* the geographically restricted mycoses (*Histoplasma capsulatum, Coccidioides immitis,* and *Blastomyces dermatitidis*), *Strongyloides stercoralis,* HIV, and hepatitis B and C. Exposures of importance within the hospital environment include those to such airborne pathogens aas *Aspergillus* species, *Legionella* species, and *Pseudomonas aeruginosa* and other gram-negative bacteria [83, 88, 91]. It is important to emphasize that such noso-

comial exposures can be of either a *domiciliary* or a *nondomiciliary* nature. Domiciliary exposures occur where the patient is housed within the hospital environment, with outbreaks being relatively easily identified because of clustering of cases in time and space. Nondomiciliary exposures occur when immunosuppressed patients are taken to such hospital facilities as radiology suites or operating theaters for essential procedures. Outbreaks due to nondomiciliary exposures are probably more common than the domiciliary variety but are far more difficult to identify because infected patients are typically cared for by different groups of physicians in widely disparate parts of the hospital environment. The essential point to remember is that immunosuppressed patients such as transplant recipients are like "sentinel chickens," quickly indicating that there is an excessive microorganism load in the environment (particularly with agents that cause opportunistic respiratory infection). Constant surveillance of infections in any transplantation unit is essential (see Chap. 5). In addition, in institutions undergoing major reconstruction, transplant recipients may benefit greatly from being housed in areas where the air quality is maintained by high-efficiency particulate air (HEPA) filters [54, 83] (see Chap. 15).

Timetable of Infection Following Organ Transplantation

Since the immunosuppressive programs utilized in patients undergoing renal, heart, liver, pancreas, lung, and heart-lung transplantation are so similar, it is not surprising that the time periods during which opportunistic and nonopportunistic infections occur, and indeed the clinical syndromes due to infection, are so similar among these patients. These time periods are shown in the timetable for the occurrence of infection in Figure 41-1 [83, 88]. There are primarily two types of differences that can be observed between the recipients of the various transplanted organs. First, there are differences related to the technical aspects of the trans-

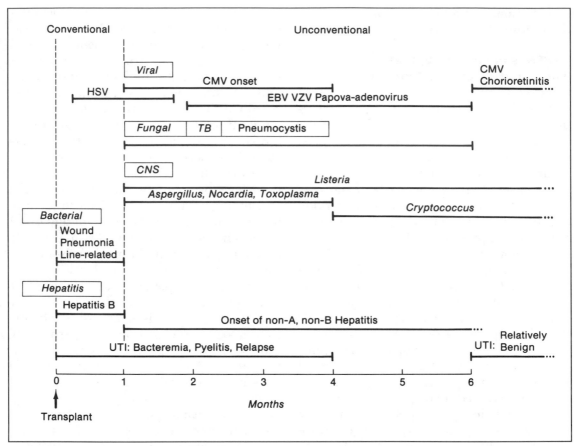

Fig. 41-1. Timetable for occurrence of infection in the organ transplant recipient. Exceptions to this timetable should initiate a search for an unusual hazard. CMV = cytomegalovirus; HSV = herpes simplex virus; EBV = Epstein-Barr virus; VZV = varicella-zoster virus; TB = tuberculosis; CNS = central nervous system; UTI = urinary tract infection. (Modified with permission from R.H. Rubin, Infection in the Renal and Liver Transplant Patient. In: R.H. Rubin and L.S. Young [Eds.], Clinical Approach to Infection in the Compromised Host [2nd ed.]. New York: Plenum, 1988. Pp. 561.)

plant procedure (i.e., the specific operation and anatomic location of the various necessary drains, the required invasive monitoring systems, and the management of the endotracheal tube and ventilatory support) and the duration of time during which the mucocutaneous host defenses are compromised by these factors. Second, differences occur as a result of the effects of systemic infection on the allograft itself. For example, clinically important CMV hepatitis occurs only in liver allograft recipients [74], and myocarditis due to CMV or *Toxoplasma gondii* occurs only in the heart allograft recipient [33, 39, 53].

In organ transplant recipients, the posttransplantation course can be divided by the types of infection observed into three time periods: the first month posttransplantation, 1 to 6 months posttransplantation, and the late period (more than 6 months posttransplantation). The timetable is useful to the clinician in two ways. First, it assists with the differential diagnosis of an infectious disease syndrome; for example, the likely etiology of pneumonia in the first month is very different from the etiology at other points in time. Second, it serves as an epidemiologic tool; for example, exceptions to the timetable are almost always due to an unusual epidemiologic exposure [83, 88].

Infection During the First Month

During the first month posttransplantation, there are three categories of infection that can occur in the organ transplant recipient: (1) infection that was present in the recipient prior to transplantation and is exacerbated by the transplant procedure or the immunosuppressive therapy; (2) infection conveyed with a contaminated allograft; and (3) bacterial and candidal infections related to technical mishaps involving the surgical wound, vascular, bladder, biliary, or pleural catheters, and endotracheal intubation.

Importance of Infection in the Recipient Prior to Transplantation

A cardinal rule of clinical transplantation is that all infectious processes should be under control prior to the transplant procedure and initiation of immunosuppressive therapy. Thus, prior to transplantation, every attempt must be made to identify and eradicate infections such as tuberculosis, localized and systemic fungal infection, and strongyloidiasis. The presence of infections due to hepatitis B and C and HIV, which are known to have the potential for causing difficulties posttransplantation and for which effective therapies are unavailable, should be regarded as relative contraindications for transplantation.

As heart, lung, and liver transplantations are being used to treat an ever-increasing number of diseases, acute bacterial infection of clinical importance may be acquired during the wait for emergency transplantation. Examples include aspiration pneumonia in the patient with advanced hepatic encephalopathy; pneumonia and line sepsis in the patient with end-stage cardiac disease who is intubated and receiving life support from pressors delivered through central venous access and cardiac assist devices; and bronchopulmonary infection or colonization with antibiotic-resistant gram-negative bacilli in the patient with end-stage pulmonary disease. For the promise of transplantation to be fulfilled for these individuals, certain guidelines should be followed:

1. For patients with chronically progressive disease of the liver, heart, and lungs, early transplantation should be considered, prior to the start of the terminal downhill spiral that accompanies the infectious complications of intensive care unit interventions. An important truism is that the patient's chances of survival posttransplantation are much improved if he or she can walk to the operating room rather than requiring life support devices to get there.

2. Whereas patients with end-stage renal disease who have important active infectious diseases can, and should, be reconstituted on dialysis prior to transplantation, there is no equivalent option for patients with other forms of end organ dysfunction. Therefore, prevention of infection in the patients with far-advanced hepatic, cardiac, and pulmonary disease is of overwhelming importance. A fundamental concern is protection of the airway, particularly in the patient with hepatic encephalopathy and mental status changes, to the point that prophylactic intubation in preparation for emergency transplantation should be seriously considered.

3. A particular problem facing the potential lung transplant recipient is the possible need for effective postoperative antibiotic prophylaxis to prevent infection secondary to the colonizing endogenous respiratory flora. Patients likely to need postoperative antibiotic prophylaxis include the increasing numbers of patients with cystic fibrosis and bronchiectasis who are coming to transplantation. Unfortunately, since these patients often have pulmonary infections and therefore have frequent exposure to antibiotic therapy before transplantation, their endogenous respiratory flora may be resistant to multiple antibiotics at the time of transplantation. Colonization with totally antibiotic-resistant organisms, particularly *P. aeruginosa,* effectively excludes such patients from consideration for transplantation. Inappropriate use of prolonged courses of broad-spectrum antibiotics in potential transplant candidates should be avoided whenever possible (see Chaps. 12, 14).

Donor as a Source of Infection

To prevent transmission of active infection with the allograft itself, the prospective donor must undergo a careful evaluation for the presence of acute infectious complications associated with preterminal intensive care unit management and long-standing infectious diseases. The major pathogens of concern are the viruses (HIV, hepatitis B and C) and systemic microbial agents that could seed the organ(s) to be transplanted and thus be transmitted to the immunosuppressed organ recipient. Transplantation of an organ from a donor infected with either HIV or hepatitis B is an extremely efficient method of transmitting these viruses to the recipient and is associated with an attack rate of infection approaching 100 percent [27, 83, 86, 94]. Recent experience with the new serologic test for hepatitis C has shown an attack rate of approximately 50 percent for clinically important hepatitis when the organ was procured from a hepatitis C antibody–positive donor [75]. In the case of such infectious agents as *M. tuberculosis, H. capsulatum,* and *Cryptococcus neoformans,* transmission via an infected allograft has been documented to occur but is relatively infrequent. The protozoan organism *T. gondii* merits special attention. Transplantation of a heart from a donor seropositive for toxoplasmosis into a seronegative recipient is associated with a high incidence of *T. gondii* myocarditis and disseminated infection. Other organs such as kidneys, liver, and lungs from seropositive donors have rarely been associated with *T. gondii* infection in the recipient. Thus, prophylaxis against toxoplasmosis (with pyrimethamine and a sulfonamide) is indicated only for seronegative heart transplant recipients who received cardiac allografts from donors who were seropositive for *T. gondii* [33, 39, 53].

A more difficult problem is the identification of immediately preterminal contamination of organs due to acute infection developing while the potential donor is in the intensive care unit. For example, our group reported a case of unsuspected *P. aeruginosa* bacteremia in an afebrile donor that resulted in seeding of both of the harvested kidneys. Both recipients developed massive retroperitoneal bleeds requiring emergent graft nephrectomy. Both recipients were found to have ruptured mycotic aneurysms at the site of the renal artery anastomosis. Intraoperative cultures grew the same *Pseudomonas* species that had been isolated from the preterminal donor blood cultures. Less commonly, organs may be secondarily contaminated during the harvesting process or during handling prior to the transplant procedure. Regardless of the route of contamination, the overriding principle is that the strictest attention must be paid to the prevention of bacterial or candidal seeding of an organ procured for transplantation [69, 83].

The following guidelines would appear to be appropriate in an effort to limit the chances of transplanting a contaminated allograft:

1. Potential donors who are seropositive by enzyme-linked immunosorbent assay (ELISA) for HIV infection should be excluded from organ donation. HIV testing must be performed on serum specimens obtained prior to administration of any transfusions, because false-negative ELISAs for HIV have been reported on serum tested after multiple transfusions. Unfortunately, in the setting of posttransfusion HIV-negative serum (subsequently corrected to HIV-positive on the basis of pretransfusion serum testing), transmission of HIV occurred following organ donation and transplantation. In addition, except in special circumstances, HIV-seronegative patients who have a history of risk factors for HIV infection (homosexuality, intravenous drug use, etc.) should also be excluded from organ donation [86, 94].

2. Potential donors whose serum tests positive for hepatitis B surface antigen or for antibody to hepatitis C should be considered as harboring transmissible virus and be excluded from organ donation [75, 83].

3. Potential donors should be carefully monitored for active actue infection prior to organ donation, with particular attention being paid to the acquisition of blood cultures. Early systemic antibiotic therapy for nonbacteremic infection in the potential donor may allow the salvage of organs for donation. Cultures should routinely be obtained from postharvest perfusate or car-

rying solutions. Positive cultures from these latter two sources usually yield non-virulent organisms such as diphtheroids or *Staphylococcus epidermidis,* and such growth probably represents insignificant contamination. It is our practice, however, to administer a 5- to 7-day course of systemic antibiotics to recipients of organs even when these cultures yield these nonvirulent organisms. A bigger concern is the presence of *Staphylococcus aureus,* gram-negative bacilli, or *Candida* species in any culture obtained pre-transplant, during harvest, or during transport. These organisms have been strongly associated with life-threatening infections in and around the allograft, and a 2- to 4-week course of systemic antimicrobial therapy should be initiated [69, 83].

4. Certain potential donors should be regarded as being at high risk for harboring infection that will be clinically important after transplantation, despite nondiagnostic surveillance cultures. These high-risk patients include victims of drowning (who may be infected with microorganisms found in water), burn victims, and patients who have been maintained on a respirator with central venous access devices and catheters for periods of more than 7 days [69, 83, 105, 120].

Technical Complications as a Risk Factor for Infection

Wound infection is the most important treatable infection occurring in the first month following transplantation (see Chap. 33). The reported incidence rates for wound infection vary widely. It is more common following liver and pancreas transplantation (reported incidence at some centers approaching 50 percent) and relatively rare following renal transplantation (most centers report an incidence rate of less than 5%). More important than the incidence of wound infection is its association with serious deep infection that may result in graft loss, systemic infection and formation of mycotic aneurysms at the site of vascular anastomoses. The major risk factor for the development of significant

wound infection is technical complications. These include the presence of devitalized tissue, wound hematomas, fluid collections such as those due to blood, urinary or bile leak, or a lymphocele, and the need for reexploration or other forms of wound manipulation following transplantation [58, 60, 67, 83, 100]. The presence of diabetes mellitus in the recipient may be an additional risk factor.

There is a consensus among many transplant surgeons that local irrigation of the wound with antibacterial solutions, such as bacitracin-neomycin, is beneficial in preventing wound infection. Another area of agreement, also in the absence of controlled studies, is the need to avoid using open drains because of the direct conduit to deep tissues that the open drain might provide to potential pathogens. Closed-suction drainage to eliminate dead space and prevent fluid collections is employed in many centers, with attention being paid to meticulous aseptic care and early removal [4, 58, 60].

There is considerable variability in the use and choice of perioperative antibiotics to prevent wound infection. Although some series report very low rates of wound infection without prophylaxis, many centers prefer to administer antibiotics in the perioperative period. Two principles apply: First, antibiotic prophylaxis is not a substitute for technically expert surgery and, second, antibiotic choice should be directed toward prevention of wound infection, not systemic sepsis. In our institution, cefazolin alone, begun on call to the operating room and continued for less than 72 hours, has provided adequate protection without providing intensive pressure for the selection of highly resistant flora. The one exception occurs in such nonrenal transplants as lung and liver, where antimicrobial choice is influenced by knowledge of the pre-existing respiratory or biliary flora. In these cases, the antibiotics selected are directed against the preexisting flora to protect the tracheal and biliary anastomoses, respectively [83, 115, 119].

Signs and symptoms of wound infection are frequently obscured by the immunosuppressive therapy. Unexplained fever is an adequate indication for either ultrasonic or computed tomographic scanning to search for fluid collections at operative sites. Presence of collections, particularly if the otherwise unexplained fever continues, mandates drainage, under coverage of broad-spectrum antibiotics. Appropriate antibiotic regimens (based on culture and sensitivity testing or isolates) are then continued for 10 to 14 days or until the patient has been afebrile for 5 to 7 days [20, 83].

Other Causes of Infection

Pneumonia, urinary tract infection, intravenous line–related bacteremia, cholangitis, infections in the pleural space, and the like indicate that the newly immunocompromised host has little ability to ward off infection when foreign bodies (such as endotracheal tubes, urinary and biliary catheters, or vascular catheters) are present. Use of these foreign bodies that also compromise natural barriers must be minimized; when such devices are necessary, meticulous attention must be paid to impeccable aseptic technique and early removal [83, 88].

Noteworthy in this discussion of infections in the first month posttransplantation is the absence of any mention of opportunistic infections. Indeed, in this 1-month "golden period," the net state of immunosuppression should not be great enough to permit infection due to such organisms as *Aspergillus fumigatus* and *Legionella pneumophila*. This observation has two important corollaries: (1) Exceptions to this rule usually mean an unsuspected environmental hazard is present; and (2) during the first month posttransplantation, the daily dose of immunosuppressive drugs is at its highest, and therefore the net state of immunosuppression is determined more by the duration of immunosuppressive therapy (analogous to the "area under the curve") than by the dosage being administered on a particular day. This latter corollary explains the biggest challenge in the use of immunosuppressive therapy: That is, increasing the dose of immunosuppressive drugs will usually result in a discernible improvement in

allograft function within 24 to 48 hours, whereas the cost of such an increase in terms of infection may not be perceived for another 2 to 4 weeks. Balancing immediate benefits with long-term side effects is the secret of successful management of transplant recipients [83, 88].

Infection 1 to 6 Months Posttransplantation

The beginning of the second posttransplantation month signifies the patient's entry into the period of greatest risk for life-threatening infection. The duration of immunosuppressive therapy is now sufficient to affect adversely the patient's ability to resist microbial invasion. In addition, this is the time when the immunomodulating viruses (HIV, the hepatitis viruses and, most notably, CMV and EBV) have their greatest clinical impact. The net effect is two categories of infection—clinical syndromes due to these viruses themselves and opportunistic infections with such organisms as *P. carinii, L. monocytogenes, N. asteroides,* and such fungal species as *Aspergillus* and *Candida*.

Two aspects of the infections that occur in this time period merit special attention: (1) the range of clinical effects that these viruses have, which is far greater than those observed with the identical organisms in the nonimmunosuppressed host; and (2) the critical role of immunosuppressive therapy in modulating the clinical events that occur during this time [83, 88].

Impact of Viral Infection on the Transplant Recipient

When clinical infection due to viral pathogens occurs in nonimmunosuppressed patients, the patient either recovers or he or she succumbs due to the direct consequences of the virus. In the transplant recipient, because there is an interaction between chronic immunosuppressive therapy and persistent infection in the presence of foreign tissue, the direct consequences of viral infection are frequently superseded by the indirect effects. Thus the possible clinical consequences of viral infection must be considered in four subgroups [83, 88, 95]:

The direct production of such infectious disease syndromes as fever, mononucleosis, pneumonia, hepatitis, and so on

The production of a state of immunosuppression over and above that induced by the antirejection therapy being administered, such that the patient is at increased risk of invasive infection with such opportunistic pathogens as *P. carinii, L. monocytogenes,* and *Aspergillus* species

The initiation of a series of events that lead to allograft injury by processes other than direct infection or classical rejection

The participation of the virus in the process of oncogenesis

Effects of Immunosuppressive Therapy on the Occurrence of Infection

Ever since the first days of clinical transplantation in humans, it has been apparent that a prime mover in the pathogenesis of infection in these patients is the immunosuppressive therapy that is administered. Over the ensuing three decades, important information has emerged regarding the relationship between immunosuppressive therapy and infection. This information may be summarized as follows:

1. Of all the immunosuppressive agents administered, the class of agents with the most global depressant effect on host defenses is corticosteroids. A major theme of modern immunosuppressive therapy is to use multiple agents, each at submaximal doses, to achieve the desired antirejection effect while limiting toxicity. (This strategy is similar to that employed in cancer chemotherapy.) Particularly important are so-called steroid-sparing regimens, as there is a limit to the amount of daily steroid therapy a patient can receive without suffering debilitating side effects, including those due to infection [83].

2. Immunosuppressive regimens need to be scrutinized not just for the effects of individual components of the regimen but for the totality of effects produced by the entire regimen. Two important examples highlight this point: In studies of renal transplant recipients, when antithymocyte globulin (ATG) was added to conventional regimens of azathioprine and prednisone to control allograft rejection, there was a marked increase in the incidence of clinical disease due to CMV and CMV viremia, as well as an attenuation of the antiviral benefits observed with prophylactic α-interferon therapy [16]. However, when the dose of azathioprine and prednisone was decreased by 50 percent while ATG was being administered, the antirejection benefits were still observed but without the increased incidence of CMV infection [87]. Recently, this experience has been extended to the anti-T-cell monoclonal antibody, OKT3. In heart transplant recipients, when OKT3 therapy was added to full-dose immunosuppressive programs consisting of cyclosporine, prednisone, and azathioprine, an excessive incidence of EBV-related lymphoproliferative disease was noted [114]. However, when OKT3 is utilized as antirejection therapy in conjunction with decreased doses of the other drugs, the incidence of the lymphoproliferative disorder falls back to baseline (a fivefold to tenfold difference) [21]. The lesson is clear: It is the net immunosuppressive effect of the entire program, rather than any one agent, that is responsible for the infectious disease complications.

3. It is now apparent that not only are the dose and duration of immunosuppressive therapies important in the pathogenesis of infection, but the temporal sequence in which they are deployed may also have important consequences on the development of infection. Studies with a murine CMV model have shown that equivalent antirejection doses of different immunosuppressive drugs have very different effects on different stages of the viral infection. Although cyclosporine and corticosteroids have no ability to reactivate latent CMV, ATG and monoclonal anti-T-cell antibodies are very powerful reactivators of CMV. In contrast, once active, replicating virus is present, ATG and the monoclonal

antibodies only moderately increase the susceptibility of the mouse of the virus, whereas cyclosporine totally blocks the host's ability to mount the virus-specific cytotoxic T-cell response necessary to control the infection. The result is that once active viral infection is present, cyclosporine-based immunosuppressive programs will amplify the effects of the virus. From this analysis, it is clear that unless antiviral prophylactic strategies are employed, the worst possible immunosuppressive regimen involves the use of OKT3 or ATG (which will permit reactivation of latent virus) followed by cyclosporine to block the host's response to the reactivated virus, a theory that has been confirmed clinically [82].

4. It is axiomatic that all forms of antirejection therapy currently in use will increase the susceptibility of the transplant patient to one or another microbial agent. It is now feasible to develop prophylactic antimicrobial strategies aimed at specific infections that occur at particular points following transplantation, so that the beneficial antirejection effects of the immunosuppressive agents can be secured more safely [84]. For example, the incidence of symptomatic CMV disease can be diminished in individuals at risk for primary infection by the use of prophylactic antiviral agents [3] or hyperimmune globulin [107, 108]. Indeed, it has been suggested that immunosuppressive regimens employed in the future will have an important antimicrobial component as well [85].

Infection More than 6 Months Posttransplantation

Patients with allografts that continue to function more than 6 months posttransplantation require maintenance immunosuppressive therapy to prevent allograft rejection and, therefore, they continue to be at risk for infection. In this time period, community-acquired diseases can have a significant impact on the health of the transplant recipient. For the most part, there are three types of community-acquired disease of importance: (1) communitywide epidemics of influenza that result in not only influenza but a high incidence of secondary pneumonias; (2) ingestion of contaminated food or water, particularly when traveling to less developed areas of the world, that not only results in gastroenteritis due to such infections as salmonellosis, listeriosis, and shigellosis but is associated with a high rate of systemic infection (a similar risk has been observed in patients infected with HIV); and (3) exposure to one of the geographically restricted systemic mycoses or tuberculosis that can result in disseminated infection in the transplant recipient. Transplant recipients are cautioned to avoid exotic travel or undue exposure to infection within the community. Disease prevention is difficult in this patient population. For example, although influenza vaccine may be administered, its efficacy is questionable, and therefore amantadine prophylaxis should be considered in the setting of a communitywide epidemic of influenza A [83].

With the exception of these special epidemiologic exposures to diseases present in the community, the infectious disease problems of the transplant recipient more than 6 months after transplantation can be grouped into three general categories [83, 88]: A few individuals, approximately 5 to 15 percent of the long-term survivors, will suffer from *progressive organ dysfunction or malignant disease* due to chronic viral infection. Examples of this include CMV-induced chorioretinitis, chronic active hepatitis and cirrhosis due to hepatitis B and C, full-blown acquired immunodeficiency syndrome (AIDS) due to HIV, and a variety of malignancies (Table 41-2). The majority of patients, who have good allograft function on minimal chronic immunosuppressive therapy and who are free from chronic viral infection, will suffer from the *same types of infection observed in the general community* (influenza, urinary tract infection, pneumococcal pneumonia, etc.). An important minority of patients, who have relatively poor allograft function but have already received a great deal of acute and chronic immunosuppressive therapy, and who frequently have chronic infection with one of the immunomodulating viruses, will suffer from a variety of *life-threatening opportunistic infections.* Indeed, the incidence of infection due to

Table 41-2. Relationships between viral infections and malignancies in organ transplant recipients

Virus	Associated malignancy
Epstein-Barr virus	B-cell lymphoproliferative disease
Hepatitis B	Hepatocellular carcinoma
Papillomavirus	Squamous cell carcinoma of the skin
Herpes simplex virus	Anogenital cancer, particularly in women
Cytomegalovirus*	?

*Although cytomegalovirus, like the other herpes viruses, must be regarded as having oncogenic potential, the relationship between CMV and malignancies such as Kaposi's sarcoma, colonic cancer, and prostatic cancer is currently unclear.

such organisms as *C. neoformans, L. monocytogenes,* and *N. asteroides* is highest among this group of patients.

Infections of Particular Importance in the Transplant Recipient
Cytomegalovirus

CMV is the single most important cause of infectious disease morbidity and mortality in transplant patients, with active infection being demonstrable in approximately 70 percent of transplant recipients (see Chap. 38). Three patterns of CMV transmission are recognized; they are primary infection, reactivated infection, and superinfection [82, 83].

Primary CMV infection occurs when a CMV-seronegative individual receives latently infected cells from a CMV-seropositive donor. More than 90 percent of the time, those cells are contained within the allograft; occasionally, viable leukocytes in blood transfusions can transmit the virus. Approximately 60 percent of individuals at risk for primary CMV infection become clinically ill [7, 52].

Reactivation CMV infection occurs when a CMV-seropositive individual reactivates endogenous latent virus. It is believed that approximately 20 percent of these individuals become ill [7, 52].

Superinfection with CMV occurs when a sero-

positive individual receives a transplant from a seropositive donor and the virus that is activated posttransplantation is of donor, rather than endogenous, origin. The true incidence of clinical disease in this circumstance remains a matter of some controversy but is probably between 20 and 40 percent [18, 37, 38].

Whichever form of CMV infection is operative, clinically overt disease presents 1 to 4 months posttransplantation, driven primarily by the immunosuppressive therapy being administered. In the laboratory, CMV can be isolated from blood, urine, respiratory secretions, and tissue biopsies, with viremia being the best noninvasive marker of potentially clinically important infection. Because of this, increasing attention in recent years has been paid to the development of rapid methods for diagnosing CMV viremia, including the shell vial cultural technique, direct detection of virally infected leukocytes in buffy coat preparations by immunofluorescent techniques, and viral detection by the polymerase chain reaction [16, 84].

The spectrum of clinical illness produced by CMV ranges from asymptomatic shedding of virus (most common in patients with reactivation infection), to a complex of symptoms that resembles infectious mononucleosis and has been termed the *CMV syndrome,* to life-threatening disease. The CMV syndrome typically refers to a prolonged episode of otherwise unexplained fever associated with constitutional symptoms in concert with such laboratory abnormalities as leukopenia (with or without thrombocytopenia), a mild atypical lymphocytosis (usually less than 10 percent of the circulating leukocytes), and a mild hepatitis. Severe CMV disease consists of severe leukopenia and thrombocytopenia, pneumonia, gastrointestinal ulcerations and perforations and, in the liver transplant patient, severe hepatitis. Not infrequently, opportunistic superinfection with other pathogens will further complicate the course of severe CMV infection. CMV chorioretinitis is a late manifestation of systemic CMV infection, presenting 4 months or more posttransplantation. Chorioretinitis may follow earlier clinical manifestations of CMV infection or be the first manifestation of CMV disease [82, 83, 89, 93].

One of the most controversial aspects of CMV infection in transplant recipients is its potential direct role in the allograft injury [10, 46, 63, 80, 104]. Increasingly, there is evidence that CMV plays a role in the pathogenesis of GVHD in bone marrow transplant recipients and in unusual forms of allograft injury in organ transplant patients. Thus CMV infection has been linked with a glomerulopathy in renal allografts [80, 97]; the disappearing bile duct syndrome [71] and an unusual form of CMV culture-negative hepatitis [74] (that is, the patient is viremic but the liver biopsy is negative for CMV) in liver allografts; both acute rejection and accelerated coronary artery atherosclerosis in cardiac allografts [34]; and obliterative bronchiolitis in lung allografts [56]. The pathogenesis of these forms of injury is not yet understood, although it is clear that the various types of tissue damage are not due to the direct effects of the virus or to deposition of immune complexes [81]. Hypotheses explaining these associations center on indirect effects of the viral infection: Cytokines elaborated in the course of CMV infection upregulate the histocompatibility antigen displayed on allografted tissue, triggering a host response and immune injury; sequence homology and immunologic cross-reactivity between a portion of the immediate early antigen of CMV and the HLA-DR beta chain may result in damage to the allograft from the expected host response to the virus; or, similarly, the production by CMV-infected cells of a glycoprotein homologous to major histocompatibility class I antigens may trigger an immune attack that will damage the allograft; and finally, there may be direct virus-mediated injury of vascular endothelium with secondary deposition of lipid and acceleration of the atherosclerotic process. Although the mechanisms of injury are not understood, it is likely that CMV infection, even if it remains asymptomatic, could have adverse effects on allograft function. These observations provide added justification for efforts to control this virus [81, 82].

In recent years, significant strides have been made in preventing CMV disease. Prophylactic regimens involving the use of either hyperimmune (anti-CMV) globulin [107, 108] or high-dose acyclovir [3] have shown some efficacy, with ability to prevent approximately 50 percent of CMV disease. Treatment with ganciclovir, particularly in conjunction with globulin, is effective in the treatment of established disease [82]. Recently, the concept of *preemptive* therapy has been defined—treating asymptomatic individuals who have an identifiable event that is associated with an increased risk of acquiring CMV disease. Thus a regimen in which ganciclovir prophylaxis is administered concurrently with OKT3 therapy appears to be particularly promising [48].

Epstein-Barr Virus

Infection due to EBV is being increasingly recognized to be of great importance in transplant recipients (see Chap. 38). Although EBV can occasionally produce a mononucleosis syndrome in transplant patients [17, 36, 64], its major significance in transplantation is as the causative agent of a B-cell lymphoproliferative disorder. The pathogenesis of this process is related to the effects of immunosuppressive therapy on the usual surveillance mechanism for preventing EBV-initiated clinical events. In normal individuals who have had previous infection with EBV (and hence are antibody-positive and latently infected with this virus), circulating cytotoxic T lymphocytes specific for EBV-induced antigens on the surface of infected B lymphocytes prevent the outgrowth of virally induced, transformed cells, which are believed to initiate the oncogenic process that ultimately culminates in lymphoproliferative disease [9, 22, 23, 128]. Immunosuppressive therapy has two effects: It not only reactivates virus from its latent state (and, as with the closely related CMV, polyclonal and monoclonal antilymphocyte antibodies appear to be particularly potent effectors of this reactivation process [14, 17, 113]), but it also blocks the surveillance mechanism. The greatest impairment of this surveillance mechanism occurs with cyclosporine, which inhibits the EBV-specific cytotoxic T-cell response in a dose-dependent fashion [9, 22, 23]. This was dramatically illustrated by Calne and colleagues [13], who reported 5 lymphomas occurring among the first 23 patients treated with cyclosporine. As lower doses of cyclosporine have been employed and close monitoring of cyclosporine blood levels has occurred, the number of cases of lymphoma has diminished but has not disappeared [8].

More recently, however, the incidence of EBV-related lymphoproliferative disease has been on the increase in association with the use of other immunosuppressive agents *in addition to full-dose cyclosporine and prednisone*. In cardiac transplant patients, the addition of OKT3 to a program of cyclosporine, azathioprine, and prednisone was associated with a tenfold increase in the incidence of lymphoproliferative disease [114]. Since OKT3 (like ATG) and, to a lesser extent, azathioprine have suppressive effects on the anti-EBV surveillance mechanisms, this observation is not surprising [21]. The increase in EBV-related lymphoproliferative disease is reminiscent of observations made with CMV infection more than a decade previously: When ATG was added to full-dose azathioprine and prednisone therapy, the incidence and severity of CMV infection was markedly increased; however, when the doses of azathioprine and prednisone were halved in association with the ATG therapy, then the antirejection benefits of the ATG were sustained without an increase in CMV infection [87]. Thus it is the effect of the entire immunosuppressive regimen on the anti-EBV surveillance mechanisms, not the contribution of any single component, that must be addressed.

Even with exquisite control of the immunosuppressive therapy, the tendency for the development of lymphoproliferative disease will remain. The incidence is highest in those with primary EBV infection posttransplantation [51] and, since primary infection is most common in children, this will remain a problem in pediatric transplantation. However, since the majority of patients receiving transplants are adults who almost always have previously been exposed to EBV, the greatest number of cases will be attributable to reactivation dis-

ease. An important question that remains unanswered is whether antiviral prophylaxis (e.g., with acyclovir) during periods of intensive antirejection therapy can prevent this condition.

Once lymphoproliferative disease develops, the first therapeutic step is to reduce drastically the amount of exogenous immunosuppression administered, particularly the dosage of cyclosporine and antilymphocyte antibody preparations [111]. High-dose acyclovir has been recommended by some groups, although fewer than 50 percent of patients so treated will have resolution of their disease. Optimal therapy remains unclear as conventional antilymphoma chemotherapy appears also to have limited efficacy. Perhaps the reason for variable responses is the likely heterogeneity of cases described in the literature. It is currently believed that the EBV-associated lymphoproliferative disease evolves from a benign EBV-dependent polyclonal B-cell hyperplasia into an EBV-independent monoclonal B-cell lymphoma. At the monoclonal stage, elimination of the virus would be without effect. Presumably, the patients whose disease responds to reduced immunosuppression are in the early polyclonal stage of the disease [32, 40–44].

HIV Infection

Transplantation of an organ or bone marrow from an HIV-infected individual into a noninfected recipient is an extremely efficient means approaching 100% of transmitting this virus (see Chap. 39). As previously discussed, careful screening of potential donors for histories of high-risk behavior and for serologic evidence of HIV infection should effectively prevent the transmission of primary HIV infection at the time of transplantation [36, 94].

A growing problem, however, is the increasing number of patients who are asymptomatic carriers of HIV and who present with end-stage renal, cardiac, liver, or lung disease for consideration as transplant candidates. Currently available information from the AIDS in Transplantation Registry [83] and from other sources suggests that if HIV carriers are transplanted, the clinical outcome will be as follows: Approximately one-third of patients die within 6 months of transplantation, usually of infection; approximately one-third of patients continue to be asymptomatic carriers of HIV and have normally functioning allografts 5 or more years posttransplantation; and approximately one-third have an intermediate result, experiencing more than the usual amount of rejection activity during the first 6 to 12 months posttransplantation (perhaps related to HIV-induced dysregulation of the immune system), followed by an asymptomatic period of 24 to 36 months, after which they develop AIDS. In the past, these individuals have died rapidly, usually within 1 month of the development of the first opportunistic infection. Recently, it has become apparent that prophylactic therapy with anti-*Pneumocystis* programs and zidovudine can extend the lives of these individuals [86, 94].

Given these data, two important questions cannot be answered completely at this time: First, should asymptomatic carriers of HIV receive a transplant, or should the limited resource of organs available for transplantation be used for the likely more successful outcome in recipients not infected with HIV? Second, if transplantation is to be offered to individuals infected with HIV, how should immunosuppressive therapy and antimicrobial prophylaxis be managed in the setting of this immunomodulating virus? Although more data are urgently needed to answer these questions, our current policy at the Massachusetts General Hospital, Boston, (subject to constant review as information becomes available) is as follows [86, 94]:

Except under unusual circumstances, we prefer to preserve life in HIV-infected patients with end-stage renal disease by maintaining them on dialysis.

HIV-infected patients with end-stage liver, heart, or lung disease remain transplant candidates, with their HIV infection regarded as a relative contraindication. However, it currently appears unwise to offer transplantation to individuals with CD4-

positive lymphocyte counts of less than 400 per cubic millimeter or with histories of opportunistic infection.

HIV-infected patients who receive a transplanted organ receive anti-*Pneumocystis* prophylaxis for life (daily low-dose trimethoprim-sulfamethoxazole, if tolerated, or monthly administration of aerosolized pentamidine) and zidovudine therapy when the CD4-positive lymphocyte count falls to fewer than 500 cells per cubic millimeter.

Again, it should be emphasized that these recommendations are tentative, subject to revision as more information becomes available.

Hepatitis Viral Infection

Both hepatitis B and hepatitis C viral infections have important effects on the outcome of organ transplantation (see Chap. 38). Once these viruses are present in the immunosuppressed transplant patient, chronic, active infection is almost the inevitable result. Such chronic infection occurs in 5 to 15 percent of organ transplant recipients, with a variety of consequences [1, 6, 57, 59, 66, 83, 109, 122, 125].

Both hepatitis B and C can be transmitted to hospital staff. It is imperative that universal precautions be employed to limit the spread of hepatitis C (and HIV) to staff and that all individuals involved in the care of transplant recipients (or who may come into contact with their blood or secretions) must be protected from hepatitis B infection either naturally or by immunization [61, 83] (see Chap. 11).

Acute hepatitis B, acquired in the peritransplant period, either from the allograft or from blood products, has a much higher rate of fulminant disease than does such infection in the normal host. Fortunately, with careful testing of prospective donors, transmission of hepatitis B has become relatively rare. Far more important are the effects of hepatitis B infection when the recipient is already a carrier of the virus at the time of transplantation. Data from renal transplant recipients (which are presumably applicable to recipients of other organs) suggests that in the first 12 to 24 months posttransplantation, chronic hepatitis B infection contributes to the net state of immunosuppression but otherwise has little impact on morbidity. After this period of time, the combination of chronic hepatitis B infection and chronic immunosuppression leads inexorably to end-stage hepatic disease from cirrhosis or hepatocellular carcinoma. For patients with end-stage renal disease who are hepatitis B carriers, some groups have suggested that patient survival is greater when the patient is maintained on dialysis rather than offered transplantation. Our view has been that because of quality-of-life issues of transplantation versus dialysis, we regard hepatitis B carriage as a relative rather than an absolute contraindication to renal transplantation [15, 24, 29, 49, 55, 62, 72, 73, 76, 103, 112, 118].

Hepatitis B infection in patients with end-stage liver disease who require liver transplantation presents a special problem. Hepatitis B infection does recur posttransplantation and may result in progressive damage to the allograft. Attempts to prevent hepatitis B infection by administering large amounts of antibody against the virus during the anhepatic phase of the liver transplant operation and postoperatively have been unsuccessful [12].

Non-A, non-B hepatitis (presumably virtually all due to hepatitis C infection) is the major cause of posttransplantation hepatic dysfunction. Typically, asymptomatic anicteric hepatitis is observed 1 to 4 months posttransplantation and is followed by chronic infection that may continue to be asymptomatic for periods of 2 to 7 years. The only sign of the chronic infection is persistent transaminase elevations. After a mean period of 4 years, patients present with evidence of end-stage liver disease—ascites, hepatic encephalopathy, spontaneous bacterial peritonitis, or hemorrhage from esophageal varices. As with hepatitis B, the progression to end-stage liver disease is both inexorable and, at present, untreatable. Thus the previously discussed preventive measures are of prime importance [59, 83].

Bacterial Infection

The bacterial infections that occur in organ transplant recipients can be divided into five general categories: (1) infections of the transplanted organ, which are primarily related to the catheters that are placed to protect the surgical anastomosis; (2) infections related to technical complications from the operative procedure; (3) infections related to the gastrointestinal tract, which may have unique systemic consequences for the transplant recipient; (4) opportunistic infection caused by *L. monocytogenes, N. asteroides,* and *Mycobacterium* species (both typical and atypical); and (5) infections that resemble those occurring in the general population, prime examples being pneumococcal pneumonia, gram-positive cellulitis beginning at sites of cutaneous injury, and late urinary tract infection (more than 4 months after renal transplantation, due to *E. coli*) [83]. The first four of these merit further comment.

Infections of the Transplanted Organ

The two main examples of infection of the transplanted organ are urinary tract infection in the renal transplant recipient and cholangitis in the liver transplant recipient. Approximately one-third of renal allograft recipients develop urinary tract infections in the first 4 to 6 months posttransplantation, with a high rate of allograft pyelonephritis, bacteremia, and relapse of urinary tract infection following conventional courses of therapy. The urinary catheter provides a portal of entry for bacteria, the surgically and immunologically traumatized kidney provides fertile ground in which infection may take hold, and the immunosuppressive therapy blocks the host's ability to control the infection [11, 35, 68, 90]. Fortunately, low-dose trimethoprim-sulfamethoxazole, trimethoprim, or ciprofloxacin prophylaxis are very effective in preventing these events. An additional benefit of trimethoprim-sulfamethoxazole prophylaxis is the prevention of infection by pathogens such as *P. carinii, L. monocytogenes,* and *N. asteroides* [31, 45, 83, 117].

The biliary catheter that is kept in place for

the first few months after liver transplantation results in colonization of the biliary tract with such organisms as *S. epidermidis, Enterococcus faecalis,* and, less commonly, aerobic gram-negative bacilli. In the absence of a biliary leak or obstruction, such colonization is of little consequence and should be ignored. Indeed, the development of symptomatic cholangitis should trigger a search for an anatomic problem related to the biliary anastomosis. However, in the presence of an intrahepatic hematoma or bile leak that may follow liver biopsy, these usually benign organisms may form liver abscesses. Similarly, cholangitis may follow manipulations of the T-tube (e.g., after cholangiography). For these reasons, antimicrobial prophylaxis directed at the colonizing flora (e.g., single doses of vancomycin and gentamicin) is recommended prior to such manipulative procedures [83].

Infections Related to Technical Complications

A cardinal rule of transplantation is that technical complications will invariably result in secondary infection with conventional bacteria or *Candida* species. Technical complications include urinary and bile leaks or obstruction, tissue infarction due to thrombosis of vascular anastomosis, lymphoceles, wound hematomas, and mismanagement of endotracheal tubes or vascular or drainage catheters [83].

Infections Stemming from the Gastrointestinal Tract

Gastrointestinal infections of two general types occur in transplant recipients—those related to compromise of bowel integrity and those related to the ingestion of virulent bacterial pathogens. In the first category, the major pathogens are CMV-induced bowel ulcerations and diverticulitis. Patients receiving corticosteroid therapy are at risk for gastrointestinal tract perforations, especially at sites of anatomic weakness such as diverticula. The clinical presentation is usually insidious—abdominal pain without overt signs of peritonitis, changes in bowel habits (either diarrhea or constipation), and fever—until far-

advanced disease lapses into septic shock. Prompt surgical exploration, with resection of the involved bowel as well as drainage, under coverage of broad-spectrum antibiotics is essential to salvage these patients [45, 77, 79, 123].

The intact gastrointestinal tract can be the portal of entry for systemic infections with such organisms as nontyphoidal salmonellae, *Campylobacter jejuni,* and *L. monocytogenes* (see Chap. 30). Whereas the normal host usually experiences a self-limited, febrile gastroenteritis syndrome following ingestion of these organisms, the transplant recipient may develop systemic infection. During *Salmonella* infection, seeding of cardiovascular sites may occur [5, 96, 106]. *Listeria* infection regularly causes fever and diarrhea and may be associated with bacteremia, meningitis, meningoencephalitis, or endocarditis [2, 70, 83, 98, 99, 110, 116, 124]. Antibiotic therapy with ampicillin-sulbactam or trimethoprim-sulfamethoxazole is recommended to prevent the consequences of *Salmonella* and *Listeria* infections [83].

Mycobacterial Infections

Infection due to *M. tuberculosis* has been less of a problem following transplantation than might have been predicted (see Chap. 29) [83]. Despite immunosuppressive therapy, reactivation and dissemination of *M. tuberculosis* has been exceedingly uncommon in individuals whose only evidence of dormant tuberculosis is a positive tuberculin test. Conversely, patients with (1) a history of active tuberculosis (treated or untreated), (2) an abnormal chest radiograph and positive tuberculin test, or (3) evidence of prior tuberculosis and current comorbid conditions such as malnutrition appear to be at higher risk of reactivated tuberculosis. For patients in these higher-risk categories, antituberculous prophylaxis with at least isoniazid is indicated. However, administration of antituberculous therapy is difficult following transplantation for two reasons. First, isoniazid and rifampicin probably interfere with cyclosporine metabolism (through the upregulation of hepatic cytochrome P450 function); and second, hepatic dysfunction is frequently already a problem in this patient population without the additional insult of potentially hepatotoxic drugs [83].

Atypical mycobacterial infection may also be observed in transplant recipients: Local or disseminated disease due to *Mycobacterium kansasii* and progressive skin infection due to *M. marinum*, *M. haemophilum*, and *M. chelonei* have been reported. These infections typically present initially at sites of cutaneous injury. Management usually involves surgery and chemotherapy based on in vitro antimicrobial susceptibility testing [83, 92].

Fungal Infections

The fungal infections that affect transplant recipients can be divided into two general categories: (1) disseminated primary or reactivated infection with one of the geographically restricted systemic mycoses (histoplasmosis, blastomycosis, and coccidioidomycosis), and (2) invasive opportunistic infections with such organisms as *Candida* species, *Aspergillus* species, *C. neoformans*, and the Mucoraceae. The first category of disease should be considered in patients with a history of recent or remote travel to an endemic region who present with one of the following clinical syndromes: subacute respiratory illness, with focal, disseminated, or miliary infiltrates on chest radiograph; a nonspecific systemic febrile illness; unexplained pancytopenia; and an illness in which metastatic aspects of the infection predominate (e.g., mucocutaneous manifestations in histoplasmosis and blastomycosis or central nervous system manifestations in coccidioidomycosis or histoplasmosis) [83, 92].

The opportunistic fungal infections have a far greater impact on the transplant patient than do the endemic mycoses. Primary infection, usually of the lungs but occasionally of the nasal sinuses, may occur in patients who inhale air contaminated with *Aspergillus* species, *C. neoformans* or, particularly in diabetic patients, Mucoraceae. In addition, secondary infection of wounds, intravenous lines, and the like by *Candida* or *Aspergillus* species may occur. Evidence of metastatic infection may

follow either primary or secondary fungal infection, with the skin and central nervous system being common sites of presentation [83, 92].

In the past, the cornerstone of antifungal therapy has been amphotericin B. However, even in the precyclosporine era, use of this nephrotoxic agent in the transplant recipient was difficult. In the postcyclosporine era, the synergistic nephrotoxicity produced by amphotericin B and cyclosporine has become more complicated. Fortunately, the new triazole antifungal agent fluconazole has been shown to be both effective and nontoxic in the treatment of invasive candidal, cryptococcal, and dermatophytic infections in the transplant recipient concurrently treated with cyclosporine [19, 47]. Preliminary experience with another new triazole, itraconazole, suggests that it may be an alternative agent to amphotericin B for the treatment of infections due to the *Aspergillus* species [25].

Pneumocystis carinii

Long considered a protozoan, *Pneumocystis carinii* was recently shown, by molecular taxonomic studies, to be more appropriately regarded as a fungus [28]. Regardless of this detail of classification, effective therapy to date has been provided by drugs having antiprotozoan (as opposed to antifungal) profiles. The incidence of *Pneumocystis* pneumonia in organ transplant patients is approximately 5 percent. Traditionally, such infections have been regarded as immunosuppression-induced reactivation of infection acquired in childhood. However, the possibility of (immunosuppressed) person–to–immunosuppressed person spread (possibly by an aerosolized route) exists. It is our policy, therefore, to isolate patients with *P. carinii* pneumonia from other immunosuppressed patients, including transplant recipients [83, 92].

In transplant recipients, *P. carinii* infection typically occurs either in the period 1 to 6 months posttransplantation, often in association with CMV infection, or in the late period, typically in the subgroup of patients with poor allograft function, excessive immunosuppression, and chronic viral infection.

When *Pneumocystis* pneumonia does develop, it is a subacute disease characterized by fever, nonproductive cough, and progressive dyspnea occurring over several days, and the presence of an interstitial infiltrate on chest radiograph. Administration of either low-dose trimethoprim-sulfamethoxazole (one single-strength tablet at bedtime) or monthly aerosolized pentamidine is effective in the prevention of *Pneumocystis* pneumonia and is routinely employed in our transplant recipients. Since treatment of confirmed *Pneumocystis* pneumonia with high-dose trimethoprim-sulfamethoxazole or parenteral pentamidine in transplant recipients is associated with a high rate of side effects, particularly bone marrow and renal toxicity [83, 92], the importance of prevention cannot be overemphasized.

Parasitic Infection

Toxoplasma gondii and *Strongyloides stercoralis* are the two major protozoan infections of concern in the transplant recipient. Toxoplasmosis, although it has been uncommonly reported in recipients of kidney, lung, and liver transplants, is a particular problem in heart transplant recipients. Transplantation of a heart from a donor who is seropositive for toxoplasmosis (connoting latent infection with *T. gondii,* particularly in the heart itself) into a seronegative recipient is associated with a high rate of disseminated toxoplasmosis in the recipient. The clinical impact of toxoplasmosis is seen predominantly in the heart and the brain. In the heart, the presentation is myocarditis, which has occasionally been misdiagnosed and treated as rejection, with disastrous consequences. In the brain, focal abscesses or diffuse encephalitis have resulted. It is now accepted practice to screen both donor and recipient of a cardiac transplant for *Toxoplasma* IgG and to administer prophylactic pyrimethamine and sulfadiazine for 3 to 6 months to recipients at risk for primary toxoplasmosis (donor seropositive, recipient seronegative) [33, 39, 53].

S. stercoralis is an intestinal nematode endemic to many regions of the world, particularly underdeveloped areas. Because of its unique autoinfection cycle, asymptomatic intestinal carriage years after the individual has left an endemic region is not uncommon. Immunosuppressive therapy, such as that administered following transplantation, can have disastrous consequences: A hyperinfection syndrome may develop, characterized by hemorrhagic pneumonia or colitis, or a disseminated infection may occur in which the *Strongyloides* larvae enter many body sites, including the central nervous system. Concomitant gram-negative bacteremia or meningitis is common. Although theoretically this severe disease can be treated with high-dose thiabendazole and antibacterial agents directed against gram-negative pathogens, emphasis should be placed on prevention. Residents or former residents of areas where *S. stercoralis* is endemic should be screened prior to transplantation by examination of Papanicolaou-stained smears of duodenal aspirates and sputum for evidence of larvae. In addition, purged stool specimens should be examined for presence of larvae. (Routine stool specimens are considered inadequate because of low sensitivity.) Therapy consists of a 3-day course of thiabendazole. Since the consequences of the hyperinfection syndrome are so disastrous, if intensive screening is not feasible, presumptive or preventive therapy is carried out on the basis of the potential exposure [26, 30, 50, 65, 78, 101, 102, 121, 126, 127].

Principles of Antimicrobial Therapy in Transplant Recipients
Problem-Directed Prophylactic Strategies

There are several challenges of antimicrobial therapy in transplant recipients: Many of the antimicrobial agents are themselves toxic and, frequently, that toxicity is exacerbated by cyclosporine, the cornerstone of current immunosuppressive regimens (see Table 41-1). Prolonged courses of therapy with these toxic agents are required to achieve adequate treatment of clinically overt disease. Once disease has occurred, the infected tissue may become vulnerable to infection with other organisms (secondary infections). The only way to avoid these difficulties is to shift the emphasis of infectious disease management of the transplant recipient to the prevention of infectious complications. This principle has led to development of prophylactic strategies directed toward specific problems, such as prevention of urinary tract infection in the renal transplant patient, prevention of procedure-related complications in the liver transplant recipient, prevention of toxoplasmosis in the heart transplant recipient, and prevention of *P. carinii* infection in all transplant recipients. All these strategies have proved to be useful approaches to disease prevention.

Preemptive Therapy

Recently, a new mode of antimicrobial therapy, called *preemptive therapy*, has been described. Traditionally, antimicrobial therapy has been administered either prophylactically to a large number of patients at risk of disease, prior to there being evidence of infection, to prevent serious disease in a few, or therapeutically to the few in whom tissue invasion and clinically overt disease are present. Typically, prophylactic regimens involve the administration of a nontoxic drug, often with less-than-ideal antimicrobial activity, for a prolonged period of time, whereas therapeutic regimens employ the most effective medications, often at toxic doses, for shorter periods of time. Preemptive therapy combines the most desirable aspects of these two options— administration of highly effective therapy over a short period of time to a relatively small number of patients who are at risk of serious infection. The short duration of therapy reduces the potential toxicity, and clinical and laboratory markers may be used to determine predictors of serious infection. For example, preemptive therapy with low-dose ganciclovir, administered in conjunction with OKT3 therapy, to CMV-seropositive renal transplant recipients appears to be a promising approach to the prevention of CMV disease [48]. These latter two agents are less toxic than ganciclovir but also less potent. Similarly, the early use of fluconazole to eradicate asymptomatic candiduria in renal transplant recipients, to prevent progression to

urinary tract obstruction and pyelonephritis, and use of fluconazole in association with surgical manipulation of a pulmonary nodule due to *Cryptococcus* to prevent cryptococcal meningitis are other examples of preemptive therapy.

Future Trends

Given the therapeutic constraints imposed by the necessary immunosuppressive regimen and the devastation that infection may cause in the transplant recipient appropriate emphasis is increasingly being placed on evaluation of predictors of serious infection. Development of clinical epidemiologic databases and appropriate laboratory markers will permit further major advances beyond the preemptive approach to infection in this ever-increasing and challenging population of patients.

References

1. Anuras, S., et al. Liver disease in renal transplant recipients. *Arch. Intern. Med.* 137:42, 1977.
2. Ascher, N.L., et al. *Listeria* infection in transplant patients; five cases and a review of the literature. *Arch. Surg.* 113:90, 1978.
3. Balfour, H.H., Jr., et al. A randomized, placebo-controlled trial of oral acyclovir for the prevention of cytomegalovirus disease in recipients of renal allografts. *N. Engl. J. Med.* 320:1381, 1989.
4. Belzer, F., et al. Prevention of wound infections by topical antibiotics in high risk patients. *Am. J. Surg.* 126:180, 1973.
5. Berk, M.R., et al. Non-typhoid *Salmonella* infections after renal transplantation. A serious clinical problem. *Nephron* 37:186, 1984.
6. Berne, T.V., et al. Hepatic dysfunction in recipients of renal allografts. *Surg. Gynecol. Obstet.* 141:171, 1975.
7. Betts, R.F., et al. Transmission of cytomegalovirus infection with renal allograft. *Kidney Int.* 8:385, 1975.
8. Bia, M.J., and Flye, M.W. Immunoblastic lymphoma in a cyclosporine-treated renal transplant recipient. *Transplantation* 39:673, 1985.
9. Bird, A.G., McLachlin, S.M., and Britton, S. Cyclosporin A promotes spontaneous outgrowth *in vitro* of Epstein-Barr virus-induced B-cell lines. *Nature* 289:300, 1981.

10. Boyce, N.W., et al. Cytomegalovirus infection complicating renal transplantation and its relationship to acute transplant glomerulopathy. *Transplantation* 45:706, 1988.
11. Burleson, R.L., Brennan, A.M., and Scruggs, B.F. Foley catheter tip cultures; a valuable diagnostic aid in the immunosuppressed patient. *Am. J. Surg.* 133:723, 1977.
12. Busuttil, R.W., et al. Liver transplantation today. *Ann. Intern. Med.* 104:377, 1986.
13. Calne, R.Y., et al. Cyclosporin A initially as the only immunosuppressant in 34 recipients of cadaveric organs: 32 kidneys, 2 pancreas, and 2 livers. *Lancet* 2:1033, 1979.
14. Chang, R.S., et al. Oropharyngeal excretion of Epstein-Barr virus by patients with lymphoproliferative disorders and by recipients of renal homografts. *Ann. Intern. Med.* 88:34, 1978.
15. Chatterjee, S.N., et al. Successful renal transplantation in patients positive for hepatitis B antigen. *N. Engl. J. Med.* 291:62, 1974.
16. Cheeseman, S.H., et al. Controlled trial of prophylactic human-leukocyte interferon in renal transplantation; effects on cytomegalovirus and herpes simplex infections. *N. Engl. J. Med.* 300:1345, 1979.
17. Cheeseman, S.H., et al. Epstein-Barr virus infection in renal transplant recipients: Effects of antithymocyte globulin and interferon. *Ann. Intern. Med.* 93:39, 1980.
18. Chou, S. Acquisition of donor strains of cytomegalovirus by renal transplant recipients. *N. Engl. J. Med.* 314:1418, 1986.
19. Conti, D.J., Tolkoff-Rubin, N.E., and Baker, G.P., Jr. Successful treatment of invasive fungal infection with fluconazole in organ transplant recipients. *Transplantation* 47:692, 1989.
20. Cosimi, A.B. Surgical Aspects of Infection in the Compromised Host. In: R.H. Rubin and L.S. Young (Eds.), *Clinical Approach to Infection in the Compromised Host* (2nd ed.). New York: Plenum, 1988. P. 649.
21. Cosimi, A.B., and Rubin, R.H. Increased incidence of lymphoproliferative disorder after immunosuppression with the monoclonal antibody OKT3 in cardiac transplant recipients. *N. Engl. J. Med.* 324:1438, 1991.
22. Crawford, D.H., et al. Long-term T-cell mediated immunity to Epstein-Barr virus in renal allograft recipients receiving cyclosporin A. *Lancet* 1:10, 1981.
23. Crawford, D.H., et al. Studies on long-term T-cell-mediated immunity to Epstein-Barr virus in immunosuppressed renal allograft recipients. *Int. J. Cancer* 28:705, 1981.
24. Dalgleish, A.G., et al. Hepatocellular carcinoma associated with hepatitis B in a renal graft recipient. *Med. J. Aust.* 2:240, 1983.
25. Denning, D.W., Tucker, R.M., Hanson, L.H.,

and Stevens, D.A. Treatment of invasive aspergillosis with itraconazole. *Am. J. Med.* 86:791, 1989.
26. DeVault, G.A., et al. Disseminated strongyloidiasis complicating acute renal allograft rejection. Prolonged thiabendazole administration and successful retransplantation. *Transplantation* 34:220, 1982.
27. Dusheiko, G., et al. Natural history of hepatitis B virus infection in renal transplant recipients—a fifteen year follow-up. *Hepatology* 3:330, 1983.
28. Edman, J.C., et al. Ribosomal RNA sequence shows *Pneumocystis carinii* to be a member of the fungi. *Nature* 334:519, 1988.
29. Fine, R.N., et al. HB_s antigenemia in renal allograft recipients. *Ann. Intern. Med.* 185:411, 1977.
30. Fowler, C.A., et al. Recurrent hyperinfestation with *Strongyloides stercoralis* in a renal allograft recipient. *Br. Med. J.* 285:1394, 1982.
31. Fox, B.C., Sollinger, H.W., Belzer, F.D., and Maki, D.G. A prospective, randomized, double-blind study of trimethoprim-sulfamethoxazole for prophylaxis of infection in renal transplantation: Clinical efficacy, absorption of trimethoprim-sulfamethoxazole, effects on the microflora, and the cost-benefit of prophylaxis. *Am. J. Med.* 89:255, 1990.
32. Frizzera, G., et al. Polymorphic diffuse B-cell hyperplasias and lymphomas in renal transplant recipients. *Cancer Res.* 41:4253, 1981.
33. Gentry, L.V., and Zeluff, B. Infection in the Cardiac Transplant Patient. In: R.H. Rubin and L.S. Young (Eds.), *Clinical Approach to Infection in the Compromised Host* (2nd ed.). New York: Plenum, 1988. p. 623–648.
34. Gratton, M.T., et al. Cytomegalovirus infection is associated with cardiac allograft rejection and atherosclerosis. *J.A.M.A.* 261:3561, 1989.
35. Griffin, P.J.A., and Salaman, J.R. Urinary tract infections after renal transplantation: Do they matter? *Br. Med. J.* 1:710, 1979.
36. Grose, C., Henle, W., and Horwitz, M.S. Primary Epstein-Barr virus infection in a renal transplant recipient. *South. Med. J.* 70:1276, 1977.
37. Grundy, J.E., et al. The source of cytomegalovirus infection in seropositive renal allograft recipients is frequently the donor kidney. *Transplant. Proc.* 19:2126, 1987.
38. Grundy, J.E., et al. Symptomatic cytomegalovirus infection in seropositive kidney recipients: Reinfection with donor virus rather than reactivation of recipient virus. *Lancet* 2:132, 1988.
39. Hakim, M., Esmore, D., Wallwork, J., and English, T.A.H. Toxoplasmosis in cardiac transplantation. *Br. Med. J.* 292:1108, 1986.
40. Hanto, D., et al. Clinical spectrum of lympho-

proliferative disorders in renal transplant recipients and evidence for the role of Epstein-Barr virus. *Cancer Res.* 41:4253, 1981.

41. Hanto, D., et al. The Epstein-Barr virus in the pathogenesis of post-transplant lymphoproliferative disorders. *Surgery* 90:204, 1981.

42. Hanto, D., et al. Epstein-Barr virus–induced B-cell lymphoma after renal transplantation. *N. Engl. J. Med.* 306:913, 1982.

43. Hanto, D.W., et al. Acyclovir therapy of Epstein-Barr virus–induced post-transplant lymphoproliferative diseases. *Transplant. Proc.* 17:89, 1985.

44. Hanto, D.W., et al. Epstein-Barr virus (EBV) induced polyclonal and monoclonal B-cell lymphoproliferative disease occurring after renal transplantation. Clinical, pathologic, and virologic findings and implications for therapy. *Ann. Surg.* 198:356, 1983.

45. Hau, T., et al. Prognostic factors of peritoneal infections in transplant patients. *Surgery* 84:403, 1978.

46. Herrera, G.A., et al. Cytomegalovirus glomerulopathy: A controversial lesion. *Kidney Int.* 29:725, 1986.

47. Hibberd, P.L., et al. New approaches to the treatment of invasive fungal infections in the solid organ transplant recipient. 1992 (submitted for publication).

48. Hibberd, P.L., et al. Symptomatic cytomegalovirus (CMV) disease in the CMV seropositive renal transplant recipient treated with muromonab-CD3 (OKT3). *Transplantation* 53:68, 1992.

49. Hillis, W.D., Hillis, A., and Walker, W.G. Hepatitis B surface antigenemia in renal transplant recipients; increased mortality risk. *J.A.M.A.* 242:329, 1979.

50. Hirschmann, J.R., Plorde, J.J., and Ochi, R.F. Fever and pulmonary infiltrates in a patient with a renal transplant. *West. J. Med.* 140:914, 1984.

51. Ho, M., et al. Epstein-Barr virus infections and DNA hybridization studies in posttransplantation lymphoma and lymphoproliferative lesions: The role of primary infection. *J. Infect. Dis.* 152:876, 1985.

52. Ho, M., et al. The transplanted kidney as a source of cytomegalovirus infection. *N. Engl. J. Med.* 293:1109, 1975.

53. Hofflin, J.M., et al. Infectious complications in heart transplant recipients receiving cyclosporine and corticosteroids. *Ann. Intern. Med.* 106:209, 1987.

54. Hopkins, C.C., Weber, D.J., Rubin, R.H. Invasive *Aspergillus* infection: Possible nonward common source within the hospital environment. *J. Hosp. Infect.* 13:19, 1989.

55. Jacobson, I.M., et al. Immunogenicity of hepatitis B vaccine in renal transplant recipients. *Transplantation* 39:393, 1985.

56. Keenan, R.J., et al. Cytomegalovirus serologic status and postoperative infection correlated with risk of developing chronic rejection after pulmonary transplantation. *Transplantation* 51:433, 1991.

57. Kirkman, R.L., et al. Late mortality and morbidity in recipients of long-term renal allografts. *Transplantation* 34:347, 1982.

58. Kyriakides, G.K., Simmons, R.L., and Najarian, J.S. Wound infections in renal transplant wounds: Pathogenetic and prognostic factors. *Ann. Surg.* 186:770, 1975.

59. LaQuaglia, M.P., et al. Impact of hepatitis on renal transplantation. *Transplantation* 32:504, 1981.

60. Lee, H.M., et al. Surgical complications in renal transplant recipients. *Surg. Clin. North Am.* 58:285, 1978.

61. Levy, B.S., et al. Hepatitis B in ward and clinical employees of a general hospital. *Am. J. Epidemiol.* 106:330, 1977.

62. London, W.T., et al. Association of graft survival with host response to hepatitis B infection in patients with kidney transplant. *N. Engl. J. Med.* 296:241, 1977.

63. Lopez, C., et al. Association of renal allograft rejection with virus infection. *Am. J. Med.* 56:280, 1974.

64. Marker, S.C., et al. Epstein-Barr virus antibody responses and clinical illness in renal transplant recipients. *Surgery* 85:433, 1979.

65. Morgan, J.S., Schaffner, W., and Stone, W.J. Opportunistic strongyloidiasis in renal transplant recipients. *Transplantation* 42:518, 1986.

66. Mozes, M.F., et al. Jaundice after renal allotransplantation. *Ann. Surg.* 188:783, 1978.

67. Muakkassa, W.F., et al. Wound infections in renal transplant patients. *J. Urol.* 130:17, 1983.

68. Murphy, J.F., et al. Factors influencing the frequency of infection in renal transplant recipients. *Arch. Intern. Med.* 136:670, 1976.

69. Nelson, P.W., et al. Unsuspected donor *Pseudomonas* infection causing arterial disruption after renal transplantation. *Transplantation* 37:313, 1984.

70. Niklasson, P.M., et al. *Listeria* encephalitis in five renal transplant recipients. *Acta Med. Scand.* 203:181, 1978.

71. O'Grady, J.G., et al. Cytomegalovirus infection and donor/recipient HLA antigens: Interdependent co-factors in pathogenesis of vanishing bile-duct syndrome after liver transplantation. *Lancet* 2:302, 1988.

72. Parfrey, P.S., et al. The clinical and pathological course of hepatitis B liver disease in renal transplant recipients. *Transplantation* 37:461, 1984.

73. Parfrey, P.S., et al. The impact of renal trans-

plantation on the course of hepatitis B liver disease. *Transplantation* 39:610, 1985.

74. Paya, C.V., et al. Cytomegalovirus hepatitis in liver transplantation: Prospective analysis of 93 consecutive orthotopic liver transplantations. *J. Infect. Dis.* 160:752, 1989.

75. Pereira, B.J.G., Milford, E.L., Kirkman, R.L., and Levey, A.S. Transmission of hepatitis C virus by organ transplantation. *N. Engl. J. Med.* 325:454, 1991.

76. Pirson, Y., Alexandre, G.P.J., and van Yper-sele de Strihou, C. Long-term effect of HB_s antigenemia on patient survival after renal transplantation. *N. Engl. J. Med.* 296:194, 1977.

77. Powis, S.J.A., et al. Ileocolonic problems after cadaveric renal transplantation. *Br. Med. J.* 1:99, 1972.

78. Purtilo, D.T., Meyers, W.M., and Connor, D.H. Fatal strongyloidiasis in immunosuppressed patients. *Am. J. Med.* 56:488, 1974.

79. ReMine, S.G., and McIlrath, D.C. Bowel perforation in steroid-treated patients. *Ann. Surg.* 192:581, 1980.

80. Richardson, W.P., et al. Glomerulopathy associated with cytomegalovirus viremia in renal allografts. *N. Engl. J. Med.* 305:57, 1981.

81. Rubin, R.H. The indirect effects of cytomegalovirus infection on the outcome of organ transplantation. *J.A.M.A.* 261:3607, 1989.

82. Rubin, R.H. Impact of cytomegalovirus infection on organ transplant recipients. *Rev. Infect. Dis.* 12 (Suppl. 7): 5754, 1990.

83. Rubin, R.H. Infection in the Renal and Liver Transplant Patient. In: R.H. Rubin and L.S. Young (Eds.), *Clinical Approach to Infection in the Compromised Host* (2nd ed.). New York: Plenum, 1988. Pp. 557–621.

84. Rubin, R.H. Preemptive therapy in the compromised host. *N. Engl. J. Med.* 324:1057, 1991.

85. Rubin, R.H., and Cosimi, A.B. Therapy, Both Immunosuppressive and Antimicrobial, for the Transplant Patient in the 1990's. In: K. Gent and R.A. Sells (Eds.), *Organ Transplantation—Current Clinical and Immunological Concepts.* London: Bailliere Tindall, 1989. Pp. 71–89.

86. Rubin, R.H., et al. The acquired immunodeficiency syndrome and transplantation. *Transplantation* 44:1, 1987.

87. Rubin, R.H., et al. Effects of antithymocyte globulin on cytomegalovirus infection in renal transplant recipients. *Transplantation* 31:143, 1981.

88. Rubin, R.H., et al. Infection in the renal transplant recipient. *Am. J. Med.* 70:405, 1981.

89. Rubin, R.H., et al. Infectious disease syndromes attributable to cytomegalovirus and their significance among renal transplant recipients. *Transplantation* 24:458, 1977.

90. Rubin, R.H., et al. Usefulness of the antibody-coated bacteria assay in the management of urinary tract infection in the renal transplant patient. *Transplantation* 27:18, 1979.

91. Rubin, R.H., and Tolkoff-Rubin, N.E. Infection: The new problem. *Transplant. Proc.* 21:1440, 1989.

92. Rubin, R.H., and Tolkoff-Rubin, N.E. Opportunistic infections in renal allograft recipients. *Transplant. Proc.* 20(Suppl. 8): 12, 1988.

93. Rubin, R.H., and Tolkoff-Rubin, N.E. The Problem of Cytomegalovirus Infection in Transplantation. In: P.J. Morris and N.L. Tilney (Eds.), *Progress in Transplantation,* Vol. 1. Edinburgh: Churchill Livingstone, 1984. Pp. 89–114.

94. Rubin, R.H., and Tolkoff-Rubin, N.E. The problem of human immunodeficiency virus (HIV) infection and transplantation. *Transpl. Int.* 1:36, 1988.

95. Rubin, R.H., and Tolkoff-Rubin, N.E. Viral infection in the renal transplant patient. *Proc. Eur. Dialysis Transplant Assoc.* 19:513, 1982.

96. Samra, Y., Shaked, Y., and Maier, M.K. Nontyphoidal salmonellosis in renal transplant recipients: Report of five cases and review of the literature. *Rev. Infect. Dis.* 8:431, 1986.

97. Schooley, R.T., et al. Association of herpesvirus infections with T-lymphocyte-subset alterations, glomerulopathy, and opportunistic infections after renal transplantation. *N. Engl. J. Med.* 308:307, 1983.

98. Schoter, G.P.J., and Weill, R., III. *Listeria monocytogenes* infection after renal transplantation. *Arch. Intern. Med.* 137:1395, 1977.

99. Schroter, G.P.J. *Listeria monocytogenes* and encephalitis. *Arch. Intern. Med.* 138:198, 1978.

100. Schweizer, R.T., Kountz, S.L., and Belzer, F.O. Wound complications in recipients of renal transplants. *Ann. Surg.* 177:58, 1973.

101. Scoggin, C.H., and Call, N.B. Acute respiratory failure due to disseminated strongyloidiasis in a renal transplant recipient. *Ann. Intern. Med.* 87:456, 1977.

102. Scowden, E.B., Schaffner, W., and Stone, W.J. Overwhelming strongyloidiasis; an unappreciated opportunistic infection. *Medicine* (Baltimore) 57:527, 1978.

103. Shons, A.R., et al. Renal transplantation in Australia antigenemia. *Am. J. Surg.* 128:699, 1974.

104. Simmons, R.L., et al. Do mild infections trigger the rejection of renal allografts? *Transplant. Proc.* 2:419, 1970.

105. Slapak, M. The immediate care of potential donors for organ transplantation. *Anaesthesia* 33:700, 1978.

106. Smith, E.J., Milligan, S.L., and Filo, R.S. *Salmonella* mycotic aneurysm after renal transplantation. *South. Med. J.* 74:1399, 1981.

107. Snydman, D.R., et al. A further analysis of primary cytomegalovirus disease prevention in renal transplant recipients with a cytomegalovirus immune globulin: Interim comparison of a randomized and an open-label trial. *Transplant. Proc.* 20(Suppl. 8): 24, 1988.

108. Snydman, D.R., et al. Use of cytomegalovirus immune globulin to prevent cytomegalovirus disease in renal transplant recipients. *N. Engl. J. Med.* 317:1049, 1987.

109. Sopko, J., and Anuras, S. Liver disease in renal transplant recipients. *Am. J. Med.* 64:139, 1978.

110. Spitzer, P.G., Hammer, S.M., and Karchiner, A.W. Treatment of *Listeria monocytogenes* infection with trimethoprim-sulfamethoxazole: Case report and review of the literature. *Rev. Infect. Dis.* 8:427, 1986.

111. Starzl, T.E., et al. Reversibility of lymphomas and lymphoproliferative lesions developing under cyclosporin-steroid therapy. *Lancet* 1: 583, 1984.

112. Stevens, C.F., et al. Hepatitis B vaccine in patients receiving hemodialysis: Immunogenicity and efficacy. *N. Engl. J. Med.* 311:496, 1984.

113. Strauch, B., et al. Oropharyngeal excretion of Epstein-Barr virus by renal transplant recipients and other patients treated with immunosuppressant drugs. *Lancet* 1:234, 1974.

114. Swinnen, L.J., et al. Increased incidence of lymphoproliferative disorder after immunosuppression with the monoclonal antibody OKT3 in cardiac transplant recipients. *N. Engl. J. Med.* 323:1723, 1990.

115. Tilney, N.L., et al. Factors contributing to the declining mortality rate in renal transplantation. *N. Engl. J. Med.* 299:1321, 1978.

116. Tilney, N.L., Kohler, T.R., and Strom, T.B. Cerebromeningitis in immunosuppressed recipients of renal allografts. *Ann. Surg.* 195: 104, 1982.

117. Tolkoff-Rubin, N.E., et al. A controlled study of trimethoprim/sulfamethoxazole prophylaxis for urinary tract infection in renal transplant patients. *Rev. Infect. Dis.* 4:614, 1982.

118. Toussaint, C., et al. Liver disease in patients undergoing hemodialysis and kidney transplantation. *Adv. Nephrol.* 8:269, 1979.

119. Townsend, T.R., et al. Prophylactic antibiotic therapy with cefamandole and tobramycin for patients undergoing renal transplantation. *Infect. Control* 1:93, 1980.

120. Van der Vliet, J.A., et al. Transplantation of contaminated organs. *Br. J. Surg.* 67:596, 1980.

121. Venizelos, P.C., et al. Respiratory failure due to strongyloidiasis stercoralis in a patient with a renal transplant. *Chest* 78:104, 1980.

122. Ware, A.J., et al. Spectrum of liver disease in renal transplant recipients. *Gastroenterology* 68:755, 1975.

123. Warshaw, A.L., Welch, J.P., and Ottinger, L.W. Acute perforation of the colon associated with chronic corticosteroid therapy. *Am. J. Surg.* 131:442, 1976.

124. Watson, G.W., et al. *Listeria* cerebritis; relapse of infection in renal transplant patients. *Arch. Intern. Med.* 138:83, 1978.

125. Weir, M.R., Kirkman, R.L., Strom, T.B., and Tilney, N.L. Liver disease in recipients of long-functioning renal allografts. *Kidney Int.* 28:839, 1985.

126. Weller, I.V.D., Copland, P., and Gabriel, R. *Strongyloides stercoralis* infection in renal transplant recipients. *Br. Med. J.* 282:524, 1981.

127. White, J.V., Garvey, G., and Hardy, M.A. Fatal strongyloidiasis after renal transplantation: A complication of immunosuppression. *Ann. Surg.* 48:39, 1982.

128. Yao, Q.Y., et al. *In vitro* analysis of the Epstein-Barr virus: Host balance in long-term renal allograft recipients. *Int. J. Cancer* 35:43, 1985.

Other Procedure-Related Infections

Robert A. Weinstein

With yards of entrails, miles of vascular network, dozens of extravascular spaces, and several organ systems, any patient is a candidate for a staggering array of diagnostic and therapeutic procedures. Although many of these procedures provide information that is essential for sophisticated patient care or to supplant more traumatic intervention or are critical for life support, most procedures also bypass natural host defenses and place patients at increased risk of nosocomial infection [99, 117]. It is not surprising, then, that the introduction of any new procedure is often followed closely by case reports of procedure-associated infections. Occasionally, epidemiologic experiments of nature, in the form of nosocomial outbreaks, provide more detailed information on certain procedure-related hazards, and eventually such hazards may be subjected to prospective study. In this chapter, we discuss a variety of procedure-associated infections that have been highlighted by retrospective or prospective investigations and that have not been discussed elsewhere in this volume.

Because of the seemingly eclectic contents of this chapter, it is important to recognize from the outset that the procedures to be discussed have certain themes in common. First, all the procedures are exquisitely vulnerable to inexperienced operators, to breaks in aseptic technique, and to contaminated, inadequately disinfected, or technically difficult to clean equipment, or ineffective antiseptics. Second, many procedure-related infection problems unfortunately reemerge as new generations of health care workers rediscover these vulnerabilities; thus, the importance of reviewing hazards that at first glance may appear remote. Third, various procedures involving many different sites have as a common site of infection the bloodstream although the risk of infection differs depending on whether the bloodstream contamination is transient or persistent as well as on host and organism-specific factors. Finally, many procedures bear the burden that the specific risks have not been defined sufficiently to determine whether certain preventive measures, such as the use of prophylactic antimicrobial therapy, are mandated.

Infections from Diagnostic Procedures Involving the Vascular System

Phlebotomy

Phlebotomy is one of the oldest and certainly the most common invasive procedure practiced in hospitals and clinics and, ever since the leech was replaced by the sterile hypodermic needle, blood drawing has been regarded by most clinicians as totally safe and simple. In the 1940s, however, it became apparent that despite sterile needles, epidemic jaundice was being transmitted by nonsterile syringes that were used commonly for phlebotomy. With a mock venous system and methylene blue as a marker, investigators showed that reflux occurred from the syringe into the test system when tourniquet pressure was released. By sterilizing syringes between uses, clinic workers abruptly halted the transmission of phlebotomy-associated hepatitis [102].

Historically, the next major risk of phlebotomy to be recognized was staphylococcal septic arthritis of the hip in neonates [8]. In the early 1960s, it was noted that this complication occasionally followed 5 to 9 days after femoral venipuncture. Localized suppuration at the puncture site and thrombosis of the femoral vein, both unusual findings with isolated septic arthritis, suggested a causal relationship between pyoarthritis and a preceding femoral venipuncture. Since it is common to strike the femoral head during femoral venipuncture in neonates (which denotes that the joint capsule has been entered), femoral "sticks" demand the same aseptic conditions used for arthrocentesis, rather than the more lax conditions under which venipuncture is

frequently performed. In light of the severe disability that may follow septic arthritis, many prediatricians now condemn the use of femoral venipuncture and recommend at least ten other sites for pediatric phlebotomy. When heel punctures are employed, the most medial or lateral portion of the heel's plantar surface should be used to avoid calcaneal puncture and osteochondritis [16].

The most recent innovation in blood drawing—the popular and ingeniously simple evacuated collection tube—has streamlined blood collection but, unfortunately, it has also reintroduced the reflux, or back flow, hazard that was first recognized in the 1940s. When commercial evacuated tubes are not sterilized routinely, they may be a source of hospital-acquired sepsis. One hospital traced an outbreak of 5 cases of "primary" *Serratia* bacteremia to contaminated commercial vacuum tubes used for blood collection. This outbreak prompted a detailed study of the back-flow phenomenon, and it was shown that reflux may occur not only when the tourniquet is released (after active flow of blood into the tube has ceased) but also when the tube is tilted upward, when blood touches the stopper, when pressure on the end of the tube compresses the stopper, or when a "short draw" occurs due to insufficient vacuum [56]. Although practices that might increase the risk of back flow are proscribed in the package insert that accompanies many commercial vacuum tubes, such inserts are not always seen by those responsible for blood drawing, and many of the recommendations, particularly those concerning the positioning of patients for phlebotomy, are difficult to follow.

Even when a sterile syringe is used to draw blood, back flow during serial inoculation of vacuum tubes and blood culture bottles can result in cross-contamination and false-positive blood cultures. Although potentially avoidable, such serial inoculation is a convenient and common practice, particularly when blood is obtained from pediatric patients for hemogram and culture, and it has resulted in two reported outbreaks of pseudo-bacteremia [51]. Although none of the patients was affected directly, false-positive cultures put them at risk of unwarranted antibiotic therapy.

More than 500 million commercial evacuated blood collection tubes are used annually in the United States and Canada. The problems cited previously, as well as culture surveys of evacuated blood collection tubes [113], have led to the routine marketing and use of sterile tubes. The preservative and diagnostic reagents present in many tubes may still pose a risk, one that is probably minimal but not fully evaluated. It is hoped that the major problem of back flow has been solved. Nevertheless, health workers should be aware of the hazard, particularly when investigating the source of an apparently primary bacteremia.

Leeches

Despite the popular appeal of highly sharpened, disposable phlebotomy needles for diagnostic bloodletting, leeches have, in fact, resurfaced as a specialized part of the reconstructive and microvascular surgeons' armamentarium [3]. However, as with many other advances discussed in this chapter, there clings an infectious dark side [1]. *Aeromonas hydrophila*, normal gut flora of the leech, has caused wound infections after as many as 20 percent of microsurgical procedures using leeches [80]. Reuse of individual leeches also carries the theoretic risk of cross-infection.

Cardiac Catheterization

Serious local and systemic infections may result from cardiac catheterization procedures, particularly when contaminated instruments or ineffective antiseptics (e.g., dilute aqueous benzalkonium chloride) are used inadvertently or when breaks in technique occur in the cardiac catheterization laboratory. The major pathogens are staphylococci and gram-negative bacteria.

Up to 50 percent of patients undergoing cardiac catheterization develop an increase in temperature of more than 1°C (1.8°F) within 24 hours after catheterization. Their fever, however, has been attributed to the use of angiocardiographic contrast material rather than to infection [97]. In fact, bacterial endocarditis has been reported very rarely in large series evaluating the complications of cardiac catheterization, and individual examples may have been due to concurrent infection that was initially undetected.

In some studies, the febrile reactions after a cardiac catheterization have been traced to pyrogenic endotoxin present in sterile catheters [91]. Reusable cardiac catheters (and disposable catheters, which many institutions now reuse in efforts to contain costs) may be exposed to contaminated distilled water during the initial phases of cleaning. Despite subsequent sterilization, usually by ethylene oxide, residual bacterial endotoxin may be present in the lumen or on the surface of the catheters and lead to sporadic as well as epidemic cases of fever and hypotension following cardiac catheterization. Single-use disposable catheters may prevent this complication. If catheters are reused, rinsing with sterile water before sterilization may lessen the problem.

Pyrogen has also been noted on sterile latex surgical gloves [61]. The incidence of febrile reactions following catheterization was reduced in one study from 11.6 to 0.6 percent when rinsing of latex gloves before catheterization was made routine [62]. One lot of surgical gloves was called to our attention because of an offensive odor left on wearers' hands. The manufacturer attributed this to "sour" talc used in preparing the gloves. The Food and Drug Administration found high levels of endotoxin on the glove surfaces. However, there are no regulations requiring testing of gloves for endotoxin, and the frequency with which commercially available surgical gloves are contaminated with endotoxin, and its side effects, are unknown.

Transient bacteremia during cardiac catheterization has been observed to occur in 4 to 18 percent of patients. In the studies reporting such an incidence, however, blood cultures were obtained from the intravascular catheter or from the vessel from which the catheter had been removed; it is therefore possible that some of the isolates represented contamination of the external part of the catheter or the site of insertion and that bacteremia was actually less frequent. In a study designed to assess this possibility, blood for culture was obtained by standard techniques from a vein distant from the site of catheter manipulation [97]. Venous blood cultures of 106 patients, the majority of whom had valvular heart disease, were obtained in this manner during cardiac catheterization, and all were sterile. Three of 38 samples that were drawn through the catheter that was placed in the heart or aorta during the procedure grew diphtheroids or microaerophilic streptococci. It was concluded that contamination of the hub end of the catheter with normal skin flora led to an overestimation of the incidence of bacteremia. Removal of organisms by lung filtration may also have accounted in part for the failure to isolate organisms from distal sites. In either case, it is clear that some contamination of the catheterization cutdown field has occurred. With rigorous application of strict aseptic technique and adoption of the working principle that cardiac catheterization is a surgical procedure, catheterization-associated infection should be very infrequent, and systemic antibiotic prophylaxis does not appear justified.

The most recently described cardiac catheterization problems relate to percutaneous transluminal angioplasty. Because catheter sheaths may be left in the catheterization site for 12 to 24 hours, there is increased risk of bacteremia and local infection.

Indwelling Arterial Catheters

Indwelling arterial catheters are used regularly in patients whose precarious cardiovascular status necessitates pressure monitoring or repeated blood gas determination (see Chap. 40). Even though they provide information that is essential for sophisticated patient care and eliminate the need for potentially traumatic repeated arterial punctures, such catheters also provide a continuing portal of entry for microbial invasion of the bloodstream.

The infectious complications of the use of arterial catheters have been studied most extensively in neonates. In different centers, the incidence of colonization of indwelling umbilical artery catheters varies from 6 to 60 percent [2, 10, 60, 90]. Unexpectedly, however, the incidence of colonization fails to increase with duration of catheterization, which suggests that catheters become contaminated initially or soon after insertion through the umbilical stump, an area that is heavily colonized and impossible to sterilize completely by local or systemic antibiotics. Indeed, the same organisms usually are isolated from both the cord and catheter in any individual patient. The most frequent contaminants are staphylococci, streptococci, and gram-negative bacilli, particularly *Pseudomonas, Proteus, Escherichia coli,* and *Klebsiella.*

The clinical significance of umbilical catheter colonization is difficult to assess, because the incidence of sepsis in most studies has been low. When serial prospective blood cultures have been obtained from catheterized neonates, however, transient catheter-related bacteremia has been noted. In a prospective study of temporary (2 to 4 hours) umbilical catheterization for exchange transfusion, investigators showed a 60 percent incidence of catheter contamination and a 10 percent incidence of transient bacteremia due to *Staphylococcus epidermidis* (and, in one case, *Proteus*) that occurred 4 to 6 hours after transfusion; this study suggests that the risk from umbilical catheterization may be greatest during the insertion and removal of catheters [5]. In this study and others, prophylactic systemic antibiotics failed to reduce the incidence of catheter contamination or bacteremia. At present, antibiotic prophylaxis does not appear to be beneficial during umbilical catheterization; instead, attention should be focused on meticulous cord preparation and care.

In adults, the rate of bacterial colonization of indwelling arterial catheters and the risk of associated sepsis have not been studied as extensively. Gardner and co-workers [43] demonstrated positive arterial catheter-tip cultures in 4 percent of 200 patients exposed to radial artery catheterization (the preferred site in adults). The source of these organisms was not evaluated, and no direct relationship with patient disease was established, but the incidence of colonization of radial catheters (in contrast to umbilical catheters) did appear to be related to longer durations of catheterization (see Chap. 40).

More recent studies in adults have emphasized the risk of endemic infections caused by arterial catheters used for hemodynamic monitoring [9, 82]. A prospective study of 95 patients (130 catheters) in a medical-surgical intensive care unit showed a 4 percent risk of arterial cannula–related septicemia; 12 percent of all sepsis in this unit was the result of intraarterial catheters [9]. These bacteremias were caused by gram-negative bacilli, enterococci, and *Candida* organisms. Risk factors for the catheter-related infections included catheter placements exceeding 4 days, placement of catheter by cutdown or in the femoral artery, and the presence of local inflammation.

Flow-directed pulmonary artery catheters carry the added risk of right-sided endocarditis related to endocardial trauma. In one autopsy study, 7 percent of 55 patients had endocarditis in association with these catheters [94].

Breaks in aseptic technique may create a greatly increased risk of arterial catheter contamination and sepsis, as was highlighted by an outbreak of *Flavobacterium* bacteremia [105]. In the affected hospital, the sterile, heparinized glass syringes used for clearing arterial lines and for withdrawing arterial blood samples were submerged routinely in ice for a few minutes before use. The ice machine in the hospital's intensive care unit was contaminated with *Flavobacterium* (an organism that can survive and grow at temperatures as low as $-38°C$ [$-36°F$]), and contamination of in-use phlebotomy syringes with this ice resulted in 14 cases of *Flavobacterium* sepsis. Control of the outbreak depended on improved aseptic technique—that is, on discontinuing the practice of cooling syringes in ice before blood withdrawal and of reinjecting blood to clear the catheter system. Ice-related bacteremia is also a potential problem if open cardiac output injectate delivery systems are used [89].

Guidelines for prevention of infections related to intravascular pressure monitoring have been formulated by the Centers for Disease Control (CDC) (Table 42-1).

Transducers

Pressure-monitoring devices (transducers or gauges connected to a closed space by a length of fluid-filled tubing) are used regularly for monitoring cardiovascular pressures of critically ill patients. These devices can provide a portal of entry for microbial invasion. Although such devices frequently are used in the setting of arterial cannulation or cardiac catheterization, we believe that the threat posed by monitoring devices is so prominent and so frequently overlooked that a separate section on transducer-related infection is warranted.

Although many hospital personnel assume that a protective pressure gradient exists between patients and transducers, contaminated monitoring devices have been the source of nosocomial infection in outbreaks of gram-negative bacteremia, candidemia, and dialysis-associated hepatitis [115]. As electronic monitoring has been used increasingly to measure cerebrospinal fluid (CSF) and intrauterine pressure, there have been occasional reports of transducer-related infections in neurosurgical and obstetric patients. In one study, epidemiologic evidence and culture suggested that contaminated intrauterine pressure transducers used during labor were a nosocomial source of group B streptococcal colonization [31].

As in infusion-related sepsis, any organism that can survive in the fluid used in the monitoring system is capable of causing monitoring-related infection. *Pseudomonas* species and members of the tribe Klebsielleae (*Klebsiella, Enterobacter,* and *Serratia*) have caused the reported bacteremias. The *Pseudomonas* species—*P. cepacia* and *P. acidovorans*—that were implicated in three outbreaks may reflect an emphasis toward unusual epidemics that are more readily recognized and evaluated. Pathogens such as *P. cepacia,* however, may have selective advantages in the hospital environment because of their ability to grow with minimal nutrients and to resist com-

Table 42-1. Guidelines for preventing infections related to intravascular pressure-monitoring systems

Category I[a]
1. Use intravascular monitoring only when clinically necessary and discontinue as soon as possible.
2. Arrange systems as simply as possible; do not assemble or fill systems with flush solution until needed.
3. Do not use glucose-containing solutions as the interface liquid between transducer head and chamber dome membrane or as flush solution (since they support growth of many microorganisms).
4. Wash hands before inserting cannulas or manipulating system; wear sterile gloves for inserting central catheters and for cutdowns.
5. Guidelines for inserting and maintaining intravascular pressure-monitoring systems are similar to those for IV cannulas (see Chap. 40).
6. During calibration of the system, contact should not occur between sterile fluid in the system and nonsterile solutions or equipment.
7. Any stopcocks should be covered; any specimens should be obtained aseptically with care to avoid contaminating any sampling ports.
8. The flush solution should be changed every 24 hours; disposable components should not be resterilized and reused.
9. After use, transducer heads (and reusable domes) should be cleaned, receive high-level disinfection or sterilization, and be stored to prevent contamination before next use.

Category II[a]
1. Disposable components, preassembled and sterile-packaged by the manufacturer, should be used.
2. Closed, rather than open (syringe and stopcock), flush systems should be used to maintain catheter patency.
3. The chamber dome, tubing, and continuous-flow device (if used) should be replaced at 48-hour intervals.[b] (It is not known whether the transducer needs periodic disinfection-sterilization during prolonged use for a single patient.)
4. The site of peripheral arterial cannulas should be changed after 4 days if possible.
5. Cannulas should not be changed over a guide wire if this is done solely for infection prophylaxis.

[a]Ranking scheme for recommendations:
  Category I. Strongly recommended for adoption
    Measures in category 1 are strongly supported by well-designed and controlled clinical studies that show effectiveness in reducing the risk of nosocomial infections or are viewed as useful by the majority of experts in the field. Measures in this category are judged to be applicable to the majority of hospitals—regardless of size, patient population, or endemic nosocomial infection rate—and are considered practical to implement.
  Category II. Moderately recommended for adoption
    Measures in category II are supported by highly suggestive clinical studies or by definitive studies in institutions that might not be representative of other hospitals. Measures that have not been adequately studied, but have a strong theoretic rationale indicating that they might be very effective are included in this category. Category II measures are judged to be practical to implement. They are *not* to be considered a standard of practice for every hospital.
[b]See text regarding totally disposable systems.
Source: Adapted from Guidelines for prevention of infections related to intravascular pressure-monitoring systems. *Infect. Control* 3:61, 1982.

monly used disinfectants, such as dilute aqueous benzalkonium chloride.

In the outbreaks that we investigated, pressure-monitoring devices were contaminated most frequently by an index patient. Just as organisms from a contaminated transducer may migrate (or be flushed) through fluid-filled monitoring lines to infect a patient, organisms in the bloodstream of a patient with preexisting bacteremia or viremia may migrate (or be refluxed) through the lines to contaminate a transducer. If the transducer is not sterilized after use, cross-infection can result.

Although we do not know how often personnel fail to sterilize transducers between uses, there are several reasons to believe that this is a relatively common error. First, many hospital personnel, failing to recognize that transducers may be a source of infection, are loath to subject such expensive and relatively delicate instruments to adequate cleaning efforts. Second, many transducers cannot withstand autoclaving, and heavy patient loads frequently may not allow time for the more lengthy gas or chemical sterilization procedures that these devices require. Finally, even when an attempt at proper care is made, the many nooks and crannies in the traditional dome-and-diaphragm transducer may hamper cleaning and sterilizing efforts.

Once transducers are sterilized for use, the many manipulations involved in using a monitoring system make extrinsic contamination of the equipment easy. As anticipated [115], the frequent use of unsterile mercury manometers for calibrating sterile transducers makes contamination likely [42]. Other potential vehicles for transducer contamination include cleaning solutions and intravenous fluids and medications, particularly those in multidose vials [111]. Infusion bacteremia caused by extrinsically contaminated intravenous fluid is rare (see Chap. 40); however, the fluid column in pressure-monitoring systems is at much greater risk of contamination (and sepsis) because it may be stagnant and subjected to frequent manipulations. In one study of 56 intensive care unit patients with 102 intra-arterial infusions, prospective cultures of the monitoring systems showed 12 episodes of contaminated fluid in the chamber domes [75]. Eight of these cases had concordant bacteremia. In all 8 cases, the transducer chamber dome had been used for more than 2 days, suggesting that with prolonged use the monitoring circuit should be replaced every 48 hours.

For reasons outlined previously, we suspect that transducer contamination is relatively common and that monitoring-related infections have been occurring sporadically since transducers were introduced into clinical medicine. As increasing use of invasive procedures places a large population at risk of monitoring-related infection, and as awareness of this problem increases, such sporadic cases and the means for preventing them should receive more attention. In each hospital, guidelines [47] need to be established for the care of transducers and for surveillance and management of monitoring-related infection (see Table 42-1). Ongoing surveillance

of transducer-related infection in patients undergoing cardiovascular monitoring, as well as possibly obtaining periodic cultures from transducers and the fluid in monitoring lines, will help each hospital assess the adequacy of its monitoring practices and sterilization procedures.

Efforts are under way to improve the ease of transducer sterilization and to simplify the aseptic use of monitoring systems [114]. More recent innovations, not yet widely used, include miniature extravascular transducers that are built into the tips of standard Luer Lok fittings and thus can be attached directly to monitoring lines (or designed for intravascular use), obviating the need for cumbersome domes; however, when sterilizing these miniature transducers, care must be taken to ensure that the area between the transducer and the Luer fitting is thoroughly cleaned and comes into full contact with the sterilizing medium. Inexpensive, disposable, pressure-monitor "isolating" devices are available also, but they allow only mean pressure readings, usually on a gauge-type manometer.

The traditional reusable transducer dome has been largely replaced by the disposable chamber dome, which has a thin membrane that abuts the transducer diaphragm and keeps the monitoring fluid within a sterile disposable circuit. The viability of this approach depends on the chamber dome not being reused and on the thin membrane reliably maintaining its integrity throughout a monitoring period [114]. Several outbreaks have documented the failure of disposable domes to prevent septicemia acquired from contaminated transducers [21, 35]. The exact way that bacteria spread from contaminated transducers to the sterile circuit is not clear; however, hand transmission of organisms from transducer heads to dome fluid was shown experimentally during assembly, calibration, and manipulation of ports. Thus sterilization, or at least high-level disinfection, of transducer heads appears necessary even when disposable chamber domes are used.

Finally, the most recently available advance in pressure monitoring is the totally dispos-

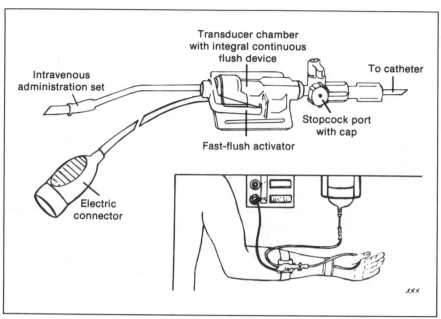

Fig. 42-1. Disposable pressure transducer with an integral flow-through continuous-flush device. *Inset.* Body mounting of radial artery transducer. (Reprinted with permission from R. L. Luskin, et al. Extended use of disposable pressure transducers. *J.A.M.A.* 255 : 916, Copyright 1986, American Medical Association.)

able transducer system (Fig. 42-1). Current guidelines for monitoring the frequency of changing systems do not apply to the disposable transducers. Based on the results of a prospective controlled trial of extended use of disposable pressure transducers, these devices can be safely used without change for 4 days, even in busy intensive care units [73]. In fact, since the publication of the CDC guidelines for preventing monitoring-related infections (see Table 42-1), a prospective study of 117 patients has called into question the need to change routinely any component of the monitoring circuit [103]. In this study, no contamination of monitoring system fluid was found despite prolonged use (25 to 439 hours). The researchers believed that by placing the continuous-flow device just distal to the transducer (Fig. 42-2), they eliminated the static in-line fluid column that, in other studies, [75] may have led to contamination. They also noted their meticulous care of stopcocks, a part of the transducer system most frequently manipulated and contaminated. Plugs were used for all stopcock sampling ports. The plugs were placed on a sterile sponge soaked with iodophor whenever the stopcock was manipulated, and the port was cleaned with iodophor before the plug was reinserted. Unless such stringent practices are adhered to uniformly, the best current approach appears to be use of the totally disposable transducer, with a 4-day change policy. The additive protective effect of using systems that employ only truly closed sampling ports, as recently suggested [73] and studied [26], could potentially extend the microbe-free life of the disposable transducer.

Transfusion-Associated Infections

This section will cover transfusion-associated infections [109] other than hepatitis, cytomegalovirus, and human immunodeficiency virus infections, which are discussed elsewhere (see Chaps. 38 and 39).

Blood Transfusion and Bacteremia
The first case reports of transfusion-related sepsis appeared in the 1940s and 1950s and involved shock syndromes produced by trans-

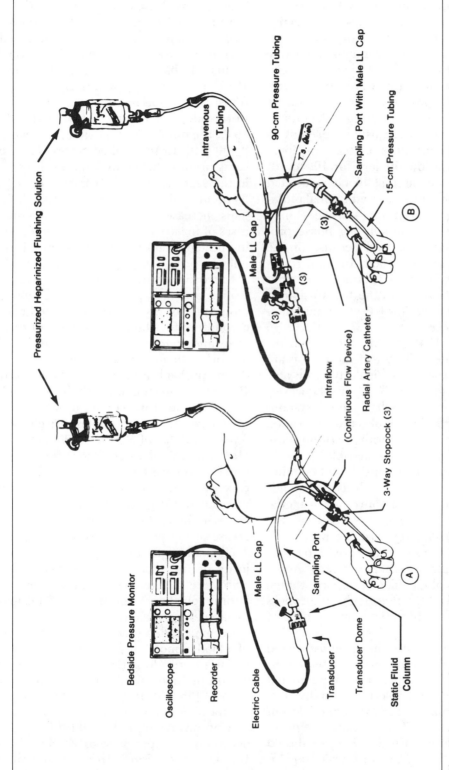

Fig. 42-2. (A, B) Components of two arterial pressure-monitoring systems using continuous-flow devices. System A has a static in-line fluid column that may increase the risk of infection; system B eliminates this column. (System A reprinted with permission from D. G. Maki and C. A. Hassemer, Endemic rate of fluid contamination and related septicemia in arterial pressure monitoring. *Am. J. Med.* 733:207, 1981. System B reprinted with permission from T. Shinozaki, et al., Bacterial contamination of arterial lines: A prospective study. *J.A.M.A.* 249:223, 1983.)

fusion of cold-stored blood contaminated with psychrophilic organisms such as *Achromobacter* and some *Pseudomonas* species. Prospective microbiologic studies soon followed these reports and documented a contamination rate of 1 to 6 percent in banked blood [55]. The majority of contaminants were normal skin flora, presumably introduced with fragments of donor skin cored out during phlebotomy. Such contaminants were usually present in extremely low concentrations (several logarithmic factors below the level of 10^6 to 10^8 organisms per milliliter of blood associated with transfusion sepsis), and additional multiplication of organisms during storage seemed unlikely because of the long lag phase produced by refrigeration and because of the antibacterial action of blood. Indeed, retrospective studies failed to document any clinical illness associated with the transfusion of blood that contained low-level contamination with skin flora [18].

Today, as in 1940, the most common organisms associated with transfusion sepsis are gram-negative bacilli, particularly those able to survive and grow at 4°C (39°F). However, with the sterile, disposable, closed systems used at present for blood collection, with good collection technique, and with the prompt use of dated, refrigerated, banked blood, problems with blood transfusions should be minimal. Nevertheless, occasionally asymptomatic patients still may be a source of bacterial contamination. For example, several cases of *Yersinia enterocolitica* septic shock have been reported in the last few years related to transfusions of red blood cells, particularly associated with units older than 25 days of storage at 1 to 6°C (34 to 43°F). Presumably the donors had asymptomatic bacteremia at the time of donation.

When an episode of transfusion-associated sepsis does occur, it is important to search for breakdowns in technique or a contaminated common source (e.g., collection sets, disinfectants, and anticoagulants [15]) that could put other patients at risk. Furthermore, the possibility of transfusion-associated sepsis should be investigated in any case of febrile transfusion reaction [107].

Blood Transfusion and Parasitemia

The increased use of blood transfusions and the increased travel to countries where malaria is endemic have led to an increased occurrence of transfusion-related malaria. It is estimated that during the period between 1911 and 1950, approximately 350 cases of transfusion-associated malaria were reported worldwide, but during the period 1950 to 1972, the number of reported cases exceeded 2,000 [19]. In the United States, 71 cases of transfusion-induced malaria were reported in the years 1958 to 1981 inclusive, of which 35 occurred between 1967 and 1972 [36, 45]. This increase has been linked to imported cases of malaria: More than 50 percent of the implicated donors had a history of recent military service in Southeast Asia [36].

Based on worldwide incidence data, *Plasmodium malariae* appears to be the most common cause of transfusion-associated malaria, accounting for almost 50 percent of cases. *P. vivax* and *P. falciparum* are second and third in worldwide incidence, respectively. This ordering probably reflects the fact that although *P. malariae* infection may persist in an asymptomatic donor for many years, the longevity of *P. vivax* malaria in humans rarely exceeds 3 years and that of *P. falciparum*, rarely a year. Hence there is greater chance for an asymptomatic donor infected with *P. malariae* to escape detection and become the source of an infected transfusion. Of note in the United States in the 1970s, however, was a relative increase in the percentage of cases due to the "malignant" species, *P. falciparum*. The majority of these cases were traced to donors who were infected in Southeast Asia, where antimicrobial-resistant strains of falciparum malaria are prevalent.

Recommended guidelines for the selection of blood donors to prevent transmission of malaria were adopted by the American Association of Blood Banks in 1970 and relaxed in 1974 [36, 45]. In the amended guidelines, prospective donors who have a definite history of malaria are deferred for 3 years after becoming asymptomatic or ceasing therapy. Immigrants or visitors from an endemic area are acceptable 3 years after departure from the area if they have been asymptomatic. Donors who have traveled to an endemic area but who have remained free of symptoms and have not taken antimalarial drugs are acceptable 6 months after their return to the United States; travelers to an endemic area who have taken antimalarials must have remained symptom-free for 3 years after discontinuation of drug therapy. Because platelet and leukocyte preparations also have been incriminated in the transmission of malaria, the guidelines must be applied to potential donors of any formed elements of blood.

Although there has been a decline in the incidence of malaria in the United States, attributed to the termination of military involvement in Southeast Asia, 26 transfusion-related cases were reported during 1972–1981. In 9 of the 18 cases in which an infected donor could be identified, the donor should have been rejected based on current recommendations but mistakenly was not [45]. When screening fails, a high index of suspicion about the recipient's disease is the best approach to rapid diagnosis and treatment of transfusion-associated malaria. The diagnosis should be considered in any patient who has received formed blood elements and who develops a fever for which no cause is determined by routine cultures. (Serologic methods are now available that accurately diagnose malaria, but they are not practical for screening donors or for rapidly diagnosing serious infection.)

Chagas' disease, or American trypanosomiasis, is prevalent through South and Central America, and there is a high potential for bloodborne transmission, because some infected individuals may become asymptomatic but still have persistent parasitemia for 10 to 30 years. Although the infectivity of blood contaminated with this parasite declines after 10 days of storage, this frequently is not a useful method for preventing transmission. Fortunately, however, carriers of Chagas' disease can be detected by complement fixation tests. In some areas of South America, 15 percent of potential blood donors are positive, and when blood from these donors has been used for transfusions, up to 25 percent of the

recipients have developed clinical Chagas' disease. Thus serologic screening has become mandatory for the acceptance of blood donors in many South American countries. The problem of transfusion-associated Chagas' disease has recently become an issue for U.S. blood banks. Political upheaval in some areas of Central America has led to increased emigration, to greater numbers of potentially infected blood donors in the United States, and to at least 2 cases of transfusion-acquired Chagas' disease [58].

Toxoplasmosis is a disease that is receiving increasing clinical attention, particularly as a cause of opportunistic infection in patients with impaired host defenses. A large portion of the general population, perhaps one-half of adults, have specific antibodies for *Toxoplasma gondii*. In one prospective survey of thalassemic patients who were frequently transfused, subclinical toxoplasmosis was detected at a rate comparable to that seen in a control group, and this was considered to be evidence against the transmission of toxoplasmosis by transfusion [57]. In another study, however, patients treated for acute leukemia developed toxoplasmosis following leukocyte transfusions from donors with chronic myelogenous leukemia; serologic data retrospectively obtained from donors revealed elevated anti-*Toxoplasma* antibody titers [104]. This inferential evidence for transfusion-associated toxoplasmosis is supported by the findings that the disease can be transmitted between animals by transfusion, that *Toxoplasma* organisms retain their viability in stored blood for up to 50 days, and that organisms can be recovered from the blood buffy-coat layers of patients with toxoplasmosis. Because it seems likely that toxoplasmosis can be transmitted if large concentrations of leukocytes are transfused, it has been recommended that blood from donors with high anti-*Toxoplasma* antibody titers not be used for leukocyte transfusion, particularly since the host defenses of recipients usually are severely compromised.

Transfusion-related babesiosis [53, 119], parvovirus B19 infection, and *Borrelia* infection have been documented or are theoretically possible.

Platelet Transfusion

The incidence of bacterial contamination of platelet concentrates has been a source of controversy. While many investigators have reported no contamination, others have consistently found bacterial contaminants in 1 to 6 percent of concentrates [20]. Because it is now recommended that platelets be stored at room temperature (rather than 4°C [39°F]) to increase in vivo half-life, there is justifiable concern over the true incidence of intrinsic contamination and the possible proliferation of contaminants during storage. It seems reasonable to assume that platelet concentrates are as susceptible to contamination during collection as is blood, which is routinely found to have a 1 to 6 percent incidence of low-level contamination. Moreover, platelet concentrates, unlike blood, have no protective antibacterial activity, and platelet transfusions are frequently obtained by pooling the contributions of several donors, which increases the risk of contamination additionally. Despite this seemingly grim picture, the majority of bacterial contaminants isolated from platelet concentrates have been normal skin flora, such as *S. epidermidis* and diphtheroids, and they have been present in extremely low concentrations (fewer than 500 organisms per milliliter). Even in the highly susceptible patient populations that normally receive platelet transfusions, such contaminants have failed to produce any documented adverse reactions [29].

Although meticulous blood-banking techniques and the widespread use of closed collection systems have made platelet transfusion relatively safe, the occurrence of outbreaks emphasizes the possibility of sporadic, significant contamination of platelets. One outbreak involved 7 cases of *Salmonella choleraesuis* sepsis that were traced to platelet transfusions from a blood donor with clinically inapparent salmonella osteomyelitis and intermittent asymptomatic bacteremia [92]. (As an interesting aside, a long incubation period in this outbreak—that is, a mean interval of 9 days between the transfusion with contaminated platelets and the signs of sepsis—was caused by coincidental administration of antibiotics

at the time of platelet transfusion in several cases, and this initially delayed recognition of platelets as the vehicle of infection.) A second outbreak involved 2 cases of transfusion-induced *Enterobacter cloacae* sepsis [20]. An investigation prompted by the occurrence of these cases revealed that 20 percent of the platelet pools prepared in the affected hospital were contaminated. Although the majority of the contaminants were nonpathogens and present only in low concentrations, 6 of 258 platelet pools were shown to harbor *Enterobacter cloacae*. The source of these unusual contaminants was not discovered. A third outbreak with *Serratia* was traced to contaminated evacuated tubes used following blood collection [15].

Albumin Infusion

Because of faith in commercial manufacturing practices and the extremely low incidence of reactions to albumin infusion, most physicians consider commercial human serum albumin to be a completely safe product. A nationwide outbreak of albumin-related *P. cepacia* sepsis, however, emphasized that any commercial product, particularly any blood component, is susceptible to contamination [106]. The outbreak involved four lots of commercial 25% normal human serum albumin. One of the lots had an estimated 1 percent contamination rate and resulted in at least 7 cases of albumin-associated sepsis in one Maryland hospital; the other three lots caused isolated cases of albumin-related disease in patients in four other states. The organisms most likely gained access to the albumin vials during a hand-filling procedure.

In addition to emphasizing the risk of infection associated with the infusion of a non-formed blood component, it is worthwhile noting that the albumin outbreak points up several general problems in the detection and evaluation of low-frequency contamination of commercial products. First, nosocomial infections caused by low-frequency contaminants may be difficult to distinguish from endemic problems in any one institution. In the Maryland hospital, the infusion-related infections became apparent only because of the enormous quantity of albumin that was used in the hospital. Second, since commercial products are usually prepared and sterilized in bulk lots, it is important to be able to trace the distribution of individual suspect lots. Although the Maryland hospital did not routinely record information on albumin distribution and use, an alert physician fortuitously noted the lot number and brand of albumin used in 1 case of suspected infusion-related sepsis. Third, sterility of an infusion product cannot be ascertained by visual inspection. Despite *P. cepacia* concentrations of 10^6 to 10^8 organisms per milliliter, the contaminated albumin was completely clear. Finally, when present in low frequency, some contaminants can be missed by the sampling schemes currently used for product quality control, and endotoxin may escape terminal filtration and be missed by currently used pyrogen tests. To facilitate the monitoring of albumin-related reactions, some hospitals distribute this product through their blood banks.

Albumin-transmitted hepatitis is discussed elsewhere (see Chap. 38).

Infection Hazards Associated with Anesthesia

As noted in previous chapters, severe bacterial infections have been well documented in association with the use of contaminated equipment for local or spinal anesthesia or the use of contaminated anesthesia machines for delivery of general anesthesia. An additional well-recognized infectious complication of general anesthesia unrelated to the use of contaminated equipment is aspiration pneumonia attributable either to the passage of an endotracheal tube or to postoperative difficulties.

Aspiration of Stomach Contents
Aspiration of stomach contents into the lungs during or following obstetric anesthesia was first described by Mendelson [79], who found the incidence of this complication to be 0.15 percent during the preantibiotic era. In approximately two-thirds of these cases,

aspiration was reported as having definitely occurred in the delivery room but, in the remainder, the complication went unrecognized until later. A common clinical pattern was that 2 to 5 hours after vomiting and aspiration, a dramatic onset of cyanosis, tachycardia, and shock was noted.

More recent investigations have shown a surprisingly high incidence of aspiration associated with general anesthesia. In one ingenious study, Evans blue dye was placed in the stomach preoperatively to be used as a marker for chemical aspiration; following anesthesia, the dye was sought by bronchoscopy [28]. Of 300 patients observed in this manner, 25 percent vomited, and aspiration was documented in 16 percent of the overall group. Interestingly, aspiration was "silent" and unnoticed by the entire operating team in one-half of those patients who did aspirate (an overall rate of 8 percent), and there were no obvious clues to the time of occurrence. No incidence of pneumonia was reported in this series, but it seems that in normal patients the aspirated inoculum is usually cleared without sequelae. Patients who have significant retention of gastric contents and preexisting pulmonary disease may be at much higher risk of developing a chemical aspiration pneumonitis and subsequent bacterial infection.

Despite these studies documenting intraoperative aspiration, it seems likely that postoperative aspiration accounts for the majority of aspiration pneumonias associated with general surgery. Surgical procedures involving the upper abdomen, thorax, or upper gastrointestinal tract have been the operations most commonly associated with aspiration pneumonia. The highest-risk patients include those undergoing emergency procedures with a full stomach and those whose condition prevents the stomach from emptying well (e.g., full-term pregnancy, marked obesity, ileus, or massive ascites).

The upper respiratory and gastrointestinal passages are colonized by vast numbers of aerobic and anaerobic organisms, and a mixture of both types of organisms is usually found when specimens from a patient with aspiration pneumonia are cultured appropriately. Among the aerobic organisms, gram-negative bacilli are now encountered more frequently than staphylococci in hospitalized patients. Penicillin is commonly used in the initial therapy for aspiration pneumonia, but an added compound with activity against gram-negative organisms would seem preferable. Use of antimicrobial agents with broader coverage of anaerobic organisms has been advocated, but there is no convincing evidence of the clinical superiority of such agents over the penicillins in therapy of aspiration pneumonia. The prophylactic use of antibiotics and steroids is of unproved value. Therapeutically, the administration of corticosteroids may be of value, but it usually is carried out too late to minimize the chemical inflammatory reaction that is the hallmark of early aspiration.

Measures to prevent anesthesia-associated aspiration have included prolonged preoperative fasting, adequate sedation, attention to problems during anesthesia, insertion of a nasogastric tube before anesthesia, and careful monitoring of the patient in the early period postoperatively. Such principles can be readily applied to elective surgical intervention. Although the insertion of a nasogastric tube is believed to reduce the incidence of aspiration during anesthesia, more than half the cases of postoperative aspiration occur in patients whose nasogastric tubes have been left in place, and a quarter of cases of postoperative aspiration pneumonia have also been associated with tracheostomy. It is difficult to interpret these data, however, since the most seriously ill and aspiration-prone patients have tracheostomies or nasogastric tubes left in place.

In emergency procedures and for the high-risk patients cited previously, measures used to prevent aspiration or ameliorate its effect include attempts to empty the stomach (with metoclopramide or a large nasogastric tube); to decrease stomach acid (with anticholinergic drugs, H_2 blockers, or antacids, although some common antacids are suspensions of particulate matter that may themselves incite pulmonary inflammation if aspirated); to use cricoid pressure to occlude the esophagus during induction of anesthesia; or to pass an endotracheal tube with inflatable balloon under topical anesthesia with the patient awake (and empty the stomach after this).

Endotracheal Intubation

Aside from aspiration, another potential hazard of anesthesia may be the occurrence of bacteremia secondary to the passage of an endotracheal tube. The organisms isolated from the blood usually are α-hemolytic streptococci, both aerobic and anaerobic diphtheroids, and other anaerobic organisms that normally colonize the upper respiratory tract. There may, however, be a higher incidence of such bacteremia following the nasotracheal route of intubation (16 percent in one series) than following the less traumatic orotracheal route [13].

Prolonged nasotracheal (or nasogastric) intubation has been associated with a 2 to 5 percent incidence of sinusitis, which may be occult [41, 67]. The maxillary and sphenoid sinuses are most commonly involved [41], and frequent pathogens include *S. aureus, Enterobacter, P. aeruginosa, Hemophilus,* pneumococci, and anaerobes [67]. Sterile and occasionally infected middle ear effusions may also be common in patients receiving endotracheal intubation and mechanical ventilation [72].

Infections of the Central Nervous System: Reservoirs and Shunts

Serious infection can complicate the insertion or prolonged use of two very important neurosurgical devices: the Ommaya-type subcutaneous reservoir, which is used for administering intrathecal therapy for fungal or neoplastic meningitis, and the ventricular shunt, which is used for decompression of hydrocephalus (see Chap. 32).

Complications have been observed frequently following the insertion or chronic use of subcutaneous intraventricular reservoirs [32, 68, 110]. In one series involving 21 reservoirs, 9 patients developed CSF bacterial infections as a result of reservoir use or insertion, and complications associated with 17 reservoirs in 12 patients either necessitated reservoir removal or prevented their later use for intrathecal therapy [32]. *S. epidermidis, Corynebacterium acnes,* and α-hemolytic streptococci were the major causes of the reservoir infections, and this predominance of normal skin flora suggests that the bacteria gained access to the CSF during repeated percutaneous injections of antifungal or antineoplastic agents into the reservoir. A more recent experience projected a 15 percent risk of infection during the first year after insertion of a reservoir [68]. Therapy of the bacterial superinfection usually is given systemically; the efficacy of antimicrobials added to the reservoir, either for prophylaxis or for treatment of superinfection, has not been established. Although in one study 80 percent of the patients who completed the treatment course were cured by systemic antimicrobial therapy alone [32], many believe that infected spinal fluid devices should be removed.

The use of valved catheters for the treatment of hydrocephalus (i.e., to shunt CSF from the lateral ventricle of the brain to the superior vena cava, the right atrium, or the peritoneum) has also been complicated by a high incidence of infections. In a number of series, the overall incidence of shunt infections has ranged from 6 to 23 percent, with a median of approximately 14 percent [74]. Most of these infections are caused by *S. aureus* or *S. epidermidis* and occur within 2 weeks to 2 months after surgery, which stresses the importance of intraoperative and perioperative shunt contamination in the pathogenesis of shunt infection. The equal risk of infection in patients with ventriculoatrial and ventriculoperitoneal shunts suggests that transient bacteremia is a less likely cause of such infections, since ventriculoperitoneal shunts are not exposed to the bloodstream [98].

Patients with infected ventricular shunts have several different clinical presentations. Some display a markedly toxic course with persistent pyrexia, progressive anemia, splenomegaly, and repeatedly positive blood cultures. More often there is a chronic, indolent course, and considerable clinical suspicion may be necessary before appropriate steps are undertaken. In certain cases, the clinical pattern may be related to the bacteriologic characteristics of the infection. Only one-third or so of infected shunts, for example, exhibit visible wound infection and necrosis but, when these occur, they are important signs of underlying infection, usually with *S. aureus.* In contrast to cases with obvious local inflammation. *S. epidermidis* is found in the great majority of other cases, and this organism is most frequently associated with bacteremic infections.

The antimicrobial treatment of the shunt infections that complicate hydrocephalus is usually unsatisfactory unless the shunt is removed [54]. Adherence of slime-producing coagulase-negative staphylococci to shunt material may be one reason for failure of antimicrobial therapy alone [120]. Although fewer than 10 percent of patients have their infection eradicated by systemic antimicrobial therapy alone, patients treated with combinations of systemic and intraventricular antibiotics may have 30 to 90 percent cure rates [78]. Repeated administration of intraventricular antibiotics has its own complications, however, and when infection is widespread, the treatment of choice appears to be the administration of appropriate systemic antibiotics and the complete removal of the shunt to a new site [46]. Preferably, some time should elapse between the removal of the infected shunt and the insertion of a new one. Despite this discouraging picture, it should be recognized that many of the antibiotics that were used to treat shunt infections in the past have been supplanted by newer agents that may prove to be more efficacious against this highly refractory infectious complication. In addition, the epidemiologic characteristics of shunt infections (e.g., perioperative acquisition of organisms) and the narrow spectrum of shunt pathogens suggest that the use of prophylactic antimicrobials at the time of shunt surgery may prove beneficial. Although one controlled study of relatively low-dose oxacillin prophylaxis failed to show that antibiotics had a significant protective effect [116], studies using larger doses of this or other drugs administered in such a way that high levels in the CSF are attained at the time of surgery may be more successful.

Transient Bacteremia from Nonvascular Procedures

The occurrence of transient bacteremia associated with relatively noninvasive manipulation of colonized mucosa is well recognized [40]. Such bacteremia usually lasts no longer than 5 to 15 minutes, may shower at its peak 100 organisms per milliliter of blood (although the peak concentration is almost always much less), and is largely asymptomatic. Hundreds of studies have reported on bacteremia following oral treatments alone [25]. In this section, we discuss bacteremia following diagnostic gastrointestinal procedures, genitourinary instrumentation, and bronchoscopy; bacteremia following endotracheal intubation and invasive vascular procedures is covered earlier in this chapter. Table 42-2 presents a summary of the characteristics of bacteremia associated with selected nonvascular procedures.

Gastrointestinal Procedures

Bacteremia has been reported as a sequel to a variety of gastrointestinal procedures, in-

Table 42-2. Characteristics of transient bacteremia associated with selected procedures

Involved system	Maximum incidence of bacteremia (%)
Dental	90
Urologic	80
Airway	30
Gastrointestinal	15
Obstetric-gynecologic	4

Concentration of bacteria per milliliter:
  < 20–130
Duration of bacteremia (minutes after
  procedure): 10–30
Predominant bacteria: anaerobes, enterococci,
  enteric gram-negative bacilli; occasionally,
  Streptococcus pneumoniae
Symptoms: usually none; fever more common
  with urologic-related bacteremia

cluding sigmoidoscopy, colonoscopy, barium enema, esophagoscopy, biopsy of mucosal masses, injection sclerotherapy of esophageal varices, endoscopic retrograde cholangiopancreatography (ERCP), liver biopsy, esophageal dilatation, and rectal examination. In one prospective study of sigmoidoscopy, transient asymptomatic bacteremia was noted in 19 of 200 procedures [64]. The majority of organisms isolated were enterococci, and bacteremia was observed more frequently 5 minutes after than 1 minute after the termination of the procedure. Of note in this study, serial blood cultures were obtained through an indwelling venous needle. Although this convenient approach may have distorted or amplified culture results and is thus open to some criticism, the temporal profile and magnitude of bacteremia, as well as the types of organisms isolated, are consistent with bacteremia arising from the site of instrumentation. Other investigators using similar methods, however, have found bacteremia to be a rare complication of their sigmoidoscopic examinations, and they have concluded that other factors, particularly the experience of the sigmoidoscopist, need to be evaluated before routine antibiotic prophylaxis can be advocated for patients undergoing sigmoidoscopy [39].

In a study of colonoscopy, careful anaerobic culturing and subsequent hourly temperature evaluation of patients showed a 27 percent incidence of transient bacteremia during the procedure and a 33 percent incidence of postprocedure fever in patients who had been bacteremic [87]. The greater trauma of colonoscopy compared to sigmoidoscopy may be responsible for the greater incidence of bacteremia and the more marked clinical response, although these are not consistently found [100]. Host factors may also influence the incidence and outcome of procedure-related bacteremia. In this regard, it is noteworthy that rare cases of symptomatic barium-enema septicemia have been reported in patients with impaired host defenses (acute leukemia) and in patients with active inflammatory bowel disease.

Although the role of antibiotic prophylaxis

for endoscopy procedures is not always certain, other preventive measures—particularly careful disinfection of endoscopes and good aseptic technique—are of definite importance. The importance of such measures is highlighted by many anecdotal reports and outbreaks [4, 23, 27, 34, 37, 38, 43, 44, 70]. In one report, 2 cases of *Pseudomonas* sepsis in leukemic patients undergoing esophagoscopy with mucosal biopsy were traced to exogenous bacteria introduced at the time of biopsy. Cultures of the esophagoscope and of the endoscopy room revealed widespread contamination with enteric organisms, including *P. aeruginosa,* and it was shown that in the routine handling of the instruments, aseptic technique was ignored [44].

In addition, several series of ERCP-related cases of bacteremia or cholangitis [4, 23, 27, 37] highlight the multiple sources of contamination in the endoscopy suite, particularly the lens irrigation bottles; the difficulty disinfecting the levers and many small-bore channels in these sophisticated instruments, even when automatic washes are used; the fact that some automatic endoscope "sterilizers," at times, are the source of endoscope contamination, particularly by *P. aeruginosa;* the fact that significant sporadic problems can be easily overlooked for prolonged periods, even with established infection control programs; and the poor level of scope disinfection in many hospitals, despite the many reported outbreaks. Interestingly, almost all of the ERCP-related cases are due to *P. aeruginosa,* and most to one particular serotype, 010, which is either very prevalent or has an unusual tropism for ERCP scopes.

Although a case of cholangitis with polymicrobial sepsis followed ERCP in a patient without biliary tract obstruction [38], most of the patients were at particular risk because of obstructions in the biliary or pancreatic ducts that trapped contaminated injectate. Any patient undergoing ERCP who has suspected ductal obstruction should receive antimicrobial prophylaxis [7]. Large series of ERCP cases have also emphasized the better results obtained with experienced operators [14].

Several cases of infection with an uncommon, non-*typhosa Salmonella* species were traced to an ineffectively cleaned endoscope [22]. Although endoscopy instruments pass through fields that are already grossly contaminated, the nosocomial organisms that may potentially be introduced by the equipment may be more invasive, more resistant, or more contagious than the patient's own flora. Clearly, any instrument that comes in contact with mucosal membranes during a procedure requires a high level of disinfection, which may be obtained if established guidelines [6] are carefully followed.

Percutaneous liver biopsy, although an invasive procedure, is not generally considered to be associated with infection risk. Two studies, however, have documented incidences of bacteremia of 6 and 14 percent following liver biopsy. In the first study, bacteremia was detectable in patients for several hours after biopsy, and it was associated in at least 1 patient with signs of gram-negative sepsis, but it may not have been attributable directly to the biopsy in all the cases [77]. In the second study, however, the bacteremias were transient, lasted for only 15 to 20 minutes after biopsy, and were asymptomatic [65]. In this study, cultures of liver biopsy specimens were positive in 7 percent of patients, and patients with positive specimens had a significantly higher incidence of bacteremia (83 percent) than did patients whose specimens were sterile (8.4 percent), which suggests a direct relationship between biopsy and bacteremia. One explanation of this relationship is that the hepatic reticuloendothelial cells that were in the process of "clearing" gut bacteria from the portal system were biopsied, resulting in a culture-positive biopsy specimen, a temporary defect in the bacterial clearance mechanisms of the biopsied area, and an associated transient bacteremia. The incidence and clinical significance of liver biopsy–associated bacteremia need additional evaluation, as does an association noted in the second study mentioned between liver biopsy and transient pneumococcal bacteremia in patients with cirrhosis. Antibiotic prophylaxis with liver biopsy is not warranted at present.

Nasogastric feeding and enteral nutrition

have been associated with bacteremia as well as with diarrhea and feeding intolerance, particularly in neonates, due to contamination introduced during collection, preparation, or administration of formula or human milk [17, 66].

Urologic and Gynecologic Instrumentation

An association among urethral instrumentation, fever, and bacteremia has been recognized for many years. In various studies, the incidence of bacteremia associated with urologic procedures has been 2 to 80 percent, with the greatest risks of bacteremia occurring in patients with preexisting urinary tract infections, patients undergoing transurethral resection of the prostate, and patients with prostatitis that is evident on histologic section of biopsy specimens [108]. In 50 to 67 percent of patients in whom bacteremia develops after instrumentation, similar organisms are recovered from both preinstrumentation urine cultures and postinstrumentation blood cultures. The available evidence suggests that the sources of the other 33 to 50 percent of postinstrumentation bacteremias include occult prostatitis, the introduction of normal urethral flora (which perhaps explains the relatively large number of blood cultures that were positive for anaerobes in one study), and the contamination of equipment or irrigating fluids before or during instrumentation. It is apparent that careful evaluation for genitourinary tract infection before instrumentation, treatment of any infection, appropriate disinfection of equipment, and careful aseptic technique are mandatory. Moreover, because of the relatively frequent occurrence of enterococcal bacteremia after urologic instrumentation and because of the association of instrumentation with gram-negative sepsis as well as with infection at distal sites (e.g., joints), a brief pulse of systemic prophylactic antibiotics at the time of instrumentation may be warranted in high-risk patients, such as those with valvular heart disease, preexisting joint disease, or impaired host defenses [24].

Endometrial biopsy and chorionic villus sampling have been associated rarely with bacteremia [11, 69].

Bronchoscopy

Although fever and bacteremia have been documented in patients after rigid-tube bronchoscopy [24], bacteremia has not yet been documented prospectively in patients undergoing flexible fiberoptic bronchoscopy. There are, however, case reports of bacteremia related to fiberoptic bronchoscopy, including one report of fatal *Pseudomonas* bacteremia in a patient with preexisting *Pseudomonas* bronchitis. Furthermore, in one series of 100 patients who were followed carefully after fiberoptic bronchoscopy, 16 developed fever, 5 developed transient parenchymal infiltrates, and 1 developed rapidly fatal pneumonia [88]. Older patients (more than 60 years old) and those with abnormalities on bronchoscopy were at greatest risk of complications. With the exception of the one fatal pneumonitis, however, all complicating infections resolved without antibiotic therapy, and prospective culturing failed to demonstrate bacteremia in any of the 100 patients [88].

Conclusions

Two conclusions can be drawn from the studies of procedure-related bacteremia just cited: The equipment used for the procedures should be adequately disinfected or sterilized before every use, and proper aseptic technique should be employed by the operator (see Chap. 15). Beyond this, it is apparent that carefully planned, prospective multicenter studies would be needed to assess the incidence and clinical significance of procedure-related transient bacteremia, to determine which hosts are at risk of associated sepsis or infection at distal sites, to determine if specific risks for certain procedures can be sufficiently defined to justify preventive measures such as antibiotic prophylaxis, and to determine which prophylactic regimens would be most efficacious. Although such studies may not be available for some time (if ever), the procedures clearly will continue, and we have tried to note situations in which it seems reasonable to "cover" patients [24, 40]. In this regard, it should be noted that for years dental patients with valvular heart disease have received endocarditis prophylaxis, largely on an empiric basis, although the specific regimens [86] and even the mechanisms by which prophylaxis may protect [49, 71] have been called into question here too.

Additional Procedures Associated with Infections

Interventional Radiology

Percutaneous radiologically guided placement of biopsy needles, catheters, and stents for diagnosis and therapy has become commonplace over the past 5 to 10 years [83]. Infectious complications—primarily bacteremia, organ perforation, and catheter site infection—vary with the particular procedure, patient risk factors, skill of the operator, and experience of the hospital, but are no more frequent than after more invasive procedures [83]. The use of prophylactic antibiotics for interventional radiographic procedures will depend on the situation [52]. In addition, when infection is suspected clinically, therapeutic antibiotics should be administered before a procedure.

Laparoscopic Surgery

Laparoscopic surgery, particularly laparoscopic cholecystectomy, has received much attention from both the public and the medical community. Recovery is much faster than after conventional surgery. For cholecystectomy, infection rates (wound, 0.9 to 2.0 percent; lung, 0.2 to 0.5 percent; urinary tract, 0.4 to 1.0 percent) are comparable to those after open surgery [118a].

Cystoscopy

In addition to the risk of bacteremia associated with cystoscopy, a significant risk of urinary tract infection is associated with this procedure. Several remarkably similar outbreaks have been reported in which the use of dilute aqueous quaternary ammonium compounds as a cystoscope disinfectant was associated with procedure-related urinary tract infections with *Pseudomonas* species, particulary *P. cepacia* (see Chap. 28). In these outbreaks, the quaternary ammonium compounds either were ineffective in decontaminating the equipment or were themselves actually harboring viable bacteria while in use as disinfectants [33].

Although the risk of infection associated with the use of dilute aqueous quaternary ammonium compounds has been known for at least 20 years, many hospital personnel persist in using these compounds as antiseptics and disinfectants. Such use has most likely resulted in many outbreaks of nosocomial urinary tract infection, as well as outbreaks of nosocomial bacteremia and occasional outbreaks of nosocomial respiratory tract and wound infection. To help decrease the risk of nosocomial urinary tract infection following cystoscopy, it is important that the equipment be thoroughly cleaned and properly disinfected between uses.

Bronchoscopy

In addition to the risks of bronchoscopy cited, several outbreaks have highlighted the problems of pulmonary infection and false-positive culture results due to inadequately cleaned fiberoptic bronchoscopes [50]. Especially worrisome is a report of the failure of povidone iodine to kill *Mycobacterium tuberculosis* on bronchoscopes [85]. Preparations of this agent that are intended for skin degerming are often used inadvisably for decontaminating equipment. This experience has reemphasized the need for higher-level disinfection (e.g., with glutaraldehyde) or sterilization of these scopes, especially after use on patients who may have tuberculosis. In addition, some parts of the scopes, such as reusable spring-operated suction valves, may require autoclaving if they become heavily contaminated with microbes that are relatively resistant to disinfection, such as mycobacteria [118].

Arthrocentesis and Thoracentesis

Although septic arthritis is caused most commonly by hematogenous spread of organisms, sporadic cases of staphylococcal arthritis and, at times, gram-negative bacillary arthritis have followed several days after invasive joint manipulations. During the mid-1960s, CDC epidemiologists investigated a cluster of cases of staphylococcal arthritis in which the infections occurred 1 to 7 days after outpatient arthrocentesis or intraarticular injection of steroids. Epidemiologic evidence suggested that the physician who had performed these procedures was a disseminator of the epidemic strain, and microbiologic investigation showed that areas of chronic dermatitis on the physician's hands harbored the epidemic organism. A similar cluster of cases of staphylococcal arthritis, in which the infections occurred 5 to 6 days after arthrographic examination of the knee joint and 3 to 4 days after knee surgery, was traced epidemiologically to the surgeon who had performed these procedures, who was a nasal carrier of staphylococci. More recently, 10 cases of *Serratia* septic arthritis were traced to contaminated benzalkonium chloride antiseptic used in a physician's office [84].

Other diagnostic taps, such as thoracentesis [12], have also been associated with nosocomial infections, which emphasizes the fact that all invasive procedures should be performed only under strict aseptic conditions, with careful skin preparation, by an appropriately scrubbed and gloved operator, and using sterile equipment. While the relative rarity of centesis-associated infections may be considered testimony that good technique is generally employed in our hospitals and clinics, the lack of such infections also may be evidence of the capacity of the local tissue response to limit bacterial invasion in uncompromised hosts [30]. When procedures are performed in patients with compromised host defenses or on tissues that may have diminished ability to limit bacterial invasion (e.g., rheumatoid joints), the risk of procedure-associated infections may be considerable, which emphasizes the need for continued vigilance.

Peritoneal Manipulation

Infectious complications of laparoscopy and amniocentesis are rare, presumably because of careful technique, sterile equipment, local host defense mechanisms, and the frequently healthy nature of the subjects. In fact, high-level disinfection of peritoneoscopes with glutaraldehyde instead of gas sterilization has appeared acceptable. In a retrospective analysis of polymicrobial bacterial ascites in 1,578 abdominal paracenteses, only 1 case of clinical peritonitis developed, presumably due to entry of the bowel by the paracentesis needle [96].

Artificial Insemination

A variety of infections have been transmitted by artificial insemination and mandate careful adherence to protocol for screening [76].

Water Baths

Contaminated water baths have led to a large number of very similar outbreaks. Warm water baths used to thaw packs of cryoprecipitate for intravenous use by hemophiliacs, to warm peritoneal dialysate, or to warm radiopaque contrast material have led to outbreaks of *P. cepacia* bacteremia, *Acinetobacter* peritonitis, and endotoxemia, respectively [93, 95, 101]. Cold ice baths used to chill the cardioplegia solution for open-heart surgery or to cool blood gas syringes have been implicated in outbreaks of mediastinitis and bacteremia [63].

The exact mechanism of bacterial transfer in these situations is often unknown but probably involves contamination of medication ports, splash onto operative fields, or hand transmission by staff. Possible preventive measures include using dry heat, using impermeable outer wraps or drying any immersed object before use, using sterile water or ice, and hand-washing after contact with water baths. The use of disinfectants in water baths has been suggested but not widely attempted.

Ophthalmologic Examination

Manipulation of the conjunctiva and cornea occurs during tonometry, instillation of eye drops, and manual ophthalmologic examination, and it can result in transmission of conjunctivitis and other eye infections. The infection most commonly transmitted is epidemic keratoconjunctivitis, a highly contagious, frequently iatrogenic disease, which usually is caused by adenovirus type 8 [48] (see Chap. 38). Transmission of the virus occurs via fomites, such as inadequately disinfected tonometers and contaminated eye droppers, as well as by indirect person-to-person spread on the hands of health workers. Similar modes of transmission have been implicated in outbreaks of other viral and bacterial eye infections. Although proper care of equipment and conscientious hand-washing between patient contacts is remarkably effective in halting the transmission of such diseases, some manufacturer recommendations for disinfection may be inadequate [59]; and ongoing community outbreaks may require extra-stringent triage and infection control to limit nosocomial spread [112].

Barium Enema

In addition to transient bacteremia, patients undergoing barium enema are at risk of two other infectious complications. First, infants may aspirate barium when faulty technique produces excessive retrograde flow of contrast material. Second, if the enema bag or tip is not replaced or is not adequately disinfected between uses, or if the barium is contaminated, the procedure may transmit enteric pathogens. This risk was highlighted by Meyers and Richards [81] when they demonstrated that attenuated poliovirus can be transferred via contaminated barium enema. At present, the use of disposable enema bags, tubing, and enema tips has largely put an end to such risks.

References

1. Abrutyn, E. Hospital-associated infection from leeches. *Ann. Intern. Med.* 109:356, 1988.
2. Adam, R.D., Edwards, L.D., Becker, C.C., and Schrom, H.M. Semiquantitative cultures and routine tip cultures on umbilical catheters. *J. Pediatr.* 100:123, 1982.
3. Adams, S.L. The medicinal leech. *Ann. Intern. Med.* 109:399, 1988.
4. Allen, J.I., et al. *Pseudomonas* infection of the biliary system resulting from use of a contaminated endoscope. *Gastroenterology* 92:759, 1987.
5. Anagnostakis, D., et al. Risk of infection associated with umbilical vein catheterization. *J. Pediatr.* 86:759, 1975.
6. Anonymous. Infection control during a gastrointestinal endoscopy. *Gastrointest. Endosc.* 34:37S, 1988.
7. Anonymous. Preparation of patients for gastrointestinal endoscopy. *Gastrointest. Endosc.* 34:32S, 1988.
8. Asnes, R.S., and Arendar, G.M. Septic arthritis of the hip. *Pediatrics* 38:837, 1966.
9. Band, J.D., and Maki, D.G. Infections caused by arterial catheters used for hemodynamic monitoring. *Am. J. Med.* 67:735, 1979.
10. Bard, H., et al. Prophylactic antibiotics in chronic umbilical artery catheterization in respiratory distress syndrome. *Arch. Dis. Child.* 48:630, 1973.
11. Barela, A.I., et al. Septic shock with renal failure after chorionic villus sampling. *Am. J. Obstet. Gynecol.* 154:1100, 1986.
12. Bayer, A.S., Necrotizing pneumonia and empyema due to *Clostridium perfringens. Am. J. Med.* 59:851, 1975.
13. Berry, F.A., Blankenbaker, W.L., and Ball, C.G. A comparison of bacteremia occurring with nasotracheal and orotracheal intubation. *Anesth. Analg.* (Cleve.) 52:873, 1973.
14. Bilbao, M.K., Dotter, C.T., Lee, T.G., and Katon, R.M. Complications of endoscopic retrograde cholangiopancreatography (ERCP). *Gastroenterology* 70:314, 1976.
15. Blajchman, M.A., et al. Platelet transfusion-induced *Serratia marcescens* sepsis due to vacuum tube contamination. *Transfusion* 19:39, 1979.
16. Blumenfeld, T.A., Turi, G.K., and Blanc, W.A. Recommended site and depth of newborn heel skin punctures based on anatomical measurements and histopathology. *Lancet* 1:230, 1979.
17. Botsford, K.B., et al. Gram-negative bacilli in human milk feedings: Quantitation and clinical consequences for premature infants. *J. Pediatr.* 109:707, 1986.
18. Braude, A.I., Sanford, J.P., Bartlett, J.E., and Mallery, O.T. Effects and clinical significance of bacterial contaminants in transfused blood. *J. Lab. Clin. Med.* 39:902, 1952.
19. Bruce-Chwatt, L.J. Blood transfusion and tropical disease. *Trop. Dis. Bull.* 69:825, 1972.
20. Buchholtz, D.H., et al. Bacterial proliferation in platelets stored at room temperature: N. *Engl. J. Med.* 285:429, 1971.
21. Buxton, A.E., Anderson, R.L., Klimek, J., and Quintiliani, R. Failure of disposable domes to prevent septicemia acquired from contaminated pressure transducers. *Chest* 74:508, 1978.
22. Chmel, H., and Armstrong, D. *Salmonella oslo:* A focal outbreak in a hospital. *Am. J. Med.* 60:203, 1976.
23. Classen, D.C., et al. Serious *Pseudomonas* infections associated with endoscopic retrograde cholangiopancreatography. *Am. J. Med.* 84:590, 1988.
24. Committee on the Prevention of Rheumatic

Fever and Bacterial Endocarditis. Prevention of bacterial endocarditis. *Circulation* 70: 1123A, 1984.

25. Crawford, J.J., et al. Bacteremia after tooth extractions studied with the aid of pre-reduced anaerobically sterilized culture media. *Appl. Microbiol.* 27:927, 1974.

26. Crow, S., Conrad, S.A., Chaney-Rowell, C., and King, J.W. Microbial contamination of arterial infusions used for hemodynamic monitoring: A randomized trial of contamination with sampling through conventional stopcocks versus a novel closed system. *Infect. Control Hosp. Epidemiol.* 10:557, 1989.

27. Cryan, E.M.J., et al. *Pseudomonas aeruginosa* cross-infection following endoscopic retrograde cholangiopancreatography. *J. Hosp. Infect.* 5:371, 1984.

28. Culver, G.A., Makel, H.P., and Beecher, H.K. Frequency of aspiration of gastric contents by the lungs during anesthesia and surgery. *Ann. Surg.* 133:289, 1951.

29. Cunningham, M., and Cash, J.D. Bacterial contamination and platelet concentrates stored at 20°C. *J. Clin. Pathol.* 26:401, 1973.

30. Dann, T.C. Routine skin preparation before injection: An unnecessary procedure. *Lancet* 2:96, 1969.

31. Davis, J.P., et al. Nasal colonization of infants with group B streptococcus associated with intrauterine pressure transducers. *J. Infect. Dis.* 138:804, 1978.

32. Diamond, R.D., and Bennett, J.E. A subcutaneous reservoir for intrathecal therapy of fungal meningitis. *N. Engl. J. Med.* 288:186, 1974.

33. Dixon, R.E., et al. Aqueous quaternary ammonium antiseptics and disinfectants: Use and mis-use. *J.A.M.A.* 236:2415, 1976.

34. Doherty, D.E., et al. *Pseudomonas aeruginosa* sepsis following retrograde cholangiopancreatography (ERCP). *Dig. Dis. Sci.* 27:169, 1982.

35. Donowitz, L.G., Marsik, F.J., Hoyt, J.W., and Wenzel, R.P. *Serratia marcescens* bacteremia from contaminated pressure transducers. *J.A.M.A.* 242:1749, 1979.

36. Dover, A.S., and Schultz, M.G. Transfusion-induced malaria. *Transfusion* 11:353, 1971.

37. Earnshaw, J.J., Clark, A.W., and Thom, B.T. Outbreak of *Pseudomonas aeruginosa* following endoscopic retrograde cholangiopancreatography. *J. Hosp. Infect.* 6:95, 1985.

38. Elson, C.O., Hattori, K., and Blackstone, M.O. Polymicrobial sepsis following endoscopic retrograde and cholangiopancreatography. *Gastroenterology* 69:507, 1975.

39. Engeling, E.R., et al. Bacteremia after sigmoidoscopy: Another view. *Ann. Intern. Med.* 85:77, 1976.

40. Everett, E.D., and Hirschmann, J.V. Tran-sient bacteremia and endocarditis prophylaxis: A review. *Medicine* 56:61, 1977.

41. Fassoulaki, A., and Pamouktsoglou, P. Prolonged nasotracheal intubation and its association with inflammation of paranasal sinuses. *Anesth. Analg.* 69:50, 1989.

42. Fisher, M.C., et al. *Pseudomonas maltophilia* bacteremia in children undergoing open heart surgery. *J.A.M.A.* 246:1571, 1981.

43. Gardner, R.M., Schwartz, R., Wong, H.C., and Burke, J.P. Percutaneous indwelling radial-artery catheters for monitoring cardiovascular function. *N. Engl. J. Med.* 290:1227, 1974.

44. Greene, W.H., et al. Esophagoscopy as a source of *P. aeruginosa* sepsis in patients with acute leukemia: The need for sterilization of endoscopes. *Gastroenterology* 67:912, 1974.

45. Guerrero, I.C., Weniger, B.C., and Schultz, M.G. Transfusion malaria in the United States, 1972–1981. *Ann. Intern. Med.* 99:221, 1983.

46. Guertin, S.R. Cerebrospinal fluid shunts. Evaluation, complications, and crisis management. *Pediatr. Clin. North Am.* 34:203, 1987.

47. Guideline for prevention of infections related to intravascular pressure-monitoring systems. *Infect. Control* 3:61, 1982.

48. Hendley, J.O. Epidemic keratoconjunctivitis and hand washing. *N. Engl. J. Med.* 289:1368, 1973.

49. Hess, J., Holloway, Y., and Dankert, J. Incidence of postextraction bacteremia under penicillin cover in children with cardiac disease. *Pediatrics* 71:554, 1983.

50. Hoffman, K.K., Weber, D.J., and Rutala, W.A. Pseudoepidemic of *Rhodotorula rubra* in patients undergoing fiberoptic bronchoscopy. *Infect. Control Hosp. Epidemiol.* 10:511, 1989.

51. Hoffman, P.C., et al. False-positive blood cultures: Association with nonsterile blood collection tubes. *J.A.M.A.* 236:2073, 1976.

52. Hunter, D.W., Simmons, R.L., and Hulbert, J.C. Antibiotics for radiologic interventional procedures. *Radiology* 166:571, 1988.

53. Jacoby, G.A., et al. Treatment of transfusion-transmitted babesiosis by exchange transfusion. *N. Engl. J. Med.* 303:1098, 1980.

54. James, H.E., et al. Prospective randomized study of therapy in cerebrospinal fluid shunt infection. *Neurosurgery* 7:459, 1980.

55. James, J.D. Bacterial contamination of preserved blood. *Vox Sang.* 4:177, 1959.

56. Katz, L., Johnson, D.L. Neufeld, P.D., and Gupta, K.G. Evacuated blood-collection tubes: The backflow hazard. *Can. Med. Assoc. J.* 113:208, 1975.

57. Kimball, A.C., Kean, B.H., and Kellner, A. The risk of transmitting toxoplasmosis by

blood transfusion. *Transfusion* 5:447, 1965.

58. Kirchhoff, L.V. Is *Trypanosoma cruzi* a threat to our blood supply? *Ann. Intern. Med.* 111: 773, 1989.

59. Koo, D., et al. Epidemic keratoconjunctivitis in a university medical center ophthalmology clinic; need for re-evaluation of the design and disinfection of instruments. *Infect. Control Hosp. Epidemiol.* 10:547, 1989.

60. Krauss, A.N., Albert, R.F., and Kannan, M.M. Contamination of umbilical catheters in the newborn infant. *J. Pediatr.* 77:965, 1970.

61. Kundsin, R.B., and Walter, C.W. Detection of endotoxin on sterile catheters used for cardiac catheterization. *J. Clin. Microbiol.* 11: 209, 1980.

62. Kure, R., Grendahl, H., and Paulssen, J. Pyrogens from surgeons' sterile latex gloves. *Acta. Pathol. Microbiol. Immunol. Scand.* 90:85, 1982.

63. Kuritsky, J.N., et al. Sternal wound infections and endocarditis due to organisms of the *Mycobacterium fortuitum* complex. *Ann. Intern. Med.* 98:938, 1983.

64. LeFrock, J.L., Ellis, C.A., Turchik, J.B., and Weinstein, L. Transient bacteremia associated with sigmoidoscopy. *N. Engl. J. Med.* 289:467, 1973.

65. LeFrock, J.L., et al. Transient bacteremia associated with percutaneous liver biopsy. *J. Infect. Dis.* 131(Suppl.): 104, 1975.

66. Levy, J. Enteral nutrition: An increasingly recognized cause of nosocomial bloodstream infection. *Infect. Control Hosp. Epidemiol.* 10: 395, 1989.

67. Linden, B.E., Aguilar, E.A., and Allen, S.J. Sinusitis in the nasotracheally intubated patient. *Arch. Otolaryngol. Head Neck Surg.* 114: 860, 1988.

68. Lishner, M., et al. Complications associated with Ommaya reservoirs in patients with cancer. *Arch. Intern. Med.* 150:173, 1990.

69. Livengood, C.H., Land, M.R., and Addison, W.A. Endometrial biopsy, bacteremia, and endocarditis, risk. *Obstet. Gynecol.* 65:678, 1985.

70. Low, D.E., Micflikier, A.B., Kennedy, J.K., and Stiver, H.G. Infectious complications of endoscopic retrograde cholangiopancreatography: A prospective assessment. *Arch. Intern. Med.* 140:1076, 1980.

71. Lowy, F.D., et al. Effect of penicillin on the adherence of *Streptococcus sanguis* in vitro and in the rabbit model of endocarditis. *J. Clin. Invest.* 71:668, 1983.

72. Lucks, D., Consiglio, A., Stankiewicz, J., and O'Keefe, P. Incidence and microbiological etiology of middle ear effusion complicating endotracheal intubation and mechanical ventilation. *J. Infect. Dis.* 157:368, 1988.

73. Luskin, R.L., et al. Extended use of disposable pressure transducers. *J.A.M.A.* 255:916, 1986.

74. Luthardt, T. Bacterial infections in ventriculo-auricular shunt systems. *Dev. Med. Child Neurol. Suppl.* 12:105, 1970.

75. Maki, D.G., and Hassemer, C.A. Endemic rate of fluid contamination and related septicemia in arterial pressure monitoring. *Am. J. Med.* 733:207, 1981.

76. Mascola, L., and Guinan, M.E. Screening to reduce transmission of sexually transmitted diseases in semen used for artificial insemination. *N. Engl. J. Med.* 314:1354, 1986.

77. McCloskey, R.V., Gold, M., and Weser, E. Bacteremia after liver biopsy. *Arch. Intern. Med.* 132:213, 1973.

78. McLaurin, R.L., and Frane, P.T. Treatment of infections of cerebrospinal fluid shunts. *Rev. Infect. Dis.* 9:595, 1987.

79. Mendelson, C.L. The aspiration of stomach contents into the lungs during obstetric anesthesia. *Am. J. Obstet. Gynecol.* 52:191, 1946.

80. Mercer, N.S., Beere, D.M., Bornemisza, A.J., and Thomas, P. Medical leeches as sources of wound infection. *Br. Med. J. [Clin. Res.]* 294: 937, 1987.

81. Meyers, P.H., and Richards, M. Transmission of polio virus vaccine by contaminated barium enema with resultant antibody rise. *Am. J. Roentgenol. Radium Ther. Nucl. Med.* 91: 864, 1964.

82. Michel, L., et al. Infection of pulmonary artery catheters in critically ill patients. *J.A.M.A.* 245:1032, 1981.

83. Mueller, P.R., and van Sonnenberg, E. Interventional radiology in the chest and abdomen. *N. Engl. J. Med.* 322:1364, 1990.

84. Nakashima, A.K., McCarthy, M.A., Martone, W.J., and Anderson, R.L. Epidemic septic arthritis caused by *Serratia marcescens* and associated with benzalkonium chloride antiseptic. *J. Clin. Microbiol.* 25:1014, 1987.

85. Nelson, K.E., Larson, P.A., Schraufnagel, D.E., and Jackson, J. Transmission of tuberculosis by flexible fiberbronchoscopes. *Am. Rev. Respir. Dis.* 127:97, 1983.

86. Oakley, C., and Somerville, W. Prevention of infective endocarditis. *Br. Heart J.* 45:233, 1981.

87. Pelican, G., Hentges, D., and Butt, J.H. Bacteremia during colonoscopy. *Gastrointest. Endosc.* 22:233, 1976.

88. Pereira, W., et al. Fever and pneumonia after flexible fiberoptic bronchoscopy. *Am. Rev. Respir. Dis.* 112:59, 1975.

89. Pien, F.D., and Bruce, A.E. Nosocomial *Ewingella americana* bacteremia in an intensive care unit. *Arch. Intern. Med.* 146:111, 1986.

90. Powers, W.F., and Tooley, W.H. Contamination of umbilical vessel catheters. *Pediatrics* 48:470, 1971.

91. Reyes, M.P., et al. Pyrogenic reactions after inadvertent infusion of endotoxin during cardiac catheterizations. *Ann. Intern. Med.* 93:32, 1980.

92. Rhame, F.S., et al. *Salmonella* septicemia from platelet transfusions. *Ann. Intern. Med.* 78:633, 1973.

93. Rhame, F.S., and McCullough, J. Follow-up on nosocomial *Pseudomonas cepacia* infection. *M.M.W.R.* 28:409, 1979.

94. Rowley, K.M., Clubb, K.S., Smith, G.J.W., and Cabin, H.S. Right-sided infective endocarditis as a consequence of flow directed pulmonary artery catheterization. *N. Engl. J. Med.* 311:1152, 1984.

95. Rubin, J., et al. Management of peritonitis and bowel perforation during chronic peritoneal dialysis. *Nephron* 16:220, 1976.

96. Runyon, B.A., Hoefs, J.C., and Canawati, H.N. Polymicrobial bacterascites. A unique entity in the spectrum of infected ascitic fluid. *Arch. Intern. Med.* 146:2173, 1986.

97. Sande, M.A., Levinson, M.E., Lukas, D.S., and Kaye, D. Bacteremia associated with cardiac catheterization. *N. Engl. J. Med.* 281:1104, 1969.

98. Schoenbaum, S.C., Gardner, P., and Shillito, J. Infections of cerebrospinal fluid shunts. *J. Infect. Dis.* 131:543, 1975.

99. Schroeder, S.A., Marton, K.I., and Strom, B.L. Frequency and morbidity of invasive procedures: Report of a pilot study from two teaching hospitals. *Arch. Intern. Med.* 138:1809, 1978.

100. Schwesinger, W.H., Levine, B.A., and Ramos, R. Complications in colonoscopy. *Surg. Gynecol. Obstet.* 148:270, 1979.

101. Sharbaugh, R.J. Suspected outbreak of endotoxemia associated with computerized axial tomography. *Am. J. Infect. Control* 8:26, 1980.

102. Sherwood, P.M. An outbreak of syringe-transmitted hepatitis with jaundice in hospitalized diabetic patients. *Ann. Intern. Med.* 33:380, 1950.

103. Shinozaki, T., et al. Bacterial contamination of arterial lines: A prospective study. *J.A.M.A.* 249:223, 1983.

104. Siegel, S.E., et al. Transmission of toxoplasmosis by leukocyte transfusion. *Blood* 37:388, 1971.

105. Stamm, W.E., Colella, J.J., Anderson, R.L., and Dixon, R.E. Indwelling arterial catheters as a source of nosocomial bacteremia. *N. Engl. J. Med.* 292:1099, 1975.

106. Steere, A.C., et al. *Pseudomonas* species bacteremia caused by contaminated normal human serum albumin. *J. Infect. Dis.* 135:729, 1977.

107. Stenhouse, M.A.E., and Milner, L.V. *Yersinia enterocolitica:* A hazard in blood transfusion. *Transfusion* 22:396, 1982.

108. Sullivan, N.M., et al. Bacteremia after genitourinary tract manipulation. *Appl. Microbiol.* 23:1101, 1972.

109. Tabor, E. *Infectious Complications of Blood Transfusions.* New York: Academic, 1982.

110. Trump, D.L., Grossman, S.A., Thompson, G., and Murray, K. CSF infections complicating the management of neoplastic meningitis. *Arch. Intern. Med.* 142:583, 1982.

111. Walton, J.R., Shapiro, B.A., and Harrison, R.A. *Serratia* bacteremia from mean arterial pressure monitors. *Anesthesiology* 43:113, 1975.

112. Warren, D., et al. A large outbreak of epidemic keratoconjunctivitis: Problems in control of nosocomial spread. *J. Infect. Dis.* 160:938, 1989.

113. Washington, J.A. The microbiology of evacuated blood collection tubes. *Ann. Intern. Med.* 86:186, 1977.

114. Weinstein, R.A. The design of pressure monitoring devices. *Med. Instrum.* 10:287, 1976.

115. Weinstein, R.A., Stamm, W.E., Kramer, L., and Corey, L. Pressure monitoring devices: Overlooked source of nosocomial infection. *J.A.M.A.* 236:936, 1976.

116. Weiss, S.R., and Raskind, R. Further experience with the ventriculoperitoneal shunt. *Int. Surg.* 53:300, 1970.

117. Wenzel, R.P., et al. Identification of procedure-related nosocomial infections in high-risk patients. *Rev. Infect. Dis.* 3:701, 1981.

118. Wheeler, P.W., Lancaster, D., and Kaiser, A.B. Bronchopulmonary cross-colonization and infection related to mycobacterial contamination of suction valves of bronchoscopes. *J. Infect. Dis.* 159:954, 1989.

118a. White, J.V. Laparoscopic cholecystectomy: The evolution of general surgery. *Ann. Intern. Med.* 115:651, 1991.

119. Wittner, M., et al. Successful chemotherapy of transfusion babesiosis. *Ann. Intern. Med.* 96:601, 1982.

120. Younger, J.J., et al. Coagulase-negative staphylococci isolated from cerebrospinal fluid shunts: Importance of slime production, species identification, and shunt removal to clinical outcome. *J. Infect. Dis.* 156:548, 1987.

Index

Index